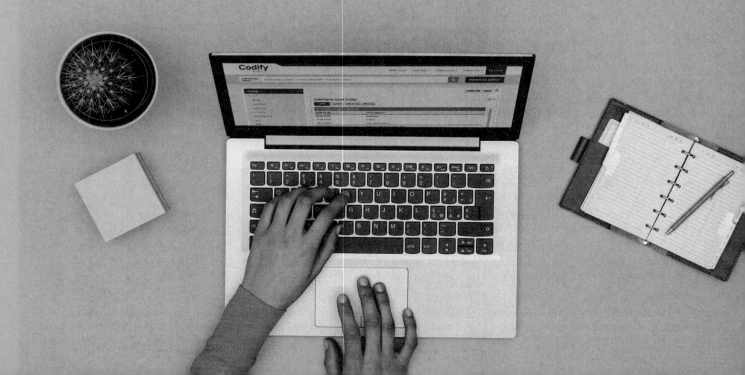

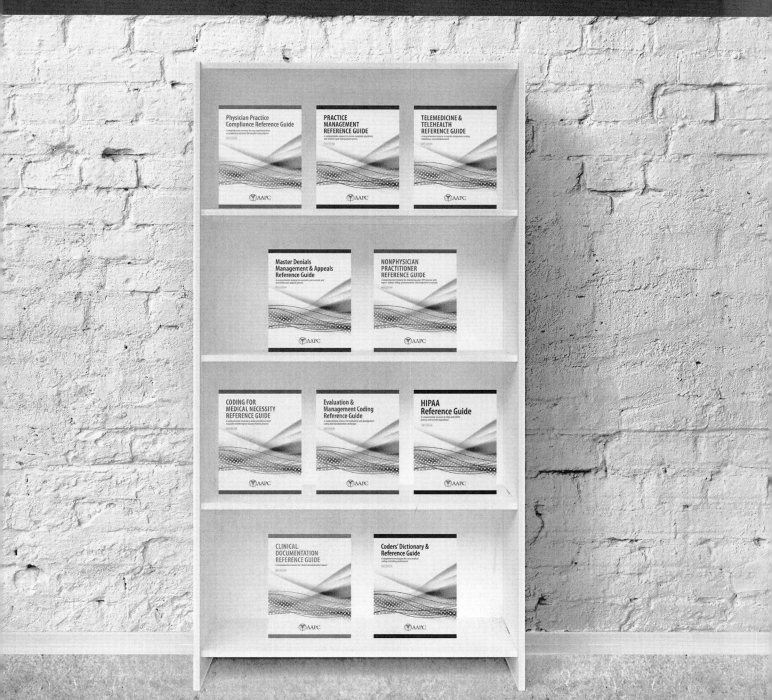

ADVANCE YOUR CREDENTIALS
ADVANCE YOUR CAREER

The more you learn, the more you can earn.

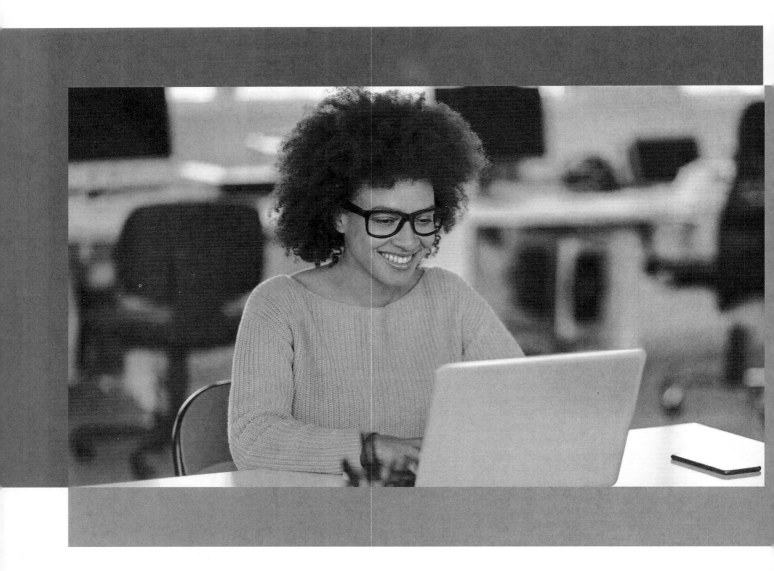

Learn more
Visit: https://www.aapc.com/training

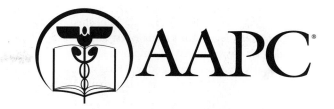

HCPCS
LEVEL II
EXPERT

Service/Supply Codes
for Caregivers & Suppliers

2021

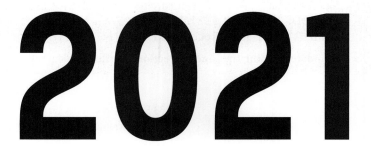

Publisher's Notice

This book was current when it was published. Every reasonable effort has been made to ensure the accuracy of the information within these pages. The ultimate responsibility lies with readers to ensure they are using the codes and following applicable guidelines correctly. AAPC employees, agents, and staff make no representation, warranty, or guarantee that this compilation of information is error-free, and will bear no responsibility or liability for the results or consequences of the use of this code book. This book is a general summary that explains guidelines and principles in profitable, efficient healthcare organizations.

U.S. Government Rights

This product includes CPT®, which is commercial technical data and/or computer data bases and/or commercial computer software and/or commercial computer software documentation, as applicable, which was developed exclusively at private expense by the American Medical Association, 515 North State Street, Chicago, Illinois, 60610. U.S. Government rights to use, modify, reproduce, release, perform, display, or disclose these technical data and/or computer data bases and/or computer software and/or computer software documentation are subject to the limited rights restrictions of DFARS 252.227-7015(b)(2) (November 1995), as applicable, for U.S. Department of Defense procurements and the limited rights restrictions of FAR 52.227-14 (June 1987) and/or subject to the restricted rights provision of FAR 52.227-14 (June 1987) and FAR 52.227-19 (June 1987), as applicable, and any applicable agency FAR Supplements, for non-Department of Defense Federal procurements.

AMA Disclaimer

CPT® copyright 2020 American Medical Association. All rights reserved.

Fee schedules, relative value units, conversion factors, and/or related components are not assigned by the AMA, are not part of CPT®, and the AMA is not recommending their use. The AMA does not directly or indirectly practice medicine or dispense medical services. The AMA assumes no liability for data contained or not contained herein.

CPT® is a registered trademark of the American Medical Association.

ACKNOWLEDGEMENT

Jaspal Arora	Himanshu Arora, BE	Chandrashekhar Boreda, CPC
Sushanta Das, MBA	Ellen Garver, BS, BA, CPC	Leesa A. Israel, BA, CPC, CUC, CEMC, CPPM, CMBS
Rahul Jain, MDSE	Prashant Kumar, MBA	Lisa Meaney, BS
Sabyasachi Nath, MS	Ganesh Prasad Sahoo	Harshita Sharma, PT, PhD
Rajendra Sharma, RN, CPC	Nikki Taylor, MSHCI, COC, CPMA, CPC, CRC	Meagan Williford, BA, MA, CPC-A

Images/Illustrations by the following artists at shutterstock.com and Adobe Photo Stock

stockshoppe - 180896807, 99671552, 180896810, 187162193, 180896855, 180896738, 177790997, 177791516, 180896873 | Blamb - 786347626, 24129706 | Alila Medical Media - 76386163, 72231811, 149230337, 149230217, 228843253, 155445671, 147789479, 228843103, 88094230, 155445686, 101696095, 96426923, 97755608, 147943922, 147943910, 155445662, 147943874, 106263593, 106263560, 125891585, 228843262, 90181147, 94216156, 93594229 | Designua - 430118209, 180938618, 135935735, 165084413 | Suwin - 405537832 | Vecton - 661087531 | Sakurra - 676139677 | stihii - 109588457, 129969767, 124562680, 121824442, 129804629, 225637774, 505306105, 505306069 | DeryaDraws - 557609659 | Naeblys - 650014342 | NatthapongSachan - 416973331, 452997697 | udaix - 502058023, 108531449, 1336924949 | ducu59us - 104022683, 125200733 | BlueRingMedia - 141161404, 141162229, 141161560, 139691554 | joshya - 261971498 | Della_Liner- 324447776 | snapgalleria - 142194094 | okili77- 156466463 | lotan - 186878060, 110661335 | Alexander_P - 404964388 | Dario Lo Presti - 140022175 | sfam_photo - 114519994, 131191925 | Kenneth Sponsler - 120523672 | Morphart Creation - 218945404 | CandyBox Images - 137790368 | Kim Reinick - 105921317 | Darren Brode - 75731074 | Mile Atanasov - 101783710 | CLIPAREA l Custom media - 110058656 | Scott L. Williams - 133285082 | Galina Mikhalishina - 99531002 | arka38 - 131293736 | Tyler Olson - 134706608 | Picsfive - 22262149 | Rob Byron - 12685576 | Ilya Andri-yanov - 71916742 | PRILL - 87388016 | Li Wa - 8657122 | Praisaeng - 107564483, 105008411 | Poznyakov - 84875050, 84875113 | Julian Rovagnati - 39613471 | Dimedrol68 - 96322862 | Andrew Mayovskyy - 128734265, 144879658 | Stocker_team - 104959208 | JPC-PROD - 154830605 | EPSTOCK - 102915110 | Alexonline - 105673283 | Hdc Photo - 97328081 | GVictoria - #1915835 | abhijith3747 - 43079699 | Rudchenko Liliia - 124770454 | hydebrink - 1059056660

Get updates, coding tips, and corrections for this book at www.aapc.com/codebook_updates.

Table of Contents

Introduction
- Features.. 3

Symbols and Conventions 4

Instructions for Using This Code Book 5

HCPCS Level II Coding Procedures 6

New/Revised/Deleted Codes for 2021 12

Deleted Codes Crosswalk........................... 25

Anatomical Illustrations............................ 29

Index to Services, Supplies, Equipment, Drugs.. 65

Tabular List.. 105
- Transportation Services Including Ambulance (A0021- A0999).......................105
- Medical and Surgical Supplies (A4206-A8004)......................................109
- Administrative, Miscellaneous and Investigational (A9150-A9999)..................131
- Enteral and Parenteral Therapy (B4034-B9999) 137
- Outpatient PPS (C1052-C9899) 141
- Durable Medical Equipment (E0100-E8002)......................................159
- Procedures / Professional Services (G0008-G9987) 189
- Alcohol and Drug Abuse Treatment (H0001-H2037) 269
- Drugs Administered Other Than Oral Method (J0120-J8999).......................273
- Chemotherapy Drugs (J9000-J9999).......301
- Durable Medical Equipment (DME) (K0001-K1012) 307
- Orthotic Procedures and Services (L0112-L4631) 315

- Prosthetic Procedures (L5000-L9900) 339
- Medical Services (M0075-M1149)............357
- Pathology and Laboratory Services (P2028-P9615) 363
- Temporary Codes (Q0035-Q9992)...........367
- Diagnostic Radiology Services (R0070-R0076) 383
- Temporary National Codes (Non-Medicare) (S0012-S9999) 385
- National Codes Established for State Medicaid Agencies (T1000-T5999)..........409
- Coronavirus Diagnostic Panel (U0001-U0005) 415
- Vision Services (V2020-V2799) 417
- Hearing Services (V5008-V5364)..............421

Appendices
- Appendix A Table of Drugs and Biologicals...427
- Appendix B HCPCS Level II Modifiers, Lay Descriptions, and Tips 447
- Appendix C List of Abbreviations..............545
- Appendix D Place of Service/ Type of Service 549
- Appendix E APC Status Indicators............553
- Appendix F ASC Payment Indicators.......555
- Appendix G Column 1 and Column 2 Correct Coding Edits 557
- Appendix H General Correct Coding Policies..567
- Appendix I Publication 100 References..575

This page intentionally left blank

Introduction

This Healthcare Common Procedure Coding System (HCPCS) Level II code book goes beyond the basics to help you to code accurately and efficiently. In addition to including a customized Alphabetic Index and Tabular List for services, supplies, durable medical equipment, and drugs which the Centers for Medicare and Medicaid Services (CMS) developed, we include the following features:

Features

We've crafted a select set of bonus features based on requests from coders in the field as well as the recommendations of our core group of veteran coding educators. Features that you'll benefit from page after page include:

- HCPCS Level II Coding Procedures guide from CMS to help you to better understand HCPCS Level II codes
- Comprehensive list of new/revised/deleted codes for 2021
- CPT® crosswalk codes for select HCPCS Level II G codes
- Deleted codes crosswalk for 2021
- 60 stick-on tabs to mark specific sections of the book
- Symbols showing which codes have restrictions based on age or sex of the patient
- Medicare coverage and reimbursement alerts
- APC status indicators and ASC payment indicators
- HCPCS Level II modifiers with lay descriptions and coding tips
- Updated and enhanced illustrations of body systems at the front of the book so you don't have to search the code book for these large color images of body systems
- Highlighted coding instructional and informational notes help you recognize important code usage guidance for specific sections
- Intuitive color-coded symbols and alerts identify new and revised codes and critical coding and reimbursement issues quickly
- Symbols in Index showing each new code
- A user-friendly page design, including dictionary-style headers, color bleed tabs, and legend keys

Additionally, our dedicated team drew on their years of experience using code books to develop this book's user friendly symbols, highlighting, color coding, and tabs, all designed to help you find the information you need quickly.

Let Us Know What You Think

Our goal for this code book is to support those involved in the business side of healthcare, helping them to do their jobs and do them well. We'd appreciate your feedback, including your suggestions for what you'll need in a HCPCS Level II resource, so we can be sure our code books serve your needs.

Symbols and Conventions

Citations to AHA's Coding Clinic® for HCPCS Level II

AHA's *Coding Clinic*®, a quarterly newsletter, is the official publication for coding guidelines and advice as designated by the four Cooperating Parties (American Hospital Association, American Health Information Management Association, Centers for Medicare and Medicaid Services (CMS), and National Center for Health Statistics) and the Editorial Advisory Board.

We've marked codes with related *Coding Clinic*® articles with a citation that includes the year and quarter of the issue.

Symbols and Conventions Used in the Code Book Include:

2021 HCPCS Level II Code Updates

- ● New code
- ▲ Revised Code
- Ⓝ 2021 New Index Entries

Symbols and Alerts Related to Medicare or Carrier Coverage and Reimbursement

When relevant, you'll see the following symbols and alerts to the left of a code or beside or under the code descriptor:

C	Carrier judgment
D	Special coverage instructions apply
I	Not payable by Medicare
M	Non-covered by Medicare
S	Non-covered by Medicare statute

A2 - Z3 = ASC Payment Indicator

A - Y = APC Status Indicator

ASC = ASC Approved Procedure

Service not separately priced by Part B

Other carrier priced

Reasonable charge

Price established using national RVUs

Price subject to national limitation amount

Price established by carriers

Statute references

BETOS code and descriptor

References to Pub 100 (non-dental codes) – Alert appears under the code descriptor.

Modifier Alerts Showing Applicable Modifiers for a HCPCS Level II Code

DME Modifier - Alert appears under the code descriptor

Symbols for Age and Sex Codes

When relevant, you'll see the following symbols to the right of a code descriptor. We based symbol use on Medicare's Outpatient Code Editor (OCE).

♀	Female code symbol
♂	Male code symbol
Ⓐ	Age

Symbols and Alerts Related to Services, Supplies, or Equipment

When relevant, you'll see the following symbols to the right of code descriptors:

DME	Paid under the DME fee schedule
MIPS	Merit-based Incentive Payment System (MIPS) code

MIPS data in this code book is from the latest update from CMS at the time this book went to print. Refer to the CMS website for the latest updates on MIPS reporting.

Instructions for Using This Code Book

Understand Code Structure to Choose the Most Specific Code

HCPCS Level II codes are made up of five alphanumeric characters, starting with a letter that represents a category of similar codes, followed by four numbers.

The Tabular List arranges codes in alphanumeric order, starting with codes beginning with the letter A.

Code descriptors identify a category of like items or services and typically do not identify specific products or brand/trade names.

Code Services, Supplies, Equipment, and Drugs With Confidence Following This Approach

➤ The first step in choosing the proper HCPCS Level II code is reading the medical documentation to identify the service, supply, equipment, or drug that the provider documents and confirms.

   • Be sure to check online or hard copy references, such as medical dictionaries and anatomy resources, to look up unfamiliar terms.

➤ Next, decide which main term you will search in the Index based on the patient's specific case. You can look under the name of the service (magnetic resonance angiography, EMG), supply (dialysis drain bag, filler), equipment (bathtub, cane), drug (hydrocortisone, ipratropium bromide), the body site involved (hip, knee), or the type of service (laboratory tests, oncology).

➤ Once you find the term in the Index, note the recommended code. Start with the main term and review any available subterms. Cross-reference all codes listed, whether it is one code, a series of codes separated by commas, or a code range separated by a hyphen. Pay attention to the Index "*see*" convention that directs you to look elsewhere in the Index to find the code or the "*see also*" convention that directs you to look in an additional place to find the code.

➤ Turn to that code in the Tabular List, and read the full code descriptor for correct code assignment.

➤ Before making your final code decision, review the surrounding codes to be sure there isn't a more appropriate code available. Pay attention to the "*see*" convention in the Tabular List that directs you to look elsewhere to find the code or the "*see also*" convention that directs you to look in an additional place to find the code.

➤ Finally, take a moment to confirm that your code choice complies with the philosophy of ethical coding. Never report a HCPCS Level II code simply because it will support reimbursement from a payer. Report only those codes the documentation supports.

➤ When searching the Table of Drugs and Biologicals, search for the name of the drug, then the unit and route to find the drug code to cross-reference to the Tabular List.

Note: When Searching the Table of Drugs and Biologicals, search for the name of the drug, then the unit and route to find the drug code to cross-reference to the Tabular List.

HCPCS Level II Coding Procedures

HEALTHCARE COMMON PROCEDURE CODING SYSTEM (HCPCS) LEVEL II CODING PROCEDURES

This information provides a description of the procedures CMS follows in processing HCPCS code applications and making coding decisions.

FOR FURTHER INFORMATION CONTACT:

Kimberlee Combs Miller	(410) 786-6707	Kimberlee.Combs@cms.hhs.gov
Irina Akelaitis	(410) 786-4602	Irina.akelaitis@cms.hhs.gov
Felicia Kyeremeh	(410) 786-1898	Felicia.kyeremeh@cms.hhs.gov
Sundus Ashar	(410) 786-0750	Sundus.ashar1@cms.hhs.gov
William Walker	(410) 786-5023	William.walker@cms.hhs.gov
Constantine Markos	(410) 786-0911	Constantine.markos@cms.hhs.gov.

A. HCPCS BACKGROUND INFORMATION

Each year in the United States, health care insurers process over 5 billion claims for payment. For Medicare and other health insurance programs to ensure that these claims are processed in an orderly and consistent manner, standardized coding systems are essential. The Healthcare Common Procedure Coding System (HCPCS) Level II Code Set is one of the standard, national medical code sets specified by the Health Insurance Portability and Accountability Act (HIPAA) for this purpose. The HCPCS is divided into two principal subsystems, referred to as Level I and Level II of the HCPCS. Level I of the HCPCS is comprised of CPT® (Current Procedural Terminology), a numeric coding system maintained by the American Medical Association (AMA). The CPT® is a uniform coding system consisting of descriptive terms and codes that are used primarily to identify medical services and procedures furnished by physicians and other health care professionals. These health care professionals use the CPT® to identify services and procedures for which they bill public or private health insurance programs. The CPT® codes are republished and updated annually by the AMA.

HCPCS Level II is a standardized coding system that is used primarily to identify products, supplies, and services not included in the CPT® code set jurisdiction, such as ambulance services and durable medical equipment, prosthetics, orthotics, and supplies (DMEPOS) when used outside a physician's office. Because Medicare and other insurers cover a variety of services, supplies, and equipment that are not identified by CPT® codes, the HCPCS Level II codes were established for submitting claims for these items. Level II codes are also referred to as alpha- numeric codes because they consist of a single alphabetical letter followed by four numeric digits, while CPT® codes primarily are identified using five numeric digits.

B. HISTORY

The development and use of Level II of the HCPCS began in the 1980s. Concurrent to the use of Level II codes, there were also Level III codes. HCPCS Level III were developed and used by Medicaid State agencies, Medicare contractors, and private insurers in their specific programs or local areas of jurisdiction. For purposes of Medicare, Level III codes were also referred to as local codes. Local codes were established when an insurer preferred that suppliers use a local code to identify a service, for which there is no Level I or Level II code, rather than use a "miscellaneous or not otherwise classified code."

HIPAA required the Secretary to adopt standards for coding systems that are used for reporting health care transactions. Thus, regulations were published in the Federal Register on August 17, 2000 (65 FR 50312), to implement standardized coding systems under HIPAA. These regulations provided for the elimination of Level III local codes by October 2002, at which time, the Level I and Level II code sets could be used. The elimination of local codes was postponed, as a result of section 532(a) of BIPA, which continued the use of local codes through December 31, 2003.

The regulation that was published on August 17, 2000 (45 CFR 162.1002), to implement the HIPAA requirement for standardized coding systems established the HCPCS Level II codes as the standardized coding system for describing and identifying health care equipment and supplies in health care transactions that are not within the CPT® code set jurisdiction. The HCPCS Level II coding system was selected as the standardized coding system because of its wide acceptance among both public and private insurers.

C. AUTHORITY

The Secretary of the Department of Health and Human Services has delegated authority under HIPAA to CMS to maintain and distribute HCPCS Level II codes. As stated in August 17, 2000 (45 CFR 162.1002), CMS establishes uniform national definitions of services, codes to represent services, and payment modifiers to the codes.

D. HCPCS LEVEL II CODES

The HCPCS Level II coding system is a comprehensive, standardized system that classifies similar products that are medical in nature into categories for the purpose of efficient claims processing. For each alpha-numeric HCPCS code, there is descriptive terminology that identifies a category of like items. These codes are used primarily for billing purposes. For example, suppliers use HCPCS Level II codes to identify items on claim forms that are being billed to a private or public health insurer. Currently, there are national HCPCS codes representing almost 8,000 separate categories of like items or services that encompass products from different manufacturers. When submitting claims, suppliers are required to use one of these codes to identify the items they are billing.

HCPCS is a system for identifying items and certain services. It is not a methodology or system for making coverage or payment determinations, and the existence of a code does not, of itself, determine coverage or non-coverage for an item or service. While these codes are used for billing purposes, decisions regarding the addition, deletion, or revision of HCPCS codes are made independent of the process for making determinations regarding coverage and payment.

With regard to the Medicare program, if specific Medicare coverage or payment indicators or values have not been established for any new HCPCS codes, this may be because a national Medicare coverage determination and/or fee schedule amounts have not yet been established for these items. This is neither an indicator of Medicare coverage or non-coverage. In these cases, until national Medicare coverage and payment guidelines have been established for these codes, the Medicare coverage and payment determinations for these items may be made based on the discretion of the Medicare contractors processing claims for these items.

E. TYPES OF HCPCS LEVEL II CODES

There are several types of HCPCS Level II codes depending on the purpose for the codes and the entity with responsibility for establishing and maintaining them.

HCPCS National Codes

National HCPCS Level II codes are maintained by CMS. CMS is responsible for making decisions about additions, revisions, and deletions to the national alpha-numeric codes. These codes are for the use of all private and public health insurers.

Within CMS, there is a CMS HCPCS Workgroup, which is an internal workgroup comprised of federal government employees who represent the major components of CMS, as well as federal employees from pertinent Federal agencies, including the Department of Veterans Affairs and the Department of Defense. Applications for a revision to the HCPCS are reviewed at a regularly scheduled meeting of the CMS HCPCS Workgroup to discuss whether coding requests warrant a change to the national codes. This Workgroup informs CMS' decisions.

The application and instructions for requesting that CMS add, revise, or discontinue a Level II code is detailed on CMS' HCPCS Level II web site at http://www.cms.gov/Medicare/Coding/Medhcpcsgeninfo/index.html. CMS also may issue codes based on the needs of its programs or other federal programs, and those programs are not required to submit an application for a code to be issued.

Dental Codes

Dental codes, or D codes, are a separate category of national codes. The Current Dental Terminology (CDT) is published, copyrighted, and licensed by the American Dental Association (ADA). The CDT lists codes for billing for dental procedures and supplies. While the CDT codes are considered HCPCS Level II codes, decisions regarding the revision, deletion, or addition of CDT codes are made by the ADA, not CMS.

Miscellaneous Codes

National codes also include "miscellaneous/not otherwise classified" codes. These codes are used when a supplier is submitting a bill for an item or service and there is no existing national code that adequately describes the item or service being billed. The importance of miscellaneous codes is that they allow suppliers to begin billing immediately for a service or item as soon as it is allowed to be marketed by the Food and Drug Administration (FDA), even though there is no distinct code that describes the service or item. A miscellaneous code may be assigned by insurers for use during the period of time a request for a new code is being considered under the HCPCS review process. The use of miscellaneous codes also helps avoid the inefficiency and administrative burden of assigning distinct codes for items or services that are rarely furnished or for which few claims are expected to be filed. Because of miscellaneous codes, the absence of a specific code for a distinct category of products does not affect the ability of a supplier to submit claims to private or public insurers.

In those cases in which a supplier or manufacturer has been advised to use a miscellaneous code because there is no existing code that describes a given product, and the supplier or manufacturer believes that a new code is needed, the supplier or manufacturer may submit a request to modify the HCPCS in accordance with the established process. The standard process for requesting a revision to the HCPCS Level II codes is explained later in this document.

Other Notable Codes

- The C codes (Pass-Through) were established to permit implementation of section 201 of the Balanced Budget Refinement Act of 1999. HCPCS C codes are utilized to report drugs, biologicals, magnetic resonance angiography (MRA), and devices used for CMS' Medicare Hospital Outpatient Prospective Payment System (HOPPS). HCPCS C codes are reported for device categories, new technology procedures, and drugs, biologicals, and radiopharmaceuticals that do not have other HCPCS code assignments. Non-OPPS hospitals, Critical Access Hospitals (CAHs), Indian Health Service hospitals (IHS), and hospitals located in American Samoa, Guam, Northern Mariana Islands, and the Virgin Islands, as well as Maryland waiver hospitals, may report these codes at their discretion.

  For information about the HOPPS pass-through process, please visit the HOPPS web site: https://www.cms.gov/Medicare/Medicare-Fee-for-Service-Payment/HospitalOutpatientPPS/index.

- The G codes are used to identify professional health care procedures and services that would otherwise be coded in CPT®-4 (the current version of CPT® codes) but for which there are no CPT®-4 codes. CMS does not have an application process for G codes, as they are established internally by CMS to support Medicare claims processing needs. As G codes are part of the national HCPCS Level II code set, they may also be used by non-Medicare insurers.

- The G codes and C codes are considered HCPCS Level II codes and as such, these codes, and changes to them, are included in CMS' HCPCS Level II Updates published by CMS. The code application procedures described in this document are not for use to apply for changes to HCPCS C codes and G codes.

- The Q codes are established to identify drugs, biologicals, and medical equipment or services not identified by national HCPCS Level II codes, but for which codes are needed for Medicare claims processing.

- The K codes are established for use by the DME MACs when current national codes do not include the codes needed to implement a DME MAC medical review policy. For example, codes other than the current, existing national codes may be needed by the DME MACs to identify certain product categories and supplies necessary for establishing appropriate regional medical review coverage policies.

Code Modifiers

HCPCS code modifiers are established internally by CMS to facilitate accurate Medicare claims processing. Modifiers are assigned for use when the information provided by a HCPCS code descriptor needs to be supplemented to identify specific circumstances that may apply to an item or service. For example, a UE modifier is used when the item identified by a HCPCS code is "used equipment;" a NU modifier is used for "new equipment." The HCPCS Level II modifiers are either alpha-numeric or two letters. HCPCS code modifiers are published as part of the HCPCS code set at https://www.cms.gov/Medicare/Coding/HCPCSReleaseCodeSets/Alpha-Numeric-HCPCS The modifiers appear at the beginning of the file, before alpha-numeric codes.

HCPCS Code Assignment Following Medicare National Coverage Determination (NCD)

Pursuant to section 1862(I)(3)(C)(iv) of the Social Security Act (added by section 731(a) of the Medicare Modernization Act), CMS identifies an appropriate existing code category and/or establishes a new code category to describe the item that is the subject of a National Coverage Determination (NCD).

Effective July 1, 2004, CMS' procedures are as follows:

1. Assignment of an existing code: When CMS determines that an item is already identified by an existing HCPCS code category, but was previously not covered, CMS will assign the item to the existing code category and ensure that the coverage indicator assigned to the code category accurately reflects Medicare policy regarding coverage for the item. Section 731 of the MMA does not require that a new code category or a product specific code be created for an item simply because a new coverage determination was made, without regard to codes available in the existing code set.

2. Assignment of a New Code: When CMS determines that a new code category is appropriate, CMS will make every effort to establish, publish, and implement the new code at the time the final coverage determination is made.

3. Assignment of a Miscellaneous Code: Under certain circumstances, the assignment of an item to a miscellaneous code may be necessary. A number of miscellaneous codes already exist under various headings throughout the HCPCS Level II code set. When a new code is appropriate, but the change cannot be implemented and incorporated into billing and claims processing systems at the time the final NCD decision memorandum is released, an unclassified code may be assigned in the interim, until a new code can be implemented, in order to ensure that claims can be processed for the item. The timing of implementation of new codes relative to the date of the coverage determination depends on a variety of factors, some of which are not within the control of the code set maintainers. One such example is when the timing of the coverage determination is such that the publication deadline for the next update is missed.

F. REQUESTING A REVISION TO THE HCPCS LEVEL II CODES

Anyone may submit a request for modifying the HCPCS Level II national code set. CMS' HCPCS Level II Code application instructions can be found on CMS' HCPCS web site at https://www.cms.gov/Medicare/Coding/MedHCPCSGenInfo/index. As part of the application, the applicant should also submit any descriptive material, including the manufacturer's product literature and information that the applicant thinks would be helpful in furthering CMS' understanding of the medical features of the item for which a coding revision is requested.

Applications that are received and determined by CMS to be complete by the deadline will be considered for inclusion in that cycle. Applications received after the deadline will be declined and the applicant should resubmit to a subsequent coding cycle. Applications received by the deadline that are determined to be incomplete will also be declined and the applicant should submit a completed application in a subsequent coding cycle. CMS will make every effort to complete the review within the applicable coding cycle for all

timely and complete code applications. However, it should be understood that on the rare occasion a particularly complex or multi-faceted decision requires additional evaluation beyond the timeframe of the coding cycle, CMS maintains the flexibility at its discretion to continue consideration of that application into the next coding cycle. Examples of circumstances under which application consideration may be extended to the next coding cycle may include but are not limited to coding considerations that require in-depth clinical or other research and complicated claims adjudication scenarios.

There are three types of coding revisions to the HCPCS that can be requested:

1. That a new code be added. This could include requests to split an existing code category into its components or into subcategories;

2. That the language used to describe an existing code be changed:

   When there is an existing code, a request can be made when a stakeholder believes that the descriptor for the code needs to be revised to provide a better description of the category of products represented by the code.

3. That an existing code be discontinued.

   When an existing code becomes obsolete or is duplicative of another code, a request can be made to discontinue the code. This could include requests to combine existing codes.

Until further notice, all applications to CMS' Level II HCPCS coding program must be submitted electronically via our secure mailbox. Paper applications sent to CMS will not be processed. Please electronically submit all HCPCS code requests to our new mailbox, using the following instructions:

- Create a PDF document, both Word and Libre Office will save documents as PDF files
- The files must be zipped with a passphrase with AES 256 encryption if they contain any proprietary or personally identifiable information
- In PKZip, set the security options to AES 256 passphrase. 7Zip can also be used to encrypt the zip files using AES 256 passphrase
- Enter the passphrase in the dialogue box to encrypt the files
- Attachments must be less than 100M. Split size will create multi part zip files which can be sent in separate messages
- Send the passphrase in a separate email from the zip files to the email address below
- The applications should be emailed to : HCPCS_Level_II_code_applications@cms.hhs.gov
- The e-mail box (above) may also be used to notify CMS staff of problems with electronic application submissions. Staff will be available to respond during normal business hours
- CMS staff will e-mail confirmation of applications received.

Evaluating HCPCS Coding Applications

CMS applies the following criteria to determine when there is not a demonstrated need for a new or modified code or the need to remove a code:

1. When an existing code adequately describes the item in a coding request, no new or modified code is established. An existing code adequately describes an item in a coding request when the existing code describes products with the following:

    -   Functions similar to the item in the coding request.
    -   No significant therapeutic distinctions from the item in the coding request.

2. When an existing code describes products that provide almost the same functionality with only minor distinctions from the item in the coding request, the item in the coding request may be grouped with that code and the code descriptor modified to reflect the distinctions.

3. A code is not established for an item that is used only in the inpatient setting or for an item that is not diagnostic or therapeutic in nature.

4. A new or modified code is not established for an item that is regulated by the FDA, unless the FDA allows the item to be marketed. Documentation of FDA approval is required to be submitted with the coding request application.

5. Applications for non-drug items that are not regulated by the FDA and also not yet available in the U.S. market will be considered incomplete and will not be processed.

6. The determination to remove a code is based on CMS' consideration of whether a code is obsolete (for example, products no longer are used, other more specific codes have been added) or duplicative and no longer useful (for example, new codes are established that better describe items identified by existing codes).

In developing its decisions, CMS uses the criteria mentioned above. Cost or pricing is not a factor.

HCPCS Coding Cycles, Timelines, Deadlines, and Final Decisions

Beginning in 2020, CMS is implementing shorter and more frequent coding cycles to further advance its initiative to unleash innovation.

DMEPOS and Other Non-drug, Non-biological Coding Cycles: no less frequently than bi-annually

2020 Coding Cycle 1 for applications for DMEPOS and other non-drug, non-biological items:

Application Deadline:	Jan. 6, 2020
Publish Preliminary Decisions by:	May 1, 2020
Public Meeting:	Mid-May 2020 (dates to be announced in Federal Register)
Publication of Final Decisions:	July

2020 Coding Cycle 2 for applications for DMEPOS and other non-drug, non-biological items:

Application Deadline:	June 29, 2020
Publish Preliminary Decisions by:	Approximately two weeks prior to the Public Meeting date
Public Meeting:	Fall (October – November) 2020 (dates to be announced in Federal Register)
Publication of Final Decisions:	January 2021 or earlier

HCPCS Public Meetings for DMEPOS and Other Non-drug, Non-biological Items:

In 2000, Congress passed the Medicare, Medicaid, and SCHIP Benefits Improvement and Protection Act of 2000 (BIPA), Public Law 106-554. Subtitle D, Section 531(b) of BIPA requires the Secretary to have procedures that permit public consultation for coding and payment determinations for new DME under Medicare Part B of title XVIII of the Social Security Act. Accordingly, CMS will host bi-annual public meetings for the 2020 Coding Cycle that provide a forum for interested parties to make oral presentations and/or to submit written comments in response to preliminary HCPCS coding for new DMEPOS as well as for other non-drug, non- biological products for which code applications have been submitted using the HCPCS coding revision process. Coding requests for other non-drug, non-biological products are addressed in these public meetings because CMS is utilizing the public meeting forum to address certain other coding requests in addition to new DME.

Agenda items for the meetings are published in advance of the public meeting on the HCPCS web site at https://www.cms.gov/Medicare/Coding/MedHCPCSGenInfo/index. The public meeting agendas include descriptions of the coding requests, the applicant, and the name of the product or service, and CMS' preliminary HCPCS coding and Medicare payment decisions and rationale.

This public meeting forum provides an opportunity for the public to become aware of coding changes under consideration for DMEPOS and other non-drug, non-biological items, as well as an opportunity for public input into final decisions. See: "Guidelines for Participation in CMS' HCPCS Public Meetings" on CMS' HCPCS web site at https://www.cms.gov/Medicare/Coding/MedHCPCSGenInfo/index.

Drugs and Biological Products Coding Cycles: no less frequently than quarterly

2020 Coding Cycle 1 for applications for drugs and biological products:

Application Deadline:	Jan. 6, 2020
Publication of Final Decisions:	April

2020 Coding Cycle 2 for applications for drugs and biological products:

Application Deadline:	April 6, 2020
Publication of Final Decisions:	July

2020 Coding Cycle 3 for applications for drugs and biological products:

Application Deadline: June 29, 2020

Publication of Final Decisions: October

2020 Coding Cycle 4 for applications for drugs and biological products:

Application Deadline: September 21, 2020

Publication of Final Decisions: January 2021 or earlier

Changes to CMS' HCPCS Coding Procedures that Enable Quarterly Coding Cycles for Drugs and Biological Products:

CMS' delivery on its important goal and stakeholder requests to implement quarterly coding cycles for drugs and biological products necessitated procedural changes that balance the need to code more quickly against the amount of time necessary to process applications, as described below.

The availability of final elements of FDA approval is critical to CMS decision-making for drug and biological codes, particularly where this shorter coding cycle makes CMS reliant upon having complete application information at the time of the application deadline. Accordingly, in implementing significantly shorter coding cycles, CMS has eliminated the 3 month deadline extension for submission of FDA clearance documentation following the application deadline (as previously offered within the annual coding cycle). Under the newly implemented shorter coding cycles, all required FDA documentation is due by the application deadline. Thus, under this new process, the overall timeframe between FDA approval and HCPCS coding will generally be significantly shorter than in the prior annual coding cycle.

In order to further achieve the additional time savings necessary to implement coding for the vast majority of drugs and biological products on a quarterly cycle, CMS will not be able to conduct public meetings for coding decisions on drugs and biological products, but for 2020 coding cycles will provide an opportunity for applicants to resubmit the application in a subsequent quarterly coding cycle. This offers an opportunity for individual applicants who are dissatisfied with CMS' coding decisions in one quarterly cycle to immediately reapply in the next or a subsequent quarterly cycle. Thus, the overall timeframe for consideration of successive applications is generally still significantly shorter than the prior, annual coding cycle. Although CMS previously included drug and biological code applications in its HCPCS Public Meeting processes, we believe that the changes above are necessary to allow CMS to provide coding on a quarterly cycle.

Requests for Separate Meetings:

The HCPCS coordinator schedules meetings with an interested party, at the party's request, as time permits to discuss the application(s) for possible changes to the HCPCS Level II codes. These meetings are held by teleconference.

These meetings are not related to the public meetings mandated by section 531(b) of BIPA; they are also not decision-making meetings or CMS HCPCS Workgroup meetings.

Final Decisions for All HCPCS Code Applications:

CMS is responsible for making the final decisions pertaining to requests for additions, deletions, and revisions to the HCPCS Level II codes. These decisions may include:

1. The request to establish new national code(s) has been approved.

2. The request to revise existing national code(s) has been approved.

3. The request to discontinue existing national code(s) has been approved.

4. A change to the national codes has been approved that reflects, completely or in part, the coding request. Examples of circumstances under which a change to coding might reflect, in part, the coding request include the addition of a single new code when the incoming request was to establish a series of related codes (e.g., for different package sizes); or addition of a new code that includes a dose descriptor reflecting the lowest common denominator that could be billed in multiples, as per CMS' longstanding coding convention, when the incoming request specified a different dose descriptor.

5. The request for a new code has not been approved because the scope of the request necessitates that additional consideration be given to the request before CMS reaches a final decision.

6. The request for a new national code has not been approved because there already is an existing code that describes the product.

7. The request for a code has not been approved because the product is not used by health care providers for diagnostic or therapeutic purposes.

8. The request for a code has not been approved because the code requested is for capital equipment.

9. The request for a code has not been approved because the product is an integral part of another service and the code for that service includes the product.

10. The request for a revision to the language that describes the current code has not been approved because it does not improve the code descriptor.

11. The request for a new code has not been approved because the product is not primarily medical in nature.

12. The request for a code has not been approved because the product is used exclusively in the inpatient hospital setting.

13. The request for a code has not been approved because it is inappropriate for inclusion in the HCPCS Level II code set and a request should be submitted independently to another coding authority (e.g. AMA for CPT® coding, ADA for CDT coding, etc.)

CMS will include the reasoning for reaching its decision, along with the decision.

For 2020 coding cycles, any applicant who is dissatisfied with CMS' final HCPCS coding decision may submit a new request in a subsequent coding cycle. Although new information is not a requirement of a new application, previously unavailable information or additional explanations that support the request may be helpful in informing CMS with regard to why CMS' prior decision should be changed.

G. AVAILABILITY OF HCPCS UPDATES

As part of CMS' ongoing efforts to improve transparency regarding HCPCS Level II coding decisions and streamline our processes, CMS has implemented additional improvements to the issuance of HCPCS coding decisions. Beginning in 2020, consistent with implementing shorter and more frequent HCPCS coding cycles, CMS will release its decisions on all coding actions on a quarterly basis in the same format as CMS previously announced its annual decisions (see timeframes above). These actions are available on CMS' web site at https://www.cms.gov/Medicare/Coding/HCPCSReleaseCodeSets/Alpha-Numeric-HCPCS.

Each payer effectuates the changes to the code sets on its own timeframes. For Medicare, unless otherwise announced or specified, the changes to the codes sets will become effective as follows:

For Quarterly Cycle 1 Drug and Biological Code Applications:

Published Decisions:	April
Effective:	July 1, 2020

For Quarterly Cycle 2 Drug and Biological Code Applications and for Bi-annual Cycle 1 DMEPOS and other Non-drug, Non-biological Code Applications:

Published Decisions:	July
Effective:	October 1, 2020

For Quarterly Cycle 3 Drug and Biological Code Applications:

Published Decisions:	October
Effective:	January 1, 2021

For Quarterly Cycle 4 Drug and Biological Code Applications and for Bi-annual Cycle 2 DMEPOS and other Non-drug, Non-biological Code Applications:

Published Decisions:	January 2021 or earlier
Effective:	April 1, 2021

Along with quarterly releases, CMS also publishes narrative statements for the HCPCS Level II coding decisions, which provide additional detailed information, including the topic and background summary of every application; CMS' preliminary HCPCS coding recommendations, where applicable; a summary of primary speaker comments at CMS' HCPCS Public Meetings, where applicable; and CMS' final coding decisions and rationale.

In early 2019, CMS created an intuitive online search feature to identify links to current and prior year's publication of narrative summaries and spreadsheets providing HCPCS code application and decision information. CMS also restored previously published information from prior years. Typically, the information in the narrative summary has also been included in the HCPCS coding decision letters written by CMS and mailed to each individual applicant. To streamline our notification processes, effective for the 2019-2020 HCPCS coding cycle, rather than issuing individual decision letters, CMS refers applicants and other stakeholders to the narrative summary and encourages stakeholders to monitor CMS' HCPCS General Information web site at https://www.cms.gov/Medicare/Coding/MedHCPCSGenInfo/index for updates.

The General Information web site also includes tools to assist stakeholders in locating files or information regarding the most recent HCPCS update, including an alphabetical index of HCPCS codes by type of service or product; an alphabetical table of drugs for which there are Level II codes; a listing of miscellaneous codes (referred to as "Not Otherwise Classified" (NOC)) codes; HCPCS Public Meeting Agendas, which list applications submitted in the current coding cycle; CMS' HCPCS code application process and instructions; HCPCS Level II Coding procedures; guidelines for participation in CMS' HCPCS Public Meeting; HCPCS Decision Tree, which illustrates CMS' code decision criteria; and notice of CMS' decisions to discontinue HCPCS codes. Electronic updates and instructions that include an updated list of codes and identify which codes have been added, revised, or deleted are sent by CMS to Medicare contractors and state Medicaid agencies.

Rev. September 16, 2020.

New/Revised/Deleted Codes for 2021

NEW CODES

Code	Code Descriptor
A9591	Fluoroestradiol f 18, diagnostic, 1 millicurie
C1052	Hemostatic agent, gastrointestinal, topical
C1062	Intravertebral body fracture augmentation with implant (e.g., metal, polymer)
C1748	Endoscope, single-use (i.e. disposable), upper gi, imaging/illumination device (insertable)
C1825	Generator, neurostimulator (implantable), non-rechargeable with carotid sinus baroreceptor stimulation lead(s)
C1849	Skin substitute, synthetic, resorbable, per square centimeter
C9065	Injection, romidepsin, non-lyophilized (e.g., liquid), 1mg
C9067	Gallium ga-68, dotatoc, diagnostic, 0.01 mci
C9068	Copper cu-64, dotatate, diagnostic, 1 millicurie
C9069	Injection, belantamab mafodontin-blmf, 0.5 mg
C9070	Injection, tafasitamab-cxix, 2 mg
C9071	Injection, viltolarsen, 10 mg
C9072	Injection, immune globulin (asceniv), 500 mg
C9073	Brexucabtagene autoleucel, up to 200 million autologous anti-cd19 car positive viable t cells, including leukapheresis and dose preparation procedures, per therapeutic dose
C9122	Mometasone furoate sinus implant, 10 micrograms (sinuva)
C9759	Transcatheter intraoperative blood vessel microinfusion(s) (e.g., intraluminal, vascular wall and/or perivascular) therapy, any vessel, including radiological supervision and interpretation, when performed
C9760	Non-randomized, non-blinded procedure for nyha class ii, iii, iv heart failure; transcatheter implantation of interatrial shunt, including right and left heart catheterization, transseptal puncture, trans-esophageal echocardiography (tee)/intracardiac echocardiography (ice), and all imaging with or without guidance (e.g., ultrasound, fluoroscopy), performed in an approved investigational device exemption (ide) study
C9761	Cystourethroscopy, with ureteroscopy and/or pyeloscopy, with lithotripsy (ureteral catheterization is included) and vacuum aspiration of the kidney, collecting system and urethra if applicable
C9762	Cardiac magnetic resonance imaging for morphology and function, quantification of segmental dysfunction; with strain imaging
C9763	Cardiac magnetic resonance imaging for morphology and function, quantification of segmental dysfunction; with stress imaging
C9764	Revascularization, endovascular, open or percutaneous, lower extremity artery(ies), except tibial/peroneal; with intravascular lithotripsy, includes angioplasty within the same vessel(s), when performed

Code	Code Descriptor
C9765	Revascularization, endovascular, open or percutaneous, lower extremity artery(ies), except tibial/peroneal; with intravascular lithotripsy, and transluminal stent placement(s), includes angioplasty within the same vessel(s), when performed
C9766	Revascularization, endovascular, open or percutaneous, lower extremity artery(ies), except tibial/peroneal; with intravascular lithotripsy and atherectomy, includes angioplasty within the same vessel(s), when performed
C9767	Revascularization, endovascular, open or percutaneous, lower extremity artery(ies), except tibial/peroneal; with intravascular lithotripsy and transluminal stent placement(s), and atherectomy, includes angioplasty within the same vessel(s), when performed
C9768	Endoscopic ultrasound-guided direct measurement of hepatic portosystemic pressure gradient by any method (list separately in addition to code for primary procedure)
C9769	Cystourethroscopy, with insertion of temporary prostatic implant/stent with fixation/anchor and incisional struts
C9770	Vitrectomy, mechanical, pars plana approach, with subretinal injection of pharmacologic/biologic agent
C9771	Nasal/sinus endoscopy, cryoablation nasal tissue(s) and/or nerve(s), unilateral or bilateral
C9772	Revascularization, endovascular, open or percutaneous, tibial/peroneal artery(ies), with intravascular lithotripsy, includes angioplasty within the same vessel (s), when performed
C9773	Revascularization, endovascular, open or percutaneous, tibial/peroneal artery(ies); with intravascular lithotripsy, and transluminal stent placement(s), includes angioplasty within the same vessel(s), when performed
C9774	Revascularization, endovascular, open or percutaneous, tibial/peroneal artery(ies); with intravascular lithotripsy and atherectomy, includes angioplasty within the same vessel (s), when performed
C9775	Revascularization, endovascular, open or percutaneous, tibial/peroneal artery(ies); with intravascular lithotripsy and transluminal stent placement(s), and atherectomy, includes angioplasty within the same vessel (s), when performed
C9803	Hospital outpatient clinic visit specimen collection for severe acute respiratory syndrome coronavirus 2 (sars-cov-2) (coronavirus disease [covid-19]), any specimen source
G0088	Professional services, initial visit, for the administration of anti-infective, pain management, chelation, pulmonary hypertension, inotropic, or other intravenous infusion drug or biological (excluding chemotherapy or other highly complex drug or biological) for each infusion drug administration calendar day in the individual's home, each 15 minutes

Code	Code Descriptor
G0089	Professional services, initial visit, for the administration of subcutaneous immunotherapy or other subcutaneous infusion drug or biological for each infusion drug administration calendar day in the individual's home, each 15 minutes
G0090	Professional services, initial visit, for the administration of intravenous chemotherapy or other highly complex infusion drug or biological for each infusion drug administration calendar day in the individual's home, each 15 minutes
G1012	Clinical decision support mechanism agilemd, as defined by the medicare appropriate use criteria program
G1013	Clinical decision support mechanism evidencecare imaging advisor, as defined by the medicare appropriate use criteria program
G1014	Clinical decision support mechanism inveniqa semantic answers in medicine, as defined by the medicare appropriate use criteria program
G1015	Clinical decision support mechanism reliant medical group, as defined by the medicare appropriate use criteria program
G1016	Clinical decision support mechanism speed of care, as defined by the medicare appropriate use criteria program
G1017	Clinical decision support mechanism healthhelp, as defined by the medicare appropriate use criteria program
G1018	Clinical decision support mechanism infinx, as defined by the medicare appropriate use criteria program
G1019	Clinical decision support mechanism logicnets, as defined by the medicare appropriate use criteria program
G1020	Clinical decision support mechanism curbside clinical augmented workflow, as defined by the medicare appropriate use criteria program
G1021	Clinical decision support mechanism ehealthline clinical decision support mechanism, as defined by the medicare appropriate use criteria program
G1022	Clinical decision support mechanism intermountain clinical decision support mechanism, as defined by the medicare appropriate use criteria program
G1023	Clinical decision support mechanism persivia clinical decision support, as defined by the medicare appropriate use criteria program
G2023	Specimen collection for severe acute respiratory syndrome coronavirus 2 (sars-cov-2) (coronavirus disease [covid-19]), any specimen source
G2024	Specimen collection for severe acute respiratory syndrome coronavirus 2 (sars-cov-2) (coronavirus disease [covid-19]) from an individual in a snf or by a laboratory on behalf of a hha, any specimen source
G2025	Payment for a telehealth distant site service furnished by a rural health clinic (rhc) or federally qualified health center (fqhc) only
G2168	Services performed by a physical therapist assistant in the home health setting in the delivery of a safe and effective physical therapy maintenance program, each 15 minutes

Code	Code Descriptor
G2169	Services performed by an occupational therapist assistant in the home health setting in the delivery of a safe and effective occupational therapy maintenance program, each 15 minutes
G2170	Percutaneous arteriovenous fistula creation (avf), direct, any site, by tissue approximation using thermal resistance energy, and secondary procedures to redirect blood flow (e.g., transluminal balloon angioplasty, coil embolization) when performed, and includes all imaging and radiologic guidance, supervision and interpretation, when performed
G2171	Percutaneous arteriovenous fistula creation (avf), direct, any site, using magnetic-guided arterial and venous catheters and radiofrequency energy, including flow-directing procedures (e.g., vascular coil embolization with radiologic supervision and interpretation, wen performed) and fistulogram(s), angiography, enography, and/or ultrasound, with radiologic supervision and interpretation, when performed
G2173	Uri episodes where the patient had a competing comorbid condition during the 12 months prior to or on the episode date (e.g., tuberculosis, neutropenia, cystic fibrosis, chronic bronchitis, pulmonary edema, respiratory failure, rheumatoid lung disease)
G2174	Uri episodes when the patient had a new or refill prescription of antibiotics (table 1) in the 30 days prior to or on the episode date
G2175	Episodes where the patient had a competing comorbid condition during the 12 months prior to or on the episode date (e.g., tuberculosis, neutropenia, cystic fibrosis, chronic bronchitis, pulmonary edema, respiratory failure, rheumatoid lung disease)
G2176	Outpatient, ed, or observation visits that result in an inpatient admission
G2177	Acute bronchitis/bronchiolitis episodes when the patient had a new or refill prescription of antibiotics (table 1) in the 30 days prior to or on the episode date
G2178	Clinician documented that patient was not an eligible candidate for lower extremity neurological exam measure, for example patient bilateral amputee; patient has condition that would not allow them to accurately respond to a neurological exam (dementia, alzheimer's, etc.); patient has previously documented diabetic peripheral neuropathy with loss of protective sensation
G2179	Clinician documented that patient had medical reason for not performing lower extremity neurological exam
G2180	Clinician documented that patient was not an eligible candidate for evaluation of footwear as patient is bilateral lower extremity amputee
G2181	Bmi not documented due to medical reason or patient refusal of height or weight measurement
G2182	Patient receiving first-time biologic disease modifying anti-rheumatic drug therapy
G2183	Documentation patient unable to communicate and informant not available
G2184	Patient does not have a caregiver
G2185	Documentation caregiver is trained and certified in dementia care

Code	Code Descriptor
G2186	Patient /caregiver dyad has been referred to appropriate resources and connection to those resources is confirmed
G2187	Patients with clinical indications for imaging of the head: head trauma
G2188	Patients with clinical indications for imaging of the head: new or change in headache above 50 years of age
G2189	Patients with clinical indications for imaging of the head: abnormal neurologic exam
G2190	Patients with clinical indications for imaging of the head: headache radiating to the neck
G2191	Patients with clinical indications for imaging of the head: positional headaches
G2192	Patients with clinical indications for imaging of the head: temporal headaches in patients over 55 years of age
G2193	Patients with clinical indications for imaging of the head: new onset headache in pre-school children or younger (<6 years of age)
G2194	Patients with clinical indications for imaging of the head: new onset headache in pediatric patients with disabilities for which headache is a concern as inferred from behavior
G2195	Patients with clinical indications for imaging of the head: occipital headache in children
G2196	Patient identified as an unhealthy alcohol user when screened for unhealthy alcohol use using a systematic screening method
G2197	Patient screened for unhealthy alcohol use using a systematic screening method and not identified as an unhealthy alcohol user
G2198	Documentation of medical reason(s) for not screening for unhealthy alcohol use using a systematic screening method (e.g., limited life expectancy, other medical reasons)
G2199	Patient not screened for unhealthy alcohol use using a systematic screening method, reason not given
G2200	Patient identified as an unhealthy alcohol user received brief counseling
G2201	Documentation of medical reason(s) for not providing brief counseling (e.g., limited life expectancy, other medical reasons)
G2202	Patient did not receive brief counseling if identified as an unhealthy alcohol user, reason not given
G2203	Documentation of medical reason(s) for not providing brief counseling if identified as an unhealthy alcohol user (e.g., limited life expectancy, other medical reasons)
G2204	Patients between 50 and 85 years of age who received a screening colonoscopy during the performance period
G2205	Patients with pregnancy during adjuvant treatment course
G2206	Patient received adjuvant treatment course including both chemotherapy and her2-targeted therapy
G2207	Reason for not administering adjuvant treatment course including both chemotherapy and her2-targeted therapy (e.g., poor performance status (ecog 3-4; karnofsky =50), cardiac contraindications, insufficient renal function, insufficient hepatic function, other active or secondary cancer diagnoses, other medical contraindications, patients who died during initial treatment course or transferred during or after initial treatment course)

Code	Code Descriptor
G2208	Patient did not receive adjuvant treatment course including both chemotherapy and her2-targeted therapy
G2209	Patient refused to participate
G2210	Risk-adjusted functional status change residual score for the neck impairment not measured because the patient did not complete the neck fs prom at initial evaluation and/or near discharge, reason not given
G2211	Visit complexity inherent to evaluation and management associated with medical care services that serve as the continuing focal point for all needed health care services and/or with medical care services that are part of ongoing care related to a patient's single, serious condition or a complex condition. (add-on code, list separately in addition to office/outpatient evaluation and management visit, new or established)
G2212	Prolonged office or other outpatient evaluation and management service(s) beyond the maximum required time of the primary procedure which has been selected using total time on the date of the primary service; each additional 15 minutes by the physician or qualified healthcare professional, with or without direct patient contact (list separately in addition to CPT® codes 99205, 99215 for office or other outpatient evaluation and management services) (do not report g2212 on the same date of service as 99354, 99355, 99358, 99359, 99415, 99416). (do not report g2212 for any time unit less than 15 minutes)
G2213	Initiation of medication for the treatment of opioid use disorder in the emergency department setting, including assessment, referral to ongoing care, and arranging access to supportive services (list separately in addition to code for primary procedure)
G2214	Initial or subsequent psychiatric collaborative care management, first 30 minutes in a month of behavioral health care manager activities, in consultation with a psychiatric consultant, and directed by the treating physician or other qualified health care professional
G2215	Take-home supply of nasal naloxone (provision of the services by a medicare-enrolled opioid treatment program); list separately in addition to code for primary procedure
G2216	Take-home supply of injectable naloxone (provision of the services by a medicare-enrolled opioid treatment program); list separately in addition to code for primary procedure
G2250	Remote assessment of recorded video and/or images submitted by an established patient (e.g., store and forward), including interpretation with follow-up with the patient within 24 business hours, not originating from a related service provided within the previous 7 days nor leading to a service or procedure within the next 24 hours or soonest available appointment
G2251	Brief communication technology-based service, e.g., virtual check-in, by a qualified health care professional who cannot report evaluation and management services, provided to an established patient, not originating from a related service provided within the previous 7 days nor leading to a service or procedure within the next 24 hours or soonest available appointment; 5-10 minutes of clinical discussion

Code	Code Descriptor
G2252	Brief communication technology-based service, e.g., virtual check-in, by a physician or other qualified health care professional who can report evaluation and management services, provided to an established patient, not originating from a related e/m service provided within the previous 7 days nor leading to an e/m service or procedure within the next 24 hours or soonest available appointment; 11-20 minutes of medical discussion
J0223	Injection, givosiran, 0.5 mg
J0591	Injection, deoxycholic acid, 1 mg
J0691	Injection, lefamulin, 1 mg
J0693	Injection, cefiderocol, 5 mg
J0742	Injection, imipenem 4 mg, cilastatin 4 mg and relebactam 2 mg
J0791	Injection, crizanlizumab-tmca, 5 mg
J0896	Injection, luspatercept-aamt, 0.25 mg
J1201	Injection, cetirizine hydrochloride, 0.5 mg
J1429	Injection, golodirsen, 10 mg
J1437	Injection, ferric derisomaltose, 10 mg
J1558	Injection, immune globulin (xembify), 100 mg
J1632	Injection, brexanolone, 1 mg
J1738	Injection, meloxicam, 1 mg
J1823	Injection, inebilizumab-cdon, 1 mg
J3032	Injection, eptinezumab-jjmr, 1 mg
J3241	Injection, teprotumumab-trbw, 10 mg
J3399	Injection, onasemnogene abeparvovec-xioi, per treatment, up to 5x10^15 vector genomes
J7169	Injection, coagulation factor xa (recombinant), inactivated-zhzo (andexxa), 10 mg
J7204	Injection, factor viii, antihemophilic factor (recombinant), (esperoct), glycopegylated-exei, per iu
J7212	Factor viia (antihemophilic factor, recombinant)-jncw (sevenfact), 1 microgram
J7333	Hyaluronan or derivative, visco-3, for intra-articular injection, per dose
J7351	Injection, bimatoprost, intracameral implant, 1 microgram
J7352	Afamelanotide implant, 1 mg
J9144	Injection, daratumumab, 10 mg and hyaluronidase-fihj
J9177	Injection, enfortumab vedotin-ejfv, 0.25 mg
J9198	Injection, gemcitabine hydrochloride, (infugem), 100 mg
J9223	Injection, lurbinectedin, 0.1 mg
J9227	Injection, isatuximab-irfc, 10 mg
J9246	Injection, melphalan (evomela), 1 mg
J9281	Mitomycin pyelocalyceal instillation, 1 mg
J9304	Injection, pemetrexed (pemfexy), 10 mg
J9316	Injection, pertuzumab, trastuzumab, and hyaluronidase-zzxf, per 10 mg
J9317	Injection, sacituzumab govitecan-hziy, 2.5 mg
J9358	Injection, fam-trastuzumab deruxtecan-nxki, 1 mg

Code	Code Descriptor
K1006	Suction pump, home model, portable or stationary, electric, any type, for use with external urine management system
K1007	Bilateral hip, knee, ankle, foot device, powered, includes pelvic component, single or double upright(s), knee joints any type, with or without ankle joints any type, includes all components and accessories, motors, microprocessors, sensors
K1009	Speech volume modulation system, any type, including all components and accessories
K1010	Indwelling intraurethral drainage device with valve, patient inserted, replacement only, each
K1011	Activation device for intraurethral drainage device with valve, replacement only, each
K1012	Charger and base station for intraurethral activation device, replacement only
M0239	Intravenous infusion, bamlanivimab-xxxx, includes infusion and post administration monitoring
M0243	Intravenous infusion, casirivimab and imdevimab includes infusion and post administration monitoring
M1145	Most favored nation (mfn) model drug add-on amount, per dose, (do not bill with line items that have the jw modifier)
M1146	Ongoing care not clinically indicated because the patient needed a home program only, referral to another provider or facility, or consultation only, as documented in the medical record
M1147	Ongoing care not medically possible because the patient was discharged early due to specific medical events, documented in the medical record, such as the patient became hospitalized or scheduled for surgery
M1148	Ongoing care not possible because the patient self-discharged early (e.g., financial or insurance reasons, transportation problems, or reason unknown)
M1149	Patient unable to complete the neck fs prom at initial evaluation and/or discharge due to blindness, illiteracy, severe mental incapacity or language incompatibility, and an adequate proxy is not available
Q0239	Injection, bamlanivimab-xxxx, 700 mg
Q0243	Injection, casirivimab and imdevimab, 2400 mg
Q4227	Amniocore, per square centimeter
Q4228	Bionextpatch, per square centimeter
Q4229	Cogenex amniotic membrane, per square centimeter
Q4230	Cogenex flowable amnion, per 0.5 cc
Q4231	Corplex p, per cc
Q4232	Corplex, per square centimeter
Q4233	Surfactor or nudyn, per 0.5 cc
Q4234	Xcellerate, per square centimeter
Q4235	Amniorepair or altiply, per square centimeter
Q4236	Carepatch, per square centimeter
Q4237	Cryo-cord, per square centimeter
Q4238	Derm-maxx, per square centimeter
Q4239	Amnio-maxx or amnio-maxx lite, per square centimeter
Q4240	Corecyte, for topical use only, per 0.5 cc
Q4241	Polycyte, for topical use only, per 0.5 cc

Code	Code Descriptor
Q4242	Amniocyte plus, per 0.5 cc
Q4244	Procenta, per 200 mg
Q4245	Amniotext, per cc
Q4246	Coretext or protext, per cc
Q4247	Amniotext patch, per square centimeter
Q4248	Dermacyte amniotic membrane allograft, per square centimeter
Q4249	Amniply, for topical use only, per square centimeter
Q4250	Amnioamp-mp, per square centimeter
Q4254	Novafix dl, per square centimeter
Q4255	Reguard, for topical use only, per square centimeter
Q5119	Injection, rituximab-pvvr, biosimilar, (ruxience), 10 mg
Q5120	Injection, pegfilgrastim-bmez, biosimilar, (ziextenzo), 0.5 mg
Q5121	Injection, infliximab-axxq, biosimilar, (avsola), 10 mg
Q5122	Injection, pegfilgrastim-apgf, biosimilar, (nyvepria), 0.5 mg
Q9001	Assessment by department of veterans affairs chaplain services
Q9002	Counseling, individual, by department of veterans affairs chaplain services
Q9003	Counseling, group, by department of veterans affairs chaplain services
S0013	Esketamine, nasal spray, 1 mg
T2047	Habilitation, prevocational, waiver; per 15 minutes
U0001	Cdc 2019 novel coronavirus (2019-ncov) real-time rt-pcr diagnostic panel
U0002	2019-ncov coronavirus, sars-cov-2/2019-ncov (covid-19), any technique, multiple types or subtypes (includes all targets), non-cdc
U0003	Infectious agent detection by nucleic acid (dna or rna); severe acute respiratory syndrome coronavirus 2 (sars-cov-2) (coronavirus disease [covid-19]), amplified probe technique, making use of high throughput technologies as described by cms-2020-01-r
U0004	2019-ncov coronavirus, sars-cov-2/2019-ncov (covid-19), any technique, multiple types or subtypes (includes all targets), non-cdc, making use of high throughput technologies as described by cms-2020-01-r
U0005	Infectious agent detection by nucleic acid (dna or rna); severe acute respiratory syndrome coronavirus 2 (sars-cov-2) (coronavirus disease [covid-19]), amplified probe technique, cdc or non-cdc, making use of high throughput technologies, completed within 2 calendar days from date of specimen collection (list separately in addition to either hcpcs code u0003 or u0004) as described by cms-2020-01-r2
V2524	Contact lens, hydrophilic, spherical, photochromic additive, per lens

REVISED CODES

Code	Code Descriptor
E0880	Traction stand, free standing, extremity traction
G0068	Professional services for the administration of anti-infective, pain management, chelation, pulmonary hypertension, inotropic, or other intravenous infusion drug or biological (excluding chemotherapy or other highly complex drug or biological) for each infusion drug administration calendar day in the individual's home, each 15 minutes
G0069	Professional services for the administration of subcutaneous immunotherapy or other subcutaneous infusion drug or biological for each infusion drug administration calendar day in the individual's home, each 15 minutes
G0070	Professional services for the administration of intravenous chemotherapy or other intravenous highly complex drug or biological infusion for each infusion drug administration calendar day in the individual's home, each 15 minutes
G0396	Alcohol and/or substance (other than tobacco) misuse structured assessment (e.g., audit, dast), and brief intervention 15 to 30 minutes
G0397	Alcohol and/or substance (other than tobacco) misuse structured assessment (e.g., audit, dast), and intervention, greater than 30 minutes
G2011	Alcohol and/or substance (other than tobacco) misuse structured assessment (e.g., audit, dast), and brief intervention, 5-14 minutes
G2061	Qualified nonphysician healthcare professional online assessment and management service, for an established patient, for up to seven days, cumulative time during the 7 days; 5-10 minutes
G2062	Qualified nonphysician healthcare professional online assessment and management service, for an established patient, for up to seven days, cumulative time during the 7 days; 11-20 minutes
G2063	Qualified nonphysician healthcare professional online assessment and management service, for an established patient, for up to seven days, cumulative time during the 7 days; 21 or more minutes
G2097	Episodes where the patient had a competing diagnosis within three days after the episode date (e.g., intestinal infection, pertussis, bacterial infection, lyme disease, otitis media, acute sinusitis, chronic sinusitis, infection of the adenoids, prostatitis, cellulitis, mastoiditis, or bone infections, acute lymphadenitis, impetigo, skin staph infections, pneumonia/gonococcal infections, venereal disease (syphilis, chlamydia, inflammatory diseases [female reproductive organs]), infections of the kidney, cystitis or uti)
G2105	Patient age 66 or older in institutional special needs plans (snp) or residing in long-term care with pos code 32, 33, 34, 54 or 56 for more than 90 consecutive days during the measurement period
G2108	Patient age 66 or older in institutional special needs plans (snp) or residing in long-term care with pos code 32, 33, 34, 54 or 56 for more than 90 consecutive days during the measurement period

Code	Code Descriptor
G2115	Patients 66 - 80 years of age with at least one claim/encounter for frailty during the measurement period and a dispensed medication for dementia during the measurement period or the year prior to the measurement period
G2116	Patients 66 - 80 years of age with at least one claim/encounter for frailty during the measurement period and either one acute inpatient encounter with a diagnosis of advanced illness or two outpatient, observation, ed or nonacute inpatient encounters on different dates of service with an advanced illness diagnosis during the measurement period or the year prior to the measurement period
G2118	Patients 81 years of age and older with at least one claim/encounter for frailty during the measurement period
G2125	Patients 81 years of age and older with at least one claim/encounter for frailty during the six months prior to the measurement period through december 31 of the measurement period
G2126	Patients 66 - 80 years of age with at least one claim/encounter for frailty during the measurement period and either one acute inpatient encounter with a diagnosis of advanced illness or two outpatient, observation, ed or nonacute inpatient encounters on different dates of service with an advanced illness diagnosis during the measurement period or the year prior to the measurement period
G2127	Patients 66 - 80 years of age with at least one claim/encounter for frailty during the measurement period and a dispensed medication for dementia during the measurement period or the year prior to the measurement period
G2151	Documentation stating patient has a diagnosis of a degenerative neurological condition such as als, ms, or parkinson's diagnosed at any time before or during the episode of care
G2152	Risk-adjusted functional status change residual score for the neck impairment successfully calculated and the score was equal to zero (0) or greater than zero (> 0)
G2167	Risk-adjusted functional status change residual score for the neck impairment successfully calculated and the score was less than zero (< 0)
G8430	Documentation of a medical reason(s) for not documenting, updating, or reviewing the patient's current medications list (e.g., patient is in an urgent or emergent medical situation)
G8601	IV alteplase not initiated within three hours (<= 180 minutes) of time last known well for reasons documented by clinician (e.g., patient enrolled in clinical trial for stroke, patient admitted for elective carotid intervention, patient received tenecteplase (tnk))
G8650	Risk-adjusted functional status change residual score for the knee impairment not measured because the patient did not complete the lepf prom at initial evaluation and/or near discharge, reason not given
G8654	Risk-adjusted functional status change residual score for the hip impairment not measured because the patient did not complete the lepf prom at initial evaluation and/or near discharge, reason not given

Code	Code Descriptor
G8658	Risk-adjusted functional status change residual score for the lower leg, foot or ankle impairment not measured because the patient did not complete the lepf prom at initial evaluation and/or near discharge, reason not given
G8694	Left ventricular ejection fraction (lvef) < 40% or documentation of moderate or severe lvsd
G8709	Uri episodes when the patient had competing diagnoses on or three days after the episode date (e.g., intestinal infection, pertussis, bacterial infection, lyme disease, otitis media, acute sinusitis, acute pharyngitis, chronic sinusitis, infection of the pharynx/larynx/tonsils/adenoids, prostatitis, cellulitis, mastoiditis, or bone infections, acute lymphadenitis, impetigo, skin staph infections, pneumonia/gonococcal infections, venereal disease (syphilis, chlamydia, inflammatory diseases [female reproductive organs]), infections of the kidney, cystitis or uti, and acne)
G8924	Spirometry test results demonstrate fev1/fvc < 70%, fev1 < 60% predicted and patient has copd symptoms (e.g., dyspnea, cough/sputum, wheezing)
G8938	Bmi is documented as being outside of normal parameters, follow-up plan is not documented, documentation the patient is not eligible
G8969	Documentation of patient reason(s) for not prescribing warfarin or another oral anticoagulant that is fda approved for the prevention of thromboembolism (e.g., patient choice of having atrial appendage device placed)
G9299	Patients who are not evaluated for venous thromboembolic and cardiovascular risk factors within 30 days prior to the procedure (e.g., history of dvt, pe, mi, arrhythmia and stroke, reason not given)
G9355	Early elective delivery by c-section, or early elective induction, not performed (less than 39 weeks gestation)
G9356	Early elective delivery by c-section, or early elective induction, performed (less than 39 week gestation)
G9401	No documentation in the patient record of a discussion between the physician or other qualfied healthcare professional and the patient that includes all of the following: treatment choices appropriate to genotype, risks and benefits, evidence of effectiveness, and patient preferences toward treatment
G9402	Patient received follow-up within 30 days after discharge
G9415	Patient did not have one dose of meningococcal vaccine (serogroups a, c, w, y) on or between the patient's 11th and 13th birthdays
G9448	Patients who were born in the years 1945 to1965
G9537	Imaging needed as part of a clinical trial; or other clinician ordered the study
G9550	Final reports for imaging studies with follow-up imaging recommended, or final reports that do not include a specific recommendation of no follow-up
G9642	Current smoker (e.g., cigarette, cigar, pipe, e-cigarette or marijuana)

Code	Code Descriptor
G9659	Patients greater than or equal to 86 years of age who underwent a screening colonoscopy and did not have a history of colorectal cancer or other valid medical reason for the colonoscopy, including: iron deficiency anemia, lower gastrointestinal bleeding, crohn's disease (i.e., regional enteritis), familial adenomatous polyposis, lynch syndrome (i.e., hereditary non-polyposis colorectal cancer), inflammatory bowel disease, ulcerative colitis, abnormal finding of gastrointestinal tract, or changes in bowel habits
G9660	Documentation of medical reason(s) for a colonoscopy performed on a patient greater than or equal to 86 years of age (e.g., iron deficiency anemia, lower gastrointestinal bleeding, crohn's disease (i.e., regional enteritis), familial history of adenomatous polyposis, lynch syndrome (i.e., hereditary non-polyposis colorectal cancer), inflammatory bowel disease, ulcerative colitis, abnormal finding of gastrointestinal tract, or changes in bowel habits)
G9661	Patients greater than or equal to 86 years of age who received a colonoscopy for an assessment of signs/symptoms of gi tract illness, and/or because the patient meets high risk criteria, and/or to follow-up on previously diagnosed advanced lesions
G9663	Any fasting or direct ldl-c laboratory test result >= 190 mg/dl
G9666	Patient's highest fasting or direct ldl-c laboratory test result in the measurement period or two years prior to the beginning of the measurement period is 70-189 mg/dl
G9703	Episodes where the patient is taking antibiotics (table 1) in the 30 days prior to the episode date
G9716	Bmi is documented as being outside of normal parameters, follow-up plan is not completed for documented reason
G9717	Documentation stating the patient has had a diagnosis of depression or has had a diagnosis of bipolar disorder
G9722	Documented history of renal failure or baseline serum creatinine >= 4.0 mg/dl; renal transplant recipients are not considered to have preoperative renal failure, unless, since transplantation the cr has been or is 4.0 or higher
G9727	Patient unable to complete the lepf prom at initial evaluation and/or discharge due to blindness, illiteracy, severe mental incapacity or language incompatibility and an adequate proxy is not available
G9729	Patient unable to complete the lepf prom at initial evaluation and/or discharge due to blindness, illiteracy, severe mental incapacity or language incompatibility and an adequate proxy is not available
G9731	Patient unable to complete the lepf prom at initial evaluation and/or discharge due to blindness, illiteracy, severe mental incapacity or language incompatibility and an adequate proxy is not available
G9898	Patients age 66 or older in institutional special needs plans (snp) or residing in long-term care with pos code 32, 33, 34, 54, or 56 for more than 90 consecutive days during the measurement period
G9901	Patient age 66 or older in institutional special needs plans (snp) or residing in long-term care with pos code 32, 33, 34, 54, or 56 for more than 90 consecutive days during the measurement period

Code	Code Descriptor
G9910	Patients age 66 or older in institutional special needs plans (snp) or residing in long-term care with pos code 32, 33, 34, 54 or 56 for more than 90 consecutive days during the measurement period
G9931	Documentation of cha2ds2-vasc risk score of 0 or 1 for men; or 0, 1, or 2 for women
G9938	Patients age 66 or older in institutional special needs plans (snp) or residing in long-term care with pos code 32, 33, 34, 54, or 56 for more than 90 consecutive days during the six months prior to the measurement period through december 31 of the measurement period
G9945	Patient had cancer, acute fracture or infection related to the lumbar spine or patient had neuromuscular, idiopathic or congenital lumbar scoliosis
J7189	Factor viia (antihemophilic factor, recombinant), (novoseven rt), 1 microgram
J7321	Hyaluronan or derivative, hyalgan or supartz, for intra-articular injection, per dose
J9245	Injection, melphalan hydrochloride, not otherwise specified, 50 mg
J9305	Injection, pemetrexed, not otherwise specified, 10 mg
L8701	Elbow, wrist, hand device, powered, with single or double upright(s), any type joint(s), includes microprocessor, sensors, all components and accessories
L8702	Elbow, wrist, hand, finger device, powered, with single or double upright(s), any type joint(s), includes microprocessor, sensors, all components and accessories
M1003	Tb screening performed and results interpreted within twelve months prior to initiation of first-time biologic disease modifying anti-rheumatic drug therapy
M1041	Patient had cancer, acute fracture or infection related to the lumbar spine or patient had neuromuscular, idiopathic or congenital lumbar scoliosis
M1045	Functional status measured by the oxford knee score (oks) at one year (9 to 15 months) postoperatively was greater than or equal to 37 or knee injury and osteoarthritis outcome score joint replacement (koos, jr.) was greater than or equal to 71
M1046	Functional status measured by the oxford knee score (oks) at one year (9 to 15 months) postoperatively was less than 37 or the knee injury and osteoarthritis outcome score joint replacement (koos, jr.) was less than 71 postoperatively
M1051	Patient had cancer, acute fracture or infection related to the lumbar spine or patient had neuromuscular, idiopathic or congenital lumbar scoliosis
M1108	Ongoing care not clinically indicated because the patient needed a home program only, referral to another provider or facility, or consultation only, as documented in the medical record
M1109	Ongoing care not medically possible because the patient was discharged early due to specific medical events, documented in the medical record, such as the patient became hospitalized or scheduled for surgery
M1110	Ongoing care not possible because the patient self-discharged early (e.g., financial or insurance reasons, transportation problems, or reason unknown)

Code	Code Descriptor
M1113	Ongoing care not clinically indicated because the patient needed a home program only, referral to another provider or facility, or consultation only, as documented in the medical record
M1114	Ongoing care not medically possible because the patient was discharged early due to specific medical events, documented in the medical record, such as the patient became hospitalized or scheduled for surgery
M1115	Ongoing care not possible because the patient self-discharged early (e.g., financial or insurance reasons, transportation problems, or reason unknown)
M1118	Ongoing care not clinically indicated because the patient needed a home program only, referral to another provider or facility, or consultation only, as documented in the medical record
M1119	Ongoing care not medically possible because the patient was discharged early due to specific medical events, documented in the medical record, such as the patient became hospitalized or scheduled for surgery
M1120	Ongoing care not possible because the patient self-discharged early (e.g., financial or insurance reasons, transportation problems, or reason unknown)
M1123	Ongoing care not clinically indicated because the patient needed a home program only, referral to another provider or facility, or consultation only, as documented in the medical record
M1124	Ongoing care not medically possible because the patient was discharged early due to specific medical events, documented in the medical record, such as the patient became hospitalized or scheduled for surgery
M1125	Ongoing care not possible because the patient self-discharged early (e.g., financial or insurance reasons, transportation problems, or reason unknown)
M1128	Ongoing care not clinically indicated because the patient needed a home program only, referral to another provider or facility, or consultation only, as documented in the medical record
M1129	Ongoing care not medically possible because the patient was discharged early due to specific medical events, documented in the medical record, such as the patient became hospitalized or scheduled for surgery
M1130	Ongoing care not possible because the patient self-discharged early (e.g., financial or insurance reasons, transportation problems, or reason unknown)
M1132	Ongoing care not clinically indicated because the patient needed a home program only, referral to another provider or facility, or consultation only, as documented in the medical record
M1133	Ongoing care not medically possible because the patient was discharged early due to specific medical events, documented in the medical record, such as the patient became hospitalized or scheduled for surgery
M1134	Ongoing care not possible because the patient self-discharged early (e.g., financial or insurance reasons, transportation problems, or reason unknown)
M1141	Functional status was not measured by the oxford knee score (oks) or the knee injury and osteoarthritis outcome score joint replacement (koos, jr.) at one year (9 to 15 months) postoperatively
Q4176	Neopatch or therion, per square centimeter

DELETED CODES

Code	Code Descriptor
C9041	Injection, coagulation factor xa (recombinant), inactivated (andexxa), 10 mg
C9053	Injection, crizanlizumab-tmca, 1 mg
C9054	Injection, lefamulin (xenleta), 1 mg
C9055	Injection, brexanolone, 1mg
C9056	Injection, givosiran, 0.5 mg
C9057	Injection, cetirizine hydrochloride, 1 mg
C9058	Injection, pegfilgrastim-bmez, biosimilar, (ziextenzo) 0.5 mg
C9059	Injection, meloxicam, 1 mg
C9060	Fluoroestradiol f18, diagnostic, 1 mci
C9061	Injection, teprotumumab-trbw, 10 mg
C9062	Injection, daratumumab 10 mg and hyaluronidase-fihj
C9063	Injection, eptinezumab-jjmr, 1 mg
C9064	Mitomycin pyelocalyceal instillation, 1 mg
C9066	Injection, sacituzumab govitecan-hziy, 2.5 mg
C9745	Nasal endoscopy, surgical; balloon dilation of eustachian tube
C9747	Ablation of prostate, transrectal, high intensity focused ultrasound (hifu), including imaging guidance
C9749	Repair of nasal vestibular lateral wall stenosis with implant(s)
C9754	Creation of arteriovenous fistula, percutaneous; direct, any site, including all imaging and radiologic supervision and interpretation, when performed and secondary procedures to redirect blood flow (e.g., transluminal balloon angioplasty, coil embolization, when performed)
C9755	Creation of arteriovenous fistula, percutaneous using magnetic-guided arterial and venous catheters and radiofrequency energy, including flow-directing procedures (e.g., vascular coil embolization with radiologic supervision and interpretation, when performed) and fistulogram(s), angiography, venography, and/or ultrasound, with radiologic supervision and interpretation, when performed
G0297	Low dose ct scan (ldct) for lung cancer screening
G1000	Clinical decision support mechanism applied pathways, as defined by the medicare appropriate use criteria program
G1005	Clinical decision support mechanism national imaging associates, as defined by the medicare appropriate use criteria program
G1006	Clinical decision support mechanism test appropriate, as defined by the medicare appropriate use criteria program
G2058	Chronic care management services, each additional 20 minutes of clinical staff time directed by a physician or other qualified health care professional, per calendar month (list separately in addition to code for primary procedure). (do not report g2058 for care management services of less than 20 minutes additional to the first 20 minutes of chronic care management services during a calendar month). (use g2058 in conjunction with 99490). (do not report 99490, g2058 in the same calendar month as 99487, 99489, 99491)).

Code	Code Descriptor
G2089	Most recent hemoglobin a1c (hba1c) level 7.0 to 9.0%
G2102	Dilated retinal eye exam with interpretation by an ophthalmologist or optometrist documented and reviewed
G2103	Seven standard field stereoscopic photos with interpretation by an ophthalmologist or optometrist documented and reviewed
G2104	Eye imaging validated to match diagnosis from seven standard field stereoscopic photos results documented and reviewed
G2114	Patients 66-80 years of age with at least one claim/encounter for frailty during the measurement period and a dispensed medication for dementia during the measurement period or the year prior to the measurement period
G2117	Patients 66-80 years of age with at least one claim/encounter for frailty during the measurement period and either one acute inpatient encounter with a diagnosis of advanced illness or two outpatient, observation, ed or nonacute inpatient encounters on different dates of service with an advanced illness diagnosis during the measurement period or the year prior to the measurement period
G2119	Within the past 2 years, calcium and/or vitamin d optimization has been ordered or performed
G2120	Within the past 2 years, calcium and/or vitamin d optimization has not been ordered or performed
G2123	Patients 66-80 years of age and had at least one claim/encounter for frailty during the measurement period and either one acute inpatient encounter with a diagnosis of advanced illness or two outpatient, observation, ed or nonacute inpatient encounters on different dates of service with an advanced illness diagnosis during the measurement period or the year prior to the measurement period
G2124	Patients 66-80 years of age and had at least one claim/encounter for frailty during the measurement period and a dispensed dementia medication
G2130	Patients age 66 or older in institutional special needs plans (snp) or residing in long-term care with pos code 32, 33, 34, 54 or 56 for more than 90 days during the measurement period
G2131	Patients 81 years and older with a diagnosis of frailty
G2132	Patients 66-80 years of age with at least one claim/encounter for frailty during the measurement period and a dispensed medication for dementia during the measurement period or the year prior to the measurement period
G2133	Patients 66-80 years of age with at least one claim/encounter for frailty during the measurement period and either one acute inpatient encounter with a diagnosis of advanced illness or two outpatient, observation, ed or nonacute inpatient encounters on different dates of service with an advanced illness diagnosis during the measurement period or the year prior to the measurement period

Code	Code Descriptor
G2134	Patients 66 years of age or older with at least one claim/encounter for frailty during the measurement period and a dispensed medication for dementia during the measurement period or the year prior to the measurement period
G2135	Patients 66 years of age or older with at least one claim/encounter for frailty during the measurement period and either one acute inpatient encounter with a diagnosis of advanced illness or two outpatient, observation, ed or nonacute inpatient encounters on different dates of service with an advanced illness diagnosis during the measurement period or the year prior to the measurement period
G2153	In hospice or using hospice services during the measurement period
G2154	Patient received at least one td vaccine or one tdap vaccine between nine years prior to the start of the measurement period and the end of the measurement period
G2155	Patient had history of at least one of the following contraindications any time during or before the measurement period: anaphylaxis due to tdap vaccine, anaphylaxis due to td vaccine or its components; encephalopathy due to tdap or td vaccination (post tetanus vaccination encephalitis, post diphtheria vaccination encephalitis or post pertussis vaccination encephalitis.)
G2156	Patient did not receive at least one td vaccine or one tdap vaccine between nine years prior to the start of the measurement period and the end of the measurement period; or have history of at least one of the following contraindications any time during or before the measurement period: anaphylaxis due to tdap vaccine, anaphylaxis due to td vaccine or its components; encephalopathy due to tdap or td vaccination (post tetanus vaccination encephalitis, post diphtheria vaccination encephalitis or post pertussis vaccination encephalitis.)
G2157	Patients received both the 13-valent pneumococcal conjugate vaccine and the 23-valent pneumococcal polysaccharide vaccine at least 12 months apart, with the first occurrence after the age of 60 before or during the measurement period
G2158	Patient had prior pneumococcal vaccine adverse reaction any time during or before the measurement period
G2159	Patient did not receive both the 13-valent pneumococcal conjugate vaccine and the 23-valent pneumococcal polysaccharide vaccine at least 12 months apart, with the first occurrence after the age of 60 before or during measurement period; or have prior pneumococcal vaccine adverse reaction any time during or before the measurement period
G2160	Patient received at least one dose of the herpes zoster live vaccine or two doses of the herpes zoster recombinant vaccine (at least 28 days apart) anytime on or after the patient's 50th birthday before or during the measurement period
G2161	Patient had prior adverse reaction caused by zoster vaccine or its components any time during or before the measurement period

Code	Code Descriptor
G2162	Patient did not receive at least one dose of the herpes zoster live vaccine or two doses of the herpes zoster recombinant vaccine (at least 28 days apart) anytime on or after the patient's 50th birthday before or during the measurement period; or have prior adverse reaction caused by zoster vaccine or its components any time during or before the measurement period
G2163	Patient received an influenza vaccine on or between july 1 of the year prior to the measurement period and june 30 of the measurement period
G2164	Patient had a prior influenza virus vaccine adverse reaction any time before or during the measurement period
G2165	Patient did not receive an influenza vaccine on or between july 1 of the year prior to the measurement period and june 30 of the measurement period; or did not have a prior influenza virus vaccine adverse reaction any time before or during the measurement period
G2166	Patient refused to participate at admission and/or discharge; patient unable to complete the neck fs prom at admission or discharge due to cognitive deficit, visual deficit, motor deficit, language barrier, or low reading level, and a suitable proxy/recorder is not available; patient self-discharged early; medical reason
G8398	Dilated macular or fundus exam not performed
G8442	Pain assessment not documented as being performed, documentation the patient is not eligible for a pain assessment using a standardized tool at the time of the encounter
G8509	Pain assessment documented as positive using a standardized tool, follow-up plan not documented, reason not given
G8571	Development of deep sternal wound infection/mediastinitis within 30 days postoperatively
G8572	No deep sternal wound infection/mediastinitis
G8573	Stroke following isolated cabg surgery
G8574	No stroke following isolated cabg surgery
G8627	Surgical procedure performed within 30 days following cataract surgery for major complications (e.g., retained nuclear fragments, endophthalmitis, dislocated or wrong power iol, retinal detachment, or wound dehiscence)
G8628	Surgical procedure not performed within 30 days following cataract surgery for major complications (e.g., retained nuclear fragments, endophthalmitis, dislocated or wrong power iol, retinal detachment, or wound dehiscence)
G8671	Risk-adjusted functional status change residual score for the neck, cranium, mandible, thoracic spine, ribs or other general orthopedic impairment successfully calculated and the score was equal to zero (0) or greater than zero (> 0)
G8672	Risk-adjusted functional status change residual score for the neck, cranium, mandible, thoracic spine, ribs or other general orthopedic impairment successfully calculated and the score was less than zero (< 0)

Code	Code Descriptor
G8674	Risk-adjusted functional status change residual score for the neck, cranium, mandible, thoracic spine, ribs or other general orthopedic impairment not measured because the patient did not complete the general orthopedic fs prom at initial evaluation and/or near discharge, reason not given
G8730	Pain assessment documented as positive using a standardized tool and a follow-up plan is documented
G8731	Pain assessment using a standardized tool is documented as negative, no follow-up plan required
G8732	No documentation of pain assessment, reason not given
G8809	Rh-immunoglobulin (rhogam) ordered
G8810	Rh-immunoglobulin (rhogam) not ordered for reasons documented by clinician (e.g., patient had prior documented receipt of rhogam within 12 weeks, patient refusal)
G8811	Documentation rh-immunoglobulin (rhogam) was not ordered, reason not given
G8872	Excised tissue evaluated by imaging intraoperatively to confirm successful inclusion of targeted lesion
G8873	Patients with needle localization specimens which are not amenable to intraoperative imaging such as mri needle wire localization, or targets which are tentatively identified on mammogram or ultrasound which do not contain a biopsy marker but which can be verified on intraoperative inspection or pathology (e.g., needle biopsy site where the biopsy marker is remote from the actual biopsy site)
G8874	Excised tissue not evaluated by imaging intraoperatively to confirm successful inclusion of targeted lesion
G8939	Pain assessment documented as positive, follow-up plan not documented, documentation the patient is not eligible at the time of the encounter
G8959	Clinician treating major depressive disorder communicates to clinician treating comorbid condition
G8960	Clinician treating major depressive disorder did not communicate to clinician treating comorbid condition, reason not given
G8973	Most recent hemoglobin (hgb) level < 10 g/dl
G8974	Hemoglobin level measurement not documented, reason not given
G8975	Documentation of medical reason(s) for patient having a hemoglobin level < 10 g/dl (e.g., patients who have non-renal etiologies of anemia [e.g., sickle cell anemia or other hemoglobinopathies, hypersplenism, primary bone marrow disease, anemia related to chemotherapy for diagnosis of malignancy, postoperative bleeding, active bloodstream or peritoneal infection], other medical reasons)
G8976	Most recent hemoglobin (hgb) level >= 10 g/dl
G9232	Clinician treating major depressive disorder did not communicate to clinician treating comorbid condition for specified patient reason (e.g., patient is unable to communicate the diagnosis of a comorbid condition; the patient is unwilling to communicate the diagnosis of a comorbid condition; or the patient is unaware of the comorbid condition, or any other specified patient reason)
G9239	Documentation of reasons for patient initiating maintenance hemodialysis with a catheter as the mode of vascular access (e.g., patient has a maturing arteriovenous fistula (avf)/arteriovenous graft (avg), time-limited trial of hemodialysis, other medical reasons, patient declined avf/avg, other patient reasons, patient followed by reporting nephrologist for fewer than 90 days, other system reasons)
G9240	Patient whose mode of vascular access is a catheter at the time maintenance hemodialysis is initiated
G9241	Patient whose mode of vascular access is not a catheter at the time maintenance hemodialysis is initiated
G9256	Documentation of patient death following cas
G9257	Documentation of patient stroke following cas
G9258	Documentation of patient stroke following cea
G9259	Documentation of patient survival and absence of stroke following cas
G9260	Documentation of patient death following cea
G9261	Documentation of patient survival and absence of stroke following cea
G9262	Documentation of patient death in the hospital following endovascular aaa repair
G9263	Documentation of patient discharged alive following endovascular aaa repair
G9264	Documentation of patient receiving maintenance hemodialysis for greater than or equal to 90 days with a catheter for documented reasons (e.g., other medical reasons, patient declined arteriovenous fistula (avf)/arteriovenous graft (avg), other patient reasons)
G9265	Patient receiving maintenance hemodialysis for greater than or equal to 90 days with a catheter as the mode of vascular access
G9266	Patient receiving maintenance hemodialysis for greater than or equal to 90 days without a catheter as the mode of vascular access
G9300	Documentation of medical reason(s) for not completely infusing the prophylactic antibiotic prior to the inflation of the proximal tourniquet (e.g., a tourniquet was not used)
G9301	Patients who had the prophylactic antibiotic completely infused prior to the inflation of the proximal tourniquet
G9302	Prophylactic antibiotic not completely infused prior to the inflation of the proximal tourniquet, reason not given
G9303	Operative report does not identify the prosthetic implant specifications including the prosthetic implant manufacturer, the brand name of the prosthetic implant and the size of each prosthetic implant, reason not given
G9304	Operative report identifies the prosthetic implant specifications including the prosthetic implant manufacturer, the brand name of the prosthetic implant and the size of each prosthetic implant
G9326	Ct studies performed not reported to a radiation dose index registry that is capable of collecting at a minimum all necessary data elements, reason not given
G9327	Ct studies performed reported to a radiation dose index registry that is capable of collecting at a minimum all necessary data elements

Code	Code Descriptor
G9329	Dicom format image data available to non-affiliated external healthcare facilities or entities on a secure, media free, reciprocally searchable basis with patient authorization for at least a 12-month period after the study not documented in final report, reason not given
G9340	Final report documented that dicom format image data available to non-affiliated external healthcare facilities or entities on a secure, media free, reciprocally searchable basis with patient authorization for at least a 12-month period after the study
G9365	One high-risk medication ordered
G9366	One high-risk medication not ordered
G9389	Unplanned rupture of the posterior capsule requiring vitrectomy during cataract surgery
G9390	No unplanned rupture of the posterior capsule requiring vitrectomy during cataract surgery
G9469	Patients who have received or are receiving corticosteroids greater than or equal to 10 mg/day of prednisone equivalents for 90 or greater consecutive days or a single prescription equating to 900 mg prednisone or greater for all fills
G9503	Patient taking tamsulosin hydrochloride
G9523	Patient discontinued from hemodialysis or peritoneal dialysis
G9524	Patient was referred to hospice care
G9525	Documentation of patient reason(s) for not referring to hospice care (e.g., patient declined, other patient reasons)
G9526	Patient was not referred to hospice care, reason not given
G9532	Patient had a head ct for trauma ordered by someone other than an emergency care provider or was ordered for a reason other than trauma
G9558	Patient treated with a beta-lactam antibiotic as definitive therapy
G9559	Documentation of medical reason(s) for not prescribing a beta-lactam antibiotic (e.g., allergy, intolerance to beta-lactam antibiotics)
G9560	Patient not treated with a beta-lactam antibiotic as definitive therapy, reason not given
G9573	Adult patients 18 years of age or older with major depression or dysthymia who did not reach remission at six months as demonstrated by a six month (+/-60 days) phq-9 or phq-9m score of less than five
G9574	Adult patients 18 years of age or older with major depression or dysthymia who did not reach remission at six months as demonstrated by a six month (+/-60 days) phq-9 or phq-9m score of less than five; either phq-9 or phq-9m score was not assessed or is greater than or equal to five
G9600	Symptomatic aaas that required urgent/emergent (non-elective) repair
G9601	Patient discharge to home no later than post-operative day #7
G9602	Patient not discharged to home by post-operative day #7
G9615	Preoperative assessment documented

Code	Code Descriptor
G9616	Documentation of reason(s) for not documenting a preoperative assessment (e.g., patient with a gynecologic or other pelvic malignancy noted at the time of surgery)
G9617	Preoperative assessment not documented, reason not given
G9701	Children who are taking antibiotics in the 30 days prior to the date of the encounter during which the diagnosis was established
G9738	Patient refused to participate
G9739	Patient unable to complete the general orthopedic fs prom at initial evaluation and/or discharge due to blindness, illiteracy, severe mental incapacity or language incompatibility and an adequate proxy is not available
G9747	Patient is undergoing palliative dialysis with a catheter
G9748	Patient approved by a qualified transplant program and scheduled to receive a living donor kidney transplant
G9749	Patient is undergoing palliative dialysis with a catheter
G9750	Patient approved by a qualified transplant program and scheduled to receive a living donor kidney transplant
G9759	History of preoperative posterior capsule rupture
G9798	Discharge(s) for ami between july 1 of the year prior measurement period to june 30 of the measurement period
G9799	Patients with a medication dispensing event indicator of a history of asthma any time during the patient's history through the end of the measure period
G9800	Patients who are identified as having an intolerance or allergy to beta-blocker therapy
G9801	Hospitalizations in which the patient was transferred directly to a non-acute care facility for any diagnosis
G9802	Patients who use hospice services any time during the measurement period
G9803	Patient prescribed at least a 135 day treatment within the 180-day measurement interval with beta-blockers post-discharge for ami
G9804	Patient was not prescribed at least a 135 day treatment within the 180-day measurement interval with beta-blockers post-discharge for ami
G9814	Death occurring during the index acute care hospitalization
G9815	Death did not occur during the index acute care hospitalization
G9816	Death occurring after discharge from the hospital but within 30 days post procedure
G9817	Death did not occur after discharge from the hospital within 30 days post procedure
G9825	Her-2/neu negative or undocumented/unknown
G9826	Patient transferred to practice after initiation of chemotherapy
G9827	Her2-targeted therapies not administered during the initial course of treatment
G9828	Her2-targeted therapies administered during the initial course of treatment
G9829	Breast adjuvant chemotherapy administered

Code	Code Descriptor
G9833	Patient transfer to practice after initiation of chemotherapy
G9834	Patient has metastatic disease at diagnosis
G9835	Trastuzumab administered within 12 months of diagnosis
G9836	Reason for not administering trastuzumab documented (e.g., patient declined, patient died, patient transferred, contraindication or other clinical exclusion, neoadjuvant chemotherapy or radiation not complete)
G9837	Trastuzumab not administered within 12 months of diagnosis
G9849	Patients who died from cancer
G9850	Patient had more than one emergency department visit in the last 30 days of life
G9851	Patient had one or less emergency department visits in the last 30 days of life
G9855	Patients who died from cancer
G9856	Patient was not admitted to hospice
G9857	Patient admitted to hospice
G9924	Documentation of medical reason(s) for not providing safety concerns screen or for not providing recommendations, orders or referrals for positive screen (e.g., patient in palliative care, other medical reason)
G9933	Adenoma(s) or colorectal cancer detected during screening colonoscopy
G9934	Documentation that neoplasm detected is only diagnosed as traditional serrated adenoma, sessile serrated polyp, or sessile serrated adenoma
G9935	Adenoma(s) or colorectal cancer not detected during screening colonoscopy
G9936	Surveillance colonoscopy - personal history of colonic polyps, colon cancer, or other malignant neoplasm of rectum, rectosigmoid junction, and anus
G9937	Diagnostic colonoscopy
G9966	Children who were screened for risk of developmental, behavioral and social delays using a standardized tool with interpretation and report
G9967	Children who were not screened for risk of developmental, behavioral and social delays using a standardized tool with interpretation and report
J9199	Injection, gemcitabine hydrochloride (infugem), 200 mg
M1015	Discharge/discontinuation of the episode of care documented in the medical record
M1023	Adolescent patients 12 to 17 years of age with major depression or dysthymia who reached remission at six months as demonstrated by a six month (+/-60 days) phq-9 or phq-9m score of less than five
M1024	Adolescent patients 12 to 17 years of age with major depression or dysthymia who did not reach remission at six months as demonstrated by a six month (+/-60 days) phq-9 or phq-9m score of less than five. either phq-9 or phq-9m score was not assessed or is greater than or equal to five
M1033	Pharmacotherapy for oud initiated after june 30th of performance period
M1061	Patient pregnancy

Code	Code Descriptor
M1062	Patient immunocompromised
M1063	Patients receiving high doses of immunosuppressive therapy
M1064	Shingrix vaccine documented as administered or previously received
M1065	Shingrix vaccine was not administered for reasons documented by clinician (e.g., patient administered vaccine other than shingrix, patient allergy or other medical reasons, patient declined or other patient reasons, vaccine not available or other system reasons)
M1066	Shingrix vaccine not documented as administered, reason not given
M1136	The start of an episode of care documented in the medical record
M1137	Documentation stating patient has a diagnosis of a degenerative neurological condition such as als, ms, or parkinson's diagnosed at any time before or during the episode of care
M1138	Ongoing care not indicated, patient seen only 1-2 visits (e.g., home program only, referred to another provider or facility, consultation only)
M1139	Ongoing care not indicated, patient self-discharged early and seen only 1-2 visits (e.g., financial or insurance reasons, transportation problems, or reason unknown)
M1140	Ongoing care not indicated, patient discharged after only 1-2 visits due to specific medical events, documented in the medical record that make the treatment episode impossible such as the patient becomes hospitalized or scheduled for surgery for surgery or hospitalized
M1144	Ongoing care not indicated, patient seen only 1-2 visits (e.g., home program only, referred to another provider or facility, consultation only

Deleted Codes Crosswalk

Deleted Code	Crosswalk Code
C9041	J7169
C9053	J0791
C9054	J0691
C9055	J1632
C9056	J0223
C9057	J1201
C9058	Q5120
C9059	J1738
C9060	A9591
C9061	J3241
C9062	J9144
C9063	J3032
C9064	J9281
C9066	J9317
C9745	69705, 69706
C9747	55880
C9749	30468
C9754	CMS does not provide crosswalk codes for this deleted code.
C9755	CMS does not provide crosswalk codes for this deleted code.
G0297	CMS does not provide crosswalk codes for this deleted code.
G1000	CMS does not provide crosswalk codes for this deleted code.
G1005	CMS does not provide crosswalk codes for this deleted code.
G1006	CMS does not provide crosswalk codes for this deleted code.
G2058	CMS does not provide crosswalk codes for this deleted code.
G2089	CMS does not provide crosswalk codes for this deleted code.
G2102	CMS does not provide crosswalk codes for this deleted code.
G2103	CMS does not provide crosswalk codes for this deleted code.
G2104	CMS does not provide crosswalk codes for this deleted code.
G2114	CMS does not provide crosswalk codes for this deleted code.
G2117	CMS does not provide crosswalk codes for this deleted code.
G2119	CMS does not provide crosswalk codes for this deleted code.
G2120	CMS does not provide crosswalk codes for this deleted code.
G2123	CMS does not provide crosswalk codes for this deleted code.

Deleted Code	Crosswalk Code
G2124	CMS does not provide crosswalk codes for this deleted code.
G2130	CMS does not provide crosswalk codes for this deleted code.
G2131	CMS does not provide crosswalk codes for this deleted code.
G2132	CMS does not provide crosswalk codes for this deleted code.
G2133	CMS does not provide crosswalk codes for this deleted code.
G2134	CMS does not provide crosswalk codes for this deleted code.
G2135	CMS does not provide crosswalk codes for this deleted code.
G2153	CMS does not provide crosswalk codes for this deleted code.
G2154	CMS does not provide crosswalk codes for this deleted code.
G2155	CMS does not provide crosswalk codes for this deleted code.
G2156	CMS does not provide crosswalk codes for this deleted code.
G2157	CMS does not provide crosswalk codes for this deleted code.
G2158	CMS does not provide crosswalk codes for this deleted code.
G2159	CMS does not provide crosswalk codes for this deleted code.
G2160	CMS does not provide crosswalk codes for this deleted code.
G2161	CMS does not provide crosswalk codes for this deleted code.
G2162	CMS does not provide crosswalk codes for this deleted code.
G2163	CMS does not provide crosswalk codes for this deleted code.
G2164	CMS does not provide crosswalk codes for this deleted code.
G2165	CMS does not provide crosswalk codes for this deleted code.
G2166	CMS does not provide crosswalk codes for this deleted code.
G8398	CMS does not provide crosswalk codes for this deleted code.
G8442	CMS does not provide crosswalk codes for this deleted code.
G8509	CMS does not provide crosswalk codes for this deleted code.
G8571	CMS does not provide crosswalk codes for this deleted code.
G8572	CMS does not provide crosswalk codes for this deleted code.

Deleted Code	Crosswalk Code	Deleted Code	Crosswalk Code
G8573	CMS does not provide crosswalk codes for this deleted code.	G9256	CMS does not provide crosswalk codes for this deleted code.
G8574	CMS does not provide crosswalk codes for this deleted code.	G9257	CMS does not provide crosswalk codes for this deleted code.
G8627	CMS does not provide crosswalk codes for this deleted code.	G9258	CMS does not provide crosswalk codes for this deleted code.
G8628	CMS does not provide crosswalk codes for this deleted code.	G9259	CMS does not provide crosswalk codes for this deleted code.
G8671	CMS does not provide crosswalk codes for this deleted code.	G9260	CMS does not provide crosswalk codes for this deleted code.
G8672	CMS does not provide crosswalk codes for this deleted code.	G9261	CMS does not provide crosswalk codes for this deleted code.
G8674	CMS does not provide crosswalk codes for this deleted code.	G9262	CMS does not provide crosswalk codes for this deleted code.
G8730	CMS does not provide crosswalk codes for this deleted code.	G9263	CMS does not provide crosswalk codes for this deleted code.
G8731	CMS does not provide crosswalk codes for this deleted code.	G9264	CMS does not provide crosswalk codes for this deleted code.
G8732	CMS does not provide crosswalk codes for this deleted code.	G9265	CMS does not provide crosswalk codes for this deleted code.
G8809	CMS does not provide crosswalk codes for this deleted code.	G9266	CMS does not provide crosswalk codes for this deleted code.
G8810	CMS does not provide crosswalk codes for this deleted code.	G9300	CMS does not provide crosswalk codes for this deleted code.
G8811	CMS does not provide crosswalk codes for this deleted code.	G9301	CMS does not provide crosswalk codes for this deleted code.
G8872	CMS does not provide crosswalk codes for this deleted code.	G9302	CMS does not provide crosswalk codes for this deleted code.
G8873	CMS does not provide crosswalk codes for this deleted code.	G9303	CMS does not provide crosswalk codes for this deleted code.
G8874	CMS does not provide crosswalk codes for this deleted code.	G9304	CMS does not provide crosswalk codes for this deleted code.
G8939	CMS does not provide crosswalk codes for this deleted code.	G9326	CMS does not provide crosswalk codes for this deleted code.
G8959	CMS does not provide crosswalk codes for this deleted code.	G9327	CMS does not provide crosswalk codes for this deleted code.
G8960	CMS does not provide crosswalk codes for this deleted code.	G9329	CMS does not provide crosswalk codes for this deleted code.
G8973	CMS does not provide crosswalk codes for this deleted code.	G9340	CMS does not provide crosswalk codes for this deleted code.
G8974	CMS does not provide crosswalk codes for this deleted code.	G9365	CMS does not provide crosswalk codes for this deleted code.
G8975	CMS does not provide crosswalk codes for this deleted code.	G9366	CMS does not provide crosswalk codes for this deleted code.
G8976	CMS does not provide crosswalk codes for this deleted code.	G9389	CMS does not provide crosswalk codes for this deleted code.
G9232	CMS does not provide crosswalk codes for this deleted code.	G9390	CMS does not provide crosswalk codes for this deleted code.
G9239	CMS does not provide crosswalk codes for this deleted code.	G9469	CMS does not provide crosswalk codes for this deleted code.
G9240	CMS does not provide crosswalk codes for this deleted code.	G9503	CMS does not provide crosswalk codes for this deleted code.
G9241	CMS does not provide crosswalk codes for this deleted code.	G9523	CMS does not provide crosswalk codes for this deleted code.

G8573 - G9523

DELETED CODES CROSSWALK

Deleted Code	Crosswalk Code	Deleted Code	Crosswalk Code
G9524	CMS does not provide crosswalk codes for this deleted code.	G9802	CMS does not provide crosswalk codes for this deleted code.
G9525	CMS does not provide crosswalk codes for this deleted code.	G9803	CMS does not provide crosswalk codes for this deleted code.
G9526	CMS does not provide crosswalk codes for this deleted code.	G9804	CMS does not provide crosswalk codes for this deleted code.
G9532	CMS does not provide crosswalk codes for this deleted code.	G9814	CMS does not provide crosswalk codes for this deleted code.
G9558	CMS does not provide crosswalk codes for this deleted code.	G9815	CMS does not provide crosswalk codes for this deleted code.
G9559	CMS does not provide crosswalk codes for this deleted code.	G9816	CMS does not provide crosswalk codes for this deleted code.
G9560	CMS does not provide crosswalk codes for this deleted code.	G9817	CMS does not provide crosswalk codes for this deleted code.
G9573	CMS does not provide crosswalk codes for this deleted code.	G9825	CMS does not provide crosswalk codes for this deleted code.
G9574	CMS does not provide crosswalk codes for this deleted code.	G9826	CMS does not provide crosswalk codes for this deleted code.
G9600	CMS does not provide crosswalk codes for this deleted code.	G9827	CMS does not provide crosswalk codes for this deleted code.
G9601	CMS does not provide crosswalk codes for this deleted code.	G9828	CMS does not provide crosswalk codes for this deleted code.
G9602	CMS does not provide crosswalk codes for this deleted code.	G9829	CMS does not provide crosswalk codes for this deleted code.
G9615	CMS does not provide crosswalk codes for this deleted code.	G9833	CMS does not provide crosswalk codes for this deleted code.
G9616	CMS does not provide crosswalk codes for this deleted code.	G9834	CMS does not provide crosswalk codes for this deleted code.
G9617	CMS does not provide crosswalk codes for this deleted code.	G9835	CMS does not provide crosswalk codes for this deleted code.
G9701	CMS does not provide crosswalk codes for this deleted code.	G9836	CMS does not provide crosswalk codes for this deleted code.
G9738	CMS does not provide crosswalk codes for this deleted code.	G9837	CMS does not provide crosswalk codes for this deleted code.
G9739	CMS does not provide crosswalk codes for this deleted code.	G9849	CMS does not provide crosswalk codes for this deleted code.
G9747	CMS does not provide crosswalk codes for this deleted code.	G9850	CMS does not provide crosswalk codes for this deleted code.
G9748	CMS does not provide crosswalk codes for this deleted code.	G9851	CMS does not provide crosswalk codes for this deleted code.
G9749	CMS does not provide crosswalk codes for this deleted code.	G9855	CMS does not provide crosswalk codes for this deleted code.
G9750	CMS does not provide crosswalk codes for this deleted code.	G9856	CMS does not provide crosswalk codes for this deleted code.
G9759	CMS does not provide crosswalk codes for this deleted code.	G9857	CMS does not provide crosswalk codes for this deleted code.
G9798	CMS does not provide crosswalk codes for this deleted code.	G9924	CMS does not provide crosswalk codes for this deleted code.
G9799	CMS does not provide crosswalk codes for this deleted code.	G9933	CMS does not provide crosswalk codes for this deleted code.
G9800	CMS does not provide crosswalk codes for this deleted code.	G9934	CMS does not provide crosswalk codes for this deleted code.
G9801	CMS does not provide crosswalk codes for this deleted code.	G9935	CMS does not provide crosswalk codes for this deleted code.

Deleted Code	Crosswalk Code
G9936	CMS does not provide crosswalk codes for this deleted code.
G9937	CMS does not provide crosswalk codes for this deleted code.
G9966	CMS does not provide crosswalk codes for this deleted code.
G9967	CMS does not provide crosswalk codes for this deleted code.
J9199	CMS does not provide crosswalk codes for this deleted code.
M1015	CMS does not provide crosswalk codes for this deleted code.
M1023	CMS does not provide crosswalk codes for this deleted code.
M1024	CMS does not provide crosswalk codes for this deleted code.
M1033	CMS does not provide crosswalk codes for this deleted code.
M1061	CMS does not provide crosswalk codes for this deleted code.
M1062	CMS does not provide crosswalk codes for this deleted code.

Deleted Code	Crosswalk Code
M1063	CMS does not provide crosswalk codes for this deleted code.
M1064	CMS does not provide crosswalk codes for this deleted code.
M1065	CMS does not provide crosswalk codes for this deleted code.
M1066	CMS does not provide crosswalk codes for this deleted code.
M1136	CMS does not provide crosswalk codes for this deleted code.
M1137	CMS does not provide crosswalk codes for this deleted code.
M1138	CMS does not provide crosswalk codes for this deleted code.
M1139	CMS does not provide crosswalk codes for this deleted code.
M1140	CMS does not provide crosswalk codes for this deleted code.
M1144	CMS does not provide crosswalk codes for this deleted code.

Anatomical Illustrations

Circulatory System — Arteries and Veins

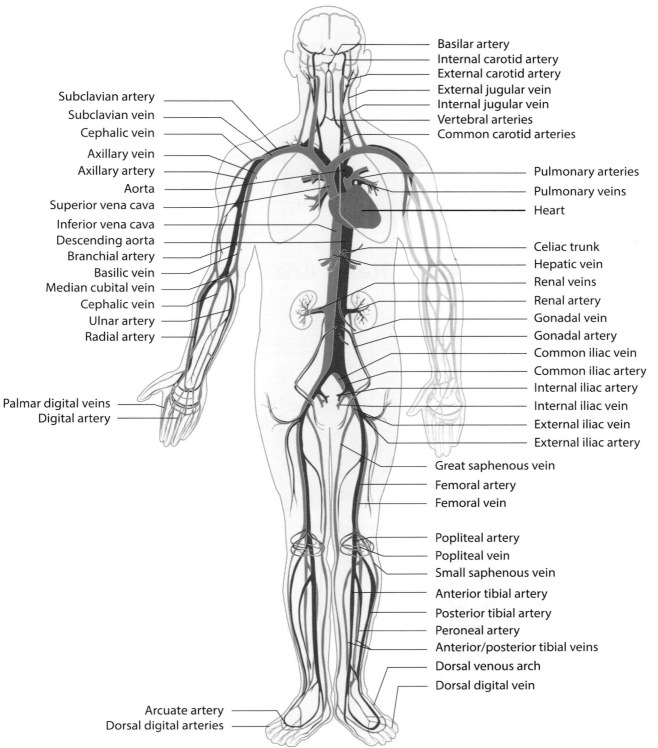

Basilar artery
Internal carotid artery
External carotid artery
External jugular vein
Internal jugular vein
Vertebral arteries
Common carotid arteries

Subclavian artery
Subclavian vein
Cephalic vein
Axillary vein
Axillary artery
Aorta
Superior vena cava
Inferior vena cava
Descending aorta
Branchial artery
Basilic vein
Median cubital vein
Cephalic vein
Ulnar artery
Radial artery

Pulmonary arteries
Pulmonary veins
Heart

Celiac trunk
Hepatic vein
Renal veins
Renal artery
Gonadal vein
Gonadal artery
Common iliac vein
Common iliac artery
Internal iliac artery
Internal iliac vein
External iliac vein
External iliac artery

Palmar digital veins
Digital artery

Great saphenous vein
Femoral artery
Femoral vein

Popliteal artery
Popliteal vein
Small saphenous vein
Anterior tibial artery
Posterior tibial artery
Peroneal artery
Anterior/posterior tibial veins
Dorsal venous arch
Dorsal digital vein

Arcuate artery
Dorsal digital arteries

Circulatory System — Artery and Vein Anatomy

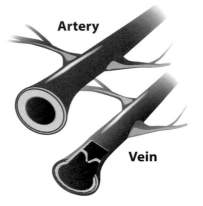

Artery

Vein

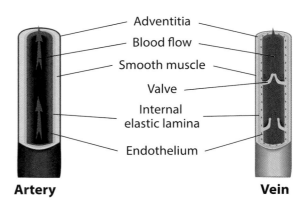

Adventitia
Blood flow
Smooth muscle
Valve
Internal elastic lamina
Endothelium

Artery

Vein

Circulatory System — Heart Anatomy and Cardiac Cycle

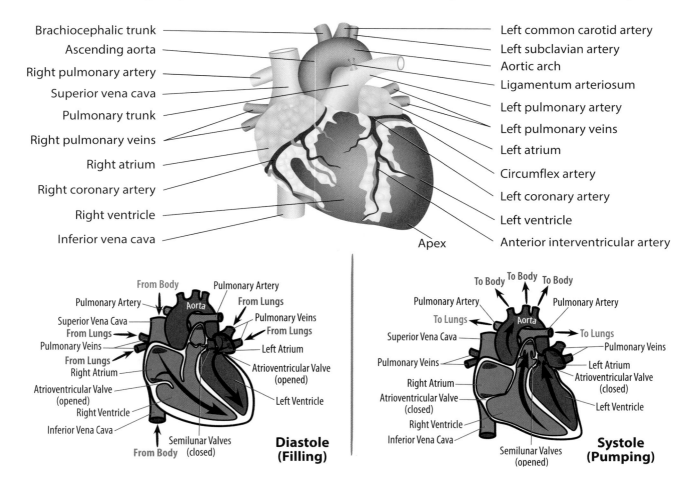

Brachiocephalic trunk
Ascending aorta
Right pulmonary artery
Superior vena cava
Pulmonary trunk
Right pulmonary veins
Right atrium
Right coronary artery
Right ventricle
Inferior vena cava

Left common carotid artery
Left subclavian artery
Aortic arch
Ligamentum arteriosum
Left pulmonary artery
Left pulmonary veins
Left atrium
Circumflex artery
Left coronary artery
Left ventricle
Apex
Anterior interventricular artery

From Body
Pulmonary Artery
Pulmonary Artery
Aorta
From Lungs
Superior Vena Cava
Pulmonary Veins
From Lungs
From Lungs
Pulmonary Veins
From Lungs
Left Atrium
Right Atrium
Atrioventricular Valve (opened)
Atrioventricular Valve (opened)
Left Ventricle
Right Ventricle
Inferior Vena Cava
Semilunar Valves (closed)
From Body

Diastole (Filling)

To Body To Body To Body
Pulmonary Artery
Pulmonary Artery
To Lungs
Aorta
To Lungs
Superior Vena Cava
Pulmonary Veins
Pulmonary Veins
Right Atrium
Left Atrium
Atrioventricular Valve (closed)
Atrioventricular Valve (closed)
Left Ventricle
Right Ventricle
Inferior Vena Cava
Semilunar Valves (opened)

Systole (Pumping)

Electrical Conducting System of the Heart

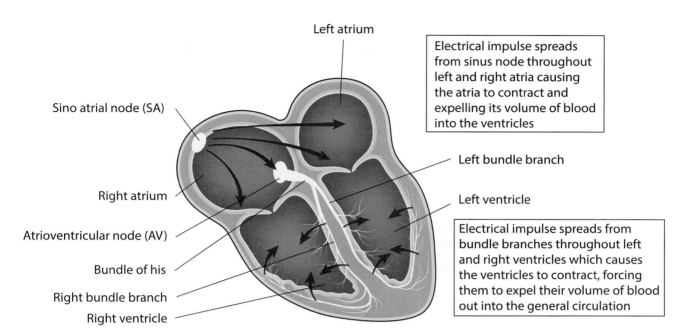

Left atrium

Sino atrial node (SA)

Right atrium

Atrioventricular node (AV)

Bundle of his

Right bundle branch

Right ventricle

Left bundle branch

Left ventricle

Electrical impulse spreads from sinus node throughout left and right atria causing the atria to contract and expelling its volume of blood into the ventricles

Electrical impulse spreads from bundle branches throughout left and right ventricles which causes the ventricles to contract, forcing them to expel their volume of blood out into the general circulation

The Pathway of Blood Flow Through the Heart

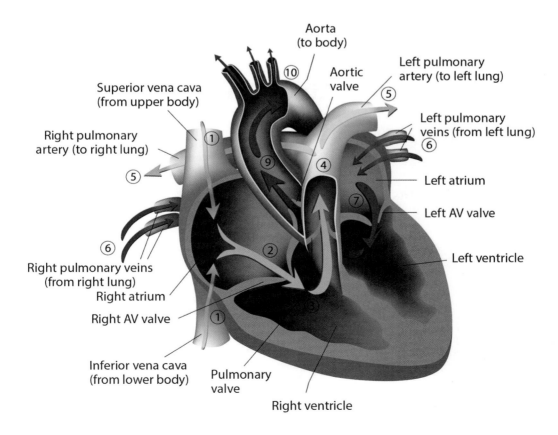

Aorta (to body)

Aortic valve

Superior vena cava (from upper body)

Right pulmonary artery (to right lung)

Right pulmonary veins (from right lung)

Right atrium

Right AV valve

Inferior vena cava (from lower body)

Pulmonary valve

Right ventricle

Left pulmonary artery (to left lung)

Left pulmonary veins (from left lung)

Left atrium

Left AV valve

Left ventricle

Digestive System Anatomy

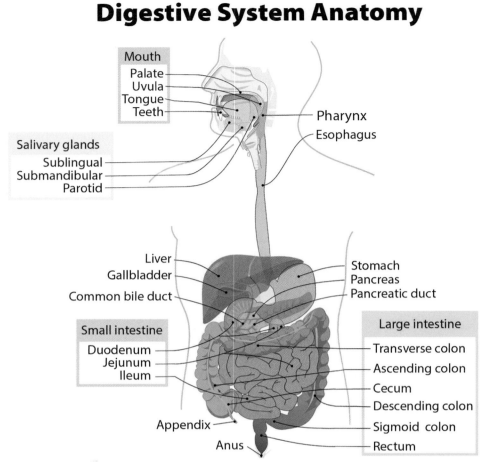

Title: Diagram of the gastrointestinal tract, **Author:** Mariana Ruiz (Lady of Hats), Jmarchn, **Source:** Own work, **License:** Public domain, **URL link:** https://en.wikiversity.org/wiki/File:Digestive_system_diagram_en.svg

Digestive System — Liver, Gallbladder, Pancreas

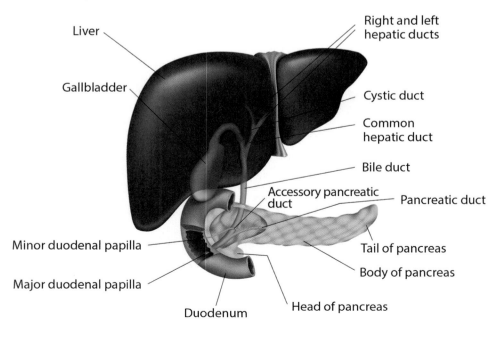

Digestive System — Mouth Anatomy

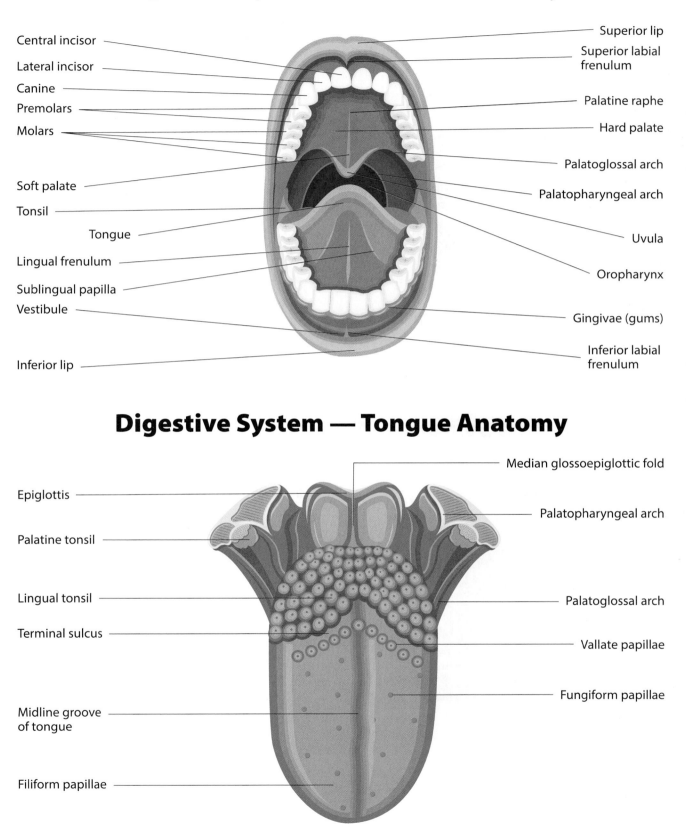

Central incisor

Lateral incisor

Canine

Premolars

Molars

Soft palate

Tonsil

Tongue

Lingual frenulum

Sublingual papilla

Vestibule

Inferior lip

Superior lip

Superior labial frenulum

Palatine raphe

Hard palate

Palatoglossal arch

Palatopharyngeal arch

Uvula

Oropharynx

Gingivae (gums)

Inferior labial frenulum

Digestive System — Tongue Anatomy

Median glossoepiglottic fold

Epiglottis

Palatine tonsil

Lingual tonsil

Terminal sulcus

Midline groove of tongue

Filiform papillae

Palatopharyngeal arch

Palatoglossal arch

Vallate papillae

Fungiform papillae

Digestive System — Stomach Anatomy

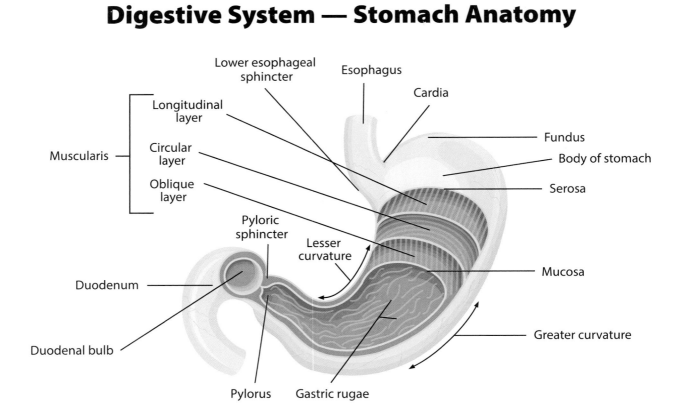

Lower esophageal sphincter

Esophagus

Cardia

Longitudinal layer

Circular layer

Oblique layer

Muscularis

Fundus

Body of stomach

Serosa

Pyloric sphincter

Lesser curvature

Mucosa

Duodenum

Duodenal bulb

Greater curvature

Pylorus

Gastric rugae

Digestive System — Small Intestine Anatomy

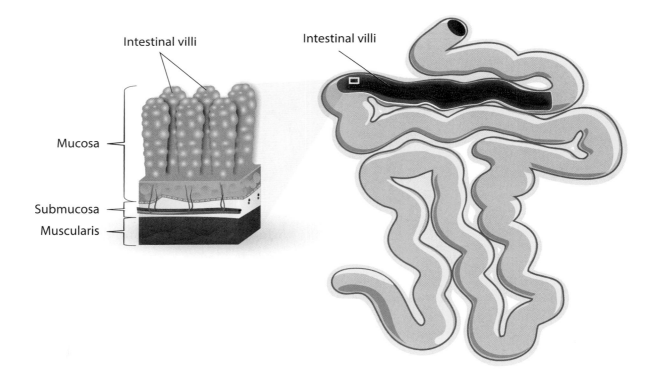

Intestinal villi

Intestinal villi

Mucosa

Submucosa

Muscularis

Digestive System — Large Intestine Anatomy

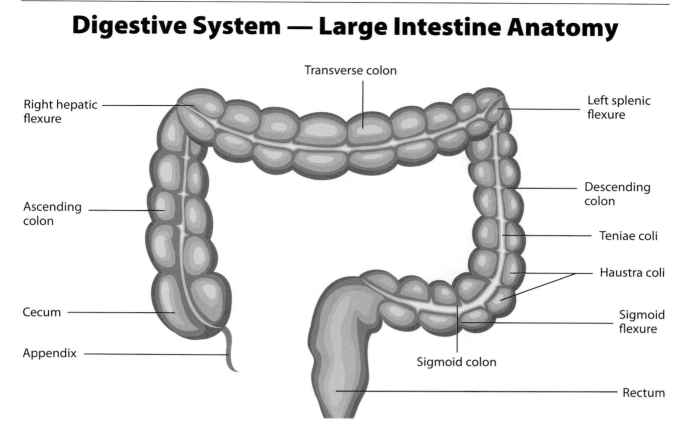

Transverse colon

Right hepatic flexure

Left splenic flexure

Ascending colon

Descending colon

Teniae coli

Haustra coli

Cecum

Sigmoid flexure

Appendix

Sigmoid colon

Rectum

Digestive System — Rectum Anatomy

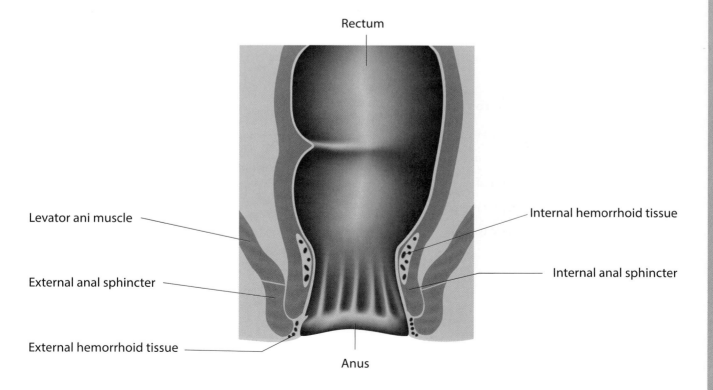

Rectum

Levator ani muscle

Internal hemorrhoid tissue

External anal sphincter

Internal anal sphincter

External hemorrhoid tissue

Anus

Ear Anatomy

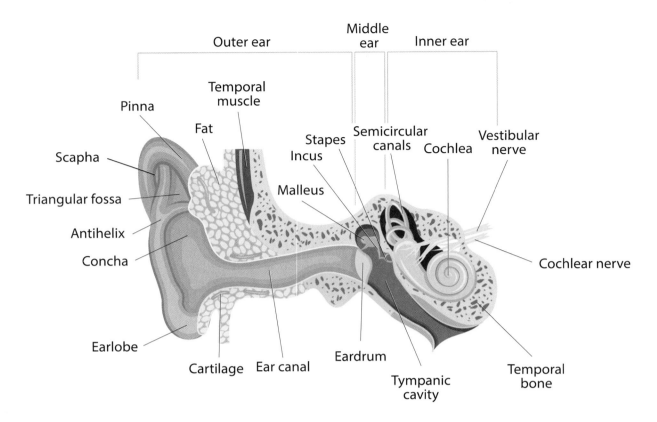

Ear Anatomy - Cochlea (Inner Ear)

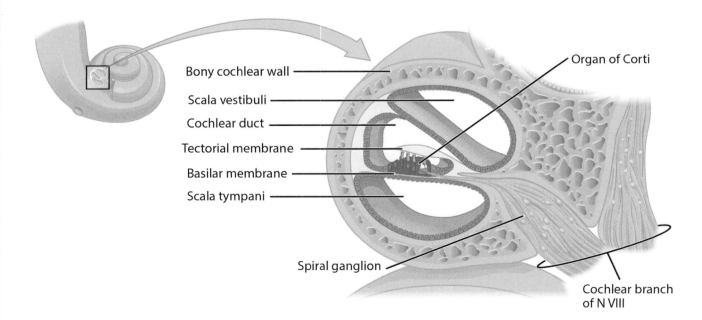

Title: 1406 Cochlea.jpg, **Author:** OpenStax, **Source:** https://cnx.org/contents/FPtK1zmh@8.25:fEI3C8Ot@10/Preface, **License/Permission:** This file is licensed under the Creative Commons Attribution 4.0 International license., **URL link:** https://en.wikiversity.org/wiki/File:1406_Cochlea.jpg

Endocrine System Anatomy and Hormones

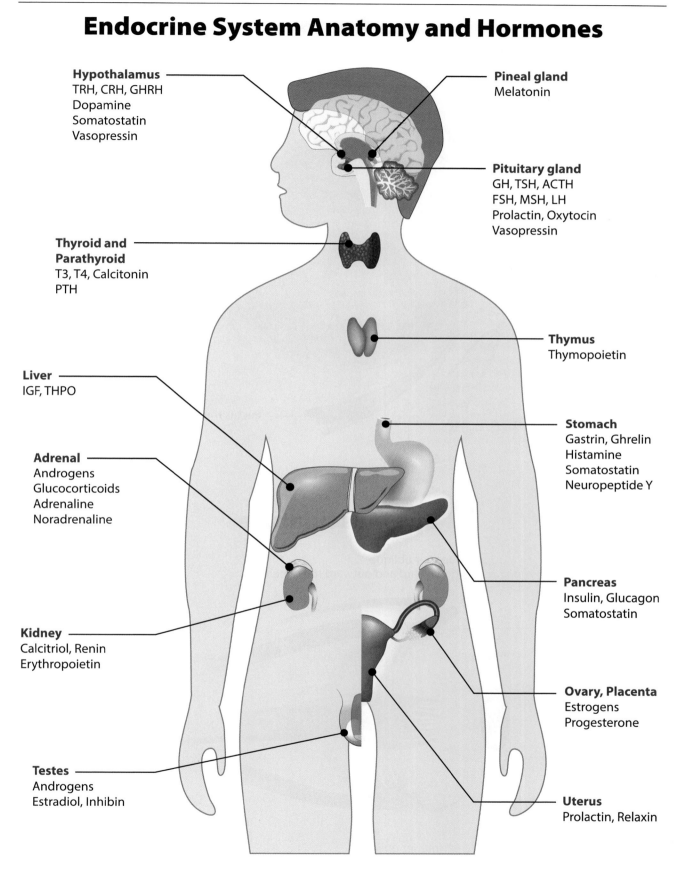

Hypothalamus
TRH, CRH, GHRH
Dopamine
Somatostatin
Vasopressin

Pineal gland
Melatonin

Pituitary gland
GH, TSH, ACTH
FSH, MSH, LH
Prolactin, Oxytocin
Vasopressin

Thyroid and Parathyroid
T3, T4, Calcitonin
PTH

Thymus
Thymopoietin

Liver
IGF, THPO

Stomach
Gastrin, Ghrelin
Histamine
Somatostatin
Neuropeptide Y

Adrenal
Androgens
Glucocorticoids
Adrenaline
Noradrenaline

Pancreas
Insulin, Glucagon
Somatostatin

Kidney
Calcitriol, Renin
Erythropoietin

Ovary, Placenta
Estrogens
Progesterone

Testes
Androgens
Estradiol, Inhibin

Uterus
Prolactin, Relaxin

Eye Anatomy

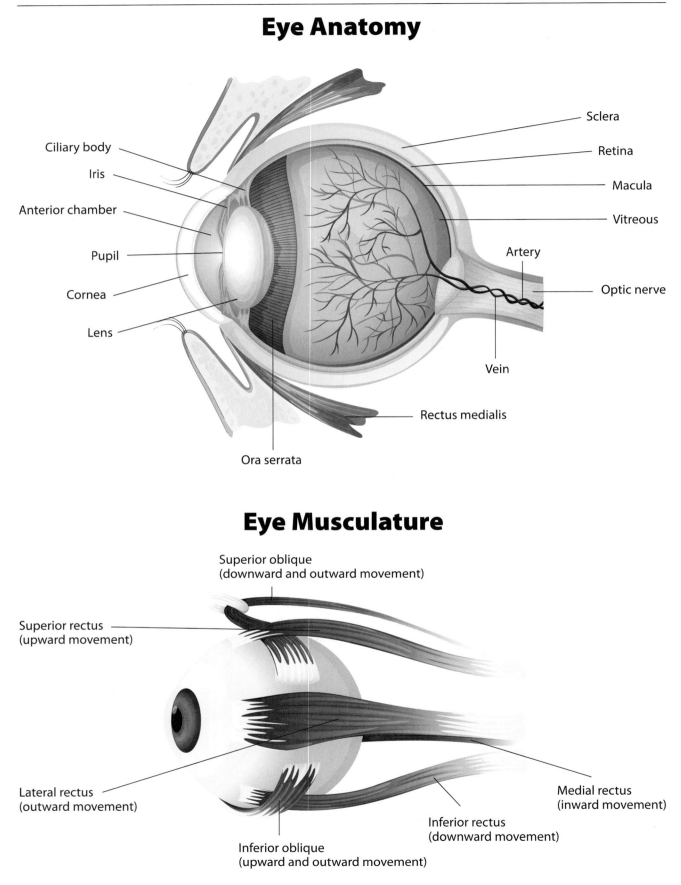

Ciliary body

Iris

Anterior chamber

Pupil

Cornea

Lens

Ora serrata

Sclera

Retina

Macula

Vitreous

Artery

Optic nerve

Vein

Rectus medialis

Eye Musculature

Superior oblique
(downward and outward movement)

Superior rectus
(upward movement)

Lateral rectus
(outward movement)

Inferior oblique
(upward and outward movement)

Inferior rectus
(downward movement)

Medial rectus
(inward movement)

Female Reproductive System Anatomy

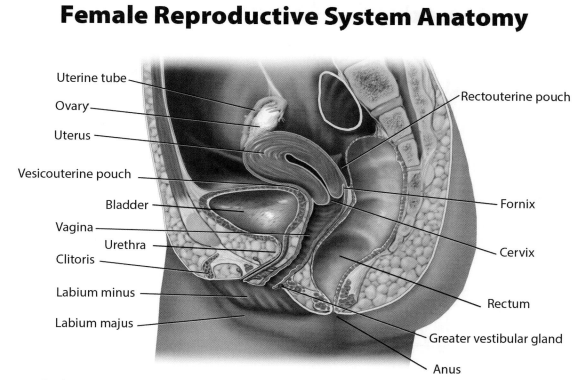

Uterine tube

Ovary

Uterus

Vesicouterine pouch

Bladder

Vagina

Urethra

Clitoris

Labium minus

Labium majus

Rectouterine pouch

Fornix

Cervix

Rectum

Greater vestibular gland

Anus

Title: Blausen 0400 FemaleReproSystem 02b.png, **Author:** BruceBlaus., **Source:** Blausen.com staff (2014). "Medical gallery of Blausen Medical 2014". *WikiJournal of Medicine* **1** (2). DOI:10.15347/wjm/2014.010. ISSN 2002-4436.Modified by User:ArnoldReinhold who released mods under CC0, **License/Permission:** This file is licensed under the Creative Commons Attribution 3.0 Unported license., **URL link:** https://commons.wikimedia.org/wiki/File:Blausen_0400_FemaleReproSystem_02b.png

Female Reproductive System — Uterus and Adnexa Anatomy

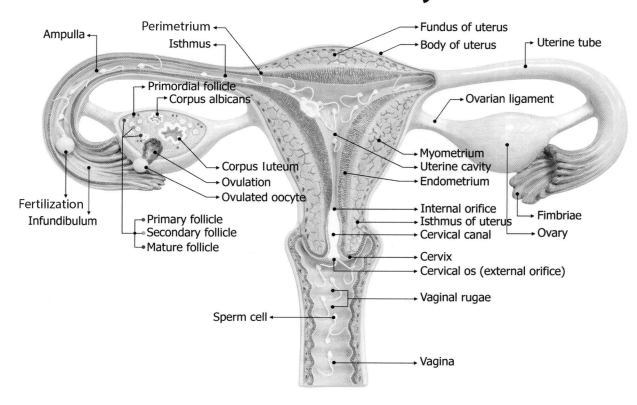

Ampulla

Perimetrium

Isthmus

Primordial follicle

Corpus albicans

Corpus luteum

Ovulation

Ovulated oocyte

Fertilization

Infundibulum

Primary follicle

Secondary follicle

Mature follicle

Sperm cell

Fundus of uterus

Body of uterus

Uterine tube

Ovarian ligament

Myometrium

Uterine cavity

Endometrium

Internal orifice

Isthmus of uterus

Cervical canal

Fimbriae

Ovary

Cervix

Cervical os (external orifice)

Vaginal rugae

Vagina

Female Reproductive System — Breast Anatomy

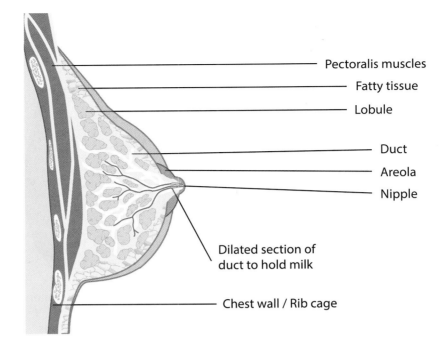

Pectoralis muscles

Fatty tissue

Lobule

Duct

Areola

Nipple

Dilated section of
duct to hold milk

Chest wall / Rib cage

Female Reproductive System — Perineum Anatomy

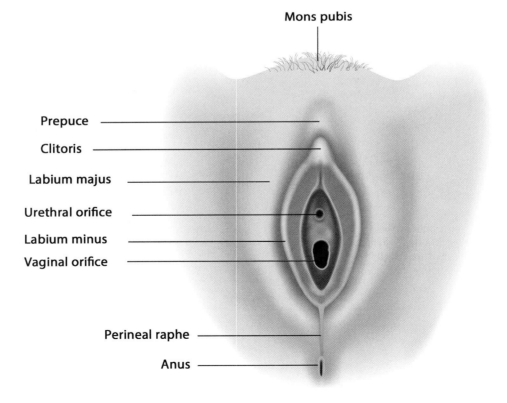

Mons pubis

Prepuce

Clitoris

Labium majus

Urethral orifice

Labium minus

Vaginal orifice

Perineal raphe

Anus

Integumentary System Anatomy

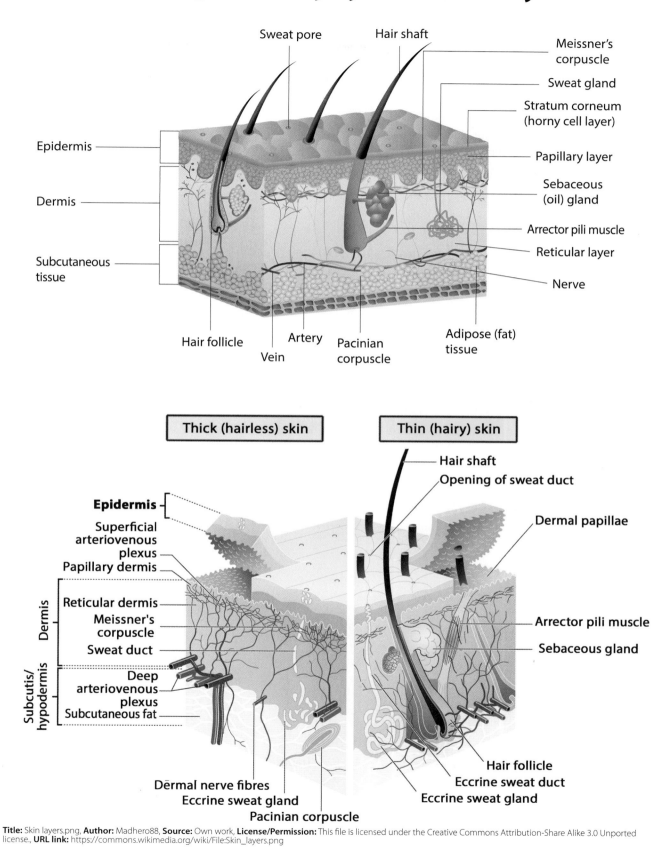

Sweat pore

Hair shaft

Meissner's corpuscle

Sweat gland

Stratum corneum (horny cell layer)

Epidermis

Papillary layer

Dermis

Sebaceous (oil) gland

Arrector pili muscle

Reticular layer

Subcutaneous tissue

Nerve

Hair follicle

Artery

Pacinian corpuscle

Adipose (fat) tissue

Vein

Thick (hairless) skin

Thin (hairy) skin

Hair shaft

Opening of sweat duct

Epidermis

Dermal papillae

Superficial arteriovenous plexus

Papillary dermis

Dermis

Reticular dermis

Meissner's corpuscle

Arrector pili muscle

Sweat duct

Sebaceous gland

Subcutis/hypodermis

Deep arteriovenous plexus

Subcutaneous fat

Dermal nerve fibres

Eccrine sweat gland

Pacinian corpuscle

Hair follicle

Eccrine sweat duct

Eccrine sweat gland

Lymphatic System Anatomy

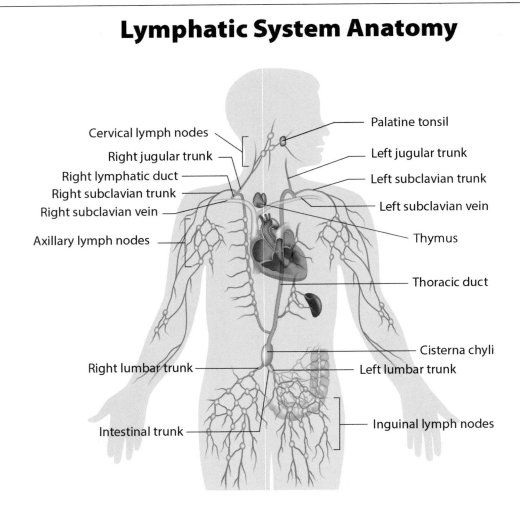

Cervical lymph nodes
Right jugular trunk
Right lymphatic duct
Right subclavian trunk
Right subclavian vein
Axillary lymph nodes

Palatine tonsil
Left jugular trunk
Left subclavian trunk
Left subclavian vein
Thymus

Thoracic duct

Cisterna chyli

Right lumbar trunk
Left lumbar trunk

Inguinal lymph nodes

Intestinal trunk

Lymphatic System — Lymph Nodes of the Head and Neck

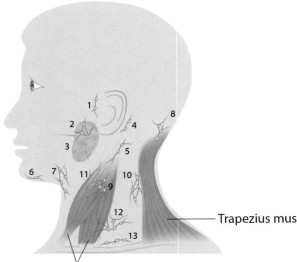

1. Preauricular
2. Superficial parotid
3. Deep parotid
4. Posterior auricular
5. Mastoid
6. Submental
7. Submandibular
8. Occipital
9. Superficial anterior cervical
10. Superficial posterior cervical
11. Superior deep cervical
12. Inferior deep cervical
13. Supraclavicular

Trapezius muscle

Sternocleidomastoid muscle

Lymphatic System — Humoral Immunity

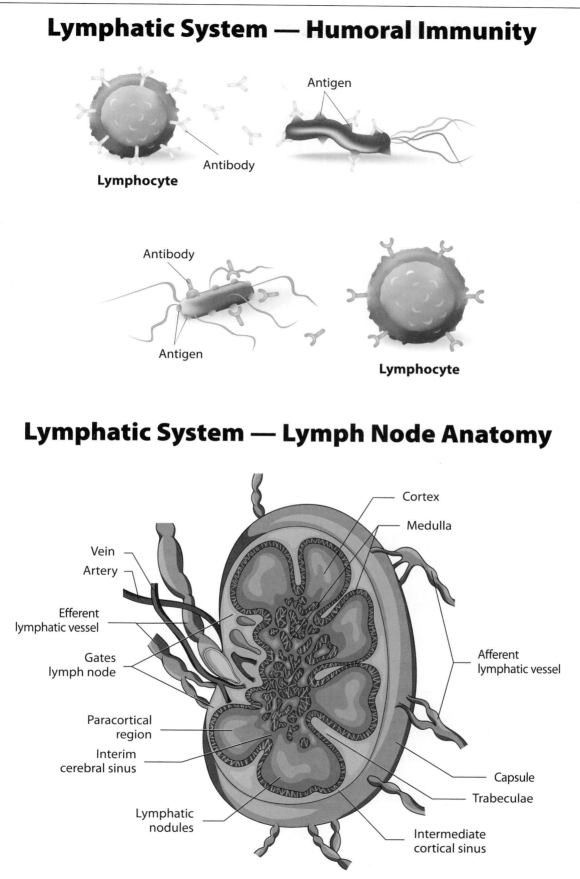

Antigen

Antibody

Lymphocyte

Antibody

Antigen

Lymphocyte

Lymphatic System — Lymph Node Anatomy

Cortex

Medulla

Vein

Artery

Efferent
lymphatic vessel

Gates
lymph node

Afferent
lymphatic vessel

Paracortical
region

Interim
cerebral sinus

Capsule

Trabeculae

Lymphatic
nodules

Intermediate
cortical sinus

Male Reproductive System Anatomy

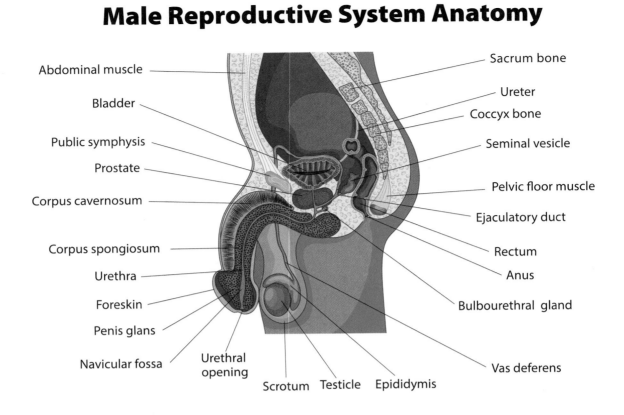

Abdominal muscle

Bladder

Public symphysis

Prostate

Corpus cavernosum

Corpus spongiosum

Urethra

Foreskin

Penis glans

Navicular fossa

Urethral opening

Scrotum

Testicle

Epididymis

Sacrum bone

Ureter

Coccyx bone

Seminal vesicle

Pelvic floor muscle

Ejaculatory duct

Rectum

Anus

Bulbourethral gland

Vas deferens

Male Reproductive System — Testicle

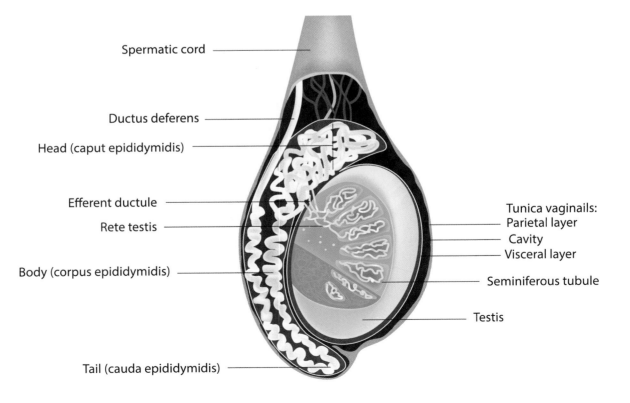

Spermatic cord

Ductus deferens

Head (caput epididymidis)

Efferent ductule

Rete testis

Body (corpus epididymidis)

Tail (cauda epididymidis)

Tunica vaginails:
Parietal layer

Cavity

Visceral layer

Seminiferous tubule

Testis

Male Reproductive System — Penis Anatomy

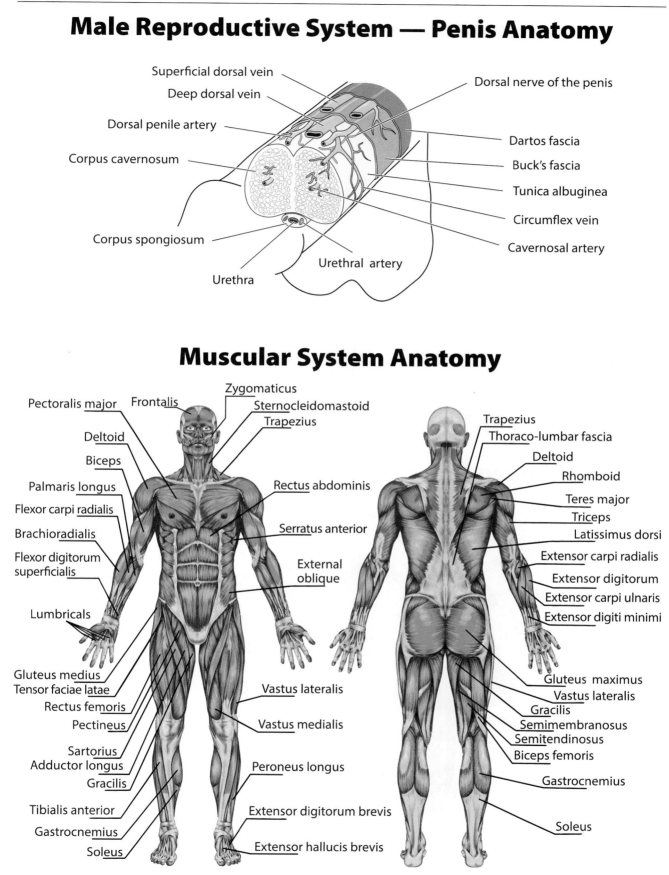

Superficial dorsal vein

Deep dorsal vein

Dorsal penile artery

Corpus cavernosum

Corpus spongiosum

Urethra

Urethral artery

Dorsal nerve of the penis

Dartos fascia

Buck's fascia

Tunica albuginea

Circumflex vein

Cavernosal artery

Muscular System Anatomy

Pectoralis major

Deltoid

Biceps

Palmaris longus

Flexor carpi radialis

Brachioradialis

Flexor digitorum superficialis

Lumbricals

Gluteus medius

Tensor faciae latae

Rectus femoris

Pectineus

Sartorius

Adductor longus

Gracilis

Tibialis anterior

Gastrocnemius

Soleus

Frontalis

Zygomaticus

Sternocleidomastoid

Trapezius

Rectus abdominis

Serratus anterior

External oblique

Vastus lateralis

Vastus medialis

Peroneus longus

Extensor digitorum brevis

Extensor hallucis brevis

Trapezius

Thoraco-lumbar fascia

Deltoid

Rhomboid

Teres major

Triceps

Latissimus dorsi

Extensor carpi radialis

Extensor digitorum

Extensor carpi ulnaris

Extensor digiti minimi

Gluteus maximus

Vastus lateralis

Gracilis

Semimembranosus

Semitendinosus

Biceps femoris

Gastrocnemius

Soleus

Muscular System — Face Muscles

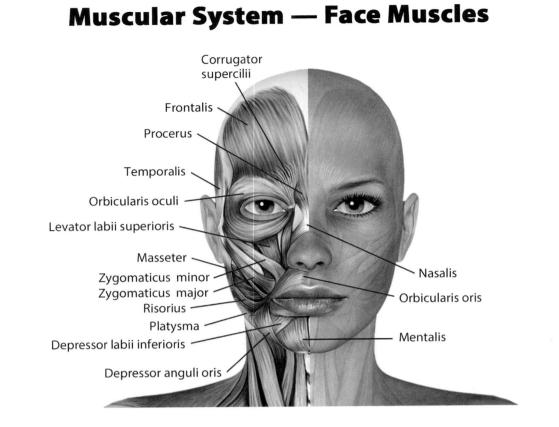

- Corrugator supercilii
- Frontalis
- Procerus
- Temporalis
- Orbicularis oculi
- Levator labii superioris
- Masseter
- Zygomaticus minor
- Zygomaticus major
- Risorius
- Platysma
- Depressor labii inferioris
- Depressor anguli oris
- Nasalis
- Orbicularis oris
- Mentalis

Muscular System — Neck, Chest, Thorax Muscles

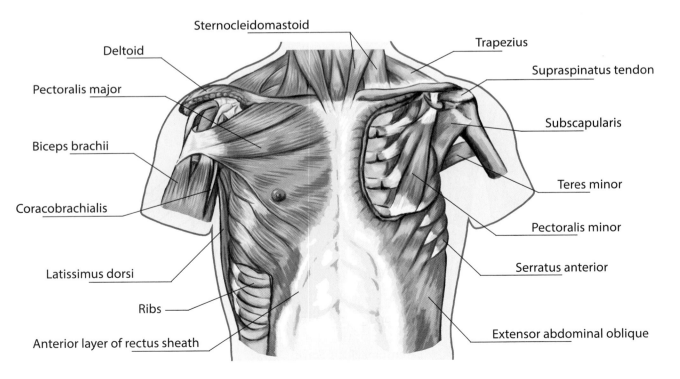

- Sternocleidomastoid
- Deltoid
- Pectoralis major
- Biceps brachii
- Coracobrachialis
- Latissimus dorsi
- Ribs
- Anterior layer of rectus sheath
- Trapezius
- Supraspinatus tendon
- Subscapularis
- Teres minor
- Pectoralis minor
- Serratus anterior
- Extensor abdominal oblique

Muscular System — Shoulder (Rotator Cuff) Muscles

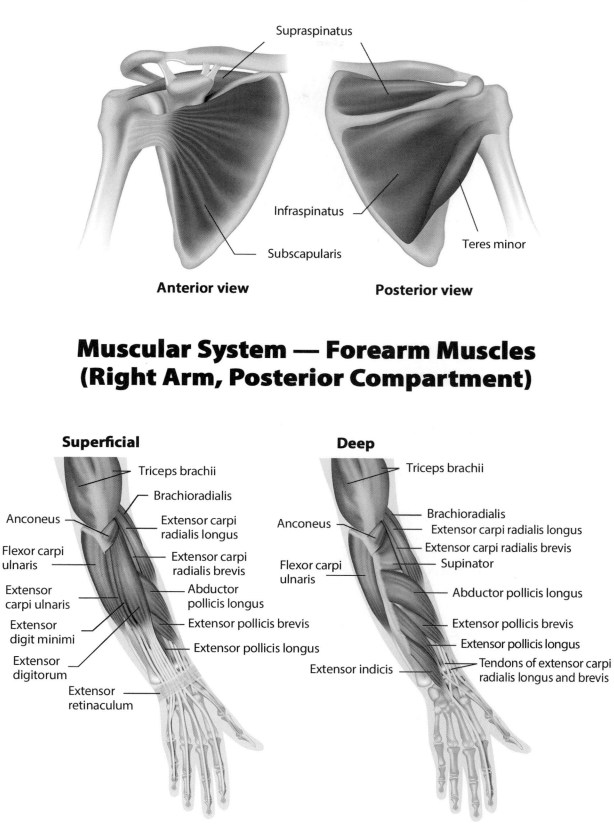

Supraspinatus

Infraspinatus

Subscapularis

Teres minor

Anterior view　　　　**Posterior view**

Muscular System — Forearm Muscles
(Right Arm, Posterior Compartment)

Superficial

Triceps brachii

Brachioradialis

Anconeus

Extensor carpi radialis longus

Flexor carpi ulnaris

Extensor carpi radialis brevis

Extensor carpi ulnaris

Abductor pollicis longus

Extensor digit minimi

Extensor pollicis brevis

Extensor digitorum

Extensor pollicis longus

Extensor retinaculum

Deep

Triceps brachii

Anconeus

Brachioradialis

Extensor carpi radialis longus

Extensor carpi radialis brevis

Flexor carpi ulnaris

Supinator

Abductor pollicis longus

Extensor pollicis brevis

Extensor pollicis longus

Extensor indicis

Tendons of extensor carpi radialis longus and brevis

Muscular System — Muscles of the Hand
(right hand, dorsal view)

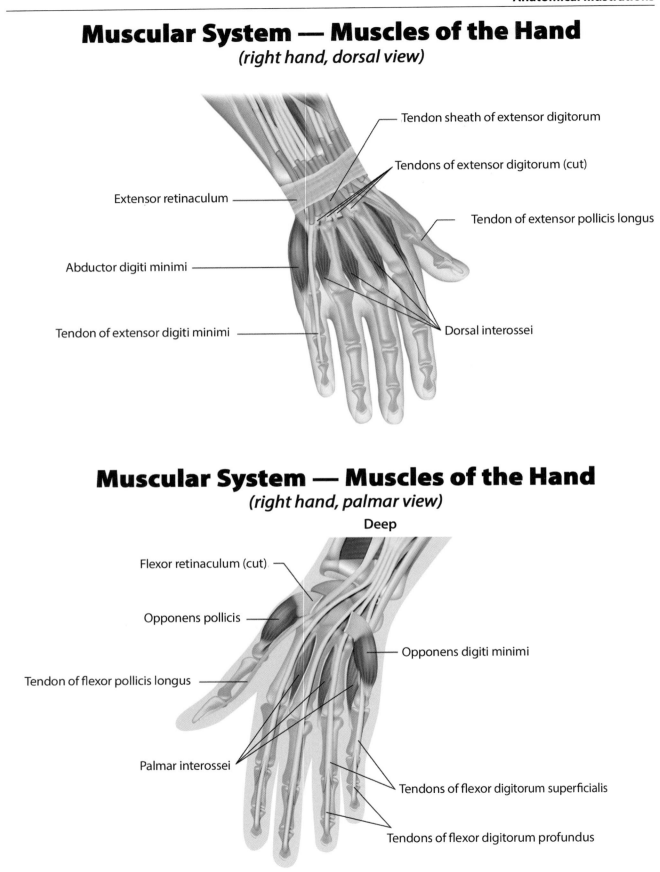

Tendon sheath of extensor digitorum

Tendons of extensor digitorum (cut)

Extensor retinaculum

Tendon of extensor pollicis longus

Abductor digiti minimi

Tendon of extensor digiti minimi

Dorsal interossei

Muscular System — Muscles of the Hand
(right hand, palmar view)

Deep

Flexor retinaculum (cut)

Opponens pollicis

Opponens digiti minimi

Tendon of flexor pollicis longus

Palmar interossei

Tendons of flexor digitorum superficialis

Tendons of flexor digitorum profundus

Muscular System — Leg Muscles

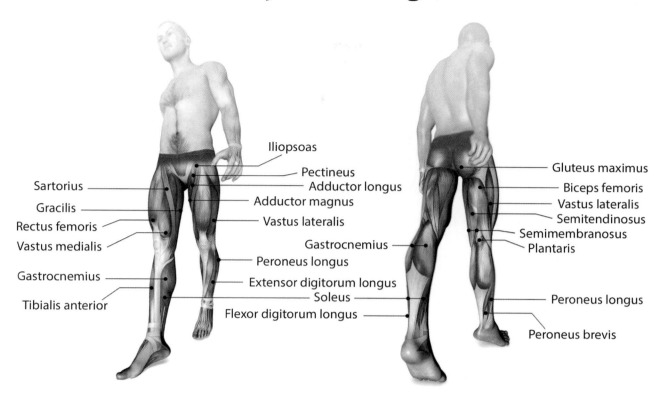

Iliopsoas
Pectineus
Adductor longus
Adductor magnus
Vastus lateralis

Sartorius
Gracilis
Rectus femoris
Vastus medialis
Gastrocnemius
Tibialis anterior

Gastrocnemius
Peroneus longus
Extensor digitorum longus
Soleus
Flexor digitorum longus

Gluteus maximus
Biceps femoris
Vastus lateralis
Semitendinosus
Semimembranosus
Plantaris

Peroneus longus

Peroneus brevis

Muscular System — Knee and Leg

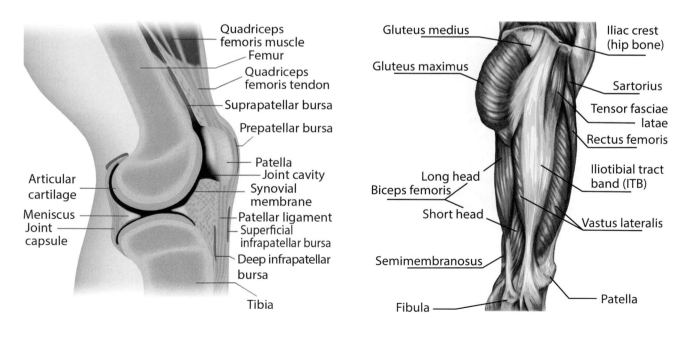

Quadriceps femoris muscle
Femur
Quadriceps femoris tendon
Suprapatellar bursa
Prepatellar bursa
Patella
Joint cavity
Synovial membrane
Patellar ligament
Superficial infrapatellar bursa
Deep infrapatellar bursa
Tibia

Articular cartilage
Meniscus
Joint capsule

Gluteus medius
Gluteus maximus
Long head
Biceps femoris
Short head
Semimembranosus
Fibula

Iliac crest (hip bone)
Sartorius
Tensor fasciae latae
Rectus femoris
Iliotibial tract band (ITB)
Vastus lateralis
Patella

Muscular System — Foot Muscles

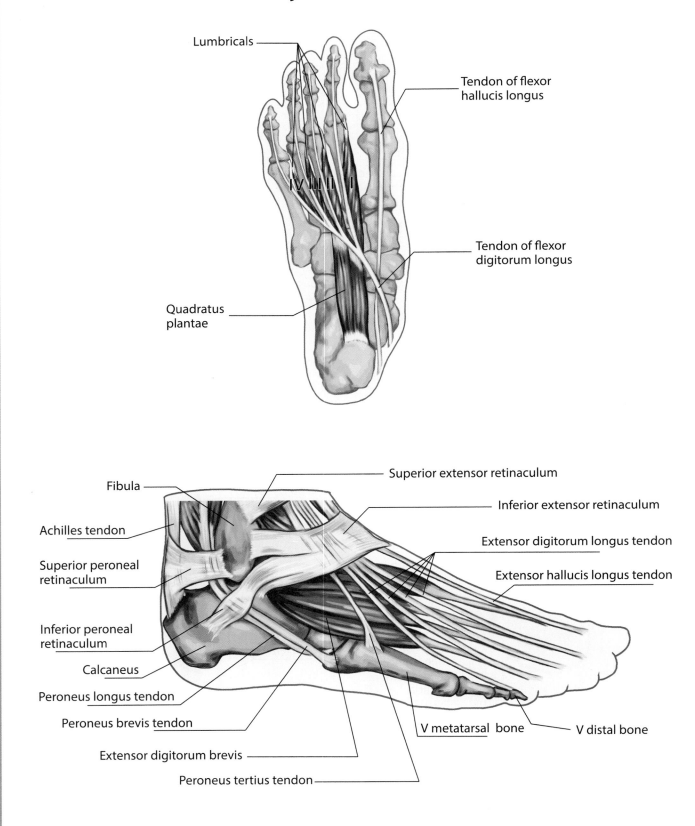

Lumbricals

Tendon of flexor hallucis longus

Tendon of flexor digitorum longus

Quadratus plantae

Fibula

Achilles tendon

Superior peroneal retinaculum

Inferior peroneal retinaculum

Calcaneus

Peroneus longus tendon

Peroneus brevis tendon

Extensor digitorum brevis

Peroneus tertius tendon

Superior extensor retinaculum

Inferior extensor retinaculum

Extensor digitorum longus tendon

Extensor hallucis longus tendon

V metatarsal bone

V distal bone

Musculoskeletal System — Shoulder Joint Structure

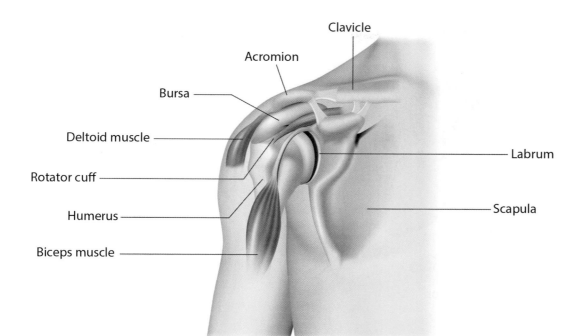

Clavicle

Acromion

Bursa

Deltoid muscle

Rotator cuff

Humerus

Biceps muscle

Labrum

Scapula

Nervous System Anatomy

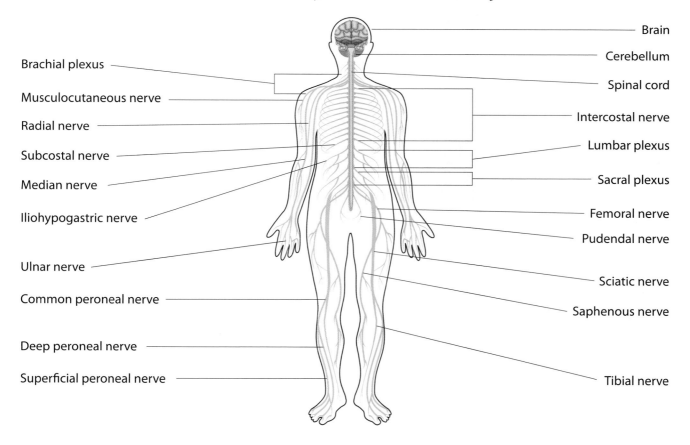

Brachial plexus

Musculocutaneous nerve

Radial nerve

Subcostal nerve

Median nerve

Iliohypogastric nerve

Ulnar nerve

Common peroneal nerve

Deep peroneal nerve

Superficial peroneal nerve

Brain

Cerebellum

Spinal cord

Intercostal nerve

Lumbar plexus

Sacral plexus

Femoral nerve

Pudendal nerve

Sciatic nerve

Saphenous nerve

Tibial nerve

Nervous System — Brain Anatomy

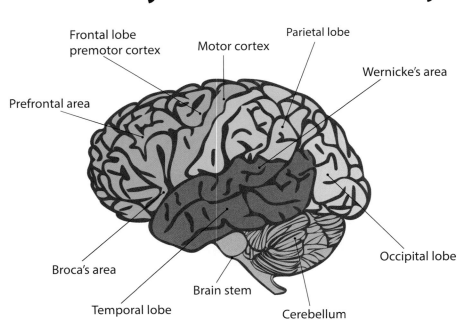

Frontal lobe premotor cortex

Motor cortex

Parietal lobe

Wernicke's area

Prefrontal area

Occipital lobe

Broca's area

Brain stem

Temporal lobe

Cerebellum

Nervous System — Median Section of the Brain

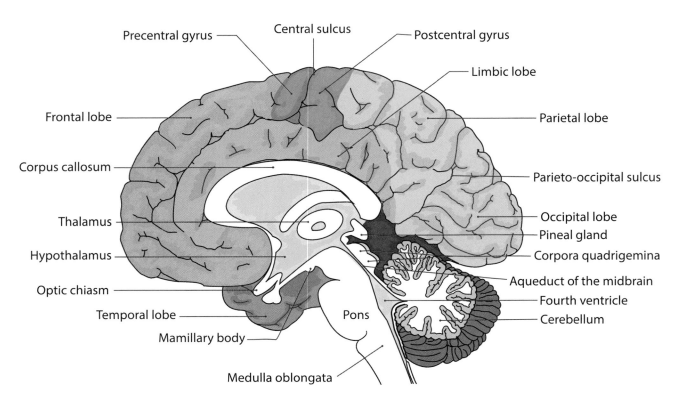

Precentral gyrus

Central sulcus

Postcentral gyrus

Limbic lobe

Frontal lobe

Parietal lobe

Corpus callosum

Parieto-occipital sulcus

Thalamus

Occipital lobe

Pineal gland

Hypothalamus

Corpora quadrigemina

Aqueduct of the midbrain

Optic chiasm

Fourth ventricle

Temporal lobe

Pons

Cerebellum

Mamillary body

Medulla oblongata

Nervous System — Cranial Nerves

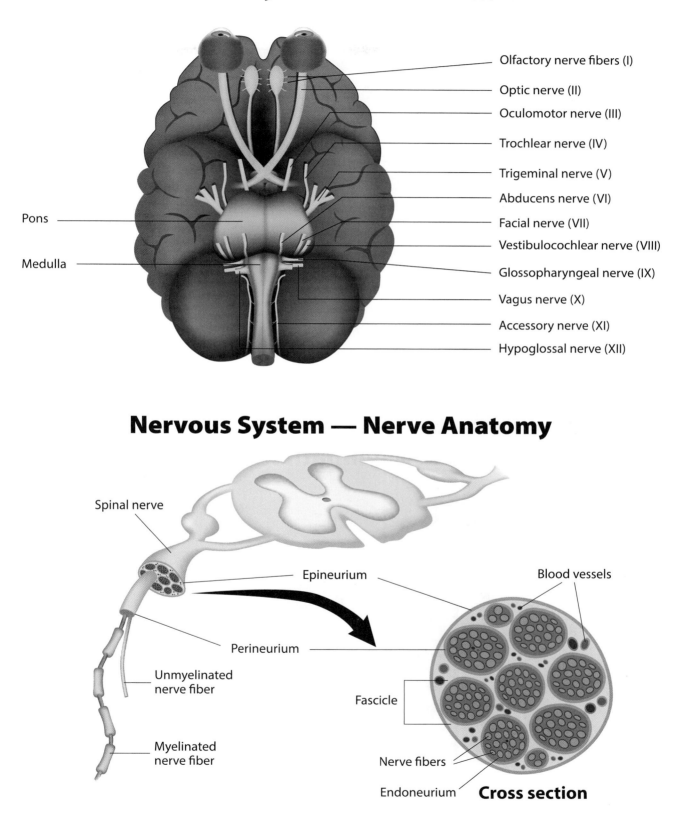

Olfactory nerve fibers (I)

Optic nerve (II)

Oculomotor nerve (III)

Trochlear nerve (IV)

Trigeminal nerve (V)

Abducens nerve (VI)

Facial nerve (VII)

Vestibulocochlear nerve (VIII)

Glossopharyngeal nerve (IX)

Vagus nerve (X)

Accessory nerve (XI)

Hypoglossal nerve (XII)

Pons

Medulla

Nervous System — Nerve Anatomy

Spinal nerve

Epineurium

Blood vessels

Perineurium

Unmyelinated nerve fiber

Fascicle

Myelinated nerve fiber

Nerve fibers

Endoneurium

Cross section

Nervous System — Parasympathetic System Anatomy

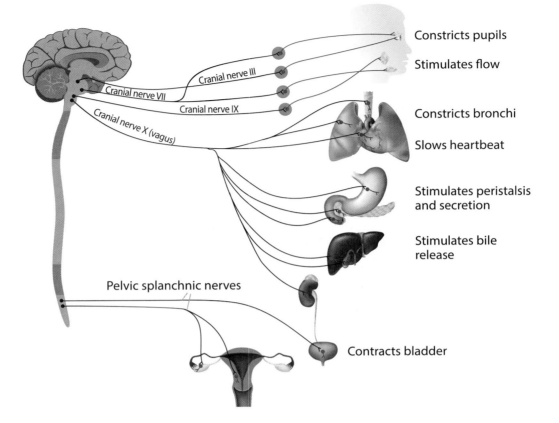

Constricts pupils

Stimulates flow

Cranial nerve III

Cranial nerve VII

Cranial nerve IX

Cranial nerve X (vagus)

Constricts bronchi

Slows heartbeat

Stimulates peristalsis and secretion

Stimulates bile release

Pelvic splanchnic nerves

Contracts bladder

Nervous System — Sympathetic System Anatomy

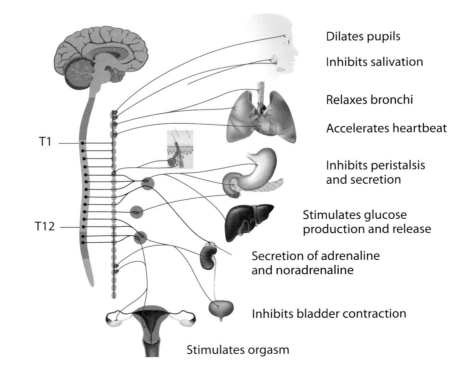

Dilates pupils

Inhibits salivation

Relaxes bronchi

Accelerates heartbeat

Inhibits peristalsis and secretion

T1

Stimulates glucose production and release

T12

Secretion of adrenaline and noradrenaline

Inhibits bladder contraction

Stimulates orgasm

Respiratory System Anatomy

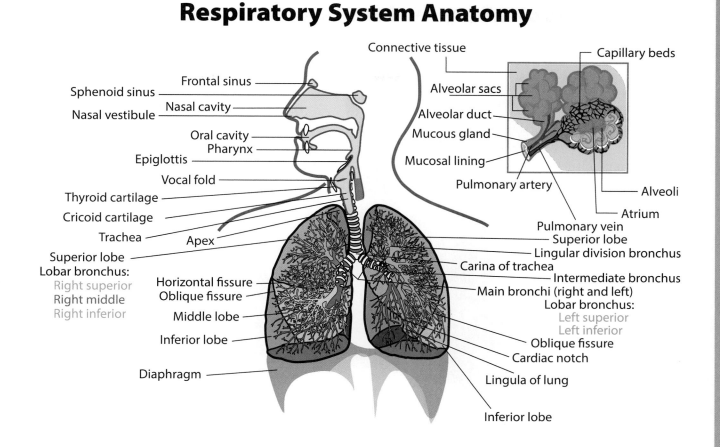

Respiratory System — Larynx Anatomy

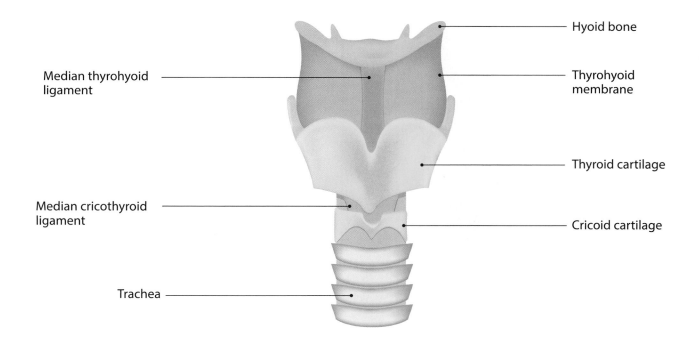

Respiratory System — Lung Anatomy

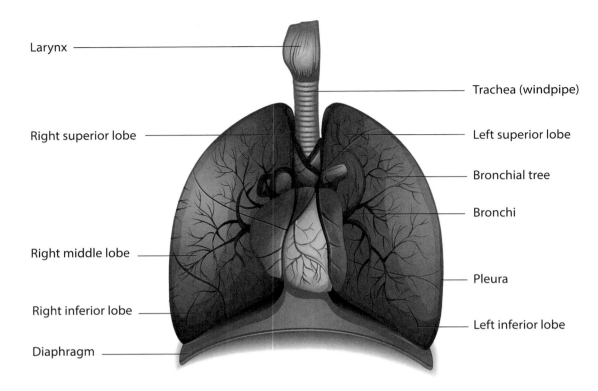

Larynx

Right superior lobe

Right middle lobe

Right inferior lobe

Diaphragm

Trachea (windpipe)

Left superior lobe

Bronchial tree

Bronchi

Pleura

Left inferior lobe

Respiratory System Function

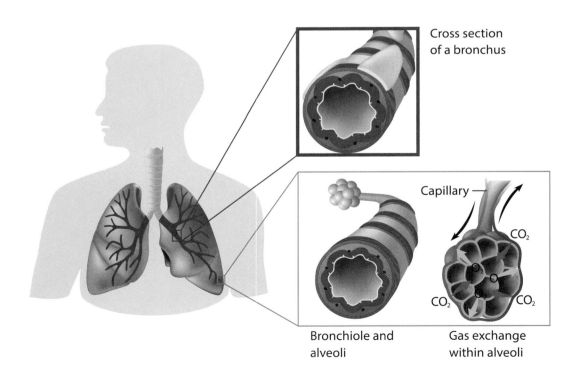

Cross section
of a bronchus

Capillary

CO_2

CO_2

CO_2

Bronchiole and
alveoli

Gas exchange
within alveoli

Respiratory System — Nose Anatomy

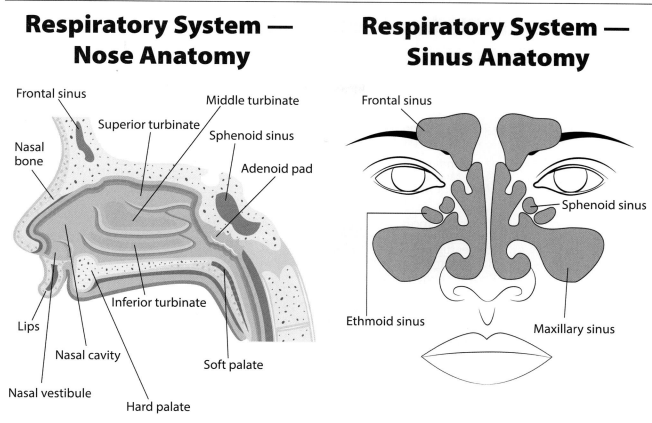

Frontal sinus

Middle turbinate

Superior turbinate

Sphenoid sinus

Nasal bone

Adenoid pad

Inferior turbinate

Lips

Nasal cavity

Soft palate

Nasal vestibule

Hard palate

Respiratory System — Sinus Anatomy

Frontal sinus

Sphenoid sinus

Ethmoid sinus

Maxillary sinus

Respiratory System — Throat Anatomy

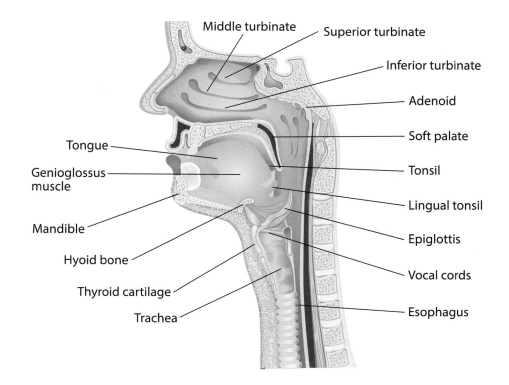

Middle turbinate

Superior turbinate

Inferior turbinate

Adenoid

Soft palate

Tonsil

Tongue

Genioglossus muscle

Lingual tonsil

Mandible

Epiglottis

Hyoid bone

Vocal cords

Thyroid cartilage

Esophagus

Trachea

Skeletal System Anatomy

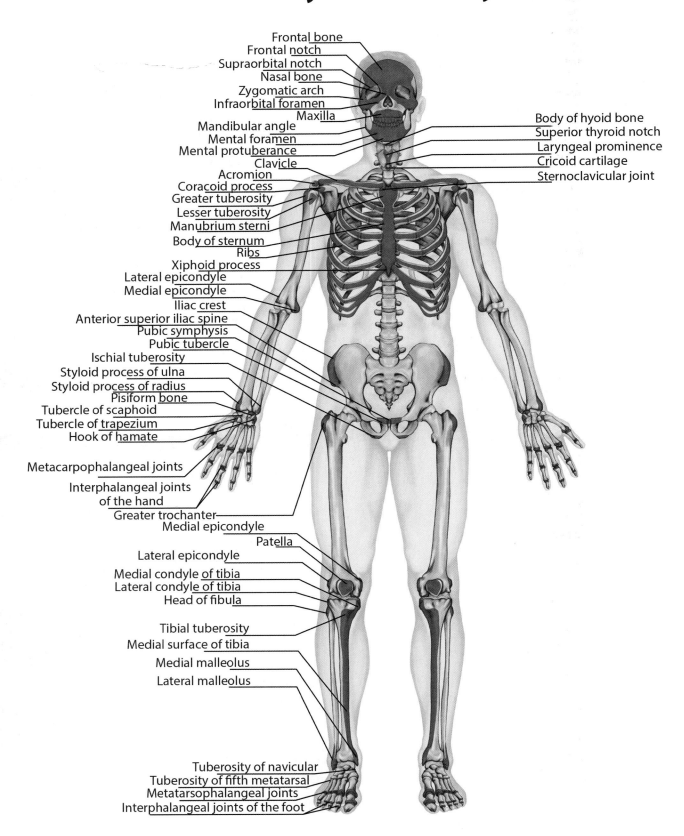

Frontal bone
Frontal notch
Supraorbital notch
Nasal bone
Zygomatic arch
Infraorbital foramen
Maxilla
Mandibular angle
Mental foramen
Mental protuberance
Clavicle
Acromion
Coracoid process
Greater tuberosity
Lesser tuberosity
Manubrium sterni
Body of sternum
Ribs
Xiphoid process
Lateral epicondyle
Medial epicondyle
Iliac crest
Anterior superior iliac spine
Pubic symphysis
Pubic tubercle
Ischial tuberosity
Styloid process of ulna
Styloid process of radius
Pisiform bone
Tubercle of scaphoid
Tubercle of trapezium
Hook of hamate

Metacarpophalangeal joints

Interphalangeal joints
of the hand
Greater trochanter
Medial epicondyle
Patella
Lateral epicondyle
Medial condyle of tibia
Lateral condyle of tibia
Head of fibula

Tibial tuberosity
Medial surface of tibia
Medial malleolus
Lateral malleolus

Body of hyoid bone
Superior thyroid notch
Laryngeal prominence
Cricoid cartilage
Sternoclavicular joint

Tuberosity of navicular
Tuberosity of fifth metatarsal
Metatarsophalangeal joints
Interphalangeal joints of the foot

Skeletal System — Bone Structure

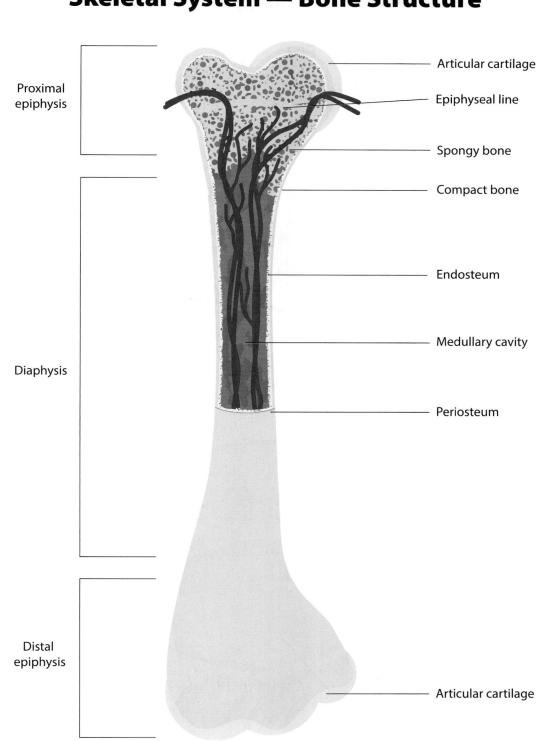

Proximal epiphysis

Diaphysis

Distal epiphysis

Articular cartilage

Epiphyseal line

Spongy bone

Compact bone

Endosteum

Medullary cavity

Periosteum

Articular cartilage

Skeletal System — Skull

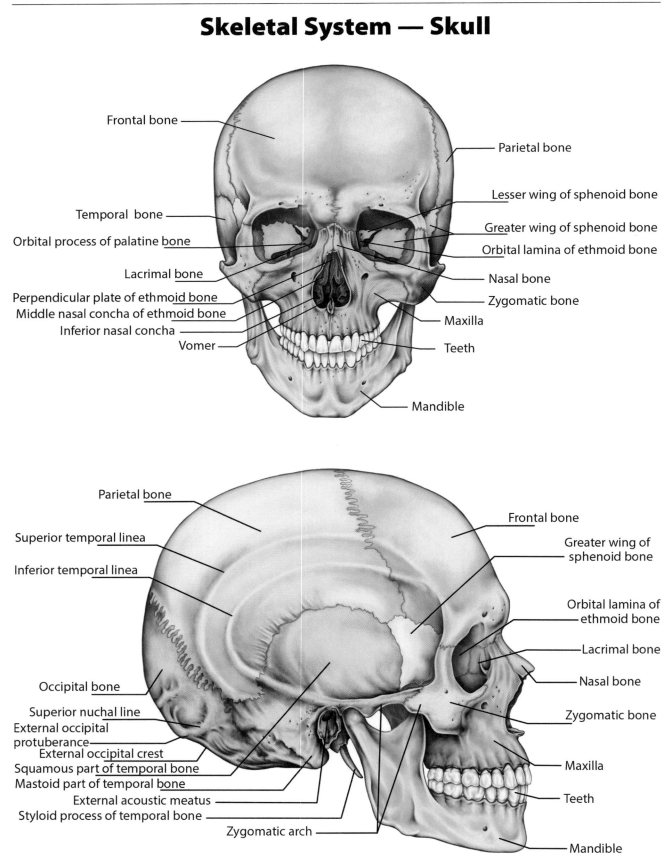

Frontal bone

Parietal bone

Lesser wing of sphenoid bone

Temporal bone

Greater wing of sphenoid bone

Orbital process of palatine bone

Orbital lamina of ethmoid bone

Lacrimal bone

Nasal bone

Perpendicular plate of ethmoid bone

Zygomatic bone

Middle nasal concha of ethmoid bone

Inferior nasal concha

Maxilla

Vomer

Teeth

Mandible

Parietal bone

Frontal bone

Superior temporal linea

Greater wing of
sphenoid bone

Inferior temporal linea

Orbital lamina of
ethmoid bone

Lacrimal bone

Nasal bone

Occipital bone

Zygomatic bone

Superior nuchal line

External occipital
protuberance

External occipital crest

Squamous part of temporal bone

Maxilla

Mastoid part of temporal bone

External acoustic meatus

Teeth

Styloid process of temporal bone

Zygomatic arch

Mandible

Skeletal System — Cervical, Thoracic, and Lumbar Spine

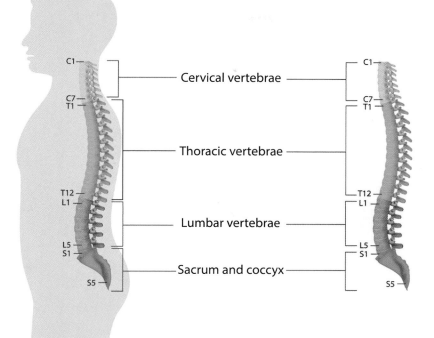

- Cervical vertebrae
- Thoracic vertebrae
- Lumbar vertebrae
- Sacrum and coccyx

Skeletal System — Pelvic Girdle

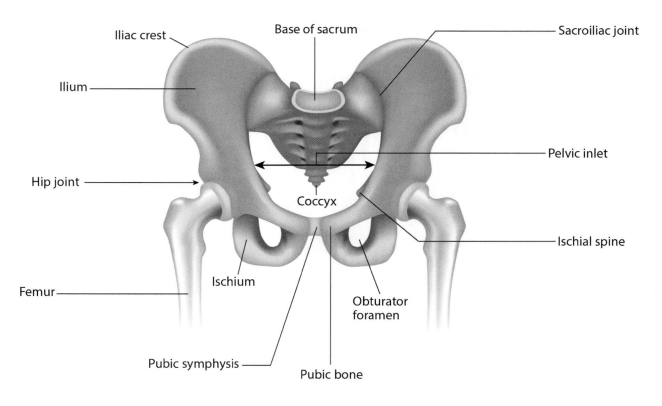

- Iliac crest
- Base of sacrum
- Sacroiliac joint
- Ilium
- Pelvic inlet
- Hip joint
- Coccyx
- Ischial spine
- Femur
- Ischium
- Obturator foramen
- Pubic symphysis
- Pubic bone

Skeletal System — Elbow Joint Structure

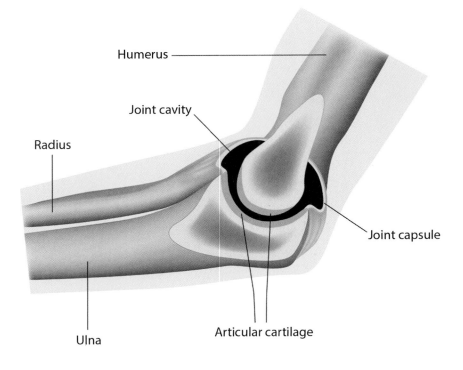

Humerus

Joint cavity

Radius

Joint capsule

Ulna

Articular cartilage

Skeletal System — Hand Bones

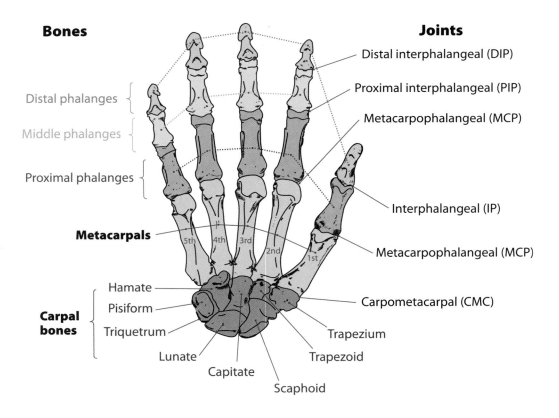

Bones

Distal phalanges

Middle phalanges

Proximal phalanges

Metacarpals

5th 4th 3rd 2nd 1st

Carpal bones

Hamate
Pisiform
Triquetrum
Lunate
Capitate
Scaphoid

Joints

Distal interphalangeal (DIP)

Proximal interphalangeal (PIP)

Metacarpophalangeal (MCP)

Interphalangeal (IP)

Metacarpophalangeal (MCP)

Carpometacarpal (CMC)

Trapezium
Trapezoid

Skeletal System — Foot Bones
(Right Foot, Lateral View)

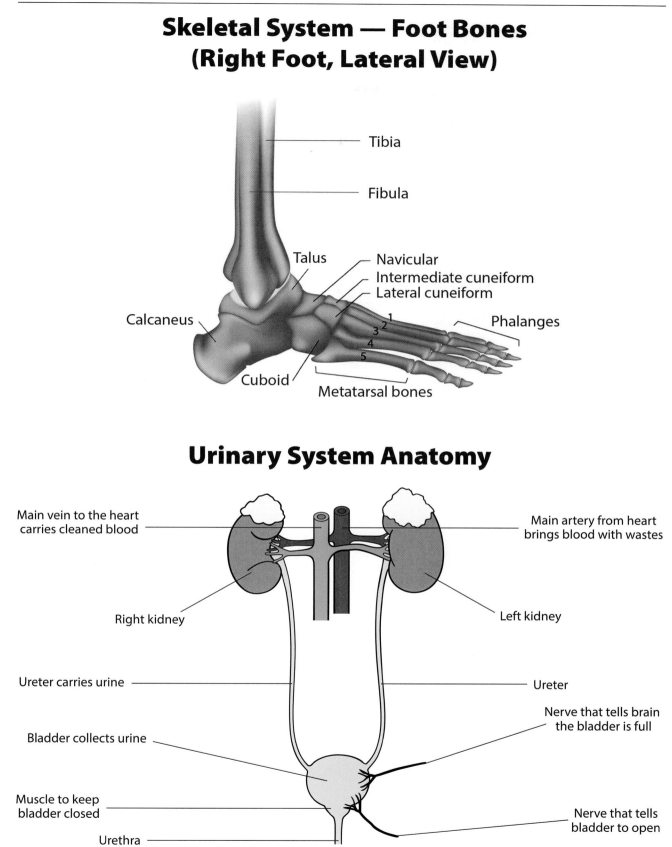

Tibia

Fibula

Talus

Navicular

Intermediate cuneiform

Lateral cuneiform

Calcaneus

1

2

3

4

5

Phalanges

Cuboid

Metatarsal bones

Urinary System Anatomy

Main vein to the heart carries cleaned blood

Main artery from heart brings blood with wastes

Right kidney

Left kidney

Ureter carries urine

Ureter

Nerve that tells brain the bladder is full

Bladder collects urine

Muscle to keep bladder closed

Nerve that tells bladder to open

Urethra

Urinary System — Kidney Anatomy

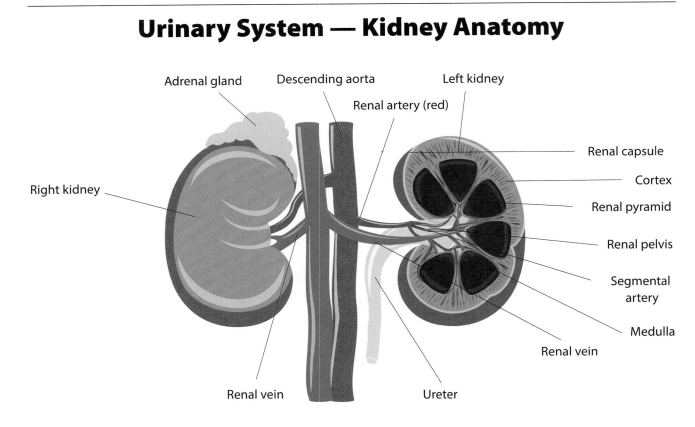

Adrenal gland

Descending aorta

Renal artery (red)

Left kidney

Renal capsule

Cortex

Right kidney

Renal pyramid

Renal pelvis

Segmental artery

Medulla

Renal vein

Renal vein

Ureter

Index to Services, Supplies, Equipment, Drugs

A

A-Hydrocort® J1710
Abatacept J0129
Abciximab J0130
Abdominal pad, TLSO L1270
Abduction
    Control, hip orthosis, hip joint
        Dynamic, adjustable L1680
        Flexible
            Frejka type L1600, L1610
            Pavlik harness L1620
        Semi-flexible, Van Rosen type L1630
        Static
            Adjustable, Ilfeld type, prefabricated L1650
            Pelvic band or spreader bar L1640
            Plastic, prefabricated L1660
    Control, lower extremity orthosis, hip joint L2624
    Pillow (miscellaneous durable medical equipment) E1399
    Restrainer, shoulder L3650
        Canvas and webbing L3660
        Vest type L3675
    Rotation bar
        Foot L3150
            Adjustable shoe-styled positioning device L3160
            Including shoes L3140
            Prefabricated, off-the-shelf, each L3170
        Lower extremity
            Hip involvement, jointed, adjustable L2300
            Straight L2310
Ablation
    Transbronchial C9751
Ablation catheter
    Electrophysiological
        3D or vector mapping C1732
        Other than 3D or vector mapping or cool-tip C1733
    Endovascular, noncardiac C1888
    Extravascular, any modality C1886
    Tissue, extravascular C1886
    Ultrasound, focused C9734
Abobotulinumtoxin type A J0586
Abortion, induced
    17 to 24 weeks S2260
    25 to 28 weeks S2265
    29 to 31 weeks S2266
    32 or greater S2267
    Drug induced, with other services S0199
Absorption dressing A6251-A6256
Access Catheters A4300-A4301
Accessories
    Ambulation devices E0153-E0159
    Beds E0271-E0280, E0300-E0316
    Dialysis E1500-E1699
    Wheelchairs E0950-E1030, E2398, E2626-E2633, K0001-K0108, K0669
Accu-Chek® or similar product
    Blood glucose meter E0607
    Test strips, box of 50 A4253
Acetaminophen J0131
Acetate concentrate for hemodialysis A4708
Acetazolamide sodium J1120

Acetylcysteine
    Inhalation solution J7604, J7608
    Injection J0132
Acid concentrate for hemodialysis A4709
Activated carbon filter for hemodialysis A4680
Activity therapy
    45 minutes or more G0176
    Per 15 minutes H2032
Acyclovir J0133
Adalimumab J0135
Adapter
    Breast pump A4282
    Electric/pneumatic ventricular assist device Q0478
    Neurostimulator C1883
    Oxygen accessory E1358
    Pacing lead C1883
    Pneumatic ventricular assist device Q0504
Addition, *see also* **Orthotic devices**
    Cushion socket
        Above knee L5648
        Below knee L5646
    Harness upper extremity
        Dual cable L6676
        Single cable L6675
    Interface replacement for halo procedure L0861
    Orthotic components, lower extremity K0672, L2750, L2760, L2780-L2861
    Prosthesis components
        Adjustable heel height L5990
        SACH foot L5970
    Torsion mechanism, upper extremity joint orthotic L3891
    Wrist unit, flexion, extension L6620
Adenosine J0153
Adhesive
    Bandage A6413
        Conforming A6442-A6447
        Padding A6441
        Self-adherent A6453, A6454, A6455
        Zinc paste impregnated A6456
    Barrier C1765
    Disc or foam pad A5126
    Dressing
        Composite
            16 sq. in. or less A6203
            More than 16 sq. in. but less than or equal to 48 sq. in. A6204
            More than 48 sq. in A6205
        Foam A6214
        Gauze
            16 sq. in. or less A6219
            More than 16 sq. in. but less than or equal to 48 sq. in. A6220
            More than 48 sq. in. A6221
        Hydrocolloid
            16 sq. in. or less A6234
            More than 16 sq. in. but less than or equal to 48 sq. in. A6238
            More than 48 sq. in. A6239
        Hydrogel
            16 sq. in. or less A6245
            More than 16 sq. in. but less than or equal to 48 sq. in. A6246
            More than 48 sq. in. A6247

Specialty
16 sq. in. or less A6254
More than 16 sq. in. but less than or equal to 48 sq. in. A6255
More than 48 sq. in. A6256
Liquid A4364
Remover A4455, A4456
Support for breast prosthesis A4280
Tape
Nonwaterproof A4450
Waterproof A4452
Tissue (wound closure) G0168
Adjustment, gastric band S2083
Administration
Aerosolized drug therapy S9061
Drug at home G0068-G0070, G0088-G0090 Ⓝ
Medication
Direct observation H0033
Oral, intramuscular and/or subcutaneous medication T1502
Other than oral and/or injectable T1503
Pain medication G9426, G9427
Vaccine G0008-G0010
Hepatitis B G0010
Influenza virus G0008
Pneumococcal G0009
Administrative, miscellaneous and investigational items A9150-A9999
Adoptive immunotherapy S2107
Ado-trastuzumab J9354
Adrenal tissue transplant S2103
Adrenalin J0171
Advance directive S0257
Aerosol
Compressor E0572
Compressor filter A7013, A7014
Mask A7015
AF, transient or reversible cause G9929
Afamelanotide implant J7352 Ⓝ
Aflibercept J0178
AFO (ankle foot orthosis) L1900-L1990
Dynamic adjustable E1815, E1830, L4397
Fracture L2106-L2116
Replace L4392, L4396
Walking boot L4631
Agalsidase beta J0180
Aggrastat J3246
Air bubble detector, dialysis E1530
Air fluidized bed E0194
Air pressure pad/mattress E0186, E0197
Air travel and nonemergency transportation A0140
Alarm, alert device A9280
Alarm, pressure, dialysis E1540
Alatrofloxacin mesylate J0200
Albumin, human
5%, 50 mL P9041
5%, 250 mL P9045
25%, 20 mL P9046
25%, 50 mL P9047
Albuterol, all formulations, inhalation solution
Concentrated
Compounded J7610
Noncompounded J7611
Unit dose
Compounded J7609
Noncompounded J7613, J7620

Alcohol (and/or drug)
Abuse and prevention services G0443, H0001-H2037, T1006-T1012
Not otherwise specified (NOS) H0047
Screening G9621, G9622, G9623, G9624
Structured, with intervention
5-14 minutes G2011
15-30 minutes G0396
Greater than 30 minutes G0397
Per pint A4244
Screening G2196-G2199 Ⓝ
Services H0047-H0050
Testing collection and handling only H0048
Unhealthy use of G2196, G2200 Ⓝ
Wipes A4245
Aldesleukin (IL2) J9015
Alefacept J0215
Alemtuzumab J0202
Alert device A9280
Alginate dressing A6196, A6197, A6198, A6199
Alglucerase J0205
Alglucosidase J0220
Alglucosidase alfa J0221
Alkaline battery
Blood glucose monitor
J cell A4234
Other than J cell A4233
Cochlear implant device replacement L8622
External infusion pump owned by patient, alkaline K0603
AlloDerm® Q4116
AlloGen® Q4212
Allogeneic cord blood harvest S2140
Allograft, small intestine and liver S2053
AlloSkin™ Q4115
Alpha-1-proteinase inhibitor, human J0256, J0257
Alphanate J7186
Alprostadil
Injection J0270
Urethral suppository J0275
ALS (advanced life support)
Disposable supplies service
Esophageal intubation A0396
IV drug therapy A0394
Level 2 A0433
Mileage A0390
Routine disposable supplies A0398
Alteplase recombinant J2997
Alternating pressure mattress/pad replacement pad A4640
Air mattress E0277
Powered pressure reducing mattress overlay/pad E0181
Replacement only E0182
Alternative communication device board E1902
Ambulance and other transport services and supplies A0021-A0999
Air A0430, A0431, A0435, A0436
Basic life support (BLS) A0428
Disposable supplies A0382-A0398
Fixed wing S9960
Mileage A0425
Nonemergency transport A0080-A0160, A0180-A0200, A0426, A0428, S0215
Oxygen A0422
Response and treatment A0998
Rotary wing S9961
Unlisted service A0999
Ambulation device E0100-E0159
Amifostine J0207
Amikacin sulfate J0278

Ⓝ New index entry

Aminocaproic acid S0017
Aminolevulinate J7309
Aminolevulinic acid HCl J7308, J7345
Aminophylline J0280
AmnioWrap2™ Q4221
Amiodarone HCl J0282
Amitriptyline HCl J1320
Ammonia N-13 A9526
Ammonia test paper A4774
Amnio wound Q4181
Amnio-maxx™ Q4239 Ⓝ
Amnioamp-mp™ Q4250 Ⓝ
Amnioarmor Q4188
Amniocore™ Q4227 Ⓝ
Amniocyte plus™ Q4242 Ⓝ
Amnioexcel®/Amnioexcel Plus ® Q4137
Amnion bio Q4211
Amniorepair® Q4235 Ⓝ
Amniotext™ Q4245, Q4247 Ⓝ
Amniotic membrane Q4198, V2790
Amniply™ Q4249 Ⓝ
Amobarbital J0300
Amphotericin B J0285
Amphotericin B injection
  Cholesteryl sulfate complex J0288
  Lipid complex J0287
  Liposome J0289
Ampicillin sodium J0290
Ampicillin sodium/sulbactam sodium J0295
Amputation after revascularization procedure G9639, G9640, G9641
Amputee
  Adapter, wheelchair E0959
  Prosthesis L5000-L7600, L7900, L8400-L8465
  Stump sock L8470-L8485
  Wheelchair E1170-E1190, E1200
Analysis
  Dose optimization S3722
  Gene analysis S3866
  Gene sequence, hypertrophic cardiomyopathy S3865
  Semen G0027
Anastrozole, oral S0170
Anchor/screw C1713
Anesthesia
  Care services G9654, G9655, G9656, G9658
  Preop no smoking instructions given G9497
Angiography
  Fluorescent, nonophthalmic C9733
  Iliac and/or femoral artery G0278
  Magnetic resonance
    Abdomen C8901
      With contrast C8900
      Without contrast followed by with contrast C8902
    Breast C8903-C8908
    Chest C8910
      With contrast C8909
      Without contrast followed by with contrast C8911
    Lower extremity C8913
      With contrast C8912
      Without contrast followed by with contrast C8914
    Pelvis C8919
      With contrast C8918
      Without contrast followed by with contrast C8920
    Spinal canal and contents C8932
      With contrast C8931
      Without contrast followed by with contrast C8933
    Upper Extremity C8935
      With contrast C8934

      Without contrast followed by with contrast C8936
    Reconstruction, aorta, CT, for vascular surgery G0288
Anidulafungin J0348
Ankle-foot orthosis (AFO) L1900-L1990
  Dynamic, adjustable E1815
  Fabricated L2112, L2114, L2116
  Fracture custom-fabricated L2106, L2108
  Replace replacement, static AFO L4392
  Static or dynamic ankle foot orthosis L4396
  Toe E1830
Annual
  Gynecological examination
    Clinical breast examination without pelvic evaluation S0613
    Established patient S0612
    New patient S0610
  Wellness visit
    Initial G0438
    Subsequent G0439
Antenna, nerve stimulation device L8696
Anti-emetic J8498, Q0161-Q0181
Anti-inflammatory medication Q5107-Q5111
Anti-platelet agents G9609, G9610, G9611
Anti-sperm antibodies test, immunobead S3655
Antibiotic
  Home infusion therapy S9494
    Every 3 hours S9497
    Every 4 hours S9504
    Every 6 hours S9503
    Every 8 hours S9502
    Every 12 hours S9501
    Every 24 hours S9500
  Intravenous for surgical site infection (SSI) G8916-G8918
    Not prescribed or dispensed G8712
  Regimen G9498, G9505
    Not prescribed within specified time period G9287
    Prescribed within specified time period G9286
  Taken within 30 days prior to episode date G9703
Anticoagulant use G9724
Anticoagulation clinic S9401
Antimicrobial prophylaxis
  Not documented G9198
  Not ordered G9196
  Ordered G9197
Antiseptic
  Chlorhexidine A4248
  Solution used to clean dialysis equipment A4674
Antithrombotic/aspirin therapy G8598, G8599, G9277, G9278
Antiviral
  Home infusion therapy S9494-S9504
Aortic aneurysm G9598, G9599
Apheresis, low density lipid (LDL) S2120
Apligraf® Q4101
Apnea monitor E0618
  Electrodes A4556
  Lead wires A4557
  With recording feature E0619
Apomorphine hydrochloride J0364
Application
  Low cost skin substitute
    Other areas C5275, C5276, C5277, C5278
    Trunk, arms, legs C5271, C5272, C5273, C5274
  Tantalum ring(s) scleral S8030
Aprepitant injection J0185
Aprotonin J0365
AquaPedic® sectional gel flotation E0196
Arbutamine HCl J0395

Arformoterol, inhalation solution J7605
Argatroban injection J0883, J0884
Argus ® II Retinal Prosthesis System, com/sup/acc misc
L8608
Aripiprazole J0400, J0401
Aripiprazole lauroxil injection J1944
Aristada initio injection J1943
Arm, wheelchair E0973
Arsenic trioxide J9017
Artacent ® Q4169, Q4189, Q4190, Q4216
Arthroereisis, subtalar S2117
Arthroscopy
  Knee
    Harvesting of cartilage S2112
    Removal foreign body G0289
  Shoulder, with capsulorrhaphy S2300
Artificial
  Cornea L8609
  Heart system com/sup/acc misc L8698
  Kidney, *see also* Dialysis
  Larynx L8500
  Pancreas device system
    Low glucose suspend feature S1034
    Receiver S1037
    Sensor S1035
    Transmitter S1036
  Saliva A9155
Ascent™ Q4213
Asparaginase J9019, J9020
Assembly
  Footrest, complete, replacement K0045
  Ratchet, replacement K0050
Assertive community treatment
  Per 15 minutes H0039
  Per diem H0040
Assessment
  Alcohol and/or substance G0396-G0397, G2011
  Alcohol or drug H0001
  Audiologic
    Conformity evaluation V5020
    Hearing aid V5010
      Fitting/orientation/checking V5011
      Repair/modification V5014
    Hearing screening V5008
  Bone loss risk G8863
  By chaplain, veterans affairs Q9001 Ⓝ
  Comp assess care plan ccm svc G0506
  Depression, self-assessment S3005
  Family H1011
  Functional outcome G9227
  Geriatric S0250
  Hearing V5008-V5020
  Home T1028
  Mental health H0031
  Nursing assessment/evaluation T1001
  Online, by qualified nonphysician healthcare professional
    G2061-G2063
  Periodic assessment G2077
  Remote recorded video G2250 Ⓝ
  Speech services
    Dysphagia screening V5364
    Language screening V5363
    Screening V5362
    Wellness S5190
Assisted living
  Per diem T2031
  Per month T2030

Assistive listening device
  Alerting V5269
  Cochlear implant assistive V5273
  FM/DM
    Accessories
      Direct audio input receiver V5285
      Ear level receiver V5284
      Neck loop induction receiver V5283
      Not otherwise specified (NOS) V5287
      Personal adapter/boot coupling V5289
      Personal Bluetooth ® receiver V5286
      Personal transmitter V5288
      Transmitter microphone V5290
    System
      Binaural V5282
      Monaural V5281
  Not otherwise specified (NOS) V5274
  Supplies and accessories not otherwise specified (NOS)
    V5267
  TDD V5272
  Telephone amplifier V5268
  Television amplifier V5270
  Television caption decoder V5271
Asthma
  Education S9441
  Kit S8097
  Reporting
    Not well-controlled, reason not given G9434
    Result documented G9432
    Well-controlled G9432
Atezolizumab injection J9022
Atropine sulfate J0461
Atropine, inhalation solution
  Concentrated J7635
  Unit dose J7636
Attendant care
  Per 15 min S5125
  Per diem S5126
Audiologic assessment
  Conformity evaluation V5020
  Fitting/orientation/checking, hearing aid V5011
  Hearing aid V5010
    Repair/modification V5014
  Hearing screening V5008
Audiometry S0618
Auditory osseointegrated device
  Abutment length replacement L8693
  Batteries L8624
  External sound processor
    Headband or other external attachment L8692
    Replacement L8691
  Internal and external components L8690
  Transducer/actuator replacement L8694
  Transmitting cable L8618
Aurothioglucose J2910
Autologous cultured chondrocytes, implant J7330
Avelumab injection J9023
Axicabtagene ciloleucel Q2041
Axobio Q4211
Axolotl Q4210, Q4215
Azacitidine J9025
Azathioprine J7500, J7501
Azithromycin J0456
Azithromycin dihydrate Q0144
Aztreonam S0073

Ⓝ **New index entry**

B

Back supports L0621-L0861
Baclofen J0475, J0476
Bacterial sensitivity study, urine P7001
Bag
  Bedside drainage A4357
  Disposable breast milk, collection and storage bag K1005
  Enema A4458
  Ostomy irrigation supply A4398
  Urinary latex A5112
  Urinary suspensory covering A5105
  Urinary, vinyl A4358
  With or without tube A4357-A4358
Ballistocardiogram S3902
Balloon
  Dilatation C1726
  Tissue dissector C1727
Bamlanivimab M0239, Q0239 Ⓝ
Bandages A6413-A6461
  By type
    Compression A6448, A6449, A6450, A6451, A6452
    Conforming A6442-A6447
    Gauze A6216-A6230, A6402, A6403, A6404
    Padding A6441, S8430
    Self-adherent A6453, A6454, A6455
    Zinc paste impregnated A6456
Barrier adhesion C1765
Basiliximab J0480
Bathing supplies E0240-E0249
Bathtub
  Chair E0240
  Rail
    Floor base E0242
    Wall E0241
  Stool or bench E0245
  Transfer bench E0247
    Heavy duty E0248
  Transfer rail E0246
Battery
  Charger
    Oxygen accessory E1357
    Power wheelchair accessory
      Dual mode E2367
      Single mode E2366
    Six volt L7362
    Twelve volt L7366
    Ventilator, patient owned A4613
  External infusion pump
    Alkaline 1.5 volt K0603
    Lithium 1.5 volt A4602
    Silver oxide
      1.5 volt K0601
      3 volt K0602
      3.6 volt K0604
      4.5 volt K0605
  Hearing device V5266
  Lithium
    Electric and/or pneumatic ventricular assist Q0495
      Replacement Q0506
    External infusion pump
      1.5 volt A4602
      3.6 volt K0604
      4.5 volt K0605
    Nonprosthetic use A4601
    Replacement L7367, L7368

Power wheelchair accessory
  Lead acid
    12 to 24 amp hour sealed K0733
    22 NF nonsealed E2360
    22 NF sealed lead E2361
    24 nonsealed E2362
    24 sealed lead E2363
    27 nonsealed E2372
    27 sealed E2371
    34 nonsealed E2358
    34 sealed E2359
    U-1 nonsealed E2364
    U-1 sealed E2365
  Lithium-based E2397
  Replacement
    Auditory osseointegrated device L8624
    Automated external defibrillator K0607
    Blood glucose monitor A4233-A4236
    Cochlear implant device L8623, L8624
    Home
      Alkaline, J cell, each A4234
      Lithium ion A4601
      Lithium, each A4235
      Other than J cell, each A4233
      Silver oxide, each A4236
  Six volt L7360
  TENS A4630
  Twelve volt L7364
  Ventilator, patient owned
    Battery cables A4612
    Battery charger A4613
    Battery, heavy duty A4611
BCG live, intravesical J9030
Becaplermin gel S0157
Beclomethasone inhalation solution J7622
Bed
  Air fluidized E0194
  Board E0273
  Cradle, any type E0280
  Hospital
    Fixed height E0250, E0291
      With mattress E0251, E0290
    Heavy-duty capacity, any type
      350 pounds to 600 pounds E0301
        With mattress E0303
      Greater than 600 pounds E0302
        With mattress E0304
    Institutional type E0270
    Pediatric E0328, E0329
    Semi-electric E0261, E0295
    Supplies E0250-E0373
      With mattress E0260, E0294
    Total electric E0266, E0297
      With mattress E0265, E0296
    Variable height E0256, E0293
      With mattress E0255, E0292
  Pan
    Fracture E0276
    Standard E0275
  Rail E0305, E0310
    Full length E0310
    Half length E0305
  Safety enclosure frame/canopy E0316
Bedside
  Drainage bag A4357
  Drainage bottle A5102
Behavioral health services G0177, G0445-G0447, G0473, H0001-H2037, S9480, S9482, T1040, T1041
Belantamab mafodontin-blmf C9069 Ⓝ

Belatacept - Breast

Belatacept J0485
Belimumab J0490
Belinostat J9032
Bellacell HD Q4220
Belt
    Extremity E0945
    Ostomy A4367
    Pelvic E0944
    Wheelchair E0978
Bench, bathtub E0245
Bendamustine HCl J9033, J9034, J9036
Benesch boot L3212, L3213, L3214
Benralizumab injection J0517
Benztropine J0515
Betadine A4246, A4247
Betamethasone acetate and betamethasone sodium phosphate J0702
Betamethasone inhalation solution J7624
Bethanechol chloride J0520
Bevacizumab J9035
Bevacizumab-awwb Q5107
Bevacizumab-bvzr Q5118
Bezlotoxumab injection J0565
Bifocal, glass or plastic V2200-V2299
Bilirubin (phototherapy) light E0202
Bimatoprost J7351 Ⓝ
Binder A4465
Bio-ConneKt® Q4161
BioDExCel™ Q4137
Biofeedback device E0746
Biologic immune response modifier G9506
Biologicals and skin substitutes Q4100-Q4255
Bionext® patch Q4228 Ⓝ
Biopsy, prostate G0416
BioWound™ Q4217
Bipolar/personality disorder G9394
Biperiden lactate J0190
Bitolterol mesylate, inhalation solution
    Concentrated J7628
    Unit dose J7629
Bivalirudin J0583
Bladder injury G9625, G9626, G9627
Blinatumomab J9039
Blinded administration convulsive therapy G2000
Blinded procedure for lumbar stenosis G0276
Blood
    Fresh frozen plasma P9017
    Glucose monitor E0607, E2100, E2101
    Glucose test A4253
    Granulocytes, pheresis P9050
    Ketone test A4252
    Leak detector, dialysis E1560
    Leukocyte poor P9016
    Leukocytes reduced P9031
    Mucoprotein P2038
    Platelets P9019
        Irradiated P9032
        Leukocytes reduced, irradiated P9033
        Pheresis P9034
            Irradiated P9036
            Leukocytes reduced P9035
            Leukocytes reduced, irradiated P9037
            Pathogen-reduced P9073
        Pathogen(s) test P9100
    Pressure monitor A4660, A4663, A4670
    Product, not otherwise specified (NOS) P9099
    Pump, dialysis E1620

    Red blood cells
        Deglycerolized P9039
        Irradiated P9038
        Leukocytes reduced P9016
        Leukocytes reduced, irradiated P9040
        Washed P9022
    Strips A4253
    Supply P9010-P9040, P9050-P9099
    Testing supplies A4770
    Tubing A4750, A4755
Blood collection devices, accessories A4257, A4652, E0620
Blood pressure G8476-G8478, G9273, G9274
BLS (basic life support)
    Mileage A0380
    Routine disposable supplies A0382
Blunt head trauma G9529, G9530, G9531, G9533, G9593, G9594, G9595, G9596, G9597
    Pediatric patient G9593, G9596, G9597
BMI (body mass index)
    Not documented G2181, G8421 Ⓝ
Body jacket, scoliosis L1300, L1310
Body sock L0984
Body worn, hearing aid
    Bilateral V5100
    Monaural, air conduction V5030
    Monaural, bone conduction V5040
Bond or cement, ostomy skin A4364
Boot
    Pelvic E0944
    Surgical, ambulatory L3260
Bortezomib J9041, J9044
Bottle, cold or hot fluid A9273
Bowel injury G9628, G9629, G9630
Brachytherapy Q3001
    Needle C1715
    Placement of endorectal intracavitary applicator C9725
    Seed administration (catheter) C1728
    Source
        Cesium-131 chloride C2644
            Nonstranded C2643
            Stranded C2642
        Gold-198 C1716
        Iodine-125
            Nonstranded C2639
                High activity C2634
            Stranded C2638
        Iridium-192
            High dose rate C1717
            Non-high-dose rate C1719
        Not otherwise specified (NOS)
            Nonstranded C2699
            Stranded C2698
        Palladium-103
            Nonstranded C2640
                High activity C2635
                Linear source C2636
            Planar C2645
            Stranded C2641
        Ytterbium-169 C2637
        Yttrium-90 C2616
    Treatment G0458
Breast
    Cancer
        Biopsy to diagnose cancer
            Attempted without diagnosis G8946
            Diagnosed G8875
            Not performed G8876, G8877

Gene expression profiling panel S3854
Stage G8881, G9704, G9705
Mammography
Digital/digital tomosynthesis (3D)
Results documented G9899
Results not documented G9900
Prosthesis
Custom postmastectomy L8035
Garment, external L8015
Implantable C1789
Silicone or equal L8600
Mastectomy bra
With integrated form, bilateral L8002
With integrated form, unilateral L8001
Without integrated form L8000
Mastectomy form L8020
Mastectomy sleeve L8010
Nipple prosthesis L8032, L8033
Not otherwise specified (NOS) L8039
Silicone or equal L8030
With integral adhesive L8031
Prosthesis, adhesive skin support A4280
Pump
Accessories A4281-A4286
Electric, any type E0603
Heavy duty, hospital grade E0604
Manual, any type E0602
Reconstruction S2066, S2067, S2068
Tomosynthesis G0279
Breastfeeding patient G9779
Breathing aids and supplies A7000-A7048, E0500-E0606, S8096-S8210
Breathing circuit A4618
Brentuximab vedotin J9042
Brexanolone J1632 Ⓝ
Brexucabtagene autoleucel ca C9073 Ⓝ
Brolucizumab-dbll J0179
Bronchitis with prior antibiotic prescription G2177 Ⓝ
Bronchodilator, prescribed G9695
Med reason not prescrib G9696
Pt reason not prescrib G9697
System reason not prescrib G9698
Not prescrib, reason NOS G9699
Brompheniramine maleate J0945
Budesonide inhalation solution
Concentrated
Compounded J7634
Noncompounded J7633
Unit dose
Compounded J7627
Noncompounded J7626
Bulking agent or material L8603-L8607
Bumetanide S0171
Bundled payment care G9187
Bupivacaine hydrochloride S0020
Buprenorphine extended-release Q9991-Q9992
Buprenorphine, take-home oral supply G2079
Buprenorphine hydrochloride J0592
Buprenorphine/naloxone J0571, J0572, J0573, J0574, J0575
Bupropion HCl, sustained release S0106
Burn documentation G8907-G8909
Burosumab-twza injection J0584
Bus, nonemergency transportation A0110
Busulfan J0594, J8510
Butorphanol tartrate J0595, S0012

C

C-1 esterase inhibitor J0596, J0597-J0599
Cabazitaxel J9043
Cabergoline, oral J8515
Caffeine citrate J0706
Calaspargase pegol-mknl J9118
Calcitonin salmon J0630
Calcitriol J0636, S0169
Calcium disodium edetate J0600
Calcium gluconate J0610
Calcium glycerophosphate and calcium lactate J0620
Calcium leucovorin J0640
Calibrator solution A4256
Canakinumab J0638
Cane
Any material, with tip E0100
Handgrip replacement A4636
Quad E0105
Tip replacement A4637
Cangrelor C9460
Canister, used with suction pump
Disposable A7000
Nondisposable A7001
Cannula
Nasal A4615
Tracheostomy, inner A4623
Capecitabine, oral J8520, J8521
Caplacizumab-yhdp C9047
Capsaicin patch J7336
Carbidopa/levodopa J7340
Carbon filter A4680
Carboplatin J9045
Cardiac
Contractility modulation generator C1824
Device evaluation G2066
Event, recorder, implantable E0616
MRI C9762, C9763 Ⓝ
Rehabilitation G0422, G0423, S9472
Cardiokymography Q0035
Cardiovascular services
Chemical endarterectomy (chelation) M0300
Fabric wrapping of abdominal aneurysm M0301
Prevention G9662-G9666, G9674, G9675, G9676
Cardioverter-defibrillator
Dual chamber (implantable) C1721
Lead C1777, C1895-C1896
Other C1882
Replacement G0448
Single chamber (implantable) C1722
Care improvement initiative G9187
Care management
Chronic care services G0506, G0511
Comprehensive services G2064-G2065
High risk disease G2064-G2065
Home care plan G0086-G0087
Home visit G0076-G0087
Ongoing care not possible M1146-M1148 Ⓝ
Psychiatric G2214 Ⓝ
Services G2021-G2025
Care plan oversight G2014, G2015
Caregiver
Certified in dementia care G2185 Ⓝ
Lack of G2184 Ⓝ
Carepatch Q4236 Ⓝ
Carfilzomib J9047
Carmustine J9050

Carotid intervention, election G9689
Carepatch Q4236 Ⓝ
Case management T1016, T1017
Casirivimab and imdevimab M0243, Q0243 Ⓝ
Caspofungin acetate J0637
Cast
    Hand restoration L6900-L6915
    Materials, special A4590
    Supplies A4580
        Body
            Fiberglass Q4002
            Plaster Q4001
        Fiberglass A4590
        Finger splint, static Q4049
        Gauntlet
            Adult, fiberglass Q4014
            Adult, plaster Q4013
            Pediatric, fiberglass Q4016
            Pediatric, plaster Q4015
        Hip spica
            Adult, fiberglass Q4026
            Adult, plaster Q4025
            Pediatric, fiberglass Q4028
            Pediatric, plaster Q4027
        Long arm
            Adult, fiberglass Q4006
            Adult, plaster Q4005
            Pediatric, fiberglass Q4008
            Pediatric, plaster Q4007
        Long arm splint
            Adult, fiberglass Q4018
            Adult, plaster Q4017
            Pediatric, fiberglass Q4020
            Pediatric, plaster Q4019
        Long leg
            Adult, fiberglass Q4030
            Adult, plaster Q4029
            Cylinder
                Adult, fiberglass Q4034
                Adult, plaster Q4033
                Pediatric, fiberglass Q4036
            Pediatric, fiberglass Q4032
            Pediatric, plaster Q4031
            Pediatric, plaster Q4035
        Long leg splint
            Adult, fiberglass Q4042
            Adult, plaster Q4041
            Pediatric, fiberglass Q4044
            Pediatric, plaster Q4043
        Miscellaneous Q4051
        Plaster A4580
        Short arm
            Adult, fiberglass Q4010
            Adult, plaster Q4009
            Pediatric, fiberglass Q4012
            Pediatric, plaster Q4011
        Short arm splint
            Adult, fiberglass Q4022
            Adult, plaster Q4021
            Pediatric, fiberglass Q4024
            Pediatric, plaster Q4023
        Short leg
            Adult, fiberglass Q4038
            Adult, plaster Q4037
            Pediatric, fiberglass Q4040
            Pediatric, plaster Q4039
        Short leg splint
            Adult, fiberglass Q4046

            Adult, plaster Q4045
            Pediatric, fiberglass Q4048
            Pediatric, plaster Q4047
        Shoulder
            Fiberglass Q4004
            Plaster Q4003
        Special casting material A4590
        Unlisted Q4050
        Thermoplastic material
            Ankle foot orthosis L2106
            Knee ankle foot orthosis L2126
Caster, wheelchair E2395, E2396
Catheter
    Access
        External A4300
        Port/reservoir A4301
    Anchoring device
        Percutaneous, adhesive skin attachment A5200
        Peritoneal dialysis A4653
        Urinary, adhesive skin attachment A4333
        Urinary, leg strap A4334
    Electrophysiology, diagnostic ablation C2630
    Guiding C1887
    Indwelling, Foley-type
        Three-way A4346
        Two-way
            All silicone A4344
            Latex with coating A4338
    Insertion tray A4354
    Intermittent, urinary, with insertion supplies A4353
    Irrigation supplies A4355
    Male external A4349
    Multiple applications C1724-C1759
    Occlusion C2628
    Oropharyngeal suction A4628
    Pressure-generating C1982
    Specialty type A4340
    Suprapubic/cystoscopic C2627
    Tip, disposable (peritoneal dialysis) A4860
    Trachea (suction) A4605, A4624
    Transluminal atherectomy, directional C1714
    Transtracheal oxygen A4608
    Vacuum drainage collection unit and tubing kit A7048
        Female, metal cup A4327
        Female, pouch A4328
        Perianal fecal A4330
Catheterization, specimen collection P9612, P9615
Cecal landmarks, postsurgical G9612, G9613, G9614
Cefazolin sodium J0690
Cefepime HCl J0692
Cefiderocol J0693 Ⓝ
Cefoperazone sodium S0021
Cefotaxime sodium J0698
Cefotetan disodium S0074
Cefoxitin sodium J0694
Ceftaroline fosamil J0712
Ceftazidime J0713
Ceftazidime and avibactam J0714
Ceftizoxime sodium J0715
Ceftolozane and tazobactam J0695
Ceftriaxone sodium J0696
Cefuroxime sodium J0697
CellCept ® J7517
Cellesta™ Q4184, Q4185, Q4214
Cellular therapy M0075
Cement, ostomy A4364
Cemiplimab-rwlc J9119

Ⓝ **New index entry**

Center for Medicare and Medicaid Innovation (CMMI) model G2001-G2015
Centrifuge E1500
Centruroides immune F(ab) J0716
Cephalin flocculation, blood P2028
Cephalothin sodium J1890
Cephapirin sodium J0710
Cerliponase alfa injection J0567
Certolizumab pegol J0717
Cerumen removal G0268
Cervical
    Halo L0810-L0830
    Head harness/halter E0942
    Orthosis L0112-L0200
    Traction E0855, E0856
Cervical cap contraceptive A4261
Cervical-thoracic-lumbar-sacral orthosis (CTLSO) L0700
    With interface material L0710
Cetirizine hydrochloride J1201 Ⓝ
Cetuximab J9055
Chair
    Adjustable, dialysis E1570
    Bath/shower E0240
    Lift E0627
    Rollabout E1031
    Sitz bath E0160, E0161, E0162
Chamber
    Pacemaker, dual C1785
    Pacemaker, single C1786
Chaplain, veterans affairs
    Assessment Q9001 Ⓝ
    Counseling Q9002, Q9003 Ⓝ
Check in by MD/QHP, brief G2012
Chelation therapy M0300
Chemical endarterectomy M0300
Chemistry and toxicology tests P2028-P3001
Chemodenervation S2340, S2341
Chemotherapy, *see also* Appendix A: Table of Drugs
    Administration (hospital reporting only) Q0083, Q0084, Q0085
    Anti-emetic Q0161-Q0181
    Drug, oral, not otherwise classified J8999
    Drugs J9000-J9999, Q5101-Q5106
    Office/clinic setting G0498
Chest
    Drain A7040, A7041
    Shell (cuirass) E0457
    Wall oscillation system E0483
        Hose, replacement A7026
        Vest, replacement A7025
    Wrap E0459
Chin cup, cervical L0150
Chlamydia screen G9820, G9821
Chlorambucil, oral S0172
Chloramphenicol sodium succinate J0720
Chlordiazepoxide HCl J1990
Chloromycetin sodium succinate J0720
Chloroprocaine HCl J2400
Chloroquine HCl J0390
Chlorothiazide sodium J1205
Chlorpromazine HCl J3230, Q0161
Choline c-11 A9515
Chorionic gonadotropin J0725
Choroid lesion destruction G0186
Christian Science practitioner services S9900, S9901
Chromic phosphate P32 suspension A9564
Chromium CR-51 sodium chromate A9553
Chronic care management services (CCM) G0506, G0511

Cidofovir J0740
Cilastatin sodium, imipenem J0743
Cimetidine hydrochloride S0023
Cinacalcet, oral J0604
Ciprofloxacin for intravenous infusion J0744
Ciprofloxacin otic suspension J7342
Cisplatin J9060
Cladribine J9065
Clamp
    Dialysis A4918
    External urethral A4356
Clarix™ Q4148, Q4156
Cleanser, wound A6260
Cleansing agent, dialysis equipment A4674
Clindamycin phosphate S0077
Clinic visit
    All-inclusive T1015
    Hospital outpatient G0463
Clinical Decision Support Mechanism (CDSM) G1001-G1004, G1007-G1023 Ⓝ
Clinical trial services S9988, S9990, S9991, S9992, S9994, S9996
Clofarabine J9027
Clonidine J0735
Clotting factors J7177-J7212 Ⓝ
Clotting time tube A4771
Clozapine S0136
Clubfoot wedge L3380
Cocaine hcl nasal solution C9046
Cochlear prosthetic implant L8614
    Batteries L8621, L8622, L8623, L8624
    Headset L8615
    Replacement L8619, L8627, L8628, L8629
    Transmitting coil/cable L8617, L8618
Codeine phosphate J0745
Cogenex
    Amniotic membrane Q4229 Ⓝ
    Flowable amnion Q4230 Ⓝ
Coil, imaging, insertable, MRI C1770
Cold pad, fluid circulating E0218
Colistimethate sodium J0770, S0142
Collagen
    Skin test Q3031
    Urinary tract implant L8603
    Wound dressing A6021, A6022, A6023, A6024
Collagenase, Clostridium histolyticum J0775
Collar, cervical
    Multiple post L0180-L0200
    Nonadjustable (foam) L0120
Coll-e-derm™ Q4193
Colonoscopy
    Advanced age G9659, G9660, G9661
    Consultation S0285
    Flexible sigmoidoscopy G0104
    Screening
        Age 50 to 85 years G2204 Ⓝ
        Barium enema G0120
        Fecal occult blood test G0328
        Individual at high risk G0105
        Not meeting criteria for high risk G0121
Coly-Mycin M® J0770
Coma stimulation s9056
Commode E0163-E0175
    Chair, mobile or stationary E0163-E0165
        With lift mechanism E0170-E0171
    Lift E0172, E0625
    Pail E0167
    Seat, wheelchair E0968

Communication board E1902
Communication device, augmentative V5336
Communication, patient unable G2183 Ⓝ
Communication services, RHC/FQHC G0071
Community support services H2000-H2037
Compensator-based beam modulation treatment G6016
Complete blood count (CBC) G0306, G0307
Composite dressing A6203, A6204, A6205
Compounded drug, not otherwise classified J7999
Comprehensive mgt and care coordination, advanced illness S0311
Compressed gas system E0424-E0480
Compression
    Bandage A6448, A6449, A6450, A6451, A6452
        Padding S8430
    Burn garment A6501-A6513
    Device, limb A4600, E0676
    Garments and stockings A6501-A6550
Compressor E0565, E0570, E0572, E0650, E0651, E0652
Computer Aided Detection, including breast MRI C8937
Conduction
    Glasses, air V5070
    Hearing aid V5030
Conductivity meter, bath, dialysis E1550
Conformer, ocular, fabrication and fitting V2628
Conformity, evaluation V5020
Congo red, blood P2029
Conivaptan hydrochloride C9488
Connective tissue C1762-C1763
Consultation, inpatient, follow-up
    15 minutes G0406
    25 minutes G0407
    35 minutes G0408
Contact layer (dressing) A6206, A6207, A6208
Contact lens supplies and services S0512, S0514, S0592, V2500-V2599
    Disposable S0500
    Gas permeable
        Bifocal, per lens V2512
        Extended wear, per lens V2513
        Spherical, per lens V2510
        Toric, prism ballast, per lens V2511
    Hydrophilic
        Bifocal, per lens V2522
        Extended wear, per lens V2523
        Spherical, per lens V2520
        Toric, or prism ballast, per lens V2521
    PMMA
        Bifocal V2502
        Color vision deficiency V2503
        Spherical V2500
        Toric or prism ballast V2501
    Scleral
        Gas impermeable, per lens V2530
        Gas permeable, per lens V2531
        Liquid bandage device S0515
Continent device A5081, A5082, A5083
Continuous glucose monitoring system
    Receiver A9278, K0554
    Sensor A9276
    Supply allowance K0553
    Transmitter A9277
Continuous passive motion exercise device E0936
Continuous positive airway pressure (CPAP) device E0601
Contraceptives
    Cervical cap A4261
    Condoms A4267, A4268
    Diaphragm A4266

Intratubal occlusion device A4264
Intrauterine device, copper J7300
Intrauterine device, Progestasert® IUD S4989
Intrauterine, levonorgestrel-releasing J7297, J7298, J7301
Levonorgestrel, implants and supplies J7297, J7298, J7301, J7306, S4981
Patch J7304
Pills S4993
Supplies A4261, A4264, A4266-A4269
Systems J7296-J7307
Spermicide A4269
Vaginal ring J7303
Contrast agents Q9950-Q9992
Contracts, maintenance, ESRD A4890
Contrast media, see also Radiopharmaceuticals
    High and low osmolar Q9959-Q9967
    High osmolar
        150-199 mg/mL Q9959
        200-249 mg/mL Q9960
        250-299 mg/mL Q9961
        300-349 mg/mL Q9962
        350-399 mg/mL Q9963
        400 or greater mg/mL Q9964
        Up to 149 mg/mL Q9958
    Injection for
        Echocardiography A9700
    Iron-based magnetic resonance Q9953, Q9954
        MRI A9576, A9577, A9578, A9579
    Low osmolar
        100-199 mg/mL Q9965
        200-299 mg/mL Q9966
        300-399 mg/mL Q9967
        400 or greater mg/mL Q9951
Coordinated care fee G9001-G9012
Copanlisib J9057
Copper cu-64, dotatate C9068 Ⓝ
CoreCyte™ Q4240 Ⓝ
Coretext™ or protext Q4246 Ⓝ
Corneal tissue processing V2785
Coronavirus
    Detection U0001-U0005 Ⓝ
    Specimen collection C9803, G2023, G2024 Ⓝ
Coronary artery bypass surgery, minimally invasive S2205, S2206, S2207, S2208, S2209
Corplex® Q4231, Q4232 Ⓝ
Corset, spinal orthosis L0970-L0976
Corticorelin ovine triflutate J0795
Corticosteroids G9468, G9470
Corticotropin J0800
Corvert® (ibutilide fumarate) J1742
Cosyntropin J0834
Cough stimulating device A7020, E0482
Counseling
    By chaplain, veterans affairs Q9002, Q9003 Ⓝ
    Hospice evaluation G0337
    Not provided G2201-G2203 Ⓝ
    Screening and prevention G0438-G0451
Cover, belt strap sleev grmnt, any A4467
Cover, wound
    Alginate dressing A6196, A6197, A6198
    Foam dressing A6209-A6214
    Hydrogel dressing A6242-A6248
    Noncontact, warming, and accessory A6000, E0231, E0232
    Specialty absorptive dressing A6251-A6256
    Synthetic resorbable dressing A6460-A6461
COVID-19
    Detection U0001-U0005 Ⓝ
    Specimen collection C9803, G2023, G2024 Ⓝ

Ⓝ New index entry

CPAP (continuous positive airway pressure), *see also*
   Positive airway pressure device
      Device E0601
      Headgear A7035
      Humidifier A7046
Cradle, bed E0280
Cranial electrotherapy stimulation (CES) system K1002
Cranial remolding orthosis S1040
Crib E0300
Crisis intervention S9484, S9485, T2034
Crizanlizumab-tmca J0791 Ⓝ
Cromolyn sodium, inhalation solution
   Compounded J7632
   Noncompounded J7631
Crotalidae immune f(ab')2 (equine) J0841
Crotalidae polyvalent immune fab J0840
Cryo-cord™ Q4237 Ⓝ
Crutches
   Accessories A4635, A4636, A4637
   Forearm
      Each E0111
      Pair E0110
   Substitute E0118
   Underarm
      Articulating E0117
      Other than wood
         Each E0116
         Pair E0114
      Wood
         Each E0113
         Pair E0112
Cryoprecipitate, each unit P9012
CTLSO L0700, L0710, L1000-L1120
Cuirass E0457
Culture sensitivity study, urine P7001
Cushion, wheelchair E2601-E2625, E2629
Customized
   DME, other than wheelchair K0900
   Item, in addition to basic item S1002
Cyanocobalamin cobalt Co57 A9559
Cycler dialysis machine E1594
Cyclophosphamide J9070
Cyclophosphamide, oral J8530
Cyclosporine J7502, J7515, J7516
Cystoscopy C9738
Cystoscopy, intraoperative G9606, G9607, G9608
Cystourethroscopy
   With insertion of transprostatic implant C9769 Ⓝ
      1 to 3 implants C9739
      4 or more implants C9740
   With ureteroscopy and/or pyeloscopy S2070
      With lithotripsy and vacuum aspiration C9761 Ⓝ
Cytarabine J9100
Cytarabine liposome J9098
Cytomegalovirus immune globulin (human) J0850

D

Dacarbazine J9130
Daclizumab J7513
Dactinomycin J9120
Dalalone J1100
Dalbavancin J0875
Dalteparin sodium J1645
Daptomycin J0878
Daratumumab and hyaluronidase-fihj J9144 Ⓝ
Daratumumab J9145

Darbepoetin alfa
   ESRD on dialysis J0882
   Non-ERSD use J0881
Daunorubicin J9150
Daunorubicin citrate J9151
Daunorubicin, cytarabine J9153
DaunoXome® (daunorubicin citrate) J9151
Day care services S5100, S5101, S5102, S5105
Decitabine J0894
Decompression procedure, intervertebral disc S2348
Decubitus care equipment E0181-E0199
Deferoxamine mesylate J0895
Defibrillator, external E0617, K0606
   Battery K0607
   Electrode K0609
   Garment K0608
Degarelix J9155
Deionizer, water purification system E1615
Delafloxacin injection C9462
Delivery or service to high risk area S9381
Delivery, home, supplies S8415
Delivery, set-up, dispensing A9901
Deluxe item S1001
Demonstration project
   ESRD G9013, G9014
   Frontier extended stay clinic G9140
   MAPCP G9151, G9152, G9153
   Oncology G9050-G9139
Denileukin diftitox J9160
Denosumab J0897
Deoxycholic acid J0591 Ⓝ
Depo-estradiol cypionate J1000
Derm-maxx Q4238 Ⓝ
Derma-gide™ Q4203
Dermacell Q4122
Dermacyte amniotic membrane allograft Q4248 Ⓝ
Dermagraft® Q4106
Desmopressin acetate J2597
Destruction
   Intraosseous basivertebral nerve C9752-C9753
Detector, blood leak, dialysis E1560
Development testing G0451
Device
   Closure, vascular C1760
   Cochlear with headset L8614, L8615
   Lower limb K1007 Ⓝ
   Other cochlear accessories L8616-L8629
Dexamethasone
   Inhalation solution
      Concentrated J7637
      Unit dose J7638
   Intraocular injection J1095
   Intravitreal implant J7312
   Ophthalmic insert J1096
   Oral J8540
Dexamethasone acetate J1094
Dexamethasone sodium phosphate J1100
Dexrazoxane hydrochloride J1190
Dextran J7100, J7110
Dextroamphetamine sulfate S0160
Dextrose S5010, S5012, S5013, S5014
   5% LR J7121
   Saline (normal) J7042
   Water J7060, J7070
Dextrostix® or similar product A4772
Diabetes
   Home management of gestational diabetes S9214
   Management program G0245, G0246, S9140, S9141,
      S9455, S9460, S9465, S9470

Diagnostic and therapeutic services - Drugs

Self-management training
    Group G0109
    Individual G0108
Supplies A4250-A4259, A9274-A9279
Diagnostic and therapeutic services G0127-G0372
Dialysate concentrate additives A4765
Dialysate solution A4728
Dialysate testing solution A4760
Dialysis, *see also* **ESRD**
    Access system (implantable) C1881
    Accessories and Systems E1510-E1699
    Air bubble detector E1530
    Bath conductivity, meter E1550
    Chemicals/antiseptics solution A4674
    Disposable cycler set A4671
    Emergency/unscheduled G0257
    Equipment A4653-A4932
    Extension line A4672, A4673
    Filter A4680
    Fluid barrier E1575
    Pressure alarm E1540
    Shunt A4740
    Supplies A4653-A4932
    Systems and Accessories E1500-E1699
    Unipuncture control system E1580
    Venous pressure clamp A4918
Diaper T4521-T4540, T4543, T4544
    Adult incontinence garment A4520
Diazepam J3360
Diazoxide J1730
Diclofenac sodium injection J1130
Dicyclomine HCl J0500
Didanosine (DDI) S0137
Diethylstilbestrol diphosphate J9165
Digoxin immune fab (ovine) J1162
Digoxin J1160
Dihydroergotamine mesylate J1110
Dimenhydrinate J1240
Dimercaprol J0470
Dimethyl sulfoxide (DMSO) J1212
Diphenhydramine HCl J1200, Q0163
Dipyridamole J1245
Direct admission/refer for hospital observation care G0379
Directional, transluminal, atherectomy C1714
Disarticulation
    Lower extremities, prosthesis L5000-L5999
    Upper extremities, prosthesis L6000-L6692
Disease management program S0315, S0316, S0317
    Telephone calls by RN S0320
Diskectomy, anterior S2350, S2351
Dispensing fee
    Bilateral V5110
    Binaural V5160
    Contralateral, monaural V5200
    Contralateral routing system, binaural V5240
    Monaural hearing aid, any type V5241
    Pharmacy
        Anti-cancer, antiemetics Q0510, Q0511, Q0512
        Compounding S9430
        Immunosuppressives Q0510
        Inhalation drug(s) G0333, Q0513, Q0514
    Unspecified hearing aid V5090
Disposable supplies, ambulance A0382, A0384, A0392-A0398
DME A9900-A9999, E0100-E8002, K0001-K1012, K0669-K0746, K0900 Ⓝ
DMSO J1212
DNA analysis, multiple endocrine neoplasia type 2 S3840
Dobutamine HCl J1250
Docetaxel J9171

Dolasetron mesylate J1260, S0174
Dome and mouthpiece (for nebulizer) A7016
Donor
    Lobectomy, living donor S2061
    Solid organs, global definition S2152
Door to puncture time G9580, G9582
Dopamine HCl J1265
Doripenem J1267
Dornase alpha, inhalation solution, unit dose form J7639
Dosimeter, radiation implantable A4650
Doxercalciferol J1270
Doxorubicin HCl J9000, Q2049, Q2050
Drainage
    Bag
        Bedside A4357
        Urinary, latex A5112
        Urinary, vinyl A4358
        With or without tube A4357-A4358
    Board, postural E0606
    Bottle, bedside A5102
    Catheter C1729
    Device, urine K1010-K1012 Ⓝ
Dressing, *see also* **Bandages by type**
    Alginate A6196, A6197, A6198, A6199
    Collagen A6021, A6022, A6023, A6024
    Composite A6203, A6204, A6205
    Contact layer A6206-A6208
    Foam A6209-A6215
    Gauze A6216-A6233, A6402, A6403, A6404
    Gel sheet A6025
    Holder/binder A4461, A4463, A4465
    Hydrocolloid A6234-A6241
    Hydrogel A6242-A6248
    Nonreusable A4461
    Packing strips A6407
    Reusable A4463
    Specialty absorptive A6251-A6256
    Synthetic resorbable A6460-A6461
    Transparent film A6257, A6258, A6259
    Tubular A6457
Dressing and Wound Supplies A4450-A4456, A4461-A4467, A6000-A6550
Dronabinol Q0167
Droperidol J1790
    With fentanyl citrate J1810
Dropper A4649
Drug abuse G9518
Drugs, *see also* **Appendix A: Table of Drugs**
    Abuse, treatment H0001-H2037
    Administered
        By injection J0120-J7175
        Through metered dose inhaler J3535
    Anti-rheumatic G2182 Ⓝ
    Cancer treatment Q5112-Q5122
    Chemotherapy J8501-J8999, J9000-J9999
        Antiemetic Q0161-Q0181
    Compounded, not otherwise classified (NOC) J7999
    Controlled dose inhalation drug delivery system K0730
    Disposable delivery system
        5 mL or less per hour A4306
        50 mL or greater per hour A4305
    Immunosuppressive J7500-J7599
    Infusion supplies A4221, A4222, A4224, A4225, A4226, A4230, A4231, A4232
    Inhalation solutions J7604-J7686
    Miscellaneous drugs, biologicals, and supplies C8957-C9488, J7308-J7401
    Non-biodegradable delivery implants
        Insertion G0516
        Removal G0517
        Removal and reinsertion G0518

Ⓝ **New index entry**

Nonprescription A9150
Not otherwise classified (NOC) J3490, J7699-J8499, Q4082
Prescription S5000, S5001
Services H0047-H0050
Take home Naloxone G2215, G2216 ⓝ
Testing, definitive
    1-7 classes G0480
    8-14 classes G0481
    15-21 classes G0482
    22 or more classes G0483
    Perf w/o rec standards, any number of classes G0659
Therapy
    Adjuvant treatment Chemotherapy and HER-2 targeted
        In pregnancy G2205 ⓝ
        Not received G2207, G2208 ⓝ
        Received G2206 ⓝ
    Anti-rheumatic G2182
    Initiation in ED G2213 ⓝ
Dry pressure pad/mattress E0184, E0199
Dual-energy X-ray absorptiometry (DXA) (DEXA) G9471
Durable medical equipment determination G0454
Durable medical equipment (DME) A9900-A9999, E0100-E8002, K0001-K1012, K0669-K0746 ⓝ
Duraclon® (clonidine) J0735
Durolane ® J7318
Durvalumab J9173
Dyphylline J1180

E

Ear mold V5264
Early periodic screening diagnosis and treatment (EPSDT) S0302
Ecallantide J1290
Echocardiography injectable contrast material A9700
Echocardiography, Transesophageal/Transthoracic C8921-C8930
Echosclerotherapy S2202
Eculizumab J1300
Edaravone J1301
Edetate calcium disodium J0600
Edetate disodium J3520
Educational services, face-to-face G0420, G0421
Eggcrate dry pressure pad/mattress E0184, E0199
Elbow
    Disarticulation, endoskeletal L6450
    Orthosis (EO) E1800, L3702-L3740, L3760, L3761, L3762
    Protector E0191
Elbow-wrist-hand-finger orthosis L3763, L3764, L3765, L3766
Electrical stimulation
    Auricular acupuncture points S8930
    Device for cancer treatment E0766
    Supplies A4595
    Treatment G0281, G0282, G0283
Electrical work, dialysis equipment A4870
Electrocardiogram (ECG), routine G0403, G0404, G0405
Electrodes A4555, A4556
Electromagnetic stimulation E0761, E0769, G0295, G0329
Electron beam CT (ultrafast CT) S8092
Electronic medication compliance management device T1505
Electrophysiology
    3D or vector mapping C1730, C1731
        Diagnostic, other than 3D mapping C1730, C1731
        Diagnostic/ablation with 3D mapping C1732
    Other than 3D or vector mapping and cool-tip C1733

Elevating leg rest
    Lower extension tube, replacement, each K0046
    Pair K0195
    Upper hanger bracket, replacement, each K0047
Elliotts B solution J9175
Elosulfase alfa J1322
Elotuzumab injection J9176
Emapalumab-lzsg J9210
Embolectomy catheter C1757
Embolization protective system C1884
Emergency and/or hospital observation services G0378-G0390
Emergency department visit G9521, G9522
    Level 1 G0380
    Level 2 G0381
    Level 3 G0382
    Level 4 G0383
    Level 5 G0384
Emergency response system S5160, S5161, S5162
Emergency stat laboratory charge S3600, S3601
Emergent cases M1142
EMG (electromyography) E0746, S3900
Emicizumab-kxwh J7170
Eminase® J0350
Enema Supplies A4458-A4459
Endarterectomy, chemical M0300
Endoscope
    Retrograde imaging colonoscope device C1749
    Sheath (disposable), each A4270
    Single use (disposable) C1748 ⓝ
Endoscopy
    Nasal/Sinus C9771 ⓝ
Endoskeletal system, addition L5848, L5856, L5857, L5925, L5969
Enfortumab vedotin-ejfv J9177 ⓝ
Enfuvirtide J1324
Enoxaparin sodium J1650
Enteral
    Additives and formulas B4100-B4162
    Feeding supplies and equipment B4034-B4088
    Feeding supply kit
        Gravity fed B4036
        Pump fed B4035
        Syringe fed B4034
    Formula
        Blenderized natural foods with intact nutrients B4149
        Complete with intact nutrients B4150
        Complete, calorically dense B4152
        Digestive enzyme(s) B4105
        Fluid and electrolyte replacement B4102
        Hydrolyzed proteins B4153
        Incomplete/modular nutrients B4155
        Pediatrics
            Complete calorically dense B4160
            Complete soy-based, intact nutrients B4159
            Complete with intact nutrients B4158
            Fluid and electrolyte replacement B4103
            Hydrolyzed/amino acids B4161
            Special metabolic needs for inherited disease of metabolism B4162
        Special metabolic needs B4154
        Special metabolic needs for inherited disease of metabolism B4157
    Nutrition infusion pump B9002
    Supplies, not otherwise classified B9998
Enterostomal therapy S9474
Enuresis alarm S8270
Envarsus XR® J7503

Eosinophil count S3630
EpiCord ® Q4187
EpiFix ® Q4186
Epinephrine J0171
Epirubicin HCl J9178
Episode of care
    Discharge/discontinuation of care M1009-M1014
    Documented M1106, M1107, M1111, M1112, M1116,
       M1117, M1121, M1122, M1126, M1127, M1131, M1135
    Episode initiated for rehab therapy, medical or chiropractic
       M1143
    Ongoing care not indicated M1108, M1109, M1110, M1113,
       M1114, M1115, M1118, M1119, M1120, M1123, M1124,
       M1125, M1128, M1129, M1130, M1132, M1133, M1134
Epoetin alpha
    ESRD on dialysis 100 units Q4081, Q5105
    Non-ERSD use J0885, Q5106
Epoetin beta J0887, J0888
Epoprostenol J1325
Eptifibatide J1327
Eptinezumab-jjmr J3032 Ⓝ
Equestrian/hippotherapy S8940
Eravacycline J0122
Ergonovine maleate J1330
Eribulin mesylate J9179
Ertapenem sodium J1335
Erythromycin lactobionate J1364
Esketamine nasal spray S0013 Ⓝ
Esketamine, visit G2082, G2083
ESRD (end-stage renal disease), *see also* Dialysis
    Emergency dialysis G0257
    Machines and accessories E1500-E1699
    Plumbing A4870
    Supplies A4651-A4929
Estradiol valerate J1380
Estrogen conjugated J1410
Estrone (5, aqueous) J1435
Etanercept J1438
Etelcalcetide injection J0606
Eteplirsen injection J1428
Ethanolamine oleate J1430
Etidronate disodium J1436
Etonogestrel implant system J7307
Etoposide J9181
Etoposide, oral J8560
Euflexxa J7323
Evaluation and assessment M1006-M1014, T1024
Evaluation and management G2082, G2083
    Complex visit G2211 Ⓝ
    Prolonged G2212 Ⓝ
Everolimus J7527
Exemestane S0156
Exercise equipment A9300
External
    Ambulatory infusion pump E0781, E0784, E0787
    Ambulatory insulin delivery system A9274
    Counterpulsation treatment G0166
    Drug infusion pump, non-insulin K0552
    Power, battery components L7360-L7368
    Power, elbow L7170-L7191
    Urinary supplies A4356, A4357, A4358, A5105
Extracorporeal shockwave lithotripsy S9034
    Global fee S0400
Extremity belt/harness E0945
Eye
    Case V2756
    Exam, routine S0620, S0621
    Lens, contact or spectacle V2100-V2615

    Miscellaneous items and services V2700-V2799
    Other miscellaneous item or service V2799
    Pad A6410, A6411
    Prosthetic
       Custom V2623
       Other type V2629
    Surgery S0800, S0810, S0812
Eye patch, occlusive A6412

F

Face tent, oxygen A4619
Faceplate, ostomy A4361
Factor VIIA coagulation factor, recombinant J7189, J7212 Ⓝ
Factor VIII, anti-hemophilic factor J7182, J7185, J7188,
    J7190, J7191, J7192, J7204, J7205, J7207, J7208, J7209,
    J7210, J7211 Ⓝ
Factor XA (recombinant), inactivated-zhzo J7169 Ⓝ
Factor IX J7193-J7195, J7200-J7203
Factor XIII, A-subunit J7181
Factor XIII, anti-hemophilic factor J7180
Fall G8907, G8910-G8911, M1069, M1070
Fam-trastuzumab deruxtecan-nxki J9358 Ⓝ
Family planning education H1010
Famotidine S0028
Fecal microbiota preparation G0455
Federally qualified health center services (FQHC) G0466,
    G0467, G0468, G0469, G0470
Fentanyl citrate and droperidol J1810
Fentanyl citrate J3010
Fern test Q0114
Ferric carboxymaltose J1439
Ferric derisomaltose J1437 Ⓝ
Ferric pyrophosphate citrate
    Powder J1444
    Solution J1443
Ferumoxytol Q0138, Q0139
Fetoscopic laser therapy S2411
Filgrastim (G-CSF) J1442
Filgrastim-aafi Q5110
Filgrastim-sndz Q5101
Filler
    Collagen meniscus implant G0428
    Dermal, injection G0429
    Wound
       Alginate dressing A6199
       Collagen based A6011
       Foam dressing A6215
       Hydrocolloid dressing A6240, A6241
       Hydrogel dressing A6248
       Not elsewhere classified (NEC) A6261, A6262
Film, transparent (for dressing) A6257, A6258, A6259
Filter
    Aerosol compressor A7014
    Dialysis carbon A4680
    Ostomy A4368
    Placement G9539, G9540, G9541, G9542, G9543, G9544
    Tracheostoma A4481
    Ultrasonic generator A7014
    Vena cava C1880
Finasteride S0138
Fistula cannulation set A4730
Fistula creation G2170, G2171 Ⓝ
Flebogamma J1572
Florbetaben Q9983
Florbetapir F18 A9586
Floweramnioflo Q4177

Floweramniopatch Q4178
Flowerderm™ Q4179
Flowmeter E0440, E0555, E0580
Floxuridine J9200
Fluciclovine f-18 A9588
Fluconazole, injection J1450
Fludarabine phosphate J8562, J9185
Fluid barrier, dialysis E1575
Fluid flow/Fluid GF Q4206
Flunisolide inhalation solution J7641
Fluocinolone acetonide J7311, J7313, J7314
Fluorodeoxyglucose F-18 FDG A9552
Fluoroestradiol f 18 A9591 Ⓝ
Fluorouracil J9190
Fluphenazine decanoate J2680
Flutamide, oral S0175
Flutemetamol Q9982
Flutter device S8185
Foam dressing A6209-A6215
Foam pad adhesive A5126
Folding walker E0135, E0143
Foley catheter A4312-A4316, A4338-A4346
Follitropin alfa S0126
Follitropin beta S0128
Follow-up interval G9862
Fomepizole J1451
Fomivirsen sodium intraocular J1452
Fondaparinux sodium J1652
Foot
    Arch support
        Nonremovable L3070-L3090
        Removable L3040-L3060
    Exam G9502, G9225, G9226
    Insert
        Formed to patient foot L3030
        High strength, lightweight material L3031
        Longitudinal/metatarsal support L3020
        Plastazote or equal L3002
        Silicone gel L3003
        Spenco® L3001
        UCB type, Berkeley shell L3000
Footdrop splint L4398
Footplate E0175, E0970, L3031
Footrest
    Complete assembly, replacement K0045
    High mount flip-up, replacement K0037
    Lower extension tube, replacement, each K0043
Footwear
    Diabetic
        Compression molded A5510
        Custom with fitting A5501
        Inserts A5512, A5513, A5514
    Orthopedic
        Custom molded shoe L3250
        Custom shoe L3230
        Ladies shoe L3215, L3216, L3217, L3224
        Men's shoe L3219, L3221, L3222, L3225
Forearm crutches E0110, E0111
Formoterol J7640
Formoterol fumarate J7606
Formula, additive, enteral B4104
Fosaprepitant J1453
Foscarnet sodium J1455
Fosnetupitant, palonoset J1454
Fosphenytoin Q2009
Fosphenytoin sodium S0078

Foster care
    Adult S5140, S5141
    Child H0041, H0042, S5145, S5146
Fracture
    Augmentation with implant C1062 Ⓝ
    Bedpan E0276
    Frame E0920, E0930, E0946, E0947, E0948
    Orthosis L2106-L2136, L3980-L3984
    Orthotic additions L2180-L2192, L3995
    Treatment G0412-G0415
Fragmin® (dalteparin sodium) J1645
Frames (spectacles) V2020, V2025
Fremanezumab-vfrm J3031
Fresh frozen plasma
    Between 8-24 hours of collection P9059
    Donor retested P9060
    Single donor, frozen within 8 hours of collection P9017
Frontier extended stay clinic G9140
Fulphila™ Q5108
Fulvestrant J9395
Functional
    Electrical stimulator, any type E0770
    Status G2090-G2152, G2210, G9916-G9918,
        M1043-M1149 Ⓝ
Furosemide J1940

G

Gadobutrol A9585
Gadofosveset trisodium A9583
Gadoxetate disodium A9581
Gait trainer E8000-E8002
Gallium (Ga67) A9556
Gallium ga-68 A9587, C9067 Ⓝ
Gallium nitrate J1457
Galsulfase J1458
Gamma globulin J1460, J1560
Gammagard® liquid J1569
Gammaplex® J1557
Gamunex® J1561
Ganciclovir sodium J1570
Ganciclovir, implant J7310
Ganirelix acetate S0132
Garamycin® J1580
Gas system
    Compressed E0424, E0425
    Gaseous E0430, E0431, E0441, E0443
    Liquid E0434-E0440, E0442, E0444
Gastrointestinal fat absorption study S3708
Gauze, *see also* **Bandages by type**
    Impregnated A6222-A6233, A6266
    Nonimpregnated A6402, A6403, A6404
Gefitinib J8565
Gel
    Conductive A4558
    Coupling A4559
    Pressure pad E0185, E0196
Gel-syn® J7328
Gelatin capsule application device L8515
Gemcitabine HCl J9198, J9201 Ⓝ
Gemtuzumab ozogamicin injection J9203
General care management, RHC/FQHC G0511
Generator, cardiac contractility modulation C1824
Generator, ultrasonic with nebulizer E0574
Genesis amniotic membrane Q4198
Genetic
    Counseling S0265
    Testing S3800-S3870
        Warfarin responsiveness G9143

Gentamicin sulfate - Hemin

Gentamicin sulfate J1580
Givosiran J0223 Ⓝ
Glasses
  Air conduction V5070
  Binaural V5120-V5150
  Bone conduction V5080
  Frames V2020, V2025
  Hearing aid V5190, V5230
Glatiramer acetate J1595
Gloves A4927, A4930
Glucagon HCl J1610
Glucose testing
  Continuous noninvasive monitoring S1030, S1031
  Disposable monitor A9275
  Monitor with lancing/blood sample collection E2101
  Monitor with voice synthesizer E2100
  Test strips
    Dialysis A4772
    Home blood glucose monitor A4253
Gluteal pad L2650
Glycopyrrolate, inhalation solution
  Concentrated J7642
  Unit dose J7643
Gold sodium thiomalate J1600
Golimumab J1602
Golodirsen J1429 Ⓝ
Gonadorelin HCl J1620
Goserelin acetate implant J9202
Grab bar, trapeze E0910, E0940
Grade-aid, wheelchair E0974
Gradient pressure aid supplies S8420-S8429
Grafix ®/Grafixpl ®
  Core Q4132
  Prime Q4133
Graft, vascular catheter C1768
Granisetron, extended release J1627
Granisetron HCl J1626, Q0166, S0091
Granulocyte colony stimulating factor (G-CSF) J1442, Q5101
Gravity traction device E0941
Gravlee jet washer A4470
Group psychotherapy G0410, G0411
Guidewire C1769
Guselkumab J1628

H

Haberman feeder, cleft palate S8265
Habilitation
  Day T2020, T2021
  Educational T2012, T2013
  Prevocational T2014, T2015, T2047 Ⓝ
  Residential T2016, T2017
  Supported employment T2018, T2019
Haegarda ® injection J0599
Hair analysis (excluding arsenic) P2031
Hallus valgus dynamic splint L3100
Hallux prosthetic implant L8642
Halo procedures L0810, L0820, L0830, L0859, L0861
Haloperidol J1630
Haloperidol decanoate J1631
Halter, cervical head E0942
Hand finger orthosis, prefabricated L3923
Hand restoration L6900-L6915
  Orthosis (WHFO) E1805, E1825, L3763-L3809, L3900-L3956
  Partial prosthesis L6000-L6020
  Rims, wheelchair, replacement E0967

Handgrip (cane, crutch, walker) A4636
Harness E0942, E0944, E0945
Harvesting of donor multivisceral organs S2055
Health club membership S9970
Health-related quality of life assessment G9634, G9635, G9636
Head Imaging
  For clinical trial G9537
Hearing aids V5030-V5060, V5120-V5267
  Binaural
    Analog V5248, V5249
      CIC V5248
      ITC V5249
    Contralateral routing device
      BTE/BTE V5221
      ITC/BTE V5215
      ITC/ITC V5214
      ITE/BTE V5213
      ITE/ITC V5212
      ITE/ITE V5211
    Contralateral routing system, glasses V5230
    Digital
      BTE V5261
      CIC V5258
      ITC V5259
      ITE V5260
    Digitally programmable
      BTE V5253
      ITC V5251
      ITE V5252
    Disposable V5263
  Monaural V5030-V5060
    Analog
      CIC (completely in ear canal) V5242
      ITC (in the canal) V5243
    Contralateral routing device
      BTE V5181
      ITC V5172
      ITE V5171
    Contralateral routing glasses V5190
    Digital
      BTE V5257
      CIC V5254
      ITC V5255
      ITE V5256
    Digitally programmable
      BTE V5247
      CIC V5244
      ITC V5245
      ITE V5246
    Disposable V5262
Hearing services and supplies L8614, V5008, V5336
Heat
  Application E0200-E0239
  Infrared heating pad system A4639, E0221
  Lamp E0200, E0205
  Pad E0210, E0215, E0249
Heater (nebulizer) E1372
Heel
  Elevator, air E0370
  Protector E0191
  Shoe L3430-L3485
  Stabilizer L3170
Helicoll™ Q4164
Helicopter, ambulance A0431
Helmets A8000-A8004
Hemin J1640

Ⓝ **New index entry**

Hemi-pelvectomy prosthesis L5280
Hemi-wheelchair E1083-E1086
Hemodialysis
    Machine E1590
    Maintenance dialysis G8956
    Short-term C1752
Hemodialyzer, portable E1635
Hemofil M J7190
Hemophilia clotting factor J7190-J7198
    Not elsewhere classified (NEC) J7199
Hemostatic agent, gastrointestinal, topical C1052 Ⓝ
Hemostick® and similar products A4773
Hep-lock (heparin lock) J1642
HepaGam B® J1571, J1573
Heparin infusion pump, dialysis E1520
Heparin lock flush J1642
Heparin sodium J1644
Hep b screen high risk indiv G0499
Hepatitis B status G9504
Hexalite® A4590
Hexaminolevulinate hydrochloride A9589
High osmolar contrast material Q9958-Q9964
High risk area, delivery or service S9381
Hip
    Core decompression S2325
    Disarticulation prosthesis L5250, L5270
    Orthosis (HO) L1600-L1690
    Total resurfacing, metal on metal S2118
Hip-knee-ankle-foot orthosis (HKAFO) L2040-L2090
History and physical, outpatient, presurgical S0260
Histrelin acetate J1675
Histrelin implant J9225
HIV antigen/antibody screening G0475, S3645
HKAFO (hip-knee-ankle-foot orthosis) L2040-L2090
Holding chamber or spacer S8100, S8101
Home care services G0076-G0087, S9097, S9098, S9110, S9122-S9131
    Chore S5120-S5121
    Companion care S5135, S5136
    Foster care S5145, S5146
    Homemaker S5130, S5131
    Infusion therapy S5497-S5523, S9325-S9379, S9490-S9504
    Injection therapy S9537, S9542, S9558, S9559, S9560, S9562
    INR monitoring G0248, G0249, G0250
    Irrigation therapy S9590
    Nurse practitioner S0274
    Other services S5165, S5170, S5175
    Pharmacy S9810
    Physical therapy G0151, G0157, G0159, G2168, G2169 Ⓝ
    Respiratory therapy S5180, S5181
    Respite care S5150, S5151, T1005
    RN, LPN visit by RHC/FQHC G0490
    Training S5108-S5116
    Transfusion S9538
Home health agency services T1022
Home therapy and management services G2168, G2169, S0270-S0272, S0280, S0281, S5522, S5523, S9208-S9379 Ⓝ
Home uterine monitor S9001
Hospice and/or home health services
    Aide G0156, T1004
    Assisted-living facility Q5002
    Care T2042-T2046
    Care coordinator G9477
    Chaplain G9473
    Clinical social worker G0155
    Dietary counselor G9474

    Hospice facility Q5010
    Inpatient hospice facility Q5006
    Inpatient hospital Q5005
    Inpatient psychiatric facility Q5008
    Long term care facility Q5007
    Long-term care facility Q5003
    Not otherwise specified (NOS) Q5009
    Nursing G0128, G0162, G0299, G0300, G0493, G0494, G0495, G0496, T1000, T1002, T1003
    Occupational therapy G0129, G0152, G0158, G0160
    Other counselor G9475
    Patient's home Q5001
    Pharmacist G9479
    Physical therapy G0151, G0157, G0159, G2168, G2169 Ⓝ
    Physician S0270, S0272, S0272, S0273
    Referral S0255
    Services G9723, G9819, M1067, T2042-T2046
    Skilled nursing facility Q5004
    Speech and language G0153, G0161
    Therapist G9478
    Volunteer G9476
Hospital services
    Admission/transfer G8907, G8914, G8915
    Inpatient admissions G9521, G9522
    Observation/ED visit G0378-G0384
Hospitalist services S0310
Housing, supported H0043, H0044
Hot or cold fluid bottle A9273
Hotline service, behavioral health H0030
Human breast milk processing T2101
Human fibrinogen concentrate J7177, J7178
Humidifier A7046, E0550-E0562
Hyalgan® J7321
Hyaluronan or derivative J7320, J7322, J7326, J7327, J7328, J7331, J7333 Ⓝ
Hyaluronidase J3470
    Ovine J3471, J3472, J3473
Hydralazine HCl J0360
Hydraulic patient lift E0630
Hydrocollator E0225, E0239
Hydrocolloid dressing A6234-A6241
Hydrocortisone
    Acetate J1700
    Sodium phosphate J1710
    Sodium succinate J1720
Hydrogel dressing A6231, A6232, A6233, A6242-A6248
Hydromorphone J1170
Hydromorphone hydrochloride S0092
Hydroxyprogesterone caproate injection
    Makena® J1726
    NOS J1729
Hydroxyurea, oral S0176
Hydroxyzine HCl J3410
Hydroxyzine pamoate Q0177
Hygienic item, device, any A9286
Hylan G-F 20 J7325
Hyoscyamine sulfate J1980
Hyperbaric oxygen treatment
    Full body chamber G0277
    Topical A4575
Hypertonic saline solution J7131

I

Ibalizumab-uiyk J1746
Ibandronate sodium J1740
Ibuprofen J1741

Ibutilide fumarate J1742
Icatibant J1744
Ice cap or collar A9273
Idarubicin HCl J9211
Idursulfase J1743
Ifosfamide J9208
Iloprost Q4074
Imaging
  Angiography G0278
  Cardiac stress G8961-G8966
  Computed tomography (CT) G9341, G9342, G9344,
    G9351-G9354, G9753, S8092
    Dose reduction technique G9637, G9638
  Echocardiography C8923-C8930
  Head G2187-G2195, G9537, M1027-M1031 Ⓝ
  Magnetic resonance (MRI) C1770, C8900-C8920,
    C8931-C8937, C9762, C9763, S8042 Ⓝ
  Magnetic source S8035
  PET scan G0219, G0235, G0252, S8085
  Studies S8030-S8092
  Ultrasound C1753, G8806, S8055, S9024
Imatinib S0088
Imiglucerase J1786
Imipenem 4 mg, cilastatin 4 mg, and relebactam 2 mg
  J0742 Ⓝ
Immune globulin
  Asceniv™ C9072 Ⓝ
  Bivigam™ J1556
  Cuvitru™ J1555
  Flebogamma® J1572
  Gammagard® liquid J1569
  Gammaplex® J1557
  Gamunex® J1561
  HepaGam ® B J1571
  Hizentra ® J1559
  HyQvia ® J1575
  Intravenous services, supplies and accessories Q2052
  Nonlyophilized, not otherwise specified (NOS) J1599
  Not otherwise specified (NOS) J1566
  Octagam ® J1568
  Privigen ® J1459
  Rho(D) J2788, J2790
  Rhophylac ® J2791
  Subcutaneous J1562
  With hyaluronidase J1575
  Xembify ® J1558 Ⓝ
Implant
  Access system A4301
  Aqueous shunt L8612
  Auditory brain stem S2235
  Autologous cultured chondrocytes J7330
  Breast L8600
  Buprenorphine J0570
  Cochlear L8614, L8619
  Collagen
    Meniscus G0428
    Urinary tract L8603
  Device, NOC C1889
  Dextranomer/hyaluronic acid copolymer L8604
  Ganciclovir J7310
  Hallux L8642
  Infusion pump, programmable E0783, E0786
  Interatrial shunt ide C9758, C9760 Ⓝ
  Interspinous implant C1821
  Joint L8630, L8641, L8658
  Lacrimal duct A4262, A4263
  Magnetic component, hearing device S2230
  Metacarpophalangeal joint L8630

  Metatarsal joint L8641
  Mometasone furoate sinus J7401
  Neurostimulator pulse generator L8679, L8681, L8685,
    L8686, L8687, L8688
    Inner ear A4638, E2120
  Not otherwise specified (NOS) L8699
  Ocular L8610
  Ossicular L8613
  Osteogenesis stimulator E0749
  Percutaneous access system A4301
  Replacement implantable intraspinal catheter E0785
  Synthetic, urinary L8606
  Urinary tract L8603, L8606
  Vascular graft L8670
Implantable orthopedic/device/drug matrix C1734
Implantable radiation dosimeter A4650
Impregnated gauze dressing A6222-A6230
Impression casting, foot S0395
Incobotulinumtoxin A J0588
Incontinence appliances and supplies
  Bedside drainage bottle A5102
  Catheter insertion tray A4310
  Disposable urethral clamp A4360
  Extension drainage tubing A4331
  Leg strap A5113, A5114
  Lubricant A4332
  Male external catheter A4349
  Pelvic floor electrical stimulator system E0740
  Rectal control system A4563
  Rectal insert A4337
  Urinary drainage bag, leg or abdomen A5112
  Urinary ostomy A5071, A5072, A5073
  Urinary suspensory with leg bag A5105
Incontinence products
  Devices and supplies A4310-A4360, A5102-A5200,
    T4521-T4545
  Disposable brief/diaper
    Adult
      Above extra large T4543
      Extra large T4524
      Large T4523
      Medium T4522
      Small T4521
    Pediatric T4529, T4530
      Large T4530
      Small/ medium T4529
    Youth T4533
  Disposable penile wrap T4545
  Disposable underpad T4541, T4542
    Large T4521
    Small T4542
  Garment A4520
  Protective brief/diaper T4543, T4544
  Protective underpad
    Bed T4537
    Chair T4540
  Protective underwear
    Adult
      Above extra large T4543
      Extra large T4524
      Large T4523
      Medium T4522
      Small T4521
    Pediatric T4531, T4532
      Large T4532
      Small/ medium T4531
    Youth T4534
  Reusable diaper/brief, any size T4539

Ⓝ **New index entry**

Indium IN-111 capromab pendetide A9507
Indium IN-111 ibritumomab tiuxetan A9542
Indium IN-111 labeled autologous platelets A9571
Indium IN-111 labeled autologous white blood cells A9570
Indium IN-111 oxyquinoline A9547
Indium IN-111 pentetate A9548
Indium IN-111 pentetreotide A9572
Indium IN-111 satumomab A4642
Induction, medical indication G9361
Inebilizumab J1823 Ⓝ
Infection control supplies S8301
Infectious agent antibody detection
    Enzyme immunoassay (EIA) technique G0432
    Enzyme-linked immunosorbent assay (ELISA) technique G0433
    Nucleic acid (DNA or RNA) G0476
    Rapid antibody test G0435
Infliximab-abda Q5104
Infliximab-dyyb Q5103
Infliximab injection J1745, Q5121 Ⓝ
Infliximab-qbtx Q5109
Inflectra® Q5103
Influenza virus vaccine
    Afluria® Q2035
    Agriflu® Q2034
    FluLaval® Q2036
    Fluvirin® Q2037
    Fluzone® Q2038
    Not otherwise specified (NOS) Q2039
Infusion
    Blood and blood products P9041-P9048
    Catheter
        Intravenous, OPPS C8957
        Other than hemodialysis C1751
    Normal saline solution
        250 cc J7050
        500 mL J7040
        1000 cc J7030
    Professional services G0068-G0070
    Pump K0455
        Ambulatory E0779-E0786
        External K0552
        Implantable/insertable device, not used C1890
        Insulin E0784, E0787
        Intravenous-pole E0776
        Mechanical, reusable E0779, E0780
        Nonprogrammable, permanent C1891
        Nonprogrammable, temporary C2626
        Parenteral E0791
        Programmable C1772
        Refill kit A4220
        Supplies A4221, A4222, A4224, A4225, A4226, A4230, A4231, A4232, E0776-E0791, K0455-K0605
        Uninterrupted parenteral administration of medication K0455
    Supplies A4222-A4231, E0776-E0791, K0552-K0605, S1015
    Therapy
        Home
            Alpha-1-proteinase inhibitor S9346
            Anti-emetic infusion, continuous or intermittent S9351
            Anti-hemophilic agent infusion S9345
            Anti-spasmodic S9363
            Anti-tumor necrosis factor S9359
            Antibiotic, antiviral, or antifungal S9494-S9504
            Anticoagulant infusion S9336
            Catheter care/maintenance S5497, S5498, S5501, S5502

            Catheter repair kit S5518
            Chelation S9355
            Chemotherapy infusion S9329
                Continuous (24 hours or more) S9330
                Intermittent S9331
            Declotting kit S5517
            Diuretic S9361
            Enzyme replacement intravenous therapy S9357
            Hydration therapy S9373, S9374, S9375, S9376, S9377
            Immunotherapy S9338
            Infusion S5497-S5523, S9325-S9379
            Insulin infusion S9353
            Midline catheter insert kit S5521
            Pain management infusion S9328
            PICC insert kit S5520
            Repair of infusion device S5036
            Routine device maintenance S5035
            Sympathomimetic/inotropic agent infusion S9349
            Total parenteral nutrition S9364, S9365, S9366, S9367, S9368
        Other than chemotherapeutic drugs Q0081
Inhalation solution, *see* **Appendix A: Table of Drugs**
Inhaler holding chamber or spacer S8100, S8101
In-home visit
    Existing patient G2006-G2013
    New patient G2001-G2005
Initial services for Medicare enrollment G0402-G0405
Injection, *see also* **Appendix A: Table of Drugs**
    Blood Factor J7175-J7209
    Sacroiliac joint G0259, G0260
    Supplies A4206-A4232
        Self-administered A4211
Inotuzumab ozogamicin J9229
Inpatient admissions
    From outpatient, ED or observation G2176 Ⓝ
INR monitoring G0248, G0249, G0250
Insertion tray
    With drainage bag
        With indwelling catheter, Foley-type
            Three-way, for continuous irrigation A4316
            Two-way, all silicone A4315
            Two-way, latex with coating A4314
        Without catheter A4354
    With indwelling catheter, Foley-type
        Three-way, for continuous irrigation A4313
        Two-way, all silicone A4312
        Two-way, latex with coating A4311
    Without catheter A4310
    Without drainage bag
Insulin
    Medication and supplies J1815, J1817, S5550-S5571
    Outpatient intravenous treatment (OIVIT) G9147
    Pump initiation S9145
    Syringes S8490
Intake activities w/medical exam G2076
Integrated keratoprosthesis C1818
Interatrial shunt ide C9758, C9760 Ⓝ
Interdisciplinary team conference G0175, S0221
Interferential current stimulator S8130, S8131
Interferon
    Alpha J9212, J9213, J9214, J9215
    Beta-1a J1826, Q3027, Q3028
    Beta-1b J1830
    Gamma J9216
Interim labor facility, global S4005
Intermittent
    Assist device with CPAP device E0470, E0471, E0472

Limb compression device A4600, E0676
Peritoneal dialysis system E1592
Positive pressure breathing (IPPB) machine E0500
Interphalangeal joint, prosthetic implant L8658, L8659
Interrogation device remote eval G2066
Interscapular thoracic prosthesis
Endoskeletal L6570
Upper limb L6350-L6370
Intracardiac echocardiography (catheter) C1759
Intradiscal catheter C1754
Intragastric hypothermia M0100
Intraocular lens
Category 4 Q1004
Category 5 Q1005
New technology C1780
Phakic S0596
Telescopic C1840
Intraoperative
Cystoscopy G9606, G9607, G9608
Fluorescence lymph mapping C9756
Neurophysiology monitoring G0453
Intrapulmonary percussive ventilation system E0481
Intraspinal catheter C1755
Intrauterine copper contraceptive J7300
Intravenous admin set, non-PVC, for unstable drugs S1016
Introducer sheaths
Guiding C1766, C1892, C1893
Other than guiding C1894, C2629
Inversion eversion correction device A9285
Iodine I-123 iobenguane A9582
Iodine I-123 ioflupane A9584
Iodine I-123 sodium iodide A9509, A9516
Iodine I-125 serum albumin A9532
Iodine I-125 sodium iodide A9527
Iodine I-125 sodium iothalamate A9554
Iodine i-131 iobenguane A9590
Iodine I-131 iodinated serum albumin A9524
Iodine I-131 sodium iodide capsule A9517, A9528
Iodine I-131 sodium iodide solution A9529, A9530, A9531
Iodine iobenguane sulfate I-131 A9508
Iodine swabs/wipes A4247
IPD system E1592
Ipilimumab J9228
IPPB machine E0500
Ipratropium bromide, inhalation solution J7644, J7645
Irinotecan J9206
Irinotecan liposome injection J9205
Iris prosthesis C1839
Iron dextran J1750
Iron sucrose J1756
Irrigation solution for bladder calculi Q2004
Irrigation supplies A4320, A4321, A4322, A4355, A4397-A4400
Ostomy
Bag A4398
Cone/catheter, with or without brush A4399
Set A4400
Sleeve A4397
Syringe, bulb or piston A4322
Therapeutic agent for urinary catheter irrigation A4321
Three-way indwelling Foley catheter A4355
Tray with bulb or piston syringe A4320
Tubing set for continuous bladder A4355
Irrigation/evacuation system, bowel
Control unit E0350
Disposable supplies for E0352
Manual pump enema A4459
Isatuximab-irfc J9227 Ⓝ
Isavuconazonium J1833

Isoetharine HCl, inhalation solution
Concentrated J7647, J7648
Unit dose J7649, J7650
Isolates B4150, B4152
Isoproterenol HCl, inhalation solution
Concentrated J7657, J7658
Unit dose J7659, J7660
Isosulfan blue Q9968
Itraconazole J1835
IV pole, each E0776, K0105
Ixabepilone J9207
IXIFI™ Q5109

J

Jacket, scoliosis L1300, L1310
Jaw motion rehabilitation systems E1700-E1702
Jenamicin J1580
Joint device C1776

K

Kanamycin sulfate J1840, J1850
Kartop® patient lift, toilet, or bathroom E0625
Keramatrix® Q4165
Kerecis™ Q4158
Ketorolac tromethamine J1885
Keroxx Q4202
Kidney
ESRD supply A4653-A4932
System E1510
Wearable artificial E1632
Kits
Enteral feeding supply
Gravity fed B4036
Pump fed B4035
Syringe fed B4034
Fistula cannulation (set) A4730
Parenteral nutrition B4220-B4224
Surgical dressing (tray) A4550
Tracheostomy A4625
Knee
Disarticulation, prosthesis L5150, L5160
Joint, miniature L5826
Orthosis (KO) E1810, L1810-L1860
Knee-ankle-foot orthosis (KAFO) L2000-L2038, L2126-L2136
Addition, high strength L2755
Replace components L4070-L4110
Kyphosis pad L1020, L1025

L

Laboratory tests
Blood and hair P2028-P2038
Cytopathology P3000, P3001, Q0091
Miscellaneous P9010-P9615, Q0111, Q0112, Q0113, Q0114, Q0115
Screening G0432-G0435
Lacrimal duct implant
Permanent A4263
Temporary A4262
Lactated Ringer's infusion J7120
Laetrile J3570
Laminotomy C9757
Lanadelumab-flyo J0593
Lancet spring-powered device
Each A4258
Per box 100 A4259

Ⓝ New index entry

Lanreotide J1930
Laparoscopic esophagomyotomy S2079
Laronidase J1931
Larynx, artificial L8500
Laser blood collection device and accessory A4257, A4652, E0620
Laser treatment, low level S8948
Laser-assisted uvulopalatoplasty S2080
Lead investigation T1029
Lead wires, per pair A4557
Left ventricular ejection fraction (LVEF) G8395, G8396
Lead, endocardial single coil C1777
Lefamulin J0691 Ⓝ
Leg
    Bag A4358, A5105, A5112
    Extensions for walker E0158
    Rest, elevating K0195
    Rest, wheelchair E0990
    Strap, replacement A5113, A5114
Legg Perthes orthosis L1700-L1755
Lens supplies and services
    Aniseikonic V2118, V2318
    Aspherical V2410-V2499
    Bifocal V2200-V2299
    Contact V2500-V2599
    Eye S0504-S0510, S0516-S0590, S0595, V2100-V2615, V2700-V2799
    Intraocular C1780, V2630, V2631, V2632
    Low vision V2600-V2615
    Progressive V2781
    Single vision V2100-V2199
    Trifocal V2300-V2399
Lepirudin J1945
Leucovorin calcium J0640
Leukocyte poor blood, each unit P9016
Leuprolide acetate
    1 mg J9218
    3.75 mg J1950
    7.5 mg J9217
    65 mg (implant) J9219
Levalbuterol and albuterol, all formulations J7612, J7613, J7614, J7615
Levalbuterol, all formulations, inhalation solution
    Compounded product J7607
    Noncompounded J7612
Levamisole hydrochloride, oral S0177
Levetiracetam J1953
Levocarnitine J1955
Levofloxacin J1956
Levoleucovorin J0641, J0642
Levonorgestrel, implants and supplies J7296, J7297, J7298, J7301, J7306
Levorphanol tartrate J1960
Lexidronam A9604
Lice treatment A9180
Lidocaine HCl J2001
Lidocaine/tetracaine patch C9285
Lifestyle modification program, cardiac S0340, S0341, S0342
Lift
    Patient (includes seat type) E0621-E0642
    Shoe L3300-L3334
Lincomycin HCl J2010
Linezolid J2020
Lipid microspheres Q9950, Q9955, Q9957
Liposomal
    Daunorubicin and cytarabine J9153
Liquid barrier, ostomy A4363

Lithium ion
    Battery, rechargeable
        Auditory Osseointegrated device L8624
        Cochlear implant speech processor L8623, L8624
        Nonprosthetic use A4601
        Prosthetic use L7367
    Charger L7368
Lobectomy, living donor S2061
Localization device, surgical implantable C1819
Lodging, recipient, escort nonemergency transport A0180, A0200
Lomustine, oral S0178
Lorazepam J2060
Low frequency ultrasonic diathermy treatment device K1004
Low osmolar contrast material
    100-199 mg/mL Q9965
    200-299 mg/mL Q9966
    300-399 mg/mL Q9967
Loxapine for inhalation J2062
Lubricant A4332, A4402
Lumbar-sacral orthosis (LSO) L0621-L0640
Lumbar spine condition M1037-M1049
Lung
    Biopsy plug with delivery system C2613
    Cancer screening, low dose CT G0296
    Volume reduction surgery (LVRS)
        Postdischarge services G0305
        Preoperative services G0302, G0303, G0304
Lurbinectedin J9223 Ⓝ
Luspatercept-aamt J0896 Ⓝ
Lutetium lu 177, dotatate A9513
Luxturna™ J3398
Lymphatic mapping, intraoperative fluorescence C9756
Lymphedema therapy S8431, S8950
Lymphocyte immune globulin J7504, J7511

M

Magnesium sulphate, injection J3475
Magnetic resonance angiography
    Abdomen C8901
        With contrast C8900
        Without contrast followed with contrast C8902
    Chest C8910
        With contrast C8909
        Without contrast followed with contrast C8911
    Lower extremity C8913
        With contrast C8912
        Without contrast followed with contrast C8914
    Pelvis C8919
        With contrast C8918
        Without contrast followed with contrast C8920
    Spinal canal and contents C8932
        With contrast C8931
        Without contrast followed with contrast C8933
    Upper extremity C8935
        With contrast C8934
        Without contrast followed with contrast C8936
Magnetic resonance imaging (MRI)
    Breast
        Bilateral
            With contrast C8906
            Without contrast followed by with contrast C8908
            Computer-aided detection C8937

Unilateral
    With contrast C8903
    Without contrast followed by
      with contrast C8905
    Cardiac C9762, C9763 Ⓝ
Maintenance contract, ESRD A4890
Major depressive disorder G9212, G9213
Mannitol
    Inhaler J7665
    Injection J2150
MAPCP demonstration project G9151, G9152, G9153
Mask, oxygen A4620
Mastectomy
    Bra L8000
    Camisole S8460
    Form L8020
    Prosthesis L8030, L8600
    Sleeve L8010
Masters two step S3904
Matrion Q4201
Mattress
    Air pressure E0186
      Pad E0197
    Alternating pressure E0277
    Dry pressure E0184
      Pad E0199
    Gel pressure E0196
      Pad E0185
    Hospital bed E0271, E0272
    Nonpowered, pressure reducing E0373
    Overlay E0371, E0372
    Powered, pressure reducing E0277
    Water pressure E0187
Measurement of hepatic portosystem C9768 Ⓝ
Mecasermin, injection J2170
Mechlorethamine HCl, injection J9230
Medicaid certified community beh hlth clinic srvcs
    Per diem T1040
    Per month T1041
Medical and surgical supplies A4206-A8004
Medical conference S0220, S0221
Medical food S9433, S9434, S9435
Medical records copying fee S9981, S9982
Medicare appropriate use criteria program, CDSM G1001-G1004, G1007-G1011
Medicare Care Choice Model (MCCM) program admission G9480
Medicare demonstration project G9013-G9140
Medicare Diabetes Prevention Program (MDPP) core session(s) G9873-G9875
    Bridge payment G9890
    Maintenance G9876-G9879, G9882-G9885
    Session reporting G9891
    Weight loss achieved G9880-G9881
Medicare-enrolled opioid treatment program G2067-G2075, G2076, G2077, G2078, G2079, G2080
Medication, *see also* **Appendix A: Table of Drugs**
    Reminder service S5185
Medication assisted treatment G2067-G2075, G2080
Medroxyprogesterone acetate J1050
Megestrol acetate, oral S0179
Melanoma G8749, G8944, G9292-G9295
Meloxicam J1738 Ⓝ
Melphalan injection J9245, J9246 Ⓝ
Melphalan, oral J8600
Menotropins S0122
Mental health services, H0046, H2000-H2037
Meperidine and promethazine HCl, injection J2180

Meperidine hydrochloride J2175
Mepivacaine HCl J0670
Mepolizumab injection J2182
Mercaptopurine, oral S0108
Merit-based Incentive Payment System (MIPS)
    Activity therapy G0176
    Adolescent depression remission
      Not reached 12 mon. M1020
      Reached 12 mo. M1019
    AF, transient or reversible cause G9929
    Alcohol (and/or drug)
      Abuse and prevention services H0002, H0004, H0017-H0019, H0031, H0034-H0037, H0039, H0040, H2000, H2001, H2010-H2020
      Screening G9621, G9622, G9623, G9624
    Amoxicillin as first-line antibiotic
      Not prescribed at the time of diagnosis
        Medical reason G9313
        Reason not documented G9314
      Prescribed at the time of diagnosis G9315
    Amputation after revascularization procedure G9639, G9640, G9641
    Androgen deprivation therapy
      Not prescribed/administered, medical reason G9895
      Not prescribed/administered, patient reason G9896
      Not prescribed/administered, reason not given G9897
      Prescribed/administered G9894
    Anesthesia care services (MAC) G9654
    Anesthetic Inhalation G9955
    Angiotensin converting enzyme (ACE) or angiotensin receptor blocker (ARB) therapy
      Not prescribed
        Reason documented G8474, G8936
        Reason not documented G8475, G8937
      Prescribed G8473, G8506, G8935
    Angiotensin converting enzyme (ACE) inhibitor or angiotensin receptor blocker (ARB) or angiotensin receptor-neprilysin inhibitor (ARNI)
      Not prescribed
        Medical reason G2093
        Patient reason G2094
        Reason not given G2096
        System reason G2095
      Prescribed G2092
    Antibiotic
      Regimen G9498, G9505
        Not prescribed within specified time period G9287
      Taken within 30 days prior to episode date G9703
      Therapy
        Not prescribed or dispensed G8708
        Prescribed or dispensed G8710, G8711, G9712
    Anticoagulation (warfarin or another oral anticoagulant)
      Not prescribed
        Medical reason G8968
        Patient reason G8969
      Prescribed G8967
    Anti-epidermal growth factor receptor monoclonal antibodies G9839-G9845
    Antimicrobial prophylaxis
      Not ordered, medical reasons G9196
      Ordered
        Documented G9197
        Not documented G9198
    Anti-TNF therapy for Hepatitis B
      Documented immunity G8869
      Hepatitis
        Hep B status assessed prior to therapy G9912
        Hep B status not assessed prior to therapy G9913

Ⓝ **New index entry**

No record HBV results G9915
Patient receiving anti-tnf agent G9914
Apnea hypopnea index
Measured G8842
Not measured
Reason documented G8843
Reason not documented G8844
Aspirin/antiplatelet therapy G9793, G9795
Not on daily aspirin or other anti-platelet, medical reason documented G2128
Assessments, patient
Disease activity, not assessed M1006
Functional outcomes, documented G8942
Psoriasis G9649, G9651, G9764
Rheumatoid arthritis encounters M1007, M1008
Asthma
Med not needed G9808
PDC achieved G9810, G9811
Reporting
Not well-controlled G9434
Well-controlled G9432
Back pain
Measured G2136-G2139
Not measured G9943, G9946
Behavioral health services
Counseling G0447, G0473
Intensive S9480
Training and educational services, G0177
Beta-blocker therapy
Documentation
Medical reason G9190
Patient reason G9191
System reason G9192
Not prescribed G8452
Reasons documented G8451
Reasons not documented G9188
Prescribed G8450, G9189
Biologic immune response modifier G9506
Biopsy results G8883, G8884, G8885, G9784-G9786
Birth year 1945 to 1965 G9448
Bladder injury G9625, G9626, G9627
Blood pressure monitoring G9788, G9789, G9790
Cardiovascular prevention G8783, G8785
No procedure-related BP taken at outpatient visit G2129
Controlling high blood pressure G8752-G8756
Blunt head trauma G9529, G9530, G9531, G9533
Pediatric patient G9593, G9594, G9595, G9597
BMI (body mass index)
Not documented G8421
Parameters
Above normal G8417
Below normal G8418
Outside normal G8419, G9716
Within normal G8420
Patient not eligible for BMI calculation G8422
Outside of normal parameters G8938
Bowel injury G9628, G9629, G9630
Breast Mammography
Digital/digital tomosynthesis (3D)
Results documented G9899
Results not documented G9900
Breast cancer
Clinically node negative G9911
Stage of breast cancer G9831, G9832
Breastfeeding pt G9779
Bronchodilator
Med reason not prescribed G9696
Prescribed G9695

Pt reason not prescribed G9697
System reason not prescribed G9698
Not prescribed, reason NOS G9699
Cardiac implantable device
Admitted G9410, G9412
Not readmitted within 180 days G9411, G9413
Readmission within 180 days G9410
Cardiac stress test imaging
Initial detection and risk assessment
Higher than low CHD risk G8966
Low CHD risk G8965
Monitoring of asymptomatic patient G8963
Performed for reason other than monitoring G8964
Performed more than 30 days before surgery G8962
Performed within 30 days of surgery G8961
Cardiac tamponade
Not within 30 days of atrial fibrillation ablation G9409
Within 30 days of atrial fibrillation ablation G9408
Cardiovascular prevention services G9662-G9666
Cataract surgery G9517, G9519, G9520
Satisfaction with care
Achieved G0916
Not achieved G0918
Visual improvement, not achieved G0915
CEA (carotid endarterectomy)
Discharged G8834
Not discharged G8838
Cecal landmarks, postsurgical G9612, G9613, G9614
CHA2DS2-VASc risk score G9931
Chemotherapy
Not received G9848
Received G9847
Clinic visit, all-inclusive T1015
Colonoscopy
Advanced age G9659, G9660, G9661
Screening
Age 50 to 85 years G2204 Ⓝ
Same physician performed biopsy and pathology G9939
Combination therapy
Not received G9958
Not received, medical reason G9957
Received G9956
Comfort care only G9930
Complications documentation
Within 30 days G9267
Within 90 days G9268
Without complications
30 days G9269
90 days G9270
COPD symptoms with spirometry test G8924
Coronary artery bypass surgery, minimally invasive S2205, S2206, S2207, S2208, S2209
Count of previous CT and myocardial perfusion studies
Documented G9321
Not documented G9322
Crisis intervention S9484, S9485
CT scan
Dose reduction technique used G9637, G9638
Current medication
Documented G8427
Not documented G8428
Depression screening
Annual screen G0444
Documented G8431
Documented as negative G8510
Documented as positive
Follow-up not documented G8511

Merit-based Incentive Payment System (MIPS)

Not documented
  Reason documented G8433
  Reason not given G8432
DEXA, DXA
  Documented G8399
  Not documented G8400
  Within past 2 years G9769
Dialysis
  Documentation (ESRD) G9231
Dilated macular exam
  Not performed, medical reason G9975
  Not performed, patient reason G9892
  Performed G9974
  Reason NOS G9893
Discharge, patient
  Follow-up within 30 days after discharge
    Not able to complete with documented reason G9403
    Not received G9404
    Received G9402
  Follow-up within 7 days from discharge
    Not able to complete with documented reason G9406
    Not received G9407
    Received G9405
  Postoperative day #2
    CAS (carotid artery stenting)
      Later than G9254
      No later than G9255
    CEA (carotid endarterectomy)
      Discharged G8834
      Not discharged G8838
    EVAR (endovascular aneurysm repair)
      Discharged G8826
      Not discharged G8833
  Postoperative day #7
    Discharged G8818
    Not discharged G8825
Documentation
  Body temperature G9771-G9773
  Bipolar disorder G9717
  Depression G8431-G8433, G8510, G8511, G9717
  Follow-up interval G9755
  Imaging G9548
  Medications G8427, G8428, G8430, G9286, G9531, G9765, G9775-G9777
  Pain G9250, G9251
  Patient-specific risk G9316, G9317
  Renal disease/transplant G9231, G9722
  Tuberculosis G9359, G9360
  Therapy G8450-G8452, G8474, G9781, G9783, G9940
  Trauma G9531, G9595
Door to puncture time G9580, G9582
During performance period
  Patient in hospice M1022, M1025, M1026
  Urgent care visits only M1021
Early elective delivery by C-section, or early induction
  Not performed G9355
  Performed G9356
Elder maltreatment
  Documented as negative G8734
  Documented as positive G8733
    Follow-up plan not documented
      No reason G8735
      Patient not eligible G8941
  No documentation
    Patient not eligible G8535
    Reason not given G8536
Embolization endpoints
  Documented G9962

Not documented G9963
  Visits G9521, G9522
Emergency surgery G9752
Emergent cases M1142
End of life
  Not offered assistance G9382
  Offered assistance G9380
Endometrial ablation/sampling G9822, G9823, G9824
Endovascular stroke treatment G9766, G9767
Episode of care
  Discharge/discontinuation of care M1009-M1014
  Documented M1106, M1107, M1111, M1112, M1116, M1117, M1121, M1122, M1126, M1127, M1131, M1135
  Episode initiated for rehab therapy, medical or chiropractic M1143
  Ongoing care not indicated M1108, M1109, M1110, M1113, M1114, M1115, M1118, M1119, M1120, M1123, M1124, M1125, M1128, M1129, M1130, M1132, M1133, M1134
ESRD (end stage renal disease) documentation G9231
Exposure to ionizing radiation
  Follow-up recommendations G9345, G9347
Filter placement G9539, G9540, G9541, G9542, G9543, G9544
Footwear evaluation
  Not an eligible candidate G8416
  Not performed G8415
  Performed G8410
Frailty, claim/encounter
  Patients age 66 years and older
    Advanced illness diagnosed G2091, G2099, G2101, G2107, G2110
    Dementia medication dispensed G2090, G2098, G2100, G2106, G2109
  Patients age 66-80 years
    Advanced illness diagnosed G2116, G2126
    Dementia medication dispensed G2115, G2127
  Patients age 81 years and older G2118, G2125
Functional outcome assessment
  Documented G8542, G9227
    Positive G8539, G8543
  Not documented
    Patient not eligible for G8540
    Reason not given G8541
Functional status
  Measured G2142-G2145, M1045, M1046
  Not measured M1043, M1049, M1141
  Not performed, reason NOS G9918
  Patient unable to complete/refuses G9726-G9737
  Performed once in last 12 months G9916
  Risk adjusted scoring G8647-G8670
Health-related quality of life assessment G9634, G9635, G9636
HCV (Hepatitis C virus) infection screening
  One time screening
    Not received
      Medical reason G9452
      Patient reason G9453
      Reason not documented G9454
    Received G9451
  Within 12 months
    Not received
      Medical reason G9384
      Patient reason G9385
      Reason not documented G9386
    Received G9383
Hepatitis B status G9504

Ⓝ **New index entry**

Hepatitis C
  Treatment options not discussed G9400
Hepatocellular cancer screening (HCC)
  Abdominal imaging G9455
    Not performed G9457
  Not ordered or performed
    Medical or patient reason G9456
High risk medication
  At least two different medications
    Not ordered G9368
    Ordered G9367
History
  Blood transfusion before 1992 G9449
  Colectomy or colorectal cancer G9711
  Hypercholesterolemia, familial or pure dx G9782
  Injection drug use G9450
Home health agency (HHA) clinical social worker services G0155
Hospice
  Services of clinical social worker G0155
  Services used during measurement pd G9687, G9688, G9690-G9694, G9700, G9702, G9707, G9709, G9710, G9713-G9715, G9718, G9720, G9725, G9740, G9741, G9758, G9760, G9761, G9768, G9805, G9809, G9858-G9861
Hospital readmission
  No unplanned G9309
  Unplanned G9310
Hospital services
  Number of ED or inpatient admissions G9521, G9522
Human epidermal growth factor receptor 2 (HER2/neu)
  Positive G9830
HPV (human papillomavirus) vaccine G9806, G9807
  Did not receive three G9763
  Received three G9762
Hypertension
  Active diagnosis G9744
  Follow-up documented G8950, G9745
  Follow-up not documented
    Reason not given G8952
Hysterectomy G9774
Imaging G9548, G9549, G9550
Imaging of head (CT or MRI) G9537, M1027-M1031
Induction, medical indication G9361
Influenza vaccination
  Administered G8482
  Not administered G8483, G8484
Institutional special needs plans (SNP) G2081, G2105, G2108, G9898, G9901, G9910, G9938
Intensive care unit (ICU)
  Admit G9853
  Not admitted G9854
Intervention, anastomosis leak
  Not required G9305
  Required G9306
Intraoperative cystoscopy G9606, G9607, G9608
LDL level G9663, G9666
Left ventricular ejection fraction (LVEF)
  Less than 40% G8451, G8694, G8923, G8934
Leg pain
  Measured G2140, G2141, G2146, G2147
  Not measured G9949, M1052
Long-term residential care T2048
Lymph node biopsy
  Not performed G8880
    Reason not documented G8882
  Performed G8878
Mastectomy G9708

Medical visit
  1 medical visit/6 month period
    Had visit G9247
    No visit G9246
  Hospital outpatient clinic visit G0463
Medication list updated or reviewed
  Documented G8427
  Not documented G8428, G8430
Meningococcal vaccine dose G9414, G9415
Metastatic disease G9838, G9842
Mitotic rate
  Patient category included G9428
  Patient category not included G9431
    Medical reason G9429
MRS score G9646, G9647, G9648
Multimodal pain management
  Not used
    Medical reason for not using documented G2149
    Performance not met G2150
  Used
    Performance met G2148
Nerve block, peripheral (PNB) G9770
Neurological examination, lower extremity G8404, G8405
Non-small-cell lung cancer
  Classification documented G9422
  Classification not documented G9425
    Medical reason G9423
  Specimen site, other than lung
    Not non-small-cell lung cancer G9424
    Not primary non-small-cell lung cancer G9420
Nutrition therapy G0270, G0271
Opioid therapy G9561, G9562, G9563, G9577, G9578, G9579, G9583, G9584, G9585
Opioid use disorders M1032-M1036
Osteoporosis
  Therapy not prescribed G8635
Otology
  Patient
    Not eligible for referral G8857
  Referral
    Not performed G8858
    Performed G8856
Pain
  Level within 48 hours
    Comfortable G9250
    Not comfortable G9251
Paranasal sinus CT
  At diagnosis
    Not ordered G9350
    Ordered G9348
    Received within 28 days G9349
Partial hospitalization services S0201
Patient admit palliative care M1017
Patient care survey, not completed G0914
Patient death G9751, G9812, G9846, G9852, G9859
Patient decision making
  Documented G9296
  Not documented G9297
Patient diagnosed
  Cancer, active or history, M1018
  Degenerative neurological condition G2151
  Lumbar spine condition M1041, M1051
  Sterile, female M1016
  With competing URI diagnosis G8709
Patient health questionnaire 9 (PHQ-9) G9509, G9510, G9511
Patient referral oth provider/specialist
  Referred G9968

Merit-based Incentive Payment System (MIPS)

Referred/report not received G9970
Referred/report received G9969
Patient refused to participate G2022, G9726, G9728, G9730, G9732, G9734, G9736
Patient survey
  Satisfaction survey G0917
  Score G9603, G9604, G9605
Patient survival G9787, G9813
Patient-specific risk assessment G9316, G9317
Patient treatment/final eval complete M1009-M1014
Patient unable to report G9727, G9729, G9731, G9733, G9735, G9737
PDC G9512, G9513
Performance met
  Multimodal pain management G2148-G2150
  Residual change score
    Equal or greater than zero G2152
    Less than zero G2167
Pharmacological therapy
  Not prescribed G8635
  Prescribed G8633
Physical examination
  Preventive G0402
Positive airway pressure therapy
  Objective measurement G8851
    Not performed G8855
      Reason given G8854
  Prescribed G8852
Postpartum
  Evaluation/screening not performed G9358
  Evaluation/screening performed G9357
Prednisone G2112, G2113
Pregnancy G9778
Pregnancy, transabdominal/transvaginal ultrasound G8806
Preoperative no smoking instructions given G9497
Primary non-small cell lung cancer
  Classification documented G9418
  Classification not documented G9421
    Medical reason G9419
Prolonged intubation
  Not required G8570
  Required G8569
Prostate cancer recurrence risk G8465, G9706
Psoriasis G9649, G9651, G9764
Psychosis, depression, anxiety, apathy, and impulse control disorder
  Assessed G2121
  Not assessed G2122
Psychotherapy, group G0410, G0411
Pulmonary nodule, incidental G9754
Radiation exposure G9500, G9501
Reexploration, postoperative mediastinal bleeding
  Not required G8578
  Required G8577
Renal failure/dialysis
  Development postoperatively G8575
  No development postoperatively G8576
Renal lesion G9547
Renal transplant documentation G9231
Retina
  Dilated macular or fundus exam performed G8397
Return to the operating room G9514, G9515, G9516, G9517
  No return G9307
  Unplanned return G9308
  Within 90 days G9514, G9515, G9516, G9517
Rhabdomyolysis dx G9780

Risk factor evaluation (venous thromboembolic and cardiovascular)
  Evaluated G9298
  Not evaluated G9299
Safety concern
  Negative G9923
  No screen, reason NOS G9925
  Positive with recommendations G9922
  Positive w/o recommendations G9926
Screening
  Negative G9920
  Not performed G9921
  Partial G9921
  Positive no recommendations G9921
  Positive with recommendations G9919
Screening Examinations G0101, G0102, G0105, G0106, G0108, G0120-G0122
Sexually transmitted disease
  Not screened
    Reason not given G9230
  Screened
    Results documented G9228
    Results not documented G9229
Sinusitis
  Due to bacterial infection G9364
Social work and psychological services G0409
Specimen site, other than
  Cutaneous location G9430
  Esophagus G8797
  Prostate G8798
Spine
  Additional procedure(s) same date as lumbar discectomy/laminotomy G9942, G9948, M1071
  Lumbar
    Acute Fracture G9945, M1041, M1051
    Cancer G9945, M1041, M1051
    Infection G9945, M1041, M1051
    Scoliosis G9945, M1041, M1051
Spirometry
  FEV1/FVC < 70%, FEV1 < 60% predicted G8924
Statin not prescribed, medical reasons G9940
Statin therapy G9796, G9797
Substance abuse G9518
Surgical, silicone oil G9756, G9757
Surgical site infection G9311, G9312
Systemic antimicrobials
  Not prescribed G9959
  Prescribed G9961
  Prescribed, medical reasons documented G9960
TB screen G9932, M1003-M1005
Tetanus, diphtheria, pertussis vaccine (Tdap)
  No vaccine G9417
  One vaccine G9416
Thyroid nodule G9552, G9554, G9555, G9556
Tobacco cessation intervention
  Identified user G9906
  Identified user, not provided, medical reason G9909
  Not provided, medical reason G9907
  Not provided, reason not given G9908
Tobacco use G9642, G9643, G9644, G9645, G9791, G9792
  Current nonuser G9459
  Tobacco cessation intervention
    Not performed G9460
    Received G9458
Tobacco user screen
  Not screened, medical reason G9904
  Not screened, reason not given G9905

Ⓝ New index entry

Screen Identified Non-user G9903
Screen Identified User G9902
tPA G8600, G8601, G8602
Treatment choices
Documentation of discussion G9399
No documentation of discussion G9401
Tuberculosis screen negative or managed positive
Documentation G9359
Not documented G9360
Ultrasound, transabdominal or transvaginal
Not performed, no reason given G8808
Not performed, reason documented G8807
Ureteral injury G9631, G9632, G9633
Uterine cancer screening G9618, G9620
Viral load G9242, G9243
Visual function
Achieved G0913
Not achieved G0915
Vomiting
Post-operative G9954
Warfarin or other anticoagulant
Not prescribed, reason documented G9927
Not prescribed, reason not given G9928
Wellness visit
Initial G0438
Subsequent G0439
Meropenem and vaborbactam J2186
Meropenem, injection J2185
Mesh (implantable) C1781
Mesna, injection J9209
Metacarpophalangeal joint, prosthetic implant L8630, L8631
Metaproterenol sulfate, inhalation solution
Concentrated J7667, J7668
Unit dose J7669, J7670
Metaraminol bitartrate, injection J0380
Metastatic disease G9838, G9842
Metatarsal joint, prosthetic implant L8641
Meter, bath conductivity, dialysis E1550
Methacholine chloride J7674
Methadone HCI, injection J1230
Methadone, oral S0109
Medthadone, take home supply G2078
Methocarbamol, injection J2800
Methotrexate sodium J9250, J9260
Methotrexate, oral J8610
Methyldopate HCI, injection J0210
Methylene blue Q9968
Methylergonovine maleate J2210
Methylnaltrexone, injection J2212
Methylprednisolone
Acetate, injection
20 mg J1020
40 mg J1030
80 mg J1040
Oral J7509
Sodium succinate J2920, J2930
Methylprednisolone acetate, injection
Metoclopramide HCI, injection J2765
Metronidazole S0030
MFN drug model add-on M1145 Ⓝ
Micafungin sodium J2248
Microinfusion, transcatheter intraoperative blood vessel C9759 Ⓝ
Midazolam HCI J2250
Mifepristone, oral S0190
Mileage, ambulance A0380, A0390
Milrinone lactate J2260

Mini-bus, nonemergency transportation A0120
Minocycline hydrochloride J2265
Minoxidil S0139
Miscellaneous therapeutic items and supplies T1999
Misoprostol, oral S0191
Mitomycin J7315, J9280, J9281 Ⓝ
Mitoxantrone HCI J9293
Mitral Stenosis G9746
Mobility, see also **Wheelchair**
Device, power operated K0800-K0812, K0899
Resource-inten svc during office visit G0501
Model participant refuses service G2022
Moderate sedation endo serv >5yrs G0500
Mogamulizumab-kpkc J9204
Moisture exchanger, mechanical ventilation A4483
Moisturizer, skin A6250
Molecular pathology G0452
Mometasone furoate sinus implant C9122 Ⓝ
Monitor
Blood glucose E0607
Blood pressure A4670
Pacemaker E0610, E0615
Monitoring feature/device A9279
Morcellator C1782
Morphine sulfate J2270, S0093
Epidural or intrathecal use J2274
Mouthpiece (for respiratory equipment) A4617
Moxetumomab pasudotox-tdfk J9313
Moxifloxacin, injection J2280
MRCP (magnetic resonance cholangiopancreatography) S8037
MRS score G9646, G9647, G9648
Mucoprotein, blood P2038
Mucus trap S8210
Multiaxial ankle prothesis L5986
Multidisciplinary services H2000-H2001, T1025, T1026
Multiple post collar, cervical L0180-L0200
Multi Podus® type AFO L4396
Muromonab-CD3 J7505
MVASI™ Q5107
Mycophenolate mofetil J7517
Mycophenolic acid J7518
MyOwn Skin™ Q4226
Myringotomy, laser-assisted S2225

N

Nabilone J8650
Nafcillin sodium S0032
Nail trimming S0390
Dystrophic G0127
Nalbuphine HCI, Injection J2300
Naloxone HCI J2310
Naltrexone J2315
Nandrolone decanoate J2320
Narrowing device, wheelchair E0969
Nasal application device A7034
Nasal endoscopy, postop debridement S2342
Nasal pillows/seals (for nasal application device) A7035
Nasal vaccine inhalation J3530
Nasogastric tubing B4081, B4082
Natalizumab J2323
National committee for quality assurance G9148, G9149, G9150
Nebulizer
Aerosol compressor E0572
Aerosol mask A7015
Corrugated tubing, disposable A7010

Filter, disposable A7013
Filter, nondisposable A7014
Glass or autoclavable plastic bottle E0580
Heater E1372
Large volume, disposable, prefilled A7008
Large volume, disposable, unfilled A7007
Not used with oxygen, durable, glass A7017
Pneumatic, administration set A7003, A7005, A7006
Pneumatic, nonfiltered A7004
Small volume A7003-A7005
Ultrasonic
    Dome and mouthpiece A7016
    Large volume E0575
    Reservoir bottle, nondisposable A7009
Ultrasonic/electronic E0574
Water collection device, large volume nebulizer A7012
With compressor and/or heater E0570, E0575, E0585
Necitumumab injection J9295
Needle A4215
Biopsy, prostate, pathology G0416
Noncoring A4212
Power bone marrow biopsy C1830
With syringe A4206-A4209
Negative pressure wound therapy pump E2402
Accessories A6550
Nelarabine, injection J9261
Neonatal transport, ambulance, base rate A0225
Neopatch™ Q4176
Neostigmine methylsulfate, injection J2710
Neox® Q4148, Q4156
Nerve stimulator with batteries E0765
Nesiritide injection J2325
Netupitant and palonosetron J8655
Neurological examination G8404, G8405
Neuromuscular
Not performed G2179 Ⓝ
Stimulation E0764, L8680
Stimulator E0745
Neurostimulator
Battery recharging system
    Replacement only L8695
Generator, nonrechargeable C1767, C1823, C1825 Ⓝ
    With rechargeable battery and charging system C1820, C1822
Implantable L8679-L8689
Lead (implantable) C1778
    Test kit C1897
Patient programmer C1787
Pulse generator replacement L8681
Receiver and/or transmitter C1816, L8682, L8683, L8684
Next Generation ACO model, image analysis G9868, G9869, G9870
Nitrogen N-13 ammonia, diagnostic A9526
Nivestym™ Q5110
Nivolumab J9299
Nonchemotherapy drug, not otherwise specified (NOS) J8499
Noncovered
Item or services A9270
Procedure G0293, G0294
Nonemergency transportation A0080-A0210
Nonimpregnated gauze dressing A6216-A6221, A6402-A6404
Nonprescription drug A9150
Non small cell lung cancer G9282-G9291
Not medically necessary service S9986
Not otherwise classified (NOC) drug J3490, J7599, J7699, J7799, J9999, Q0181

Novachor Q4194
Novafix™ Q4208, Q4254 Ⓝ
NPH insulin J1815
NTIOL (new technology intraocular lens)
Category 4 Q1004
Category 5 Q1005
Nursing care, in home T1030, T1031
Nursing services T1000-T1005, T1030, T1031
NuShield® Q4160
Nusinersen injection J2326
Nutrition
Enteral infusion pump B9002
Parenteral infusion pump B9004, B9006
Parenteral solution B4164-B5200
Therapy G0270, G0271

O

O&P (orthotics and prosthetics) L0112-L9900
Component L9900
Obizur® J7188
Observation service G0378, G0379
Occipital/mandibular support, cervical L0160
Occlusive device placement G0269
Ocrelizumab injection J2350
Ocriplasmin J7316
Octafluoropropane Q9956
Octagam® J1568
Octreotide acetate J2353, J2354
Ocular
Device, intraoperative, detached retina C1784
Implant, aqueous drainage assist device C1783
Prosthetic implant L8610
Ocularist evaluation S9150
Ofatumumab, injection J9302
Ofloxacin S0034
Olanzapine, injection J2358, S0166
Olaratumab injection J9285
Omacetaxine mepesuccinate J9262
Omadacycline J0121
Omalizumab J2357
Omnicardiogram/cardiointegram S9025
Onabotulinumtoxin A J0585
Onasemnogene abeparvovec-xioi J3399 Ⓝ
Oncology G9050-G9139, G9678
Ondansetron HCl J2405
Ondansetron oral Q0162, S0119
One arm drive attachment, manual wheelchair E0958
Online assessment by qualified nonphysician healthcare professional G2061-G2063
Opioid therapy G9561, G9562, G9563, G9577, G9578, G9579, G9583, G9584, G9585
Opioid Use Disorder
Evaluation and Treatment G2076-G2080
Treatment (Office Based) G2086-G2088
Oprelvekin, injection J2355
Oral device/appliance E0485, E0486
Oral interface A7047
Oral/nasal mask A7027
Nasal pillows A7029
Oral cushion A7028
Oritavancin J2407
Oropharyngeal suction catheter A4628
Orphenadrine citrate, injection J2360
Orthopedic shoes
Arch support L3040-L3090
Footwear L3201-L3265

Insert L3000-L3030
Joint L3956
Lift L3300-L3334
Miscellaneous additions L3500-L3595, L3649
Positioning device L3140-L3170
Transfer L3600-L3649
Wedge L3340-L3420
Orthotic additions
Carbon/graphite lamination L2755
Fracture
Lower extremity L2180-L2192
Upper extremity L3980-L3999, L3995
Halo L0859
Knee joint L2405-L2492
Lower extremity L2200-L2999
Ratchet lock L2430
Scoliosis L1010-L1120, L1210-L1290
Shoe L3300-L3595, L3649
Spinal L0970-L0999
Upper limb E2631, E2632, E2633, L3995
Orthotic devices, *see also* **Orthopedic shoes**
Ankle-foot (AFO) E1815, E1816, E1830, L1900-L1990, L2106-L2116, L3160, L4361
Anterior-posterior-lateral L0700, L0710
Cervical L0112-L0200
Cervical-thoracic-lumbar-sacral (CTLSO) L0700, L0710
Elbow (EO) E1801, L3702-L3762
Elbow-wrist-hand-finger (EWHFO) L3763-L3766
Finger L3925, L3927, L3933, L3935
Fracture L2106-L2136, L3917, L3980-L3999
Halo L0810-L0861
Hand L3917-L3919
Hand-finger L3912, L3913, L3921, L3923, L3924, L3929, L3930
Hip (HO) L1600-L1690
Hip-knee-ankle-foot (HKAFO) L2040-L2090
Interface material, replacement E1820
Knee (KO) L1810-L1860
Knee-ankle-foot (KAFO) L2000-L2038, L2126-L2136
Legg Perthes L1700-L1755
Lumbar L0625-L0627, L0641, L0642
Lumber-Sacral L0628-L0640, L0643-L0651
Multiple post collar, cervical L0180-L0200
Not otherwise specified (NOS) L0999, L1499, L2999, L3999, L5999, L7499, L8039
Pneumatic splint L4350-L4370
Pronation/supination E1818
Repair or replacement L4000-L4210
Replacement, soft interface material L4392, L4394
Sacral L0621-L0624
Scoliosis L1000-L1120, L1300-L1499
Shoulder (SO) L3650-L3678
Shoulder-elbow-wrist-hand (SEWHO) L3960-L3978
Side bar disconnect L2768
Spinal, cervical L0120-L0200
Thoracic-lumbar-sacral (TLSO) L0220, L0450-L0492, L0970-L0999, L1200-L1290
Toe E1830, E1831
Wrist-hand L3905-L3908, L3915, L3916
Wrist-hand-finger (WHFO) E1805, E1825, L3806-L3904, L3931
Orthotic and prosthetic services L8690-L9900
Orthovisc® J7324
Ossicular prosthetic implant L8613
Osteogenesis stimulator E0747-E0749, E0760
Osteotomy, periacetabular S2115
Ostomy
Absorbent material sheet A4422

Belt A4396
Convex insert, accessory A5093
Incontinence supply, miscellaneous A4335
Miscellaneous supply A4421
Pouches and supplies A4361-A4435, A5051-A5093
Skin barrier A4405-A4435
Otologic evaluation/active drainage G8559-G8568
Outpatient PPS hospital services C1713-C9899
Oxacillin sodium, injection J2700
Oxaliplatin, injection J9263
Oximeter device A4606, E0445
Oxygen
Ambulance supply A0422
Battery charger E1357
Battery pack/cartridge E1356
Chamber, hyperbaric, topical A4575
Concentrator E1390, E1391, E1392
Contents S8120, S8121
DC power adapter E1358
Delivery systems and supplies E0424-E0487, E1352-E1406
Liquid oxygen system, portable, rental E0433
Mask A4620
Portable E0447, K0738
Probe A4606
Rack/stand E1355
Regulator E1352, E1353
Respiratory equipment/supplies A4611-A4627, E0424-E0480
Tent E0455
Tubing, per foot A4616
Water vapor enriching system E1405, E1406
Wheeled cart E1354
Oxymorphone HCl, injection J2410
Oxytetracycline HCl, injection J2460
Oxytocin, injection J2590

P

Pacemaker
Lead
Combination (implantable) C1899
Other C1898
Transvenous VDD C1779
Monitor
Audible and visible check systems E0610
Digital/visible check systems E0615
Non-rate-responsive (implantable)
Dual chamber C2619
Single chamber C2620
Other than single or dual chamber (implantable) C2621
Rate-responsive (implantable)
Dual chamber C1785
Single chamber C1786
Pacemaker monitor E0610, E0615
Paclitaxel protein-bound particles, injection J9264
Paclitaxel, injection J9267
Pad
Cold, fluid circulating with pump E0218
Gel pressure E0185, E0196
Heat
Electric E0210, E0215
Replacement E0249
Water circulating with pump E0217
Orthotic device interface E1820
Sheepskin E0188, E0189
Pail or pan, for use with commode chair E0167

Palifermin, injection J2425
Paliperidone palmitate, injection J2426
Palonosetron HCl, injection J2469
Pamidronate disodium, injection J2430
Panitumumab, injection J9303
Pantoprazole sodium S0164
Papanicolaou (Pap) screening smear P3000, P3001, Q0091
Papaverine HC, injection J2440
Paraffin bath unit E0235
Paraffin, per pound A4265
Paramedic intercept A0432, S0207, S0208
Parenteral nutrition B4164-B5200
    Additives B4216
    Administration kit B4224
    Infusion pump
        Enteral nutrition, any type B9002
        Portable B9004
        Stationary B9006
    Solution and supplies B4164-B4199, B5000-B5200
        Amino acid
            3.5% B4168
            5.5% through 7% B4172
            7% through 8.5% B4176
            Greater than 8.5% B4178
        Carbohydrates
            50% or less B4164
            Greater than 50% B4180
        Compounded amino acid and carbohydrates
            10 to 51 grams B4189
            52 to 73 grams B4193
            74 to 100 grams B4197
            Hepatic B5100
            Renal B5000
            Stress B5200
        Lipids B4185
        Omegaven B4187
    Supplies, not otherwise classified (NOC) B9999
    Supply kit
        Home mix, per day B4222
        Premix, per day B4220
Paricalcitol, injection J2501
Parking fee, nonemergency transport A0170
Partial hospitalization services S0201
Pasireotide J2502
Paste, conductive A4558
Pathology and laboratory
    Services P2028-P9615
    Tests, miscellaneous P9010-P9615
Patient diagnosed
    With competing comorbid condition G2175 Ⓝ
Patient education
    Back school S9117
    Classes S9436-S9454
    Face-to-face for CKD G0420,G0421
Patient not ambulatory G9719, G9721, M1068
Patient not eligible for exam G2178, G2180 Ⓝ
Patient support system E0636
Patient survey G0917, G9603, G9604, G9605
Patient transfer system E1035, E1036
Patisiran injection J0222
PDC G9512, G9513
PEFR (peak expiratory flow rate)
    Meter A4614, S8096
    Physician services S8110
Pegademase bovine, injection J2504
Pegaptanib, injection J2503
Pegaspargase, injection J9266

Pegfilgrastim, injection J2505, Q5108, Q5111, Q5120, Q5122 Ⓝ
Peginesatide, injection J0890
Pegloticase, injection J2507
Pegylated interferon alfa-2a S0145
Pegylated interferon alfa-2b S0148
Pelvic
    Belt/harness/boot E0944
    Bone fracture treatment G0412, G0413, G0414, G0415
Pembrolizumab J9271
Pemetrexed, injection J9304, J9305 Ⓝ
Penicillin G
    Benzathine J0561
    Benzathine and procaine J0558
    Potassium J2540
    Procaine, aqueous J2510
Penile prosthesis
    Inflatable C1813
    Noninflatable C2622
Pentamidine isethionate
    Inhalation solution J2545, J7676
    Injection S0080
Pentastarch, 10% solution, injection J2513
Pentazocine HCl, injection J3070
Pentobarbital sodium, injection J2515
Pentostatin, injection J9268
Peramivir J2547
Percussor, electric or pneumatic E0480
Percutaneous access system A4301
Percutaneous transluminal coronary atherectomy
    Each additional branch C9603
    Single major coronary artery C9602
Percutaneous transluminal revascularization
    Acute occlusion, single vessel C9606
    Chronic total occlusion, single vessel C9607
        Each additional coronary artery or branch C9608
    Each additional branch C9605
    Single vessel C9604
Perflexane lipid microspheres, injection Q9955
Perflutren lipid microspheres, injection Q9957
Peroneal strap L0980
Peroxide or alcohol A4244
Perphenazine
    Injection J3310
    Oral Q0175
Personal care
    Item, not otherwise specified (NOS) S5199
    Services T1019, T1020, T1021
Pertuzumab, injection J9306, J9316 Ⓝ
Pessary
    Nonrubber A4562
    Rubber A4561
Pharmacy fees Q0510-Q0514
PET scan G0219, G0235, G0252, S8085
Phenobarbital sodium, injection J2560
Phentolamine mesylate, injection J2760
Phenylephrine and ketorolac J1097
Phenylephrine HCl, injection J2370
Phenytoin sodium, injection J1165
pHisoHex® solution A4246
Photofrin® (porfimer sodium) J9600
Phototherapy light E0202
PHQ-9 (patient health questionnaire 9) score G9393, G9395, G9396, G9509, G9510, G9511
Physical examination
    Preventive G0402
    School, college S0622
Physical therapy, maintenance S8990

Ⓝ **New index entry**

Physician
Certification/recertification G0179, G0180
Remote eval image from patient G2010
Remote in home E/M
CMS Innovation Center demonstration project
G9481-G9489, G9490
Bundled Payments for Care Improvement Advanced
(BPCI Advanced) model G9978-G9982,
G9983-G9986, G9987
Service for a power mobility device G0372
Supervision G0181, G0182
Phytonadione J3430
Pinworm examination Q0113
Piperacillin sodium S0081
Piperacillin sodium/tazobactam sodium J2543
Placement, intracoronary stent, drug eluting
Each additional branch C9601
Single major coronary artery or branch C9600
Plasma
Multiple donor, pooled, frozen P9023, P9070, P9071
Single donor, fresh frozen P9017
Plastazote L3002, L3252, L3253, L3265, L5654-L5658
Platelet
Concentrate, each unit P9019
Rich plasma, each unit P9020
Platform attachment
Forearm crutch E0153
Walker E0154
Plazomicin injection J0291
Plerixafor J2562
Plicamycin J9270
Plumbing, for home ESRD equipment A4870
Pneumatic
Appliance E0655-E0673, L4350-L4370
Compressor, compression device E0650-E0652, E0675
Splint L4370
Ventricular assist device Q0480-Q0506
Pneumatic nebulizer, small volume
Administration set
Filtered A7006
Nonfiltered A7003, A7005
Nonfiltered, disposable A7004
Pneumocystis jiroveci G9223
Pneumococcal screening G9279
Polatuzumab vedotin-piiq J9309
Polycyte™ Q4241 Ⓝ
Porfimer, injection J9600
Port, indwelling C1788
Portable
Hemodialyzer system E1635
Liquid oxygen system E0433
X-ray equipment Q0092
X-ray equipment transfer R0070-R0076
Positioning hardware, wheelchair back E2398
Positioning seat T5001
Positive airway pressure device, accessories
Chin strap A7036
Cushion, nasal mask interface A7032
Exhalation port A7045
Filter
Disposable A7038
Nondisposable A7039
Full face mask A7030
Interface replacement A7031
Head gear A7035
Humidifier E0561, E0562
Nasal interface, mask or cannula A7034
Oral interface A7044
Pillow, nasal cannula interface A7033
Tubing A7037
Positive airway pressure therapy G8850
Positive expiratory pressure device E0484
Post-coital examination Q0115
Postural drainage board E0606
Potassium chloride J3480
Potassium hydroxide (KOH) preparation Q0112
Pouch
Fecal collection A4330
Ostomy A4375-A4378, A5051-A5054, A5061-A5073
Urinary A4379-A4383, A5071-A5073
Power operated vehicles K0800-K0812
Pralatrexate J9307
Pralidoxime chloride J2730
Pre-admission screening T2010, T2011
Prednisolone
Acetate J2650
Oral J7510
Prednisone G2112, G2113, J7512
Prefabricated splint
Digit S8450
Elbow S8452
Wrist or ankle S8451
Pregnancy, home management S9208-S9214
Prehensile actuator L7040
Prenatal care services H1000-H1005
Home delivery, supplies S8415
Preparatory prosthesis L5510-L5595
Prescription, *see also* **Appendix A: Table of Drugs**
Chemotherapeutic, not otherwise specified (NOS) J8999
Nonchemotherapeutic, not otherwise specified (NOS)
J8499
Pressure
Alarm, dialysis E1540
Mattress, pads, and other supplies A4640, E0181-E0199
Pump for pressure pad E0182
Sensor, pulmonary artery, implantable wireless C2624
Preventive services, prolonged G0513, G0514
Privigen® J1459
Probe
Cryoablation C2618
Percutaneous lumbar discectomy C2614
Robotic, water-jet C2596
Procainamide HCl J2690
Procarbazine hydrochloride, oral S0182
Procenta® Q4244 Ⓝ
Prochlorperazine J0780
Prochlorperazine maleate Q0164
Non-Medicare S0183
Proctoscopy, screening S0601
Procuren® or similar product S9055
ProgenaMatrix™ Q4222
Progestasert® IUD S4989
Progesterone, injection J2675
Prolonged preventive services G0513, G0514
Prolotherapy M0076
Promazine HCl J2950
Promethazine and meperidine J2180
Promethazine HCl
Injection J2550
Oral Q0169
Propofol J2704
Propranolol HCl J1800
Prostate, risk of recurrence G8465
Prosthesis
Artificial larynx battery/accessory L8505
Breast C1789, L8000-L8039, L8600

Donning sleeve L7600
Ear L8613-L8629
Eye L8608-L8612, V2623-V2629
Facial/external ear L8040-L8049
Fitting L5400-L5460, L6380-L6388
Foot/ankle L5000-L5020, L5968-L5999, L8641, L8642
Hand/wrist L6000-L6026, L6050-L6055, L8630, L8631,
    L8658, L8659
    Electric L7007, L7008
Hip L5250, L5270
Hook, electric L7009, L7045
Implants L8600-L8690
Iris C1839
Knee L5100-L5230, L5500, L5505
Larynx L8500
Lower extremity L5280-L5341, L5700-L5999, L8641, L8642
Maxillofacial, provided by a nonphysician L8040-L8048
Miscellaneous service L8499
Penile C1813, L7900, L7902
Preparatory L5510-L5600, L6580-L6590
Protective covers L5704-L5707
Repair L7510, L7520, L8049
Replacement socket L5700-L5703, L6883-L6885
Services, unlisted L8499
Socks (shrinker, sheath, stump sock) L8400-L8485
Tracheo-esophageal L8507, L8509
Upper extremity L6000-L6570, L7499
Vacuum erection system L7900
Voice L8500-L8515
Prosthetic additions
Lower extremity L5610-L5699, L5710-L5966
Upper extremity L6600-L7405
Prosthetic and orthotic services L8690-L9900
Prosthetic socket insert, gasket or seal L7700
Protamine sulfate J2720
Protectant, skin A6250
Protector, heel or elbow E0191
Protein C concentrate J2724
Protirelin J2725
Psoriasis G9649, G9651, G9764
Psychiatric collaborative care model, RHC/FQHC G0512
Psychological services G0409-G0411
Pulmonary nodule, incidental G9754
Pulmonary rehabilitation G0424, S9473
Pulse generator system, inner ear A4638, E2120
Pump
Alternating pressure pad E0182
Ambulatory infusion E0779, E0781
Ambulatory insulin E0784, E0787
    Supplies A4230, A4232
Blood, dialysis E1620
Breast E0602-E0604
Enteral infusion B9002
Heparin infusion E1520
Implantable infusion E0782, E0783
    Refill kit A4220
Negative pressure wound therapy E2402
Parenteral infusion B9004, B9006
Suction, respiratory E0600
Suction, urine K1005
Water circulating pad E0236
Pumps, monitors, and supplies E2000-E2120, K0455-K0605
PuraPly® Q4195-Q4197
Purification system, water E1610, E1615
Pyridoxine HCl J3415

Q

Quad cane E0105
Qualified nonphysician healthcare professional online assessment G2061-G2063
Quality of life assessment G9634, G9635, G9636
Quinupristin/dalfopristin J2770

R

Rack/stand, oxygen E1355
Radiation
Exposure G9500, G9501
Intensity modulated G6015
Intra-fraction localization and tracking G6017
Therapy services G6001-G6017
Treatment delivery
    1 area G6003, G6004, G6005, G6006
    2 areas G6007, G6008, G6009, G6010
    3 or more areas G6011, G6012, G6013, G6014
Radiesse® Q2026
Radioelements for brachytherapy Q3001
Radiology, portable equipment transport R0070-R0076
Radiopharmaceuticals A4641, A4642, A9500-A9700
Not otherwise classified A4641, A9698
Rail
Bathtub E0241, E0242, E0246
Bed side, full length E0310
Bed side, half length E0305
Toilet E0243
Ramucirumab J9308
Range of motion assist device
Powered L8701-L8702
Ranibizumab J2778
Ranitidine hydrochloride J2780
Rasburicase J2783
Ras Testing G9843
Not performed G9841
Performed G9840
Ravulizumab-cwvz J1303
Reaching/grabbing device A9281
Reagent strip
Blood glucose A4253
Blood ketone A4252
Urine A4250
Reciprocating peritoneal dialysis system E1630
Rectal control system A4563
Recorder, event, cardiac C1764
Red blood cells P9021, P9022
Red congo, blood P2029
Referral to appropriate resources G2186 Ⓝ
Refusal to participate, patient G2209 Ⓝ
Regadenoson J2785
Reguard Q4255 Ⓝ
Regular insulin J1815
Regulator, oxygen E1353
Rehabilitation
Cardiac G0422, G0423, S9472
Devices, extension/flexion E1800-E1841
Program H2001
Psychosocial rehabilitation services H2017, H2018
Pulmonary G0424, S9473
Vestibular S9476
Remission G9509, G9510
Renal dialysis
Acute kidney injury G0491-G0492
Renflexis® Q5104

Ⓝ **New index entry**

Repair
    Contract, ESRD A4890
    Device, urinary A4890
        With sling graft C1771
    DME (durable medical equipment)
        Other than oxygen equipment K0739
        Oxygen equipment K0740
    Fetal
        In utero procedures S2400, S2401, S2402, S2403,
            S2404, S2409
        Sacrococcygeal teratoma S2405
    Maxillofacial prosthesis
        Labor component L8049
Replacement
    Batteries A4233-A4236, A4601, A4602, A4630
    Orthotic components L4000-L4130
    Pad (alternating pressure) A4640
    Parts A4630-A4640
    Temporary, pt owned equipment K0462
    Tip for cane, crutches, walker A4637
    Underarm pad for crutches A4635
Reproductive medicine services S4011-S4989
Reslizumab injection J2786
Respiratory procedures, therapeutic G0237, G0238, G0239
Residential care, long-term T2048
Respiratory supplies and equipment A4611-A4629
Respite care services H0045
Restorigin™ Q4191, Q4192
Restraint, any type E0710
Resuscitation bag S8999
Retacrit® Q5105-Q5106
Reteplase J2993
Retinal
    Diabetic indicator eye exam S3000
    Prosthesis C1841, C1842
    Tamponade device C1814
Retrieval device, insertable C1773
Return to the operating room G9514, G9515, G9516, G9517
Revascularization of tibial/peroneal arteries
    With intravascular lithotripsy and angioplasty C9772, C9764 Ⓝ
        With arthrectomy C9774, C9766 Ⓝ
        With stent C9773, C9765 Ⓝ
            With arthrectomy C9775, C9767 Ⓝ
Revefenacin inhalation solution J7677
Revita® Q4180
Rhabdomyolysis dx G9780
Rho(D) immune globulin, human J2788, J2790, J2791, J2792
Rib belt, thoracic L0220
Riboflavin 5'-phosphate, ophthalmic solution J2787
Rilonacept J2793
RimabotulinumtoxinB J0587
Ring, ostomy A4404
Ringers lactate infusion J7120
Risperidone J2794, J2798
Rituximab J9312, Q5115, Q5119 Ⓝ
Rituximab and hyaluronidase J9311
Robin-Aids® hand L6000, L6010, L6020, L6708, L6709
Robotic surgical system techniques S2900
Rocking bed E0462
Rolapitant
    Injection J2797
    Oral J8670
Rollabout chair E1031
Romidepsin C9065, J9315 Ⓝ
Romiplostim J2796
Romosozumab-aqqg J3111
Ropivacaine HCl J2795
Routine foot care S0390

    Diabetic patient G0247
    Exam G9502
Rubidium-82 (Rb-82) A9555
Rural Health Clinic or Federally Qualified Health Center (RHC/FQHC) only G0511, G0512

S

Sacituzumab govitecan-hziy J9317 Ⓝ
Sacral nerve stimulation test lead A4290
Safety equipment E0700-E0710
    Vest, wheelchair E0980
Sales tax S9999
Saline solution A4216, J7030-J7050
    Metered dose dispenser A4218
Saliva
    Artificial A9155
    Test, hormone level S3650, S3652
Samarium SM 153 lexidronam A9604
Saquinavir S0140
Sargramostim (GM-CSF) J2820
SARS-COV-2
    Detection U0001-U0005 Ⓝ
    Specimen collection C9803, G2023, G2024 Ⓝ
School-based education program T1018
Scintimammography S8080
Scoliosis, orthoses and procedures L1000-L1499
    Additions L1010-L1290
Score
    MRS G9646, G9647, G9648
    PHQ-9M G9509, G9511
    PHQ-9 score G9393, G9395, G9396, G9509, G9510, G9511
Screening
    Alcohol G0442, G2196-G2199 Ⓝ
    Cancer
        Abdominopelvic G0101-G0105
        Cervical or vaginal G0101
        Colorectal
            Barium enema G0106, G0120, G0122
            Colonoscopy G0105, G0121
            Fecal occult blood test G0328
            Flexible sigmoidoscopy G0104
            Proctoscopy S0601
        Lung, computed tomography G0296
        Prostate, rectal, digital exam G0102
            PSA (prostate specific antigen) test G0103
        Uterine G9618, G9620
    Cytopathology, cervical/vaginal G0123, G0124, G0141, G0143, G0144, G0145, G0147, G0148
    Depression G0444
    Dysphagia V5364
    Glaucoma G0117, G0118
    Hearing V5008
    HCV (Hepatitis C virus) infection G0472
    HIV G0475
    Language V5363
    Lung cancer G0296
    Miscellaneous T1023
    Newborn metabolic panel S3620
    Papanicolaou smear Q0091
        Performed under physician supervision P3000
        Requiring interpretation by physician P3001
    Preadmission
        Level I T2010
        Level II T2011
    Speech V5362-V5364
    TB M1003-M1005

Tobacco user
Identified Non-user G9903
Identified User G9902
Not screened, medical reason G9904
Not screened, reason not given G9905
Sculptra® Q2028
Sealant
Skin A6250
Pulmonary, liquid C2615
Seat
Attachment, walker E0156
Insert, wheelchair E0992
Lift E0621, E0627-E0629
Upholstery E0981, E1297
Sebelipase alfa injection J2840
Secretin J2850
Semen analysis G0027
Sensitivity study, urinary tract infection P7001
Sensory nerve conduction test (SNCT) G0255
Septal defect implant system, intracardiac C1817
Sermorelin acetate Q0515
Serum clotting time tube A4771
Severe acute respiratory syndrome coronavirus 2
Detection U0001-U0005 Ⓝ
Specimen collection C9803, G2023, G2024 Ⓝ
Services provided outside the USA S9989
SEWHO (shoulder, elbow, wrist, hand orthosis) L3960-L3973
SEXA (bone density study) G0130
Sexual activity G9818
Sheath, prosthetic L8400-L8417
Sheepskin pad E0188, E0189
Shoes
Arch support
Nonremovable
Longitudinal L3070
Longitudinal/metatarsal L3090
Metatarsal L3080
Removable
Longitudinal L3040
Longitudinal/metatarsal L3060
Metatarsal L3050
Diabetic
Deluxe feature A5508
Fitting A5500, A5501
Modification A5503, A5504, A5505, A5506
Not otherwise specified (NOS) modification A5507
Insert, removable
Formed to patient foot L3030
Longitudinal arch support, each L3010
Longitudinal/metatarsal support, each L3020
Plastazote or equal, each L3002
Silicone gel, each L3003
Spenco®, each L3001
UCB type, Berkeley shell, each L3000
Lift L3300-L3334
Orthopedic L3201-L3265
Additions
Shoes L3500-L3595
High-top
Child L3206
Infant L3204
Junior L3207
Oxford
Child L3202
Infant L3201
Junior L3203
Positioning device L3140, L3150, L3160, L3170
Transfer, orthosis L3600-L3649

Shoulder
Disarticulation, prosthetic L6300-L6320, L6550
Orthosis (SO) L3650-L3674, L3677, L3678
Spinal, cervical L0120-L0200
Shoulder sling A4566
Shoulder-elbow-wrist-hand orthosis (SEWHO) L3960-L3973
Shrinker L8440-L8465
Shunt
Accessory for dialysis A4740
Interatrial shunt investigational device exemption (IDE) C9758, C9760 Ⓝ
Aqueous, for glaucoma L8612
Sigmoidoscopy, cancer screening G0104, G0106
Sign language/oral interpretive services T1013
Sildenafil citrate S0090
Siltuximab J2860
Sincalide J2805
Sipuleucel-T Q2043
Sirolimus J7520
Sitz bath
Chair E0162
With or without commode E0160
With faucet attachment E0161
Skills training and development H2014
Skin
Barrier, ostomy A4362, A4363, A4369-A4373, A4385, A5120
Adhesive, liquid or equal A4364
Sealant, protectant, moisturizer A6250
Substitutes and biologics C1849, J3590, Q4100-Q4255 Ⓝ
Sleep apnea/symptoms G8839-G8841, G8845, G8846, G8849
Sleep study test, home (HST) G0398, G0399, G0400
Sleeve A4600, L7600
Sling A4565
Patient lift E0621, E0630, E0635
Smoker
Current G9642
Smoking cessation services and supplies
Counseling G9016
Supplies S4990, S4991, S4995
Social work and psychological services G0409
Sock L8417-L8435, L8470-L8485
Body L0984
Prosthetic
Above knee L8430
Below knee L8420
Upper limb L8435
Stump
Above knee L8480
Below knee L8470
Upper limb L8485
Sodium
Ferric gluconate complex in sucrose J2916
Fluoride F-18 A9580
Hyaluronan J7325
Synvisc®, Synvisc One® J7325
Hyaluronate
Euflexxa® J7323
Hyalgan® J7321
Orthovisc® J7324
Supartz® J7321
VISCO-3TM J7333 Ⓝ
Phosphate P32 A9563
Succinate J1720
Solution
Calibrator A4256
Dialysate, test kit A4760

Elliotts B J9175
Enteral formula B4149-B4162
Parenteral nutrition B4164-B5200
Somatrem J2940
Somatropin J2941
Sorbent cartridge, ESRD E1636
Sotalol hydrochloride iv C9482
Specialty absorptive dressing A6251-A6256
Specimen collection C9803, G0471, G2023, G2024 Ⓝ
Spectinomycin HCl J3320
Speech assessment V5362, V5363, V5364
Speech generating device
  Accessory
    Mounting system E2512
    Not otherwise classified E2599
  Digitized speech, pre-recorded messages
    Less than or equal to 8 minutes E2500
    More than 8 minutes, less than or equal to 20 minutes E2502
    More than 20 minutes but less than or equal to 40 minutes E2504
    More than 40 minutes E2506
  Synthesized speech
    Message formulation by spelling E2508
    Multiple methods of message formulation E2510
Speech generating software program E2511
Speech volume modulation system K1009 Ⓝ
Speech therapy
  In home S9128
  Re-evaluation S9152
Sperm procurement and cryopreservation S4030, S4031
Spinal orthosis
  Cervical L0120-L0200
    Multiple post collar L0180-L0200
  Cervical-thoracic-lumbar-sacral (CTLSO) L0700, L0710
  Halo L0810-L0830
  Scoliosis L1000-L1499
Spine/lumbar disc surgery C9757
Spirometer A9284, E0487
Splint A4570
  Dynamic adjustable extension/flexion device
    Ankle E1815
    Elbow/forearm E1800, E1802
    Finger E1825
    Knee E1810, E1812
    Toe E1830
    Wrist E1805
  Finger, static Q4049
  Flexion/abduction/rotation device, shoulder E1840
  Footdrop L4394, L4398
  Hallus-valgus L3100
  Static progressive stretch device
    Shoulder E1841
    Toe E1831
  Supplies, miscellaneous Q4051
Stat laboratory charge S3600, S3601
Static progressive stretch device
  Ankle E1816
  Elbow E1801
  Forearm E1818
  Knee E1811
  Replacement, soft interface material/cuffs E1821
  Wrist E1806
Statin therapy G8815, G8816, G8817, G9507, G9508
Stent C1874-C1877, C2617, C2625
Stereoscopic X-ray guidance G6002
Stereotactic radiosurgery G0339, G0340

Sterile cefuroxime sodium J0697
Sterile diluent for epoprostenol S0155
Sterile water A4216, A4217
Stimulation devices E0720-E0770
Stimulators
  Neuromuscular E0744, E0745
  Osteogenesis
    Electrical E0747, E0748, E0749
    Ultrasound, low intensity E0760
  Salivary reflex E0755
Stocking, gradient compression
  Below knee
    18-30 mmHg A6530
    30-40 mmHg A6531
    40-50 mmHg A6532
  Full length/chap style
    18-30 mmHg A6536
    30-40 mmHg A6537
    40-50 mmHg A6538
  Garter belt A6544
  Not otherwise specified (NOS) A6549
  Thigh length
    18-30 mmHg A6533
    30-40 mmHg A6534
    40-50 mmHg A6535
  Waist length
    18-30 mmHg A6539
    30-40 mmHg A6540
    40-50 mmHg A6541
Stoma absorptive cover A5083
Stomach tube B4083
Stravix ®/Stravixpl ® Q4133
Streptokinase J2995
Streptomycin J3000
Streptozocin J9320
Strip
  Blood glucose test A4253, A4772
  Blood ketone test A4252
  Urine reagent A4250
Strontium-89 chloride A9600
Stump sock L8470, L8480, L8485
Stylet A4212
Substance abuse G9518, S9475
Succinylcholine chloride J0330
Suction pump
  Gastric E2000
  Respiratory E0600
  Urine K1006 Ⓝ
  Wounds, home model K0743
Sulfamethoxazole and trimethoprim S0039
Sulfur hexafluoride lipid microspheres Q9950
Sumatriptan succinate J3030
Supartz® J7321
Supplies, various medical A4450-A4608
  Miscellaneous DME A9900-A9999
  Not otherwise specified (NOS) T5999
Support
  Arch L3040-L3090
  Cervical L0120-L0200
  Stockings A6530-A6549
Supported housing H0043, H0044
SureDerm® Q4220
Surface electromyography (EMG) S3900
Surfactor® Q4233 Ⓝ
Surgical
  Boot L3208-L3211
  Dressing A4461-A4467, A6196-A6403
  Pathology, prostate needle biopsy G0416

SOMATREM - SURGICAL

INDEX TO SERVICES, SUPPLIES, EQUIPMENT, DRUGS

Stocking
  Above knee length A4490
  Below knee length A4500
  Full length A4510
  Thigh length A4495
Silicone oil G9756, G9757
Supplies, miscellaneous A4649
Tray A4550
Surgicord Q4218
Surgigraft Q4183, Q4219
Surgraft® Q4209
Suture removal S0630
Swabs, betadine or iodine A4247
Swivel adapter S8186
Synthetic resorbable dressing A6460-A6461
Synvisc®, Synvisc One® J7325
Syringe A4213
  With needle A4206, A4207, A4208, A4209

T

Tables, for bed E0274, E0315
Tacrine hydrochloride S0014
Tacrolimus
  Extended release J7503
  Oral J7507, J7508
  Parenteral J7525
Tafasitamab-cxix C9070 Ⓝ
Tagraxofusp-erzs J9269
Taliglucerase alfa J3060
Talimogene laherparepvec J9325
Tamoxifen citrate S0187
Tape
  Nonwaterproof A4450
  Waterproof A4452
Targeted
  Case management
    Each 15 minutes T1017
    Per month T2023
Taxi, nonemergency transportation A0100
TBO-filgrastim J1447
Technetium TC 99m
  Apcitide A9504
  Arcitumomab A9568
  Bicisate A9557
  Depreotide A9536
  Disofenin A9510
  Exametazime A9521
  Exametazime labeled autologous white blood cells A9569
  Fanolesomab A9566
  Gluceptate A9550
  Highly enriched Q9969
  Labeled red blood cells A9560
  Macroaggregated albumin A9540
  Mebrofenin A9537
  Medronate A9503
  Mertiatide A9562
  Oxidronate A9561
  Pentetate A9539, A9567
  Pertechnetate A9512
  Pyrophosphate A9538
  Sestamibi A9500
  Sodium gluceptate A9550
  Succimer A9551
  Sulfur colloid A9541
  Teboroxime A9501
  Tetrofosmin A9502
  Tilmanocept A9520

Tedizolid phosphate J3090
Telavancin J3095
Telehealth services G0071
  Consultation G0406-G0408, G0425-G0427, G0508, G0509
  Inpatient pharmacologic management G0459
  Originating site fee Q3014
  Payment G2025 Ⓝ
  Transmission T1014
Temozolomide
  Injection J9328
  Oral J8700
Temsirolimus J9330
Tenecteplase J3101
Teniposide Q2017
TENS (transcutaneous electric nerve stimulation) A4595, E0720-E0749
Tension ring, vacuum erection device L7902
Tent, oxygen E0455
Teprotumumab-trbw J3241 Ⓝ
Terbutaline sulfate
  Inhalation solution, concentrated J7680
  Inhalation solution, unit dose J7681
  Injection J3105
Teriparatide J3110
Terminal devices
  Hook or hand, heavy duty L6721, L6722
  Hook, mechanical, voluntary closing L6707, L6709
    Pediatric L6712, L6714
  Hook, mechanical, voluntary opening L6706, L6708
    Pediatric L6711, L6713
  Multiple articulating digit L6715
  Passive hand/mitt L6703
  Sport/recreational/work attachment L6704
Testosterone
  Cypionate and estradiol cypionate J1071
  Enanthate J3121
  Pellet S0189
  Undecanoate J3145
Tetanus immune globulin, human J1670
Tetracycline J0120
Thallous chloride TI-201 A9505
Theophylline J2810
Therapeutic lightbox A4634, E0203
Therapeutic services and supplies C9725-C9899, G0127-G0372, T1999
Therapies, heat, cold, and light E0200-E0239
TheraSkin® Q4121
Thermometer A4931, A4932
Thiamine HCl J3411
Thickener, food B4100
Thiethylperazine maleate J3280, Q0174
Thiotepa J9340
Thoracic rib belt L0220
Thoracic-lumbar-sacral orthosis (TLSO) L1200
  Additions L1210-L1290
  Spinal L0450, L0452-L0492
Thrombectomy catheter C1757
Thromboembolism risk factor
  None or one moderate risk factor G8970
Thymol turbidity, blood P2033
Thyroid nodule G9552, G9553, G9554, G9555, G9556, G9557
Thyrotropin alfa J3240
Ticarcillin disodium and clavulanate potassium S0040
Tigecycline J3243
Tildrakizumab J3245
Tinzaparin sodium J1655
Tip (cane/crutch/walker) replacement A4637

Ⓝ New index entry

Tire, wheelchair, pneumatic E2381-E2385
Tirofiban J3246
Tisagenlecleucel, therapeutic dose Q2042
Tissue marker A4648
Tissue, connective
    Human C1762
    Nonhuman C1763
TLSO (thoracic-lumbar-sacral orthosis) L0452-L0492, L1200-L1290
Tobacco cessation intervention
    Identified user G9906
    Identified user, not provided, medical reason G9909
    Not provided, medical reason G9907
    Not provided, reason not given G9908
Tobacco use G9275, G9276, G9458, G9459, G9642, G9791, G9792, G9902-G9909
Tobramycin sulfate J3260
Tobramycin, inhalation solution, unit dose J7682, J7685
Tocilizumab J3262
Toilet and accessories
    Commode chair
        Electric E0170
        Extra wide E0168
        Nonelectric E0171
        With integrated lift E0170-E0171
    Footrest E0175
    Pan/pail E0167
    Patient lift E0625
    Rail E0243
    Raised seat E0244
    Seat lift E0172
Tolazoline HCl J2670
Toll, nonemergency transport A0170
Tomosynthesis, breast G0279
Topical hyperbaric oxygen chamber A4575
Topographic brain mapping S8040
Topotecan
    Injection J9351
    Oral J8705
Torsemide J3265
Trabectedin injection J9352
Tracheostoma heat moisture exchange system A7501-A7509
Tracheostomy
    Care kit A4629
    Filter A4481
    Speaking valve L8501
    Supplies A7501-A7527, S8189
    Tube A7520-A7522
Tracheotomy mask or collar A7525, A7526
Traction device, ambulatory E0830
Traction equipment E0830-E0948
Training
    Alcohol and/or drug training service H0021
    Child development, family T1027
    Diabetes self management G0108, G0109
    Medication training and support H0034
    Skills training and development H2014
Transcatheter occlusion or embolization S2095
Transcutaneous electrical nerve stimulator (TENS)
    Conductive garment E0731
    Electrical stimulator supplies A4595
    Four-lead or more E0730
    Two-lead E0720
Transcyte Q4182
Transducer protector, dialysis E1575

Transesophageal
    Doppler measurement G9157
    Echocardiography
        For congenital cardiac anomalies C8926
            For monitoring purposes C8927
        Real time with 2D image documentation C8925
    Pacing (catheter) C1756
Transfer (shoe orthosis) L3600-L3640
Transfer system with seat E1035
Transluminal angioplasty
    Laser catheter C1885
    Nonlaser catheter C1725, C2623
Transluminal, atherectomy
    Directional catheter C1714
    Rotational catheter C1724
Transparent film (for dressing) A6257-A6259
Transplant
    Bone marrow S2150
    Islet cell S2102
        Laparoscopy G0342
        Laparotomy G0343
        Percutaneous G0341
    Kidney and pancreas, simultaneous S2065
    Lobar lung S2060
    Multiple visceral organs S2054
    Related lodging, meals, transportation S9975, S9976
    Stem cells, cord blood derived S2142
Transport chairs E1037-E1039
Transportation
    Ambulance A0021-A0999
    Conventional air A0430, A0431
    Corneal tissue V2785
    EKG equipment, portable R0076
    Neonatal, emergency ambulance service A0225
    Nonemergency A0080-A0210, T2001-T2005
        Air A0140, T2007
        Ancillary
            Lodging A0180, A0200
            Meals A0190, A0210, S9977
            Out-of-state ambulance transport A0021
            Parking fees/tolls A0170
        Bus A0110
        Case worker or social worker A0160
        Mini-bus A0120
        Stretcher van T2005, T2049
        Taxi A0100
        Vehicle provided by
            Individual A0090
            Volunteer A0080
        Wheelchair van A0130, S0209
    X-ray equipment, portable R0070, R0075
    Services T2001-T2007
Transtracheal oxygen catheter A4608
Trapeze bar E0910, E0911, E0912, E0940
Trastuzumab J9316, J9355, Q5112-Q5114, Q5116, Q5117
Trastuzumab and hyaluronidase J9316, J9356
Trauma response team G0390
Travel allowance for specimen collection P9603, P9604
Tray
    Insertion A4310-A4316
    Irrigation A4320
    Surgical A4550
    Wheelchair E0950
Treatment, acute care at NF G9679-G9685
Treatment in place (TIP) G2021
Treatment planning and care coordination S0353, S0354
Treprostinil J3285
Tretinoin, topical S0117

Triamcinolone - Viltolarsen

Triamcinolone J3301-J3303
  Acetonide
    Not otherwise specified (NOS) J3301
    Preservative free J3300, J3304
  Diacetate J3302
  Hexacetonide J3303
  Inhalation solution
    Concentrated J7683
    Unit dose J7684
Triflupromazine HCl J3400
Trifocal, glass or plastic V2300-V2399
Trimethobenzamide HCl
  Injection J3250
  Oral Q0173
Trimetrexate glucuronate J3305
Trimming, routine foot care
  Corns/calluses/nails S0390
Triptorelin extended release J3316
Triptorelin pamoate J3315
TriVisc™ J7329
Truss L8300, L8310, L8320, L8330
Tube/Tubing
  Anchoring device A5200
  Blood A4750, A4755
  Calibrated microcapillary A4651
  Drainage extension A4331
  Gastrostomy/Jejunostomy B4087, B4088
  Irrigation A4355
  Nasogastric B4081, B4082
  Oxygen A4616
  Sealant, microcapillary tube A4652
  Serum clotting time A4771
  Stomach B4083
  Suction pump, each A7002
  Urinary drainage A4331
  With heating element A4604
Tumor
  Category documented G8721
  Not included in pathology report
    Medical reason G8722
    Reason not given G8724
  Specimen site
    Other than anatomic location G8723

U

Ultrafiltration monitor S9007
Ultrasonic diathermy treatment device, low frequency K1004
Ultrasonic nebulizer E0575
Ultrasound
  Catheter, intravascular C1753
  Gel A4559
  Guidance for placement of radiation therapy fields G6001
  Intravascular C1753
Ultraviolet light therapy system A4633, E0691-E0694
Unclassified biological J3590
Unclassified drug J3490
Unclassified drug or biological. ESRD J3591
Underpads
  Non-disposable A4553
  Disposable A4554
Unipuncture control system, dialysis E1580
Unspecified oral dosage form Q0181
Upper extremity addition, locking elbow L6693
Upper extremity orthosis L3980-L3999
  Addition of joint L3956
Upper limb prosthesis L6000-L7499

Urea J3350
Ureteral
  Catheter C1758
  Injury G9631, G9632, G9633
Ureterostomy supplies A4450-A4554
Urethral suppository J0275
Urgent care center
  Global fee S9083
  Services S9088
URI
  Child with competing diagnosis G2097
  With prior antibiotic prescription G2174 ⓝ
  With prior comorbid condition G2173 ⓝ
Urinal
  Jug-type, female E0326
  Jug-type, male E0325
Urinary
  Catheter A4338-A4346, A4351-A4353
  Collection and retention (supplies) A4310-A4360
  Drainage device K1010-K1012 ⓝ
  Management system pump K1005
  Repair device without sling graft C2631
  Sphincter prosthesis C1815
  Tract implant
    Collagen L8603
    Synthetic L8606
Urine
  Culture, bacterial P7001
  Tests A4250
Urofollitropin J3355
Urokinase J3364, J3365
Ustekinumab J3357, J3358
UV lens V2755

V

Vabra aspirator A4480
Vaccination
  Administration
    Hepatitis B G0010
    Influenza virus G0008
    Pneumococcal G0009, G9280, G8864-G8867
  Screening performed G9281
Vaccine
  Influenza Q2034-Q2039
Vancomycin HCl J3370
Vaporizer E0605
Vascular
  Catheter and supplies A4300-A4306
  Graft material, synthetic L8670
Vedolizumab J3380
Velaglucerase alfa J3385
Velcade ® J9041
Venipuncture S9529
Venous pressure clamp, dialysis A4918
Ventilator
  Battery A4611, A4612, A4613
  Home
    Any type E0465, E0466
    Multi-function E0467
  Moisture exchanger A4483
Ventricular assist device Q0477-Q0509
Vertebral axial decompression S9090
Verteporfin J3396
Vest, safety, wheelchair E0980
Vestibular rehabilitation program S9476
Vestronidase alfa-vjbk J3397
Viltolarsen C9071 ⓝ

ⓝ New index entry

Vinblastine sulfate J9360
Vincristine sulfate J9370, J9371
Vinorelbine tartrate J9390
Virtual check-in G2251, G2252 Ⓝ
VISCO-3TM J7333 Ⓝ
Vision service V2700-V2799
Vision supplies S0500-S0596, V2600-V2615
Visual acuity improvement G9517, G9519, G9520
Vitamins
   B-12 cyanocobalamin J3420
   Dialysis stress supplement S0194
   K J3430
   Not otherwise specified A9152-A9153
   Prenatal S0197
Vivectomy C9770 Ⓝ
Voice amplifier L8510
Voice prosthesis L8511-L8514
Volume management G8955, G8958
Von Willebrand factor complex J7183, J7187
Voretigene neparvovec-rzyl J3398
Voriconazole J3465

W

Waiver T2012-T2041
Walking aids E0100-E0149
   Accessories A4636, A4637
   Attachments E0153-E0159
Walking boot
   Custom L4387
   Off-the-shelf L4386
Warfarin or other anticoagulant
   Not prescribed, reason documented G9927
   Not prescribed, reason not given G9928
Warfarin responsiveness G9143
Water
   Distilled, for nebulizer A7018
   Pressure pad/mattress E0187, E0198
   Purification system (ESRD) E1610, E1615
   Softening system (ESRD) E1625
   Sterile A4714
Wedges, shoe L3340-L3420
Well-child visit G9964, G9965
Wet mount Q0111
Wheel attachment, rigid pickup walker E0155
Wheelchair E0950-E1298, K0001-K0108
   Accessories E0950-E1036, E2201-E2398, E2626-E2633, K0669
     Interface, head or extremity control E2328, E2329
   Amputee E1170-E1200
   Back E1226, E2291, E2293
   Component or accessory K0001-K0195
   Cushions, seat and back E2601-E2625
     Custom fabricated E2617
     General use
       Width 22 inches or greater E2612
       Width less than 22 inches E2611
     Positioning
       Posterior, width 22 inches or greater E2614
       Posterior, width less than 22 inches E2613
       Posterior-lateral, width 22 inches or greater E2616
       Posterior-lateral, width less than 22 inches E2615
   Fully-reclining
     Detachable arms/detachable footrests E1070
     Detachable arms/detachable leg rests E1060
     Fixed arms/detachable leg rests E1050

   Group 2
     Extra heavy duty, single power option, sling/solid seat/back K0840
     Heavy duty, single power option
       Captain's chair K0838
       Sling/solid seat/back K0837
     Very heavy duty, single power option sling/solid seat/back K0839
   Group 3
     Extra heavy duty captain's chair K0855
       Sling/solid seat/back K0854
     Heavy duty captain's chair K0851
       Sling/solid seat/back K0850
     Very heavy duty captain's chair K0853
       Sling/solid seat/back K0852
   Heavy duty E1092, E1093, E1280-E1298
   Hemi
     Detachable arms/detachable footrests E1070
     Detachable arms/detachable leg rests E1084
     Fixed arms/detachable footrest E1085, E1086
     Fixed arms/detachable leg rest E1083
     Standard, low seat K0002
   Lightweight E1240-E1270
     High-strength E1087-E1090
     Portable motorized K0012
   Narrowing device E0969
   Pediatric E1229-E1239
     Folding E1236
     Not otherwise specified (NOS) E1229
     Power operated E1239
   Power add-on E0983-E0984
   Power operated E1230, E1239, K0813-K0899
   Reclining E1050-E1070, E1100-E1110
   Seat E2292, E2294
   Shock absorber E1015-E1018
   Specially sized E1220, E1230
   Standard K0001, E1130-E1161
     Hemi, low seat K0002
     Weight frame motorized K0010
     With programmable control parameters K0011
   Stump support system E1020
   Tire, pneumatic E2381-E2385
   Transfer board or device E0705
   Tray E0950
   Van, nonemergency A0130
Wheelchair evaluation G9156
WHFO (wrist hand finger orthosis) L3807
Whirlpool E1300, E1310, K1003
WHO, wrist extension L3908
Wig A9282
Wipes A4245, A4247
Wood
   Canes, all materials E0100
   Crutches
     Other than wood E0114, E0116
     Wood E0112, E0113
Wound
   Cleanser A6260
   Cover
     Alginate dressing A6196-A6198
     Collagen dressing A6021-A6024
     Foam dressing A6209-A6214
       Hydrocolloid dressing A6234-A6239
     Hydrogel dressing A6242-A6247
     Specialty absorptive dressing A6251-A6256
     Wound warming device, noncontact E0231, E0232
   Dressing K0744, K0745, K0746, L3254, L3255

Filler
    Adhesive tissue G0168
    Alginate dressing A6199
    Collagen based A6010
    Foam dressing per gram A6215
    Hydrocolloid dressing A6240, A6241
    Hydrogel dressing A6248
    Not elsewhere classified (NEC) A6261, A6262
Pouch A6154
Supplies and dressings A4450-A4456, A4461-A4467,
    A6000-A6550
Suction A9272, K0743
Treatment
    Autologous platelet rich plasma G0460
    Biologicals and skin substitutes C1849, Q4100-Q4255,
        S9055 Ⓝ
    Compression burn mask A6513
    Electric or electromagnetic stimulation E0769, G0295,
        G0329
    Gel sheet A6025
    Packing strips A6407
WoundEx® Q4162, Q4163
WoundFix™ Q4217
Wrap, chest E0459
Wrap, heat and/or cold A9273
Wrist
    Disarticulation prosthesis L6050, L6055
    Electronic wrist rotator L7259
    Hand/finger orthosis (WHFO) E1805, E1825, L3808,
        L3809, L3900, L3901, L3904
Wrong site/side/patient/procedure/implant G8907,
    G8912-G8913

X

Xcellerate® Q4234 Ⓝ
Xenon (Xe) 133 A9558
Xwrap® Q4204
X-ray equipment, portable Q0092, R0070, R0075

Y

Yttrium-90 (Y-90) ibritumomab A9543

Z

Ziconotide J2278
Zidovudine J3485, S0104
Ziprasidone mesylate J3486
Zoledronic acid J3489

Ⓝ **New index entry**

CMS includes parenthetical coding guidelines for several codes throughout the Tabular List, which are effective for 2021. Some of these guidelines include deleted CPT® or HCPCS codes, even though the guidelines were from the latest updates from CMS for 2021. Please check the CMS website for further updates or guideline changes.

Generic and brand-name drugs found throughout the Tabular List are from the latest CMS updates. Please check the CMS website and the FDA website for further information on valid or discontinued drugs.

TRANSPORTATION SERVICES INCLUDING AMBULANCE (A0021-A0999)

HCPCS Level II codes for ambulance services (A0021-A0999) must be reported with modifiers indicating pick-up origins and destinations. The modifier describing the arrangement (QM, QN) is listed first. The modifiers describing the origin and destination are listed second. Origin and destination modifiers are created by combining two alpha characters from the following list. Each alpha character, with the exception of X, represents either an origin or destination. Each pair of the alpha characters creates one modifier. The first position represents the origin and the second the destination. The modifiers most commonly used are:

D   Diagnostic or therapeutic site other than P or H when these are used as origin codes

E   Residential, domiciliary, custodial facility (other than 1819 facility)

G   Hospital-based dialysis facility

H   Hospital

I   Site of transfer (e.g., airport or helicopter pad) between modes of ambulance transport

J   Free standing ESRD facility

N   Skilled nursing facility (SNF)

P   Physician's office

R   Residence

S   Scene of accident or acute event

X   Intermediate stop at physician's office on way to hospital (destination code only)

AMBULANCE AND OTHER TRANSPORT SERVICES AND SUPPLIES (A0021-A0999)

A0021   Ambulance service, outside state per mile, transport (Medicaid only)   E1
     BETOS: O1A   Ambulance
     Service not separately priced by Part B

A0080   Non-emergency transportation, per mile - vehicle provided by volunteer (individual or organization), with no vested interest   E1
     BETOS: O1A   Ambulance
     Service not separately priced by Part B

A0090   Non-emergency transportation, per mile - vehicle provided by individual (family member, self, neighbor) with vested interest   E1
     BETOS: O1A   Ambulance
     Service not separately priced by Part B

A0100   Non-emergency transportation; taxi   E1
     BETOS: O1A   Ambulance
     Service not separately priced by Part B

A0110   Non-emergency transportation and bus, intra- or inter-state carrier   E1
     BETOS: O1A   Ambulance
     Service not separately priced by Part B

A0120   Non-emergency transportation: mini-bus, mountain area transports, or other transportation systems   E1
     BETOS: O1A   Ambulance
     Service not separately priced by Part B

A0130   Non-emergency transportation: wheelchair van   E1
     BETOS: O1A   Ambulance
     Service not separately priced by Part B

A0140   Non-emergency transportation and air travel (private or commercial) intra- or inter-state   E1
     BETOS: O1A   Ambulance
     Service not separately priced by Part B

A0160   Non-emergency transportation: per mile - case worker or social worker   E1
     BETOS: O1A   Ambulance
     Service not separately priced by Part B

A0170   Transportation ancillary: parking fees, tolls, other   E1
     BETOS: O1A   Ambulance
     Service not separately priced by Part B

A0180   Non-emergency transportation: ancillary: lodging-recipient   E1
     BETOS: O1A   Ambulance
     Service not separately priced by Part B

A0190   Non-emergency transportation: ancillary: meals-recipient   E1
     BETOS: O1A   Ambulance
     Service not separately priced by Part B

A0200   Non-emergency transportation: ancillary: lodging escort   E1
     BETOS: O1A   Ambulance
     Service not separately priced by Part B

A0210   Non-emergency transportation: ancillary: meals-escort   E1
     BETOS: O1A   Ambulance
     Service not separately priced by Part B

A0225   Ambulance service, neonatal transport, base rate, emergency transport, one-way   Ⓐ E1
     BETOS: O1A   Ambulance
     Service not separately priced by Part B

A0380   BLS mileage (per mile)   E1
     BETOS: O1A   Ambulance
     Service not separately priced by Part B
     Pub: 100-4, Chapter-15, 30.2

♂ Male only   ♀ Female only   Ⓐ Age   A2 - Z3 = ASC Payment indicator   A - Y = APC Status indicator
ASC = ASC Approved Procedure   **DME** Paid under the DME fee schedule   **MIPS** MIPS code

CPT® is a registered trademark of the American Medical Association. All rights reserved.

105

A0382 BLS routine disposable supplies E1
BETOS: O1A Ambulance
Service not separately priced by Part B

A0384 BLS specialized service disposable supplies; defibrillation (used by ALS ambulances and BLS ambulances in jurisdictions where defibrillation is permitted in BLS ambulances) E1
BETOS: O1A Ambulance
Service not separately priced by Part B

A0390 ALS mileage (per mile) E1
BETOS: O1A Ambulance
Service not separately priced by Part B
Pub: 100-4, Chapter-15, 30.2

A0392 ALS specialized service disposable supplies; defibrillation (to be used only in jurisdictions where defibrillation cannot be performed in BLS ambulances) E1
BETOS: O1A Ambulance
Service not separately priced by Part B

A0394 ALS specialized service disposable supplies; IV drug therapy E1
BETOS: O1A Ambulance
Service not separately priced by Part B

A0396 ALS specialized service disposable supplies; esophageal intubation E1
BETOS: O1A Ambulance
Service not separately priced by Part B

A0398 ALS routine disposable supplies E1
BETOS: O1A Ambulance
Service not separately priced by Part B

Waiting Time Units for Ambulance Services	
Units	Total Time
1	1/2 to 1 hour
2	1 to 1-1/2 hours
3	1-1/2 to 2 hours
4	2 to 2-1/2 hours
5	2-1/2 to 3 hours
6	3 to 3-1/2 hours
7	3-1/2 to 4 hours
8	4 to 4-1/2 hours
9	4-1/2 to 5 hours
10	5 to 5-1/2 hours

A0420 Ambulance waiting time (ALS or BLS), one half (1/2) hour increments E1
BETOS: O1A Ambulance
Service not separately priced by Part B

A0422 Ambulance (ALS or BLS) oxygen and oxygen supplies, life sustaining situation E1
BETOS: O1A Ambulance
Service not separately priced by Part B

A0424 Extra ambulance attendant, ground (ALS or BLS) or air (fixed or rotary winged); (requires medical review) E1
BETOS: O1A Ambulance
Service not separately priced by Part B

A0425 Ground mileage, per statute mile A
BETOS: O1A Ambulance
Reasonable charge
Coding Clinic: 2012, Q4
Pub: 100-4, Chapter-15, 20.6; 100-4, Chapter-15, 30.2; 100-4, Chapter-15, 30.2.1

A0426 Ambulance service, advanced life support, non-emergency transport, level 1 (ALS 1) A
BETOS: O1A Ambulance
Reasonable charge
Coding Clinic: 2012, Q4
Pub: 100-4, Chapter-15, 30.2; 100-4, Chapter-15, 30.2.1

A0427 Ambulance service, advanced life support, emergency transport, level 1 (ALS 1-emergency) A
BETOS: O1A Ambulance
Reasonable charge
Coding Clinic: 2012, Q4
Pub: 100-4, Chapter-15, 30.2.1; 100-4, Chapter-15, 30.2

A0428 Ambulance service, basic life support, non-emergency transport, (BLS) A
BETOS: O1A Ambulance
Reasonable charge
Coding Clinic: 2012, Q4
Pub: 100-4, Chapter-15, 20.6; 100-4, Chapter-15, 30.2; 100-4, Chapter-15, 30.2.1

A0429 Ambulance service, basic life support, emergency transport (BLS-emergency) A
BETOS: O1A Ambulance
Reasonable charge
Coding Clinic: 2012, Q4
Pub: 100-4, Chapter-15, 30.2; 100-4, Chapter-15, 30.2.1

A0430 Ambulance service, conventional air services, transport, one-way (fixed wing) A
BETOS: O1A Ambulance
Reasonable charge
Coding Clinic: 2012, Q4
Pub: 100-4, Chapter-15, 30.2.1; 100-4, Chapter-15, 30.2; 100-4, Chapter-15, 20.3

A0431 Ambulance service, conventional air services, transport, one-way (rotary wing) A
BETOS: O1A Ambulance
Reasonable charge
Coding Clinic: 2012, Q4
Pub: 100-4, Chapter-15, 20.3; 100-4, Chapter-15, 30.2; 100-4, Chapter-15, 30.2.1

C **A0432** Paramedic intercept (PI), rural area, transport furnished by a volunteer ambulance company which is prohibited by state law from billing third party payers   A
BETOS: O1A   Ambulance
Reasonable charge
Coding Clinic: 2012, Q4
Pub: 100-4, Chapter-15, 30.2; 100-4, Chapter-15, 30.2.1

C **A0433** Advanced life support, level 2 (ALS 2)   A
BETOS: O1A   Ambulance
Reasonable charge
Coding Clinic: 2012, Q4
Pub: 100-4, Chapter-15, 30.2; 100-4, Chapter-15, 30.2.1

C **A0434** Specialty care transport (SCT)   A
BETOS: O1A   Ambulance
Reasonable charge
Coding Clinic: 2012, Q4
Pub: 100-4, Chapter-15, 30.2.1; 100-4, Chapter-15, 30.2

C **A0435** Fixed wing air mileage, per statute mile   A
BETOS: O1A   Ambulance
Reasonable charge
Coding Clinic: 2012, Q4
Pub: 100-4, Chapter-15, 20.3; 100-4, Chapter-15, 30.2; 100-4, Chapter-15, 30.2.1

C **A0436** Rotary wing air mileage, per statute mile   A
BETOS: O1A   Ambulance
Reasonable charge
Coding Clinic: 2012, Q4
Pub: 100-4, Chapter-15, 20.3; 100-4, Chapter-15, 30.2; 100-4, Chapter-15, 30.2.1

M **A0888** Noncovered ambulance mileage, per mile (e.g., for miles traveled beyond closest appropriate facility)   E1
BETOS: O1A   Ambulance
Service not separately priced by Part B
Pub: 100-4, Chapter-15, 30.2.4

I **A0998** Ambulance response and treatment, no transport   E1
BETOS: O1A   Ambulance
Service not separately priced by Part B

D **A0999** Unlisted ambulance service   A
BETOS: O1A   Ambulance
Other carrier priced
Coding Clinic: 2009, Q2

NOTES

MEDICAL AND SURGICAL SUPPLIES
(A4206-A8004)

INJECTION AND INFUSION SUPPLIES (A4206-A4232)

C A4206 Syringe with needle, sterile, 1 cc or less, each   N
BETOS: D1A   Medical/surgical supplies
Service not separately priced by Part B

C A4207 Syringe with needle, sterile 2 cc, each   N
BETOS: D1A   Medical/surgical supplies
Service not separately priced by Part B

C A4208 Syringe with needle, sterile 3 cc, each   N
BETOS: D1A   Medical/surgical supplies
Service not separately priced by Part B

C A4209 Syringe with needle, sterile 5 cc or greater, each   N
BETOS: D1A   Medical/surgical supplies
Service not separately priced by Part B

M A4210 Needle-free injection device, each   E1
BETOS: D1A   Medical/surgical supplies
Service not separately priced by Part B

D A4211 Supplies for self-administered injections   N
BETOS: D1A   Medical/surgical supplies
Service not separately priced by Part B

C A4212 Non-coring needle or stylet with or without catheter   N
BETOS: D1A   Medical/surgical supplies
Other carrier priced

C A4213 Syringe, sterile, 20 cc or greater, each   N
BETOS: D1A   Medical/surgical supplies
Service not separately priced by Part B

C A4215 Needle, sterile, any size, each   N
BETOS: D1A   Medical/surgical supplies
Service not separately priced by Part B

D A4216 Sterile water, saline and/or dextrose, diluent/ flush, 10 ml   DME   N
BETOS: D1F   Prosthetic/Orthotic devices

D A4217 Sterile water/saline, 500 ml   DME   N
BETOS: D1F   Prosthetic/Orthotic devices
DME Modifier: AU

D A4218 Sterile saline or water, metered dose dispenser, 10 ml   N
BETOS: O1E   Other drugs

D A4220 Refill kit for implantable infusion pump   N
BETOS: D1A   Medical/surgical supplies
Other carrier priced

C A4221 Supplies for maintenance of non-insulin drug infusion catheter, per week (list drugs separately)   DME   N
BETOS: D1E   Other DME

C A4222 Infusion supplies for external drug infusion pump, per cassette or bag (list drugs separately)   DME   N
BETOS: D1E   Other DME

C A4223 Infusion supplies not used with external infusion pump, per cassette or bag (list drugs separately)   N
BETOS: D1A   Medical/surgical supplies
Service not separately priced by Part B

C A4224 Supplies for maintenance of insulin infusion catheter, per week   DME   N
BETOS: D1E   Other DME

D A4225 Supplies for external insulin infusion pump, syringe type cartridge, sterile, each   DME   N
BETOS: D1E   Other DME

I A4226 Supplies for maintenance of insulin infusion pump with dosage rate adjustment using therapeutic continuous glucose sensing, per week   E1
BETOS: Z2   Undefined codes
Service not separately priced by Part B

D A4230 Infusion set for external insulin pump, non needle cannula type   N
BETOS: D1E   Other DME

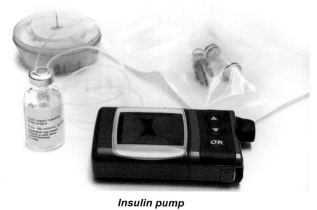

Insulin pump

D A4231 Infusion set for external insulin pump, needle type   N
BETOS: D1E   Other DME

I A4232 Syringe with needle for external insulin pump, sterile, 3 cc   E1
BETOS: D1E   Other DME
Service not separately priced by Part B

REPLACEMENT BATTERIES (A4233-A4236)

C A4233 Replacement battery, alkaline (other than J cell), for use with medically necessary home blood glucose monitor owned by patient, each   DME   E1
BETOS: D1E   Other DME
DME Modifier: NU

C **A4234** Replacement battery, alkaline, J cell, for use with medically necessary home blood glucose monitor owned by patient, each DME E1
BETOS: D1E Other DME
DME Modifier: NU

C **A4235** Replacement battery, lithium, for use with medically necessary home blood glucose monitor owned by patient, each DME E1
BETOS: D1E Other DME
DME Modifier: NU

C **A4236** Replacement battery, silver oxide, for use with medically necessary home blood glucose monitor owned by patient, each DME E1
BETOS: D1E Other DME
DME Modifier: NU

OTHER SUPPLIES INCLUDING DIABETES SUPPLIES AND CONTRACEPTIVES (A4244-A4290)

C **A4244** Alcohol or peroxide, per pint N
BETOS: D1A Medical/surgical supplies
Service not separately priced by Part B

C **A4245** Alcohol wipes, per box N
BETOS: D1A Medical/surgical supplies
Service not separately priced by Part B

C **A4246** Betadine or pHisoHex solution, per pint N
BETOS: D1A Medical/surgical supplies
Service not separately priced by Part B

C **A4247** Betadine or iodine swabs/wipes, per box N
BETOS: D1A Medical/surgical supplies
Service not separately priced by Part B

C **A4248** Chlorhexidine containing antiseptic, 1 ml N
BETOS: P9B Dialysis services (non-Medicare fee schedule)
Service not separately priced by Part B

M **A4250** Urine test or reagent strips or tablets (100 tablets or strips) E1
BETOS: T1E Lab tests - glucose
Service not separately priced by Part B

S **A4252** Blood ketone test or reagent strip, each E1
BETOS: D1E Other DME
Service not separately priced by Part B
Statute: 1861(n)

D **A4253** Blood glucose test or reagent strips for home blood glucose monitor, per 50 strips DME N
BETOS: D1E Other DME
DME Modifier: NU

D **A4255** Platforms for home blood glucose monitor, 50 per box DME N
BETOS: D1E Other DME

D **A4256** Normal, low and high calibrator solution/chips DME N
BETOS: D1E Other DME

C **A4257** Replacement lens shield cartridge for use with laser skin piercing device, each DME E1
BETOS: D1E Other DME
Coding Clinic: 2002, Q1

D **A4258** Spring-powered device for lancet, each DME N
BETOS: D1E Other DME

D **A4259** Lancets, per box of 100 DME N
BETOS: D1E Other DME

S **A4261** Cervical cap for contraceptive use ♀ E1
BETOS: Z2 Undefined codes
Service not separately priced by Part B
Statute: 1862a1

D **A4262** Temporary, absorbable lacrimal duct implant, each N
BETOS: D1A Medical/surgical supplies
Service not separately priced by Part B

D **A4263** Permanent, long term, non-dissolvable lacrimal duct implant, each N
BETOS: Y1 Other - Medicare fee schedule
Price established using national RVUs

I **A4264** Permanent implantable contraceptive intratubal occlusion device(s) and delivery system ♀ E1
BETOS: Z2 Undefined codes
Service not separately priced by Part B

D **A4265** Paraffin, per pound DME N
BETOS: D1E Other DME

I **A4266** Diaphragm for contraceptive use ♀ E1
BETOS: Z2 Undefined codes
Service not separately priced by Part B

I **A4267** Contraceptive supply, condom, male, each ♂ E1
BETOS: Z2 Undefined codes
Service not separately priced by Part B

I **A4268** Contraceptive supply, condom, female, each ♀ E1
BETOS: Z2 Undefined codes
Service not separately priced by Part B

I **A4269** Contraceptive supply, spermicide (e.g., foam, gel), each ♀ E1
BETOS: Z2 Undefined codes
Service not separately priced by Part B

C **A4270** Disposable endoscope sheath, each N
BETOS: P8D Endoscopy - colonoscopy
Service not separately priced by Part B

C **A4280** Adhesive skin support attachment for use with external breast prosthesis, each DME N
BETOS: D1F Prosthetic/Orthotic devices

C **A4281** Tubing for breast pump, replacement ♀ Ⓐ E1
BETOS: Z2 Undefined codes
Service not separately priced by Part B

● New code   ▲ Revised code   C Carrier judgment   D Special coverage instructions apply
I Not payable by Medicare   M Non-covered by Medicare   S Non-covered by Medicare statute   AHA Coding Clinic®

C **A4282** Adapter for breast pump, replacement ♀ ⒶⒺ1

BETOS: Z2 Undefined codes

Service not separately priced by Part B

C **A4283** Cap for breast pump bottle, replacement ♀ ⒶⒺ1

BETOS: Z2 Undefined codes

Service not separately priced by Part B

C **A4284** Breast shield and splash protector for use with breast pump, replacement ♀ ⒶⒺ1

BETOS: Z2 Undefined codes

Service not separately priced by Part B

C **A4285** Polycarbonate bottle for use with breast pump, replacement ♀ ⒶⒺ1

BETOS: Z2 Undefined codes

Service not separately priced by Part B

C **A4286** Locking ring for breast pump, replacement ♀ ⒶⒺ1

BETOS: Z2 Undefined codes

Service not separately priced by Part B

C **A4290** Sacral nerve stimulation test lead, each N

BETOS: Z2 Undefined codes

Service not separately priced by Part B

Coding Clinic: 2002, Q1

ACCESS CATHETERS AND DRUG DELIVERY SYSTEMS (A4300-A4306)

D **A4300** Implantable access catheter, (e.g., venous, arterial, epidural subarachnoid, or peritoneal, etc.) external access N

BETOS: Y1 Other - Medicare fee schedule

Price established using national RVUs

C **A4301** Implantable access total catheter, port/ reservoir (e.g., venous, arterial, epidural, subarachnoid, peritoneal, etc.) N

BETOS: D1A Medical/surgical supplies

Service not separately priced by Part B

C **A4305** Disposable drug delivery system, flow rate of 50 ml or greater per hour N

BETOS: D1A Medical/surgical supplies

Service not separately priced by Part B

C **A4306** Disposable drug delivery system, flow rate of less than 50 ml per hour N

BETOS: D1A Medical/surgical supplies

Service not separately priced by Part B

INCONTINENCE DEVICES AND SUPPLIES (A4310-A4360), SEE ALSO INCONTINENCE DEVICES AND SUPPLIES (A5102-A5200)

D **A4310** Insertion tray without drainage bag and without catheter (accessories only) DME N

BETOS: D1F Prosthetic/Orthotic devices

D **A4311** Insertion tray without drainage bag with indwelling catheter, Foley-type, two-way latex with coating (Teflon, silicone, silicone elastomer or hydrophilic, etc.) DME N

BETOS: D1F Prosthetic/Orthotic devices

D **A4312** Insertion tray without drainage bag with indwelling catheter, Foley-type, two-way, all silicone DME N

BETOS: D1F Prosthetic/Orthotic devices

D **A4313** Insertion tray without drainage bag with indwelling catheter, Foley-type, three-way, for continuous irrigation DME N

BETOS: D1F Prosthetic/Orthotic devices

D **A4314** Insertion tray with drainage bag with indwelling catheter, Foley-type, two-way latex with coating (Teflon, silicone, silicone elastomer or hydrophilic, etc.) DME N

BETOS: D1F Prosthetic/Orthotic devices

D **A4315** Insertion tray with drainage bag with indwelling catheter, Foley-type, two-way, all silicone DME N

BETOS: D1F Prosthetic/Orthotic devices

D **A4316** Insertion tray with drainage bag with indwelling catheter, Foley-type, three-way, for continuous irrigation DME N

BETOS: D1F Prosthetic/Orthotic devices

D **A4320** Irrigation tray with bulb or piston syringe, any purpose DME N

BETOS: D1A Medical/surgical supplies

D **A4321** Therapeutic agent for urinary catheter irrigation DME N

BETOS: D1F Prosthetic/Orthotic devices

D **A4322** Irrigation syringe, bulb or piston, each DME N

BETOS: D1F Prosthetic/Orthotic devices

D **A4326** Male external catheter with integral collection chamber, any type, each ♂ DME N

BETOS: D1F Prosthetic/Orthotic devices

D **A4327** Female external urinary collection device; meatal cup, each ♀ DME N

BETOS: D1F Prosthetic/Orthotic devices

D **A4328** Female external urinary collection device; pouch, each ♀ DME N

BETOS: D1F Prosthetic/Orthotic devices

D **A4330** Perianal fecal collection pouch with adhesive, each DME N

BETOS: D1F Prosthetic/Orthotic devices

D **A4331** Extension drainage tubing, any type, any length, with connector/adaptor, for use with urinary leg bag or urostomy pouch, each DME N

BETOS: D1F Prosthetic/Orthotic devices

D **A4332** Lubricant, individual sterile packet, each DME N

BETOS: D1F Prosthetic/Orthotic devices

D **A4333** Urinary catheter anchoring device, adhesive skin attachment, each DME N
BETOS: D1F   Prosthetic/Orthotic devices

D **A4334** Urinary catheter anchoring device, leg strap, each DME N
BETOS: D1F   Prosthetic/Orthotic devices

D **A4335** Incontinence supply; miscellaneous N
BETOS: D1F   Prosthetic/Orthotic devices

D **A4336** Incontinence supply, urethral insert, any type, each DME N
BETOS: D1F   Prosthetic/Orthotic devices

D **A4337** Incontinence supply, rectal insert, any type, each N
BETOS: D1F   Prosthetic/Orthotic devices

D **A4338** Indwelling catheter; Foley-type, two-way latex with coating (Teflon, silicone, silicone elastomer, or hydrophilic, etc.), each DME N
BETOS: D1F   Prosthetic/Orthotic devices

D **A4340** Indwelling catheter; specialty type, (e.g., Coude, mushroom, wing, etc.), each DME N
BETOS: D1F   Prosthetic/Orthotic devices

D **A4344** Indwelling catheter, Foley-type, two-way, all silicone, each DME N
BETOS: D1F   Prosthetic/Orthotic devices

D **A4346** Indwelling catheter; Foley-type, three-way for continuous irrigation, each DME N
BETOS: D1F   Prosthetic/Orthotic devices

Foley catheter

D **A4349** Male external catheter, with or without adhesive, disposable, each ♂ DME N
BETOS: D1A   Medical/surgical supplies

D **A4351** Intermittent urinary catheter; straight tip, with or without coating (Teflon, silicone, silicone elastomer, or hydrophilic, etc.), each DME N
BETOS: D1F   Prosthetic/Orthotic devices

D **A4352** Intermittent urinary catheter; Coude (curved) tip, with or without coating (Teflon, silicone, silicone elastomeric, or hydrophilic, etc.), each DME N
BETOS: D1F   Prosthetic/Orthotic devices

D **A4353** Intermittent urinary catheter, with insertion supplies DME N
BETOS: D1F   Prosthetic/Orthotic devices

D **A4354** Insertion tray with drainage bag but without catheter DME N
BETOS: D1F   Prosthetic/Orthotic devices

D **A4355** Irrigation tubing set for continuous bladder irrigation through a three-way indwelling Foley catheter, each DME N
BETOS: D1F   Prosthetic/Orthotic devices

D **A4356** External urethral clamp or compression device (not to be used for catheter clamp), each DME N
BETOS: D1F   Prosthetic/Orthotic devices

D **A4357** Bedside drainage bag, day or night, with or without anti-reflux device, with or without tube, each DME N
BETOS: D1F   Prosthetic/Orthotic devices

D **A4358** Urinary drainage bag, leg or abdomen, vinyl, with or without tube, with straps, each DME N
BETOS: D1F   Prosthetic/Orthotic devices

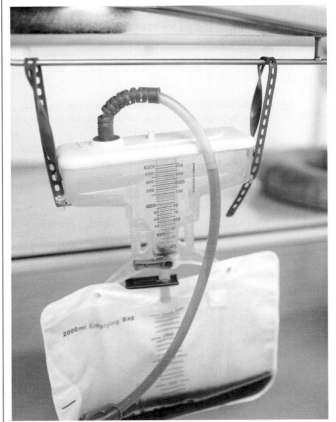

Urinary drainage bag

D **A4360** Disposable external urethral clamp or compression device, with pad and/or pouch, each DME N
BETOS: D1F   Prosthetic/Orthotic devices

OSTOMY POUCHES AND SUPPLIES (A4361-A4435), SEE ALSO OSTOMY POUCHES AND SUPPLIES (A5051-A5093)

D **A4361** Ostomy faceplate, each **DME** N
BETOS: D1F   Prosthetic/Orthotic devices

D **A4362** Skin barrier; solid, 4 x 4 or equivalent; each **DME** N
BETOS: D1F   Prosthetic/Orthotic devices

D **A4363** Ostomy clamp, any type, replacement only, each **DME** E1
BETOS: D1F   Prosthetic/Orthotic devices

D **A4364** Adhesive, liquid or equal, any type, per oz. **DME** N
BETOS: D1F   Prosthetic/Orthotic devices

C **A4366** Ostomy vent, any type, each **DME** N
BETOS: D1F   Prosthetic/Orthotic devices

D **A4367** Ostomy belt, each **DME** N
BETOS: D1F   Prosthetic/Orthotic devices

C **A4368** Ostomy filter, any type, each **DME** N
BETOS: D1F   Prosthetic/Orthotic devices

D **A4369** Ostomy skin barrier, liquid (spray, brush, etc.), per oz. **DME** N
BETOS: D1F   Prosthetic/Orthotic devices

D **A4371** Ostomy skin barrier, powder, per oz. **DME** N
BETOS: D1F   Prosthetic/Orthotic devices

D **A4372** Ostomy skin barrier, solid 4 x 4 or equivalent, standard wear, with built-in convexity, each **DME** N
BETOS: D1F   Prosthetic/Orthotic devices

D **A4373** Ostomy skin barrier, with flange (solid, flexible or accordion), with built-in convexity, any size, each **DME** N
BETOS: D1F   Prosthetic/Orthotic devices

D **A4375** Ostomy pouch, drainable, with faceplate attached, plastic, each **DME** N
BETOS: D1F   Prosthetic/Orthotic devices

D **A4376** Ostomy pouch, drainable, with faceplate attached, rubber, each **DME** N
BETOS: D1F   Prosthetic/Orthotic devices

D **A4377** Ostomy pouch, drainable, for use on faceplate, plastic, each **DME** N
BETOS: D1F   Prosthetic/Orthotic devices

D **A4378** Ostomy pouch, drainable, for use on faceplate, rubber, each **DME** N
BETOS: D1F   Prosthetic/Orthotic devices

D **A4379** Ostomy pouch, urinary, with faceplate attached, plastic, each **DME** N
BETOS: D1F   Prosthetic/Orthotic devices

D **A4380** Ostomy pouch, urinary, with faceplate attached, rubber, each **DME** N
BETOS: D1F   Prosthetic/Orthotic devices

D **A4381** Ostomy pouch, urinary, for use on faceplate, plastic, each **DME** N
BETOS: D1F   Prosthetic/Orthotic devices

D **A4382** Ostomy pouch, urinary, for use on faceplate, heavy plastic, each **DME** N
BETOS: D1F   Prosthetic/Orthotic devices

D **A4383** Ostomy pouch, urinary, for use on faceplate, rubber, each **DME** N
BETOS: D1F   Prosthetic/Orthotic devices

D **A4384** Ostomy faceplate equivalent, silicone ring, each **DME** N
BETOS: D1F   Prosthetic/Orthotic devices

D **A4385** Ostomy skin barrier, solid 4 x 4 or equivalent, extended wear, without built-in convexity, each **DME** N
BETOS: D1F   Prosthetic/Orthotic devices

D **A4387** Ostomy pouch, closed, with barrier attached, with built-in convexity (1 piece), each **DME** N
BETOS: D1F   Prosthetic/Orthotic devices

D **A4388** Ostomy pouch, drainable, with extended wear barrier attached, (1 piece), each **DME** N
BETOS: D1F   Prosthetic/Orthotic devices

D **A4389** Ostomy pouch, drainable, with barrier attached, with built-in convexity (1 piece), each **DME** N
BETOS: D1F   Prosthetic/Orthotic devices

D **A4390** Ostomy pouch, drainable, with extended wear barrier attached, with built-in convexity (1 piece), each **DME** N
BETOS: D1F   Prosthetic/Orthotic devices

D **A4391** Ostomy pouch, urinary, with extended wear barrier attached (1 piece), each **DME** N
BETOS: D1F   Prosthetic/Orthotic devices

D **A4392** Ostomy pouch, urinary, with standard wear barrier attached, with built-in convexity (1 piece), each **DME** N
BETOS: D1F   Prosthetic/Orthotic devices

D **A4393** Ostomy pouch, urinary, with extended wear barrier attached, with built-in convexity (1 piece), each **DME** N
BETOS: D1F   Prosthetic/Orthotic devices

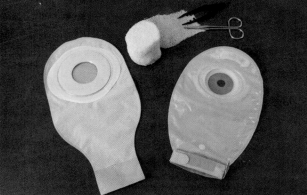

Ostomy pouch

♂ Male only   ♀ Female only   Ⓐ Age   A2 - Z3 = ASC Payment indicator   A - Y = APC Status indicator
ASC = ASC Approved Procedure   **DME** Paid under the DME fee schedule   **MIPS** MIPS code

D A4394 Ostomy deodorant, with or without lubricant, for use in ostomy pouch, per fluid ounce [DME] N
BETOS: D1F   Prosthetic/Orthotic devices

D A4395 Ostomy deodorant for use in ostomy pouch, solid, per tablet [DME] N
BETOS: D1F   Prosthetic/Orthotic devices

D A4396 Ostomy belt with peristomal hernia support [DME] N
BETOS: D1F   Prosthetic/Orthotic devices

D A4397 Irrigation supply; sleeve, each [DME] N
BETOS: D1F   Prosthetic/Orthotic devices

D A4398 Ostomy irrigation supply; bag, each [DME] N
BETOS: D1F   Prosthetic/Orthotic devices

D A4399 Ostomy irrigation supply; cone/catheter, with or without brush [DME] N
BETOS: D1F   Prosthetic/Orthotic devices

D A4400 Ostomy irrigation set [DME] N
BETOS: D1F   Prosthetic/Orthotic devices

D A4402 Lubricant, per ounce [DME] N
BETOS: D1F   Prosthetic/Orthotic devices

D A4404 Ostomy ring, each [DME] N
BETOS: D1F   Prosthetic/Orthotic devices

D A4405 Ostomy skin barrier, non-pectin based, paste, per ounce [DME] N
BETOS: D1F   Prosthetic/Orthotic devices

D A4406 Ostomy skin barrier, pectin-based, paste, per ounce [DME] N
BETOS: D1F   Prosthetic/Orthotic devices

D A4407 Ostomy skin barrier, with flange (solid, flexible, or accordion), extended wear, with built-in convexity, 4 x 4 inches or smaller, each [DME] N
BETOS: D1F   Prosthetic/Orthotic devices

D A4408 Ostomy skin barrier, with flange (solid, flexible or accordion), extended wear, with built-in convexity, larger than 4 x 4 inches, each [DME] N
BETOS: D1F   Prosthetic/Orthotic devices

D A4409 Ostomy skin barrier, with flange (solid, flexible or accordion), extended wear, without built-in convexity, 4 x 4 inches or smaller, each [DME] N
BETOS: D1F   Prosthetic/Orthotic devices

D A4410 Ostomy skin barrier, with flange (solid, flexible or accordion), extended wear, without built-in convexity, larger than 4 x 4 inches, each [DME] N
BETOS: D1F   Prosthetic/Orthotic devices

D A4411 Ostomy skin barrier, solid 4 x 4 or equivalent, extended wear, with built-in convexity, each [DME] N
BETOS: D1F   Prosthetic/Orthotic devices

D A4412 Ostomy pouch, drainable, high output, for use on a barrier with flange (2 piece system), without filter, each [DME] N
BETOS: D1F   Prosthetic/Orthotic devices

D A4413 Ostomy pouch, drainable, high output, for use on a barrier with flange (2 piece system), with filter, each [DME] N
BETOS: D1F   Prosthetic/Orthotic devices

D A4414 Ostomy skin barrier, with flange (solid, flexible or accordion), without built-in convexity, 4 x 4 inches or smaller, each [DME] N
BETOS: D1F   Prosthetic/Orthotic devices

D A4415 Ostomy skin barrier, with flange (solid, flexible or accordion), without built-in convexity, larger than 4 x 4 inches, each [DME] N
BETOS: D1F   Prosthetic/Orthotic devices

C A4416 Ostomy pouch, closed, with barrier attached, with filter (1 piece), each [DME] N
BETOS: D1F   Prosthetic/Orthotic devices

C A4417 Ostomy pouch, closed, with barrier attached, with built-in convexity, with filter (1 piece), each [DME] N
BETOS: D1F   Prosthetic/Orthotic devices

C A4418 Ostomy pouch, closed; without barrier attached, with filter (1 piece), each [DME] N
BETOS: D1F   Prosthetic/Orthotic devices

C A4419 Ostomy pouch, closed; for use on barrier with non-locking flange, with filter (2 piece), each [DME] N
BETOS: D1F   Prosthetic/Orthotic devices

C A4420 Ostomy pouch, closed; for use on barrier with locking flange (2 piece), each [DME] N
BETOS: D1F   Prosthetic/Orthotic devices

C A4421 Ostomy supply; miscellaneous N
BETOS: D1F   Prosthetic/Orthotic devices

D A4422 Ostomy absorbent material (sheet/pad/crystal packet) for use in ostomy pouch to thicken liquid stomal output, each [DME] N
BETOS: D1F   Prosthetic/Orthotic devices

C A4423 Ostomy pouch, closed; for use on barrier with locking flange, with filter (2 piece), each [DME] N
BETOS: D1F   Prosthetic/Orthotic devices

C A4424 Ostomy pouch, drainable, with barrier attached, with filter (1 piece), each [DME] N
BETOS: D1F   Prosthetic/Orthotic devices

C A4425 Ostomy pouch, drainable; for use on barrier with non-locking flange, with filter (2 piece system), each [DME] N
BETOS: D1F   Prosthetic/Orthotic devices

C A4426 Ostomy pouch, drainable; for use on barrier with locking flange (2 piece system), each [DME] N
BETOS: D1F   Prosthetic/Orthotic devices

● New code   ▲ Revised code   **C** Carrier judgment   **D** Special coverage instructions apply
I Not payable by Medicare   **M** Non-covered by Medicare   **S** Non-covered by Medicare statute   *AHA Coding Clinic®*

C A4427 Ostomy pouch, drainable; for use on barrier with locking flange, with filter (2 piece system), each   **DME** N
   BETOS: D1F Prosthetic/Orthotic devices

C A4428 Ostomy pouch, urinary, with extended wear barrier attached, with faucet-type tap with valve (1 piece), each   **DME** N
   BETOS: D1F Prosthetic/Orthotic devices

C A4429 Ostomy pouch, urinary, with barrier attached, with built-in convexity, with faucet-type tap with valve (1 piece), each   **DME** N
   BETOS: D1F Prosthetic/Orthotic devices

C A4430 Ostomy pouch, urinary, with extended wear barrier attached, with built-in convexity, with faucet-type tap with valve (1 piece), each   **DME** N
   BETOS: D1F Prosthetic/Orthotic devices

C A4431 Ostomy pouch, urinary; with barrier attached, with faucet-type tap with valve (1 piece), each   **DME** N
   BETOS: D1F Prosthetic/Orthotic devices

C A4432 Ostomy pouch, urinary; for use on barrier with non-locking flange, with faucet-type tap with valve (2 piece), each   **DME** N
   BETOS: D1F Prosthetic/Orthotic devices

C A4433 Ostomy pouch, urinary; for use on barrier with locking flange (2 piece), each   **DME** N
   BETOS: D1F Prosthetic/Orthotic devices

C A4434 Ostomy pouch, urinary; for use on barrier with locking flange, with faucet-type tap with valve (2 piece), each   **DME** N
   BETOS: D1F Prosthetic/Orthotic devices

C A4435 Ostomy pouch, drainable, high output, with extended wear barrier (one-piece system), with or without filter, each   **DME** N
   BETOS: D1F Prosthetic/Orthotic devices

VARIOUS MEDICAL SUPPLIES INCLUDING TAPES AND SURGICAL DRESSINGS (A4450-A4608)

D A4450 Tape, non-waterproof, per 18 square inches   **DME** N
   BETOS: D1F Prosthetic/Orthotic devices
   DME Modifier: AU,AV,AW

D A4452 Tape, waterproof, per 18 square inches   **DME** N
   BETOS: D1F Prosthetic/Orthotic devices
   DME Modifier: AU,AV,AW

D A4455 Adhesive remover or solvent (for tape, cement or other adhesive), per ounce   **DME** N
   BETOS: D1F Prosthetic/Orthotic devices

D A4456 Adhesive remover, wipes, any type, each   **DME** N
   BETOS: D1F Prosthetic/Orthotic devices

C A4458 Enema bag with tubing, reusable   N
   BETOS: Z2 Undefined codes
   Service not separately priced by Part B

C A4459 Manual pump-operated enema system, includes balloon, catheter and all accessories, reusable, any type   N
   BETOS: Z2 Undefined codes
   Service not separately priced by Part B

C A4461 Surgical dressing holder, non-reusable, each   **DME** N
   BETOS: D1A Medical/surgical supplies

C A4463 Surgical dressing holder, reusable, each   **DME** N
   BETOS: D1A Medical/surgical supplies

C A4465 Non-elastic binder for extremity   N
   BETOS: D1A Medical/surgical supplies
   Service not separately priced by Part B

M A4467 Belt, strap, sleeve, garment, or covering, any type   E1
   BETOS: Z2 Undefined codes
   Service not separately priced by Part B

D A4470 Gravlee jet washer   ♀ N
   BETOS: D1A Medical/surgical supplies
   Service not separately priced by Part B

D A4480 Vabra aspirator   ♀ N
   BETOS: D1A Medical/surgical supplies
   Service not separately priced by Part B

D A4481 Tracheostoma filter, any type, any size, each   **DME** N
   BETOS: D1F Prosthetic/Orthotic devices

D A4483 Moisture exchanger, disposable, for use with invasive mechanical ventilation   **DME** N
   BETOS: D1F Prosthetic/Orthotic devices

M A4490 Surgical stockings above knee length, each   E1
   BETOS: D1A Medical/surgical supplies
   Service not separately priced by Part B

M A4495 Surgical stockings thigh length, each   E1
   BETOS: D1A Medical/surgical supplies
   Service not separately priced by Part B

M A4500 Surgical stockings below knee length, each   E1
   BETOS: D1A Medical/surgical supplies
   Service not separately priced by Part B

M A4510 Surgical stockings full length, each   E1
   BETOS: D1A Medical/surgical supplies
   Service not separately priced by Part B

M A4520 Incontinence garment, any type, (e.g., brief, diaper), each   E1
   BETOS: D1A Medical/surgical supplies
   Service not separately priced by Part B

D **A4550** Surgical trays   B
    BETOS: Y1   Other - Medicare fee schedule
    Price established using national RVUs

M **A4553** Non-disposable underpads, all sizes   E1
    BETOS: D1A   Medical/surgical supplies
    Service not separately priced by Part B

M **A4554** Disposable underpads, all sizes   E1
    BETOS: D1A   Medical/surgical supplies
    Service not separately priced by Part B

I **A4555** Electrode/transducer for use with electrical stimulation device used for cancer treatment, replacement only   E1
    BETOS: D1E   Other DME
    Service not separately priced by Part B

C **A4556** Electrodes, (e.g., apnea monitor), per pair   DME N
    BETOS: D1E   Other DME

C **A4557** Lead wires, (e.g., apnea monitor), per pair   DME N
    BETOS: D1E   Other DME

C **A4558** Conductive gel or paste, for use with electrical device (e.g., TENS, NMES), per oz.   DME N
    BETOS: D1E   Other DME

C **A4559** Coupling gel or paste, for use with ultrasound device, per oz.   DME N
    BETOS: D1E   Other DME

C **A4561** Pessary, rubber, any type   ♀ DME N
    BETOS: D1F   Prosthetic/Orthotic devices

Pessary

C **A4562** Pessary, non rubber, any type   ♀ DME N
    BETOS: D1F   Prosthetic/Orthotic devices

C **A4563** Rectal control system for vaginal insertion, for long term use, includes pump and all supplies and accessories, any type each   ♀ DME A
    BETOS: D1F   Prosthetic/Orthotic devices

C **A4565** Slings   DME N
    BETOS: D1A   Medical/surgical supplies

I **A4566** Shoulder sling or vest design, abduction restrainer, with or without swathe control, prefabricated, includes fitting and adjustment   E1
    BETOS: Z2   Undefined codes
    Service not separately priced by Part B

I **A4570** Splint   E1
    BETOS: D1A   Medical/surgical supplies
    Reasonable charge

C **A4575** Topical hyperbaric oxygen chamber, disposable   A
    BETOS: D1A   Medical/surgical supplies
    Service not separately priced by Part B

I **A4580** Cast supplies (e.g., plaster)   E1
    BETOS: D1A   Medical/surgical supplies
    Service not separately priced by Part B

I **A4590** Special casting material (e.g., fiberglass)   E1
    BETOS: D1A   Medical/surgical supplies
    Service not separately priced by Part B

D **A4595** Electrical stimulator supplies, 2 lead, per month, (e.g., TENS, NMES)   DME N
    BETOS: D1E   Other DME

C **A4600** Sleeve for intermittent limb compression device, replacement only, each   E1
    BETOS: D1E   Other DME

C **A4601** Lithium ion battery, rechargeable, for non-prosthetic use, replacement   E1
    BETOS: D1E   Other DME

C **A4602** Replacement battery for external infusion pump owned by patient, lithium, 1.5 volt, each   DME N
    BETOS: D1E   Other DME
    DME Modifier: NU

C **A4604** Tubing with integrated heating element for use with positive airway pressure device   DME N
    BETOS: D1E   Other DME
    DME Modifier: NU
    Pub: 100-4, Chapter-36, 50.14

C **A4605** Tracheal suction catheter, closed system, each   DME N
    BETOS: D1E   Other DME
    DME Modifier: NU

C **A4606** Oxygen probe for use with oximeter device, replacement   N
    BETOS: D1E   Other DME
    Service not separately priced by Part B

C **A4608** Transtracheal oxygen catheter, each   DME N
    BETOS: D1C   Oxygen and supplies
    Service not separately priced by Part B

● New code   ▲ Revised code   **C** Carrier judgment   **D** Special coverage instructions apply
I Not payable by Medicare   **M** Non-covered by Medicare   **S** Non-covered by Medicare statute   AHA Coding Clinic®

RESPIRATORY SUPPLIES AND EQUIPMENT (A4611-A4629)

S A4611 Battery, heavy duty; replacement for patient owned ventilator   E1
BETOS: D1E   Other DME
Service not separately priced by Part B
Statute: 1834a3A

S A4612 Battery cables; replacement for patient-owned ventilator   E1
BETOS: D1E   Other DME
Service not separately priced by Part B
Statute: 1834a3A

S A4613 Battery charger; replacement for patient-owned ventilator   E1
BETOS: D1E   Other DME
Service not separately priced by Part B
Statute: 1834a3A

C A4614 Peak expiratory flow rate meter, Hand-held   DME N
BETOS: Z2   Undefined codes

D A4615 Cannula, nasal   DME N
BETOS: D1C   Oxygen and supplies
Service not separately priced by Part B

Nasal cannula

D A4616 Tubing (oxygen), per foot   DME N
BETOS: D1C   Oxygen and supplies
Service not separately priced by Part B

D A4617 Mouth piece   DME N
BETOS: D1C   Oxygen and supplies
Service not separately priced by Part B

D A4618 Breathing circuits   DME N
BETOS: D1E   Other DME
DME Modifier: NU,RR,UE

D A4619 Face tent   DME N
BETOS: D1E   Other DME
DME Modifier: NU

D A4620 Variable concentration mask   DME N
BETOS: D1C   Oxygen and supplies
Service not separately priced by Part B

D A4623 Tracheostomy, inner cannula   DME N
BETOS: D1F   Prosthetic/Orthotic devices

C A4624 Tracheal suction catheter, any type other than closed system, each   DME N
BETOS: D1E   Other DME
DME Modifier: NU

D A4625 Tracheostomy care kit for new tracheostomy   DME N
BETOS: D1F   Prosthetic/Orthotic devices

D A4626 Tracheostomy cleaning brush, each   DME N
BETOS: D1F   Prosthetic/Orthotic devices

M A4627 Spacer, bag or reservoir, with or without mask, for use with metered dose inhaler   E1
BETOS: D1A   Medical/surgical supplies
Service not separately priced by Part B

C A4628 Oropharyngeal suction catheter, each   DME N
BETOS: D1E   Other DME
DME Modifier: NU

D A4629 Tracheostomy care kit for established tracheostomy   DME N
BETOS: D1F   Prosthetic/Orthotic devices

REPLACEMENT PARTS (A4630-A4640)

D A4630 Replacement batteries, medically necessary, transcutaneous electrical stimulator, owned by patient   DME E1
BETOS: D1E   Other DME
DME Modifier: NU

C A4633 Replacement bulb/lamp for ultraviolet light therapy system, each   DME E1
BETOS: D1E   Other DME
DME Modifier: NU

C A4634 Replacement bulb for therapeutic light box, tabletop model   N
BETOS: D1E   Other DME
Service not separately priced by Part B

D A4635 Underarm pad, crutch, replacement, each   DME E1
BETOS: D1E   Other DME
DME Modifier: NU,RR,UE

D A4636 Replacement, handgrip, cane, crutch, or walker, each   DME E1
BETOS: D1E   Other DME
DME Modifier: KE,NU,RR,UE
Pub: 100-4, Chapter-36, 50.15

D A4637 Replacement, tip, cane, crutch, walker, each.   DME E1
BETOS: D1E   Other DME
DME Modifier: KE,NU,RR,UE
Pub: 100-4, Chapter-36, 50.15

C A4638 Replacement battery for patient-owned ear pulse generator, each   DME E1
BETOS: D1E   Other DME
DME Modifier: NU,RR,UE

♂ Male only   ♀ Female only   **A** Age   A2 - Z3 = ASC Payment indicator   A - Y = APC Status indicator
ASC = ASC Approved Procedure   **DME** Paid under the DME fee schedule   **MIPS** MIPS code

C **A4639** Replacement pad for infrared heating pad system, each   DME E1
   BETOS: D1E   Other DME
   DME Modifier: RR
   Pub: 100-4, Chapter-5, 20.4

D **A4640** Replacement pad for use with medically necessary alternating pressure pad owned by patient   DME E1
   BETOS: D1E   Other DME
   DME Modifier: NU,RR,UE

DIAGNOSTIC RADIOPHARMACEUTICALS (A4641-A4642), SEE ALSO DIAGNOSTIC AND THERAPEUTIC RADIOPHARMACEUTICALS (A9500-A9700)

C **A4641** Radiopharmaceutical, diagnostic, not otherwise classified   N
   BETOS: I1E   Standard imaging - nuclear medicine
   Coding Clinic: 2005, Q4
   Pub: 100-4, Chapter-13, 60.3

C **A4642** Indium In-111 satumomab pendetide, diagnostic, per study dose, up to 6 millicuries   N
   BETOS: I1E   Standard imaging - nuclear medicine
   Coding Clinic: 2002, Q2; 2005, Q4

OTHER SUPPLIES (A4648-A4652)

C **A4648** Tissue marker, implantable, any type, each   N
   BETOS: I1E   Standard imaging - nuclear medicine
   Other carrier priced
   Coding Clinic: 2013, Q3; 2018, Q2

C **A4649** Surgical supply; miscellaneous   N
   BETOS: D1A   Medical/surgical supplies

C **A4650** Implantable radiation dosimeter, each   N
   BETOS: I1E   Standard imaging - nuclear medicine
   Other carrier priced

D **A4651** Calibrated microcapillary tube, each   N
   BETOS: P9B   Dialysis services (non-Medicare fee schedule)
   Service not separately priced by Part B
   Coding Clinic: 2002, Q1

D **A4652** Microcapillary tube sealant   N
   BETOS: P9B   Dialysis services (non-Medicare fee schedule)
   Service not separately priced by Part B
   Coding Clinic: 2002, Q1

DIALYSIS EQUIPMENT AND SUPPLIES (A4653-A4932)

C **A4653** Peritoneal dialysis catheter anchoring device, belt, each   N
   BETOS: P9B   Dialysis services (non-Medicare fee schedule)
   Service not separately priced by Part B

D **A4657** Syringe, with or without needle, each   N
   BETOS: P9B   Dialysis services (non-Medicare fee schedule)
   Service not separately priced by Part B
   Coding Clinic: 2002, Q1
   Pub: 100-4, Chapter-8, 60.4; 100-4, Chapter-8, 60.4.6.3; 100-4, Chapter-8, 60.6

D **A4660** Sphygmomanometer/blood pressure apparatus with cuff and stethoscope   N
   BETOS: P9B   Dialysis services (non-Medicare fee schedule)
   Service not separately priced by Part B

D **A4663** Blood pressure cuff only   N
   BETOS: P9B   Dialysis services (non-Medicare fee schedule)
   Service not separately priced by Part B

M **A4670** Automatic blood pressure monitor   E1
   BETOS: P9B   Dialysis services (non-Medicare fee schedule)
   Service not separately priced by Part B

Blood pressure cuff

D **A4671** Disposable cycler set used with cycler dialysis machine, each   B
   BETOS: P9B   Dialysis services (non-Medicare fee schedule)
   Service not separately priced by Part B

● New code   ▲ Revised code   **C** Carrier judgment   **D** Special coverage instructions apply
I Not payable by Medicare   **M** Non-covered by Medicare   **S** Non-covered by Medicare statute   AHA Coding Clinic®

D **A4672** Drainage extension line, sterile, for dialysis, each B

BETOS: P9B Dialysis services (non-Medicare fee schedule)

Service not separately priced by Part B

D **A4673** Extension line with easy lock connectors, used with dialysis B

BETOS: P9B Dialysis services (non-Medicare fee schedule)

Service not separately priced by Part B

D **A4674** Chemicals/antiseptics solution used to clean/sterilize dialysis equipment, per 8 oz. B

BETOS: P9B Dialysis services (non-Medicare fee schedule)

Service not separately priced by Part B

D **A4680** Activated carbon filter for hemodialysis, each N

BETOS: P9B Dialysis services (non-Medicare fee schedule)

Service not separately priced by Part B

D **A4690** Dialyzer (artificial kidneys), all types, all sizes, for hemodialysis, each N

BETOS: P9B Dialysis services (non-Medicare fee schedule)

Service not separately priced by Part B

D **A4706** Bicarbonate concentrate, solution, for hemodialysis, per gallon N

BETOS: P9B Dialysis services (non-Medicare fee schedule)

Service not separately priced by Part B

Coding Clinic: 2002, Q1

D **A4707** Bicarbonate concentrate, powder, for hemodialysis, per packet N

BETOS: P9B Dialysis services (non-Medicare fee schedule)

Service not separately priced by Part B

Coding Clinic: 2002, Q1

D **A4708** Acetate concentrate solution, for hemodialysis, per gallon N

BETOS: P9B Dialysis services (non-Medicare fee schedule)

Service not separately priced by Part B

Coding Clinic: 2002, Q1

D **A4709** Acid concentrate, solution, for hemodialysis, per gallon N

BETOS: P9B Dialysis services (non-Medicare fee schedule)

Service not separately priced by Part B

Coding Clinic: 2002, Q1

D **A4714** Treated water (deionized, distilled, or reverse osmosis) for peritoneal dialysis, per gallon N

BETOS: P9B Dialysis services (non-Medicare fee schedule)

Service not separately priced by Part B

D **A4719** "Y set" tubing for peritoneal dialysis N

BETOS: P9B Dialysis services (non-Medicare fee schedule)

Service not separately priced by Part B

Coding Clinic: 2002, Q1

D **A4720** Dialysate solution, any concentration of dextrose, fluid volume greater than 249 cc, but less than or equal to 999 cc, for peritoneal dialysis N

BETOS: P9B Dialysis services (non-Medicare fee schedule)

Service not separately priced by Part B

Coding Clinic: 2002, Q1

D **A4721** Dialysate solution, any concentration of dextrose, fluid volume greater than 999 cc but less than or equal to 1999 cc, for peritoneal dialysis N

BETOS: P9B Dialysis services (non-Medicare fee schedule)

Service not separately priced by Part B

Coding Clinic: 2002, Q1

D **A4722** Dialysate solution, any concentration of dextrose, fluid volume greater than 1999 cc but less than or equal to 2999 cc, for peritoneal dialysis N

BETOS: P9B Dialysis services (non-Medicare fee schedule)

Service not separately priced by Part B

Coding Clinic: 2002, Q1

D **A4723** Dialysate solution, any concentration of dextrose, fluid volume greater than 2999 cc but less than or equal to 3999 cc, for peritoneal dialysis N

BETOS: P9B Dialysis services (non-Medicare fee schedule)

Service not separately priced by Part B

Coding Clinic: 2002, Q1

D **A4724** Dialysate solution, any concentration of dextrose, fluid volume greater than 3999 cc but less than or equal to 4999 cc, for peritoneal dialysis N

BETOS: P9B Dialysis services (non-Medicare fee schedule)

Service not separately priced by Part B

Coding Clinic: 2002, Q1

D **A4725** Dialysate solution, any concentration of dextrose, fluid volume greater than 4999 cc but less than or equal to 5999 cc, for peritoneal dialysis N

BETOS: P9B Dialysis services (non-Medicare fee schedule)

Service not separately priced by Part B

Coding Clinic: 2002, Q1

D **A4726** Dialysate solution, any concentration of dextrose, fluid volume greater than 5999 cc, for peritoneal dialysis N

BETOS: P9B Dialysis services (non-Medicare fee schedule)

Service not separately priced by Part B

Coding Clinic: 2002, Q1

C A4728 Dialysate solution, non-dextrose containing, 500 ml · B
BETOS: P9B Dialysis services (non-Medicare fee schedule)
Service not separately priced by Part B

D A4730 Fistula cannulation set for hemodialysis, each · N
BETOS: P9B Dialysis services (non-Medicare fee schedule)
Service not separately priced by Part B

D A4736 Topical anesthetic, for dialysis, per gram · N
BETOS: P9B Dialysis services (non-Medicare fee schedule)
Service not separately priced by Part B
Coding Clinic: 2002, Q1

D A4737 Injectable anesthetic, for dialysis, per 10 ml · N
BETOS: P9B Dialysis services (non-Medicare fee schedule)
Service not separately priced by Part B
Coding Clinic: 2002, Q1

D A4740 Shunt accessory, for hemodialysis, any type, each · N
BETOS: P9B Dialysis services (non-Medicare fee schedule)
Service not separately priced by Part B

D A4750 Blood tubing, arterial or venous, for hemodialysis, each · N
BETOS: P9B Dialysis services (non-Medicare fee schedule)
Service not separately priced by Part B

D A4755 Blood tubing, arterial and venous combined, for hemodialysis, each · N
BETOS: P9B Dialysis services (non-Medicare fee schedule)
Service not separately priced by Part B

D A4760 Dialysate solution test kit, for peritoneal dialysis, any type, each · N
BETOS: P9B Dialysis services (non-Medicare fee schedule)
Service not separately priced by Part B

D A4765 Dialysate concentrate, powder, additive for peritoneal dialysis, per packet · N
BETOS: P9B Dialysis services (non-Medicare fee schedule)
Service not separately priced by Part B

D A4766 Dialysate concentrate, solution, additive for peritoneal dialysis, per 10 ml · N
BETOS: P9B Dialysis services (non-Medicare fee schedule)
Service not separately priced by Part B
Coding Clinic: 2002, Q1

D A4770 Blood collection tube, vacuum, for dialysis, per 50 · N
BETOS: P9B Dialysis services (non-Medicare fee schedule)
Service not separately priced by Part B

D A4771 Serum clotting time tube, for dialysis, per 50 · N
BETOS: P9B Dialysis services (non-Medicare fee schedule)
Service not separately priced by Part B

D A4772 Blood glucose test strips, for dialysis, per 50 · N
BETOS: P9B Dialysis services (non-Medicare fee schedule)
Service not separately priced by Part B

D A4773 Occult blood test strips, for dialysis, per 50 · N
BETOS: P9B Dialysis services (non-Medicare fee schedule)
Service not separately priced by Part B

D A4774 Ammonia test strips, for dialysis, per 50 · N
BETOS: P9B Dialysis services (non-Medicare fee schedule)
Service not separately priced by Part B

D A4802 Protamine sulfate, for hemodialysis, per 50 mg · N
BETOS: P9B Dialysis services (non-Medicare fee schedule)
Service not separately priced by Part B
Coding Clinic: 2002, Q1

D A4860 Disposable catheter tips for peritoneal dialysis, per 10 · N
BETOS: P9B Dialysis services (non-Medicare fee schedule)
Service not separately priced by Part B

D A4870 Plumbing and/or electrical work for home hemodialysis equipment · N
BETOS: P9B Dialysis services (non-Medicare fee schedule)
Service not separately priced by Part B

D A4890 Contracts, repair and maintenance, for hemodialysis equipment · N
BETOS: P9B Dialysis services (non-Medicare fee schedule)
Service not separately priced by Part B

D A4911 Drain bag/bottle, for dialysis, each · N
BETOS: P9B Dialysis services (non-Medicare fee schedule)
Service not separately priced by Part B
Coding Clinic: 2002, Q1

D A4913 Miscellaneous dialysis supplies, not otherwise specified · N
BETOS: P9B Dialysis services (non-Medicare fee schedule)
Service not separately priced by Part B

D A4918 Venous pressure clamp, for hemodialysis, each · N
BETOS: P9B Dialysis services (non-Medicare fee schedule)
Service not separately priced by Part B

● New code   ▲ Revised code   **C** Carrier judgment   **D** Special coverage instructions apply
I Not payable by Medicare   **M** Non-covered by Medicare   **S** Non-covered by Medicare statute   AHA Coding Clinic®

D **A4927** Gloves, non-sterile, per 100　　　　N
　　　BETOS: P9B　Dialysis services (non-Medicare fee schedule)
　　　Service not separately priced by Part B

D **A4928** Surgical mask, per 20　　　　N
　　　BETOS: P9B　Dialysis services (non-Medicare fee schedule)
　　　Service not separately priced by Part B
　　　Coding Clinic: 2002, Q1

D **A4929** Tourniquet for dialysis, each　　　　N
　　　BETOS: P9B　Dialysis services (non-Medicare fee schedule)
　　　Service not separately priced by Part B
　　　Coding Clinic: 2002, Q1

D **A4930** Gloves, sterile, per pair　　　　N
　　　BETOS: P9B　Dialysis services (non-Medicare fee schedule)
　　　Service not separately priced by Part B

C **A4931** Oral thermometer, reusable, any type, each　N
　　　BETOS: P9B　Dialysis services (non-Medicare fee schedule)
　　　Service not separately priced by Part B

C **A4932** Rectal thermometer, reusable, any type, each　　　　N
　　　BETOS: Z2　Undefined codes
　　　Service not separately priced by Part B

OSTOMY POUCHES AND SUPPLIES (A5051-A5093), SEE ALSO OSTOMY POUCHES AND SUPPLIES (A4361-A4435)

D **A5051** Ostomy pouch, closed; with barrier attached (1 piece), each　DME N
　　　BETOS: D1F　Prosthetic/Orthotic devices

D **A5052** Ostomy pouch, closed; without barrier attached (1 piece), each　DME N
　　　BETOS: D1F　Prosthetic/Orthotic devices

D **A5053** Ostomy pouch, closed; for use on faceplate, each　DME N
　　　BETOS: D1F　Prosthetic/Orthotic devices

D **A5054** Ostomy pouch, closed; for use on barrier with flange (2 piece), each　DME N
　　　BETOS: D1F　Prosthetic/Orthotic devices

D **A5055** Stoma cap　DME N
　　　BETOS: D1F　Prosthetic/Orthotic devices

D **A5056** Ostomy pouch, drainable, with extended wear barrier attached, with filter, (1 piece), each　DME N
　　　BETOS: D1F　Prosthetic/Orthotic devices

D **A5057** Ostomy pouch, drainable, with extended wear barrier attached, with built in convexity, with filter, (1 piece), each　DME N
　　　BETOS: D1F　Prosthetic/Orthotic devices

C **A5061** Ostomy pouch, drainable; with barrier attached, (1 piece), each　DME N
　　　BETOS: D1F　Prosthetic/Orthotic devices

D **A5062** Ostomy pouch, drainable; without barrier attached (1 piece), each　DME N
　　　BETOS: D1F　Prosthetic/Orthotic devices

D **A5063** Ostomy pouch, drainable; for use on barrier with flange (2 piece system), each　DME N
　　　BETOS: D1F　Prosthetic/Orthotic devices

D **A5071** Ostomy pouch, urinary; with barrier attached (1 piece), each　DME N
　　　BETOS: D1F　Prosthetic/Orthotic devices

D **A5072** Ostomy pouch, urinary; without barrier attached (1 piece), each　DME N
　　　BETOS: D1F　Prosthetic/Orthotic devices

D **A5073** Ostomy pouch, urinary; for use on barrier with flange (2 piece), each　DME N
　　　BETOS: D1F　Prosthetic/Orthotic devices

D **A5081** Stoma plug or seal, any type　DME N
　　　BETOS: D1F　Prosthetic/Orthotic devices

D **A5082** Continent device; catheter for continent stoma　DME N
　　　BETOS: D1F　Prosthetic/Orthotic devices

C **A5083** Continent device, stoma absorptive cover for continent stoma　DME N
　　　BETOS: D1F　Prosthetic/Orthotic devices

D **A5093** Ostomy accessory; convex insert　DME N
　　　BETOS: D1F　Prosthetic/Orthotic devices

INCONTINENCE DEVICES AND SUPPLIES (A5102-A5200), SEE ALSO INCONTINENCE DEVICES AND SUPPLIES (A4310-A4360)

D **A5102** Bedside drainage bottle with or without tubing, rigid or expandable, each　DME N
　　　BETOS: D1F　Prosthetic/Orthotic devices

D **A5105** Urinary suspensory with leg bag, with or without tube, each　DME N
　　　BETOS: D1F　Prosthetic/Orthotic devices

D **A5112** Urinary drainage bag, leg or abdomen, latex, with or without tube, with straps, each　DME N
　　　BETOS: D1F　Prosthetic/Orthotic devices

D **A5113** Leg strap; latex, replacement only, per set　DME E1
　　　BETOS: D1F　Prosthetic/Orthotic devices

D **A5114** Leg strap; foam or fabric, replacement only, per set　DME E1
　　　BETOS: D1F　Prosthetic/Orthotic devices

D **A5120** Skin barrier, wipes or swabs, each　DME N
　　　BETOS: D1F　Prosthetic/Orthotic devices
　　　DME Modifier: AU,AV

D **A5121** Skin barrier; solid, 6 x 6 or equivalent, each　DME N
　　　BETOS: D1F　Prosthetic/Orthotic devices

D **A5122** Skin barrier; solid, 8 x 8 or equivalent, each　DME N
　　　BETOS: D1F　Prosthetic/Orthotic devices

D **A5126** Adhesive or non-adhesive; disk or foam pad `DME` N
BETOS: D1F   Prosthetic/Orthotic devices

D **A5131** Appliance cleaner, incontinence and ostomy appliances, per 16 oz. `DME` N
BETOS: D1F   Prosthetic/Orthotic devices

D **A5200** Percutaneous catheter/tube anchoring device, adhesive skin attachment `DME` N
BETOS: D1F   Prosthetic/Orthotic devices

DIABETIC FOOTWEAR (A5500-A5514)

D **A5500** For diabetics only, fitting (including follow-up), custom preparation and supply of off-the-shelf depth-inlay shoe manufactured to accommodate multi-density insert(s), per shoe `DME` Y
BETOS: D1F   Prosthetic/Orthotic devices

D **A5501** For diabetics only, fitting (including follow-up), custom preparation and supply of shoe molded from cast(s) of patient's foot (custom molded shoe), per shoe `DME` Y
BETOS: D1F   Prosthetic/Orthotic devices

D **A5503** For diabetics only, modification (including fitting) of off-the-shelf depth-inlay shoe or custom-molded shoe with roller or rigid rocker bottom, per shoe `DME` Y
BETOS: D1F   Prosthetic/Orthotic devices

D **A5504** For diabetics only, modification (including fitting) of off-the-shelf depth-inlay shoe or custom-molded shoe with wedge(s), per shoe `DME` Y
BETOS: D1F   Prosthetic/Orthotic devices

D **A5505** For diabetics only, modification (including fitting) of off-the-shelf depth-inlay shoe or custom-molded shoe with metatarsal bar, per shoe `DME` Y
BETOS: D1F   Prosthetic/Orthotic devices

D **A5506** For diabetics only, modification (including fitting) of off-the-shelf depth-inlay shoe or custom-molded shoe with off-set heel(s), per shoe `DME` Y
BETOS: D1F   Prosthetic/Orthotic devices

D **A5507** For diabetics only, not otherwise specified modification (including fitting) of off-the-shelf depth-inlay shoe or custom-molded shoe, per shoe `DME` Y
BETOS: D1F   Prosthetic/Orthotic devices

D **A5508** For diabetics only, deluxe feature of off-the-shelf depth-inlay shoe or custom-molded shoe, per shoe Y
BETOS: D1F   Prosthetic/Orthotic devices

D **A5510** For diabetics only, direct formed, compression molded to patient's foot without external heat source, multiple-density insert(s) prefabricated, per shoe N
BETOS: D1F   Prosthetic/Orthotic devices
Coding Clinic: 2002, Q1

D **A5512** For diabetics only, multiple density insert, direct formed, molded to foot after external heat source of 230 degrees Fahrenheit or higher, total contact with patient's foot, including arch, base layer minimum of 1/4 inch material of shore a 35 durometer or 3/16 inch material of shore a 40 durometer (or higher), prefabricated, each `DME` Y
BETOS: D1F   Prosthetic/Orthotic devices

D **A5513** For diabetics only, multiple density insert, custom molded from model of patient's foot, total contact with patient's foot, including arch, base layer minimum of 3/16 inch material of shore a 35 durometer (or higher), includes arch filler and other shaping material, custom fabricated, each `DME` Y
BETOS: D1F   Prosthetic/Orthotic devices

D **A5514** For diabetics only, multiple density insert, made by direct carving with cam technology from a rectified cad model created from a digitized scan of the patient, total contact with patient's foot, including arch, base layer minimum of 3/16 inch material of shore a 35 durometer (or higher), includes arch filler and other shaping material, custom fabricated, each `DME` Y
BETOS: D1F   Prosthetic/Orthotic devices

MISCELLANEOUS DRESSING AND WOUND SUPPLIES (A6000-A6208)

M **A6000** Non-contact wound warming wound cover for use with the non-contact wound warming device and warming card E1
BETOS: D1E   Other DME
Service not separately priced by Part B
Coding Clinic: 2002, Q1

D **A6010** Collagen based wound filler, dry form, sterile, per gram of collagen `DME` N
BETOS: D1A   Medical/surgical supplies
Coding Clinic: 2002, Q1

D **A6011** Collagen based wound filler, gel/paste, per gram of collagen `DME` N
BETOS: D1A   Medical/surgical supplies

D **A6021** Collagen dressing, sterile, size 16 sq. in. or less, each `DME` N
BETOS: D1A   Medical/surgical supplies

D **A6022** Collagen dressing, sterile, size more than 16 sq. in. but less than or equal to 48 sq. in., each `DME` N
BETOS: D1A   Medical/surgical supplies

D **A6023** Collagen dressing, sterile, size more than 48 sq. in., each `DME` N
BETOS: D1A   Medical/surgical supplies

D **A6024** Collagen dressing wound filler, sterile, per 6 inches `DME` N
BETOS: D1A   Medical/surgical supplies

● New code   ▲ Revised code   **C** Carrier judgment   **D** Special coverage instructions apply
I Not payable by Medicare   **M** Non-covered by Medicare   **S** Non-covered by Medicare statute   AHA Coding Clinic®

C **A6025** Gel sheet for dermal or epidermal application, (e.g., silicone, hydrogel, other), each   N
> **BETOS:** D1A   Medical/surgical supplies
> Service not separately priced by Part B

D **A6154** Wound pouch, each   DME N
> **BETOS:** D1A   Medical/surgical supplies

D **A6196** Alginate or other fiber gelling dressing, wound cover, sterile, pad size 16 sq. in. or less, each dressing   DME N
> **BETOS:** D1A   Medical/surgical supplies

D **A6197** Alginate or other fiber gelling dressing, wound cover, sterile, pad size more than 16 sq. in. but less than or equal to 48 sq. in., each dressing   DME N
> **BETOS:** D1A   Medical/surgical supplies

D **A6198** Alginate or other fiber gelling dressing, wound cover, sterile, pad size more than 48 sq. in., each dressing   N
> **BETOS:** D1A   Medical/surgical supplies

D **A6199** Alginate or other fiber gelling dressing, wound filler, sterile, per 6 inches   DME N
> **BETOS:** D1A   Medical/surgical supplies

D **A6203** Composite dressing, sterile, pad size 16 sq. in. or less, with any size adhesive border, each dressing   DME N
> **BETOS:** D1A   Medical/surgical supplies

D **A6204** Composite dressing, sterile, pad size more than 16 sq. in. but less than or equal to 48 sq. in., with any size adhesive border, each dressing   DME N
> **BETOS:** D1A   Medical/surgical supplies

D **A6205** Composite dressing, sterile, pad size more than 48 sq. in., with any size adhesive border, each dressing   N
> **BETOS:** D1A   Medical/surgical supplies

D **A6206** Contact layer, sterile, 16 sq. in. or less, each dressing   N
> **BETOS:** D1A   Medical/surgical supplies

D **A6207** Contact layer, sterile, more than 16 sq. in. but less than or equal to 48 sq. in., each dressing   DME N
> **BETOS:** D1A   Medical/surgical supplies

D **A6208** Contact layer, sterile, more than 48 sq. in., each dressing   N
> **BETOS:** D1A   Medical/surgical supplies

FOAM DRESSINGS (A6209-A6215)

D **A6209** Foam dressing, wound cover, sterile, pad size 16 sq. in. or less, without adhesive border, each dressing   DME N
> **BETOS:** D1A   Medical/surgical supplies

D **A6210** Foam dressing, wound cover, sterile, pad size more than 16 sq. in. but less than or equal to 48 sq. in., without adhesive border, each dressing   DME N
> **BETOS:** D1A   Medical/surgical supplies

D **A6211** Foam dressing, wound cover, sterile, pad size more than 48 sq. in., without adhesive border, each dressing   DME N
> **BETOS:** D1A   Medical/surgical supplies

D **A6212** Foam dressing, wound cover, sterile, pad size 16 sq. in. or less, with any size adhesive border, each dressing   DME N
> **BETOS:** D1A   Medical/surgical supplies

D **A6213** Foam dressing, wound cover, sterile, pad size more than 16 sq. in. but less than or equal to 48 sq. in., with any size adhesive border, each dressing   N
> **BETOS:** D1A   Medical/surgical supplies

D **A6214** Foam dressing, wound cover, sterile, pad size more than 48 sq. in., with any size adhesive border, each dressing   DME N
> **BETOS:** D1A   Medical/surgical supplies

D **A6215** Foam dressing, wound filler, sterile, per gram   N
> **BETOS:** D1A   Medical/surgical supplies

GAUZE DRESSINGS (A6216-A6233)

D **A6216** Gauze, non-impregnated, non-sterile, pad size 16 sq. in. or less, without adhesive border, each dressing   DME N
> **BETOS:** D1A   Medical/surgical supplies

D **A6217** Gauze, non-impregnated, non-sterile, pad size more than 16 sq. in. but less than or equal to 48 sq. in., without adhesive border, each dressing   DME N
> **BETOS:** D1A   Medical/surgical supplies

D **A6218** Gauze, non-impregnated, non-sterile, pad size more than 48 sq. in., without adhesive border, each dressing   N
> **BETOS:** D1A   Medical/surgical supplies

D **A6219** Gauze, non-impregnated, sterile, pad size 16 sq. in. or less, with any size adhesive border, each dressing   DME N
> **BETOS:** D1A   Medical/surgical supplies

D **A6220** Gauze, non-impregnated, sterile, pad size more than 16 sq. in. but less than or equal to 48 sq. in., with any size adhesive border, each dressing   DME N
> **BETOS:** D1A   Medical/surgical supplies

D **A6221** Gauze, non-impregnated, sterile, pad size more than 48 sq. in., with any size adhesive border, each dressing   N
> **BETOS:** D1A   Medical/surgical supplies

D **A6222** Gauze, impregnated with other than water, normal saline, or hydrogel, sterile, pad size 16 sq. in. or less, without adhesive border, each dressing DME N

BETOS: D1A Medical/surgical supplies

D **A6223** Gauze, impregnated with other than water, normal saline, or hydrogel, sterile, pad size more than 16 sq. in., but less than or equal to 48 sq. in., without adhesive border, each dressing DME N

BETOS: D1A Medical/surgical supplies

D **A6224** Gauze, impregnated with other than water, normal saline, or hydrogel, sterile, pad size more than 48 sq. in., without adhesive border, each dressing DME N

BETOS: D1A Medical/surgical supplies

D **A6228** Gauze, impregnated, water or normal saline, sterile, pad size 16 sq. in. or less, without adhesive border, each dressing N

BETOS: D1A Medical/surgical supplies

D **A6229** Gauze, impregnated, water or normal saline, sterile, pad size more than 16 sq. in. but less than or equal to 48 sq. in., without adhesive border, each dressing DME N

BETOS: D1A Medical/surgical supplies

D **A6230** Gauze, impregnated, water or normal saline, sterile, pad size more than 48 sq. in., without adhesive border, each dressing N

BETOS: D1A Medical/surgical supplies

D **A6231** Gauze, impregnated, hydrogel, for direct wound contact, sterile, pad size 16 sq. in. or less, each dressing DME N

BETOS: D1A Medical/surgical supplies

D **A6232** Gauze, impregnated, hydrogel, for direct wound contact, sterile, pad size greater than 16 sq. in., but less than or equal to 48 sq. in., each dressing DME N

BETOS: D1A Medical/surgical supplies

D **A6233** Gauze, impregnated, hydrogel, for direct wound contact, sterile, pad size more than 48 sq. in., each dressing DME N

BETOS: D1A Medical/surgical supplies

HYDROCOLLOID DRESSINGS (A6234-A6241)

D **A6234** Hydrocolloid dressing, wound cover, sterile, pad size 16 sq. in. or less, without adhesive border, each dressing DME N

BETOS: D1A Medical/surgical supplies

D **A6235** Hydrocolloid dressing, wound cover, sterile, pad size more than 16 sq. in. but less than or equal to 48 sq. in., without adhesive border, each dressing DME N

BETOS: D1A Medical/surgical supplies

D **A6236** Hydrocolloid dressing, wound cover, sterile, pad size more than 48 sq. in., without adhesive border, each dressing DME N

BETOS: D1A Medical/surgical supplies

D **A6237** Hydrocolloid dressing, wound cover, sterile, pad size 16 sq. in. or less, with any size adhesive border, each dressing DME N

BETOS: D1A Medical/surgical supplies

D **A6238** Hydrocolloid dressing, wound cover, sterile, pad size more than 16 sq. in. but less than or equal to 48 sq. in., with any size adhesive border, each dressing DME N

BETOS: D1A Medical/surgical supplies

D **A6239** Hydrocolloid dressing, wound cover, sterile, pad size more than 48 sq. in., with any size adhesive border, each dressing N

BETOS: D1A Medical/surgical supplies

D **A6240** Hydrocolloid dressing, wound filler, paste, sterile, per ounce DME N

BETOS: D1A Medical/surgical supplies

D **A6241** Hydrocolloid dressing, wound filler, dry form, sterile, per gram DME N

BETOS: D1A Medical/surgical supplies

HYDROGEL DRESSINGS (A6242-A6248)

D **A6242** Hydrogel dressing, wound cover, sterile, pad size 16 sq. in. or less, without adhesive border, each dressing DME N

BETOS: D1A Medical/surgical supplies

D **A6243** Hydrogel dressing, wound cover, sterile, pad size more than 16 sq. in. but less than or equal to 48 sq. in., without adhesive border, each dressing DME N

BETOS: D1A Medical/surgical supplies

D **A6244** Hydrogel dressing, wound cover, sterile, pad size more than 48 sq. in., without adhesive border, each dressing DME N

BETOS: D1A Medical/surgical supplies

D **A6245** Hydrogel dressing, wound cover, sterile, pad size 16 sq. in. or less, with any size adhesive border, each dressing DME N

BETOS: D1A Medical/surgical supplies

D **A6246** Hydrogel dressing, wound cover, sterile, pad size more than 16 sq. in. but less than or equal to 48 sq. in., with any size adhesive border, each dressing DME N

BETOS: D1A Medical/surgical supplies

D **A6247** Hydrogel dressing, wound cover, sterile, pad size more than 48 sq. in., with any size adhesive border, each dressing DME N

BETOS: D1A Medical/surgical supplies

D **A6248** Hydrogel dressing, wound filler, gel, per fluid ounce DME N

BETOS: D1A Medical/surgical supplies

● New code   ▲ Revised code   **C** Carrier judgment   **D** Special coverage instructions apply

I Not payable by Medicare   **M** Non-covered by Medicare   **S** Non-covered by Medicare statute   AHA Coding Clinic®

OTHER DRESSINGS, COVERINGS, AND WOUND TREATMENT SUPPLIES (A6250-A6412)

D A6250 Skin sealants, protectants, moisturizers, ointments, any type, any size   N
BETOS: D1A   Medical/surgical supplies
Service not separately priced by Part B

D A6251 Specialty absorptive dressing, wound cover, sterile, pad size 16 sq. in. or less, without adhesive border, each dressing   **DME** N
BETOS: D1A   Medical/surgical supplies

D A6252 Specialty absorptive dressing, wound cover, sterile, pad size more than 16 sq. in. but less than or equal to 48 sq. in., without adhesive border, each dressing   **DME** N
BETOS: D1A   Medical/surgical supplies

D A6253 Specialty absorptive dressing, wound cover, sterile, pad size more than 48 sq. in., without adhesive border, each dressing   **DME** N
BETOS: D1A   Medical/surgical supplies

D A6254 Specialty absorptive dressing, wound cover, sterile, pad size 16 sq. in. or less, with any size adhesive border, each dressing   **DME** N
BETOS: D1A   Medical/surgical supplies

D A6255 Specialty absorptive dressing, wound cover, sterile, pad size more than 16 sq. in. but less than or equal to 48 sq. in., with any size adhesive border, each dressing   **DME** N
BETOS: D1A   Medical/surgical supplies

D A6256 Specialty absorptive dressing, wound cover, sterile, pad size more than 48 sq. in., with any size adhesive border, each dressing   N
BETOS: D1A   Medical/surgical supplies

D A6257 Transparent film, sterile, 16 sq. in. or less, each dressing   **DME** N
BETOS: D1A   Medical/surgical supplies

D A6258 Transparent film, sterile, more than 16 sq. in. but less than or equal to 48 sq. in., each dressing   **DME** N
BETOS: D1A   Medical/surgical supplies

D A6259 Transparent film, sterile, more than 48 sq. in., each dressing   **DME** N
BETOS: D1A   Medical/surgical supplies

D A6260 Wound cleansers, any type, any size   N
BETOS: D1A   Medical/surgical supplies
Service not separately priced by Part B

D A6261 Wound filler, gel/paste, per fluid ounce, not otherwise specified   N
BETOS: D1A   Medical/surgical supplies

D A6262 Wound filler, dry form, per gram, not otherwise specified   N
BETOS: D1A   Medical/surgical supplies

D A6266 Gauze, impregnated, other than water, normal saline, or zinc paste, sterile, any width, per linear yard   **DME** N
BETOS: D1A   Medical/surgical supplies

D A6402 Gauze, non-impregnated, sterile, pad size 16 sq. in. or less, without adhesive border, each dressing   **DME** N
BETOS: D1A   Medical/surgical supplies

D A6403 Gauze, non-impregnated, sterile, pad size more than 16 sq. in. less than or equal to 48 sq. in., without adhesive border, each dressing   **DME** N
BETOS: D1A   Medical/surgical supplies

D A6404 Gauze, non-impregnated, sterile, pad size more than 48 sq. in., without adhesive border, each dressing   N
BETOS: D1A   Medical/surgical supplies

C A6407 Packing strips, non-impregnated, sterile, up to 2 inches in width, per linear yard   **DME** N
BETOS: D1A   Medical/surgical supplies

D A6410 Eye pad, sterile, each   **DME** N
BETOS: D1A   Medical/surgical supplies

D A6411 Eye pad, non-sterile, each   **DME** N
BETOS: D1A   Medical/surgical supplies

C A6412 Eye patch, occlusive, each   N
BETOS: Z2   Undefined codes
Service not separately priced by Part B

BANDAGES (A6413-A6461)

S A6413 Adhesive bandage, first-aid type, any size, each   E1
BETOS: D1A   Medical/surgical supplies
Service not separately priced by Part B
Statute: 1861(s)(5)

C A6441 Padding bandage, non-elastic, non-woven/non-knitted, width greater than or equal to three inches and less than five inches, per yard   **DME** N
BETOS: D1A   Medical/surgical supplies

C A6442 Conforming bandage, non-elastic, knitted/woven, non-sterile, width less than three inches, per yard   **DME** N
BETOS: D1A   Medical/surgical supplies

C A6443 Conforming bandage, non-elastic, knitted/woven, non-sterile, width greater than or equal to three inches and less than five inches, per yard   **DME** N
BETOS: D1A   Medical/surgical supplies

C A6444 Conforming bandage, non-elastic, knitted/woven, non-sterile, width greater than or equal to 5 inches, per yard   **DME** N
BETOS: D1A   Medical/surgical supplies

C A6445 Conforming bandage, non-elastic, knitted/woven, sterile, width less than three inches, per yard   **DME** N
BETOS: D1A   Medical/surgical supplies

♂ Male only   ♀ Female only   🅐 Age   A2 - Z3 = ASC Payment indicator   A - Y = APC Status indicator
ASC = ASC Approved Procedure   **DME** Paid under the DME fee schedule   **MIPS** MIPS code

CPT® is a registered trademark of the American Medical Association. All rights reserved.   **125**

C A6446 Conforming bandage, non-elastic, knitted/ woven, sterile, width greater than or equal to three inches and less than five inches, per yard DME N

    BETOS: D1A Medical/surgical supplies

C A6447 Conforming bandage, non-elastic, knitted/ woven, sterile, width greater than or equal to five inches, per yard DME N

    BETOS: D1A Medical/surgical supplies

C A6448 Light compression bandage, elastic, knitted/ woven, width less than three inches, per yard DME N

    BETOS: D1A Medical/surgical supplies

C A6449 Light compression bandage, elastic, knitted/ woven, width greater than or equal to three inches and less than five inches, per yard DME N

    BETOS: D1A Medical/surgical supplies

C A6450 Light compression bandage, elastic, knitted/ woven, width greater than or equal to five inches, per yard DME N

    BETOS: D1A Medical/surgical supplies

C A6451 Moderate compression bandage, elastic, knitted/woven, load resistance of 1.25 to 1.34 foot pounds at 50% maximum stretch, width greater than or equal to three inches and less than five inches, per yard DME N

    BETOS: D1A Medical/surgical supplies

Elastic ACE compression bandage

C A6452 High compression bandage, elastic, knitted/ woven, load resistance greater than or equal to 1.35 foot pounds at 50% maximum stretch, width greater than or equal to three inches and less than five inches, per yard DME N

    BETOS: D1A Medical/surgical supplies

C A6453 Self-adherent bandage, elastic, non-knitted/ non-woven, width less than three inches, per yard DME N

    BETOS: D1A Medical/surgical supplies

C A6454 Self-adherent bandage, elastic, non-knitted/ non-woven, width greater than or equal to three inches and less than five inches, per yard DME N

    BETOS: D1A Medical/surgical supplies

C A6455 Self-adherent bandage, elastic, non-knitted/ non-woven, width greater than or equal to five inches, per yard DME N

    BETOS: D1A Medical/surgical supplies

C A6456 Zinc paste impregnated bandage, non-elastic, knitted/woven, width greater than or equal to three inches and less than five inches, per yard DME N

    BETOS: D1A Medical/surgical supplies

C A6457 Tubular dressing with or without elastic, any width, per linear yard DME N

    BETOS: D1A Medical/surgical supplies

C A6460 Synthetic resorbable wound dressing, sterile, pad size 16 sq. in. or less, without adhesive border, each dressing N

    BETOS: D1A Medical/surgical supplies

C A6461 Synthetic resorbable wound dressing, sterile, pad size more than 16 sq. in. but less than or equal to 48 sq. in., without adhesive border, each dressing N

    BETOS: D1A Medical/surgical supplies

COMPRESSION GARMENTS AND STOCKINGS (A6501-A6550)

D A6501 Compression burn garment, bodysuit (head to foot), custom fabricated DME N

    BETOS: D1A Medical/surgical supplies

D A6502 Compression burn garment, chin strap, custom fabricated DME N

    BETOS: D1A Medical/surgical supplies

D A6503 Compression burn garment, facial hood, custom fabricated DME N

    BETOS: D1A Medical/surgical supplies

D A6504 Compression burn garment, glove to wrist, custom fabricated DME N

    BETOS: D1A Medical/surgical supplies

D A6505 Compression burn garment, glove to elbow, custom fabricated DME N

    BETOS: D1A Medical/surgical supplies

D A6506 Compression burn garment, glove to axilla, custom fabricated DME N

    BETOS: D1A Medical/surgical supplies

D A6507 Compression burn garment, foot to knee length, custom fabricated DME N

    BETOS: D1A Medical/surgical supplies

D A6508 Compression burn garment, foot to thigh length, custom fabricated DME N

    BETOS: D1A Medical/surgical supplies

D A6509 Compression burn garment, upper trunk to waist including arm openings (vest), custom fabricated DME N

    BETOS: D1A Medical/surgical supplies

D A6510 Compression burn garment, trunk, including arms down to leg openings (leotard), custom fabricated DME N

    BETOS: D1A Medical/surgical supplies

● New code ▲ Revised code **C** Carrier judgment **D** Special coverage instructions apply
I Not payable by Medicare **M** Non-covered by Medicare **S** Non-covered by Medicare statute AHA Coding Clinic®

D **A6511** Compression burn garment, lower trunk including leg openings (panty), custom fabricated DME N

  BETOS: D1A Medical/surgical supplies

D **A6512** Compression burn garment, not otherwise classified N

  BETOS: D1A Medical/surgical supplies

C **A6513** Compression burn mask, face and/or neck, plastic or equal, custom fabricated DME B

  BETOS: D1A Medical/surgical supplies

  Service not separately priced by Part B

M **A6530** Gradient compression stocking, below knee, 18-30 mmHg, each E1

  BETOS: D1A Medical/surgical supplies

  Service not separately priced by Part B

D **A6531** Gradient compression stocking, below knee, 30-40 mmHg, each DME N

  BETOS: D1A Medical/surgical supplies

  DME Modifier: AW

D **A6532** Gradient compression stocking, below knee, 40-50 mmHg, each DME N

  BETOS: D1A Medical/surgical supplies

  DME Modifier: AW

M **A6533** Gradient compression stocking, thigh length, 18-30 mmHg, each E1

  BETOS: D1A Medical/surgical supplies

  Service not separately priced by Part B

M **A6534** Gradient compression stocking, thigh length, 30-40 mmHg, each E1

  BETOS: D1A Medical/surgical supplies

  Service not separately priced by Part B

M **A6535** Gradient compression stocking, thigh length, 40-50 mmHg, each E1

  BETOS: D1A Medical/surgical supplies

  Service not separately priced by Part B

M **A6536** Gradient compression stocking, full length/chap style, 18-30 mmHg, each E1

  BETOS: D1A Medical/surgical supplies

  Service not separately priced by Part B

M **A6537** Gradient compression stocking, full length/chap style, 30-40 mmHg, each E1

  BETOS: D1A Medical/surgical supplies

  Service not separately priced by Part B

M **A6538** Gradient compression stocking, full length/chap style, 40-50 mmHg, each E1

  BETOS: D1A Medical/surgical supplies

  Service not separately priced by Part B

M **A6539** Gradient compression stocking, waist length, 18-30 mmHg, each E1

  BETOS: D1A Medical/surgical supplies

  Service not separately priced by Part B

M **A6540** Gradient compression stocking, waist length, 30-40 mmHg, each E1

  BETOS: D1A Medical/surgical supplies

  Service not separately priced by Part B

M **A6541** Gradient compression stocking, waist length, 40-50 mmHg, each E1

  BETOS: D1A Medical/surgical supplies

  Service not separately priced by Part B

M **A6544** Gradient compression stocking, garter belt E1

  BETOS: D1A Medical/surgical supplies

  Service not separately priced by Part B

D **A6545** Gradient compression wrap, non-elastic, below knee, 30-50 mmHg, each DME N

  BETOS: D1A Medical/surgical supplies

  DME Modifier: AW

  Coding Clinic: 2008, Q4

M **A6549** Gradient compression stocking/sleeve, not otherwise specified E1

  BETOS: D1A Medical/surgical supplies

  Service not separately priced by Part B

C **A6550** Wound care set, for negative pressure wound therapy electrical pump, includes all supplies and accessories DME N

  BETOS: D1E Other DME

BREATHING AIDS (A7000-A7048), SEE ALSO INTERMITTENT POSITIVE PRESSURE BREATHING DEVICES (E0500); OTHER BREATHING AIDS (E0605, E0606); ASSISTED BREATHING SUPPLIES (S8096-S8210)

C **A7000** Canister, disposable, used with suction pump, each DME Y

  BETOS: D1E Other DME

  DME Modifier: KE,NU

C **A7001** Canister, non-disposable, used with suction pump, each DME Y

  BETOS: D1E Other DME

  DME Modifier: NU

C **A7002** Tubing, used with suction pump, each DME Y

  BETOS: D1E Other DME

  DME Modifier: NU

C **A7003** Administration set, with small volume nonfiltered pneumatic nebulizer, disposable DME Y

  BETOS: D1E Other DME

  DME Modifier: NU

C **A7004** Small volume nonfiltered pneumatic nebulizer, disposable DME Y

  BETOS: D1E Other DME

  DME Modifier: NU

C **A7005** Administration set, with small volume nonfiltered pneumatic nebulizer, non-disposable DME Y

  BETOS: D1E Other DME

  DME Modifier: NU

C **A7006** Administration set, with small volume filtered pneumatic nebulizer DME Y

  BETOS: D1E Other DME

  DME Modifier: NU

♂ Male only ♀ Female only Ⓐ Age A2 - Z3 = ASC Payment indicator A - Y = APC Status indicator

ASC = ASC Approved Procedure DME Paid under the DME fee schedule MIPS MIPS code

A7007 - A7036

MEDICAL AND SURGICAL SUPPLIES (A4206-A8004)

C A7007 Large volume nebulizer, disposable, unfilled, used with aerosol compressor **DME** Y
BETOS: D1E   Other DME
DME Modifier: NU

C A7008 Large volume nebulizer, disposable, prefilled, used with aerosol compressor **DME** Y
BETOS: D1E   Other DME
DME Modifier: NU

C A7009 Reservoir bottle, non-disposable, used with large volume ultrasonic nebulizer **DME** Y
BETOS: D1E   Other DME
DME Modifier: NU

C A7010 Corrugated tubing, disposable, used with large volume nebulizer, 100 feet **DME** Y
BETOS: D1E   Other DME
DME Modifier: NU

C A7012 Water collection device, used with large volume nebulizer **DME** Y
BETOS: D1E   Other DME
DME Modifier: NU

C A7013 Filter, disposable, used with aerosol compressor or ultrasonic generator **DME** Y
BETOS: D1E   Other DME
DME Modifier: NU

C A7014 Filter, nondisposable, used with aerosol compressor or ultrasonic generator **DME** Y
BETOS: D1E   Other DME
DME Modifier: NU

C A7015 Aerosol mask, used with DME nebulizer **DME** Y
BETOS: D1E   Other DME
DME Modifier: NU

C A7016 Dome and mouthpiece, used with small volume ultrasonic nebulizer **DME** Y
BETOS: D1E   Other DME
DME Modifier: NU

D A7017 Nebulizer, durable, glass or autoclavable plastic, bottle type, not used with oxygen **DME** Y
BETOS: D1E   Other DME
DME Modifier: NU,RR,UE

C A7018 Water, distilled, used with large volume nebulizer, 1000 ml **DME** Y
BETOS: D1E   Other DME

C A7020 Interface for cough stimulating device, includes all components, replacement only **DME** Y
BETOS: D1E   Other DME
DME Modifier: NU

C A7025 High frequency chest wall oscillation system vest, replacement for use with patient owned equipment, each **DME** N
BETOS: D1E   Other DME
DME Modifier: RR

C A7026 High frequency chest wall oscillation system hose, replacement for use with patient owned equipment, each **DME** Y
BETOS: D1E   Other DME
DME Modifier: NU

C A7027 Combination oral/nasal mask, used with continuous positive airway pressure device, each **DME** Y
BETOS: D1E   Other DME
DME Modifier: NU

C A7028 Oral cushion for combination oral/nasal mask, replacement only, each **DME** Y
BETOS: D1E   Other DME
DME Modifier: NU

C A7029 Nasal pillows for combination oral/nasal mask, replacement only, pair **DME** Y
BETOS: D1E   Other DME
DME Modifier: NU

C A7030 Full face mask used with positive airway pressure device, each **DME** Y
BETOS: D1E   Other DME
DME Modifier: NU
Pub: 100-4, Chapter-36, 50.14

C A7031 Face mask interface, replacement for full face mask, each **DME** Y
BETOS: D1E   Other DME
DME Modifier: NU
Pub: 100-4, Chapter-36, 50.14

C A7032 Cushion for use on nasal mask interface, replacement only, each **DME** Y
BETOS: D1E   Other DME
DME Modifier: NU
Pub: 100-4, Chapter-36, 50.14

C A7033 Pillow for use on nasal cannula type interface, replacement only, pair **DME** Y
BETOS: D1E   Other DME
DME Modifier: NU
Pub: 100-4, Chapter-36, 50.14

C A7034 Nasal interface (mask or cannula type) used with positive airway pressure device, with or without head strap **DME** Y
BETOS: D1E   Other DME
DME Modifier: NU
Pub: 100-4, Chapter-36, 50.14

C A7035 Headgear used with positive airway pressure device **DME** Y
BETOS: D1E   Other DME
DME Modifier: NU
Pub: 100-4, Chapter-36, 50.14

C A7036 Chinstrap used with positive airway pressure device **DME** Y
BETOS: D1E   Other DME
DME Modifier: NU
Pub: 100-4, Chapter-36, 50.14

● New code   ▲ Revised code   **C** Carrier judgment   **D** Special coverage instructions apply
I Not payable by Medicare   **M** Non-covered by Medicare   **S** Non-covered by Medicare statute   AHA Coding Clinic®

C **A7037** Tubing used with positive airway pressure device DME Y

BETOS: D1E   Other DME

DME Modifier: NU

Pub: 100-4, Chapter-36, 50.14

C **A7038** Filter, disposable, used with positive airway pressure device DME Y

BETOS: D1E   Other DME

DME Modifier: NU

Pub: 100-4, Chapter-36, 50.14

C **A7039** Filter, non disposable, used with positive airway pressure device DME Y

BETOS: D1E   Other DME

DME Modifier: NU

Pub: 100-4, Chapter-36, 50.14

C **A7040** One-way chest drain valve DME N

BETOS: D1F   Prosthetic/Orthotic devices

C **A7041** Water seal drainage container and tubing for use with implanted chest tube DME N

BETOS: D1F   Prosthetic/Orthotic devices

C **A7044** Oral interface used with positive airway pressure device, each DME Y

BETOS: D1E   Other DME

DME Modifier: NU

Pub: 100-4, Chapter-36, 50.14

D **A7045** Exhalation port with or without swivel used with accessories for positive airway devices, replacement only DME Y

BETOS: D1E   Other DME

DME Modifier: NU,RR,UE

Pub: 100-4, Chapter-36, 50.14

D **A7046** Water chamber for humidifier, used with positive airway pressure device, replacement, each DME Y

BETOS: D1E   Other DME

DME Modifier: NU

Pub: 100-4, Chapter-36, 50.14

C **A7047** Oral interface used with respiratory suction pump, each DME N

BETOS: D1E   Other DME

DME Modifier: NU

C **A7048** Vacuum drainage collection unit and tubing kit, including all supplies needed for collection unit change, for use with implanted catheter, each DME N

BETOS: D1F   Prosthetic/Orthotic devices

TRACHEOSTOMY SUPPLIES (A7501-A7527)

D **A7501** Tracheostoma valve, including diaphragm, each DME N

BETOS: D1F   Prosthetic/Orthotic devices

D **A7502** Replacement diaphragm/faceplate for tracheostoma valve, each DME N

BETOS: D1F   Prosthetic/Orthotic devices

D **A7503** Filter holder or filter cap, reusable, for use in a tracheostoma heat and moisture exchange system, each DME N

BETOS: D1F   Prosthetic/Orthotic devices

D **A7504** Filter for use in a tracheostoma heat and moisture exchange system, each DME N

BETOS: D1F   Prosthetic/Orthotic devices

D **A7505** Housing, reusable without adhesive, for use in a heat and moisture exchange system and/or with a tracheostoma valve, each DME N

BETOS: D1F   Prosthetic/Orthotic devices

D **A7506** Adhesive disc for use in a heat and moisture exchange system and/or with tracheostoma valve, any type each DME N

BETOS: D1F   Prosthetic/Orthotic devices

D **A7507** Filter holder and integrated filter without adhesive, for use in a tracheostoma heat and moisture exchange system, each DME N

BETOS: D1F   Prosthetic/Orthotic devices

D **A7508** Housing and integrated adhesive, for use in a tracheostoma heat and moisture exchange system and/or with a tracheostoma valve, each DME N

BETOS: D1F   Prosthetic/Orthotic devices

D **A7509** Filter holder and integrated filter housing, and adhesive, for use as a tracheostoma heat and moisture exchange system, each DME N

BETOS: D1F   Prosthetic/Orthotic devices

C **A7520** Tracheostomy/laryngectomy tube, non-cuffed, polyvinylchloride (PVC), silicone or equal, each DME N

BETOS: D1F   Prosthetic/Orthotic devices

C **A7521** Tracheostomy/laryngectomy tube, cuffed, polyvinylchloride (PVC), silicone or equal, each DME N

BETOS: D1F   Prosthetic/Orthotic devices

C **A7522** Tracheostomy/laryngectomy tube, stainless steel or equal (sterilizable and reusable), each DME N

BETOS: D1F   Prosthetic/Orthotic devices

C **A7523** Tracheostomy shower protector, each N

BETOS: D1F   Prosthetic/Orthotic devices

C **A7524** Tracheostoma stent/stud/button, each DME N

BETOS: D1F   Prosthetic/Orthotic devices

C **A7525** Tracheostomy mask, each DME N

BETOS: D1F   Prosthetic/Orthotic devices

C **A7526** Tracheostomy tube collar/holder, each DME N

BETOS: D1F   Prosthetic/Orthotic devices

C **A7527** Tracheostomy/laryngectomy tube plug/stop, each DME N

BETOS: D1A   Medical/surgical supplies

♂ Male only   ♀ Female only   🅐 Age   A2 - Z3 = ASC Payment indicator   A - Y = APC Status indicator

ASC = ASC Approved Procedure   DME Paid under the DME fee schedule   MIPS MIPS code

HELMETS (A8000-A8004)

C **A8000** Helmet, protective, soft, prefabricated, includes all components and accessories **DME** Y
BETOS: D1E   Other DME
DME Modifier: NU,RR,UE

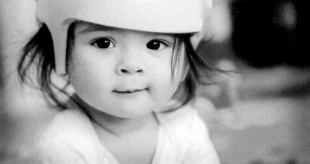

Helmet

C **A8001** Helmet, protective, hard, prefabricated, includes all components and accessories **DME** Y
BETOS: D1E   Other DME
DME Modifier: NU,RR,UE

C **A8002** Helmet, protective, soft, custom fabricated, includes all components and accessories **DME** Y
BETOS: D1E   Other DME
DME Modifier: NU,RR,UE

C **A8003** Helmet, protective, hard, custom fabricated, includes all components and accessories **DME** Y
BETOS: D1E   Other DME
DME Modifier: NU,RR,UE

C **A8004** Soft interface for helmet, replacement only **DME** Y
BETOS: D1E   Other DME
DME Modifier: NU,RR,UE

ADMINISTRATIVE, MISCELLANEOUS AND INVESTIGATIONAL (A9150-A9999)

MISCELLANEOUS SUPPLIES AND EQUIPMENT (A9150-A9300)

D **A9150** Non-prescription drugs   B
BETOS: O1E   Other drugs
Other carrier priced

I **A9152** Single vitamin/mineral/trace element, oral, per dose, not otherwise specified   E1
BETOS: Z2   Undefined codes
Service not separately priced by Part B

I **A9153** Multiple vitamins, with or without minerals and trace elements, oral, per dose, not otherwise specified   E1
BETOS: Z2   Undefined codes
Service not separately priced by Part B

C **A9155** Artificial saliva, 30 ml   B
BETOS: Z2   Undefined codes
Other carrier priced

I **A9180** Pediculosis (lice infestation) treatment, topical, for administration by patient/caretaker   E1
BETOS: Z2   Undefined codes
Service not separately priced by Part B

M **A9270** Non-covered item or service   E1
BETOS: Z2   Undefined codes
Service not separately priced by Part B
Pub: 100-4, Chapter-11, 100.1

S **A9272** Wound suction, disposable, includes dressing, all accessories and components, any type, each   E1
BETOS: D1A   Medical/surgical supplies
Service not separately priced by Part B
Statute: 1861(n)

M **A9273** Cold or hot fluid bottle, ice cap or collar, heat and/or cold wrap, any type   E1
BETOS: Z2   Undefined codes
Service not separately priced by Part B

S **A9274** External ambulatory insulin delivery system, disposable, each, includes all supplies and accessories   E1
BETOS: D1A   Medical/surgical supplies
Service not separately priced by Part B
Statute: 1861(n)

M **A9275** Home glucose disposable monitor, includes test strips   E1
BETOS: T1E   Lab tests - glucose
Service not separately priced by Part B

S **A9276** Sensor; invasive (e.g., subcutaneous), disposable, for use with interstitial continuous glucose monitoring system, one unit = 1 day supply   E1
BETOS: D1E   Other DME
Service not separately priced by Part B
Statute: 1861(n)

S **A9277** Transmitter; external, for use with interstitial continuous glucose monitoring system   E1
BETOS: D1E   Other DME
Service not separately priced by Part B
Statute: 1861(n)

S **A9278** Receiver (monitor); external, for use with interstitial continuous glucose monitoring system   E1
BETOS: D1E   Other DME
Service not separately priced by Part B
Statute: 1861(n)

S **A9279** Monitoring feature/device, stand-alone or integrated, any type, includes all accessories, components and electronics, not otherwise classified   E1
BETOS: T2D   Other tests - other
Service not separately priced by Part B
Statute: 1861(n)

S **A9280** Alert or alarm device, not otherwise classified   E1
BETOS: Z2   Undefined codes
Service not separately priced by Part B
Statute: 1861

S **A9281** Reaching/grabbing device, any type, any length, each   E1
BETOS: D1E   Other DME
Service not separately priced by Part B
Statute: 1862 SSA

S **A9282** Wig, any type, each   E1
BETOS: Z2   Undefined codes
Service not separately priced by Part B
Statute: 1861SSA

S **A9283** Foot pressure off loading/supportive device, any type, each   E1
BETOS: D1E   Other DME
Service not separately priced by Part B
Statute: 1862a(i)13

D **A9284** Spirometer, non-electronic, includes all accessories   N
BETOS: Z2   Undefined codes
Service not separately priced by Part B
Coding Clinic: 2008, Q4

C **A9285** Inversion/eversion correction device   A
BETOS: Z2   Undefined codes
Service not separately priced by Part B

S **A9286** Hygienic item or device, disposable or non-disposable, any type, each   E1
BETOS: D1A   Medical/surgical supplies
Service not separately priced by Part B
Statute: 1834

M **A9300** Exercise equipment   E1
BETOS: Z2   Undefined codes
Service not separately priced by Part B

♂ Male only   ♀ Female only   **A** Age   A2 - Z3 = ASC Payment indicator   A - Y = APC Status indicator
ASC = ASC Approved Procedure   **DME** Paid under the DME fee schedule   **MIPS** MIPS code

DIAGNOSTIC AND THERAPEUTIC RADIOPHARMACEUTICALS (A9500-A9700), SEE ALSO DIAGNOSTIC RADIOPHARMACEUTICALS (A4641-A4642)

C A9500 Technetium Tc-99m sestamibi, diagnostic, per study dose   N1 ASC N
BETOS: I1E   Standard imaging - nuclear medicine
Other carrier priced
Coding Clinic: 2005, Q4; 2006, Q2

C A9501 Technetium Tc-99m teboroxime, diagnostic, per study dose   N1 ASC N
BETOS: I1E   Standard imaging - nuclear medicine
Other carrier priced
Coding Clinic: 2008, Q1

C A9502 Technetium Tc-99m tetrofosmin, diagnostic, per study dose   N1 ASC N
BETOS: I1E   Standard imaging - nuclear medicine
Other carrier priced
Coding Clinic: 2005, Q4; 2006, Q2

C A9503 Technetium Tc-99m medronate, diagnostic, per study dose, up to 30 millicuries N1 ASC N
BETOS: I1E   Standard imaging - nuclear medicine
Other carrier priced
Coding Clinic: 2002, Q2; 2004, Q3; 2005, Q4

C A9504 Technetium Tc-99m apcitide, diagnostic, per study dose, up to 20 millicuries   N1 ASC N
BETOS: I1E   Standard imaging - nuclear medicine
Other carrier priced
Coding Clinic: 2001, Q4; 2002, Q2

C A9505 Thallium Tl-201 thallous chloride, diagnostic, per millicurie   N1 ASC N
BETOS: I1E   Standard imaging - nuclear medicine
Other carrier priced
Coding Clinic: 2002, Q2; 2004, Q3; 2005, Q4

C A9507 Indium In-111 capromab pendetide, diagnostic, per study dose, up to 10 millicuries   N1 ♂ ASC N
BETOS: I1E   Standard imaging - nuclear medicine
Other carrier priced
Coding Clinic: 2005, Q4

C A9508 Iodine I-131 iobenguane sulfate, diagnostic, per 0.5 millicurie   N1 ASC N
BETOS: I1E   Standard imaging - nuclear medicine
Coding Clinic: 2002, Q2; 2005, Q4

C A9509 Iodine I-123 sodium iodide, diagnostic, per millicurie   N1 ASC N
BETOS: I1E   Standard imaging - nuclear medicine
Other carrier priced
Coding Clinic: 2008, Q1

C A9510 Technetium Tc-99m disofenin, diagnostic, per study dose, up to 15 millicuries   N1 ASC N
BETOS: I1E   Standard imaging - nuclear medicine
Coding Clinic: 2005, Q4

C A9512 Technetium Tc-99m pertechnetate, diagnostic, per millicurie   N1 ASC N
BETOS: I1E   Standard imaging - nuclear medicine
Other carrier priced
Coding Clinic: 2005, Q4

D A9513 Lutetium Lu 177, dotatate, therapeutic, 1 millicurie   K
BETOS: I1E   Standard imaging - nuclear medicine
Other carrier priced
Drugs: LUTATHERA
Coding Clinic: 2005, Q4; 2019, Q1

C A9515 Choline C-11, diagnostic, per study dose up to 20 millicuries   N1 ASC N
BETOS: I1E   Standard imaging - nuclear medicine
Other carrier priced
Coding Clinic: 2005, Q4

C A9516 Iodine I-123 sodium iodide, diagnostic, per 100 microcuries, up to 999 microcuries   N1 ASC N
BETOS: I1E   Standard imaging - nuclear medicine
Other carrier priced
Coding Clinic: 2005, Q4

C A9517 Iodine I-131 sodium iodide capsule(s), therapeutic, per millicurie   K
BETOS: I1E   Standard imaging - nuclear medicine
Other carrier priced
Coding Clinic: 2005, Q4; 2008, Q3

C A9520 Technetium Tc-99m, tilmanocept, diagnostic, up to 0.5 millicuries   N1 ASC N
BETOS: I1E   Standard imaging - nuclear medicine
Other carrier priced
Coding Clinic: 2005, Q4; 2013, Q4

C A9521 Technetium Tc-99m exametazime, diagnostic, per study dose, up to 25 millicuries   N1 ASC N
BETOS: I1E   Standard imaging - nuclear medicine
Other carrier priced
Coding Clinic: 2005, Q4

C A9524 Iodine I-131 iodinated serum albumin, diagnostic, per 5 microcuries   N1 ASC N
BETOS: I1E   Standard imaging - nuclear medicine
Other carrier priced
Coding Clinic: 2005, Q4

C **A9526** Nitrogen N-13 ammonia, diagnostic, per study dose, up to 40 millicuries   N1 ASC N
BETOS: I1E   Standard imaging - nuclear medicine
Coding Clinic: 2005, Q4
Pub: 100-4, Chapter-13, 60.3

C **A9527** Iodine I-125, sodium iodide solution, therapeutic, per millicurie   H2 ASC U
BETOS: I1E   Standard imaging - nuclear medicine
Other carrier priced
Coding Clinic: 2007, Q2; 2016, Q3; 2016, Q3

C **A9528** Iodine I-131 sodium iodide capsule(s), diagnostic, per millicurie   N1 ASC N
BETOS: I1E   Standard imaging - nuclear medicine
Other carrier priced
Coding Clinic: 2005, Q4

C **A9529** Iodine I-131 sodium iodide solution, diagnostic, per millicurie   N1 ASC N
BETOS: I1E   Standard imaging - nuclear medicine
Other carrier priced
Coding Clinic: 2005, Q4

C **A9530** Iodine I-131 sodium iodide solution, therapeutic, per millicurie   K
BETOS: I1E   Standard imaging - nuclear medicine
Other carrier priced
Coding Clinic: 2005, Q4

C **A9531** Iodine I-131 sodium iodide, diagnostic, per microcurie (up to 100 microcuries)   N1 ASC N
BETOS: I1E   Standard imaging - nuclear medicine
Other carrier priced
Coding Clinic: 2005, Q4

C **A9532** Iodine I-125 serum albumin, diagnostic, per 5 microcuries   N1 ASC N
BETOS: I1E   Standard imaging - nuclear medicine
Other carrier priced
Coding Clinic: 2005, Q4

C **A9536** Technetium Tc-99m depreotide, diagnostic, per study dose, up to 35 millicuries   N1 ASC N
BETOS: I1E   Standard imaging - nuclear medicine
Other carrier priced
Coding Clinic: 2005, Q4

C **A9537** Technetium Tc-99m mebrofenin, diagnostic, per study dose, up to 15 millicuries   N1 ASC N
BETOS: I1E   Standard imaging - nuclear medicine
Other carrier priced
Coding Clinic: 2005, Q4

C **A9538** Technetium Tc-99m pyrophosphate, diagnostic, per study dose, up to 25 millicuries   N1 ASC N
BETOS: I1E   Standard imaging - nuclear medicine
Other carrier priced
Coding Clinic: 2005, Q4

C **A9539** Technetium Tc-99m pentetate, diagnostic, per study dose, up to 25 millicuries   N1 ASC N
BETOS: I1E   Standard imaging - nuclear medicine
Other carrier priced
Coding Clinic: 2005, Q4

C **A9540** Technetium Tc-99m macroaggregated albumin, diagnostic, per study dose, up to 10 millicuries   N1 ASC N
BETOS: I1E   Standard imaging - nuclear medicine
Other carrier priced
Coding Clinic: 2005, Q4

C **A9541** Technetium Tc-99m sulfur colloid, diagnostic, per study dose, up to 20 millicuries   N1 ASC N
BETOS: I1E   Standard imaging - nuclear medicine
Other carrier priced
Coding Clinic: 2005, Q4

C **A9542** Indium In-111 ibritumomab tiuxetan, diagnostic, per study dose, up to 5 millicuries   N1 ASC N
BETOS: I1E   Standard imaging - nuclear medicine
Coding Clinic: 2005, Q4

C **A9543** Yttrium Y-90 ibritumomab tiuxetan, therapeutic, per treatment dose, up to 40 millicuries   K
BETOS: I1E   Standard imaging - nuclear medicine
Drugs: ZEVALIN Y-90
Coding Clinic: 2005, Q4

C **A9546** Cobalt Co-57/58, cyanocobalamin, diagnostic, per study dose, up to 1 microcurie   N1 ASC N
BETOS: I1E   Standard imaging - nuclear medicine
Coding Clinic: 2005, Q4

C **A9547** Indium In-111 oxyquinoline, diagnostic, per 0.5 millicurie   N1 ASC N
BETOS: I1E   Standard imaging - nuclear medicine
Coding Clinic: 2005, Q4

C **A9548** Indium In-111 pentetate, diagnostic, per 0.5 millicurie   N1 ASC N
BETOS: I1E   Standard imaging - nuclear medicine
Coding Clinic: 2005, Q4

C **A9550** Technetium Tc-99m sodium gluceptate, diagnostic, per study dose, up to 25 millicurie N1 ASC N
BETOS: I1E Standard imaging - nuclear medicine
Coding Clinic: 2005, Q4

C **A9551** Technetium Tc-99m succimer, diagnostic, per study dose, up to 10 millicuries N1 ASC N
BETOS: I1E Standard imaging - nuclear medicine
Coding Clinic: 2005, Q4

C **A9552** Fluorodeoxyglucose F-18 FDG, diagnostic, per study dose, up to 45 millicuries N1 ASC N
BETOS: I1E Standard imaging - nuclear medicine
Coding Clinic: 2005, Q4; 2008, Q3
Pub: 100-4, Chapter-13, 60.16

C **A9553** Chromium Cr-51 sodium chromate, diagnostic, per study dose, up to 250 microcuries N1 ASC N
BETOS: I1E Standard imaging - nuclear medicine
Coding Clinic: 2005, Q4

C **A9554** Iodine I-125 sodium iothalamate, diagnostic, per study dose, up to 10 microcuries N1 ASC N
BETOS: I1E Standard imaging - nuclear medicine
Coding Clinic: 2005, Q4

C **A9555** Rubidium Rb-82, diagnostic, per study dose, up to 60 millicuries N1 ASC N
BETOS: I1E Standard imaging - nuclear medicine
Value not established
Coding Clinic: 2005, Q4

C **A9556** Gallium Ga-67 citrate, diagnostic, per millicurie N1 ASC N
BETOS: I1E Standard imaging - nuclear medicine
Other carrier priced
Coding Clinic: 2005, Q4

C **A9557** Technetium Tc-99m bicisate, diagnostic, per study dose, up to 25 millicuries N1 ASC N
BETOS: I1E Standard imaging - nuclear medicine
Other carrier priced
Coding Clinic: 2005, Q4

C **A9558** Xenon Xe-133 gas, diagnostic, per 10 millicuries N1 ASC N
BETOS: I1E Standard imaging - nuclear medicine
Other carrier priced
Coding Clinic: 2005, Q4

C **A9559** Cobalt Co-57 cyanocobalamin, oral, diagnostic, per study dose, up to 1 microcurie N1 ASC N
BETOS: I1E Standard imaging - nuclear medicine
Other carrier priced
Coding Clinic: 2005, Q4

C **A9560** Technetium Tc-99m labeled red blood cells, diagnostic, per study dose, up to 30 millicuries N1 ASC N
BETOS: I1E Standard imaging - nuclear medicine
Other carrier priced
Coding Clinic: 2005, Q4; 2008, Q3

C **A9561** Technetium Tc-99m oxidronate, diagnostic, per study dose, up to 30 millicuries N1 ASC N
BETOS: I1E Standard imaging - nuclear medicine
Other carrier priced
Coding Clinic: 2005, Q4

C **A9562** Technetium Tc-99m mertiatide, diagnostic, per study dose, up to 15 millicuries N1 ASC N
BETOS: I1E Standard imaging - nuclear medicine
Other carrier priced
Coding Clinic: 2005, Q4

C **A9563** Sodium phosphate P-32, therapeutic, per millicurie K
BETOS: I1E Standard imaging - nuclear medicine
Other carrier priced
Coding Clinic: 2005, Q4

C **A9564** Chromic phosphate P-32 suspension, therapeutic, per millicurie E1
BETOS: I1E Standard imaging - nuclear medicine
Other carrier priced
Coding Clinic: 2005, Q4

C **A9566** Technetium Tc-99m fanolesomab, diagnostic, per study dose, up to 25 millicuries N1 ASC N
BETOS: I1E Standard imaging - nuclear medicine
Other carrier priced
Coding Clinic: 2005, Q4

C **A9567** Technetium Tc-99m pentetate, diagnostic, aerosol, per study dose, up to 75 millicuries N1 ASC N
BETOS: I1E Standard imaging - nuclear medicine
Other carrier priced
Coding Clinic: 2005, Q4

C **A9568** Technetium Tc-99m arcitumomab, diagnostic, per study dose, up to 45 millicuries N1 ASC N
BETOS: I1E Standard imaging - nuclear medicine

● New code ▲ Revised code C Carrier judgment D Special coverage instructions apply
I Not payable by Medicare M Non-covered by Medicare S Non-covered by Medicare statute AHA Coding Clinic®

C **A9569** Technetium Tc-99m exametazime labeled autologous white blood cells, diagnostic, per study dose N1 ASC N

BETOS: I1E Standard imaging - nuclear medicine

Other carrier priced

Coding Clinic: 2008, Q1

C **A9570** Indium In-111 labeled autologous white blood cells, diagnostic, per study dose N1 ASC N

BETOS: I1E Standard imaging - nuclear medicine

Other carrier priced

Coding Clinic: 2008, Q1

C **A9571** Indium In-111 labeled autologous platelets, diagnostic, per study dose N1 ASC N

BETOS: I1E Standard imaging - nuclear medicine

Other carrier priced

Coding Clinic: 2008, Q1

C **A9572** Indium In-111 pentetreotide, diagnostic, per study dose, up to 6 millicuries N1 ASC N

BETOS: I1E Standard imaging - nuclear medicine

Other carrier priced

Coding Clinic: 2008, Q1

C **A9575** Injection, gadoterate meglumine, 0.1 ml N1 ASC N

BETOS: I1E Standard imaging - nuclear medicine

Other carrier priced

Drugs: CLARISCAN, DOTAREM

Coding Clinic: 2014, Q1

C **A9576** Injection, gadoteridol, (ProHance multipack), per ml N1 ASC N

BETOS: I1E Standard imaging - nuclear medicine

Drugs: PROHANCE MULTIPACK

Coding Clinic: 2008, Q1

C **A9577** Injection, gadobenate dimeglumine (MultiHance), per ml N1 ASC N

BETOS: I1E Standard imaging - nuclear medicine

Drugs: MULTIHANCE

Coding Clinic: 2008, Q1

C **A9578** Injection, gadobenate dimeglumine (MultiHance multipack), per ml N1 ASC N

BETOS: I1E Standard imaging - nuclear medicine

Drugs: MULTIHANCE MULTIPACK

Coding Clinic: 2008, Q1

C **A9579** Injection, gadolinium-based magnetic resonance contrast agent, not otherwise specified (NOS), per ml N1 ASC N

BETOS: I1E Standard imaging - nuclear medicine

Drugs: MAGNEVIST 46.9%, NOVAPLUS® OMNISCAN, OMNISCAN, OPTIMARK, PROHANCE, PROHANCE PREFILLED SYRINGES

Coding Clinic: 2008, Q1

C **A9580** Sodium fluoride F-18, diagnostic, per study dose, up to 30 millicuries N1 ASC N

BETOS: I1E Standard imaging - nuclear medicine

Other carrier priced

Coding Clinic: 2009, Q1; 2008, Q4

Pub: 100-4, Chapter-13, 60.18

C **A9581** Injection, gadoxetate disodium, 1 ml N1 ASC N

BETOS: I2D Advanced imaging - MRI/MRA: other

Drugs: EOVIST, GADOXETATE DISODIUM

C **A9582** Iodine I-123 iobenguane, diagnostic, per study dose, up to 15 millicuries N1 ASC N

BETOS: I1E Standard imaging - nuclear medicine

C **A9583** Injection, gadofosveset trisodium, 1 ml N1 ASC N

BETOS: I1E Standard imaging - nuclear medicine

C **A9584** Iodine 1-123 ioflupane, diagnostic, per study dose, up to 5 millicuries N1 ASC N

BETOS: I1E Standard imaging - nuclear medicine

Other carrier priced

C **A9585** Injection, gadobutrol, 0.1 ml N1 ASC N

BETOS: I1E Standard imaging - nuclear medicine

Other carrier priced

Drugs: GADAVIST

Coding Clinic: 2012, Q1

D **A9586** Florbetapir F18, diagnostic, per study dose, up to 10 millicuries N1 ASC N

BETOS: I1E Standard imaging - nuclear medicine

Service not separately priced by Part B

Coding Clinic: 2014, Q1; 2014, Q3

C **A9587** Gallium Ga-68, dotatate, diagnostic, 0.1 millicurie N1 ASC N

BETOS: I1E Standard imaging - nuclear medicine

Other carrier priced

Coding Clinic: 2017, Q1

C **A9588** Fluciclovine F-18, diagnostic, 1 millicurie N1 ASC N

BETOS: I1E Standard imaging - nuclear medicine

Other carrier priced

Coding Clinic: 2017, Q1

C **A9589** Instillation, hexaminolevulinate hydrochloride, 100 mg   N
BETOS: I1E   Standard imaging - nuclear medicine
Other carrier priced
Drugs: CYSVIEW
Coding Clinic: 2019, Q1

C **A9590** Iodine I-131, iobenguane, 1 millicurie   K2 ASC G
BETOS: I1E   Standard imaging - nuclear medicine
Drugs: AZEDRA DOSIMETRIC, AZEDRA THERAPEUTIC

● C **A9591** Fluoroestradiol f 18, diagnostic, 1 millicurie   K2 ASC G
BETOS: I1E   Standard imaging - nuclear medicine
Other carrier priced
Drugs: CERIANNA

C **A9597** Positron emission tomography radiopharmaceutical, diagnostic, for tumor identification, not otherwise classified   N1 ASC N
BETOS: I1E   Standard imaging - nuclear medicine
Other carrier priced
Coding Clinic: 2017, Q1; 2017, Q1
Pub: 100-4, Chapter-13, 60.3.2

C **A9598** Positron emission tomography radiopharmaceutical, diagnostic, for non-tumor identification, not otherwise classified   N1 ASC N
BETOS: I1E   Standard imaging - nuclear medicine
Other carrier priced
Coding Clinic: 2017, Q1; 2017, Q1
Pub: 100-4, Chapter-13, 60.3.2

C **A9600** Strontium Sr-89 chloride, therapeutic, per millicurie   K
BETOS: I1E   Standard imaging - nuclear medicine
Other carrier priced
Drugs: METASTRON, STRONTIUM CHLORIDE SR 89
Coding Clinic: 2002, Q2; 2005, Q4

C **A9604** Samarium Sm-153 lexidronam, therapeutic, per treatment dose, up to 150 millicuries   K
BETOS: I1E   Standard imaging - nuclear medicine
Other carrier priced
Drugs: QUADRAMET

C **A9606** Radium Ra-223 dichloride, therapeutic, per microcurie   ♂ K
BETOS: I1E   Standard imaging - nuclear medicine
Other carrier priced
Drugs: XOFIGO
Coding Clinic: 2014, Q4

D **A9698** Non-radioactive contrast imaging material, not otherwise classified, per study   N1 ASC N
BETOS: I1E   Standard imaging - nuclear medicine
Coding Clinic: 2005, Q4; 2017, Q1

C **A9699** Radiopharmaceutical, therapeutic, not otherwise classified   N
BETOS: I1E   Standard imaging - nuclear medicine
Other carrier priced
Coding Clinic: 2005, Q4

D **A9700** Supply of injectable contrast material for use in echocardiography, per study   N1 ASC N
BETOS: I1E   Standard imaging - nuclear medicine
Other carrier priced
Coding Clinic: 2001, Q4; 2003, Q2; 2017, Q1
Pub: 100-4, Chapter-12, 30.4

MISCELLANEOUS DME SUPPLIES AND SERVICES (A9900-A9999)

C **A9900** Miscellaneous DME supply, accessory, and/or service component of another HCPCS code   Y
BETOS: D1E   Other DME

C **A9901** DME delivery, set up, and/or dispensing service component of another HCPCS code   A
BETOS: D1E   Other DME

C **A9999** Miscellaneous DME supply or accessory, not otherwise specified   Y
BETOS: D1F   Prosthetic/Orthotic devices

● New code   ▲ Revised code   C Carrier judgment   D Special coverage instructions apply   I Not payable by Medicare   M Non-covered by Medicare   S Non-covered by Medicare statute   AHA Coding Clinic®

136   *CPT® is a registered trademark of the American Medical Association. All rights reserved.*

ENTERAL AND PARENTERAL THERAPY (B4034-B9999)

ENTERAL FEEDING SUPPLIES AND EQUIPMENT (B4034-B4088)

D B4034 Enteral feeding supply kit; syringe fed, per day, includes but not limited to feeding/flushing syringe, administration set tubing, dressings, tape Y
BETOS: O1C Enteral and parenteral

D B4035 Enteral feeding supply kit; pump fed, per day, includes but not limited to feeding/flushing syringe, administration set tubing, dressings, tape Y
BETOS: O1C Enteral and parenteral

D B4036 Enteral feeding supply kit; gravity fed, per day, includes but not limited to feeding/flushing syringe, administration set tubing, dressings, tape Y
BETOS: O1C Enteral and parenteral

D B4081 Nasogastric tubing with stylet Y
BETOS: O1C Enteral and parenteral

D B4082 Nasogastric tubing without stylet Y
BETOS: O1C Enteral and parenteral

D B4083 Stomach tube - Levine type Y
BETOS: O1C Enteral and parenteral

C B4087 Gastrostomy/jejunostomy tube, standard, any material, any type, each Y
BETOS: O1C Enteral and parenteral

C B4088 Gastrostomy/jejunostomy tube, low-profile, any material, any type, each Y
BETOS: O1C Enteral and parenteral

ENTERAL FORMULAS AND ADDITIVES (B4100-B4162)

M B4100 Food thickener, administered orally, per ounce E1
BETOS: Z2 Undefined codes
Service not separately priced by Part B

D B4102 Enteral formula, for adults, used to replace fluids and electrolytes (e.g., clear liquids), 500 ml = 1 unit Ⓐ Y
BETOS: O1C Enteral and parenteral

D B4103 Enteral formula, for pediatrics, used to replace fluids and electrolytes (e.g., clear liquids), 500 ml = 1 unit Ⓐ Y
BETOS: O1C Enteral and parenteral

D B4104 Additive for enteral formula (e.g., fiber) E1
BETOS: O1C Enteral and parenteral
Service not separately priced by Part B

C B4105 In-line cartridge containing digestive enzyme(s) for enteral feeding, each Y
BETOS: O1C Enteral and parenteral

D B4149 Enteral formula, manufactured blenderized natural foods with intact nutrients, includes proteins, fats, carbohydrates, vitamins and minerals, may include fiber, administered through an enteral feeding tube, 100 calories = 1 unit Y
BETOS: O1C Enteral and parenteral

D B4150 Enteral formula, nutritionally complete with intact nutrients, includes proteins, fats, carbohydrates, vitamins and minerals, may include fiber, administered through an enteral feeding tube, 100 calories = 1 unit Y
BETOS: O1C Enteral and parenteral

D B4152 Enteral formula, nutritionally complete, calorically dense (equal to or greater than 1.5 kcal/ml) with intact nutrients, includes proteins, fats, carbohydrates, vitamins and minerals, may include fiber, administered through an enteral feeding tube, 100 calories = 1 unit Y
BETOS: O1C Enteral and parenteral

D B4153 Enteral formula, nutritionally complete, hydrolyzed proteins (amino acids and peptide chain), includes fats, carbohydrates, vitamins and minerals, may include fiber, administered through an enteral feeding tube, 100 calories = 1 unit Y
BETOS: O1C Enteral and parenteral

D B4154 Enteral formula, nutritionally complete, for special metabolic needs, excludes inherited disease of metabolism, includes altered composition of proteins, fats, carbohydrates, vitamins and/or minerals, may include fiber, administered through an enteral feeding tube, 100 calories = 1 unit Y
BETOS: O1C Enteral and parenteral

D B4155 Enteral formula, nutritionally incomplete/modular nutrients, includes specific nutrients, carbohydrates (e.g., glucose polymers), proteins/amino acids (e.g., glutamine, arginine), fat (e.g., medium chain triglycerides) or combination, administered through an enteral feeding tube, 100 calories = 1 unit Y
BETOS: O1C Enteral and parenteral

D B4157 Enteral formula, nutritionally complete, for special metabolic needs for inherited disease of metabolism, includes proteins, fats, carbohydrates, vitamins and minerals, may include fiber, administered through an enteral feeding tube, 100 calories = 1 unit Y
BETOS: O1C Enteral and parenteral

D B4158 Enteral formula, for pediatrics, nutritionally complete with intact nutrients, includes proteins, fats, carbohydrates, vitamins and minerals, may include fiber and/or iron, administered through an enteral feeding tube, 100 calories = 1 unit Ⓐ Y
BETOS: O1C Enteral and parenteral

B4159 Enteral formula, for pediatrics, nutritionally complete soy based with intact nutrients, includes proteins, fats, carbohydrates, vitamins and minerals, may include fiber and/or iron, administered through an enteral feeding tube, 100 calories = 1 unit Ⓐ Y
BETOS: O1C   Enteral and parenteral

B4160 Enteral formula, for pediatrics, nutritionally complete calorically dense (equal to or greater than 0.7 kcal/ml) with intact nutrients, includes proteins, fats, carbohydrates, vitamins and minerals, may include fiber, administered through an enteral feeding tube, 100 calories = 1 unit Ⓐ Y
BETOS: O1C   Enteral and parenteral

B4161 Enteral formula, for pediatrics, hydrolyzed/ amino acids and peptide chain proteins, includes fats, carbohydrates, vitamins and minerals, may include fiber, administered through an enteral feeding tube, 100 calories = 1 unit Ⓐ Y
BETOS: O1C   Enteral and parenteral

B4162 Enteral formula, for pediatrics, special metabolic needs for inherited disease of metabolism, includes proteins, fats, carbohydrates, vitamins and minerals, may include fiber, administered through an enteral feeding tube, 100 calories = 1 unit Ⓐ Y
BETOS: O1C   Enteral and parenteral

PARENTERAL SOLUTIONS AND SUPPLIES (B4164-B5200)

B4164 Parenteral nutrition solution: carbohydrates (dextrose), 50% or less (500 ml = 1 unit) - home mix Y
BETOS: O1C   Enteral and parenteral

B4168 Parenteral nutrition solution; amino acid, 3.5%, (500 ml = 1 unit) - home mix Y
BETOS: O1C   Enteral and parenteral

B4172 Parenteral nutrition solution; amino acid, 5.5% through 7%, (500 ml = 1 unit) - home mix Y
BETOS: O1C   Enteral and parenteral

B4176 Parenteral nutrition solution; amino acid, 7% through 8.5%, (500 ml = 1 unit) - home mix Y
BETOS: O1C   Enteral and parenteral

B4178 Parenteral nutrition solution: amino acid, greater than 8.5% (500 ml = 1 unit) - home mix Y
BETOS: O1C   Enteral and parenteral

B4180 Parenteral nutrition solution; carbohydrates (dextrose), greater than 50% (500 ml = 1 unit) - home mix Y
BETOS: O1C   Enteral and parenteral

B4185 Parenteral nutrition solution, not otherwise specified, 10 grams lipids B
BETOS: O1C   Enteral and parenteral

B4187 Omegaven, 10 grams lipids Ⓐ B
BETOS: O1C   Enteral and parenteral

B4189 Parenteral nutrition solution; compounded amino acid and carbohydrates with electrolytes, trace elements, and vitamins, including preparation, any strength, 10 to 51 grams of protein - premix Y
BETOS: O1C   Enteral and parenteral

B4193 Parenteral nutrition solution; compounded amino acid and carbohydrates with electrolytes, trace elements, and vitamins, including preparation, any strength, 52 to 73 grams of protein - premix Y
BETOS: O1C   Enteral and parenteral

B4197 Parenteral nutrition solution; compounded amino acid and carbohydrates with electrolytes, trace elements and vitamins, including preparation, any strength, 74 to 100 grams of protein - premix Y
BETOS: O1C   Enteral and parenteral

B4199 Parenteral nutrition solution; compounded amino acid and carbohydrates with electrolytes, trace elements and vitamins, including preparation, any strength, over 100 grams of protein - premix Y
BETOS: O1C   Enteral and parenteral

B4216 Parenteral nutrition; additives (vitamins, trace elements, heparin, electrolytes) homemix, per day Y
BETOS: O1C   Enteral and parenteral

B4220 Parenteral nutrition supply kit; premix, per day Y
BETOS: O1C   Enteral and parenteral

B4222 Parenteral nutrition supply kit; home mix, per day Y
BETOS: O1C   Enteral and parenteral

B4224 Parenteral nutrition administration kit, per day Y
BETOS: O1C   Enteral and parenteral

B5000 Parenteral nutrition solution compounded amino acid and carbohydrates with electrolytes, trace elements, and vitamins, including preparation, any strength, renal-Aminosyn RF, NephrAmine, RenAmine-premix Y
BETOS: O1C   Enteral and parenteral

B5100 Parenteral nutrition solution compounded amino acid and carbohydrates with electrolytes, trace elements, and vitamins, including preparation, any strength, hepatic, HepAtamine-premix Y
BETOS: O1C   Enteral and parenteral

● New code   ▲ Revised code   Ⓒ Carrier judgment   Ⓓ Special coverage instructions apply
Ⓘ Not payable by Medicare   Ⓜ Non-covered by Medicare   Ⓢ Non-covered by Medicare statute   AHA Coding Clinic®

D **B5200** Parenteral nutrition solution compounded amino acid and carbohydrates with electrolytes, trace elements, and vitamins, including preparation, any strength, stress-branch chain amino acids-FreAmineHBC-premix   Y

    BETOS: O1C   Enteral and parenteral

NUTRITION INFUSION PUMPS AND SUPPLIES NOT OTHERWISE CLASSIFIED (NOC) (B9002-B9999)

D **B9002** Enteral nutrition infusion pump, any type   Y

    BETOS: O1C   Enteral and parenteral

D **B9004** Parenteral nutrition infusion pump, portable   Y

    BETOS: O1C   Enteral and parenteral

D **B9006** Parenteral nutrition infusion pump, stationary   Y

    BETOS: O1C   Enteral and parenteral

D **B9998** NOC for enteral supplies   Y

    BETOS: O1C   Enteral and parenteral
    Other carrier priced

D **B9999** NOC for parenteral supplies   Y

    BETOS: O1C   Enteral and parenteral
    Other carrier priced
    Coding Clinic: 2009, Q2

♂ Male only   ♀ Female only   **A** Age   A2 - Z3 = ASC Payment indicator   A - Y = APC Status indicator

ASC = ASC Approved Procedure   **DME** Paid under the DME fee schedule   **MIPS** MIPS code

NOTES

OUTPATIENT PPS (C1052-C9899)

OTHER THERAPEUTIC PROCEDURES (C1052-C1062)

- **D C1052** Hemostatic agent, gastrointestinal, topical   J7 ASC H
  BETOS: D1A   Medical/surgical supplies
  Statute: 1833(T)

- **D C1062** Intravertebral body fracture augmentation with implant (e.g., metal, polymer)   J7 ASC H
  BETOS: D1A   Medical/surgical supplies
  Statute: 1833(T)

ASSORTED DEVICES AND SUPPLIES (C1713-C1715)

- **D C1713** Anchor/screw for opposing bone-to-bone or soft tissue-to-bone (implantable)   N1 ASC N
  BETOS: D1A   Medical/surgical supplies
  Statute: 1833(T)
  Coding Clinic: 2001, Q1; 2002, Q3; 2010, Q1; 2016, Q3; 2016, Q3; 2018, Q1; 2018, Q2

- **D C1714** Catheter, transluminal atherectomy, directional   N1 ASC N
  BETOS: D1A   Medical/surgical supplies
  Statute: 1833(T)
  Coding Clinic: 2001, Q1; 2002, Q3; 2003, Q4; 2004, Q4; 2016, Q3

- **D C1715** Brachytherapy needle   N1 ASC N
  BETOS: D1A   Medical/surgical supplies
  Statute: 1833(T)
  Coding Clinic: 2001, Q1; 2002, Q3; 2016, Q3

BRACHYTHERAPY SOURCES (C1716-C1719), SEE ALSO BRACHYTHERAPY SOURCES (C2616), (C2634-C2699)

- **D C1716** Brachytherapy source, non-stranded, gold-198, per source   H2 ASC U
  BETOS: I4B   Imaging/procedure - other
  Statute: 1833(T)
  Coding Clinic: 2001, Q1; 2002, Q3; 2004, Q4; 2004, Q2; 2007, Q2; 2016, Q3; 2016, Q3; 2016, Q3

- **D C1717** Brachytherapy source, non-stranded, high dose rate iridium-192, per source   H2 ASC U
  BETOS: I4B   Imaging/procedure - other
  Statute: 1833(T)
  Coding Clinic: 2001, Q1; 2002, Q3; 2004, Q4; 2004, Q2; 2007, Q2; 2016, Q3; 2016, Q3; 2016, Q3

- **D C1719** Brachytherapy source, non-stranded, non-high dose rate iridium-192, per source   H2 ASC U
  BETOS: I4B   Imaging/procedure - other
  Statute: 1833(T)
  Coding Clinic: 2001, Q1; 2002, Q3; 2004, Q4; 2004, Q2; 2007, Q2; 2016, Q3; 2016, Q3; 2016, Q3

CARDIOVERTER-DEFIBRILLATORS (C1721-C1722)

- **D C1721** Cardioverter-defibrillator, dual chamber (implantable)   N1 ASC N
  BETOS: D1A   Medical/surgical supplies
  Statute: 1833(T)
  Coding Clinic: 2001, Q1; 2002, Q3; 2004, Q4; 2006, Q4; 2016, Q3

- **D C1722** Cardioverter-defibrillator, single chamber (implantable)   N1 ASC N
  BETOS: D1A   Medical/surgical supplies
  Statute: 1833(T)
  Coding Clinic: 2001, Q1; 2002, Q3; 2004, Q4; 2006, Q4; 2006, Q2; 2016, Q3; 2017, Q2

CATHETERS FOR MULTIPLE APPLICATIONS (C1724-C1759)

- **D C1724** Catheter, transluminal atherectomy, rotational   N1 ASC N
  BETOS: D1A   Medical/surgical supplies
  Statute: 1833(T)
  Coding Clinic: 2001, Q1; 2002, Q3; 2003, Q4; 2004, Q4; 2016, Q3; 2016, Q3

- **D C1725** Catheter, transluminal angioplasty, non-laser (may include guidance, infusion/perfusion capability)   N1 ASC N
  BETOS: D1A   Medical/surgical supplies
  Statute: 1833(T)
  Coding Clinic: 2001, Q1; 2002, Q3; 2003, Q4; 2004, Q4; 2016, Q3; 2016, Q3

- **D C1726** Catheter, balloon dilatation, non-vascular   N1 ASC N
  BETOS: D1A   Medical/surgical supplies
  Statute: 1833(T)
  Coding Clinic: 2001, Q1; 2002, Q3; 2016, Q3; 2016, Q3

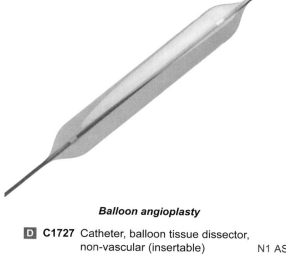

Balloon angioplasty

- **D C1727** Catheter, balloon tissue dissector, non-vascular (insertable)   N1 ASC N
  BETOS: D1A   Medical/surgical supplies
  Statute: 1833(T)
  Coding Clinic: 2001, Q1; 2002, Q3; 2016, Q3; 2016, Q3

♂ Male only   ♀ Female only   **A** Age   A2 - Z3 = ASC Payment indicator   A - Y = APC Status indicator
ASC = ASC Approved Procedure   **DME** Paid under the DME fee schedule   **MIPS** MIPS code

D **C1728** Catheter, brachytherapy seed administration   N1 ASC N
  BETOS: D1A Medical/surgical supplies
  Statute: 1833(T)
  Coding Clinic: 2001, Q1; 2002, Q3; 2016, Q3

D **C1729** Catheter, drainage   N1 ASC N
  BETOS: D1A Medical/surgical supplies
  Statute: 1833(T)
  Coding Clinic: 2001, Q1; 2002, Q3; 2016, Q3; 2016, Q3

D **C1730** Catheter, electrophysiology, diagnostic, other than 3D mapping (19 or fewer electrodes)   N1 ASC N
  BETOS: D1A Medical/surgical supplies
  Statute: 1833(T)
  Coding Clinic: 2001, Q3; 2001, Q1; 2002, Q3; 2004, Q4; 2016, Q3; 2016, Q3

D **C1731** Catheter, electrophysiology, diagnostic, other than 3D mapping (20 or more electrodes)   N1 ASC N
  BETOS: D1A Medical/surgical supplies
  Statute: 1833(T)
  Coding Clinic: 2001, Q1; 2002, Q3; 2004, Q4; 2016, Q3; 2016, Q3

D **C1732** Catheter, electrophysiology, diagnostic/ablation, 3D or vector mapping   N1 ASC N
  BETOS: D1A Medical/surgical supplies
  Statute: 1833(T)
  Coding Clinic: 2001, Q3; 2001, Q1; 2002, Q3; 2004, Q4; 2016, Q3; 2016, Q3

D **C1733** Catheter, electrophysiology, diagnostic/ablation, other than 3D or vector mapping, other than cool-tip   N1 ASC N
  BETOS: D1A Medical/surgical supplies
  Statute: 1833(T)
  Coding Clinic: 2001, Q3; 2001, Q1; 2002, Q3; 2004, Q4; 2016, Q3; 2016, Q3

D **C1734** Orthopedic/device/drug matrix for opposing bone-to-bone or soft tissue-to bone (implantable)   J7 ASC H
  BETOS: D1A Medical/surgical supplies
  Statute: 1833(T)
  Coding Clinic: 2020, Q1

● **D** **C1748** Endoscope, single-use (i.e., disposable), upper GI, imaging/illumination device (insertable)   J7 ASC H
  BETOS: D1A Medical/surgical supplies
  Statute: 1833(t)
  Coding Clinic: 2020, Q2

D **C1749** Endoscope, retrograde imaging/illumination colonoscope device (implantable)   N1 ASC N
  BETOS: D1A Medical/surgical supplies
  Statute: 1833(t)
  Coding Clinic: 2016, Q3

D **C1750** Catheter, hemodialysis/peritoneal, long-term   N1 ASC N
  BETOS: D1A Medical/surgical supplies
  Statute: 1833(T)
  Coding Clinic: 2001, Q1; 2002, Q3; 2003, Q4; 2012, Q4

D **C1751** Catheter, infusion, inserted peripherally, centrally or midline (other than hemodialysis)   N1 ASC N
  BETOS: D1A Medical/surgical supplies
  Statute: 1833(T)
  Coding Clinic: 2001, Q3; 2001, Q1; 2002, Q3; 2003, Q4; 2004, Q4; 2014, Q3; 2016, Q3; 2019, Q2

D **C1752** Catheter, hemodialysis/peritoneal, short-term   N1 ASC N
  BETOS: D1A Medical/surgical supplies
  Statute: 1833(T)
  Coding Clinic: 2001, Q1; 2002, Q3; 2003, Q4; 2016, Q3

D **C1753** Catheter, intravascular ultrasound   N1 ASC N
  BETOS: D1A Medical/surgical supplies
  Statute: 1833(T)
  Coding Clinic: 2001, Q1; 2002, Q3; 2003, Q4; 2016, Q3

D **C1754** Catheter, intradiscal   N1 ASC N
  BETOS: D1A Medical/surgical supplies
  Statute: 1833(T)
  Coding Clinic: 2001, Q1; 2002, Q3; 2003, Q4; 2016, Q3

D **C1755** Catheter, intraspinal   N1 ASC N
  BETOS: D1A Medical/surgical supplies
  Statute: 1833(T)
  Coding Clinic: 2001, Q1; 2002, Q3; 2003, Q4; 2016, Q3

D **C1756** Catheter, pacing, transesophageal   N1 ASC N
  BETOS: D1A Medical/surgical supplies
  Statute: 1833(T)
  Coding Clinic: 2001, Q1; 2002, Q3; 2003, Q4

D **C1757** Catheter, thrombectomy/embolectomy   N1 ASC N
  BETOS: D1A Medical/surgical supplies
  Statute: 1833(T)
  Coding Clinic: 2001, Q1; 2002, Q3; 2003, Q4; 2016, Q3

D **C1758** Catheter, ureteral   N1 ASC N
  BETOS: D1A Medical/surgical supplies
  Statute: 1833(T)
  Coding Clinic: 2001, Q1; 2002, Q3; 2003, Q4; 2016, Q3

D **C1759** Catheter, intracardiac echocardiography   N1 ASC N
  BETOS: D1A Medical/surgical supplies
  Statute: 1833(T)
  Coding Clinic: 2001, Q3; 2001, Q1; 2002, Q3; 2003, Q4; 2016, Q3

● New code   ▲ Revised code   **C** Carrier judgment   **D** Special coverage instructions apply
I Not payable by Medicare   **M** Non-covered by Medicare   **S** Non-covered by Medicare statute   *AHA Coding Clinic®*

ASSORTED DEVICES, IMPLANTS, AND SYSTEMS
(C1760-C2615)

D **C1760** Closure device, vascular (implantable/
insertable) N1 ASC N

BETOS: D1A Medical/surgical supplies
Statute: 1833(T)
Coding Clinic: 2001, Q1; 2002, Q3; 2003,
Q4; 2016, Q3; 2016, Q3

D **C1762** Connective tissue, human (includes fascia
lata) N1 ASC N

BETOS: D1A Medical/surgical supplies
Statute: 1833(T)
Coding Clinic: 2001, Q1; 2002, Q3; 2003,
Q4; 2003, Q3; 2010, Q1; 2016, Q3; 2016,
Q3; 2016, Q3

D **C1763** Connective tissue, non-human (includes
synthetic) N1 ASC N

BETOS: D1A Medical/surgical supplies
Statute: 1833(T)
Coding Clinic: 2001, Q1; 2002, Q3; 2003,
Q4; 2003, Q3; 2010, Q1; 2010, Q4; 2016,
Q3; 2016, Q3; 2016, Q3

D **C1764** Event recorder, cardiac
(implantable) N1 ASC N

BETOS: D1A Medical/surgical supplies
Statute: 1833(T)
Coding Clinic: 2001, Q1; 2002, Q3; 2003,
Q4; 2016, Q3

D **C1765** Adhesion barrier N1 ASC N

BETOS: D1A Medical/surgical supplies
Statute: 1833(T)
Coding Clinic: 2016, Q3; 2016, Q3

D **C1766** Introducer/sheath, guiding, intracardiac
electrophysiological, steerable, other than
peel-away N1 ASC N

BETOS: D1A Medical/surgical supplies
Statute: 1833(T)
Coding Clinic: 2001, Q3; 2002, Q3; 2004,
Q4; 2016, Q3

D **C1767** Generator, neurostimulator (implantable),
non-rechargeable N1 ASC N

BETOS: D1A Medical/surgical supplies
Statute: 1833(T)
Coding Clinic: 2001, Q1; 2002, Q3; 2002,
Q1; 2003, Q4; 2004, Q4; 2006, Q4; 2006,
Q1; 2007, Q1; 2016, Q3

D **C1768** Graft, vascular N1 ASC N

BETOS: D1A Medical/surgical supplies
Statute: 1833(T)
Coding Clinic: 2001, Q1; 2002, Q3; 2003,
Q4; 2016, Q3

D **C1769** Guide wire N1 ASC N

BETOS: D1A Medical/surgical supplies
Statute: 1833(T)
Coding Clinic: 2001, Q3; 2001, Q1; 2002,
Q3; 2003, Q4; 2007, Q2; 2014, Q3; 2016,
Q3; 2016, Q3; 2019, Q2; 2019, Q3

D **C1770** Imaging coil, magnetic resonance
(insertable) N1 ASC N

BETOS: D1A Medical/surgical supplies
Statute: 1833(T)
Coding Clinic: 2001, Q1; 2002, Q3; 2003,
Q4; 2016, Q3

D **C1771** Repair device, urinary, incontinence,
with sling graft N1 ASC N

BETOS: D1A Medical/surgical supplies
Statute: 1833(T)
Coding Clinic: 2001, Q3; 2001, Q1; 2002,
Q3; 2003, Q4; 2008, Q3; 2016, Q3; 2016, Q3

D **C1772** Infusion pump, programmable
(implantable) N1 ASC N

BETOS: D1A Medical/surgical supplies
Statute: 1833(T)
Coding Clinic: 2001, Q1; 2002, Q3; 2004,
Q4; 2016, Q3

D **C1773** Retrieval device, insertable (used to retrieve
fractured medical devices) N1 ASC N

BETOS: D1A Medical/surgical supplies
Statute: 1833(T)
Coding Clinic: 2001, Q1; 2002, Q3; 2003,
Q4; 2016, Q3; 2016, Q3

D **C1776** Joint device (implantable) N1 ASC N

BETOS: D1A Medical/surgical supplies
Statute: 1833(T)
Coding Clinic: 2001, Q3; 2001, Q1; 2002,
Q3; 2008, Q4; 2010, Q3; 2016, Q3; 2016,
Q3; 2016, Q3; 2018, Q3; 2020, Q1

D **C1777** Lead, cardioverter-defibrillator, endocardial
single coil (implantable) N1 ASC N

BETOS: D1A Medical/surgical supplies
Statute: 1833(T)
Coding Clinic: 2001, Q1; 2002, Q3; 2004,
Q4; 2006, Q4; 2006, Q2; 2016, Q3; 2017, Q2

D **C1778** Lead, neurostimulator
(implantable) N1 ASC N

BETOS: D1A Medical/surgical supplies
Statute: 1833(T)
Coding Clinic: 2001, Q1; 2002, Q3; 2002,
Q1; 2006, Q4; 2007, Q1; 2011, Q4; 2016,
Q3; 2019, Q1

D **C1779** Lead, pacemaker, transvenous VDD single
pass N1 ASC N

BETOS: D1A Medical/surgical supplies
Statute: 1833(T)
Coding Clinic: 2001, Q1; 2002, Q3; 2004,
Q4; 2006, Q4; 2016, Q3; 2016, Q3

D **C1780** Lens, intraocular (new technology) N1 ASC N

BETOS: D1A Medical/surgical supplies
Statute: 1833(T)
Coding Clinic: 2001, Q1; 2002, Q3; 2016,
Q3; 2016, Q3

D **C1781** Mesh (implantable) N1 ASC N

BETOS: D1A Medical/surgical supplies
Statute: 1833(T)
Coding Clinic: 2001, Q1; 2002, Q3; 2012,
Q2; 2010, Q1; 2016, Q3; 2016, Q3; 2019, Q1

♂ Male only   ♀ Female only   **A** Age   A2 - Z3 = ASC Payment indicator   A - Y = APC Status indicator

ASC = ASC Approved Procedure   **DME** Paid under the DME fee schedule   **MIPS** MIPS code

OUTPATIENT PPS (C1052-C9899)

D C1782 Morcellator N1 ASC N
BETOS: D1A Medical/surgical supplies
Statute: 1833(T)
Coding Clinic: 2001, Q1; 2002, Q3; 2016, Q3; 2016, Q3

D C1783 Ocular implant, aqueous drainage assist device N1 ASC N
BETOS: D1A Medical/surgical supplies
Statute: 1833(T)
Coding Clinic: 2016, Q3; 2017, Q1

D C1784 Ocular device, intraoperative, detached retina N1 ASC N
BETOS: D1A Medical/surgical supplies
Statute: 1833(T)
Coding Clinic: 2001, Q1; 2002, Q3; 2016, Q3; 2016, Q3

D C1785 Pacemaker, dual chamber, rate-responsive (implantable) N1 ASC N
BETOS: D1A Medical/surgical supplies
Statute: 1833(T)
Coding Clinic: 2001, Q1; 2002, Q3; 2003, Q4; 2006, Q4; 2016, Q3

D C1786 Pacemaker, single chamber, rate-responsive (implantable) N1 ASC N
BETOS: D1A Medical/surgical supplies
Statute: 1833(T)
Coding Clinic: 2001, Q1; 2002, Q3; 2003, Q4; 2004, Q4; 2006, Q4; 2016, Q3

Single chamber

Subclavian vein
Pulse generator
Lead

Dual chamber *Biventricular*

Coronary sinus vein LV lead
RA lead
RV lead

Pacemaker insertion

D C1787 Patient programmer, neurostimulator N1 ASC N
BETOS: D1A Medical/surgical supplies
Statute: 1833(T)
Coding Clinic: 2001, Q1; 2002, Q3; 2003, Q4; 2016, Q3; 2016, Q3

D C1788 Port, indwelling (implantable) N1 ASC N
BETOS: D1A Medical/surgical supplies
Statute: 1833(T)
Coding Clinic: 2001, Q3; 2001, Q1; 2002, Q3; 2003, Q4; 2004, Q4; 2014, Q3; 2016, Q3; 2019, Q2

D C1789 Prosthesis, breast (implantable) N1 ○ ASC N
BETOS: D1A Medical/surgical supplies
Statute: 1833(T)
Coding Clinic: 2001, Q1; 2002, Q3; 2003, Q4; 2016, Q3

D C1813 Prosthesis, penile, inflatable N1 ♂ ASC N
BETOS: D1A Medical/surgical supplies
Statute: 1833(T)
Coding Clinic: 2001, Q1; 2002, Q3; 2003, Q4; 2016, Q3

D C1814 Retinal tamponade device, silicone oil N1 ASC N
BETOS: D1A Medical/surgical supplies
Statute: 1833t
Coding Clinic: 2006, Q2; 2016, Q3; 2016, Q3

D C1815 Prosthesis, urinary sphincter (implantable) N1 ASC N
BETOS: D1A Medical/surgical supplies
Statute: 1833(T)
Coding Clinic: 2001, Q1; 2002, Q3; 2003, Q4; 2016, Q3

D C1816 Receiver and/or transmitter, neurostimulator (implantable) N1 ASC N
BETOS: D1A Medical/surgical supplies
Statute: 1833(T)
Coding Clinic: 2001, Q1; 2002, Q3; 2003, Q4; 2016, Q3

D C1817 Septal defect implant system, intracardiac N1 ASC N
BETOS: D1A Medical/surgical supplies
Statute: 1833(T)
Coding Clinic: 2001, Q1; 2002, Q3; 2003, Q4; 2016, Q3; 2016, Q3

D C1818 Integrated keratoprosthesis N1 ASC N
BETOS: D1A Medical/surgical supplies
Statute: 1833T
Coding Clinic: 2016, Q3; 2016, Q3

D C1819 Surgical tissue localization and excision device (implantable) N1 ASC N
BETOS: D1A Medical/surgical supplies
Statute: 1833T
Coding Clinic: 2004, Q1; 2016, Q3

D C1820 Generator, neurostimulator (implantable), with rechargeable battery and charging system N1 ASC N
BETOS: D1A Medical/surgical supplies
Statute: 1833(T)
Coding Clinic: 2006, Q4; 2006, Q1; 2006, Q1; 2016, Q1; 2016, Q2; 2016, Q3

● New code ▲ Revised code **C** Carrier judgment **D** Special coverage instructions apply
I Not payable by Medicare **M** Non-covered by Medicare **S** Non-covered by Medicare statute AHA Coding Clinic®

D C1821 Interspinous process distraction device
(implantable)   N1 ASC N
    BETOS: D1A   Medical/surgical supplies
    Statute: 1833(T)
    Coding Clinic: 2007, Q1; 2009, Q2; 2016, Q3

D C1822 Generator, neurostimulator (implantable),
high frequency, with rechargeable battery
and charging system   N1 ASC N
    BETOS: D1A   Medical/surgical supplies
    Statute: 1833(T)
    Coding Clinic: 2016, Q1; 2016, Q2; 2016, Q3

D C1823 Generator, neurostimulator (implantable),
non-rechargeable, with transvenous sensing
and stimulation leads   J7 ASC H
    BETOS: D1A   Medical/surgical supplies
    Statute: 1833(t)
    Coding Clinic: 2019, Q1

D C1824 Generator, cardiac contractility modulation
(implantable)   J7 ASC H
    BETOS: D1A   Medical/surgical supplies
    Statute: 1833(T)
    Coding Clinic: 2020, Q1

● **D C1825** Generator, neurostimulator (implantable),
non-rechargeable with carotid sinus
baroreceptor stimulation lead(s)   J7 ASC H
    BETOS: D1A   Medical/surgical supplies
    Statute: 1833(T)

D C1830 Powered bone marrow biopsy
needle   N1 ASC N
    BETOS: D1A   Medical/surgical supplies
    Statute: 1833(t)
    Coding Clinic: 2011, Q4; 2016, Q3

D C1839 Iris prosthesis   J7 ASC H
    BETOS: D1A   Medical/surgical supplies
    Statute: 1833(T)
    Coding Clinic: 2020, Q1

D C1840 Lens, intraocular (telescopic)   N1 ASC N
    BETOS: D1A   Medical/surgical supplies
    Statute: 1833(t)
    Coding Clinic: 2011, Q4; 2012, Q1; 2012,
    Q3; 2016, Q3

D C1841 Retinal prosthesis, includes all internal and
external components   J7 ASC N
    BETOS: D1E   Other DME
    Statute: 1833(t)
    Coding Clinic: 2016, Q3; 2017, Q1

D C1842 Retinal prosthesis, includes all internal
and external components; add-on to
C1841   J7 ASC E1
    BETOS: D1E   Other DME
    Statute: 1833(t)
    Coding Clinic: 2017, Q1

● **D C1849** Skin substitute, synthetic, resorbable,
per square centimeter   N1 ASC N
    BETOS: D1A   Medical/surgical supplies
    Statute: 1833(t)
    Coding Clinic: 2020, Q2

D C1874 Stent, coated/covered, with delivery
system   N1 ASC N
    BETOS: D1A   Medical/surgical supplies
    Statute: 1833(T)
    Coding Clinic: 2001, Q3; 2001, Q1; 2002,
    Q3; 2002, Q3; 2003, Q4; 2004, Q4; 2004,
    Q3; 2016, Q3; 2016, Q3

D C1875 Stent, coated/covered, without delivery
system   N1 ASC N
    BETOS: D1A   Medical/surgical supplies
    Statute: 1833(T)
    Coding Clinic: 2001, Q1; 2002, Q3; 2002,
    Q3; 2003, Q4; 2004, Q4; 2016, Q3; 2016,
    Q3; 2020, Q2

D C1876 Stent, non-coated/non-covered, with delivery
system   N1 ASC N
    BETOS: D1A   Medical/surgical supplies
    Statute: 1833(T)
    Coding Clinic: 2001, Q3; 2001, Q1; 2002,
    Q3; 2002, Q3; 2003, Q4; 2004, Q4; 2016,
    Q3; 2016, Q3

D C1877 Stent, non-coated/non-covered, without
delivery system   N1 ASC N
    BETOS: D1A   Medical/surgical supplies
    Statute: 1833(T)
    Coding Clinic: 2001, Q3; 2001, Q1; 2002,
    Q3; 2002, Q3; 2003, Q4; 2004, Q4; 2016, Q3

D C1878 Material for vocal cord medialization,
synthetic (implantable)   N1 ASC N
    BETOS: D1A   Medical/surgical supplies
    Statute: 1833(T)
    Coding Clinic: 2001, Q1; 2002, Q3; 2016,
    Q3; 2016, Q3

D C1880 Vena cava filter   N1 ASC N
    BETOS: D1A   Medical/surgical supplies
    Statute: 1833(T)
    Coding Clinic: 2001, Q1; 2002, Q3; 2003,
    Q4; 2016, Q3

D C1881 Dialysis access system
(implantable)   N1 ASC N
    BETOS: D1A   Medical/surgical supplies
    Statute: 1833(T)
    Coding Clinic: 2001, Q1; 2002, Q3; 2003,
    Q4; 2016, Q3

D C1882 Cardioverter-defibrillator, other than single or
dual chamber (implantable)   N1 ASC N
    BETOS: D1A   Medical/surgical supplies
    Statute: 1833(T)
    Coding Clinic: 2001, Q1; 2002, Q3; 2004,
    Q4; 2006, Q4; 2006, Q2; 2012, Q2; 2016,
    Q3; 2016, Q3

D C1883 Adapter/extension, pacing lead or
neurostimulator lead (implantable) N1 ASC N
    BETOS: D1A   Medical/surgical supplies
    Statute: 1833(T)
    Coding Clinic: 2001, Q1; 2002, Q3; 2002,
    Q1; 2007, Q1; 2016, Q3; 2016, Q3

♂ Male only   ♀ Female only   Ⓐ Age   A2 - Z3 = ASC Payment indicator   A - Y = APC Status indicator
ASC = ASC Approved Procedure   **DME** Paid under the DME fee schedule   **MIPS** MIPS code

C1884 - C2596

D C1884 Embolization protective system   N1 ASC N
     BETOS: D1A   Medical/surgical supplies
     Statute: 1833T
     Coding Clinic: 2014, Q3; 2016, Q3; 2016, Q3

D C1885 Catheter, transluminal angioplasty, laser   N1 ASC N
     BETOS: D1A   Medical/surgical supplies
     Statute: 1833(T)
     Coding Clinic: 2001, Q1; 2002, Q3; 2003, Q4; 2004, Q4; 2016, Q1; 2016, Q3; 2016, Q3

D C1886 Catheter, extravascular tissue ablation, any modality (insertable)   N1 ASC N
     BETOS: D1A   Medical/surgical supplies
     Statute: 1833(t)
     Coding Clinic: 2016, Q3

D C1887 Catheter, guiding (may include infusion/perfusion capability)   N1 ASC N
     BETOS: D1A   Medical/surgical supplies
     Statute: 1833(T)
     Coding Clinic: 2001, Q3; 2001, Q1; 2002, Q3; 2004, Q4; 2016, Q3

D C1888 Catheter, ablation, non-cardiac, endovascular (implantable)   N1 ASC N
     BETOS: D1A   Medical/surgical supplies
     Statute: 1833(T)
     Coding Clinic: 2016, Q3; 2016, Q3

D C1889 Implantable/insertable device, not otherwise classified   N1 ASC N
     BETOS: D1A   Medical/surgical supplies
     Statute: 1833(T)

D C1890 No implantable/insertable device used with device-intensive procedures   J7 ASC E1
     BETOS: D1E   Other DME
     Statute: 1833(t)
     Coding Clinic: 2019, Q1

D C1891 Infusion pump, non-programmable, permanent (implantable)   N1 ASC N
     BETOS: D1A   Medical/surgical supplies
     Statute: 1833(T)
     Coding Clinic: 2001, Q1; 2002, Q3; 2003, Q4; 2004, Q4; 2016, Q3

D C1892 Introducer/sheath, guiding, intracardiac electrophysiological, fixed-curve, peel-away   N1 ASC N
     BETOS: D1A   Medical/surgical supplies
     Statute: 1833(T)
     Coding Clinic: 2001, Q1; 2002, Q3; 2004, Q4; 2016, Q3; 2016, Q3

D C1893 Introducer/sheath, guiding, intracardiac electrophysiological, fixed-curve, other than peel-away   N1 ASC N
     BETOS: D1A   Medical/surgical supplies
     Statute: 1833(T)
     Coding Clinic: 2001, Q3; 2001, Q1; 2002, Q3; 2004, Q4; 2016, Q3

D C1894 Introducer/sheath, other than guiding, other than intracardiac electrophysiological, non-laser   N1 ASC N
     BETOS: D1A   Medical/surgical supplies
     Statute: 1833(T)
     Coding Clinic: 2001, Q1; 2002, Q3; 2016, Q3; 2016, Q3; 2019, Q2

D C1895 Lead, cardioverter-defibrillator, endocardial dual coil (implantable)   N1 ASC N
     BETOS: D1A   Medical/surgical supplies
     Statute: 1833(T)
     Coding Clinic: 2001, Q1; 2002, Q3; 2004, Q4; 2006, Q4; 2006, Q2; 2016, Q3

D C1896 Lead, cardioverter-defibrillator, other than endocardial single or dual coil (implantable)   N1 ASC N
     BETOS: D1A   Medical/surgical supplies
     Statute: 1833(T)
     Coding Clinic: 2001, Q1; 2002, Q3; 2004, Q4; 2006, Q4; 2006, Q2; 2016, Q3

D C1897 Lead, neurostimulator test kit (implantable)   N1 ASC N
     BETOS: D1A   Medical/surgical supplies
     Statute: 1833(T)
     Coding Clinic: 2001, Q1; 2002, Q3; 2002, Q1; 2006, Q4; 2007, Q1; 2016, Q3

D C1898 Lead, pacemaker, other than transvenous VDD single pass   N1 ASC N
     BETOS: D1A   Medical/surgical supplies
     Statute: 1833(T)
     Coding Clinic: 2001, Q3; 2001, Q1; 2002, Q3; 2002, Q3; 2006, Q4; 2016, Q3

D C1899 Lead, pacemaker/cardioverter-defibrillator combination (implantable)   N1 ASC N
     BETOS: D1A   Medical/surgical supplies
     Statute: 1833(T)
     Coding Clinic: 2001, Q1; 2002, Q3; 2004, Q4; 2006, Q4; 2016, Q3

D C1900 Lead, left ventricular coronary venous system   N1 ASC N
     BETOS: D1A   Medical/surgical supplies
     Statute: 1833(T)
     Coding Clinic: 2004, Q4; 2006, Q4; 2016, Q3; 2016, Q3

D C1982 Catheter, pressure-generating, one-way valve, intermittently occlusive   J7 ASC H
     BETOS: D1A   Medical/surgical supplies
     Statute: 1833(T)
     Coding Clinic: 2020, Q1

D C2596 Probe, image-guided, robotic, waterjet ablation   J7 ASC H
     BETOS: D1A   Medical/surgical supplies
     Statute: 1833(T)
     Coding Clinic: 2020, Q1

● New code   ▲ Revised code   **C** Carrier judgment   **D** Special coverage instructions apply
I Not payable by Medicare   **M** Non-covered by Medicare   **S** Non-covered by Medicare statute   AHA Coding Clinic®

D **C2613** Lung biopsy plug with delivery system   N1 ASC N
    BETOS: D1A   Medical/surgical supplies
    Statute: 1833(t)
    Coding Clinic: 2016, Q3

D **C2614** Probe, percutaneous lumbar discectomy   N1 ASC N
    BETOS: D1A   Medical/surgical supplies
    Statute: 1833(T)
    Coding Clinic: 2016, Q3

D **C2615** Sealant, pulmonary, liquid   N1 ASC N
    BETOS: D1A   Medical/surgical supplies
    Statute: 1833(T)
    Coding Clinic: 2001, Q1; 2002, Q3; 2003, Q4; 2016, Q3; 2016, Q3

BRACHYTHERAPY SOURCES (C2616), SEE ALSO BRACHYTHERAPY SOURCES (C1716-C1719); BRACHYTHERAPY SOURCES (C2634-C2699)

D **C2616** Brachytherapy source, non-stranded, Yttrium-90, per source   H2 ASC U
    BETOS: I4B   Imaging/procedure - other
    Statute: 1833(T)
    Coding Clinic: 2002, Q3; 2003, Q3; 2004, Q4; 2004, Q2; 2007, Q2; 2016, Q3; 2016, Q3; 2016, Q3

ASSORTED CARDIOVASCULAR AND GENITOURINARY DEVICES (C2617-C2631)

D **C2617** Stent, non-coronary, temporary, without delivery system   N1 ASC N
    BETOS: D1A   Medical/surgical supplies
    Statute: 1833(T)
    Coding Clinic: 2001, Q1; 2002, Q3; 2003, Q4; 2004, Q4; 2016, Q3; 2016, Q3; 2016, Q3; 2018, Q1

D **C2618** Probe/needle, cryoablation   N1 ASC N
    BETOS: D1A   Medical/surgical supplies
    Statute: 1833(T)
    Coding Clinic: 2001, Q1; 2002, Q3; 2003, Q4; 2004, Q4; 2016, Q3

D **C2619** Pacemaker, dual chamber, non rate-responsive (implantable)   N1 ASC N
    BETOS: D1A   Medical/surgical supplies
    Statute: 1833(T)
    Coding Clinic: 2001, Q3; 2001, Q1; 2002, Q3; 2006, Q4; 2016, Q3

D **C2620** Pacemaker, single chamber, non rate-responsive (implantable)   N1 ASC N
    BETOS: D1A   Medical/surgical supplies
    Statute: 1833(T)
    Coding Clinic: 2001, Q1; 2002, Q3; 2003, Q4; 2004, Q4; 2006, Q4; 2016, Q3

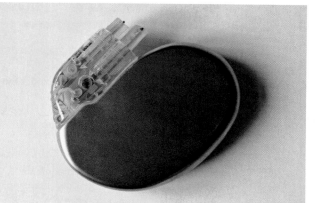

Pacemaker

D **C2621** Pacemaker, other than single or dual chamber (implantable)   N1 ASC N
    BETOS: D1A   Medical/surgical supplies
    Statute: 1833(T)
    Coding Clinic: 2001, Q1; 2002, Q3; 2002, Q3; 2003, Q4; 2006, Q4; 2016, Q3; 2016, Q3

D **C2622** Prosthesis, penile, non-inflatable   N1 ♂ ASC N
    BETOS: D1A   Medical/surgical supplies
    Statute: 1833(T)
    Coding Clinic: 2001, Q1; 2002, Q3; 2003, Q4; 2016, Q3

D **C2623** Catheter, transluminal angioplasty, drug-coated, non-laser   N1 ASC N
    BETOS: D1A   Medical/surgical supplies
    Statute: 1833(t)
    Coding Clinic: 2016, Q3

D **C2624** Implantable wireless pulmonary artery pressure sensor with delivery catheter, including all system components   N1 ASC N
    BETOS: D1A   Medical/surgical supplies
    Statute: 1833(t)
    Coding Clinic: 2016, Q3

D **C2625** Stent, non-coronary, temporary, with delivery system   N1 ASC N
    BETOS: D1A   Medical/surgical supplies
    Statute: 1833(T)
    Coding Clinic: 2001, Q1; 2002, Q3; 2003, Q4; 2004, Q4; 2016, Q3; 2016, Q3

D **C2626** Infusion pump, non-programmable, temporary (implantable)   N1 ASC N
    BETOS: D1A   Medical/surgical supplies
    Statute: 1833(T)
    Coding Clinic: 2001, Q1; 2002, Q3; 2004, Q4; 2016, Q3; 2016, Q3

D **C2627** Catheter, suprapubic/cystoscopic   N1 ASC N
    BETOS: D1A   Medical/surgical supplies
    Statute: 1833(T)
    Coding Clinic: 2001, Q1; 2002, Q3; 2003, Q4; 2016, Q3; 2016, Q3

C2628 Catheter, occlusion   N1 ASC N
BETOS: D1A   Medical/surgical supplies
Statute: 1833(T)
Coding Clinic: 2001, Q1; 2002, Q3; 2003, Q4; 2004, Q4; 2016, Q3

C2629 Introducer/sheath, other than guiding, other than intracardiac electrophysiological, laser   N1 ASC N
BETOS: D1A   Medical/surgical supplies
Statute: 1833(T)
Coding Clinic: 2001, Q1; 2002, Q3; 2016, Q3

C2630 Catheter, electrophysiology, diagnostic/ablation, other than 3D or vector mapping, cool-tip   N1 ASC N
BETOS: D1A   Medical/surgical supplies
Statute: 1833(T)
Coding Clinic: 2001, Q1; 2002, Q3; 2009, Q2; 2016, Q3; 2016, Q3

C2631 Repair device, urinary, incontinence, without sling graft   N1 ASC N
BETOS: D1A   Medical/surgical supplies
Statute: 1833(T)
Coding Clinic: 2001, Q1; 2002, Q3; 2003, Q4; 2016, Q3; 2016, Q3

BRACHYTHERAPY SOURCES (C2634-C2699), SEE ALSO BRACHYTHERAPY SOURCES (C1716-C1719), (C2616)

C2634 Brachytherapy source, non-stranded, high activity, Iodine-125, greater than 1.01 mCi (NIST), per source   H2 ASC U
BETOS: I4B   Imaging/procedure - other
Statute: 1833(T)
Coding Clinic: 2004, Q4; 2005, Q2; 2007, Q2; 2009, Q2; 2016, Q3; 2016, Q3

C2635 Brachytherapy source, non-stranded, high activity, Palladium-103, greater than 2.2 mCi (NIST), per source   H2 ASC U
BETOS: I4B   Imaging/procedure - other
Statute: 1833(T)
Coding Clinic: 2004, Q4; 2005, Q2; 2007, Q2; 2016, Q3; 2016, Q3

C2636 Brachytherapy linear source, non-stranded, Palladium-103, per 1 mm   H2 ASC U
BETOS: I4B   Imaging/procedure - other
Statute: 1833(T)
Coding Clinic: 2004, Q4; 2007, Q2; 2016, Q3; 2016, Q3

C2637 Brachytherapy source, non-stranded, Ytterbium-169, per source   B
BETOS: I4B   Imaging/procedure - other
Statute: 1833(T)
Coding Clinic: 2005, Q3; 2007, Q2; 2016, Q3; 2016, Q3

C2638 Brachytherapy source, stranded, Iodine-125, per source   H2 ASC U
BETOS: I4B   Imaging/procedure - other

Statute: 1833(t)(2)
Coding Clinic: 2007, Q2; 2016, Q3; 2016, Q3

C2639 Brachytherapy source, non-stranded, Iodine-125, per source   H2 ASC U
BETOS: I4B   Imaging/procedure - other
Statute: 1833(t)(2)
Coding Clinic: 2007, Q2; 2016, Q3; 2016, Q3

C2640 Brachytherapy source, stranded, Palladium-103, per source   H2 ASC U
BETOS: I4B   Imaging/procedure - other
Statute: 1833(t)(2)
Coding Clinic: 2007, Q2; 2016, Q3; 2016, Q3

C2641 Brachytherapy source, non-stranded, Palladium-103, per source   H2 ASC U
BETOS: I4B   Imaging/procedure - other
Statute: 1833(t)(2)
Coding Clinic: 2007, Q2; 2016, Q3; 2016, Q3

C2642 Brachytherapy source, stranded, Cesium-131, per source   H2 ASC U
BETOS: I4B   Imaging/procedure - other
Statute: 1833(t)(2)
Coding Clinic: 2007, Q2; 2016, Q3; 2016, Q3

C2643 Brachytherapy source, non-stranded, Cesium-131, per source   H2 ASC U
BETOS: I4B   Imaging/procedure - other
Statute: 1833(t)(2)
Coding Clinic: 2007, Q2; 2016, Q3; 2016, Q3

C2644 Brachytherapy source, Cesium-131 chloride solution, per millicurie   K5 ASC E2
BETOS: I4B   Imaging/procedure - other
Statute: 1833(t)
Coding Clinic: 2016, Q3; 2016, Q3

C2645 Brachytherapy planar source, Palladium-103, per square millimeter   H2 ASC U
BETOS: I4B   Imaging/procedure - other
Statute: 1833(T)
Coding Clinic: 2016, Q3; 2016, Q3

C2698 Brachytherapy source, stranded, not otherwise specified, per source H2 ASC U
BETOS: I4B   Imaging/procedure - other
Statute: 1833(t)(2)
Coding Clinic: 2007, Q3; 2007, Q2; 2016, Q3; 2016, Q3

C2699 Brachytherapy source, non-stranded, not otherwise specified, per source H2 ASC U
BETOS: I4B   Imaging/procedure - other
Statute: 1833(t)(2)
Coding Clinic: 2007, Q3; 2007, Q2; 2009, Q2; 2016, Q3; 2016, Q3

● New code   ▲ Revised code   **C** Carrier judgment   **D** Special coverage instructions apply
I Not payable by Medicare   **M** Non-covered by Medicare   **S** Non-covered by Medicare statute   AHA Coding Clinic®

SKIN SUBSTITUTE GRAFT APPLICATION (C5271-C5278)

D **C5271** Application of low cost skin substitute graft to trunk, arms, legs, total wound surface area up to 100 sq cm; first 25 sq cm or less wound surface area G2 ASC T

BETOS: P5A   Ambulatory procedures - skin
Statute: 1833(t)
Coding Clinic: 2013, Q4

D **C5272** Application of low cost skin substitute graft to trunk, arms, legs, total wound surface area up to 100 sq cm; each additional 25 sq cm wound surface area, or part thereof (list separately in addition to code for primary procedure) N1 ASC N

BETOS: P5A   Ambulatory procedures - skin
Statute: 1833(t)
Coding Clinic: 2013, Q4

D **C5273** Application of low cost skin substitute graft to trunk, arms, legs, total wound surface area greater than or equal to 100 sq cm; first 100 sq cm wound surface area, or 1% of body area of infants and children G2 ASC T

BETOS: P5A   Ambulatory procedures - skin
Statute: 1833(t)
Coding Clinic: 2013, Q4

D **C5274** Application of low cost skin substitute graft to trunk, arms, legs, total wound surface area greater than or equal to 100 sq cm; each additional 100 sq cm wound surface area, or part thereof, or each additional 1% of body area of infants and children, or part thereof (list separately in addition to code for primary procedure) N1 ASC N

BETOS: P5A   Ambulatory procedures - skin
Statute: 1833(t)
Coding Clinic: 2013, Q4

D **C5275** Application of low cost skin substitute graft to face, scalp, eyelids, mouth, neck, ears, orbits, genitalia, hands, feet, and/or multiple digits, total wound surface area up to 100 sq cm; first 25 sq cm or less wound surface area G2 ASC T

BETOS: P5A   Ambulatory procedures - skin
Statute: 1833(t)
Coding Clinic: 2013, Q4

D **C5276** Application of low cost skin substitute graft to face, scalp, eyelids, mouth, neck, ears, orbits, genitalia, hands, feet, and/or multiple digits, total wound surface area up to 100 sq cm; each additional 25 sq cm wound surface area, or part thereof (list separately in addition to code for primary procedure) N1 ASC N

BETOS: P5A   Ambulatory procedures - skin
Statute: 1833(t)
Coding Clinic: 2013, Q4

D **C5277** Application of low cost skin substitute graft to face, scalp, eyelids, mouth, neck, ears, orbits, genitalia, hands, feet, and/or multiple digits, total wound surface area greater than or equal to 100 sq cm; first 100 sq cm wound surface area, or 1% of body area of infants and children G2 ASC T

BETOS: P5A   Ambulatory procedures - skin
Statute: 1833(t)
Coding Clinic: 2013, Q4

D **C5278** Application of low cost skin substitute graft to face, scalp, eyelids, mouth, neck, ears, orbits, genitalia, hands, feet, and/or multiple digits, total wound surface area greater than or equal to 100 sq cm; each additional 100 sq cm wound surface area, or part thereof, or each additional 1% of body area of infants and children, or part thereof (list separately in addition to code for primary procedure) N1 ASC N

BETOS: P5A   Ambulatory procedures - skin
Statute: 1833(t)
Coding Clinic: 2013, Q4

MAGNETIC RESONANCE ANGIOGRAPHY, TRUNK AND LOWER EXTREMITIES (C8900-C8920)

D **C8900** Magnetic resonance angiography with contrast, abdomen Z2 ASC S

BETOS: I2D   Advanced imaging - MRI/MRA: other
Statute: 1833(t)(2)
Coding Clinic: 2009, Q2
Pub: 100-4, Chapter-13, 40.1.2

D **C8901** Magnetic resonance angiography without contrast, abdomen Z2 ASC S

BETOS: I2D   Advanced imaging - MRI/MRA: other
Statute: 1833(t)(2)

D **C8902** Magnetic resonance angiography without contrast followed by with contrast, abdomen Z2 ASC S

BETOS: I2D   Advanced imaging - MRI/MRA: other
Statute: 1833(t)(2)
Pub: 100-4, Chapter-13, 40.1.2

D **C8903** Magnetic resonance imaging with contrast, breast; unilateral Z2 ASC S

BETOS: I2D   Advanced imaging - MRI/MRA: other
Statute: 1833(t)(2)

D **C8905** Magnetic resonance imaging without contrast followed by with contrast, breast; unilateral Z2 ASC S

BETOS: I2D   Advanced imaging - MRI/MRA: other
Statute: 1833(t)(2)

D C8906 Magnetic resonance imaging with contrast, breast; bilateral   Z2 ASC S

BETOS: I2D Advanced imaging - MRI/MRA: other

Statute: 1833(t)(2)

D C8908 Magnetic resonance imaging without contrast followed by with contrast, breast; bilateral   Z2 ASC S

BETOS: I2D Advanced imaging - MRI/MRA: other

Statute: 1833(t)(2)

D C8909 Magnetic resonance angiography with contrast, chest (excluding myocardium)   Z2 ASC S

BETOS: I2D Advanced imaging - MRI/MRA: other

Statute: 1833(t)(2)

Pub: 100-4, Chapter-13, 40.1.2

D C8910 Magnetic resonance angiography without contrast, chest (excluding myocardium)   Z2 ASC S

BETOS: I2D Advanced imaging - MRI/MRA: other

Statute: 1833(t)(2)

D C8911 Magnetic resonance angiography without contrast followed by with contrast, chest (excluding myocardium)   Z2 ASC S

BETOS: I2D Advanced imaging - MRI/MRA: other

Statute: 1833(t)(2)

Pub: 100-4, Chapter-13, 40.1.2

D C8912 Magnetic resonance angiography with contrast, lower extremity   Z2 ASC S

BETOS: I2D Advanced imaging - MRI/MRA: other

Statute: 1833(t)(2)

Pub: 100-4, Chapter-13, 40.1.2

D C8913 Magnetic resonance angiography without contrast, lower extremity   Z2 ASC S

BETOS: I2D Advanced imaging - MRI/MRA: other

Statute: 1833(t)(2)

D C8914 Magnetic resonance angiography without contrast followed by with contrast, lower extremity   Z2 ASC S

BETOS: I2D Advanced imaging - MRI/MRA: other

Statute: 1833(t)(2)

Pub: 100-4, Chapter-13, 40.1.2

D C8918 Magnetic resonance angiography with contrast, pelvis   Z2 ASC S

BETOS: I2D Advanced imaging - MRI/MRA: other

Statute: 430 BIPA

Pub: 100-4, Chapter-13, 40.1.2

D C8919 Magnetic resonance angiography without contrast, pelvis   Z2 ASC S

BETOS: I2D Advanced imaging - MRI/MRA: other

Statute: 430 BIPA

D C8920 Magnetic resonance angiography without contrast followed by with contrast, pelvis   Z2 ASC S

BETOS: I2D Advanced imaging - MRI/MRA: other

Statute: 430 BIPA

Coding Clinic: 2009, Q2

Pub: 100-4, Chapter-13, 40.1.2

TRANSESOPHAGEAL/TRANSTHORACIC ECHOCARDIOGRAPHY (C8921-C8930)

D C8921 Transthoracic echocardiography with contrast, or without contrast followed by with contrast, for congenital cardiac anomalies; complete   S

BETOS: I3C Echography/ultrasonography - heart

Statute: 1833(t)(2)

Coding Clinic: 2007, Q4; 2008, Q2; 2009, Q2; 2012, Q3

Pub: 100-4, Chapter-4, 200.7.2

D C8922 Transthoracic echocardiography with contrast, or without contrast followed by with contrast, for congenital cardiac anomalies; follow-up or limited study   S

BETOS: I3C Echography/ultrasonography - heart

Statute: 1833(t)(2)

Coding Clinic: 2007, Q4; 2008, Q2

Pub: 100-4, Chapter-4, 200.7.2

D C8923 Transthoracic echocardiography with contrast, or without contrast followed by with contrast, real-time with image documentation (2D), includes M-mode recording, when performed, complete, without spectral or color doppler echocardiography   S

BETOS: I3C Echography/ultrasonography - heart

Statute: 1833(t)(2)

Coding Clinic: 2007, Q4; 2008, Q2

Pub: 100-4, Chapter-4, 200.7.2

D C8924 Transthoracic echocardiography with contrast, or without contrast followed by with contrast, real-time with image documentation (2D), includes M-mode recording, when performed, follow-up or limited study   S

BETOS: I3C Echography/ultrasonography - heart

Statute: 1833(t)(2)

Coding Clinic: 2007, Q4; 2008, Q2

Pub: 100-4, Chapter-4, 200.7.2

● New code   ▲ Revised code   **C** Carrier judgment   **D** Special coverage instructions apply

I Not payable by Medicare   **M** Non-covered by Medicare   **S** Non-covered by Medicare statute   AHA Coding Clinic®

D **C8925** Transesophageal echocardiography (TEE) with contrast, or without contrast followed by with contrast, real time with image documentation (2D) (with or without M-mode recording); including probe placement, image acquisition, interpretation and report　　S

BETOS: I3C　Echography/ultrasonography - heart

Statute: 1833(t)(2)

Coding Clinic: 2007, Q4; 2008, Q2

Pub: 100-4, Chapter-4, 200.7.2

D **C8926** Transesophageal echocardiography (TEE) with contrast, or without contrast followed by with contrast, for congenital cardiac anomalies; including probe placement, image acquisition, interpretation and report　S

BETOS: I3C　Echography/ultrasonography - heart

Statute: 1833(t)(2)

Coding Clinic: 2007, Q4; 2008, Q2

Pub: 100-4, Chapter-4, 200.7.2

D **C8927** Transesophageal echocardiography (TEE) with contrast, or without contrast followed by with contrast, for monitoring purposes, including probe placement, real time 2-dimensional image acquisition and interpretation leading to ongoing (continuous) assessment of (dynamically changing) cardiac pumping function and to therapeutic measures on an immediate time basis　　S

BETOS: I3C　Echography/ultrasonography - heart

Statute: 1833(t)(2)

Coding Clinic: 2007, Q4; 2008, Q2

Pub: 100-4, Chapter-4, 200.7.2

D **C8928** Transthoracic echocardiography with contrast, or without contrast followed by with contrast, real-time with image documentation (2D), includes M-mode recording, when performed, during rest and cardiovascular stress test using treadmill, bicycle exercise and/or pharmacologically induced stress, with interpretation and report　　S

BETOS: I3C　Echography/ultrasonography - heart

Statute: 1833(t)(2)

Coding Clinic: 2007, Q4; 2008, Q2

Pub: 100-4, Chapter-4, 200.7.2

D **C8929** Transthoracic echocardiography with contrast, or without contrast followed by with contrast, real-time with image documentation (2D), includes M-mode recording, when performed, complete, with spectral doppler echocardiography, and with color flow doppler echocardiography　　S

BETOS: I3C　Echography/ultrasonography - heart

Statute: 1833(t)(2)

Coding Clinic: 2008, Q4

Pub: 100-4, Chapter-4, 200.7.2

D **C8930** Transthoracic echocardiography, with contrast, or without contrast followed by with contrast, real-time with image documentation (2D), includes M-mode recording, when performed, during rest and cardiovascular stress test using treadmill, bicycle exercise and/or pharmacologically induced stress, with interpretation and report; including performance of continuous electrocardiographic monitoring, with physician supervision　　S

BETOS: I3C　Echography/ultrasonography - heart

Statute: 1833(t)(2)

Coding Clinic: 2008, Q4; 2012, Q3

Pub: 100-4, Chapter-4, 200.7.2

MAGNETIC RESONANCE ANGIOGRAPHY, SPINE AND UPPER EXTREMITIES (C8931-C8936)

D **C8931** Magnetic resonance angiography with contrast, spinal canal and contents　Z2 ASC S

BETOS: I2D　Advanced imaging - MRI/MRA: other

Statute: 1833(t)

D **C8932** Magnetic resonance angiography without contrast, spinal canal and contents　Z2 ASC S

BETOS: I2D　Advanced imaging - MRI/MRA: other

Statute: 1833(t)

D **C8933** Magnetic resonance angiography without contrast followed by with contrast, spinal canal and contents　　Z2 ASC S

BETOS: I2D　Advanced imaging - MRI/MRA: other

Statute: 1833(t)

D **C8934** Magnetic resonance angiography with contrast, upper extremity　Z2 ASC S

BETOS: I2D　Advanced imaging - MRI/MRA: other

Statute: 1833(t)

D **C8935** Magnetic resonance angiography without contrast, upper extremity　Z2 ASC S

BETOS: I2D　Advanced imaging - MRI/MRA: other

Statute: 1833(t)

D **C8936** Magnetic resonance angiography without contrast followed by with contrast, upper extremity　　Z2 ASC S

BETOS: I2D　Advanced imaging - MRI/MRA: other

Statute: 1833(t)

♂ Male only　　♀ Female only　　**A** Age　　A2 - Z3 = ASC Payment indicator　　A - Y = APC Status indicator

ASC = ASC Approved Procedure　　**DME** Paid under the DME fee schedule　　**MIPS** MIPS code

BREAST MRI - COMPUTER AIDED DETECTION (C8937)

D C8937 Computer-aided detection, including computer algorithm analysis of breast MRI image data for lesion detection/ characterization, pharmacokinetic analysis, with further physician review for interpretation (list separately in addition to code for primary procedure)   N
BETOS: I2D   Advanced imaging - MRI/MRA: other
Statute: 1833(t)

MISCELLANEOUS DRUGS, BIOLOGICALS, AND SUPPLIES (C8957-C9488)

D C8957 Intravenous infusion for therapy/diagnosis; initiation of prolonged infusion (more than 8 hours), requiring use of portable or implantable pump   S
BETOS: P6D   Minor procedures - other (non-Medicare fee schedule)
Value not established
Statute: 1833(t)
Coding Clinic: 2005, Q4; 2006, Q4; 2008, Q3
Pub: 100-4, Chapter-4, 230.2

D C9046 Cocaine hydrochloride nasal solution for topical administration, 1 mg   K2 ASC G
BETOS: O1E   Other drugs
Statute: 1833(t)
Drugs: COCAINE HCL (GOPRELTO AUTH. GENERIC), GOPRELTO
Coding Clinic: 2019, Q2; 2019, Q2

D C9047 Injection, caplacizumab-yhdp, 1 mg   K2 ASC G
BETOS: O1E   Other drugs
Statute: 1833(t)
Drugs: CABLIVI
Coding Clinic: 2019, Q3

● D C9065 Injection, romidepsin, non-lyophilized (e.g. liquid), 1mg   K2 ASC G
BETOS: O1D   Chemotherapy
Statute: 1833(t)
Drugs: ROMIDEPSIN

● D C9067 Gallium ga-68, dotatoc, diagnostic, 0.01 mci   K2 ASC G
BETOS: O1E   Other drugs
Statute: 1833(t)
Drugs: DOTATOC GA 68

● D C9068 Copper cu-64, dotatate, diagnostic, 1 millicurie   K2 ASC G
BETOS: I1E   Standard imaging - nuclear medicine
Statute: 1833(T)
Drugs: DETECTNET

● D C9069 Injection, belantamab mafodontin-blmf, 0.5 mg   K2 Ⓐ ASC G
BETOS: O1D   Chemotherapy

Statute: 1833(T)
Drugs: BLENREP

● D C9070 Injection, tafasitamab-cxix, 2 mg   K2 Ⓐ ASC G
BETOS: O1D   Chemotherapy
Statute: 1833(T)
Drugs: MONJUVI

● D C9071 Injection, viltolarsen, 10 mg   K2 Ⓐ ASC G
BETOS: O1D   Chemotherapy
Statute: 1833(T)
Drugs: VILTEPSO

● D C9072 Injection, immune globulin (asceniv), 500 mg   K2 Ⓐ ASC G
BETOS: O1E   Other drugs
Statute: 1833(T)
Drugs: ASCENIV

● D C9073 Brexucabtagene autoleucel, up to 200 million autologous anti-cd19 car positive viable T cells, including leukapheresis and dose preparation procedures, per therapeutic dose   K2 Ⓐ ASC G
BETOS: O1E   Other drugs
Statute: 1833(T)
Drugs: TECARTUS

D C9113 Injection, Pantoprazole sodium, per vial   N1 ASC N
BETOS: O1E   Other drugs
Statute: 1833(T)
Coding Clinic: 2002, Q1

● D C9122 Mometasone furoate sinus implant, 10 micrograms (sinuva)   K2 ASC G
BETOS: O1E   Other drugs
Statute: 1833(t)
Drugs: SINUVA
Coding Clinic: 2020, Q2

D C9132 Prothrombin complex concentrate (human), kcentra, per IU of Factor IX activity   K2 ASC K
BETOS: O1E   Other drugs
Statute: 1833(t)
Drugs: KCENTRA

D C9248 Injection, Clevidipine butyrate, 1 mg   K2 ASC K
BETOS: O1E   Other drugs
Statute: 1833(t)
Drugs: CLEVIPREX
Coding Clinic: 2009, Q1; 2008, Q4

D C9250 Human plasma fibrin sealant, vapor-heated, solvent-detergent (Artiss), 2 ml   K2 ASC K
BETOS: O1E   Other drugs
Statute: 621MMA
Drugs: ARTISS
Coding Clinic: 2009, Q3

D C9254 Injection, Lacosamide, 1 mg   N1 ASC N
BETOS: O1E   Other drugs
Statute: 621MMA

● New code   ▲ Revised code   C Carrier judgment   D Special coverage instructions apply
I Not payable by Medicare   M Non-covered by Medicare   S Non-covered by Medicare statute   AHA Coding Clinic®

D **C9257** Injection, Bevacizumab, 0.25 mg   K2 ASC K
  BETOS: O1E   Other drugs
  Statute: 1833(t)
  Drugs: AVASTIN
  Coding Clinic: 2013, Q3

D **C9285** Lidocaine 70 mg/Tetracaine 70 mg,
  per patch   N1 ASC N
  BETOS: O1E   Other drugs
  Statute: 1833(t)

D **C9290** Injection, Bupivacaine liposome,
  1 mg   K2 ASC N
  BETOS: O1E   Other drugs
  Statute: 1833(t)
  Drugs: EXPAREL
  Coding Clinic: 2012, Q2

D **C9293** Injection, Glucarpidase, 10 units   K5 ASC E2
  BETOS: O1E   Other drugs
  Statute: 1833(t)

D **C9352** Microporous collagen implantable tube
  (NeuraGen Nerve Guide), per centimeter
  length   N1 ASC N
  BETOS: D1A   Medical/surgical supplies
  Statute: 621MMA
  Coding Clinic: 2008, Q1

D **C9353** Microporous collagen implantable slit tube
  (NeuraWrap Nerve Protector), per centimeter
  length   N1 ASC N
  BETOS: D1A   Medical/surgical supplies
  Statute: 621MMA
  Coding Clinic: 2008, Q1

D **C9354** Acellular pericardial tissue matrix of
  non-human origin (Veritas), per square
  centimeter   N1 ASC N
  BETOS: D1A   Medical/surgical supplies
  Statute: 621MMA
  Coding Clinic: 2008, Q1

D **C9355** Collagen nerve cuff (NeuroMatrix),
  per 0.5 centimeter length   N1 ASC N
  BETOS: D1A   Medical/surgical supplies
  Statute: 621MMA
  Coding Clinic: 2008, Q1

D **C9356** Tendon, porous matrix of cross-linked
  collagen and glycosaminoglycan matrix
  (TenoGlide Tendon Protector Sheet),
  per square centimeter   N1 ASC N
  BETOS: D1A   Medical/surgical supplies
  Statute: 621 MMA
  Coding Clinic: 2008, Q3

D **C9358** Dermal substitute, native, non-denatured
  collagen, fetal bovine origin (SurgiMend
  Collagen Matrix), per 0.5 square
  centimeters   N1 ASC N
  BETOS: D1A   Medical/surgical supplies
  Statute: 621 MMA
  Coding Clinic: 2009, Q3; 2008, Q3; 2012,
  Q2

D **C9359** Porous purified collagen matrix bone void
  filler (Integra Mozaik Osteoconductive
  Scaffold Putty, Integra Os Osteoconductive
  Scaffold Putty), per 0.5 cc   N1 ASC N
  BETOS: D1A   Medical/surgical supplies
  Statute: 1833(T)
  Coding Clinic: 2009, Q3

D **C9360** Dermal substitute, native, non-denatured
  collagen, neonatal bovine origin (SurgiMend
  Collagen Matrix), per 0.5 square
  centimeters   N1 ASC N
  BETOS: D1A   Medical/surgical supplies
  Statute: 621MMA
  Coding Clinic: 2009, Q3; 2012, Q2

D **C9361** Collagen matrix nerve wrap (NeuroMend
  Collagen Nerve Wrap), per 0.5 centimeter
  length   N1 ASC N
  BETOS: D1A   Medical/surgical supplies
  Statute: 621MMA
  Coding Clinic: 2009, Q3

D **C9362** Porous purified collagen matrix bone void
  filler (Integra Mozaik Osteoconductive
  Scaffold Strip), per 0.5 cc   N1 ASC N
  BETOS: D1A   Medical/surgical supplies
  Statute: 621MMA
  Coding Clinic: 2009, Q3; 2010, Q1

D **C9363** Skin substitute, Integra Meshed
  Bilayer Wound Matrix, per square
  centimeter   N1 ASC N
  BETOS: D1A   Medical/surgical supplies
  Statute: 621MMA
  Coding Clinic: 2009, Q3; 2012, Q2; 2010,
  Q1

D **C9364** Porcine implant, Permacol, per square
  centimeter   N1 ASC N
  BETOS: D1A   Medical/surgical supplies
  Statute: 621MMA
  Coding Clinic: 2009, Q3

D **C9399** Unclassified drugs or biologicals   K7 ASC A
  BETOS: O1E   Other drugs
  Statute: 621MMA
  Coding Clinic: 2004, Q4; 2005, Q4; 2008,
  Q1; 2009, Q1; 2009, Q3; 2011, Q4; 2013,
  Q1; 2010, Q3; 2014, Q2; 2014, Q4; 2016,
  Q4; 2017, Q1; 2017, Q1
  Pub: 100-4, Chapter-17, 90.3

D **C9460** Injection, Cangrelor, 1 mg   K2 ASC K
  BETOS: O1E   Other drugs
  Statute: 1833(t)
  Drugs: KENGREAL
  Coding Clinic: 2016, Q1

D **C9462** Injection, Delafloxacin, 1 mg   K2 Ⓐ ASC K
  BETOS: O1E   Other drugs
  Statute: 1833(t)
  Drugs: BAXDELA
  Coding Clinic: 2018, Q2

♂ Male only   ♀ Female only   Ⓐ Age   A2 - Z3 = ASC Payment indicator   A - Y = APC Status indicator
ASC = ASC Approved Procedure   **DME** Paid under the DME fee schedule   **MIPS** MIPS code

D **C9482** Injection, Sotalol hydrochloride,
1 mg   K2 ASC K
BETOS: O1E   Other drugs
Statute: 1833(t)
Drugs: SOTALOL
Coding Clinic: 2016, Q4

D **C9488** Injection, Conivaptan hydrochloride,
1 mg   K2 ASC K
BETOS: O1E   Other drugs
Statute: 1833(t)
Drugs: VAPRISOL

PERCUTANEOUS TRANSCATHETER/TRANSLUMINAL CORONARY PROCEDURES (C9600-C9608)

D **C9600** Percutaneous transcatheter placement of drug-eluting intracoronary stent(s), with coronary angioplasty when performed; single major coronary artery or branch   J8 ASC J1
BETOS: P2F   Major procedure, cardiovascular-Other
Statute: 1833(t)
Coding Clinic: 2012, Q4

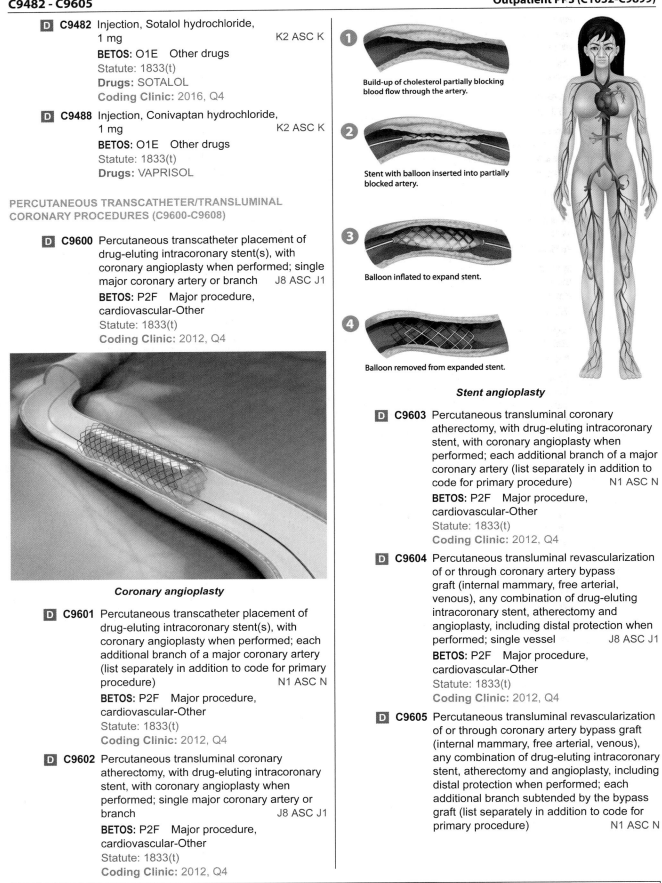

Coronary angioplasty

Stent angioplasty

D **C9601** Percutaneous transcatheter placement of drug-eluting intracoronary stent(s), with coronary angioplasty when performed; each additional branch of a major coronary artery (list separately in addition to code for primary procedure)   N1 ASC N
BETOS: P2F   Major procedure, cardiovascular-Other
Statute: 1833(t)
Coding Clinic: 2012, Q4

D **C9602** Percutaneous transluminal coronary atherectomy, with drug-eluting intracoronary stent, with coronary angioplasty when performed; single major coronary artery or branch   J8 ASC J1
BETOS: P2F   Major procedure, cardiovascular-Other
Statute: 1833(t)
Coding Clinic: 2012, Q4

D **C9603** Percutaneous transluminal coronary atherectomy, with drug-eluting intracoronary stent, with coronary angioplasty when performed; each additional branch of a major coronary artery (list separately in addition to code for primary procedure)   N1 ASC N
BETOS: P2F   Major procedure, cardiovascular-Other
Statute: 1833(t)
Coding Clinic: 2012, Q4

D **C9604** Percutaneous transluminal revascularization of or through coronary artery bypass graft (internal mammary, free arterial, venous), any combination of drug-eluting intracoronary stent, atherectomy and angioplasty, including distal protection when performed; single vessel   J8 ASC J1
BETOS: P2F   Major procedure, cardiovascular-Other
Statute: 1833(t)
Coding Clinic: 2012, Q4

D **C9605** Percutaneous transluminal revascularization of or through coronary artery bypass graft (internal mammary, free arterial, venous), any combination of drug-eluting intracoronary stent, atherectomy and angioplasty, including distal protection when performed; each additional branch subtended by the bypass graft (list separately in addition to code for primary procedure)   N1 ASC N

● New code   ▲ Revised code   **C** Carrier judgment   **D** Special coverage instructions apply
I Not payable by Medicare   **M** Non-covered by Medicare   **S** Non-covered by Medicare statute   AHA Coding Clinic®

BETOS: P2F   Major procedure, cardiovascular-Other
Statute: 1833(t)
Coding Clinic: 2012, Q4

D **C9606** Percutaneous transluminal revascularization of acute total/subtotal occlusion during acute myocardial infarction, coronary artery or coronary artery bypass graft, any combination of drug-eluting intracoronary stent, atherectomy and angioplasty, including aspiration thrombectomy when performed, single vessel   C
BETOS: P2F   Major procedure, cardiovascular-Other
Statute: 1833(t)
Coding Clinic: 2012, Q4; 2019, Q1

D **C9607** Percutaneous transluminal revascularization of chronic total occlusion, coronary artery, coronary artery branch, or coronary artery bypass graft, any combination of drug-eluting intracoronary stent, atherectomy and angioplasty; single vessel   J8 ASC J1
BETOS: P2F   Major procedure, cardiovascular-Other
Statute: 1833(t)
Coding Clinic: 2012, Q4

D **C9608** Percutaneous transluminal revascularization of chronic total occlusion, coronary artery, coronary artery branch, or coronary artery bypass graft, any combination of drug-eluting intracoronary stent, atherectomy and angioplasty; each additional coronary artery, coronary artery branch, or bypass graft (list separately in addition to code for primary procedure)   N1 ASC N
BETOS: P2F   Major procedure, cardiovascular-Other
Statute: 1833(t)

OTHER THERAPEUTIC SERVICES AND SUPPLIES (C9725-C9899)

D **C9725** Placement of endorectal intracavitary applicator for high intensity brachytherapy   G2 ASC T
BETOS: P7A   Oncology - radiation therapy
Statute: 1833(T)
Coding Clinic: 2005, Q3

D **C9726** Placement and removal (if performed) of applicator into breast for intraoperative radiation therapy, add-on to primary breast procedure   N1 ♀ ASC N
BETOS: P7A   Oncology - radiation therapy
Statute: 1833(T)
Coding Clinic: 2006, Q1; 2007, Q2

D **C9727** Insertion of implants into the soft palate; minimum of three implants   G2 ASC J1

BETOS: P6D   Minor procedures - other (non-Medicare fee schedule)
Statute: 1833(T)

D **C9728** Placement of interstitial device(s) for radiation therapy/surgery guidance (e.g., fiducial markers, dosimeter), for other than the following sites (any approach): abdomen, pelvis, prostate, retroperitoneum, thorax, single or multiple   J8 ASC S
BETOS: P5E   Ambulatory procedures - other
Statute: 1833(T)
Coding Clinic: 2007, Q2; 2018, Q2

D **C9733** Non-ophthalmic fluorescent vascular angiography   N
BETOS: I4B   Imaging/procedure - other
Statute: 1833(t)

D **C9734** Focused ultrasound ablation/therapeutic intervention, other than uterine leiomyomata, with magnetic resonance (MR) guidance ♀ J1
BETOS: P5E   Ambulatory procedures - other
Statute: 1833(t)
Coding Clinic: 2013, Q3

D **C9738** Adjunctive blue light cystoscopy with fluorescent imaging agent (list separately in addition to code for primary procedure)   N1 ASC N
BETOS: I1F   Standard imaging - other
Statute: 1833(t)

D **C9739** Cystourethroscopy, with insertion of transprostatic implant; 1 to 3 implants   J8 ♂ ASC J1
BETOS: P5E   Ambulatory procedures - other
Statute: 1833(t)
Coding Clinic: 2014, Q2

D **C9740** Cystourethroscopy, with insertion of transprostatic implant; 4 or more implants   J8 ♂ ASC J1
BETOS: P5E   Ambulatory procedures - other
Statute: 1833(t)
Coding Clinic: 2014, Q2

D **C9751** Bronchoscopy, rigid or flexible, transbronchial ablation of lesion(s) by microwave energy, including fluoroscopic guidance, when performed, with computed tomography acquisition(s) and 3-D rendering, computer-assisted, image-guided navigation, and endobronchial ultrasound (EBUS) guided transtracheal and/or transbronchial sampling (e.g., aspiration[s]/ biopsy[ies]) and all mediastinal and/or hilar lymph node stations or structures and therapeutic intervention(s)   G2 ASC T
BETOS: P8F   Endoscopy - bronchoscopy
Statute: 1833(t)
Coding Clinic: 2019, Q1

♂ Male only   ♀ Female only   **Ⓐ** Age   A2 - Z3 = ASC Payment indicator   A - Y = APC Status indicator
ASC = ASC Approved Procedure   **DME** Paid under the DME fee schedule   **MIPS** MIPS code

D C9752 Destruction of intraosseous basivertebral nerve, first two vertebral bodies, including imaging guidance (e.g., fluoroscopy), lumbar/sacrum   J8 ASC J1
    BETOS: P5B   Ambulatory procedures - musculoskeletal
    Statute: 1833(t)
    Coding Clinic: 2019, Q1; 2020, Q3

D C9753 Destruction of intraosseous basivertebral nerve, each additional vertebral body, including imaging guidance (e.g., fluoroscopy), lumbar/sacrum (list separately in addition to code for primary procedure)   N1 ASC N
    BETOS: P5B   Ambulatory procedures - musculoskeletal
    Statute: 1833(t)
    Coding Clinic: 2019, Q1

D C9756 Intraoperative near-infrared fluorescence lymphatic mapping of lymph node(s) (sentinel or tumor draining) with administration of indocyanine green (ICG) (list separately in addition to code for primary procedure)   N
    BETOS: I4B   Imaging/procedure - other
    Statute: 1833(t)
    Coding Clinic: 2019, Q3

D C9757 Laminotomy (hemilaminectomy), with decompression of nerve root(s), including partial facetectomy, foraminotomy and excision of herniated intervertebral disc, and repair of annular defect with implantation of bone anchored annular closure device, including annular defect measurement, alignment and sizing assessment, and image guidance; 1 interspace, lumbar   J8 ASC J1
    BETOS: P6B   Minor procedures - musculoskeletal
    Statute: 1833(T)
    Coding Clinic: 2020, Q1

D C9758 Blinded procedure for NYHA class III/IV heart failure; transcatheter implantation of interatrial shunt or placebo control, including right heart catheterization, trans-esophageal echocardiography (TEE)/intracardiac echocardiography (ICE), and all imaging with or without guidance (e.g., ultrasound, fluoroscopy), performed in an approved investigational device exemption (IDE) study   G2 ASC T
    BETOS: P2F   Major procedure, cardiovascular-Other
    Statute: 1833(T)

● D C9759 Transcatheter intraoperative blood vessel microinfusion(s) (e.g., intraluminal, vascular wall and/or perivascular) therapy, any vessel, including radiological supervision and interpretation, when performed   N1 ASC N
    BETOS: P2F   Major procedure, cardiovascular-Other

Statute: 1833(t)
Coding Clinic: 2020, Q2

● D C9760 Non-randomized, non-blinded procedure for NYHA class II, III, IV heart failure; transcatheter implantation of interatrial shunt, including right and left heart catheterization, transeptal puncture, trans-esophageal echocardiography (TEE)/intracardiac echocardiography (ICE), and all imaging with or without guidance (e.g., ultrasound, fluoroscopy), performed in an approved investigational device exemption (IDE) study   T
    BETOS: P2F   Major procedure, cardiovascular-Other
    Statute: 1833(t)
    Coding Clinic: 2020, Q2

● D C9761 Cystourethroscopy, with ureteroscopy and/or pyeloscopy, with lithotripsy (ureteral catheterization is included) and vacuum aspiration of the kidney, collecting system and urethra if applicable   J8 ASC J1
    BETOS: P5E   Ambulatory procedures - other
    Statute: 1833(t)

● D C9762 Cardiac magnetic resonance imaging for morphology and function, quantification of segmental dysfunction; with strain imaging   Z2 ASC S
    BETOS: I2D   Advanced imaging - MRI/MRA: other
    Statute: 1833(t)
    Coding Clinic: 2020, Q2

● D C9763 Cardiac magnetic resonance imaging for morphology and function, quantification of segmental dysfunction; with stress imaging   Z2 ASC S
    BETOS: I2D   Advanced imaging - MRI/MRA: other
    Statute: 1833(t)
    Coding Clinic: 2020, Q2

● D C9764 Revascularization, endovascular, open or percutaneous, lower extremity artery(ies), except tibial/peroneal; with intravascular lithotripsy, includes angioplasty within the same vessel(s), when performed   G2 ASC J1
    BETOS: P2F   Major procedure, cardiovascular-Other
    Statute: 1833(t)
    Coding Clinic: 2020, Q2

● D C9765 Revascularization, endovascular, open or percutaneous, lower extremity artery(ies), except tibial/peroneal; with intravascular lithotripsy, and transluminal stent placement(s), includes angioplasty within the same vessel(s), when performed   J8 ASC J1
    BETOS: P2F   Major procedure, cardiovascular-Other
    Statute: 1833(t)
    Coding Clinic: 2020, Q2

● New code   ▲ Revised code   **C** Carrier judgment   **D** Special coverage instructions apply
I Not payable by Medicare   **M** Non-covered by Medicare   **S** Non-covered by Medicare statute   AHA Coding Clinic®

● **D** **C9766** Revascularization, endovascular, open or percutaneous, lower extremity artery(ies), except tibial/peroneal; with intravascular lithotripsy and atherectomy, includes angioplasty within the same vessel(s), when performed G2 ASC J1
BETOS: P2F Major procedure, cardiovascular-Other
Statute: 1833(t)
Coding Clinic: 2020, Q2

● **D** **C9767** Revascularization, endovascular, open or percutaneous, lower extremity artery(ies), except tibial/peroneal; with intravascular lithotripsy and transluminal stent placement(s), and atherectomy, includes angioplasty within the same vessel(s), when performed J8 ASC J1
BETOS: P2F Major procedure, cardiovascular-Other
Statute: 1833(t)
Coding Clinic: 2020, Q2

● **D** **C9768** Endoscopic ultrasound-guided direct measurement of hepatic portosystemic pressure gradient by any method (list separately in addition to code for primary procedure) N
BETOS: P8B Endoscopy - upper gastrointestinal
Statute: 1833(t)

● **D** **C9769** Cystourethroscopy, with insertion of temporary prostatic implant/stent with fixation/anchor and incisional struts J8 ASC J1
BETOS: P5E Ambulatory procedures - other
Statute: 1833(t)

● **D** **C9770** Vitrectomy, mechanical, pars plana approach, with subretinal injection of pharmacologic/biologic agent G2 ASC T
BETOS: P4E Eye procedure - other
Statute: 1833(T)

● **D** **C9771** Nasal/sinus endoscopy, cryoablation nasal tissue(s) and/or nerve(s), unilateral or bilateral J8 ASC J1
BETOS: P5E Ambulatory procedures - other
Statute: 1833(T)

● **D** **C9772** Revascularization, endovascular, open or percutaneous, tibial/peroneal artery(ies), with intravascular lithotripsy, includes angioplasty within the same vessel (s), when performed J8 ASC J1
BETOS: P2F Major procedure, cardiovascular-Other
Statute: 1833(T)

● **D** **C9773** Revascularization, endovascular, open or percutaneous, tibial/peroneal artery(ies); with intravascular lithotripsy, and transluminal stent placement(s), includes angioplasty within the same vessel(s), when performed J8 ASC J1
BETOS: P2F Major procedure, cardiovascular-Other
Statute: 1833(T)

● **D** **C9774** Revascularization, endovascular, open or percutaneous, tibial/peroneal artery(ies); with intravascular lithotripsy and atherectomy, includes angioplasty within the same vessel (s), when performed J8 ASC J1
BETOS: P2F Major procedure, cardiovascular-Other
Statute: 1833(T)

● **D** **C9775** Revascularization, endovascular, open or percutaneous, tibial/peroneal artery(ies); with intravascular lithotripsy and transluminal stent placement(s), and atherectomy, includes angioplasty within the same vessel (s), when performed J8 ASC J1
BETOS: P2F Major procedure, cardiovascular-Other
Statute: 1833(T)

● **D** **C9803** Hospital outpatient clinic visit specimen collection for severe acute respiratory syndrome coronavirus 2 (sars-cov-2) (coronavirus disease [covid-19]), any specimen source N
BETOS: T1G Lab tests - other (Medicare fee schedule)
Statute: 1833(t)
Coding Clinic: 2020, Q2

D **C9898** Radiolabeled product provided during a hospital inpatient stay N
BETOS: Z2 Undefined codes
Service not separately priced by Part B
Statute: NA

D **C9899** Implanted prosthetic device, payable only for inpatients who do not have inpatient coverage A
BETOS: Z2 Undefined codes
Statute: 1833(t)
Coding Clinic: 2008, Q4

♂ Male only ♀ Female only **A** Age A2 - Z3 = ASC Payment indicator A - Y = APC Status indicator
ASC = ASC Approved Procedure **DME** Paid under the DME fee schedule **MIPS** MIPS code

NOTES

DURABLE MEDICAL EQUIPMENT (E0100-E8002)

WALKING AIDS AND ATTACHMENTS (E0100-E0159)

D E0100 Cane, includes canes of all materials, adjustable or fixed, with tip **DME** Y
BETOS: D1E   Other DME
DME Modifier: NU,RR,UE
Coding Clinic: 2009, Q2

D E0105 Cane, quad or three prong, includes canes of all materials, adjustable or fixed, with tips **DME** Y
BETOS: D1E   Other DME
DME Modifier: NU,RR,UE

D E0110 Crutches, forearm, includes crutches of various materials, adjustable or fixed, pair, complete with tips and handgrips **DME** Y
BETOS: D1E   Other DME
DME Modifier: NU,RR,UE

D E0111 Crutch forearm, includes crutches of various materials, adjustable or fixed, each, with tip and handgrips **DME** Y
BETOS: D1E   Other DME
DME Modifier: NU,RR,UE

D E0112 Crutches underarm, wood, adjustable or fixed, pair, with pads, tips and handgrips **DME** Y
BETOS: D1E   Other DME
DME Modifier: NU,RR,UE

D E0113 Crutch underarm, wood, adjustable or fixed, each, with pad, tip and handgrip **DME** Y
BETOS: D1E   Other DME
DME Modifier: NU,RR,UE

D E0114 Crutches underarm, other than wood, adjustable or fixed, pair, with pads, tips and handgrips **DME** Y
BETOS: D1E   Other DME
DME Modifier: NU,RR,UE
Coding Clinic: 2002, Q2

D E0116 Crutch, underarm, other than wood, adjustable or fixed, with pad, tip, handgrip, with or without shock absorber, each **DME** Y
BETOS: D1E   Other DME
DME Modifier: NU,RR,UE

D E0117 Crutch, underarm, articulating, spring assisted, each **DME** Y
BETOS: D1E   Other DME
DME Modifier: RR

C E0118 Crutch substitute, lower leg platform, with or without wheels, each   E1
BETOS: D1E   Other DME

D E0130 Walker, rigid (pickup), adjustable or fixed height **DME** Y
BETOS: D1E   Other DME

DME Modifier: NU,RR,UE
Pub: 100-4, Chapter-36, 50.15

D E0135 Walker, folding (pickup), adjustable or fixed height **DME** Y
BETOS: D1E   Other DME
DME Modifier: NU,RR,UE
Pub: 100-4, Chapter-36, 50.15

D E0140 Walker, with trunk support, adjustable or fixed height, any type **DME** Y
BETOS: D1E   Other DME
DME Modifier: RR
Pub: 100-4, Chapter-36, 50.15

D E0141 Walker, rigid, wheeled, adjustable or fixed height **DME** Y
BETOS: D1E   Other DME
DME Modifier: NU,RR,UE
Pub: 100-4, Chapter-36, 50.15

D E0143 Walker, folding, wheeled, adjustable or fixed height **DME** Y
BETOS: D1E   Other DME
DME Modifier: NU,RR,UE
Pub: 100-4, Chapter-36, 50.15

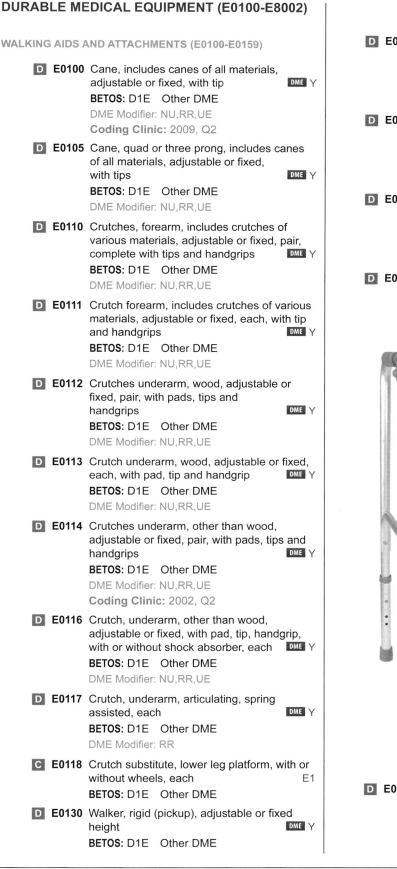

Walker

D E0144 Walker, enclosed, four sided framed, rigid or folding, wheeled with posterior seat **DME** Y
BETOS: D1E   Other DME
DME Modifier: RR
Pub: 100-4, Chapter-36, 50.15

D **E0147** Walker, heavy duty, multiple braking system, variable wheel resistance **DME** Y
BETOS: D1E   Other DME
DME Modifier: NU,RR,UE
Pub: 100-4, Chapter-36, 50.15

C **E0148** Walker, heavy duty, without wheels, rigid or folding, any type, each **DME** Y
BETOS: D1E   Other DME
DME Modifier: NU,RR,UE
Pub: 100-4, Chapter-36, 50.15

C **E0149** Walker, heavy duty, wheeled, rigid or folding, any type **DME** Y
BETOS: D1E   Other DME
DME Modifier: RR
Pub: 100-4, Chapter-36, 50.15

C **E0153** Platform attachment, forearm crutch, each **DME** Y
BETOS: D1E   Other DME
DME Modifier: NU,RR,UE

C **E0154** Platform attachment, walker, each **DME** Y
BETOS: D1E   Other DME
Pub: 100-4, Chapter-36, 50.14; 100-4, Chapter-36, 50.15

C **E0155** Wheel attachment, rigid pick-up walker, per pair **DME** Y
BETOS: D1E   Other DME
DME Modifier: NU,RR,UE
Pub: 100-4, Chapter-36, 50.15

C **E0156** Seat attachment, walker **DME** Y
BETOS: D1E   Other DME
DME Modifier: NU,RR,UE
Pub: 100-4, Chapter-36, 50.14; 100-4, Chapter-36, 50.15

C **E0157** Crutch attachment, walker, each **DME** Y
BETOS: D1E   Other DME
DME Modifier: NU,RR,UE
Pub: 100-4, Chapter-36, 50.15; 100-4, Chapter-36, 50.14

C **E0158** Leg extensions for walker, per set of four (4) **DME** Y
BETOS: D1E   Other DME
DME Modifier: NU,RR,UE
Pub: 100-4, Chapter-36, 50.14; 100-4, Chapter-36, 50.15

C **E0159** Brake attachment for wheeled walker, replacement, each **DME** Y
BETOS: D1E   Other DME
DME Modifier: NU,RR,UE
Pub: 100-4, Chapter-36, 50.15

SITZ BATH/EQUIPMENT (E0160-E0162)

D **E0160** Sitz type bath or equipment, portable, used with or without commode **DME** Y
BETOS: D1E   Other DME
DME Modifier: NU,RR,UE

D **E0161** Sitz type bath or equipment, portable, used with or without commode, with faucet attachment/s **DME** Y
BETOS: D1E   Other DME
DME Modifier: NU,RR,UE
Coding Clinic: 2009, Q2

D **E0162** Sitz bath chair **DME** Y
BETOS: D1E   Other DME
DME Modifier: NU,RR,UE

COMMODE CHAIR AND SUPPLIES (E0163-E0175)

D **E0163** Commode chair, mobile or stationary, with fixed arms **DME** Y
BETOS: D1E   Other DME
DME Modifier: NU,RR,UE

D **E0165** Commode chair, mobile or stationary, with detachable arms **DME** Y
BETOS: D1E   Other DME
DME Modifier: RR

D **E0167** Pail or pan for use with commode chair, replacement only **DME** Y
BETOS: D1E   Other DME
DME Modifier: NU,RR,UE

C **E0168** Commode chair, extra wide and/or heavy duty, stationary or mobile, with or without arms, any type, each **DME** Y
BETOS: D1E   Other DME
DME Modifier: NU,RR,UE

C **E0170** Commode chair with integrated seat lift mechanism, electric, any type **DME** Y
BETOS: D1E   Other DME
DME Modifier: RR

C **E0171** Commode chair with integrated seat lift mechanism, non-electric, any type **DME** Y
BETOS: D1E   Other DME
DME Modifier: RR

S **E0172** Seat lift mechanism placed over or on top of toilet, any type   E1
BETOS: D1E   Other DME
Service not separately priced by Part B
Statute: 1861SSA

C **E0175** Foot rest, for use with commode chair, each **DME** Y
BETOS: D1E   Other DME
DME Modifier: NU,RR,UE

● New code   ▲ Revised code   **C** Carrier judgment   **D** Special coverage instructions apply
I Not payable by Medicare   **M** Non-covered by Medicare   **S** Non-covered by Medicare statute   AHA Coding Clinic®

PRESSURE MATTRESSES, PADS, AND OTHER SUPPLIES (E0181-E0199)

D **E0181** Powered pressure reducing mattress overlay/pad, alternating, with pump, includes heavy duty　　DME Y
BETOS: D1E　Other DME
DME Modifier: RR

D **E0182** Pump for alternating pressure pad, for replacement only　　DME Y
BETOS: D1E　Other DME
DME Modifier: RR

D **E0184** Dry pressure mattress　　DME Y
BETOS: D1E　Other DME
DME Modifier: NU,RR,UE

D **E0185** Gel or gel-like pressure pad for mattress, standard mattress length and width　　DME Y
BETOS: D1E　Other DME
DME Modifier: NU,RR,UE

D **E0186** Air pressure mattress　　DME Y
BETOS: D1E　Other DME
DME Modifier: RR

D **E0187** Water pressure mattress　　DME Y
BETOS: D1E　Other DME
DME Modifier: RR

D **E0188** Synthetic sheepskin pad　　DME Y
BETOS: D1E　Other DME
DME Modifier: NU,RR,UE

D **E0189** Lambswool sheepskin pad, any size　　DME Y
BETOS: D1E　Other DME
DME Modifier: NU,RR,UE

D **E0190** Positioning cushion/pillow/wedge, any shape or size, includes all components and accessories　　E1
BETOS: D1E　Other DME
Service not separately priced by Part B

C **E0191** Heel or elbow protector, each　　DME Y
BETOS: D1E　Other DME
DME Modifier: NU,RR,UE

C **E0193** Powered air flotation bed (low air loss therapy)　　DME Y
BETOS: D1E　Other DME
DME Modifier: RR

D **E0194** Air fluidized bed　　DME Y
BETOS: D1E　Other DME
DME Modifier: RR

D **E0196** Gel pressure mattress　　DME Y
BETOS: D1E　Other DME
DME Modifier: RR

D **E0197** Air pressure pad for mattress, standard mattress length and width　　DME Y
BETOS: D1E　Other DME
DME Modifier: RR

D **E0198** Water pressure pad for mattress, standard mattress length and width　　DME Y
BETOS: D1E　Other DME
DME Modifier: RR

D **E0199** Dry pressure pad for mattress, standard mattress length and width　　DME Y
BETOS: D1E　Other DME
DME Modifier: NU,RR,UE

HEAT, COLD, AND LIGHT THERAPIES (E0200-E0239), SEE ALSO ULTRAVIOLET LIGHT THERAPY SYSTEMS (E0691-E0694)

D **E0200** Heat lamp, without stand (table model), includes bulb, or infrared element　　DME Y
BETOS: D1E　Other DME
DME Modifier: NU,RR,UE

C **E0202** Phototherapy (bilirubin) light with photometer　　DME Y
BETOS: D1E　Other DME
DME Modifier: RR

M **E0203** Therapeutic lightbox, minimum 10,000 lux, table top model　　E1
BETOS: D1E　Other DME
Service not separately priced by Part B

D **E0205** Heat lamp, with stand, includes bulb, or infrared element　　DME Y
BETOS: D1E　Other DME
DME Modifier: NU,RR,UE

D **E0210** Electric heat pad, standard　　DME Y
BETOS: D1E　Other DME
DME Modifier: NU,RR,UE

D **E0215** Electric heat pad, moist　　DME Y
BETOS: D1E　Other DME
DME Modifier: NU,RR,UE

D **E0217** Water circulating heat pad with pump　　DME Y
BETOS: D1E　Other DME
DME Modifier: NU,RR,UE

D **E0218** Fluid circulating cold pad with pump, any type　　Y
BETOS: D1E　Other DME

C **E0221** Infrared heating pad system　　Y
BETOS: D1E　Other DME
Service not separately priced by Part B
Coding Clinic: 2002, Q1
Pub: 100-4, Chapter-5, 20.4

D **E0225** Hydrocollator unit, includes pads　　DME Y
BETOS: D1E　Other DME
DME Modifier: NU,RR,UE

M **E0231** Non-contact wound warming device (temperature control unit, AC adapter and power cord) for use with warming card and wound cover　　E1
BETOS: D1E　Other DME
Service not separately priced by Part B
Coding Clinic: 2002, Q1

♂ Male only　　♀ Female only　　Ⓐ Age　　A2 - Z3 = ASC Payment indicator　　A - Y = APC Status indicator
ASC = ASC Approved Procedure　　DME Paid under the DME fee schedule　　MIPS MIPS code

M E0232 Warming card for use with the non contact wound warming device and non contact wound warming wound cover　E1
BETOS: D1E　Other DME
Service not separately priced by Part B
Coding Clinic: 2002, Q1

D E0235 Paraffin bath unit, portable (see medical supply code A4265 for paraffin)　DME Y
BETOS: D1E　Other DME
DME Modifier: RR

D E0236 Pump for water circulating pad　DME Y
BETOS: D1E　Other DME
DME Modifier: RR

D E0239 Hydrocollator unit, portable　DME Y
BETOS: D1E　Other DME
DME Modifier: NU,RR,UE

BATHING SUPPLIES (E0240-E0249)

M E0240 Bath/shower chair, with or without wheels, any size　E1
BETOS: D1E　Other DME
Service not separately priced by Part B

M E0241 Bath tub wall rail, each　E1
BETOS: D1E　Other DME
Service not separately priced by Part B

M E0242 Bath tub rail, floor base　E1
BETOS: D1E　Other DME
Service not separately priced by Part B

M E0243 Toilet rail, each　E1
BETOS: D1E　Other DME
Service not separately priced by Part B

M E0244 Raised toilet seat　E1
BETOS: D1E　Other DME
Service not separately priced by Part B

M E0245 Tub stool or bench　E1
BETOS: D1E　Other DME
Service not separately priced by Part B

C E0246 Transfer tub rail attachment　E1
BETOS: D1E　Other DME
Service not separately priced by Part B

D E0247 Transfer bench for tub or toilet with or without commode opening　E1
BETOS: D1E　Other DME
Service not separately priced by Part B

D E0248 Transfer bench, heavy duty, for tub or toilet with or without commode opening　E1
BETOS: D1E　Other DME
Service not separately priced by Part B

D E0249 Pad for water circulating heat unit, for replacement only　DME Y
BETOS: D1E　Other DME
DME Modifier: NU,RR,UE

HOSPITAL BEDS AND ASSOCIATED SUPPLIES (E0250-E0373)

D E0250 Hospital bed, fixed height, with any type side rails, with mattress　DME Y
BETOS: D1B　Hospital beds
DME Modifier: RR

D E0251 Hospital bed, fixed height, with any type side rails, without mattress　DME Y
BETOS: D1B　Hospital beds
DME Modifier: RR

D E0255 Hospital bed, variable height, hi-lo, with any type side rails, with mattress　DME Y
BETOS: D1B　Hospital beds
DME Modifier: RR

D E0256 Hospital bed, variable height, hi-lo, with any type side rails, without mattress　DME Y
BETOS: D1B　Hospital beds
DME Modifier: RR

D E0260 Hospital bed, semi-electric (head and foot adjustment), with any type side rails, with mattress　DME Y
BETOS: D1B　Hospital beds
DME Modifier: RR

D E0261 Hospital bed, semi-electric (head and foot adjustment), with any type side rails, without mattress　DME Y
BETOS: D1B　Hospital beds
DME Modifier: RR

D E0265 Hospital bed, total electric (head, foot and height adjustments), with any type side rails, with mattress　DME Y
BETOS: D1B　Hospital beds
DME Modifier: RR

D E0266 Hospital bed, total electric (head, foot and height adjustments), with any type side rails, without mattress　DME Y
BETOS: D1B　Hospital beds
DME Modifier: RR

M E0270 Hospital bed, institutional type includes: oscillating, circulating and stryker frame, with mattress　E1
BETOS: D1B　Hospital beds
Service not separately priced by Part B

D E0271 Mattress, innerspring　DME Y
BETOS: D1B　Hospital beds
DME Modifier: NU,RR,UE
Pub: 100-4, Chapter-36, 50.14

D E0272 Mattress, foam rubber　DME Y
BETOS: D1B　Hospital beds
DME Modifier: NU,RR,UE
Pub: 100-4, Chapter-36, 50.14

M E0273 Bed board　E1
BETOS: D1B　Hospital beds
Service not separately priced by Part B

● New code　▲ Revised code　C Carrier judgment　D Special coverage instructions apply
I Not payable by Medicare　M Non-covered by Medicare　S Non-covered by Medicare statute　AHA Coding Clinic®

M **E0274** Over-bed table   E1
    BETOS: D1B   Hospital beds
    Service not separately priced by Part B

D **E0275** Bed pan, standard, metal or plastic   DME Y
    BETOS: D1E   Other DME
    DME Modifier: NU,RR,UE

D **E0276** Bed pan, fracture, metal or plastic   DME Y
    BETOS: D1E   Other DME
    DME Modifier: NU,RR,UE

D **E0277** Powered pressure-reducing air mattress   DME Y
    BETOS: D1E   Other DME
    DME Modifier: RR

C **E0280** Bed cradle, any type   DME Y
    BETOS: D1B   Hospital beds
    DME Modifier: NU,RR,UE
    Pub: 100-4, Chapter-36, 50.14

D **E0290** Hospital bed, fixed height, without side rails, with mattress   DME Y
    BETOS: D1B   Hospital beds
    DME Modifier: RR

D **E0291** Hospital bed, fixed height, without side rails, without mattress   DME Y
    BETOS: D1B   Hospital beds
    DME Modifier: RR

D **E0292** Hospital bed, variable height, hi-lo, without side rails, with mattress   DME Y
    BETOS: D1B   Hospital beds
    DME Modifier: RR

D **E0293** Hospital bed, variable height, hi-lo, without side rails, without mattress   DME Y
    BETOS: D1B   Hospital beds
    DME Modifier: RR

D **E0294** Hospital bed, semi-electric (head and foot adjustment), without side rails, with mattress   DME Y
    BETOS: D1B   Hospital beds
    DME Modifier: RR

D **E0295** Hospital bed, semi-electric (head and foot adjustment), without side rails, without mattress   DME Y
    BETOS: D1B   Hospital beds
    DME Modifier: RR

D **E0296** Hospital bed, total electric (head, foot and height adjustments), without side rails, with mattress   DME Y
    BETOS: D1B   Hospital beds
    DME Modifier: RR

D **E0297** Hospital bed, total electric (head, foot and height adjustments), without side rails, without mattress   DME Y
    BETOS: D1B   Hospital beds
    DME Modifier: RR

C **E0300** Pediatric crib, hospital grade, fully enclosed, with or without top enclosure   DME A Y
    BETOS: D1B   Hospital beds
    DME Modifier: RR

D **E0301** Hospital bed, heavy duty, extra wide, with weight capacity greater than 350 pounds, but less than or equal to 600 pounds, with any type side rails, without mattress   DME Y
    BETOS: D1B   Hospital beds
    DME Modifier: RR

D **E0302** Hospital bed, extra heavy duty, extra wide, with weight capacity greater than 600 pounds, with any type side rails, without mattress   DME Y
    BETOS: D1B   Hospital beds
    DME Modifier: RR

D **E0303** Hospital bed, heavy duty, extra wide, with weight capacity greater than 350 pounds, but less than or equal to 600 pounds, with any type side rails, with mattress   DME Y
    BETOS: D1B   Hospital beds
    DME Modifier: RR

D **E0304** Hospital bed, extra heavy duty, extra wide, with weight capacity greater than 600 pounds, with any type side rails, with mattress   DME Y
    BETOS: D1B   Hospital beds
    DME Modifier: RR

D **E0305** Bed side rails, half length   DME Y
    BETOS: D1B   Hospital beds
    DME Modifier: RR

D **E0310** Bed side rails, full length   DME Y
    BETOS: D1B   Hospital beds
    DME Modifier: NU,RR,UE
    Pub: 100-4, Chapter-36, 50.14

M **E0315** Bed accessory: board, table, or support device, any type   E1
    BETOS: D1B   Hospital beds
    Service not separately priced by Part B

C **E0316** Safety enclosure frame/canopy for use with hospital bed, any type   DME Y
    BETOS: D1B   Hospital beds
    DME Modifier: RR
    Coding Clinic: 2002, Q1

D **E0325** Urinal; male, jug-type, any material   ♂ DME Y
    BETOS: D1E   Other DME
    DME Modifier: NU,RR,UE

D **E0326** Urinal; female, jug-type, any material   ♀ DME Y
    BETOS: D1E   Other DME
    DME Modifier: NU,RR,UE

♂ Male only   ♀ Female only   A Age   A2 - Z3 = ASC Payment indicator   A - Y = APC Status indicator
ASC = ASC Approved Procedure   DME Paid under the DME fee schedule   MIPS MIPS code

C **E0328** Hospital bed, pediatric, manual, 360 degree side enclosures, top of headboard, footboard and side rails up to 24 inches above the spring, includes mattress   Ⓐ Y
BETOS: D1B   Hospital beds

C **E0329** Hospital bed, pediatric, electric or semi-electric, 360 degree side enclosures, top of headboard, footboard and side rails up to 24 inches above the spring, includes mattress   Ⓐ Y
BETOS: D1B   Hospital beds

C **E0350** Control unit for electronic bowel irrigation/evacuation system   E1
BETOS: Z2   Undefined codes
Other carrier priced

C **E0352** Disposable pack (water reservoir bag, speculum, valving mechanism and collection bag/box) for use with the electronic bowel irrigation/evacuation system   E1
BETOS: Z2   Undefined codes
Other carrier priced

C **E0370** Air pressure elevator for heel   E1
BETOS: D1E   Other DME
Service not separately priced by Part B

C **E0371** Nonpowered advanced pressure reducing overlay for mattress, standard mattress length and width   DME Y
BETOS: D1E   Other DME
DME Modifier: RR

C **E0372** Powered air overlay for mattress, standard mattress length and width   DME Y
BETOS: D1E   Other DME
DME Modifier: RR

C **E0373** Nonpowered advanced pressure reducing mattress   DME Y
BETOS: D1E   Other DME
DME Modifier: RR

OXYGEN DELIVERY SYSTEMS AND RELATED SUPPLIES (E0424-E0487)

D **E0424** Stationary compressed gaseous oxygen system, rental; includes container, contents, regulator, flowmeter, humidifier, nebulizer, cannula or mask, and tubing   DME Y
BETOS: D1C   Oxygen and supplies
DME Modifier: QB,QF,RR

D **E0425** Stationary compressed gas system, purchase; includes regulator, flowmeter, humidifier, nebulizer, cannula or mask, and tubing   E1
BETOS: D1C   Oxygen and supplies
Service not separately priced by Part B

D **E0430** Portable gaseous oxygen system, purchase; includes regulator, flowmeter, humidifier, cannula or mask, and tubing   E1
BETOS: D1C   Oxygen and supplies
Service not separately priced by Part B

D **E0431** Portable gaseous oxygen system, rental; includes portable container, regulator, flowmeter, humidifier, cannula or mask, and tubing   DME Y
BETOS: D1C   Oxygen and supplies
DME Modifier: QB,QF,RR

C **E0433** Portable liquid oxygen system, rental; home liquefier used to fill portable liquid oxygen containers, includes portable containers, regulator, flowmeter, humidifier, cannula or mask and tubing, with or without supply reservoir and contents gauge   DME Y
BETOS: D1C   Oxygen and supplies
DME Modifier: QB,QF,RR

D **E0434** Portable liquid oxygen system, rental; includes portable container, supply reservoir, humidifier, flowmeter, refill adaptor, contents gauge, cannula or mask, and tubing   DME Y
BETOS: D1C   Oxygen and supplies
DME Modifier: QB,QF,RR

D **E0435** Portable liquid oxygen system, purchase; includes portable container, supply reservoir, flowmeter, humidifier, contents gauge, cannula or mask, tubing and refill adaptor   E1
BETOS: D1C   Oxygen and supplies
Service not separately priced by Part B

D **E0439** Stationary liquid oxygen system, rental; includes container, contents, regulator, flowmeter, humidifier, nebulizer, cannula or mask, & tubing   DME Y
BETOS: D1C   Oxygen and supplies
DME Modifier: QB,QF,RR

D **E0440** Stationary liquid oxygen system, purchase; includes use of reservoir, contents indicator, regulator, flowmeter, humidifier, nebulizer, cannula or mask, and tubing   E1
BETOS: D1C   Oxygen and supplies
Service not separately priced by Part B

D **E0441** Stationary oxygen contents, gaseous, 1 month's supply = 1 unit   DME Y
BETOS: D1C   Oxygen and supplies

D **E0442** Stationary oxygen contents, liquid, 1 month's supply = 1 unit   DME Y
BETOS: D1C   Oxygen and supplies

D **E0443** Portable oxygen contents, gaseous, 1 month's supply = 1 unit   DME Y
BETOS: D1C   Oxygen and supplies

D **E0444** Portable oxygen contents, liquid, 1 month's supply = 1 unit   DME Y
BETOS: D1C   Oxygen and supplies

C **E0445** Oximeter device for measuring blood oxygen levels non-invasively   N
BETOS: Z2   Undefined codes
Service not separately priced by Part B

● New code   ▲ Revised code   C Carrier judgment   D Special coverage instructions apply
I Not payable by Medicare   M Non-covered by Medicare   S Non-covered by Medicare statute   AHA Coding Clinic®

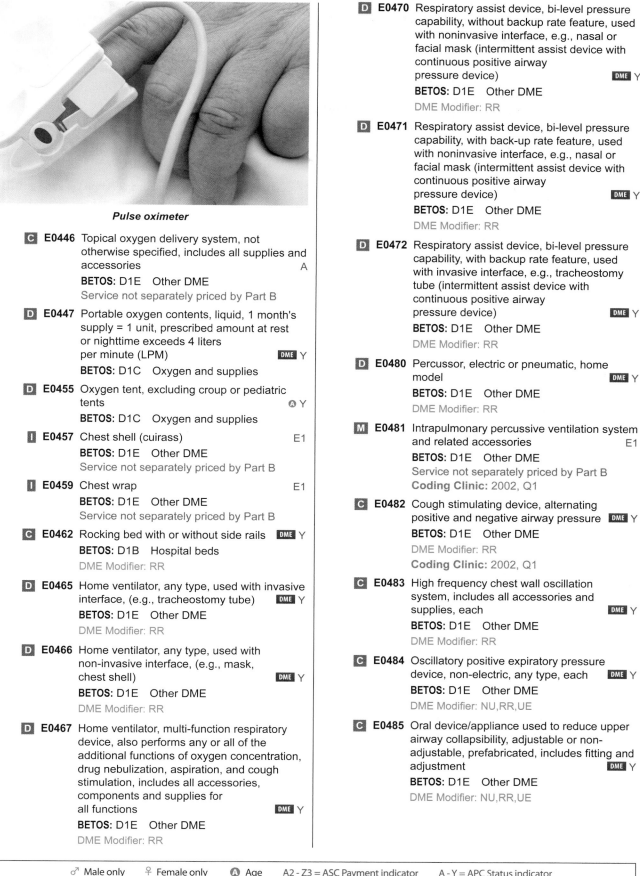

Pulse oximeter

C **E0446** Topical oxygen delivery system, not otherwise specified, includes all supplies and accessories A

BETOS: D1E   Other DME

Service not separately priced by Part B

D **E0447** Portable oxygen contents, liquid, 1 month's supply = 1 unit, prescribed amount at rest or nighttime exceeds 4 liters per minute (LPM) **DME** Y

BETOS: D1C   Oxygen and supplies

D **E0455** Oxygen tent, excluding croup or pediatric tents **A** Y

BETOS: D1C   Oxygen and supplies

I **E0457** Chest shell (cuirass) E1

BETOS: D1E   Other DME

Service not separately priced by Part B

I **E0459** Chest wrap E1

BETOS: D1E   Other DME

Service not separately priced by Part B

C **E0462** Rocking bed with or without side rails **DME** Y

BETOS: D1B   Hospital beds

DME Modifier: RR

D **E0465** Home ventilator, any type, used with invasive interface, (e.g., tracheostomy tube) **DME** Y

BETOS: D1E   Other DME

DME Modifier: RR

D **E0466** Home ventilator, any type, used with non-invasive interface, (e.g., mask, chest shell) **DME** Y

BETOS: D1E   Other DME

DME Modifier: RR

D **E0467** Home ventilator, multi-function respiratory device, also performs any or all of the additional functions of oxygen concentration, drug nebulization, aspiration, and cough stimulation, includes all accessories, components and supplies for all functions **DME** Y

BETOS: D1E   Other DME

DME Modifier: RR

D **E0470** Respiratory assist device, bi-level pressure capability, without backup rate feature, used with noninvasive interface, e.g., nasal or facial mask (intermittent assist device with continuous positive airway pressure device) **DME** Y

BETOS: D1E   Other DME

DME Modifier: RR

D **E0471** Respiratory assist device, bi-level pressure capability, with back-up rate feature, used with noninvasive interface, e.g., nasal or facial mask (intermittent assist device with continuous positive airway pressure device) **DME** Y

BETOS: D1E   Other DME

DME Modifier: RR

D **E0472** Respiratory assist device, bi-level pressure capability, with backup rate feature, used with invasive interface, e.g., tracheostomy tube (intermittent assist device with continuous positive airway pressure device) **DME** Y

BETOS: D1E   Other DME

DME Modifier: RR

D **E0480** Percussor, electric or pneumatic, home model **DME** Y

BETOS: D1E   Other DME

DME Modifier: RR

M **E0481** Intrapulmonary percussive ventilation system and related accessories E1

BETOS: D1E   Other DME

Service not separately priced by Part B

Coding Clinic: 2002, Q1

C **E0482** Cough stimulating device, alternating positive and negative airway pressure **DME** Y

BETOS: D1E   Other DME

DME Modifier: RR

Coding Clinic: 2002, Q1

C **E0483** High frequency chest wall oscillation system, includes all accessories and supplies, each **DME** Y

BETOS: D1E   Other DME

DME Modifier: RR

C **E0484** Oscillatory positive expiratory pressure device, non-electric, any type, each **DME** Y

BETOS: D1E   Other DME

DME Modifier: NU,RR,UE

C **E0485** Oral device/appliance used to reduce upper airway collapsibility, adjustable or non-adjustable, prefabricated, includes fitting and adjustment **DME** Y

BETOS: D1E   Other DME

DME Modifier: NU,RR,UE

♂ Male only   ♀ Female only   **A** Age   A2 - Z3 = ASC Payment indicator   A - Y = APC Status indicator
ASC = ASC Approved Procedure   **DME** Paid under the DME fee schedule   **MIPS** MIPS code

C **E0486** Oral device/appliance used to reduce upper airway collapsibility, adjustable or non-adjustable, custom fabricated, includes fitting and adjustment DME Y
BETOS: D1E   Other DME
DME Modifier: NU,RR,UE

D **E0487** Spirometer, electronic, includes all accessories N
BETOS: Z2   Undefined codes
Service not separately priced by Part B
Coding Clinic: 2008, Q4

INTERMITTENT POSITIVE PRESSURE BREATHING DEVICES (E0500), SEE ALSO BREATHING AIDS (A7000-A7048); OTHER BREATHING AIDS (E0605, E0606); ASSISTED BREATHING SUPPLIES (S8096-S8210)

D **E0500** IPPB machine, all types, with built-in nebulization; manual or automatic valves; internal or external power source DME Y
BETOS: D1E   Other DME
DME Modifier: RR

HUMIDIFIERS AND NEBULIZERS WITH RELATED EQUIPMENT (E0550-E0601)

D **E0550** Humidifier, durable for extensive supplemental humidification during IPPB treatments or oxygen delivery DME Y
BETOS: D1E   Other DME
DME Modifier: RR

D **E0555** Humidifier, durable, glass or autoclavable plastic bottle type, for use with regulator or flowmeter Y
BETOS: D1C   Oxygen and supplies

D **E0560** Humidifier, durable for supplemental humidification during IPPB treatment or oxygen delivery DME Y
BETOS: D1E   Other DME
DME Modifier: NU,RR,UE

C **E0561** Humidifier, non-heated, used with positive airway pressure device DME Y
BETOS: D1E   Other DME
DME Modifier: NU,RR,UE
Pub: 100-4, Chapter-36, 50.14

C **E0562** Humidifier, heated, used with positive airway pressure device DME Y
BETOS: D1E   Other DME
DME Modifier: NU,RR,UE
Pub: 100-4, Chapter-36, 50.14

C **E0565** Compressor, air power source for equipment which is not self-contained or cylinder driven DME Y
BETOS: D1E   Other DME
DME Modifier: RR

D **E0570** Nebulizer, with compressor DME Y
BETOS: D1E   Other DME
DME Modifier: RR

C **E0572** Aerosol compressor, adjustable pressure, light duty for intermittent use DME Y
BETOS: D1E   Other DME
DME Modifier: RR

C **E0574** Ultrasonic/electronic aerosol generator with small volume nebulizer DME Y
BETOS: D1E   Other DME
DME Modifier: RR

D **E0575** Nebulizer, ultrasonic, large volume DME Y
BETOS: D1E   Other DME
DME Modifier: RR

D **E0580** Nebulizer, durable, glass or autoclavable plastic, bottle type, for use with regulator or flowmeter DME Y
BETOS: D1E   Other DME
DME Modifier: NU,RR,UE

D **E0585** Nebulizer, with compressor and heater DME Y
BETOS: D1E   Other DME
DME Modifier: RR

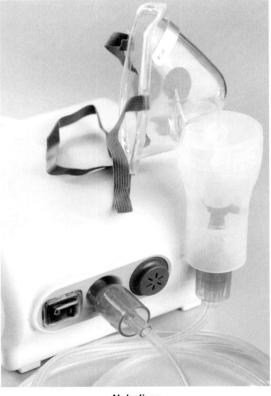

Nebulizer

D **E0600** Respiratory suction pump, home model, portable or stationary, electric DME Y
BETOS: D1E   Other DME
DME Modifier: RR

● New code   ▲ Revised code   C Carrier judgment   D Special coverage instructions apply
I Not payable by Medicare   M Non-covered by Medicare   S Non-covered by Medicare statute   AHA Coding Clinic®

D **E0601** Continuous positive airway pressure (CPAP) device **DME** Y
BETOS: D1E Other DME
DME Modifier: RR

BREAST PUMPS (E0602-E0604)

C **E0602** Breast pump, manual, any type ♀ **DME** **A** Y
BETOS: D1E Other DME
DME Modifier: NU,RR,UE

C **E0603** Breast pump, electric (AC and/or DC), any type ♀ **A** N
BETOS: Z2 Undefined codes
Service not separately priced by Part B
Coding Clinic: 2002, Q1

C **E0604** Breast pump, hospital grade, electric (AC and / or DC), any type ♀ **A** A
BETOS: Z2 Undefined codes
Service not separately priced by Part B
Coding Clinic: 2002, Q1

OTHER BREATHING AIDS (E0605, E0606), SEE ALSO BREATHING AIDS (A7000-A7048); INTERMITTENT POSITIVE PRESSURE BREATHING DEVICES (E0500); ASSISTED BREATHING SUPPLIES (S8096-S8210)

D **E0605** Vaporizer, room type **DME** Y
BETOS: D1E Other DME
DME Modifier: NU,RR,UE

D **E0606** Postural drainage board **DME** Y
BETOS: D1E Other DME
DME Modifier: RR

MONITORING EQUIPMENT (E0607-E0620)

D **E0607** Home blood glucose monitor **DME** Y
BETOS: D1E Other DME
DME Modifier: NU,RR,UE

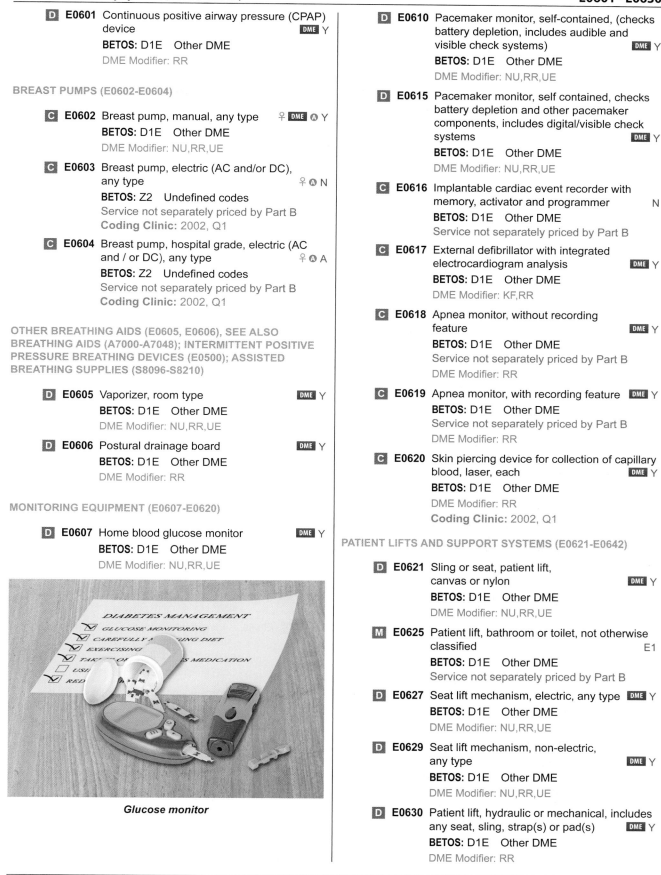

Glucose monitor

D **E0610** Pacemaker monitor, self-contained, (checks battery depletion, includes audible and visible check systems) **DME** Y
BETOS: D1E Other DME
DME Modifier: NU,RR,UE

D **E0615** Pacemaker monitor, self contained, checks battery depletion and other pacemaker components, includes digital/visible check systems **DME** Y
BETOS: D1E Other DME
DME Modifier: NU,RR,UE

C **E0616** Implantable cardiac event recorder with memory, activator and programmer N
BETOS: D1E Other DME
Service not separately priced by Part B

C **E0617** External defibrillator with integrated electrocardiogram analysis **DME** Y
BETOS: D1E Other DME
DME Modifier: KF,RR

C **E0618** Apnea monitor, without recording feature **DME** Y
BETOS: D1E Other DME
Service not separately priced by Part B
DME Modifier: RR

C **E0619** Apnea monitor, with recording feature **DME** Y
BETOS: D1E Other DME
Service not separately priced by Part B
DME Modifier: RR

C **E0620** Skin piercing device for collection of capillary blood, laser, each **DME** Y
BETOS: D1E Other DME
DME Modifier: RR
Coding Clinic: 2002, Q1

PATIENT LIFTS AND SUPPORT SYSTEMS (E0621-E0642)

D **E0621** Sling or seat, patient lift, canvas or nylon **DME** Y
BETOS: D1E Other DME
DME Modifier: NU,RR,UE

M **E0625** Patient lift, bathroom or toilet, not otherwise classified E1
BETOS: D1E Other DME
Service not separately priced by Part B

D **E0627** Seat lift mechanism, electric, any type **DME** Y
BETOS: D1E Other DME
DME Modifier: NU,RR,UE

D **E0629** Seat lift mechanism, non-electric, any type **DME** Y
BETOS: D1E Other DME
DME Modifier: NU,RR,UE

D **E0630** Patient lift, hydraulic or mechanical, includes any seat, sling, strap(s) or pad(s) **DME** Y
BETOS: D1E Other DME
DME Modifier: RR

♂ Male only   ♀ Female only   **A** Age   A2 - Z3 = ASC Payment indicator   A - Y = APC Status indicator
ASC = ASC Approved Procedure   **DME** Paid under the DME fee schedule   **MIPS** MIPS code

E0635 - E0671

D **E0635** Patient lift, electric with seat or sling **DME** Y
    BETOS: D1E   Other DME
    DME Modifier: RR

C **E0636** Multipositional patient support system, with integrated lift, patient accessible controls **DME** Y
    BETOS: D1E   Other DME
    DME Modifier: RR

M **E0637** Combination sit to stand frame/table system, any size including pediatric, with seat lift feature, with or without wheels **Ⓐ** E1
    BETOS: D1E   Other DME
    Service not separately priced by Part B

M **E0638** Standing frame/table system, one position (e.g., upright, supine or prone stander), any size including pediatric, with or without wheels **Ⓐ** E1
    BETOS: D1E   Other DME
    Service not separately priced by Part B

C **E0639** Patient lift, moveable from room to room with disassembly and reassembly, includes all components/accessories **DME** E1
    BETOS: Y2   Other - non-Medicare fee schedule
    Service not separately priced by Part B
    DME Modifier: RR

C **E0640** Patient lift, fixed system, includes all components/accessories **DME** E1
    BETOS: Y2   Other - non-Medicare fee schedule
    Service not separately priced by Part B
    DME Modifier: RR

M **E0641** Standing frame/table system, multi-position (e.g., 3-way stander), any size including pediatric, with or without wheels **Ⓐ** E1
    BETOS: D1E   Other DME
    Service not separately priced by Part B

M **E0642** Standing frame/table system, mobile (dynamic stander), any size including pediatric **Ⓐ** E1
    BETOS: D1E   Other DME
    Service not separately priced by Part B

PNEUMATIC COMPRESSORS AND APPLIANCES (E0650-E0676)

D **E0650** Pneumatic compressor, non-segmental home model **DME** Y
    BETOS: D1E   Other DME
    DME Modifier: NU,RR,UE

D **E0651** Pneumatic compressor, segmental home model without calibrated gradient pressure **DME** Y
    BETOS: D1E   Other DME
    DME Modifier: NU,RR,UE

D **E0652** Pneumatic compressor, segmental home model with calibrated gradient pressure **DME** Y
    BETOS: D1E   Other DME
    DME Modifier: NU,RR,UE

D **E0655** Non-segmental pneumatic appliance for use with pneumatic compressor, half arm **DME** Y
    BETOS: D1E   Other DME
    DME Modifier: NU,RR,UE

D **E0656** Segmental pneumatic appliance for use with pneumatic compressor, trunk **DME** Y
    BETOS: D1E   Other DME
    DME Modifier: RR
    Coding Clinic: 2008, Q4

D **E0657** Segmental pneumatic appliance for use with pneumatic compressor, chest **DME** Y
    BETOS: D1E   Other DME
    DME Modifier: RR
    Coding Clinic: 2008, Q4

D **E0660** Non-segmental pneumatic appliance for use with pneumatic compressor, full leg **DME** Y
    BETOS: D1E   Other DME
    DME Modifier: NU,RR,UE

D **E0665** Non-segmental pneumatic appliance for use with pneumatic compressor, full arm **DME** Y
    BETOS: D1E   Other DME
    DME Modifier: NU,RR,UE

D **E0666** Non-segmental pneumatic appliance for use with pneumatic compressor, half leg **DME** Y
    BETOS: D1E   Other DME
    DME Modifier: NU,RR,UE

D **E0667** Segmental pneumatic appliance for use with pneumatic compressor, full leg **DME** Y
    BETOS: D1E   Other DME
    DME Modifier: NU,RR,UE

D **E0668** Segmental pneumatic appliance for use with pneumatic compressor, full arm **DME** Y
    BETOS: D1E   Other DME
    DME Modifier: NU,RR,UE

D **E0669** Segmental pneumatic appliance for use with pneumatic compressor, half leg **DME** Y
    BETOS: D1E   Other DME
    DME Modifier: NU,RR,UE

D **E0670** Segmental pneumatic appliance for use with pneumatic compressor, integrated, 2 full legs and trunk **DME** Y
    BETOS: D1E   Other DME
    DME Modifier: NU,RR,UE

D **E0671** Segmental gradient pressure pneumatic appliance, full leg **DME** Y
    BETOS: D1E   Other DME
    DME Modifier: NU,RR,UE

● New code   ▲ Revised code   **C** Carrier judgment   **D** Special coverage instructions apply
I Not payable by Medicare   **M** Non-covered by Medicare   **S** Non-covered by Medicare statute   AHA Coding Clinic®

DURABLE MEDICAL EQUIPMENT (E0100-E8002)

D **E0672** Segmental gradient pressure pneumatic appliance, full arm `DME` Y
BETOS: D1E Other DME
DME Modifier: NU,RR,UE

D **E0673** Segmental gradient pressure pneumatic appliance, half leg `DME` Y
BETOS: D1E Other DME
DME Modifier: NU,RR,UE

C **E0675** Pneumatic compression device, high pressure, rapid inflation/deflation cycle, for arterial insufficiency (unilateral or bilateral system) `DME` Y
BETOS: D1E Other DME
DME Modifier: RR

C **E0676** Intermittent limb compression device (includes all accessories), not otherwise specified Y
BETOS: D1E Other DME
Service not separately priced by Part B

ULTRAVIOLET LIGHT THERAPY SYSTEMS (E0691-E0694), SEE ALSO HEAT, COLD, AND LIGHT THERAPIES (E0200-E0239)

C **E0691** Ultraviolet light therapy system, includes bulbs/lamps, timer and eye protection; treatment area 2 square feet or less `DME` Y
BETOS: D1E Other DME
DME Modifier: NU,RR,UE

C **E0692** Ultraviolet light therapy system panel, includes bulbs/lamps, timer and eye protection, 4 foot panel `DME` Y
BETOS: D1E Other DME
DME Modifier: NU,RR,UE

C **E0693** Ultraviolet light therapy system panel, includes bulbs/lamps, timer and eye protection, 6 foot panel `DME` Y
BETOS: D1E Other DME
DME Modifier: NU,RR,UE

C **E0694** Ultraviolet multidirectional light therapy system in 6 foot cabinet, includes bulbs/lamps, timer and eye protection `DME` Y
BETOS: D1E Other DME
DME Modifier: NU,RR,UE

SAFETY DEVICES (E0700-E0710)

C **E0700** Safety equipment, device or accessory, any type E1
BETOS: D1E Other DME
Service not separately priced by Part B

D **E0705** Transfer device, any type, each `DME` B
BETOS: D1E Other DME
DME Modifier: KU,NU,RR,UE

C **E0710** Restraints, any type (body, chest, wrist or ankle) E1
BETOS: Z2 Undefined codes
Other carrier priced

STIMULATION DEVICES (E0720-E0770)

D **E0720** Transcutaneous electrical nerve stimulation (TENS) device, two lead, localized stimulation `DME` Y
BETOS: D1E Other DME
DME Modifier: NU

D **E0730** Transcutaneous electrical nerve stimulation (TENS) device, four or more leads, for multiple nerve stimulation `DME` Y
BETOS: D1E Other DME
DME Modifier: NU

D **E0731** Form fitting conductive garment for delivery of TENS or NMES (with conductive fibers separated from the patient's skin by layers of fabric) `DME` Y
BETOS: D1E Other DME
DME Modifier: NU

D **E0740** Non-implanted pelvic floor electrical stimulator, complete system `DME` Y
BETOS: D1E Other DME
DME Modifier: RR

C **E0744** Neuromuscular stimulator for scoliosis `DME` Y
BETOS: D1E Other DME
DME Modifier: RR

D **E0745** Neuromuscular stimulator, electronic shock unit `DME` Y
BETOS: D1E Other DME
DME Modifier: RR

D **E0746** Electromyography (EMG), biofeedback device N
BETOS: D1E Other DME
Reasonable charge

D **E0747** Osteogenesis stimulator, electrical, non-invasive, other than spinal applications `DME` Y
BETOS: D1E Other DME
DME Modifier: KF,NU,RR,UE

D **E0748** Osteogenesis stimulator, electrical, non-invasive, spinal applications `DME` Y
BETOS: D1E Other DME
DME Modifier: KF,NU,RR,UE

D **E0749** Osteogenesis stimulator, electrical, surgically implanted `DME` N
BETOS: D1E Other DME
DME Modifier: KF,RR

C **E0755** Electronic salivary reflex stimulator (intra-oral/non-invasive) E1
BETOS: Z2 Undefined codes
Reasonable charge

C **E0760** Osteogenesis stimulator, low intensity ultrasound, non-invasive `DME` Y
BETOS: D1E Other DME
DME Modifier: KF,NU,RR,UE
Pub: 100-4, Chapter-32, 110.5

♂ Male only   ♀ Female only   **A** Age   A2 - Z3 = ASC Payment indicator   A - Y = APC Status indicator
ASC = ASC Approved Procedure   `DME` Paid under the DME fee schedule   `MIPS` MIPS code

Ultrasound diagnostic equipment

D E0761 Non-thermal pulsed high frequency radiowaves, high peak power electromagnetic energy treatment device   E1
BETOS: D1E   Other DME
Service not separately priced by Part B

C E0762 Transcutaneous electrical joint stimulation device system, includes all accessories   DME B
BETOS: D1E   Other DME
DME Modifier: RR

D E0764 Functional neuromuscular stimulation, transcutaneous stimulation of sequential muscle groups of ambulation with computer control, used for walking by spinal cord injured, entire system, after completion of training program   DME Y
BETOS: D1F   Prosthetic/Orthotic devices
DME Modifier: KF,RR

C E0765 FDA-approved nerve stimulator, with replaceable batteries, for treatment of nausea and vomiting   DME Y
BETOS: D1E   Other DME
DME Modifier: NU,RR,UE

C E0766 Electrical stimulation device used for cancer treatment, includes all accessories, any type   DME Y
BETOS: D1E   Other DME
DME Modifier: KF,RR

D E0769 Electrical stimulation or electromagnetic wound treatment device, not otherwise classified   B
BETOS: Y2   Other - non-Medicare fee schedule
Service not separately priced by Part B

D E0770 Functional electrical stimulator, transcutaneous stimulation of nerve and/or muscle groups, any type, complete system, not otherwise specified   Y
BETOS: D1E   Other DME
Coding Clinic: 2008, Q4

INFUSION PUMPS AND SUPPLIES (E0776-E0791)

C E0776 IV pole   DME Y
BETOS: D1E   Other DME
DME Modifier: NU,RR,UE

C E0779 Ambulatory infusion pump, mechanical, reusable, for infusion 8 hours or greater   DME Y
BETOS: D1E   Other DME
DME Modifier: RR

C E0780 Ambulatory infusion pump, mechanical, reusable, for infusion less than 8 hours DME Y
BETOS: D1E   Other DME
DME Modifier: NU

D E0781 Ambulatory infusion pump, single or multiple channels, electric or battery operated, with administrative equipment, worn by patient   DME Y
BETOS: D1E   Other DME
DME Modifier: RR

D E0782 Infusion pump, implantable, non-programmable (includes all components, e.g., pump, catheter, connectors, etc.) DME N
BETOS: D1E   Other DME
DME Modifier: KF,NU,RR,UE

D E0783 Infusion pump system, implantable, programmable (includes all components, e.g., pump, catheter, connectors, etc.) DME N
BETOS: D1E   Other DME
DME Modifier: KF,NU,RR,UE

D E0784 External ambulatory infusion pump, insulin   DME Y
BETOS: D1E   Other DME
DME Modifier: RR

D **E0785** Implantable intraspinal (epidural/intrathecal) catheter used with implantable infusion pump, replacement **DME** N
  BETOS: D1E   Other DME
  DME Modifier: KF

D **E0786** Implantable programmable infusion pump, replacement (excludes implantable intraspinal catheter) **DME** N
  BETOS: D1E   Other DME
  DME Modifier: KF,NU,RR,UE

I **E0787** External ambulatory infusion pump, insulin, dosage rate adjustment using therapeutic continuous glucose sensing E1
  BETOS: Z2   Undefined codes
  Service not separately priced by Part B

D **E0791** Parenteral infusion pump, stationary, single or multi-channel **DME** Y
  BETOS: D1E   Other DME
  DME Modifier: RR

TRACTION AND OTHER ORTHOPEDIC DEVICES (E0830-E0948)

D **E0830** Ambulatory traction device, all types, each N
  BETOS: D1E   Other DME
  Service not separately priced by Part B

D **E0840** Traction frame, attached to headboard, cervical traction **DME** Y
  BETOS: D1E   Other DME
  DME Modifier: NU,RR,UE

C **E0849** Traction equipment, cervical, free-standing stand/frame, pneumatic, applying traction force to other than mandible **DME** Y
  BETOS: D1E   Other DME
  DME Modifier: RR

D **E0850** Traction stand, free standing, cervical traction **DME** Y
  BETOS: D1E   Other DME
  DME Modifier: NU,RR,UE

C **E0855** Cervical traction equipment not requiring additional stand or frame **DME** Y
  BETOS: D1E   Other DME
  DME Modifier: RR

C **E0856** Cervical traction device, with inflatable air bladder(s) **DME** Y
  BETOS: D1E   Other DME
  DME Modifier: RR

D **E0860** Traction equipment, overdoor, cervical **DME** Y
  BETOS: D1E   Other DME
  DME Modifier: NU,RR,UE

D **E0870** Traction frame, attached to footboard, extremity traction, (e.g., Buck's) **DME** Y
  BETOS: D1E   Other DME
  DME Modifier: NU,RR,UE

▲ **D** **E0880** Traction stand, free standing, extremity traction **DME** Y
  BETOS: D1E   Other DME
  DME Modifier: NU,RR,UE

D **E0890** Traction frame, attached to footboard, pelvic traction **DME** Y
  BETOS: D1E   Other DME
  DME Modifier: NU,RR,UE

D **E0900** Traction stand, free standing, pelvic traction, (e.g., Buck's) **DME** Y
  BETOS: D1E   Other DME
  DME Modifier: NU,RR,UE

D **E0910** Trapeze bars, also known as Patient Helper, attached to bed, with grab bar **DME** Y
  BETOS: D1E   Other DME
  DME Modifier: RR

D **E0911** Trapeze bar, heavy duty, for patient weight capacity greater than 250 pounds, attached to bed, with grab bar **DME** Y
  BETOS: D1B   Hospital beds
  DME Modifier: RR

D **E0912** Trapeze bar, heavy duty, for patient weight capacity greater than 250 pounds, free standing, complete with grab bar **DME** Y
  BETOS: D1B   Hospital beds
  DME Modifier: RR

D **E0920** Fracture frame, attached to bed, includes weights **DME** Y
  BETOS: D1E   Other DME
  DME Modifier: RR

D **E0930** Fracture frame, free standing, includes weights **DME** Y
  BETOS: D1E   Other DME
  DME Modifier: RR

D **E0935** Continuous passive motion exercise device for use on knee only **DME** Y
  BETOS: D1E   Other DME
  DME Modifier: RR

M **E0936** Continuous passive motion exercise device for use other than knee E1
  BETOS: D1E   Other DME
  Service not separately priced by Part B

D **E0940** Trapeze bar, free standing, complete with grab bar **DME** Y
  BETOS: D1B   Hospital beds
  DME Modifier: RR

D **E0941** Gravity assisted traction device, any type **DME** Y
  BETOS: D1E   Other DME
  DME Modifier: RR

C **E0942** Cervical head harness/halter **DME** Y
  BETOS: D1E   Other DME
  DME Modifier: NU,RR,UE

C **E0944** Pelvic belt/harness/boot `DME` Y
BETOS: D1E   Other DME
DME Modifier: NU,RR,UE

C **E0945** Extremity belt/harness `DME` Y
BETOS: D1E   Other DME
DME Modifier: NU,RR,UE

D **E0946** Fracture, frame, dual with cross bars, attached to bed, (e.g., Balken, 4 poster) `DME` Y
BETOS: D1E   Other DME
DME Modifier: RR

D **E0947** Fracture frame, attachments for complex pelvic traction `DME` Y
BETOS: D1E   Other DME
DME Modifier: NU,RR,UE

D **E0948** Fracture frame, attachments for complex cervical traction `DME` Y
BETOS: D1E   Other DME
DME Modifier: NU,RR,UE

WHEELCHAIR ACCESSORIES (E0950-E1036)

D **E0950** Wheelchair accessory, tray, each `DME` Y
BETOS: D1D   Wheelchairs
DME Modifier: KE,KU,NU,RR,UE

C **E0951** Heel loop/holder, any type, with or without ankle strap, each `DME` Y
BETOS: D1D   Wheelchairs
Service not separately priced by Part B
DME Modifier: KE,KU,NU,RR,UE

D **E0952** Toe loop/holder, any type, each `DME` Y
BETOS: D1D   Wheelchairs
Service not separately priced by Part B
DME Modifier: KE,KU,NU,RR,UE

C **E0953** Wheelchair accessory, lateral thigh or knee support, any type including fixed mounting hardware, each `DME` Y
BETOS: D1D   Wheelchairs
DME Modifier: KE,KU,NU,RR,UE

C **E0954** Wheelchair accessory, foot box, any type, includes attachment and mounting hardware, each foot `DME` Y
BETOS: D1D   Wheelchairs
DME Modifier: KE,KU,NU,RR,UE

C **E0955** Wheelchair accessory, headrest, cushioned, any type, including fixed mounting hardware, each `DME` Y
BETOS: D1D   Wheelchairs
DME Modifier: KE,KU,RR

C **E0956** Wheelchair accessory, lateral trunk or hip support, any type, including fixed mounting hardware, each `DME` Y
BETOS: D1D   Wheelchairs
DME Modifier: KE,KU,NU,RR,UE

C **E0957** Wheelchair accessory, medial thigh support, any type, including fixed mounting hardware, each `DME` Y
BETOS: D1D   Wheelchairs
DME Modifier: KE,KU,NU,RR,UE

D **E0958** Manual wheelchair accessory, one-arm drive attachment, each `DME` Y
BETOS: D1D   Wheelchairs
Service not separately priced by Part B
DME Modifier: KU,RR

C **E0959** Manual wheelchair accessory, adapter for amputee, each `DME` B
BETOS: D1D   Wheelchairs
Service not separately priced by Part B
DME Modifier: KU,NU,RR,UE

C **E0960** Wheelchair accessory, shoulder harness/straps or chest strap, including any type mounting hardware `DME` Y
BETOS: D1D   Wheelchairs
DME Modifier: KE,KU,NU,RR,UE

C **E0961** Manual wheelchair accessory, wheel lock brake extension (handle), each `DME` B
BETOS: D1D   Wheelchairs
Service not separately priced by Part B
DME Modifier: KU,NU,RR,UE

C **E0966** Manual wheelchair accessory, headrest extension, each `DME` B
BETOS: D1D   Wheelchairs
Service not separately priced by Part B
DME Modifier: KU,NU,RR,UE

D **E0967** Manual wheelchair accessory, hand rim with projections, any type, replacement only, each `DME` Y
BETOS: D1D   Wheelchairs
DME Modifier: KU,NU,RR,UE

D **E0968** Commode seat, wheelchair `DME` Y
BETOS: D1D   Wheelchairs
DME Modifier: RR

D **E0969** Narrowing device, wheelchair `DME` Y
BETOS: D1D   Wheelchairs
DME Modifier: NU,RR,UE

I **E0970** No. 2 footplates, except for elevating leg rest `E1`
BETOS: D1D   Wheelchairs
Service not separately priced by Part B

C **E0971** Manual wheelchair accessory, anti-tipping device, each `DME` B
BETOS: D1D   Wheelchairs
Service not separately priced by Part B
DME Modifier: KU,NU,RR,UE

D **E0973** Wheelchair accessory, adjustable height, detachable armrest, complete assembly, each `DME` B
BETOS: D1D   Wheelchairs

Service not separately priced by Part B
DME Modifier: KE,KU,NU,RR,UE

D **E0974** Manual wheelchair accessory, anti-rollback device, each   `DME` B
BETOS: D1D   Wheelchairs
Service not separately priced by Part B
DME Modifier: KU,NU,RR,UE

C **E0978** Wheelchair accessory, positioning belt/safety belt/pelvic strap, each   `DME` B
BETOS: D1D   Wheelchairs
DME Modifier: KE,KU,NU,RR,UE

C **E0980** Safety vest, wheelchair   `DME` Y
BETOS: D1D   Wheelchairs
DME Modifier: NU,RR,UE

C **E0981** Wheelchair accessory, seat upholstery, replacement only, each   `DME` Y
BETOS: D1D   Wheelchairs
DME Modifier: KE,KU,NU,RR,UE

C **E0982** Wheelchair accessory, back upholstery, replacement only, each   `DME` Y
BETOS: D1D   Wheelchairs
DME Modifier: KE,KU,NU,RR,UE

C **E0983** Manual wheelchair accessory, power add-on to convert manual wheelchair to motorized wheelchair, joystick control   `DME` Y
BETOS: D1D   Wheelchairs
DME Modifier: RR

C **E0984** Manual wheelchair accessory, power add-on to convert manual wheelchair to motorized wheelchair, tiller control   `DME` Y
BETOS: D1D   Wheelchairs
DME Modifier: RR

C **E0985** Wheelchair accessory, seat lift mechanism   `DME` Y
BETOS: D1D   Wheelchairs
DME Modifier: KU,RR

C **E0986** Manual wheelchair accessory, push-rim activated power assist system   `DME` Y
BETOS: D1D   Wheelchairs
DME Modifier: RR

C **E0988** Manual wheelchair accessory, lever-activated, wheel drive, pair   `DME` Y
BETOS: D1D   Wheelchairs
DME Modifier: RR

C **E0990** Wheelchair accessory, elevating leg rest, complete assembly, each   `DME` B
BETOS: D1D   Wheelchairs
Service not separately priced by Part B
DME Modifier: KE,KU,NU,RR,UE

C **E0992** Manual wheelchair accessory, solid seat insert   `DME` B
BETOS: D1D   Wheelchairs
DME Modifier: KU,NU,RR,UE

D **E0994** Arm rest, each   `DME` Y
BETOS: D1D   Wheelchairs
DME Modifier: NU,RR,UE

C **E0995** Wheelchair accessory, calf rest/pad, replacement only, each   `DME` B
BETOS: D1D   Wheelchairs
Service not separately priced by Part B
DME Modifier: KE,KU,NU,RR,UE

C **E1002** Wheelchair accessory, power seating system, tilt only   `DME` Y
BETOS: D1D   Wheelchairs
DME Modifier: KE,KU,RR

C **E1003** Wheelchair accessory, power seating system, recline only, without shear reduction   `DME` Y
BETOS: D1D   Wheelchairs
DME Modifier: KE,KU,RR

C **E1004** Wheelchair accessory, power seating system, recline only, with mechanical shear reduction   `DME` Y
BETOS: D1D   Wheelchairs
DME Modifier: KE,KU,RR

C **E1005** Wheelchair accessory, power seating system, recline only, with power shear reduction   `DME` Y
BETOS: D1D   Wheelchairs
DME Modifier: KE,KU,RR

C **E1006** Wheelchair accessory, power seating system, combination tilt and recline, without shear reduction   `DME` Y
BETOS: D1D   Wheelchairs
DME Modifier: KE,KU,RR

C **E1007** Wheelchair accessory, power seating system, combination tilt and recline, with mechanical shear reduction   `DME` Y
BETOS: D1D   Wheelchairs
DME Modifier: KE,KU,RR

C **E1008** Wheelchair accessory, power seating system, combination tilt and recline, with power shear reduction   `DME` Y
BETOS: D1D   Wheelchairs
DME Modifier: KE,KU,RR

C **E1009** Wheelchair accessory, addition to power seating system, mechanically linked leg elevation system, including pushrod and leg rest, each   `DME` Y
BETOS: D1D   Wheelchairs
DME Modifier: NU,RR,UE

C **E1010** Wheelchair accessory, addition to power seating system, power leg elevation system, including leg rest, pair   `DME` Y
BETOS: D1D   Wheelchairs
DME Modifier: KE,KU,RR

D **E1011** Modification to pediatric size wheelchair, width adjustment package (not to be dispensed with initial chair) **DME** Ⓐ Y
  BETOS: D1D   Wheelchairs
  DME Modifier: NU,RR,UE

C **E1012** Wheelchair accessory, addition to power seating system, center mount power elevating leg rest/platform, complete system, any type, each **DME** Y
  BETOS: D1D   Wheelchairs
  DME Modifier: KU,RR

D **E1014** Reclining back, addition to pediatric size wheelchair **DME** Ⓐ Y
  BETOS: D1D   Wheelchairs
  DME Modifier: RR

D **E1015** Shock absorber for manual wheelchair, each **DME** Y
  BETOS: D1D   Wheelchairs
  DME Modifier: KU,NU,RR,UE

D **E1016** Shock absorber for power wheelchair, each **DME** Y
  BETOS: D1D   Wheelchairs
  DME Modifier: KE,KU,NU,RR,UE

D **E1017** Heavy duty shock absorber for heavy duty or extra heavy duty manual wheelchair, each **DME** Y
  BETOS: D1D   Wheelchairs
  DME Modifier: NU,RR,UE

D **E1018** Heavy duty shock absorber for heavy duty or extra heavy duty power wheelchair, each **DME** Y
  BETOS: D1D   Wheelchairs
  DME Modifier: NU,RR,UE

D **E1020** Residual limb support system for wheelchair, any type **DME** Y
  BETOS: D1D   Wheelchairs
  DME Modifier: KE,KU,RR

C **E1028** Wheelchair accessory, manual swing away, retractable or removable mounting hardware for joystick, other control interface or positioning accessory **DME** Y
  BETOS: D1D   Wheelchairs
  DME Modifier: KE,KU,RR

C **E1029** Wheelchair accessory, ventilator tray, fixed **DME** Y
  BETOS: D1D   Wheelchairs
  DME Modifier: KE,KU,RR

C **E1030** Wheelchair accessory, ventilator tray, gimbaled **DME** Y
  BETOS: D1D   Wheelchairs
  DME Modifier: KE,KU,RR

D **E1031** Rollabout chair, any and all types with casters 5" or greater **DME** Y
  BETOS: D1D   Wheelchairs
  DME Modifier: RR

D **E1035** Multi-positional patient transfer system, with integrated seat, operated by care giver, patient weight capacity up to and including 300 lbs **DME** Y
  BETOS: D1D   Wheelchairs
  DME Modifier: RR

C **E1036** Multi-positional patient transfer system, extra-wide, with integrated seat, operated by caregiver, patient weight capacity greater than 300 lbs **DME** Y
  BETOS: D1D   Wheelchairs
  DME Modifier: RR

TRANSPORT CHAIRS (E1037-E1039)

D **E1037** Transport chair, pediatric size **DME** Ⓐ Y
  BETOS: D1D   Wheelchairs
  DME Modifier: RR

D **E1038** Transport chair, adult size, patient weight capacity up to and including 300 pounds **DME** Ⓐ Y
  BETOS: D1D   Wheelchairs
  DME Modifier: RR

C **E1039** Transport chair, adult size, heavy duty, patient weight capacity greater than 300 pounds **DME** Ⓐ Y
  BETOS: D1D   Wheelchairs
  DME Modifier: RR

FULLY RECLINING WHEELCHAIRS (E1050-E1070)

D **E1050** Fully-reclining wheelchair, fixed full length arms, swing away detachable elevating leg rests **DME** Y
  BETOS: D1D   Wheelchairs
  DME Modifier: RR

D **E1060** Fully-reclining wheelchair, detachable arms, desk or full length, swing away detachable elevating leg rests **DME** Y
  BETOS: D1D   Wheelchairs
  DME Modifier: RR

D **E1070** Fully-reclining wheelchair, detachable arms (desk or full length) swing away detachable foot rest **DME** Y
  BETOS: D1D   Wheelchairs
  DME Modifier: RR

HEMI-WHEELCHAIRS (E1083-E1086)

D **E1083** Hemi-wheelchair, fixed full length arms, swing away detachable elevating leg rest **DME** Y
  BETOS: D1D   Wheelchairs
  DME Modifier: RR

D **E1084** Hemi-wheelchair, detachable arms desk or full length arms, swing away detachable elevating leg rests **DME** Y

BETOS: D1D   Wheelchairs
DME Modifier: RR

I **E1085**   Hemi-wheelchair, fixed full length arms, swing away detachable foot rests   E1
BETOS: D1D   Wheelchairs
Service not separately priced by Part B

I **E1086**   Hemi-wheelchair detachable arms desk or full length, swing away detachable foot rests   E1
BETOS: D1D   Wheelchairs
Service not separately priced by Part B

LIGHTWEIGHT, HIGH-STRENGTH WHEELCHAIRS (E1087-E1090)

D **E1087**   High strength lightweight wheelchair, fixed full length arms, swing away detachable elevating leg rests   DME Y
BETOS: D1D   Wheelchairs
DME Modifier: RR

D **E1088**   High strength lightweight wheelchair, detachable arms desk or full length, swing away detachable elevating leg rests   DME Y
BETOS: D1D   Wheelchairs
DME Modifier: RR

I **E1089**   High strength lightweight wheelchair, fixed length arms, swing away detachable foot rest   E1
BETOS: D1D   Wheelchairs
Service not separately priced by Part B

I **E1090**   High strength lightweight wheelchair, detachable arms desk or full length, swing away detachable foot rests   E1
BETOS: D1D   Wheelchairs
Service not separately priced by Part B

HEAVY DUTY, WIDE WHEELCHAIRS (E1092, E1093)

D **E1092**   Wide heavy duty wheel chair, detachable arms (desk or full length), swing away detachable elevating leg rests   DME Y
BETOS: D1D   Wheelchairs
DME Modifier: RR

D **E1093**   Wide heavy duty wheelchair, detachable arms desk or full length arms, swing away detachable foot rests   DME Y
BETOS: D1D   Wheelchairs
DME Modifier: RR

SEMI-RECLINING WHEELCHAIRS (E1100, E1110)

D **E1100**   Semi-reclining wheelchair, fixed full length arms, swing away detachable elevating leg rests   DME Y
BETOS: D1D   Wheelchairs
DME Modifier: RR

D **E1110**   Semi-reclining wheelchair, detachable arms (desk or full length) elevating leg rest   DME Y
BETOS: D1D   Wheelchairs
DME Modifier: RR

STANDARD WHEELCHAIRS (E1130-E1161)

I **E1130**   Standard wheelchair, fixed full length arms, fixed or swing away detachable foot rests   E1
BETOS: D1D   Wheelchairs
Service not separately priced by Part B

I **E1140**   Wheelchair, detachable arms, desk or full length, swing away detachable foot rests   E1
BETOS: D1D   Wheelchairs
Service not separately priced by Part B

D **E1150**   Wheelchair, detachable arms, desk or full length swing away detachable elevating leg rests   DME Y
BETOS: D1D   Wheelchairs
DME Modifier: RR

D **E1160**   Wheelchair, fixed full length arms, swing away detachable elevating leg rests   DME Y
BETOS: D1D   Wheelchairs
DME Modifier: RR

C **E1161**   Manual adult size wheelchair, includes tilt in space   DME A Y
BETOS: D1D   Wheelchairs
DME Modifier: RR

AMPUTEE WHEELCHAIRS (E1170-E1200)

D **E1170**   Amputee wheelchair, fixed full length arms, swing away detachable elevating leg rests   DME Y
BETOS: D1D   Wheelchairs
DME Modifier: RR

D **E1171**   Amputee wheelchair, fixed full length arms, without foot rests or leg rest   DME Y
BETOS: D1D   Wheelchairs
DME Modifier: RR

D **E1172**   Amputee wheelchair, detachable arms (desk or full length) without foot rests or leg rest   DME Y
BETOS: D1D   Wheelchairs
DME Modifier: RR

D **E1180**   Amputee wheelchair, detachable arms (desk or full length) swing away detachable foot rests   DME Y
BETOS: D1D   Wheelchairs
DME Modifier: RR

D **E1190**   Amputee wheelchair, detachable arms (desk or full length) swing away detachable elevating leg rests   DME Y
BETOS: D1D   Wheelchairs
DME Modifier: RR

D **E1195** Heavy duty wheelchair, fixed full length arms, swing away detachable elevating leg rests   DME Y
    BETOS: D1D   Wheelchairs
    DME Modifier: RR

D **E1200** Amputee wheelchair, fixed full length arms, swing away detachable foot rest   DME Y
    BETOS: D1D   Wheelchairs
    DME Modifier: RR

OTHER WHEELCHAIRS AND ACCESSORIES (E1220-E1228)

D **E1220** Wheelchair; specially sized or constructed, (indicate brand name, model number, if any) and justification   Y
    BETOS: D1D   Wheelchairs

D **E1221** Wheelchair with fixed arm, foot rests   DME Y
    BETOS: D1D   Wheelchairs
    DME Modifier: RR

D **E1222** Wheelchair with fixed arm, elevating leg rests   DME Y
    BETOS: D1D   Wheelchairs
    DME Modifier: RR

D **E1223** Wheelchair with detachable arms, foot rests   DME Y
    BETOS: D1D   Wheelchairs
    DME Modifier: RR

D **E1224** Wheelchair with detachable arms, elevating leg rests   DME Y
    BETOS: D1D   Wheelchairs
    DME Modifier: RR

D **E1225** Wheelchair accessory, manual semi-reclining back, (recline greater than 15 degrees, but less than 80 degrees), each   DME Y
    BETOS: D1D   Wheelchairs
    DME Modifier: KU,RR

D **E1226** Wheelchair accessory, manual fully reclining back, (recline greater than 80 degrees), each   DME B
    BETOS: D1D   Wheelchairs
    Service not separately priced by Part B
    DME Modifier: KU,NU,RR,UE

D **E1227** Special height arms for wheelchair   DME Y
    BETOS: D1D   Wheelchairs
    DME Modifier: NU,RR,UE

D **E1228** Special back height for wheelchair   DME Y
    BETOS: D1D   Wheelchairs
    DME Modifier: RR

PEDIATRIC WHEELCHAIRS (E1229-E1239)

C **E1229** Wheelchair, pediatric size, not otherwise specified   Ⓐ Y
    BETOS: D1D   Wheelchairs

D **E1230** Power operated vehicle (three or four wheel nonhighway) specify brand name and model number   DME Y
    BETOS: D1D   Wheelchairs
    DME Modifier: NU,RR,UE

D **E1231** Wheelchair, pediatric size, tilt-in-space, rigid, adjustable, with seating system   DME Ⓐ Y
    BETOS: D1D   Wheelchairs
    DME Modifier: NU,RR,UE

D **E1232** Wheelchair, pediatric size, tilt-in-space, folding, adjustable, with seating system   DME Ⓐ Y
    BETOS: D1D   Wheelchairs
    DME Modifier: RR

D **E1233** Wheelchair, pediatric size, tilt-in-space, rigid, adjustable, without seating system   DME Ⓐ Y
    BETOS: D1D   Wheelchairs
    DME Modifier: RR

D **E1234** Wheelchair, pediatric size, tilt-in-space, folding, adjustable, without seating system   DME Ⓐ Y
    BETOS: D1D   Wheelchairs
    DME Modifier: RR

D **E1235** Wheelchair, pediatric size, rigid, adjustable, with seating system   DME Ⓐ Y
    BETOS: D1D   Wheelchairs
    DME Modifier: RR

D **E1236** Wheelchair, pediatric size, folding, adjustable, with seating system   DME Ⓐ Y
    BETOS: D1D   Wheelchairs
    DME Modifier: RR

D **E1237** Wheelchair, pediatric size, rigid, adjustable, without seating system   DME Ⓐ Y
    BETOS: D1D   Wheelchairs
    DME Modifier: RR

D **E1238** Wheelchair, pediatric size, folding, adjustable, without seating system   DME Ⓐ Y
    BETOS: D1D   Wheelchairs
    DME Modifier: RR

C **E1239** Power wheelchair, pediatric size, not otherwise specified   Ⓐ Y
    BETOS: D1D   Wheelchairs
    Coding Clinic: 2006, Q1

LIGHTWEIGHT WHEELCHAIRS (E1240-E1270)

D **E1240** Lightweight wheelchair, detachable arms, (desk or full length) swing away detachable, elevating leg rest   DME Y
    BETOS: D1D   Wheelchairs
    DME Modifier: RR

I **E1250** Lightweight wheelchair, fixed full length arms, swing away detachable foot rest   E1
    BETOS: D1D   Wheelchairs
    Service not separately priced by Part B

I E1260 Lightweight wheelchair, detachable arms (desk or full length) swing away detachable foot rest   E1
     BETOS: D1D   Wheelchairs
     Service not separately priced by Part B

D E1270 Lightweight wheelchair, fixed full length arms, swing away detachable elevating leg rests   DME   Y
     BETOS: D1D   Wheelchairs
     DME Modifier: RR

HEAVY DUTY AND SPECIAL WHEELCHAIRS (E1280-E1298)

D E1280 Heavy duty wheelchair, detachable arms (desk or full length) elevating leg rests   DME   Y
     BETOS: D1D   Wheelchairs
     DME Modifier: RR

I E1285 Heavy duty wheelchair, fixed full length arms, swing away detachable foot rest   E1
     BETOS: D1D   Wheelchairs
     Service not separately priced by Part B

I E1290 Heavy duty wheelchair, detachable arms (desk or full length) swing away detachable foot rest   E1
     BETOS: D1D   Wheelchairs
     Service not separately priced by Part B

D E1295 Heavy duty wheelchair, fixed full length arms, elevating leg rest   DME   Y
     BETOS: D1D   Wheelchairs
     DME Modifier: RR

D E1296 Special wheelchair seat height from floor   DME   Y
     BETOS: D1D   Wheelchairs
     DME Modifier: NU,RR,UE

D E1297 Special wheelchair seat depth, by upholstery   DME   Y
     BETOS: D1D   Wheelchairs
     DME Modifier: NU,RR,UE

D E1298 Special wheelchair seat depth and/or width, by construction   DME   Y
     BETOS: D1D   Wheelchairs
     DME Modifier: NU,RR,UE

WHIRLPOOL BATHS (E1300, E1310)

M E1300 Whirlpool, portable (overtub-type)   E1
     BETOS: D1E   Other DME
     Service not separately priced by Part B

D E1310 Whirlpool, non-portable (built-in type)   DME   Y
     BETOS: D1E   Other DME
     DME Modifier: NU,RR,UE

ACCESSORIES FOR OXYGEN DELIVERY DEVICES (E1352-E1406)

C E1352 Oxygen accessory, flow regulator capable of positive inspiratory pressure   Y
     BETOS: D1C   Oxygen and supplies
     Service not separately priced by Part B

D E1353 Regulator   DME   Y
     BETOS: D1C   Oxygen and supplies
     Service not separately priced by Part B

C E1354 Oxygen accessory, wheeled cart for portable cylinder or portable concentrator, any type, replacement only, each   Y
     BETOS: D1C   Oxygen and supplies
     Service not separately priced by Part B
     Coding Clinic: 2008, Q4

D E1355 Stand/rack   DME   Y
     BETOS: D1C   Oxygen and supplies
     Service not separately priced by Part B

C E1356 Oxygen accessory, battery pack/cartridge for portable concentrator, any type, replacement only, each   Y
     BETOS: D1C   Oxygen and supplies
     Service not separately priced by Part B
     Coding Clinic: 2008, Q4

C E1357 Oxygen accessory, battery charger for portable concentrator, any type, replacement only, each   Y
     BETOS: D1C   Oxygen and supplies
     Service not separately priced by Part B
     Coding Clinic: 2008, Q4

D E1358 Oxygen accessory, DC power adapter for portable concentrator, any type, replacement only, each   Y
     BETOS: D1C   Oxygen and supplies
     Service not separately priced by Part B
     Coding Clinic: 2008, Q4

D E1372 Immersion external heater for nebulizer   DME   Y
     BETOS: D1E   Other DME
     DME Modifier: NU,RR,UE

D E1390 Oxygen concentrator, single delivery port, capable of delivering 85 percent or greater oxygen concentration at the prescribed flow rate   DME   Y
     BETOS: D1C   Oxygen and supplies
     DME Modifier: QB,QF,RR

D E1391 Oxygen concentrator, dual delivery port, capable of delivering 85 percent or greater oxygen concentration at the prescribed flow rate, each   DME   Y
     BETOS: D1C   Oxygen and supplies
     DME Modifier: QB,QF,RR

D E1392 Portable oxygen concentrator, rental   DME   Y
     BETOS: D1C   Oxygen and supplies
     DME Modifier: QB,QF,RR

E1260 - E1392

DURABLE MEDICAL EQUIPMENT (E0100-E8002)

C **E1399** Durable medical equipment, miscellaneous Y
BETOS: D1E   Other DME
Pub: 100-4, Chapter-32, 110.5

D **E1405** Oxygen and water vapor enriching system
with heated delivery   DME Y
BETOS: D1C   Oxygen and supplies
DME Modifier: RR

D **E1406** Oxygen and water vapor enriching system
without heated delivery   DME Y
BETOS: D1C   Oxygen and supplies
DME Modifier: RR

DIALYSIS SYSTEMS AND ACCESSORIES (E1500-E1699)

D **E1500** Centrifuge, for dialysis   A
BETOS: P9B   Dialysis services (non-Medicare fee schedule)
Service not separately priced by Part B
Coding Clinic: 2002, Q1

D **E1510** Kidney, dialysate delivery system, kidney
machine, pump recirculating, air removal
system, flowrate meter, power off, heater
and temperature control with alarm, IV poles,
pressure gauge, concentrate container   A
BETOS: P9B   Dialysis services (non-Medicare fee schedule)
Service not separately priced by Part B

D **E1520** Heparin infusion pump for hemodialysis   A
BETOS: P9B   Dialysis services (non-Medicare fee schedule)
Service not separately priced by Part B

D **E1530** Air bubble detector for hemodialysis, each,
replacement   A
BETOS: P9B   Dialysis services (non-Medicare fee schedule)
Service not separately priced by Part B

D **E1540** Pressure alarm for hemodialysis, each,
replacement   A
BETOS: P9B   Dialysis services (non-Medicare fee schedule)
Service not separately priced by Part B

D **E1550** Bath conductivity meter for hemodialysis,
each   A
BETOS: P9B   Dialysis services (non-Medicare fee schedule)
Service not separately priced by Part B

D **E1560** Blood leak detector for hemodialysis, each,
replacement   A
BETOS: P9B   Dialysis services (non-Medicare fee schedule)
Service not separately priced by Part B

D **E1570** Adjustable chair, for ESRD patients   A
BETOS: P9B   Dialysis services (non-Medicare fee schedule)
Service not separately priced by Part B

D **E1575** Transducer protectors/fluid barriers, for
hemodialysis, any size, per 10   A
BETOS: P9B   Dialysis services
(non-Medicare fee schedule)
Service not separately priced by Part B

D **E1580** Unipuncture control system for
hemodialysis   A
BETOS: P9B   Dialysis services
(non-Medicare fee schedule)
Service not separately priced by Part B

D **E1590** Hemodialysis machine   A
BETOS: P9B   Dialysis services
(non-Medicare fee schedule)
Service not separately priced by Part B

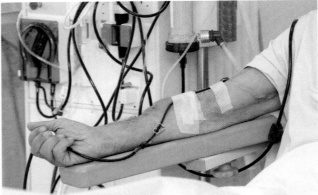

Dialysis medical device

D **E1592** Automatic intermittent peritoneal dialysis
system   A
BETOS: P9B   Dialysis services
(non-Medicare fee schedule)
Service not separately priced by Part B

D **E1594** Cycler dialysis machine for peritoneal
dialysis   A
BETOS: P9B   Dialysis services
(non-Medicare fee schedule)
Service not separately priced by Part B

D **E1600** Delivery and/or installation charges for
hemodialysis equipment   A
BETOS: P9B   Dialysis services
(non-Medicare fee schedule)
Service not separately priced by Part B

D **E1610** Reverse osmosis water purification system,
for hemodialysis   A
BETOS: P9B   Dialysis services
(non-Medicare fee schedule)
Service not separately priced by Part B

D **E1615** Deionizer water purification system, for
hemodialysis   A
BETOS: P9B   Dialysis services
(non-Medicare fee schedule)
Service not separately priced by Part B

● New code   ▲ Revised code   **C** Carrier judgment   **D** Special coverage instructions apply
I Not payable by Medicare   **M** Non-covered by Medicare   **S** Non-covered by Medicare statute   AHA Coding Clinic®

D **E1620** Blood pump for hemodialysis, replacement A
BETOS: P9B   Dialysis services (non-Medicare fee schedule)
Service not separately priced by Part B

D **E1625** Water softening system, for hemodialysis A
BETOS: P9B   Dialysis services (non-Medicare fee schedule)
Service not separately priced by Part B

C **E1630** Reciprocating peritoneal dialysis system A
BETOS: P9B   Dialysis services (non-Medicare fee schedule)
Service not separately priced by Part B

D **E1632** Wearable artificial kidney, each A
BETOS: P9B   Dialysis services (non-Medicare fee schedule)
Service not separately priced by Part B

D **E1634** Peritoneal dialysis clamps, each B
BETOS: P9B   Dialysis services (non-Medicare fee schedule)
Service not separately priced by Part B

D **E1635** Compact (portable) travel hemodialyzer system A
BETOS: P9B   Dialysis services (non-Medicare fee schedule)
Service not separately priced by Part B

D **E1636** Sorbent cartridges, for hemodialysis, per 10 A
BETOS: P9B   Dialysis services (non-Medicare fee schedule)
Service not separately priced by Part B

D **E1637** Hemostats, each A
BETOS: P9B   Dialysis services (non-Medicare fee schedule)
Service not separately priced by Part B
Coding Clinic: 2002, Q1

D **E1639** Scale, each A
BETOS: P9B   Dialysis services (non-Medicare fee schedule)
Service not separately priced by Part B
Coding Clinic: 2002, Q1

D **E1699** Dialysis equipment, not otherwise specified A
BETOS: P9B   Dialysis services (non-Medicare fee schedule)
Service not separately priced by Part B

JAW MOTION REHABILITATION SYSTEMS (E1700-E1702)

C **E1700** Jaw motion rehabilitation system DME Y
BETOS: D1E   Other DME
DME Modifier: RR

C **E1701** Replacement cushions for jaw motion rehabilitation system, pkg. of 6 DME Y
BETOS: D1E   Other DME

C **E1702** Replacement measuring scales for jaw motion rehabilitation system, pkg. of 200 DME Y
BETOS: D1E   Other DME

EXTENSION/FLEXION REHABILITATION DEVICES (E1800-E1841)

C **E1800** Dynamic adjustable elbow extension/flexion device, includes soft interface material DME Y
BETOS: D1E   Other DME
DME Modifier: RR

C **E1801** Static progressive stretch elbow device, extension and/or flexion, with or without range of motion adjustment, includes all components and accessories DME Y
BETOS: D1E   Other DME
DME Modifier: RR
Coding Clinic: 2002, Q1

C **E1802** Dynamic adjustable forearm pronation/ supination device, includes soft interface material DME Y
BETOS: D1E   Other DME
DME Modifier: RR

C **E1805** Dynamic adjustable wrist extension / flexion device, includes soft interface material DME Y
BETOS: D1E   Other DME
DME Modifier: RR

C **E1806** Static progressive stretch wrist device, flexion and/or extension, with or without range of motion adjustment, includes all components and accessories DME Y
BETOS: D1E   Other DME
DME Modifier: RR
Coding Clinic: 2002, Q1

C **E1810** Dynamic adjustable knee extension / flexion device, includes soft interface material DME Y
BETOS: D1E   Other DME
DME Modifier: RR

C **E1811** Static progressive stretch knee device, extension and/or flexion, with or without range of motion adjustment, includes all components and accessories DME Y
BETOS: D1E   Other DME
DME Modifier: RR
Coding Clinic: 2002, Q1

C **E1812** Dynamic knee, extension/flexion device with active resistance control DME Y
BETOS: D1E   Other DME
DME Modifier: RR

C **E1815** Dynamic adjustable ankle extension/flexion device, includes soft interface material DME Y
BETOS: D1E   Other DME
DME Modifier: RR

E1816 - E2205 *(side tab)*

DURABLE MEDICAL EQUIPMENT (E0100-E8002) *(side tab)*

C **E1816** Static progressive stretch ankle device, flexion and/or extension, with or without range of motion adjustment, includes all components and accessories   DME   Y
    BETOS: D1E   Other DME
    DME Modifier: RR
    Coding Clinic: 2002, Q1

C **E1818** Static progressive stretch forearm pronation/supination device, with or without range of motion adjustment, includes all components and accessories   DME   Y
    BETOS: D1E   Other DME
    DME Modifier: RR
    Coding Clinic: 2002, Q1

C **E1820** Replacement soft interface material, dynamic adjustable extension/flexion device   DME   Y
    BETOS: D1E   Other DME
    DME Modifier: NU,RR,UE

C **E1821** Replacement soft interface material/cuffs for bi-directional static progressive stretch device   DME   Y
    BETOS: D1E   Other DME
    DME Modifier: NU,RR,UE
    Coding Clinic: 2002, Q1

C **E1825** Dynamic adjustable finger extension/flexion device, includes soft interface material   DME   Y
    BETOS: D1E   Other DME
    DME Modifier: RR

C **E1830** Dynamic adjustable toe extension/flexion device, includes soft interface material   DME   Y
    BETOS: D1E   Other DME
    DME Modifier: RR

C **E1831** Static progressive stretch toe device, extension and/or flexion, with or without range of motion adjustment, includes all components and accessories   DME   Y
    BETOS: D1E   Other DME
    DME Modifier: RR

C **E1840** Dynamic adjustable shoulder flexion / abduction / rotation device, includes soft interface material   DME   Y
    BETOS: D1E   Other DME
    DME Modifier: RR
    Coding Clinic: 2002, Q1

C **E1841** Static progressive stretch shoulder device, with or without range of motion adjustment, includes all components and accessories   DME   Y
    BETOS: D1E   Other DME
    DME Modifier: RR

COMMUNICATION BOARDS (E1902)

C **E1902** Communication board, non-electronic augmentative or alternative communication device   Y
    BETOS: Z2   Undefined codes
    Service not separately priced by Part B
    Coding Clinic: 2002, Q1

MISCELLANEOUS PUMPS AND MONITORS (E2000-E2120)

C **E2000** Gastric suction pump, home model, portable or stationary, electric   DME   Y
    BETOS: D1E   Other DME
    DME Modifier: RR
    Coding Clinic: 2002, Q1

D **E2100** Blood glucose monitor with integrated voice synthesizer   DME   Y
    BETOS: D1E   Other DME
    DME Modifier: NU,RR,UE
    Coding Clinic: 2002, Q1

D **E2101** Blood glucose monitor with integrated lancing/blood sample   DME   Y
    BETOS: D1E   Other DME
    DME Modifier: NU,RR,UE
    Coding Clinic: 2002, Q1

C **E2120** Pulse generator system for tympanic treatment of inner ear endolymphatic fluid   DME   Y
    BETOS: D1E   Other DME
    DME Modifier: RR

MANUAL WHEELCHAIR ACCESSORIES (E2201-E2295)

C **E2201** Manual wheelchair accessory, nonstandard seat frame, width greater than or equal to 20 inches and less than 24 inches   DME   Y
    BETOS: D1D   Wheelchairs
    DME Modifier: KU,NU,RR,UE

C **E2202** Manual wheelchair accessory, nonstandard seat frame width, 24-27 inches   DME   Y
    BETOS: D1D   Wheelchairs
    DME Modifier: KU,NU,RR,UE

C **E2203** Manual wheelchair accessory, nonstandard seat frame depth, 20 to less than 22 inches   DME   Y
    BETOS: D1D   Wheelchairs
    DME Modifier: KU,NU,RR,UE

C **E2204** Manual wheelchair accessory, nonstandard seat frame depth, 22 to 25 inches   DME   Y
    BETOS: D1D   Wheelchairs
    DME Modifier: KU,NU,RR,UE

C **E2205** Manual wheelchair accessory, handrim without projections (includes ergonomic or contoured), any type, replacement only, each   DME   Y
    BETOS: D1D   Wheelchairs
    DME Modifier: KU,NU,RR,UE

● New code   ▲ Revised code   **C** Carrier judgment   **D** Special coverage instructions apply
I Not payable by Medicare   **M** Non-covered by Medicare   **S** Non-covered by Medicare statute   AHA Coding Clinic®

C E2206 Manual wheelchair accessory, wheel lock assembly, complete, replacement only, each   **DME** Y

    BETOS: D1D   Wheelchairs

    DME Modifier: KU,NU,RR,UE

C E2207 Wheelchair accessory, crutch and cane holder, each   **DME** Y

    BETOS: D1D   Wheelchairs

    DME Modifier: KU,NU,RR,UE

C E2208 Wheelchair accessory, cylinder tank carrier, each   **DME** Y

    BETOS: D1D   Wheelchairs

    DME Modifier: KE,KU,NU,RR,UE

C E2209 Accessory, arm trough, with or without hand support, each   **DME** Y

    BETOS: D1D   Wheelchairs

    DME Modifier: KE,KU,NU,RR,UE

C E2210 Wheelchair accessory, bearings, any type, replacement only, each   **DME** Y

    BETOS: D1D   Wheelchairs

    DME Modifier: KE,KU,NU,RR,UE

C E2211 Manual wheelchair accessory, pneumatic propulsion tire, any size, each   **DME** Y

    BETOS: D1D   Wheelchairs

    DME Modifier: KU,NU,RR,UE

C E2212 Manual wheelchair accessory, tube for pneumatic propulsion tire, any size, each   **DME** Y

    BETOS: D1D   Wheelchairs

    DME Modifier: KU,NU,RR,UE

C E2213 Manual wheelchair accessory, insert for pneumatic propulsion tire (removable), any type, any size, each   **DME** Y

    BETOS: D1D   Wheelchairs

    DME Modifier: KU,NU,RR,UE

C E2214 Manual wheelchair accessory, pneumatic caster tire, any size, each   **DME** Y

    BETOS: D1D   Wheelchairs

    DME Modifier: KU,NU,RR,UE

C E2215 Manual wheelchair accessory, tube for pneumatic caster tire, any size, each   **DME** Y

    BETOS: D1D   Wheelchairs

    DME Modifier: KU,NU,RR,UE

C E2216 Manual wheelchair accessory, foam filled propulsion tire, any size, each   **DME** Y

    BETOS: D1D   Wheelchairs

    DME Modifier: KU,NU,RR,UE

C E2217 Manual wheelchair accessory, foam filled caster tire, any size, each   **DME** Y

    BETOS: D1D   Wheelchairs

    DME Modifier: KU,NU,RR,UE

C E2218 Manual wheelchair accessory, foam propulsion tire, any size, each   **DME** Y

    BETOS: D1D   Wheelchairs

    DME Modifier: KU,NU,RR,UE

C E2219 Manual wheelchair accessory, foam caster tire, any size, each   **DME** Y

    BETOS: D1D   Wheelchairs

    DME Modifier: KU,NU,RR,UE

C E2220 Manual wheelchair accessory, solid (rubber/plastic) propulsion tire, any size, replacement only, each   **DME** Y

    BETOS: D1D   Wheelchairs

    DME Modifier: KU,NU,RR,UE

C E2221 Manual wheelchair accessory, solid (rubber/plastic) caster tire (removable), any size, replacement only, each   **DME** Y

    BETOS: D1D   Wheelchairs

    DME Modifier: KU,NU,RR,UE

C E2222 Manual wheelchair accessory, solid (rubber/plastic) caster tire with integrated wheel, any size, replacement only, each   **DME** Y

    BETOS: D1D   Wheelchairs

    DME Modifier: KU,NU,RR,UE

C E2224 Manual wheelchair accessory, propulsion wheel excludes tire, any size, replacement only, each   **DME** Y

    BETOS: D1D   Wheelchairs

    DME Modifier: KU,NU,RR,UE

C E2225 Manual wheelchair accessory, caster wheel excludes tire, any size, replacement only, each   **DME** Y

    BETOS: D1D   Wheelchairs

    DME Modifier: KU,NU,RR,UE

C E2226 Manual wheelchair accessory, caster fork, any size, replacement only, each   **DME** Y

    BETOS: D1D   Wheelchairs

    DME Modifier: KU,NU,RR,UE

C E2227 Manual wheelchair accessory, gear reduction drive wheel, each   **DME** Y

    BETOS: D1D   Wheelchairs

    DME Modifier: RR

C E2228 Manual wheelchair accessory, wheel braking system and lock, complete, each   **DME** Y

    BETOS: D1D   Wheelchairs

    DME Modifier: KU,RR

C E2230 Manual wheelchair accessory, manual standing system   Y

    BETOS: D1D   Wheelchairs

    Service not separately priced by Part B

    Coding Clinic: 2008, Q4

C E2231 Manual wheelchair accessory, solid seat support base (replaces sling seat), includes any type mounting hardware   **DME** Y

    BETOS: D1D   Wheelchairs

    DME Modifier: KU,NU,RR,UE

    Coding Clinic: 2008, Q4

♂ Male only   ♀ Female only   **A** Age   A2 - Z3 = ASC Payment indicator   A - Y = APC Status indicator

ASC = ASC Approved Procedure   **DME** Paid under the DME fee schedule   **MIPS** MIPS code

C E2291 Back, planar, for pediatric size wheelchair including fixed attaching hardware Ⓐ Y
BETOS: D1D   Wheelchairs

C E2292 Seat, planar, for pediatric size wheelchair including fixed attaching hardware Ⓐ Y
BETOS: D1D   Wheelchairs

C E2293 Back, contoured, for pediatric size wheelchair including fixed attaching hardware Ⓐ Y
BETOS: D1D   Wheelchairs

C E2294 Seat, contoured, for pediatric size wheelchair including fixed attaching hardware Ⓐ Y
BETOS: D1D   Wheelchairs

C E2295 Manual wheelchair accessory, for pediatric size wheelchair, dynamic seating frame, allows coordinated movement of multiple positioning features Ⓐ Y
BETOS: D1D   Wheelchairs
Coding Clinic: 2008, Q4

POWER WHEELCHAIR ACCESSORIES (E2300-E2398)

C E2300 Wheelchair accessory, power seat elevation system, any type Y
BETOS: D1D   Wheelchairs

C E2301 Wheelchair accessory, power standing system, any type Y
BETOS: D1D   Wheelchairs
Service not separately priced by Part B

C E2310 Power wheelchair accessory, electronic connection between wheelchair controller and one power seating system motor, including all related electronics, indicator feature, mechanical function selection switch, and fixed mounting hardware DME Y
BETOS: D1D   Wheelchairs
DME Modifier: KE,KU,RR

C E2311 Power wheelchair accessory, electronic connection between wheelchair controller and two or more power seating system motors, including all related electronics, indicator feature, mechanical function selection switch, and fixed mounting hardware DME Y
BETOS: D1D   Wheelchairs
DME Modifier: KE,KU,RR

C E2312 Power wheelchair accessory, hand or chin control interface, mini-proportional remote joystick, proportional, including fixed mounting hardware DME Y
BETOS: D1D   Wheelchairs
DME Modifier: KC,RR

C E2313 Power wheelchair accessory, harness for upgrade to expandable controller, including all fasteners, connectors and mounting hardware, each DME Y
BETOS: D1D   Wheelchairs
DME Modifier: RR

C E2321 Power wheelchair accessory, hand control interface, remote joystick, nonproportional, including all related electronics, mechanical stop switch, and fixed mounting hardware DME Y
BETOS: D1D   Wheelchairs
DME Modifier: KC,KE,KU,RR

C E2322 Power wheelchair accessory, hand control interface, multiple mechanical switches, nonproportional, including all related electronics, mechanical stop switch, and fixed mounting hardware DME Y
BETOS: D1D   Wheelchairs
DME Modifier: KC,KE,KU,RR

C E2323 Power wheelchair accessory, specialty joystick handle for hand control interface, prefabricated DME Y
BETOS: D1D   Wheelchairs
DME Modifier: KE,KU,NU,RR,UE

C E2324 Power wheelchair accessory, chin cup for chin control interface DME Y
BETOS: D1D   Wheelchairs
DME Modifier: KE,KU,NU,RR,UE

C E2325 Power wheelchair accessory, sip and puff interface, nonproportional, including all related electronics, mechanical stop switch, and manual swingaway mounting hardware DME Y
BETOS: D1D   Wheelchairs
DME Modifier: KE,KU,RR

C E2326 Power wheelchair accessory, breath tube kit for sip and puff interface DME Y
BETOS: D1D   Wheelchairs
DME Modifier: KE,KU,RR

C E2327 Power wheelchair accessory, head control interface, mechanical, proportional, including all related electronics, mechanical direction change switch, and fixed mounting hardware DME Y
BETOS: D1D   Wheelchairs
DME Modifier: KC,KE,KU,RR

C E2328 Power wheelchair accessory, head control or extremity control interface, electronic, proportional, including all related electronics and fixed mounting hardware DME Y
BETOS: D1D   Wheelchairs
DME Modifier: KE,KU,RR

C E2329 Power wheelchair accessory, head control interface, contact switch mechanism, nonproportional, including all related electronics, mechanical stop switch, mechanical direction change switch, head array, and fixed mounting hardware DME Y
BETOS: D1D   Wheelchairs
DME Modifier: KE,KU,RR

C **E2330** Power wheelchair accessory, head control interface, proximity switch mechanism, nonproportional, including all related electronics, mechanical stop switch, mechanical direction change switch, head array, and fixed mounting hardware **DME** Y
BETOS: D1D   Wheelchairs
DME Modifier: KE,KU,RR

C **E2331** Power wheelchair accessory, attendant control, proportional, including all related electronics and fixed mounting hardware   Y
BETOS: D1D   Wheelchairs

C **E2340** Power wheelchair accessory, nonstandard seat frame width, 20-23 inches **DME** Y
BETOS: D1D   Wheelchairs
DME Modifier: NU,RR,UE

C **E2341** Power wheelchair accessory, nonstandard seat frame width, 24-27 inches **DME** Y
BETOS: D1D   Wheelchairs
DME Modifier: NU,RR,UE

C **E2342** Power wheelchair accessory, nonstandard seat frame depth, 20 or 21 inches **DME** Y
BETOS: D1D   Wheelchairs
DME Modifier: NU,RR,UE

C **E2343** Power wheelchair accessory, nonstandard seat frame depth, 22-25 inches **DME** Y
BETOS: D1D   Wheelchairs
DME Modifier: NU,RR,UE

C **E2351** Power wheelchair accessory, electronic interface to operate speech generating device using power wheelchair control interface **DME** Y
BETOS: D1D   Wheelchairs
DME Modifier: KE,KU,NU,RR,UE

C **E2358** Power wheelchair accessory, group 34 non-sealed lead acid battery, each   Y
BETOS: D1D   Wheelchairs

C **E2359** Power wheelchair accessory, group 34 sealed lead acid battery, each (e.g., gel cell, absorbed glassmat) **DME** Y
BETOS: D1D   Wheelchairs
DME Modifier: KU,NU,RR,UE

C **E2360** Power wheelchair accessory, 22 NF non-sealed lead acid battery, each **DME** Y
BETOS: D1D   Wheelchairs
DME Modifier: KU,NU,RR,UE

C **E2361** Power wheelchair accessory, 22 NF sealed lead acid battery, each, (e.g., gel cell, absorbed glassmat) **DME** Y
BETOS: D1D   Wheelchairs
DME Modifier: KE,KU,NU,RR,UE

C **E2362** Power wheelchair accessory, group 24 non-sealed lead acid battery, each **DME** Y
BETOS: D1D   Wheelchairs
DME Modifier: KU,NU,RR,UE

C **E2363** Power wheelchair accessory, group 24 sealed lead acid battery, each (e.g., gel cell, absorbed glassmat) **DME** Y
BETOS: D1D   Wheelchairs
DME Modifier: KE,KU,NU,RR,UE

C **E2364** Power wheelchair accessory, U-1 non-sealed lead acid battery, each **DME** Y
BETOS: D1D   Wheelchairs
DME Modifier: KU,NU,RR,UE

C **E2365** Power wheelchair accessory, U-1 sealed lead acid battery, each (e.g., gel cell, absorbed glassmat) **DME** Y
BETOS: D1D   Wheelchairs
DME Modifier: KE,KU,NU,RR,UE

C **E2366** Power wheelchair accessory, battery charger, single mode, for use with only one battery type, sealed or non-sealed, each **DME** Y
BETOS: D1D   Wheelchairs
DME Modifier: KE,KU,NU,RR,UE

C **E2367** Power wheelchair accessory, battery charger, dual mode, for use with either battery type, sealed or non-sealed, each **DME** Y
BETOS: D1D   Wheelchairs
DME Modifier: KE,KU,NU,RR,UE

C **E2368** Power wheelchair component, drive wheel motor, replacement only **DME** Y
BETOS: D1D   Wheelchairs
DME Modifier: KE,KU,RR

C **E2369** Power wheelchair component, drive wheel gear box, replacement only **DME** Y
BETOS: D1D   Wheelchairs
DME Modifier: KE,KU,RR

C **E2370** Power wheelchair component, integrated drive wheel motor and gear box combination, replacement only **DME** Y
BETOS: D1D   Wheelchairs
DME Modifier: KE,KU,RR

C **E2371** Power wheelchair accessory, group 27 sealed lead acid battery, (e.g., gel cell, absorbed glassmat), each **DME** Y
BETOS: D1D   Wheelchairs
DME Modifier: KE,KU,NU,RR,UE

C **E2372** Power wheelchair accessory, group 27 non-sealed lead acid battery, each **DME** Y
BETOS: D1D   Wheelchairs
DME Modifier: NU,RR,UE

C **E2373** Power wheelchair accessory, hand or chin control interface, compact remote joystick, proportional, including fixed mounting hardware **DME** Y
BETOS: D1D   Wheelchairs
DME Modifier: KC,KE,KU,RR

D **E2374** Power wheelchair accessory, hand or chin control interface, standard remote joystick (not including controller), proportional, including all related electronics and fixed mounting hardware, replacement only **DME** Y

    BETOS: D1D   Wheelchairs

    DME Modifier: KE,KU,RR

D **E2375** Power wheelchair accessory, non-expandable controller, including all related electronics and mounting hardware, replacement only **DME** Y

    BETOS: D1D   Wheelchairs

    DME Modifier: KE,KU,RR

D **E2376** Power wheelchair accessory, expandable controller, including all related electronics and mounting hardware, replacement only **DME** Y

    BETOS: D1D   Wheelchairs

    DME Modifier: KE,KU,RR

D **E2377** Power wheelchair accessory, expandable controller, including all related electronics and mounting hardware, upgrade provided at initial issue **DME** Y

    BETOS: D1D   Wheelchairs

    DME Modifier: KE,KU,RR

C **E2378** Power wheelchair component, actuator, replacement only **DME** Y

    BETOS: D1D   Wheelchairs

    DME Modifier: KU,RR

D **E2381** Power wheelchair accessory, pneumatic drive wheel tire, any size, replacement only, each **DME** Y

    BETOS: D1D   Wheelchairs

    DME Modifier: KE,KU,NU,RR,UE

D **E2382** Power wheelchair accessory, tube for pneumatic drive wheel tire, any size, replacement only, each **DME** Y

    BETOS: D1D   Wheelchairs

    DME Modifier: KE,KU,NU,RR,UE

D **E2383** Power wheelchair accessory, insert for pneumatic drive wheel tire (removable), any type, any size, replacement only, each **DME** Y

    BETOS: D1D   Wheelchairs

    DME Modifier: KE,KU,NU,RR,UE

D **E2384** Power wheelchair accessory, pneumatic caster tire, any size, replacement only, each **DME** Y

    BETOS: D1D   Wheelchairs

    DME Modifier: KE,KU,NU,RR,UE

D **E2385** Power wheelchair accessory, tube for pneumatic caster tire, any size, replacement only, each **DME** Y

    BETOS: D1D   Wheelchairs

    DME Modifier: KE,KU,NU,RR,UE

D **E2386** Power wheelchair accessory, foam filled drive wheel tire, any size, replacement only, each **DME** Y

    BETOS: D1D   Wheelchairs

    DME Modifier: KE,KU,NU,RR,UE

D **E2387** Power wheelchair accessory, foam filled caster tire, any size, replacement only, each **DME** Y

    BETOS: D1D   Wheelchairs

    DME Modifier: KE,KU,NU,RR,UE

D **E2388** Power wheelchair accessory, foam drive wheel tire, any size, replacement only, each **DME** Y

    BETOS: D1D   Wheelchairs

    DME Modifier: KE,KU,NU,RR,UE

D **E2389** Power wheelchair accessory, foam caster tire, any size, replacement only, each **DME** Y

    BETOS: D1D   Wheelchairs

    DME Modifier: KE,KU,NU,RR,UE

D **E2390** Power wheelchair accessory, solid (rubber/plastic) drive wheel tire, any size, replacement only, each **DME** Y

    BETOS: D1D   Wheelchairs

    DME Modifier: KE,KU,NU,RR,UE

D **E2391** Power wheelchair accessory, solid (rubber/plastic) caster tire (removable), any size, replacement only, each **DME** Y

    BETOS: D1D   Wheelchairs

    DME Modifier: KE,KU,NU,RR,UE

D **E2392** Power wheelchair accessory, solid (rubber/plastic) caster tire with integrated wheel, any size, replacement only, each **DME** Y

    BETOS: D1D   Wheelchairs

    DME Modifier: KE,KU,NU,RR,UE

D **E2394** Power wheelchair accessory, drive wheel excludes tire, any size, replacement only, each **DME** Y

    BETOS: D1D   Wheelchairs

    DME Modifier: KE,KU,NU,RR,UE

D **E2395** Power wheelchair accessory, caster wheel excludes tire, any size, replacement only, each **DME** Y

    BETOS: D1D   Wheelchairs

    DME Modifier: KE,KU,NU,RR,UE

D **E2396** Power wheelchair accessory, caster fork, any size, replacement only, each **DME** Y

    BETOS: D1D   Wheelchairs

    DME Modifier: KE,KU,NU,RR,UE

C **E2397** Power wheelchair accessory, lithium-based battery, each **DME** Y

    BETOS: D1D   Wheelchairs

    DME Modifier: KU,NU,RR,UE

C **E2398** Wheelchair accessory, dynamic positioning hardware for back Y

    BETOS: D1D   Wheelchairs

● New code   ▲ Revised code   **C** Carrier judgment   **D** Special coverage instructions apply

I Not payable by Medicare   **M** Non-covered by Medicare   **S** Non-covered by Medicare statute   AHA Coding Clinic®

WOUND THERAPY PUMPS (E2402)

C **E2402** Negative pressure wound therapy electrical pump, stationary or portable `DME` Y
BETOS: D1E   Other DME
DME Modifier: RR

SPEECH GENERATING DEVICES, SOFTWARE, AND ACCESSORIES (E2500-E2599)

D **E2500** Speech generating device, digitized speech, using pre-recorded messages, less than or equal to 8 minutes recording time `DME` Y
BETOS: D1E   Other DME
DME Modifier: NU,RR,UE

D **E2502** Speech generating device, digitized speech, using pre-recorded messages, greater than 8 minutes but less than or equal to 20 minutes recording time `DME` Y
BETOS: D1E   Other DME
DME Modifier: NU,RR,UE

D **E2504** Speech generating device, digitized speech, using pre-recorded messages, greater than 20 minutes but less than or equal to 40 minutes recording time `DME` Y
BETOS: D1E   Other DME
DME Modifier: NU,RR,UE

D **E2506** Speech generating device, digitized speech, using pre-recorded messages, greater than 40 minutes recording time `DME` Y
BETOS: D1E   Other DME
DME Modifier: NU,RR,UE

D **E2508** Speech generating device, synthesized speech, requiring message formulation by spelling and access by physical contact with the device `DME` Y
BETOS: D1E   Other DME
DME Modifier: NU,RR,UE

D **E2510** Speech generating device, synthesized speech, permitting multiple methods of message formulation and multiple methods of device access `DME` Y
BETOS: D1E   Other DME
DME Modifier: NU,RR,UE

D **E2511** Speech generating software program, for personal computer or personal digital assistant `DME` Y
BETOS: D1E   Other DME
DME Modifier: NU,RR,UE

D **E2512** Accessory for speech generating device, mounting system `DME` Y
BETOS: D1E   Other DME
DME Modifier: NU,RR,UE

D **E2599** Accessory for speech generating device, not otherwise classified Y
BETOS: D1E   Other DME

WHEELCHAIR SEAT AND BACK CUSHIONS (E2601-E2625)

C **E2601** General use wheelchair seat cushion, width less than 22 inches, any depth `DME` Y
BETOS: D1D   Wheelchairs
DME Modifier: KE,KU,NU,RR,UE

C **E2602** General use wheelchair seat cushion, width 22 inches or greater, any depth `DME` Y
BETOS: D1D   Wheelchairs
DME Modifier: KE,KU,NU,RR,UE

C **E2603** Skin protection wheelchair seat cushion, width less than 22 inches, any depth `DME` Y
BETOS: D1D   Wheelchairs
DME Modifier: KE,KU,NU,RR,UE

C **E2604** Skin protection wheelchair seat cushion, width 22 inches or greater, any depth `DME` Y
BETOS: D1D   Wheelchairs
DME Modifier: KE,KU,NU,RR,UE

C **E2605** Positioning wheelchair seat cushion, width less than 22 inches, any depth `DME` Y
BETOS: D1D   Wheelchairs
DME Modifier: KE,KU,NU,RR,UE

C **E2606** Positioning wheelchair seat cushion, width 22 inches or greater, any depth `DME` Y
BETOS: D1D   Wheelchairs
DME Modifier: KE,KU,NU,RR,UE

C **E2607** Skin protection and positioning wheelchair seat cushion, width less than 22 inches, any depth `DME` Y
BETOS: D1D   Wheelchairs
DME Modifier: KE,KU,NU,RR,UE

C **E2608** Skin protection and positioning wheelchair seat cushion, width 22 inches or greater, any depth `DME` Y
BETOS: D1D   Wheelchairs
DME Modifier: KE,KU,NU,RR,UE

C **E2609** Custom fabricated wheelchair seat cushion, any size Y
BETOS: D1D   Wheelchairs

C **E2610** Wheelchair seat cushion, powered B
BETOS: D1D   Wheelchairs

C **E2611** General use wheelchair back cushion, width less than 22 inches, any height, including any type mounting hardware `DME` Y
BETOS: D1D   Wheelchairs
DME Modifier: KE,KU,NU,RR,UE

C **E2612** General use wheelchair back cushion, width 22 inches or greater, any height, including any type mounting hardware `DME` Y
BETOS: D1D   Wheelchairs
DME Modifier: KE,KU,NU,RR,UE

♂ Male only   ♀ Female only   **A** Age   A2 - Z3 = ASC Payment indicator   A - Y = APC Status indicator
ASC = ASC Approved Procedure   `DME` Paid under the DME fee schedule   `MIPS` MIPS code

C E2613 Positioning wheelchair back cushion, posterior, width less than 22 inches, any height, including any type mounting hardware `DME` Y
   BETOS: D1D   Wheelchairs
   DME Modifier: KE,KU,NU,RR,UE

C E2614 Positioning wheelchair back cushion, posterior, width 22 inches or greater, any height, including any type mounting hardware `DME` Y
   BETOS: D1D   Wheelchairs
   DME Modifier: KE,KU,NU,RR,UE

C E2615 Positioning wheelchair back cushion, posterior-lateral, width less than 22 inches, any height, including any type mounting hardware `DME` Y
   BETOS: D1D   Wheelchairs
   DME Modifier: KE,KU,NU,RR,UE

C E2616 Positioning wheelchair back cushion, posterior-lateral, width 22 inches or greater, any height, including any type mounting hardware `DME` Y
   BETOS: D1D   Wheelchairs
   DME Modifier: KE,KU,NU,RR,UE

C E2617 Custom fabricated wheelchair back cushion, any size, including any type mounting hardware   Y
   BETOS: D1D   Wheelchairs

C E2619 Replacement cover for wheelchair seat cushion or back cushion, each `DME` Y
   BETOS: D1D   Wheelchairs
   DME Modifier: KE,KU,NU,RR,UE

C E2620 Positioning wheelchair back cushion, planar back with lateral supports, width less than 22 inches, any height, including any type mounting hardware `DME` Y
   BETOS: D1D   Wheelchairs
   DME Modifier: KE,KU,NU,RR,UE

C E2621 Positioning wheelchair back cushion, planar back with lateral supports, width 22 inches or greater, any height, including any type mounting hardware `DME` Y
   BETOS: D1D   Wheelchairs
   DME Modifier: KE,KU,NU,RR,UE

C E2622 Skin protection wheelchair seat cushion, adjustable, width less than 22 inches, any depth `DME` Y
   BETOS: D1D   Wheelchairs
   DME Modifier: KE,KU,NU,RR,UE

C E2623 Skin protection wheelchair seat cushion, adjustable, width 22 inches or greater, any depth `DME` Y
   BETOS: D1D   Wheelchairs
   DME Modifier: KE,KU,NU,RR,UE

C E2624 Skin protection and positioning wheelchair seat cushion, adjustable, width less than 22 inches, any depth `DME` Y
   BETOS: D1D   Wheelchairs
   DME Modifier: KE,KU,NU,RR,UE

C E2625 Skin protection and positioning wheelchair seat cushion, adjustable, width 22 inches or greater, any depth `DME` Y
   BETOS: D1D   Wheelchairs
   DME Modifier: KE,KU,NU,RR,UE

WHEELCHAIR MOBILE ARM SUPPORTS (E2626-E2633)

C E2626 Wheelchair accessory, shoulder elbow, mobile arm support attached to wheelchair, balanced, adjustable `DME` Y
   BETOS: D1D   Wheelchairs
   DME Modifier: KU,NU,RR,UE

C E2627 Wheelchair accessory, shoulder elbow, mobile arm support attached to wheelchair, balanced, adjustable rancho type `DME` Y
   BETOS: D1D   Wheelchairs
   DME Modifier: KU,NU,RR,UE

C E2628 Wheelchair accessory, shoulder elbow, mobile arm support attached to wheelchair, balanced, reclining `DME` Y
   BETOS: D1D   Wheelchairs
   DME Modifier: KU,NU,RR,UE

C E2629 Wheelchair accessory, shoulder elbow, mobile arm support attached to wheelchair, balanced, friction arm support (friction dampening to proximal and distal joints) `DME` Y
   BETOS: D1D   Wheelchairs
   DME Modifier: KU,NU,RR,UE

C E2630 Wheelchair accessory, shoulder elbow, mobile arm support, mono suspension arm and hand support, overhead elbow forearm hand sling support, yoke type suspension support `DME` Y
   BETOS: D1D   Wheelchairs
   DME Modifier: KU,NU,RR,UE

C E2631 Wheelchair accessory, addition to mobile arm support, elevating proximal arm `DME` Y
   BETOS: D1D   Wheelchairs
   DME Modifier: KU,NU,RR,UE

C E2632 Wheelchair accessory, addition to mobile arm support, offset or lateral rocker arm with elastic balance control `DME` Y
   BETOS: D1D   Wheelchairs
   DME Modifier: KU,NU,RR,UE

C E2633 Wheelchair accessory, addition to mobile arm support, supinator `DME` Y
   BETOS: D1D   Wheelchairs
   DME Modifier: KU,NU,RR,UE

● New code   ▲ Revised code   **C** Carrier judgment   **D** Special coverage instructions apply
I Not payable by Medicare   **M** Non-covered by Medicare   **S** Non-covered by Medicare statute   AHA Coding Clinic®

CPT® is a registered trademark of the American Medical Association. All rights reserved.

PEDIATRIC GAIT TRAINERS (E8000-E8002)

E8000 Gait trainer, pediatric size, posterior support, includes all accessories and components   Ⓐ E1

       BETOS: Z2   Undefined codes
       Service not separately priced by Part B

E8001 Gait trainer, pediatric size, upright support, includes all accessories and components   Ⓐ E1

       BETOS: Z2   Undefined codes
       Service not separately priced by Part B

E8002 Gait trainer, pediatric size, anterior support, includes all accessories and components   Ⓐ E1

       BETOS: Z2   Undefined codes
       Service not separately priced by Part B

♂ Male only   ♀ Female only   Ⓐ Age   A2 - Z3 = ASC Payment indicator   A - Y = APC Status indicator

ASC = ASC Approved Procedure   **DME** Paid under the DME fee schedule   **MIPS** MIPS code

NOTES

PROCEDURES / PROFESSIONAL SERVICES (G0008-G9987)

VACCINE ADMINISTRATION (G0008-G0010)

[C] G0008 Administration of influenza virus vaccine   S

CPT® Crosswalk: 90460, 90461, 90471, 90472, 90473, 90474, 90630, 90644, 90647, 90648, 90653, 90654, 90655, 90656, 90657, 90658, 90660, 90661, 90662, 90664, 90666, 90667, 90668, 90672, 90673, 90674, 90682, 90685, 90686, 90687, 90688, 90689, 90697, 90749, 90756

BETOS: O1G   Immunizations/Vaccinations
Coding Clinic: 2003, Q2; 2006, Q2; 2009, Q2; 2016, Q4; 2018, Q3
Pub: 100-4, Chapter-18, 10.4.3; 100-4, Chapter-18, 10.4.1; 100-4, Chapter-18, 10.3.1.1; 100-4, Chapter-18, 10.2.5.2; 100-4, Chapter-18, 10.2.1; 100-2, Chapter-12, 40.11

[C] G0009 Administration of pneumococcal vaccine   S

CPT® Crosswalk: 90460, 90461, 90471, 90472, 90473, 90474, 90670, 90732, 90749

BETOS: O1G   Immunizations/Vaccinations
Coding Clinic: 2003, Q2; 2009, Q2; 2016, Q4; 2018, Q3
Pub: 100-4, Chapter-18, 10.4.3; 100-4, Chapter-18, 10.4.1; 100-4, Chapter-18, 10.3.1.1; 100-4, Chapter-18, 10.2.5.2; 100-4, Chapter-18, 10.2.1; 100-2, Chapter-12, 40.11

[C] G0010 Administration of Hepatitis B vaccine   S

CPT® Crosswalk: 90460, 90461, 90471, 90472, 90636, 90697, 90723, 90739, 90740, 90743, 90744, 90746, 90747, 90748, 90749

BETOS: O1G   Immunizations/Vaccinations
Coding Clinic: 2016, Q4; 2018, Q3
Pub: 100-4, Chapter-18, 10.3.1.1; 100-4, Chapter-18, 10.2.5.2; 100-4, Chapter-18, 10.2.1; 100-2, Chapter-12, 40.11

ANALYSIS OF SEMEN SPECIMEN (G0027)

[C] G0027 Semen analysis; presence and/or motility of sperm excluding huhner   ♂ N

BETOS: T1H   Lab tests - other (non-Medicare fee schedule)
Price subject to national limitation amount

PROFESSIONAL SERVICES FOR DRUG INFUSION (G0068-G0070)

▲ [D] G0068 Professional services for the administration of anti-infective, pain management, chelation, pulmonary hypertension, inotropic, or other intravenous infusion drug or biological (excluding chemotherapy or other highly complex drug or biological) for each infusion drug administration calendar day in the individual's home, each 15 minutes   A

BETOS: M4A   Home visit
Price established using national RVUs

▲ [D] G0069 Professional services for the administration of subcutaneous immunotherapy or other subcutaneous infusion drug or biological for each infusion drug administration calendar day in the individual's home, each 15 minutes   A

BETOS: M4A   Home visit
Price established using national RVUs

▲ [D] G0070 Professional services for the administration of intravenous chemotherapy or other intravenous highly complex drug or biological infusion for each infusion drug administration calendar day in the individual's home, each 15 minutes   A

BETOS: M4A   Home visit
Price established using national RVUs

TELEMED SERVICES (G0071)

[C] G0071 Payment for communication technology-based services for 5 minutes or more of a virtual (non-face-to-face) communication between an rural health clinic (RHC) or federally qualified health center (FQHC) practitioner and RHC or FQHC patient, or 5 minutes or more of remote evaluation of recorded video and/or images by an RHC or FQHC practitioner, occurring in lieu of an office visit; RHC or FQHC only   A

BETOS: M5D   Specialist - other
Price established by carriers

HOME CARE MANAGEMENT SERVICES (G0076-G0087)

[C] G0076 Brief (20 minutes) care management home visit for a new patient. For use only in a Medicare-approved CMMI model. (services must be furnished within a beneficiary's home, domiciliary, rest home, assisted living and/or nursing facility)   B

BETOS: M4A   Home visit
Price established by carriers

[C] G0077 Limited (30 minutes) care management home visit for a new patient. For use only in a Medicare-approved CMMI model. (services must be furnished within a beneficiary's home, domiciliary, rest home, assisted living and/or nursing facility)   B

BETOS: M4A   Home visit
Price established by carriers

[C] G0078 Moderate (45 minutes) care management home visit for a new patient. For use only in a Medicare-approved CMMI model. (services must be furnished within a beneficiary's home, domiciliary, rest home, assisted living and/or nursing facility)   B

BETOS: M4A   Home visit
Price established by carriers

♂ Male only   ♀ Female only   Ⓐ Age   A2 - Z3 = ASC Payment indicator   A - Y = APC Status indicator
ASC = ASC Approved Procedure   **DME** Paid under the DME fee schedule   **MIPS** MIPS code

G **G0079** Comprehensive (60 minutes) care management home visit for a new patient. For use only in a Medicare-approved CMMI model. (services must be furnished within a beneficiary's home, domiciliary, rest home, assisted living and/or nursing facility)   B
     BETOS: M4A   Home visit
     Price established by carriers

G **G0080** Extensive (75 minutes) care management home visit for a new patient. For use only in a Medicare-approved CMMI model. (services must be furnished within a beneficiary's home, domiciliary, rest home, assisted living and/or nursing facility)   B
     BETOS: M4A   Home visit
     Price established by carriers

G **G0081** Brief (20 minutes) care management home visit for an existing patient. For use only in a Medicare-approved CMMI model. (services must be furnished within a beneficiary's home, domiciliary, rest home, assisted living and/or nursing facility)   B
     BETOS: M4A   Home visit
     Price established by carriers

G **G0082** Limited (30 minutes) care management home visit for an existing patient. For use only in a Medicare-approved CMMI model. (services must be furnished within a beneficiary's home, domiciliary, rest home, assisted living and/or nursing facility)   B
     BETOS: M4A   Home visit
     Price established by carriers

G **G0083** Moderate (45 minutes) care management home visit for an existing patient. For use only in a Medicare-approved CMMI model. (services must be furnished within a beneficiary's home, domiciliary, rest home, assisted living and/or nursing facility)   B
     BETOS: M4A   Home visit
     Price established by carriers

G **G0084** Comprehensive (60 minutes) care management home visit for an existing patient. For use only in a Medicare-approved CMMI model. (services must be furnished within a beneficiary's home, domiciliary, rest home, assisted living and/or nursing facility)   B
     BETOS: M4A   Home visit
     Price established by carriers

G **G0085** Extensive (75 minutes) care management home visit for an existing patient. For use only in a Medicare-approved CMMI model. (services must be furnished within a beneficiary's home, domiciliary, rest home, assisted living and/or nursing facility)   B
     BETOS: M4A   Home visit
     Price established by carriers

G **G0086** Limited (30 minutes) care management home care plan oversight. For use only in a Medicare-approved CMMI model. (services must be furnished within a beneficiary's home, domiciliary, rest home, assisted living and/or nursing facility)   B
     BETOS: M4A   Home visit
     Price established by carriers

G **G0087** Comprehensive (60 minutes) care management home care plan oversight. For use only in a Medicare-approved CMMI model. (services must be furnished within a beneficiary's home, domiciliary, rest home, assisted living and/or nursing facility)   B
     BETOS: M4A   Home visit
     Price established by carriers

INITIAL VISIT FOR PROFESSIONAL SERVICES (G0088-G0090)

● **D** **G0088** Professional services, initial visit, for the administration of anti-infective, pain management, chelation, pulmonary hypertension, inotropic, or other intravenous infusion drug or biological (excluding chemotherapy or other highly complex drug or biological) for each infusion drug administration calendar day in the individual's home, each 15 minutes   A
     BETOS: M4A   Home visit
     Price established using national RVUs

● **D** **G0089** Professional services, initial visit, for the administration of subcutaneous immunotherapy or other subcutaneous infusion drug or biological for each infusion drug administration calendar day in the individual's home, each 15 minutes   A
     BETOS: M4A   Home visit
     Price established using national RVUs

● **D** **G0090** Professional services, initial visit, for the administration of intravenous chemotherapy or other highly complex infusion drug or biological for each infusion drug administration calendar day in the individual's home, each 15 minutes   A
     BETOS: M4A   Home visit
     Price established using national RVUs

SCREENING EXAMINATIONS AND DISEASE MANAGEMENT TRAINING (G0101-G0124)

D **G0101** Cervical or vaginal cancer screening; pelvic and clinical breast examination   ♀ S **MIPS**
     CPT® Crosswalk: 99384, 99385, 99386, 99387, 99394, 99395, 99396, 99397, 0009U, 0045U, 0422T
     BETOS: M1A   Office visits - new
     Price established using national RVUs
     Coding Clinic: 2001, Q3; 2002, Q4; 2008, Q3

● New code   ▲ Revised code   **C** Carrier judgment   **D** Special coverage instructions apply
I Not payable by Medicare   **M** Non-covered by Medicare   **S** Non-covered by Medicare statute   AHA Coding Clinic®

D **G0102** Prostate cancer screening; digital rectal examination　　　　　　　♂ N MIPS

BETOS: Y1　Other - Medicare fee schedule
Price established using national RVUs

D **G0103** Prostate cancer screening; prostate specific antigen test (PSA)　　　　　　♂ A

CPT® Crosswalk: 81539, 81541, 81551, 84152, 84153, 84154, 86316, 0005U, 0021U, 0047U, 0053U, 0421T, 0443T

BETOS: T1H　Lab tests - other (non-Medicare fee schedule)
Price subject to national limitation amount

D **G0104** Colorectal cancer screening; flexible sigmoidoscopy　　　　　　　P3 ASC T

CPT® Crosswalk: 00811, 00813, 45330, 45331, 45332, 45333, 45334, 45335, 45337, 45338, 45340, 45341, 45342, 45346, 45347, 45349, 45350, 45378, 45990, 81327, 82270, 82272, 91299

BETOS: P8C　Endoscopy - sigmoidoscopy
Price established using national RVUs
Coding Clinic: 2009, Q2; 2011, Q2
Pub: 100-4, Chapter-18, 60.6; 100-4, Chapter-18, 60.1; 100-4, Chapter-1, 30.3.1

D **G0105** Colorectal cancer screening; colonoscopy on individual at high risk　　　A2 ASC T MIPS

CPT® Crosswalk: 00731, 00732, 00811, 00812, 00813, 44404, 44408, 45330, 45378

BETOS: P8D　Endoscopy - colonoscopy
Price established using national RVUs
Coding Clinic: 2009, Q2; 2018, Q2
Pub: 100-4, Chapter-1, 30.3.1; 100-4, Chapter-18, 60.1; 100-4, Chapter-18, 60.6

D **G0106** Colorectal cancer screening; alternative to G0104, screening sigmoidoscopy, barium enema　　　　　　　　　　S MIPS

CPT® Crosswalk: 45330, 74270, 91299

BETOS: I1D　Standard imaging - contrast gastrointestinal
Price established using national RVUs
Coding Clinic: 2009, Q2; 2011, Q2
Pub: 100-4, Chapter-18, 60.1; 100-4, Chapter-18, 60.6

C **G0108** Diabetes outpatient self-management training services, individual, per 30 minutes　　　　　　　　　A MIPS

BETOS: Y1　Other - Medicare fee schedule
Price established using national RVUs
Coding Clinic: 2019, Q3
Pub: 100-2, Chapter-15, 300.3; 100-4, Chapter-9, 70.5; 100-4, Chapter-12, 190.3.6; 100-4, Chapter-18, 120.1

C **G0109** Diabetes outpatient self-management training services, group session (2 or more), per 30 minutes　　　　　A

BETOS: Y1　Other - Medicare fee schedule
Price established using national RVUs
Coding Clinic: 2019, Q3

Pub: 100-4, Chapter-18, 120.1; 100-4, Chapter-12, 190.3.6; 100-4, Chapter-9, 70.5; 100-2, Chapter-15, 300.3

C **G0117** Glaucoma screening for high risk patients furnished by an optometrist or ophthalmologist　　　　　　S

CPT® Crosswalk: 92285, 0333T, 0464T

BETOS: T2D　Other tests - other
Price established using national RVUs
Coding Clinic: 2001, Q3; 2002, Q1; 2002, Q1
Pub: 100-2, Chapter-15, 280.1

C **G0118** Glaucoma screening for high risk patient furnished under the direct supervision of an optometrist or ophthalmologist　　　S

CPT® Crosswalk: 92285, 0333T, 0464T

BETOS: T2D　Other tests - other
Price established using national RVUs
Coding Clinic: 2001, Q3; 2002, Q1; 2002, Q1
Pub: 100-2, Chapter-15, 280.1

D **G0120** Colorectal cancer screening; alternative to G0105, screening colonoscopy, barium enema.　　　　　　S MIPS

CPT® Crosswalk: 45330, 45378, 45990, 91299

BETOS: I1D　Standard imaging - contrast gastrointestinal
Price established using national RVUs
Pub: 100-4, Chapter-18, 60.1; 100-4, Chapter-18, 60.6

D **G0121** Colorectal cancer screening; colonoscopy on individual not meeting criteria for high risk　　　　　A2 ASC T MIPS

CPT® Crosswalk: 00812, 00813, 44404, 44408, 45330, 45378, 91299

BETOS: I1D　Standard imaging - contrast gastrointestinal
Price established using national RVUs
Coding Clinic: 2001, Q3; 2018, Q2
Pub: 100-4, Chapter-18, 60.6; 100-4, Chapter-18, 60.1; 100-4, Chapter-1, 30.3.1

M **G0122** Colorectal cancer screening; barium enema　　　　　　　　E1 MIPS

CPT® Crosswalk: 45330, 45378, 45990, 74270, 91299

BETOS: I1D　Standard imaging - contrast gastrointestinal
Service not separately priced by Part B
Pub: 100-4, Chapter-18, 60.6

D **G0123** Screening cytopathology, cervical or vaginal (any reporting system), collected in preservative fluid, automated thin layer preparation, screening by cytotechnologist under physician supervision　　　♀ A

BETOS: T1H　Lab tests - other (non-Medicare fee schedule)
Price subject to national limitation amount

♂ Male only　♀ Female only　**A** Age　A2 - Z3 = ASC Payment indicator　A - Y = APC Status indicator
ASC = ASC Approved Procedure　**DME** Paid under the DME fee schedule　**MIPS** MIPS code

D **G0124** Screening cytopathology, cervical or vaginal (any reporting system), collected in preservative fluid, automated thin layer preparation, requiring interpretation by physician   ♀ B
    BETOS: T1H   Lab tests - other (non-Medicare fee schedule)
    Price established using national RVUs

MISCELLANEOUS DIAGNOSTIC AND THERAPEUTIC SERVICES (G0127-G0372)

D **G0127** Trimming of dystrophic nails, any number   N
    BETOS: P5A   Ambulatory procedures - skin
    Price established using national RVUs

D **G0128** Direct (face-to-face with patient) skilled nursing services of a registered nurse provided in a comprehensive outpatient rehabilitation facility, each 10 minutes beyond the first 5 minutes   B
    BETOS: Y2   Other - non-Medicare fee schedule
    Value not established
    Statute: 1833(a)
    Pub: 100-2, Chapter-12, 30.1; 100-2, Chapter-12, 40.8; 100-4, Chapter-5, 20.4

C **G0129** Occupational therapy services requiring the skills of a qualified occupational therapist, furnished as a component of a partial hospitalization treatment program, per session (45 minutes or more)   P
    BETOS: Y1   Other - Medicare fee schedule
    Service not separately priced by Part B
    Coding Clinic: 2012, Q4

D **G0130** Single energy X-ray absorptiometry (SEXA) bone density study, one or more sites; appendicular skeleton (peripheral) (e.g., radius, wrist, heel)   Z3 ASC S
    BETOS: I4B   Imaging/procedure - other
    Price established using national RVUs

C **G0141** Screening cytopathology smears, cervical or vaginal, performed by automated system, with manual rescreening, requiring interpretation by physician   ♀ B
    BETOS: T1H   Lab tests - other (non-Medicare fee schedule)
    Price established using national RVUs

C **G0143** Screening cytopathology, cervical or vaginal (any reporting system), collected in preservative fluid, automated thin layer preparation, with manual screening and rescreening by cytotechnologist under physician supervision   ♀ A
    BETOS: T1H   Lab tests - other (non-Medicare fee schedule)
    Price subject to national limitation amount

C **G0144** Screening cytopathology, cervical or vaginal (any reporting system), collected in preservative fluid, automated thin layer preparation, with screening by automated system, under physician supervision   ♀ A
    BETOS: T1H   Lab tests - other (non-Medicare fee schedule)
    Price subject to national limitation amount

C **G0145** Screening cytopathology, cervical or vaginal (any reporting system), collected in preservative fluid, automated thin layer preparation, with screening by automated system and manual rescreening under physician supervision   ♀ A
    CPT® Crosswalk: 88141, 88142, 88143, 88147, 88148, 88150, 88152, 88153, 88155, 88160, 88161, 88162, 88164, 88165, 88166, 88167, 88172, 88173, 88174, 88175, 88177, 88199
    BETOS: T1H   Lab tests - other (non-Medicare fee schedule)
    Price subject to national limitation amount

C **G0147** Screening cytopathology smears, cervical or vaginal, performed by automated system under physician supervision   ♀ A
    BETOS: T1H   Lab tests - other (non-Medicare fee schedule)
    Price subject to national limitation amount

C **G0148** Screening cytopathology smears, cervical or vaginal, performed by automated system with manual rescreening   ♀ A
    BETOS: T1H   Lab tests - other (non-Medicare fee schedule)
    Price subject to national limitation amount

C **G0151** Services performed by a qualified physical therapist in the home health or hospice setting, each 15 minutes   B
    BETOS: Y2   Other - non-Medicare fee schedule
    Service not separately priced by Part B
    Pub: 100-4, Chapter-10, 40.2; 100-4, Chapter-11, 30.3

C **G0152** Services performed by a qualified occupational therapist in the home health or hospice setting, each 15 minutes   B
    BETOS: Y2   Other - non-Medicare fee schedule
    Service not separately priced by Part B
    Pub: 100-4, Chapter-11, 30.3; 100-4, Chapter-10, 40.2

C **G0153** Services performed by a qualified speech-language pathologist in the home health or hospice setting, each 15 minutes   B
    BETOS: Y2   Other - non-Medicare fee schedule
    Service not separately priced by Part B
    Pub: 100-4, Chapter-10, 40.2; 100-4, Chapter-11, 30.3

● New code   ▲ Revised code   **C** Carrier judgment   **D** Special coverage instructions apply
I Not payable by Medicare   **M** Non-covered by Medicare   **S** Non-covered by Medicare statute   AHA Coding Clinic®

C G0155 Services of clinical social worker in home health or hospice settings, each 15 minutes   B MIPS
  BETOS: Y2   Other - non-Medicare fee schedule
  Service not separately priced by Part B
  Pub: 100-4, Chapter-10, 40.2; 100-4, Chapter-11, 30.3

C G0156 Services of home health/hospice aide in home health or hospice settings, each 15 minutes   B
  BETOS: Y2   Other - non-Medicare fee schedule
  Service not separately priced by Part B
  Pub: 100-4, Chapter-11, 30.3; 100-4, Chapter-10, 40.2

C G0157 Services performed by a qualified physical therapist assistant in the home health or hospice setting, each 15 minutes   B
  BETOS: Y2   Other - non-Medicare fee schedule
  Service not separately priced by Part B
  Pub: 100-4, Chapter-10, 40.2

C G0158 Services performed by a qualified occupational therapist assistant in the home health or hospice setting, each 15 minutes   B
  BETOS: Y2   Other - non-Medicare fee schedule
  Service not separately priced by Part B
  Pub: 100-4, Chapter-10, 40.2

C G0159 Services performed by a qualified physical therapist, in the home health setting, in the establishment or delivery of a safe and effective physical therapy maintenance program, each 15 minutes   B
  BETOS: Y2   Other - non-Medicare fee schedule
  Service not separately priced by Part B
  Pub: 100-4, Chapter-10, 40.2

C G0160 Services performed by a qualified occupational therapist, in the home health setting, in the establishment or delivery of a safe and effective occupational therapy maintenance program, each 15 minutes   B
  BETOS: Y2   Other - non-Medicare fee schedule
  Service not separately priced by Part B
  Pub: 100-4, Chapter-10, 40.2

C G0161 Services performed by a qualified speech-language pathologist, in the home health setting, in the establishment or delivery of a safe and effective speech-language pathology maintenance program, each 15 minutes   B
  BETOS: Y2   Other - non-Medicare fee schedule
  Service not separately priced by Part B
  Pub: 100-4, Chapter-10, 40.2

C G0162 Skilled services by a registered nurse (RN) for management and evaluation of the plan of care; each 15 minutes (the patient's underlying condition or complication requires an RN to ensure that essential non-skilled care achieves its purpose in the home health or hospice setting)   B
  BETOS: Y2   Other - non-Medicare fee schedule
  Service not separately priced by Part B
  Pub: 100-4, Chapter-10, 40.2

D G0166 External counterpulsation, per treatment session   N
  BETOS: P6C   Minor procedures - other (Medicare fee schedule)
  Price established using national RVUs
  Pub: 100-4, Chapter-32, 130.1

C G0168 Wound closure utilizing tissue adhesive(s) only   B
  BETOS: P6C   Minor procedures - other (Medicare fee schedule)
  Service not separately priced by Part B
  Coding Clinic: 2001, Q4; 2001, Q3; 2005, Q1

C G0175 Scheduled interdisciplinary team conference (minimum of three exclusive of patient care nursing staff) with patient present   V
  BETOS: M6   Consultations
  Service not separately priced by Part B
  Coding Clinic: 2001, Q3; 2006, Q4

D G0176 Activity therapy, such as music, dance, art or play therapies not for recreation, related to the care and treatment of patient's disabling mental health problems, per session (45 minutes or more)   P MIPS
  BETOS: Y2   Other - non-Medicare fee schedule
  Service not separately priced by Part B
  Coding Clinic: 2012, Q4

D G0177 Training and educational services related to the care and treatment of patient's disabling mental health problems per session (45 minutes or more)   N MIPS
  BETOS: Y2   Other - non-Medicare fee schedule
  Service not separately priced by Part B
  Coding Clinic: 2012, Q4

C G0179 Physician re-certification for Medicare-covered home health services under a home health plan of care (patient not present), including contacts with home health agency and review of reports of patient status required by physicians to affirm the initial implementation of the plan of care that meets patient's needs, per re-certification period   M
  BETOS: Y1   Other - Medicare fee schedule
  Price established using national RVUs

C **G0180** Physician certification for Medicare-covered home health services under a home health plan of care (patient not present), including contacts with home health agency and review of reports of patient status required by physicians to affirm the initial implementation of the plan of care that meets patient's needs, per certification period   M
BETOS: Y1   Other - Medicare fee schedule
Price established using national RVUs

C **G0181** Physician supervision of a patient receiving Medicare-covered services provided by a participating home health agency (patient not present) requiring complex and multidisciplinary care modalities involving regular physician development and/or revision of care plans, review of subsequent reports of patient status, review of laboratory and other studies, communication (including telephone calls) with other health care professionals involved in the patient's care, integration of new information into the medical treatment plan and/or adjustment of medical therapy, within a calendar month, 30 minutes or more   M
BETOS: Y1   Other - Medicare fee schedule
Price established using national RVUs

C **G0182** Physician supervision of a patient under a Medicare-approved hospice (patient not present) requiring complex and multidisciplinary care modalities involving regular physician development and/or revision of care plans, review of subsequent reports of patient status, review of laboratory and other studies, communication (including telephone calls) with other health care professionals involved in the patient's care, integration of new information into the medical treatment plan and/or adjustment of medical therapy, within a calendar month, 30 minutes or more   M
BETOS: Y1   Other - Medicare fee schedule
Price established using national RVUs

C **G0186** Destruction of localized lesion of choroid (for example, choroidal neovascularization); photocoagulation, feeder vessel technique (one or more sessions)   R2 ASC T
BETOS: P4D   Eye procedure - treatment of retinal lesions
Service not separately priced by Part B

M **G0219** PET imaging whole body; melanoma for non-covered indications   E1
CPT® Crosswalk: 78813, 78816
BETOS: I4B   Imaging/procedure - other
Service not separately priced by Part B
Coding Clinic: 2001, Q2; 2002, Q1; 2002, Q1; 2007, Q1
Pub: 100-4, Chapter-13, 60.3

M **G0235** PET imaging, any site, not otherwise specified   Z2 ASC S
CPT® Crosswalk: 78811, 78812, 78813, 78814
BETOS: T2D   Other tests - other
Service not separately priced by Part B
Coding Clinic: 2007, Q1
Pub: 100-4, Chapter-13, 60.14; 100-4, Chapter-13, 60.3

C **G0237** Therapeutic procedures to increase strength or endurance of respiratory muscles, face to face, one on one, each 15 minutes (includes monitoring)   S
BETOS: P6C   Minor procedures - other (Medicare fee schedule)
Price established using national RVUs
Coding Clinic: 2002, Q1
Pub: 100-2, Chapter-12, 30.1; 100-2, Chapter-12, 40.5; 100-4, Chapter-5, 20

C **G0238** Therapeutic procedures to improve respiratory function, other than described by G0237, one on one, face to face, per 15 minutes (includes monitoring)   S
BETOS: P6C   Minor procedures - other (Medicare fee schedule)
Price established using national RVUs
Coding Clinic: 2002, Q1
Pub: 100-2, Chapter-12, 30.1; 100-2, Chapter-12, 40.5; 100-4, Chapter-5, 20

C **G0239** Therapeutic procedures to improve respiratory function or increase strength or endurance of respiratory muscles, two or more individuals (includes monitoring)   S
BETOS: P6C   Minor procedures - other (Medicare fee schedule)
Price established using national RVUs
Coding Clinic: 2002, Q1
Pub: 100-4, Chapter-5, 20; 100-2, Chapter-12, 40.5; 100-2, Chapter-12, 30.1

D **G0245** Initial physician evaluation and management of a diabetic patient with diabetic sensory neuropathy resulting in a loss of protective sensation (LOPS) which must include: (1) the diagnosis of LOPS, (2) a patient history, (3) a physical examination that consists of at least the following elements: (a) visual inspection of the forefoot, hindfoot and toe web spaces, (b) evaluation of a protective sensation, (c) evaluation of foot structure and biomechanics, (d) evaluation of vascular status and skin integrity, and (e) evaluation and recommendation of footwear and (4) patient education   V
BETOS: M1A   Office visits - new
Price established using national RVUs
Coding Clinic: 2002, Q4; 2002, Q3
Pub: 100-4, Chapter-32, 80.2; 100-4, Chapter-32, 80.8

● New code   ▲ Revised code   **C** Carrier judgment   **D** Special coverage instructions apply
I Not payable by Medicare   **M** Non-covered by Medicare   **S** Non-covered by Medicare statute   AHA Coding Clinic®

D **G0246** Follow-up physician evaluation and management of a diabetic patient with diabetic sensory neuropathy resulting in a loss of protective sensation (LOPS) to include at least the following: (1) a patient history, (2) a physical examination that includes: (a) visual inspection of the forefoot, hindfoot and toe web spaces, (b) evaluation of protective sensation, (c) evaluation of foot structure and biomechanics, (d) evaluation of vascular status and skin integrity, and (e) evaluation and recommendation of footwear, and (3) patient education   V

   BETOS: M1B   Office visits - established
   Price established using national RVUs
   Coding Clinic: 2002, Q4
   Pub: 100-4, Chapter-32, 80.2; 100-4, Chapter-32, 80.8

D **G0247** Routine foot care by a physician of a diabetic patient with diabetic sensory neuropathy resulting in a loss of protective sensation (LOPS) to include, the local care of superficial wounds (i.e., superficial to muscle and fascia) and at least the following if present: (1) local care of superficial wounds, (2) debridement of corns and calluses, and (3) trimming and debridement of nails   N

   BETOS: M1B   Office visits - established
   Price established using national RVUs
   Coding Clinic: 2002, Q4
   Pub: 100-4, Chapter-32, 80.8; 100-4, Chapter-32, 80.2

D **G0248** Demonstration, prior to initiation of home INR monitoring, for patient with either mechanical heart valve(s), chronic atrial fibrillation, or venous thromboembolism who meets Medicare coverage criteria, under the direction of a physician; includes: face-to-face demonstration of use and care of the INR monitor, obtaining at least one blood sample, provision of instructions for reporting home INR test results, and documentation of patient's ability to perform testing and report results   V

   BETOS: M1A   Office visits - new
   Price established using national RVUs
   Coding Clinic: 2002, Q4

D **G0249** Provision of test materials and equipment for home INR monitoring of patient with either mechanical heart valve(s), chronic atrial fibrillation, or venous thromboembolism who meets Medicare coverage criteria; includes: provision of materials for use in the home and reporting of test results to physician; testing not occurring more frequently than once a week; testing materials, billing units of service include 4 tests   V

   BETOS: Y1   Other - Medicare fee schedule
   Price established using national RVUs
   Coding Clinic: 2002, Q4

D **G0250** Physician review, interpretation, and patient management of home INR testing for patient with either mechanical heart valve(s), chronic atrial fibrillation, or venous thromboembolism who meets Medicare coverage criteria; testing not occurring more frequently than once a week; billing units of service include 4 tests   M

   BETOS: M1B   Office visits - established
   Price established using national RVUs
   Coding Clinic: 2002, Q4; 2002, Q3

M **G0252** PET imaging, full and partial-ring PET scanners only, for initial diagnosis of breast cancer and/or surgical planning for breast cancer (e.g., initial staging of axillary lymph nodes)   E1

   CPT® Crosswalk: 78811, 78812, 78813, 0422T

   BETOS: I2D   Advanced imaging - MRI/MRA: other
   Service not separately priced by Part B
   Coding Clinic: 2002, Q4; 2006, Q1; 2007, Q1
   Pub: 100-4, Chapter-13, 60.3

M **G0255** Current perception threshold/sensory nerve conduction test, (SNCT) per limb, any nerve   E1

   BETOS: T2D   Other tests - other
   Service not separately priced by Part B
   Coding Clinic: 2002, Q4

D **G0257** Unscheduled or emergency dialysis treatment for an ESRD patient in a hospital outpatient department that is not certified as an ESRD facility   S

   BETOS: P6D   Minor procedures - other (non-Medicare fee schedule)
   Service not separately priced by Part B
   Coding Clinic: 2002, Q4; 2003, Q1; 2014, Q3
   Pub: 100-4, Chapter-4, 200.2; 100-4, Chapter-8, 60.4.7

D **G0259** Injection procedure for sacroiliac joint; arthrography   N

   BETOS: O1E   Other drugs
   Service not separately priced by Part B
   Coding Clinic: 2002, Q4

D **G0260** Injection procedure for sacroiliac joint; provision of anesthetic, steroid and/or other therapeutic agent, with or without arthrography   A2 ASC T

   BETOS: O1E   Other drugs
   Service not separately priced by Part B
   Coding Clinic: 2002, Q4

C **G0268** Removal of impacted cerumen (one or both ears) by physician on same date of service as audiologic function testing   N

   CPT® Crosswalk: 00124, 69209, 69210

   BETOS: P6C   Minor procedures - other (Medicare fee schedule)
   Price established using national RVUs
   Coding Clinic: 2003, Q1; 2016, Q2

♂ Male only   ♀ Female only   **A** Age   A2 - Z3 = ASC Payment indicator   A - Y = APC Status indicator

ASC = ASC Approved Procedure   **DME** Paid under the DME fee schedule   **MIPS** MIPS code

D **G0269** Placement of occlusive device into either a venous or arterial access site, post surgical or interventional procedure (e.g., angioseal plug, vascular plug)   N
    CPT® Crosswalk: 34808
    BETOS: P6D   Minor procedures - other (non-Medicare fee schedule)
    Service not separately priced by Part B
    Coding Clinic: 2010, Q4; 2012, Q4

C **G0270** Medical nutrition therapy; reassessment and subsequent intervention(s) following second referral in same year for change in diagnosis, medical condition or treatment regimen (including additional hours needed for renal disease), individual, face to face with the patient, each 15 minutes   A MIPS
    BETOS: M5D   Specialist - other
    Price established using national RVUs
    Coding Clinic: 2019, Q3
    Pub: 100-4, Chapter-9, 70.5

C **G0271** Medical nutrition therapy, reassessment and subsequent intervention(s) following second referral in same year for change in diagnosis, medical condition, or treatment regimen (including additional hours needed for renal disease), group (2 or more individuals), each 30 minutes   A MIPS
    BETOS: M5D   Specialist - other
    Price established using national RVUs
    Pub: 100-4, Chapter-9, 70.5

D **G0276** Blinded procedure for lumbar stenosis, percutaneous image-guided lumbar decompression (PILD) or placebo-control, performed in an approved coverage with evidence development (CED) clinical trial   G2 ASC J1
    BETOS: P6D   Minor procedures - other (non-Medicare fee schedule)
    Price established by carriers

D **G0277** Hyperbaric oxygen under pressure, full body chamber, per 30 minute interval   S
    BETOS: P5E   Ambulatory procedures - other
    Price established by carriers

C **G0278** Iliac and/or femoral artery angiography, non-selective, bilateral or ipsilateral to catheter insertion, performed at the same time as cardiac catheterization and/or coronary angiography, includes positioning or placement of the catheter in the distal aorta or ipsilateral femoral or iliac artery, injection of dye, production of permanent images, and radiologic supervision and interpretation (list separately in addition to primary procedure)   N
    BETOS: I4A   Imaging/procedure - heart including cardiac catheterization
    Price established using national RVUs
    Coding Clinic: 2006, Q4

C **G0279** Diagnostic digital breast tomosynthesis, unilateral or bilateral (list separately in addition to 77065 or 77066)   A
    CPT® Crosswalk: 77061, 77062, 0422T
    BETOS: I1C   Standard imaging - breast
    Price established by carriers

C **G0281** Electrical stimulation, (unattended), to one or more areas, for chronic Stage III and Stage IV pressure ulcers, arterial ulcers, diabetic ulcers, and venous stasis ulcers not demonstrating measurable signs of healing after 30 days of conventional care, as part of a therapy plan of care   A
    BETOS: P5E   Ambulatory procedures - other
    Price established using national RVUs
    Coding Clinic: 2003, Q2; 2003, Q1
    Pub: 100-4, Chapter-32, 11.1

M **G0282** Electrical stimulation, (unattended), to one or more areas, for wound care other than described in G0281   E1
    BETOS: P5E   Ambulatory procedures - other
    Service not separately priced by Part B
    Coding Clinic: 2003, Q2; 2003, Q1

C **G0283** Electrical stimulation (unattended), to one or more areas for indication(s) other than wound care, as part of a therapy plan of care   A
    BETOS: P5E   Ambulatory procedures - other
    Price established using national RVUs
    Coding Clinic: 2003, Q2; 2003, Q1; 2009, Q2

C **G0288** Reconstruction, computed tomographic angiography of aorta for surgical planning for vascular surgery   N
    BETOS: I2B   Advanced imaging - CAT/CT/CTA: other
    Price established using national RVUs

C **G0289** Arthroscopy, knee, surgical, for removal of loose body, foreign body, debridement/shaving of articular cartilage (chondroplasty) at the time of other surgical knee arthroscopy in a different compartment of the same knee   N
    BETOS: P8A   Endoscopy - arthroscopy
    Price established using national RVUs
    Coding Clinic: 2003, Q2; 2011, Q2; 2011, Q2

D **G0293** Noncovered surgical procedure(s) using conscious sedation, regional, general or spinal anesthesia in a Medicare qualifying clinical trial, per day   N
    BETOS: Y2   Other - non-Medicare fee schedule
    Service not separately priced by Part B
    Coding Clinic: 2002, Q4

D **G0294** Noncovered procedure(s) using either no anesthesia or local anesthesia only, in a Medicare qualifying clinical trial, per day   N

● New code   ▲ Revised code   **C** Carrier judgment   **D** Special coverage instructions apply
I Not payable by Medicare   **M** Non-covered by Medicare   **S** Non-covered by Medicare statute   AHA Coding Clinic®

BETOS: Y2   Other - non-Medicare fee schedule
Service not separately priced by Part B
Coding Clinic: 2002, Q4

M G0295 Electromagnetic therapy, to one or more areas, for wound care other than described in G0329 or for other uses   E1
BETOS: I2B   Advanced imaging - CAT/CT/CTA: other
Service not separately priced by Part B
Coding Clinic: 2003, Q1

C G0296 Counseling visit to discuss need for lung cancer screening using low dose CT scan (LDCT) (service is for eligibility determination and shared decision making)   S
BETOS: M6   Consultations
Price established by carriers
Coding Clinic: 2005, Q2; 2019, Q3
Pub: 100-4, Chapter-13, 60.3

C G0299 Direct skilled nursing services of a registered nurse (RN) in the home health or hospice setting, each 15 minutes   B
BETOS: M5D   Specialist - other
Service not separately priced by Part B
Coding Clinic: 2003, Q4; 2006, Q2; 2008, Q2
Pub: 100-4, Chapter-11, 30.3

C G0300 Direct skilled nursing services of a licensed practical nurse (LPN) in the home health or hospice setting, each 15 minutes   B
BETOS: M5D   Specialist - other
Service not separately priced by Part B
Coding Clinic: 2003, Q4; 2007, Q1; 2008, Q2
Pub: 100-4, Chapter-11, 30.3

C G0302 Pre-operative pulmonary surgery services for preparation for LVRS, complete course of services, to include a minimum of 16 days of services   S
BETOS: T2D   Other tests - other
Service not separately priced by Part B

C G0303 Pre-operative pulmonary surgery services for preparation for LVRS, 10 to 15 days of services   S
BETOS: T2D   Other tests - other
Service not separately priced by Part B

C G0304 Pre-operative pulmonary surgery services for preparation for LVRS, 1 to 9 days of services   S
BETOS: T2D   Other tests - other
Service not separately priced by Part B

C G0305 Post-discharge pulmonary surgery services after LVRS, minimum of 6 days of services   S
BETOS: T2D   Other tests - other
Service not separately priced by Part B

C G0306 Complete CBC, automated (HgB, HCT, RBC, WBC, without platelet count) and automated WBC differential count   N
BETOS: T1D   Lab tests - blood counts
Price subject to national limitation amount

C G0307 Complete (CBC), automated (HgB, HCT, RBC, WBC; without platelet count)   N
BETOS: T1D   Lab tests - blood counts
Price subject to national limitation amount

D G0328 Colorectal cancer screening; fecal occult blood test, immunoassay, 1-3 simultaneous   A
CPT® Crosswalk: 81327, 82274
BETOS: T1H   Lab tests - other (non-Medicare fee schedule)
Price subject to national limitation amount
Coding Clinic: 2012, Q2
Pub: 100-4, Chapter-18, 60.1; 100-4, Chapter-18, 60.6

C G0329 Electromagnetic therapy, to one or more areas for chronic Stage III and Stage IV pressure ulcers, arterial ulcers, diabetic ulcers and venous stasis ulcers not demonstrating measurable signs of healing after 30 days of conventional care as part of a therapy plan of care   A
BETOS: I2B   Advanced imaging - CAT/CT/CTA: other
Service not separately priced by Part B
Pub: 100-4, Chapter-32, 11.2

D G0333 Pharmacy dispensing fee for inhalation drug(s); initial 30-day supply as a beneficiary   M
BETOS: D1E   Other DME

C G0337 Hospice evaluation and counseling services, pre-election   B
BETOS: M5D   Specialist - other
Price established using national RVUs
Pub: 100-4, Chapter-11, 10.1

C G0339 Image-guided robotic linear accelerator-based stereotactic radiosurgery, complete course of therapy in one session or first session of fractionated treatment   B
CPT® Crosswalk: 01922, 61796, 61797, 61798, 61799, 63620, 63621, 77372
BETOS: P5E   Ambulatory procedures - other
Price established by carriers
Coding Clinic: 2004, Q1

C G0340 Image-guided robotic linear accelerator-based stereotactic radiosurgery, delivery including collimator changes and custom plugging, fractionated treatment, all lesions, per session, second through fifth sessions, maximum five sessions per course of treatment   B
BETOS: P5E   Ambulatory procedures - other
Price established by carriers
Coding Clinic: 2004, Q1

♂ Male only   ♀ Female only   **A** Age   A2 - Z3 = ASC Payment indicator   A - Y = APC Status indicator
ASC = ASC Approved Procedure   **DME** Paid under the DME fee schedule   **MIPS** MIPS code

CPT® is a registered trademark of the American Medical Association. All rights reserved.   **197**

G0341 – G0382

PROCEDURES / PROFESSIONAL SERVICES (G0008-G9987)

D **G0341** Percutaneous islet cell transplant, includes portal vein catheterization and infusion C
BETOS: P1G Major procedure - Other
Price established by carriers

D **G0342** Laparoscopy for islet cell transplant, includes portal vein catheterization and infusion C
BETOS: P1G Major procedure - Other
Price established by carriers

D **G0343** Laparotomy for islet cell transplant, includes portal vein catheterization and infusion C
BETOS: P1G Major procedure - Other
Price established by carriers

D **G0372** Physician service required to establish and document the need for a power mobility device M
BETOS: M5D Specialist - other
Price established by carriers
Pub: 100-4, Chapter-12, 30.6.15.4

HOSPITAL OBSERVATION AND EMERGENCY SERVICES (G0378-G0384)

D **G0378** Hospital observation service, per hour N
BETOS: M2A Hospital visit - initial
Service not separately priced by Part B
Coding Clinic: 2005, Q4; 2005, Q4; 2005, Q4; 2006, Q3; 2007, Q1
Pub: 100-4, Chapter-4, 290.5.2; 100-4, Chapter-4, 290.5.1; 100-4, Chapter-4, 290.4.3; 100-4, Chapter-4, 290.4.2; 100-4, Chapter-4, 290.4.1; 100-4, Chapter-4, 290.2.2; 100-4, Chapter-1, 50.3.2; 100-2, Chapter-6, 20.6

D **G0379** Direct admission of patient for hospital observation care J2
BETOS: M2A Hospital visit - initial
Service not separately priced by Part B
Coding Clinic: 2005, Q4; 2005, Q4; 2005, Q4; 2007, Q1
Pub: 100-4, Chapter-4, 290.5.2; 100-4, Chapter-4, 290.5.1; 100-4, Chapter-4, 290.4.3; 100-4, Chapter-4, 290.4.2; 100-4, Chapter-4, 290.4.1

C **G0380** Level 1 hospital emergency department visit provided in a type B emergency department; (the ED must meet at least one of the following requirements: (1) it is licensed by the state in which it is located under applicable state law as an emergency room or emergency department; (2) it is held out to the public (by name, posted signs, advertising, or other means) as a place that provides care for emergency medical conditions on an urgent basis without requiring a previously scheduled appointment; or (3) during the calendar year immediately preceding the calendar year in which a determination under 42 CFR 489.24 is being made, based on a representative sample of patient visits that occurred during that calendar year, it provides at least one-third of all of its outpatient visits for the treatment of emergency medical conditions on an urgent basis without requiring a previously scheduled appointment) J2
BETOS: M3 Emergency room visit
Service not separately priced by Part B
Coding Clinic: 2006, Q4; 2007, Q4; 2007, Q2; 2009, Q1; 2013, Q4

C **G0381** Level 2 hospital emergency department visit provided in a type B emergency department; (the ED must meet at least one of the following requirements: (1) it is licensed by the state in which it is located under applicable state law as an emergency room or emergency department; (2) it is held out to the public (by name, posted signs, advertising, or other means) as a place that provides care for emergency medical conditions on an urgent basis without requiring a previously scheduled appointment; or (3) during the calendar year immediately preceding the calendar year in which a determination under 42 CFR 489.24 is being made, based on a representative sample of patient visits that occurred during that calendar year, it provides at least one-third of all of its outpatient visits for the treatment of emergency medical conditions on an urgent basis without requiring a previously scheduled appointment) J2
BETOS: M3 Emergency room visit
Service not separately priced by Part B
Coding Clinic: 2006, Q4; 2007, Q4; 2013, Q4

C **G0382** Level 3 hospital emergency department visit provided in a type B emergency department; (the ED must meet at least one of the following requirements: (1) it is licensed by the state in which it is located under applicable state law as an emergency room or emergency department; (2) it is held out to the public (by name, posted signs, advertising, or other means) as a place that provides care for emergency medical conditions on an urgent basis without requiring a previously scheduled appointment; or (3) during the calendar year immediately preceding the calendar year in which a determination under 42 CFR 489.24 is being made, based on a representative sample of patient visits that occurred during that calendar year, it provides at least one-third of all of its outpatient visits for the treatment of emergency medical conditions on an urgent basis without requiring a previously scheduled appointment) J2
BETOS: M3 Emergency room visit
Service not separately priced by Part B
Coding Clinic: 2006, Q4; 2007, Q4; 2013, Q4

● New code   ▲ Revised code   **C** Carrier judgment   **D** Special coverage instructions apply
I Not payable by Medicare   **M** Non-covered by Medicare   **S** Non-covered by Medicare statute   AHA Coding Clinic®

C **G0383** Level 4 hospital emergency department visit provided in a type B emergency department; (the ED must meet at least one of the following requirements: (1) it is licensed by the state in which it is located under applicable state law as an emergency room or emergency department; (2) it is held out to the public (by name, posted signs, advertising, or other means) as a place that provides care for emergency medical conditions on an urgent basis without requiring a previously scheduled appointment; or (3) during the calendar year immediately preceding the calendar year in which a determination under 42 CFR 489.24 is being made, based on a representative sample of patient visits that occurred during that calendar year, it provides at least one-third of all of its outpatient visits for the treatment of emergency medical conditions on an urgent basis without requiring a previously scheduled appointment)   J2
BETOS: M3   Emergency room visit
Service not separately priced by Part B
Coding Clinic: 2007, Q4; 2013, Q4

C **G0384** Level 5 hospital emergency department visit provided in a type B emergency department; (the ED must meet at least one of the following requirements: (1) it is licensed by the state in which it is located under applicable state law as an emergency room or emergency department; (2) it is held out to the public (by name, posted signs, advertising, or other means) as a place that provides care for emergency medical conditions on an urgent basis without requiring a previously scheduled appointment; or (3) during the calendar year immediately preceding the calendar year in which a determination under 42 CFR 489.24 is being made, based on a representative sample of patient visits that occurred during that calendar year, it provides at least one-third of all of its outpatient visits for the treatment of emergency medical conditions on an urgent basis without requiring a previously scheduled appointment)   J2
BETOS: M3   Emergency room visit
Service not separately priced by Part B
Coding Clinic: 2006, Q4; 2007, Q2; 2009, Q1; 2013, Q4
Pub: 100-4, Chapter-4, 290.5.1

OTHER EMERGENCY SERVICES (G0390)

D **G0390** Trauma response team associated with hospital critical care service   S
BETOS: M5D   Specialist - other
Service not separately priced by Part B
Coding Clinic: 2006, Q4; 2007, Q2
Pub: 100-4, Chapter-4, 160.1

ALCOHOL AND SUBSTANCE ABUSE ASSESSMENTS (G0396, G0397)

▲ C **G0396** Alcohol and/or substance (other than tobacco) misuse structured assessment (e.g., AUDIT, DAST), and brief intervention 15 to 30 minutes   S
BETOS: M5D   Specialist - other
Price established using national RVUs
Coding Clinic: 2007, Q4; 2019, Q3
Pub: 100-4, Chapter-4, 200.6

▲ C **G0397** Alcohol and/or substance (other than tobacco) misuse structured assessment (e.g., AUDIT, DAST), and intervention, greater than 30 minutes   S
BETOS: M5D   Specialist - other
Price established using national RVUs
Coding Clinic: 2019, Q3
Pub: 100-4, Chapter-4, 200.6

SLEEP STUDIES, IN HOME (G0398-G0400)

C **G0398** Home sleep study test (HST) with type II portable monitor, unattended; minimum of 7 channels: EEG, EOG, EMG, ECG/heart rate, airflow, respiratory effort and oxygen saturation   S
BETOS: T2D   Other tests - other
Price established by carriers
Coding Clinic: 2008, Q3

C **G0399** Home sleep test (HST) with type III portable monitor, unattended; minimum of 4 channels: 2 respiratory movement/airflow, 1 ECG/heart rate and 1 oxygen saturation   S
BETOS: T2D   Other tests - other
Price established by carriers
Coding Clinic: 2008, Q3

C **G0400** Home sleep test (HST) with type IV portable monitor, unattended; minimum of 3 channels   S
BETOS: T2D   Other tests - other
Price established by carriers
Coding Clinic: 2008, Q3

INITIAL SERVICES FOR MEDICARE ENROLLMENT (G0402-G0405)

C **G0402** Initial preventive physical examination; face-to-face visit, services limited to new beneficiary during the first 12 months of Medicare enrollment   V MIPS
CPT® Crosswalk: 99381, 99382, 99383, 99384, 99385, 99386, 99387, 99401, 99402, 99403, 99404, 99411, 99412, 99429
BETOS: M1A   Office visits - new
Price established using national RVUs
Coding Clinic: 2009, Q4; 2008, Q4
Pub: 100-4, Chapter-18, 140.6; 100-4, Chapter-18, 80.4; 100-4, Chapter-18, 80.3.3; 100-4, Chapter-18, 80.2; 100-4, Chapter-18, 80.1; 100-4, Chapter-12, 100.1.1; 100-4, Chapter-9, 70.6

♂ Male only   ♀ Female only   Ⓐ Age   A2 - Z3 = ASC Payment indicator   A - Y = APC Status indicator
ASC = ASC Approved Procedure   **DME** Paid under the DME fee schedule   **MIPS** MIPS code

G0403 - G0414

PROCEDURES / PROFESSIONAL SERVICES (G0008-G9987)

C **G0403** Electrocardiogram, routine ECG with 12 leads; performed as a screening for the initial preventive physical examination with interpretation and report M

CPT® Crosswalk: 93000, 93010, 93040, 93042, 99429

BETOS: T2C Other tests - EKG monitoring

Price established using national RVUs

Coding Clinic: 2008, Q4

Pub: 100-4, Chapter-18, 80.1; 100-4, Chapter-18, 80.2

C **G0404** Electrocardiogram, routine ECG with 12 leads; tracing only, without interpretation and report, performed as a screening for the initial preventive physical examination S

BETOS: T2C Other tests - EKG monitoring

Price established using national RVUs

Coding Clinic: 2008, Q4

Pub: 100-4, Chapter-18, 80.3.3; 100-4, Chapter-18, 80.2; 100-4, Chapter-18, 80.1

C **G0405** Electrocardiogram, routine ECG with 12 leads; interpretation and report only, performed as a screening for the initial preventive physical examination B

BETOS: T2C Other tests - EKG monitoring

Price established using national RVUs

Coding Clinic: 2008, Q4

Pub: 100-4, Chapter-18, 80.1; 100-4, Chapter-18, 80.2

FOLLOW-UP TELEHEALTH CONSULTATIONS (G0406-G0408), SEE ALSO INITIAL TELEHEALTH CONSULTATIONS (G0425-G0427)

C **G0406** Follow-up inpatient consultation, limited, physicians typically spend 15 minutes communicating with the patient via telehealth B

BETOS: M6 Consultations

Price established by carriers

Coding Clinic: 2008, Q4; 2019, Q3

Pub: 100-4, Chapter-12, 190.3.3

C **G0407** Follow-up inpatient consultation, intermediate, physicians typically spend 25 minutes communicating with the patient via telehealth B

BETOS: M6 Consultations

Price established using national RVUs

Coding Clinic: 2008, Q4; 2019, Q3

Pub: 100-4, Chapter-12, 190.3.3

C **G0408** Follow-up inpatient consultation, complex, physicians typically spend 35 minutes communicating with the patient via telehealth B

BETOS: M6 Consultations

Price established using national RVUs

Coding Clinic: 2008, Q4; 2019, Q3

Pub: 100-4, Chapter-12, 190.3.3

PSYCHOLOGICAL SERVICES (G0409-G0411)

C **G0409** Social work and psychological services, directly relating to and/or furthering the patient's rehabilitation goals, each 15 minutes, face-to-face; individual (services provided by a CORF-qualified social worker or psychologist in a CORF) B MIPS

BETOS: M5D Specialist - other

Price established by carriers

Coding Clinic: 2008, Q4

Pub: 100-4, Chapter-5, 100.11; 100-4, Chapter-5, 100.4; 100-2, Chapter-12, 30.1

C **G0410** Group psychotherapy other than of a multiple-family group, in a partial hospitalization setting, approximately 45 to 50 minutes P MIPS

BETOS: P6D Minor procedures - other (non-Medicare fee schedule)

Price established by carriers

Coding Clinic: 2009, Q4; 2008, Q4; 2012, Q4

C **G0411** Interactive group psychotherapy, in a partial hospitalization setting, approximately 45 to 50 minutes P MIPS

BETOS: P6D Minor procedures - other (non-Medicare fee schedule)

Price established by carriers

Coding Clinic: 2009, Q4; 2008, Q4; 2012, Q4

FRACTURE TREATMENT (G0412-G0415)

C **G0412** Open treatment of iliac spine(s), tuberosity avulsion, or iliac wing fracture(s), unilateral or bilateral for pelvic bone fracture patterns which do not disrupt the pelvic ring includes internal fixation, when performed J1

CPT® Crosswalk: 01120, 27215

BETOS: P3D Major procedure, orthopedic - other

Price established by carriers

Coding Clinic: 2008, Q4

C **G0413** Percutaneous skeletal fixation of posterior pelvic bone fracture and/or dislocation, for fracture patterns which disrupt the pelvic ring, unilateral or bilateral, (includes ilium, sacroiliac joint and/or sacrum) J1

CPT® Crosswalk: 01120, 27216

BETOS: P3D Major procedure, orthopedic - other

Price established by carriers

Coding Clinic: 2008, Q4

C **G0414** Open treatment of anterior pelvic bone fracture and/or dislocation for fracture patterns which disrupt the pelvic ring, unilateral or bilateral, includes internal fixation when performed (includes pubic symphysis and/or superior/inferior rami) J1

CPT® Crosswalk: 01120, 27217

● New code ▲ Revised code **C** Carrier judgment **D** Special coverage instructions apply
I Not payable by Medicare **M** Non-covered by Medicare **S** Non-covered by Medicare statute AHA Coding Clinic®

BETOS: P3D   Major procedure, orthopedic - other
Price established by carriers
Coding Clinic: 2008, Q4

G0415 Open treatment of posterior pelvic bone fracture and/or dislocation, for fracture patterns which disrupt the pelvic ring, unilateral or bilateral, includes internal fixation, when performed (includes ilium, sacroiliac joint and/or sacrum)   J1
BETOS: P3D   Major procedure, orthopedic - other
Price established by carriers
Coding Clinic: 2008, Q4

GROSS AND MICROSCOPIC EXAMINATIONS, PROSTATE BIOPSY (G0416)

G0416 Surgical pathology, gross and microscopic examinations, for prostate needle biopsy, any method   ♂ N
BETOS: T1G   Lab tests - other (Medicare fee schedule)
Price established by carriers
Coding Clinic: 2008, Q4

FACE-TO-FACE EDUCATIONAL SERVICES (G0420, G0421)

G0420 Face-to-face educational services related to the care of chronic kidney disease; individual, per session, per one hour   A
BETOS: M1B   Office visits - established
Price established using national RVUs
Coding Clinic: 2019, Q3
Pub: 100-2, Chapter-15, 310.3

G0421 Face-to-face educational services related to the care of chronic kidney disease; group, per session, per one hour   A
BETOS: M1B   Office visits - established
Price established using national RVUs
Coding Clinic: 2019, Q3
Pub: 100-2, Chapter-15, 310.3

CARDIAC AND PULMONARY REHABILITATION SERVICES (G0422-G0424)

G0422 Intensive cardiac rehabilitation; with or without continuous ECG monitoring with exercise, per session   S
CPT® Crosswalk: 93797, 93798, 93799
BETOS: M5D   Specialist - other
Price established using national RVUs
Pub: 100-4, Chapter-32, 140.3.1

G0423 Intensive cardiac rehabilitation; with or without continuous ECG monitoring; without exercise, per session   S
BETOS: M5D   Specialist - other
Price established using national RVUs
Pub: 100-4, Chapter-32, 140.3.1

G0424 Pulmonary rehabilitation, including exercise (includes monitoring), one hour, per session, up to two sessions per day   S
BETOS: M5D   Specialist - other
Price established using national RVUs
Pub: 100-4, Chapter-32, 140.4.1

INITIAL TELEHEALTH CONSULTATIONS (G0425-G0427), SEE ALSO FOLLOW-UP TELEHEALTH CONSULTATIONS (G0406-G0408)

G0425 Telehealth consultation, emergency department or initial inpatient, typically 30 minutes communicating with the patient via telehealth   B
BETOS: M6   Consultations
Price established by carriers
Coding Clinic: 2019, Q3
Pub: 100-4, Chapter-12, 190.3.2

G0426 Telehealth consultation, emergency department or initial inpatient, typically 50 minutes communicating with the patient via telehealth   B
BETOS: M6   Consultations
Price established by carriers
Coding Clinic: 2019, Q3
Pub: 100-4, Chapter-12, 190.3.2

G0427 Telehealth consultation, emergency department or initial inpatient, typically 70 minutes or more communicating with the patient via telehealth   B
BETOS: M6   Consultations
Price established by carriers
Coding Clinic: 2019, Q3
Pub: 100-4, Chapter-12, 190.3.2

FILLER PROCEDURES (G0428, G0429)

G0428 Collagen meniscus implant procedure for filling meniscal defects (e.g., CMI, collagen scaffold, Menaflex)   E1
BETOS: P1G   Major procedure - Other
Service not separately priced by Part B

G0429 Dermal filler injection(s) for the treatment of facial lipodystrophy syndrome (LDS) (e.g., as a result of highly active antiretroviral therapy)   P3 ASC T
CPT® Crosswalk: 00300, 11950, 11951, 11952, 11954
BETOS: P6A   Minor procedures - skin
Price established by carriers
Coding Clinic: 2010, Q3
Pub: 100-4, Chapter-32, 260.2.1; 100-4, Chapter-32, 260.2.2

LABORATORY SCREENING TESTS (G0432-G0435)

G0432 Infectious agent antibody detection by enzyme immunoassay (EIA) technique, HIV-1 and/or HIV-2, screening   A
CPT® Crosswalk: 86701, 86702, 86703, 87389, 87390, 87391

♂ Male only   ♀ Female only   Ⓐ Age   A2 - Z3 = ASC Payment indicator   A - Y = APC Status indicator
ASC = ASC Approved Procedure   **DME** Paid under the DME fee schedule   **MIPS** MIPS code

BETOS: T1H   Lab tests - other (non-Medicare fee schedule)
Price subject to national limitation amount
Coding Clinic: 2010, Q1
Pub: 100-4, Chapter-18, 130.1; 100-4, Chapter-18, 130.2; 100-4, Chapter-18, 130.3; 100-4, Chapter-18, 130.4

C G0433 Infectious agent antibody detection by enzyme-linked immunosorbent assay (ELISA) technique, HIV-1 and/or HIV-2, screening   A
CPT® Crosswalk: 86701, 86702, 86703, 87389, 87390, 87391
BETOS: T1H   Lab tests - other (non-Medicare fee schedule)
Price subject to national limitation amount
Coding Clinic: 2010, Q1
Pub: 100-4, Chapter-18, 130.4; 100-4, Chapter-18, 130.3; 100-4, Chapter-18, 130.2; 100-4, Chapter-18, 130.1

C G0435 Infectious agent antibody detection by rapid antibody test, HIV-1 and/or HIV-2, screening   A
CPT® Crosswalk: 86689, 86701, 86702, 86703, 87389, 87390, 87391
BETOS: T1H   Lab tests - other (non-Medicare fee schedule)
Price subject to national limitation amount
Coding Clinic: 2010, Q1
Pub: 100-4, Chapter-18, 130.1; 100-4, Chapter-18, 130.2; 100-4, Chapter-18, 130.3; 100-4, Chapter-18, 130.4

COUNSELING, SCREENING, AND PREVENTION SERVICES (G0438-G0451)

C G0438 Annual wellness visit; includes a personalized prevention plan of service (PPPS), initial visit   A MIPS
CPT® Crosswalk: 99381, 99382, 99383, 99384, 99385, 99386, 99387, 99401, 99402, 99403, 99404, 99406, 99407, 99408, 99409, 99429
BETOS: M5D   Specialist - other
Price established by carriers
Coding Clinic: 2019, Q3
Pub: 100-4, Chapter-18, 140.6; 100-4, Chapter-18, 140.1; 100-4, Chapter-12, 100.1.1

C G0439 Annual wellness visit, includes a personalized prevention plan of service (PPPS), subsequent visit   A MIPS
CPT® Crosswalk: 99391, 99392, 99393, 99394, 99395, 99396, 99397, 99401, 99402, 99403, 99404, 99406, 99407, 99408, 99409, 99429
BETOS: M5D   Specialist - other
Price established by carriers
Coding Clinic: 2019, Q3
Pub: 100-4, Chapter-12, 100.1.1; 100-4, Chapter-18, 140.1; 100-4, Chapter-18, 140.6

C G0442 Annual alcohol misuse screening, 15 minutes   S
BETOS: Y1   Other - Medicare fee schedule
Price established by carriers
Coding Clinic: 2012, Q1; 2019, Q3
Pub: 100-4, Chapter-18, 180.5; 100-4, Chapter-18, 180.4; 100-4, Chapter-18, 180.3; 100-4, Chapter18, 180.2; 100-4, Chapter-18, 180.1

C G0443 Brief face-to-face behavioral counseling for alcohol misuse, 15 minutes   S
BETOS: Y1   Other - Medicare fee schedule
Price established by carriers
Coding Clinic: 2012, Q1; 2019, Q3
Pub: 100-4, Chapter-18, 180.1; 100-4, Chapter18, 180.2; 100-4, Chapter-18, 180.3; 100-4, Chapter-18, 180.4; 100-4, Chapter-18, 180.5

C G0444 Annual depression screening, 15 minutes   S MIPS
CPT® Crosswalk: 96160, 96161, 99401
BETOS: Y1   Other - Medicare fee schedule
Price established by carriers
Coding Clinic: 2019, Q3
Pub: 100-4, Chapter-18, 190.3; 100-4, Chapter-18, 190.2; 100-4, Chapter-18, 190.1

C G0445 High intensity behavioral counseling to prevent sexually transmitted infection; face-to-face, individual, includes: education, skills training and guidance on how to change sexual behavior; performed semi-annually, 30 minutes   S
BETOS: Y1   Other - Medicare fee schedule
Price established by carriers
Coding Clinic: 2019, Q3
Pub: 100-4, Chapter-18, 170.1; 100-4, Chapter-18, 170.3; 100-4, Chapter-18, 170.4; 100-4, Chapter-18, 170.4.1

C G0446 Annual, face-to-face intensive behavioral therapy for cardiovascular disease, individual, 15 minutes   S
BETOS: Y1   Other - Medicare fee schedule
Price established by carriers
Coding Clinic: 2012, Q2; 2019, Q3
Pub: 100-4, Chapter-18, 160.5; 100-4, Chapter-18, 160.4; 100-4, Chapter-18, 160.3; 100-4, Chapter-18, 160.2.2; 100-4, Chapter-18, 160.2.1; 100-4, Chapter-18, 160.1

C G0447 Face-to-face behavioral counseling for obesity, 15 minutes   S MIPS
BETOS: Y1   Other - Medicare fee schedule
Price established by carriers
Coding Clinic: 2012, Q1; 2019, Q3
Pub: 100-4, Chapter-18, 200.1; 100-4, Chapter-18, 200.2; 100-4, Chapter-18, 200.3; 100-4, Chapter-18, 200.4; 100-4, Chapter-18, 200.5

● New code   ▲ Revised code   C Carrier judgment   D Special coverage instructions apply
I Not payable by Medicare   M Non-covered by Medicare   S Non-covered by Medicare statute   AHA Coding Clinic®

202   CPT® is a registered trademark of the American Medical Association. All rights reserved.

C **G0448** Insertion or replacement of a permanent pacing cardioverter-defibrillator system with transvenous lead(s), single or dual chamber with insertion of pacing electrode, cardiac venous system, for left ventricular pacing   B
CPT® Crosswalk: 00534, 33230, 33231, 33240, 33241, 33249, 33262, 33263, 33264, 33270, 33999
BETOS: Y1   Other - Medicare fee schedule
Price established by carriers

C **G0451** Development testing, with interpretation and report, per standardized instrument form   S
BETOS: M5D   Specialist - other
Price established by carriers

MISCELLANEOUS SERVICES (G0452-G0463)

C **G0452** Molecular pathology procedure; physician interpretation and report   B
BETOS: T2D   Other tests - other
Price established by carriers

C **G0453** Continuous intraoperative neurophysiology monitoring, from outside the operating room (remote or nearby), per patient, (attention directed exclusively to one patient) each 15 minutes (list in addition to primary procedure)   N
BETOS: T2D   Other tests - other
Price established by carriers

C **G0454** Physician documentation of face-to-face visit for durable medical equipment determination performed by nurse practitioner, physician assistant or clinical nurse specialist   B
BETOS: M5D   Specialist - other
Price established by carriers

C **G0455** Preparation with instillation of fecal microbiota by any method, including assessment of donor specimen   N
BETOS: T2D   Other tests - other
Price established by carriers
Coding Clinic: 2013, Q3

C **G0458** Low dose rate (LDR) prostate brachytherapy services, composite rate   ♂ B
BETOS: P7A   Oncology - radiation therapy
Service not separately priced by Part B

C **G0459** Inpatient telehealth pharmacologic management, including prescription, use, and review of medication with no more than minimal medical psychotherapy   B
CPT® Crosswalk: 90863
BETOS: M5D   Specialist - other
Price established by carriers
Coding Clinic: 2019, Q3

C **G0460** Autologous platelet rich plasma for chronic wounds/ulcers, including phlebotomy, centrifugation, and all other preparatory procedures, administration and dressings, per treatment   T

BETOS: P5E   Ambulatory procedures - other
Price established by carriers
Pub: 100-4, Chapter-32, 11.3.6; 100-4, Chapter-32, 11.3.2

C **G0463** Hospital outpatient clinic visit for assessment and management of a patient   J2 MIPS
BETOS: M1B   Office visits - established
Service not separately priced by Part B
Coding Clinic: 2013, Q4; 2014, Q4; 2020, Q2
Pub: 100-4, Chapter-4, 290.5.1

FEDERALLY QUALIFIED HEALTH CENTER (FQHC) VISITS (G0466-G0470)

C **G0466** Federally qualified health center (FQHC) visit, new patient; a medically-necessary, face-to-face encounter (one-on-one) between a new patient and a FQHC practitioner during which time one or more FQHC services are rendered and includes a typical bundle of Medicare-covered services that would be furnished per diem to a patient receiving a FQHC visit   A
BETOS: M1A   Office visits - new
Price established by carriers
Pub: 100-4, Chapter-9, 70.5

C **G0467** Federally qualified health center (FQHC) visit, established patient; a medically-necessary, face-to-face encounter (one-on-one) between an established patient and a FQHC practitioner during which time one or more FQHC services are rendered and includes a typical bundle of Medicare-covered services that would be furnished per diem to a patient receiving a FQHC visit   A
BETOS: M1B   Office visits - established
Price established by carriers
Pub: 100-4, Chapter-9, 70.5

C **G0468** Federally qualified health center (FQHC) visit, IPPE or AWV; a FQHC visit that includes an initial preventive physical examination (IPPE) or annual wellness visit (AWV) and includes a typical bundle of Medicare-covered services that would be furnished per diem to a patient receiving an IPPE or AWV   A
BETOS: M1B   Office visits - established
Price established by carriers
Pub: 100-4, Chapter-9, 70.6

C **G0469** Federally qualified health center (FQHC) visit, mental health, new patient; a medically-necessary, face-to-face mental health encounter (one-on-one) between a new patient and a FQHC practitioner during which time one or more FQHC services are rendered and includes a typical bundle of Medicare-covered services that would be furnished per diem to a patient receiving a mental health visit   A
BETOS: M1A   Office visits - new
Price established by carriers

♂ Male only   ♀ Female only   Ⓐ Age   A2 - Z3 = ASC Payment indicator   A - Y = APC Status indicator
ASC = ASC Approved Procedure   DME Paid under the DME fee schedule   MIPS MIPS code

CPT® is a registered trademark of the American Medical Association. All rights reserved.

203

C G0470 Federally qualified health center (FQHC) visit, mental health, established patient; a medically-necessary, face-to-face mental health encounter (one-on-one) between an established patient and a FQHC practitioner during which time one or more FQHC services are rendered and includes a typical bundle of Medicare-covered services that would be furnished per diem to a patient receiving a mental health visit   A

BETOS: M1B   Office visits - established
Price established by carriers

OTHER SERVICES (G0471-G0659)

C G0471 Collection of venous blood by venipuncture or urine sample by catheterization from an individual in a skilled nursing facility (SNF) or by a laboratory on behalf of a home health agency (HHA)   A
CPT® Crosswalk: 36400, 36405, 36406, 36410, 36415, 51701
BETOS: Z2   Undefined codes
Price subject to national limitation amount
Pub: 100-4, Chapter-16, 60.1.4

D G0472 Hepatitis C antibody screening, for individual at high risk and other covered indication(s)   A
BETOS: P5E   Ambulatory procedures - other
Price established by carriers
Statute: 1861SSA

C G0473 Face-to-face behavioral counseling for obesity, group (2-10), 30 minutes   S MIPS
CPT® Crosswalk: 99078, 99411
BETOS: M1B   Office visits - established
Price established by carriers
Pub: 100-4, Chapter-18, 200.5; 100-4, Chapter-18, 200.4; 100-4, Chapter-18, 200.3; 100-4, Chapter-18, 200.2; 100-4, Chapter-18, 200.1

C G0475 HIV antigen/antibody, combination assay, screening   A
CPT® Crosswalk: 86701, 86702, 86703, 87389, 87390, 87391
BETOS: T2D   Other tests - other
Price established by carriers
Pub: 100-4, Chapter-18, 130.2; 100-4, Chapter-18, 130.3; 100-4, Chapter-18, 130.4

C G0476 Infectious agent detection by nucleic acid (DNA or RNA); human papillomavirus (HPV), high-risk types (e.g., 16, 18, 31, 33, 35, 39, 45, 51, 52, 56, 58, 59, 68) for cervical cancer screening, must be performed in addition to pap test   ♀ A
CPT® Crosswalk: 87624, 87625, 0500T
BETOS: T2D   Other tests - other
Price established by carriers

C G0480 Drug test(s), definitive, utilizing (1) drug identification methods able to identify individual drugs and distinguish between structural isomers (but not necessarily stereoisomers), including, but not limited to GC/MS (any type, single or tandem) and LC/MS (any type, single or tandem and excluding immunoassays (e.g., IA, EIA, ELISA, EMIT, FPIA) and enzymatic methods (e.g., alcohol dehydrogenase)), (2) stable isotope or other universally recognized internal standards in all samples (e.g., to control for matrix effects, interferences and variations in signal strength), and (3) method or drug-specific calibration and matrix-matched quality control material (e.g., to control for instrument variations and mass spectral drift); qualitative or quantitative, all sources, includes specimen validity testing, per day; 1-7 drug class(es), including metabolite(s) if performed   N
BETOS: T1H   Lab tests - other (non-Medicare fee schedule)
Price subject to national limitation amount
Coding Clinic: 2018, Q1

C G0481 Drug test(s), definitive, utilizing (1) drug identification methods able to identify individual drugs and distinguish between structural isomers (but not necessarily stereoisomers), including, but not limited to GC/MS (any type, single or tandem) and LC/MS (any type, single or tandem and excluding immunoassays (e.g., IA, EIA, ELISA, EMIT, FPIA) and enzymatic methods (e.g., alcohol dehydrogenase)), (2) stable isotope or other universally recognized internal standards in all samples (e.g., to control for matrix effects, interferences and variations in signal strength), and (3) method or drug-specific calibration and matrix-matched quality control material (e.g., to control for instrument variations and mass spectral drift); qualitative or quantitative, all sources, includes specimen validity testing, per day; 8-14 drug class(es), including metabolite(s) if performed   N
BETOS: T1H   Lab tests - other (non-Medicare fee schedule)
Price subject to national limitation amount
Coding Clinic: 2018, Q1

C G0482 Drug test(s), definitive, utilizing (1) drug identification methods able to identify individual drugs and distinguish between structural isomers (but not necessarily stereoisomers), including, but not limited to GC/MS (any type, single or tandem) and LC/MS (any type, single or tandem and excluding immunoassays (e.g., IA, EIA, ELISA, EMIT, FPIA) and enzymatic methods (e.g., alcohol dehydrogenase)), (2) stable isotope or other universally recognized

---

● New code   ▲ Revised code   **C** Carrier judgment   **D** Special coverage instructions apply
I Not payable by Medicare   **M** Non-covered by Medicare   **S** Non-covered by Medicare statute   AHA Coding Clinic®

internal standards in all samples (e.g., to control for matrix effects, interferences and variations in signal strength), and (3) method or drug-specific calibration and matrix-matched quality control material (e.g., to control for instrument variations and mass spectral drift); qualitative or quantitative, all sources, includes specimen validity testing, per day; 15-21 drug class(es), including metabolite(s) if performed   N

BETOS: T1H   Lab tests - other (non-Medicare fee schedule)

Price subject to national limitation amount

Coding Clinic: 2018, Q1

C G0483 Drug test(s), definitive, utilizing (1) drug identification methods able to identify individual drugs and distinguish between structural isomers (but not necessarily stereoisomers), including, but not limited to GC/MS (any type, single or tandem) and LC/MS (any type, single or tandem and excluding immunoassays (e.g., IA, EIA, ELISA, EMIT, FPIA) and enzymatic methods (e.g., alcohol dehydrogenase)), (2) stable isotope or other universally recognized internal standards in all samples (e.g., to control for matrix effects, interferences and variations in signal strength), and (3) method or drug-specific calibration and matrix-matched quality control material (e.g., to control for instrument variations and mass spectral drift); qualitative or quantitative, all sources, includes specimen validity testing, per day; 22 or more drug class(es), including metabolite(s) if performed   N

BETOS: T1H   Lab tests - other (non-Medicare fee schedule)

Price subject to national limitation amount

Coding Clinic: 2018, Q1

C G0490 Face-to-face home health nursing visit by a rural health clinic (RHC) or federally qualified health center (FQHC) in an area with a shortage of home health agencies; (services limited to RN or LPN only)   A

BETOS: M4A   Home visit

Price established by carriers

C G0491 Dialysis procedure at a Medicare certified ESRD facility for acute kidney injury without ESRD   B

BETOS: P9A   Dialysis services (Medicare fee schedule)

Price established by carriers

C G0492 Dialysis procedure with single evaluation by a physician or other qualified health care professional for acute kidney injury without ESRD   B

BETOS: P9A   Dialysis services (Medicare fee schedule)

Price established by carriers

C G0493 Skilled services of a registered nurse (RN) for the observation and assessment of the patient's condition, each 15 minutes (the change in the patient's condition requires skilled nursing personnel to identify and evaluate the patient's need for possible modification of treatment in the home health or hospice setting)   B

BETOS: Y2   Other - non-Medicare fee schedule

Service not separately priced by Part B

C G0494 Skilled services of a licensed practical nurse (LPN) for the observation and assessment of the patient's condition, each 15 minutes (the change in the patient's condition requires skilled nursing personnel to identify and evaluate the patient's need for possible modification of treatment in the home health or hospice setting)   B

BETOS: Y2   Other - non-Medicare fee schedule

Service not separately priced by Part B

C G0495 Skilled services of a registered nurse (RN), in the training and/or education of a patient or family member, in the home health or hospice setting, each 15 minutes   B

BETOS: Y2   Other - non-Medicare fee schedule

Service not separately priced by Part B

C G0496 Skilled services of a licensed practical nurse (LPN), in the training and/or education of a patient or family member, in the home health or hospice setting, each 15 minutes   B

BETOS: Y2   Other - non-Medicare fee schedule

Service not separately priced by Part B

C G0498 Chemotherapy administration, intravenous infusion technique; initiation of infusion in the office/clinic setting using office/clinic pump/supplies, with continuation of the infusion in the community setting (e.g., home, domiciliary, rest home or assisted living) using a portable pump provided by the office/clinic, includes follow-up office/clinic visit at the conclusion of the infusion   S

BETOS: P7B   Oncology - other

Price established by carriers

Coding Clinic: 2017, Q2

C G0499 Hepatitis B screening in non-pregnant, high risk individual includes Hepatitis B surface antigen (HBsAg), antibodies to HBsAg (anti-HBS) and antibodies to Hepatitis B core antigen (anti-HBC), and is followed by a neutralizing confirmatory test, when performed, only for an initially reactive HBsAg result   A

BETOS: T1H   Lab tests - other (non-Medicare fee schedule)

Price established by carriers

♂ Male only   ♀ Female only   **A** Age   A2 - Z3 = ASC Payment indicator   A - Y = APC Status indicator

ASC = ASC Approved Procedure   **DME** Paid under the DME fee schedule   **MIPS** MIPS code

C **G0500** Moderate sedation services provided by the same physician or other qualified health care professional performing a gastrointestinal endoscopic service that sedation supports, requiring the presence of an independent trained observer to assist in the monitoring of the patient's level of consciousness and physiological status; initial 15 minutes of intra-service time; patient age 5 years or older (additional time may be reported with 99153, as appropriate) **Ⓐ N**

CPT® Crosswalk: 99151, 99152, 99153

BETOS: P0   Anesthesia
Price established by carriers

C **G0501** Resource-intensive services for patients for whom the use of specialized mobility-assistive technology (such as adjustable height chairs or tables, patient lift, and adjustable padded leg supports) is medically necessary and used during the provision of an office/outpatient, evaluation and management visit (list separately in addition to primary service) **N**

BETOS: M5D   Specialist - other
Price established by carriers

C **G0506** Comprehensive assessment of and care planning for patients requiring chronic care management services (list separately in addition to primary monthly care management service) **N**

BETOS: M5D   Specialist - other
Price established by carriers
Coding Clinic: 2019, Q3

C **G0508** Telehealth consultation, critical care, initial, physicians typically spend 60 minutes communicating with the patient and providers via telehealth **B**

BETOS: M5D   Specialist - other
Price established by carriers
Coding Clinic: 2019, Q3

C **G0509** Telehealth consultation, critical care, subsequent, physicians typically spend 50 minutes communicating with the patient and providers via telehealth **B**

BETOS: M5D   Specialist - other
Price established by carriers
Coding Clinic: 2019, Q3

D **G0511** Rural health clinic or federally qualified health center (RHC or FQHC) only, general care management, 20 minutes or more of clinical staff time for chronic care management services or behavioral health integration services directed by an RHC or FQHC practitioner (physician, NP, PA, or CNM), per calendar month **A**

BETOS: M5D   Specialist - other
Price established by carriers

D **G0512** Rural health clinic or federally qualified health center (RHC or FQHC) only, psychiatric collaborative care model (psychiatric COCM), 60 minutes or more of clinical staff time for psychiatric cocm services directed by an RHC or FQHC practitioner (physician, NP, PA, or CNM) and including services furnished by a behavioral health care manager and consultation with a psychiatric consultant, per calendar month **A**

BETOS: M5D   Specialist - other
Price established by carriers

C **G0513** Prolonged preventive service(s) (beyond the typical service time of the primary procedure), in the office or other outpatient setting requiring direct patient contact beyond the usual service; first 30 minutes (list separately in addition to code for preventive service) **N**

CPT® Crosswalk: 99354

BETOS: M5D   Specialist - other
Price established by carriers
Coding Clinic: 2019, Q3

C **G0514** Prolonged preventive service(s) (beyond the typical service time of the primary procedure), in the office or other outpatient setting requiring direct patient contact beyond the usual service; each additional 30 minutes (list separately in addition to code G0513 for additional 30 minutes of preventive service) **N**

CPT® Crosswalk: 99355

BETOS: M5D   Specialist - other
Price established by carriers
Coding Clinic: 2019, Q3

C **G0516** Insertion of non-biodegradable drug delivery implants, 4 or more (services for subdermal rod implant) **N1 ASC N**

CPT® Crosswalk: 11981, 0278T

BETOS: P6C   Minor procedures - other (Medicare fee schedule)
Price established by carriers

C **G0517** Removal of non-biodegradable drug delivery implants, 4 or more (services for subdermal implants) **N1 ASC N**

CPT® Crosswalk: 11982

BETOS: P6C   Minor procedures - other (Medicare fee schedule)
Price established by carriers

C **G0518** Removal with reinsertion, non-biodegradable drug delivery implants, 4 or more (services for subdermal implants) **N1 ASC N**

CPT® Crosswalk: 11983, 0278T

BETOS: P6C   Minor procedures - other (Medicare fee schedule)
Price established by carriers

● New code   ▲ Revised code   **C** Carrier judgment   **D** Special coverage instructions apply
I Not payable by Medicare   **M** Non-covered by Medicare   **S** Non-covered by Medicare statute   AHA Coding Clinic®

C **G0659** Drug test(s), definitive, utilizing drug identification methods able to identify individual drugs and distinguish between structural isomers (but not necessarily stereoisomers), including but not limited to GC/MS (any type, single or tandem) and LC/MS (any type, single or tandem), excluding immunoassays (e.g., IA, EIA, ELISA, EMIT, FPIA) and enzymatic methods (e.g., alcohol dehydrogenase), performed without method or drug-specific calibration, without matrix-matched quality control material, or without use of stable isotope or other universally recognized internal standard(s) for each drug, drug metabolite or drug class per specimen; qualitative or quantitative, all sources, includes specimen validity testing, per day, any number of drug classes   N

    BETOS: T1H   Lab tests - other (non-Medicare fee schedule)
    Price subject to national limitation amount

QUALITY MEASURES FOR CATARACT SURGERY (G0913-G0918)

C **G0913** Improvement in visual function achieved within 90 days following cataract surgery   M MIPS

    BETOS: M5D   Specialist - other
    Service not separately priced by Part B

C **G0914** Patient care survey was not completed by patient   M MIPS

    BETOS: M5D   Specialist - other
    Service not separately priced by Part B

C **G0915** Improvement in visual function not achieved within 90 days following cataract surgery   M MIPS

    BETOS: M5D   Specialist - other
    Service not separately priced by Part B

C **G0916** Satisfaction with care achieved within 90 days following cataract surgery   M MIPS

    BETOS: M5D   Specialist - other
    Service not separately priced by Part B

C **G0917** Patient satisfaction survey was not completed by patient   M MIPS

    BETOS: M5D   Specialist - other
    Service not separately priced by Part B

C **G0918** Satisfaction with care not achieved within 90 days following cataract surgery   M MIPS

    BETOS: M5D   Specialist - other
    Service not separately priced by Part B

CLINICAL DECISION SUPPORT MECHANISM (G1001-G1023)

C **G1001** Clinical decision support mechanism eviCore, as defined by the Medicare Appropriate Use Criteria Program   E1

    BETOS: Z2   Undefined codes
    Service not separately priced by Part B

C **G1002** Clinical decision support mechanism MedCurrent, as defined by the Medicare Appropriate Use Criteria Program   E1

    BETOS: Z2   Undefined codes
    Service not separately priced by Part B

C **G1003** Clinical decision support mechanism Medicalis, as defined by the Medicare Appropriate Use Criteria Program   E1

    BETOS: Z2   Undefined codes
    Service not separately priced by Part B

C **G1004** Clinical decision support mechanism national decision support company, as defined by the Medicare Appropriate Use Criteria Program   E1

    BETOS: Z2   Undefined codes
    Service not separately priced by Part B

C **G1007** Clinical decision support mechanism aim specialty health, as defined by the Medicare Appropriate Use Criteria Program   E1

    BETOS: Z2   Undefined codes
    Service not separately priced by Part B

C **G1008** Clinical decision support mechanism cranberry peak, as defined by the Medicare Appropriate Use Criteria Program   E1

    BETOS: Z2   Undefined codes
    Service not separately priced by Part B

C **G1009** Clinical decision support mechanism sage health management solutions, as defined by the Medicare Appropriate Use Criteria Program   E1

    BETOS: Z2   Undefined codes
    Service not separately priced by Part B

C **G1010** Clinical decision support mechanism stanson, as defined by the Medicare Appropriate Use Criteria Program   E1

    BETOS: Z2   Undefined codes
    Service not separately priced by Part B

C **G1011** Clinical decision support mechanism, qualified tool not otherwise specified, as defined by the Medicare Appropriate Use Criteria Program   E1

    BETOS: Z2   Undefined codes
    Service not separately priced by Part B

● C **G1012** Clinical decision support mechanism agilemd, as defined by the Medicare appropriate use criteria program   E1

    BETOS: Z2   Undefined codes
    Service not separately priced by Part B

● C **G1013** Clinical decision support mechanism evidencecare imaging advisor, as defined by the medicare appropriate use criteria program   E1

    BETOS: Z2   Undefined codes
    Service not separately priced by Part B

- **C** **G1014** Clinical decision support mechanism inveniqa semantic answers in medicine, as defined by the medicare appropriate use criteria program   E1

    BETOS: Z2   Undefined codes
    Service not separately priced by Part B

- **C** **G1015** Clinical decision support mechanism reliant medical group, as defined by the medicare appropriate use criteria program   E1

    BETOS: Z2   Undefined codes
    Service not separately priced by Part B

- **C** **G1016** Clinical decision support mechanism speed of care, as defined by the medicare appropriate use criteria program   E1

    BETOS: Z2   Undefined codes
    Service not separately priced by Part B

- **C** **G1017** Clinical decision support mechanism healthhelp, as defined by the medicare appropriate use criteria program   E1

    BETOS: Z2   Undefined codes
    Service not separately priced by Part B

- **C** **G1018** Clinical decision support mechanism infinx, as defined by the medicare appropriate use criteria program   E1

    BETOS: Z2   Undefined codes
    Service not separately priced by Part B

- **C** **G1019** Clinical decision support mechanism logicnets, as defined by the medicare appropriate use criteria program   E1

    BETOS: Z2   Undefined codes
    Service not separately priced by Part B

- **C** **G1020** Clinical decision support mechanism curbside clinical augmented workflow, as defined by the medicare appropriate use criteria program   E1

    CPT® Crosswalk: 96130, 96131, 96132, 96133, 96156, 97161, 97162, 97163, 97165, 97166, 97167, 97169, 97170, 97171

    BETOS: Z2   Undefined codes
    Service not separately priced by Part B

- **C** **G1021** Clinical decision support mechanism ehealthline clinical decision support mechanism, as defined by the medicare appropriate use criteria program   E1

    CPT® Crosswalk: 96130, 96131, 96132, 96133, 96156, 97161, 97162, 97163, 97165, 97166, 97167, 97169, 97170, 97171

    BETOS: Z2   Undefined codes
    Service not separately priced by Part B

- **C** **G1022** Clinical decision support mechanism intermountain clinical decision support mechanism, as defined by the medicare appropriate use criteria program   E1

    CPT® Crosswalk: 96130, 96131, 96132, 96133, 96156, 97161, 97162, 97163, 97165, 97166, 97167, 97169, 97170, 97171

    BETOS: Z2   Undefined codes
    Service not separately priced by Part B

- **C** **G1023** Clinical decision support mechanism persivia clinical decision support, as defined by the medicare appropriate use criteria program   E1

    CPT® Crosswalk: 96130, 96131, 96132, 96133, 96156, 97161, 97162, 97163, 97165, 97166, 97167, 97169, 97170, 97171

    BETOS: Z2   Undefined codes
    Service not separately priced by Part B

CONVULSIVE THERAPY PROCEDURE (G2000)

- **C** **G2000** Blinded administration of convulsive therapy procedure, either electroconvulsive therapy (ECT, current covered gold standard) or magnetic seizure therapy (MST, non-covered experimental therapy), performed in an approved IDE-based clinical trial, per treatment session   S

    BETOS: P6D   Minor procedures - other (non-Medicare fee schedule)
    Service not separately priced by Part B

OTHER EVALUATION AND MANAGEMENT SERVICES (G2001-G2015)

- **C** **G2001** Brief (20 minutes) in-home visit for a new patient post-discharge. For use only in a Medicare-approved CMMI model. (Services must be furnished within a beneficiary's home, domiciliary, rest home, assisted living and/or nursing facility within 90 days following discharge from an inpatient facility and no more than 9 times.)   B

    BETOS: M4A   Home visit
    Price established by carriers

- **C** **G2002** Limited (30 minutes) in-home visit for a new patient post-discharge. For use only in a Medicare-approved CMMI model. (Services must be furnished within a beneficiary's home, domiciliary, rest home, assisted living and/or nursing facility within 90 days following discharge from an inpatient facility and no more than 9 times.)   B

    BETOS: M4A   Home visit
    Price established by carriers

- **C** **G2003** Moderate (45 minutes) in-home visit for a new patient post-discharge. For use only in a Medicare-approved CMMI model. (Services must be furnished within a beneficiary's home, domiciliary, rest home, assisted living and/or nursing facility within 90 days following discharge from an inpatient facility and no more than 9 times.)   B

    BETOS: M4A   Home visit
    Price established by carriers

- **C** **G2004** Comprehensive (60 minutes) in-home visit for a new patient post-discharge. For use only in a Medicare-approved CMMI model. (Services must be furnished within a beneficiary's home, domiciliary, rest home, assisted living and/or nursing facility within

---

90 days following discharge from an inpatient facility and no more than 9 times.)　　B

BETOS: M4A　Home visit
Price established by carriers

C **G2005** Extensive (75 minutes) in-home visit for a new patient post-discharge. For use only in a Medicare-approved CMMI model. (Services must be furnished within a beneficiary's home, domiciliary, rest home, assisted living and/or nursing facility within 90 days following discharge from an inpatient facility and no more than 9 times.)　　B

BETOS: M4A　Home visit
Price established by carriers

C **G2006** Brief (20 minutes) in-home visit for an existing patient post-discharge. For use only in a Medicare-approved CMMI model. (Services must be furnished within a beneficiary's home, domiciliary, rest home, assisted living and/or nursing facility within 90 days following discharge from an inpatient facility and no more than 9 times.)　　B

BETOS: M4A　Home visit
Price established by carriers

C **G2007** Limited (30 minutes) in-home visit for an existing patient post-discharge. For use only in a Medicare-approved CMMI model. (Services must be furnished within a beneficiary's home, domiciliary, rest home, assisted living and/or nursing facility within 90 days following discharge from an inpatient facility and no more than 9 times.)　　B

BETOS: M4A　Home visit
Price established by carriers

C **G2008** Moderate (45 minutes) in-home visit for an existing patient post-discharge. For use only in a Medicare-approved CMMI model. (Services must be furnished within a beneficiary's home, domiciliary, rest home, assisted living and/or nursing facility within 90 days following discharge from an inpatient facility and no more than 9 times.)　　B

BETOS: M4A　Home visit
Price established by carriers

C **G2009** Comprehensive (60 minutes) in-home visit for an existing patient post-discharge. For use only in a Medicare-approved CMMI model. (Services must be furnished within a beneficiary's home, domiciliary, rest home, assisted living and/or nursing facility within 90 days following discharge from an inpatient facility and no more than 9 times.)　　B

BETOS: M4A　Home visit
Price established by carriers

C **G2010** Remote evaluation of recorded video and/ or images submitted by an established patient (e.g., store and forward), including interpretation with follow-up with the patient within 24 business hours, not originating

from a related E/M service provided within the previous 7 days nor leading to an E/M service or procedure within the next 24 hours or soonest available appointment　　A

BETOS: M5D　Specialist - other
Price established by carriers

▲ **C** **G2011** Alcohol and/or substance (other than tobacco) misuse structured assessment (e.g., AUDIT, DAST), and brief intervention, 5-14 minutes　　S

BETOS: M1B　Office visits - established
Price established by carriers

C **G2012** Brief communication technology-based service, e.g. virtual check-in, by a physician or other qualified health care professional who can report evaluation and management services, provided to an established patient, not originating from a related E/M service provided within the previous 7 days nor leading to an e/m service or procedure within the next 24 hours or soonest available appointment; 5-10 minutes of medical discussion　　A

BETOS: M5D　Specialist - other
Price established by carriers

C **G2013** Extensive (75 minutes) in-home visit for an existing patient post-discharge. For use only in a Medicare-approved CMMI model. (Services must be furnished within a beneficiary's home, domiciliary, rest home, assisted living and/or nursing facility within 90 days following discharge from an inpatient facility and no more than 9 times.)　　B

BETOS: M4A　Home visit
Price established by carriers

C **G2014** Limited (30 minutes) care plan oversight. For use only in a Medicare-approved CMMI model. (Services must be furnished within a beneficiary's home, domiciliary, rest home, assisted living and/or nursing facility within 90 days following discharge from an inpatient facility and no more than 9 times.)　　B

BETOS: M4A　Home visit
Price established by carriers

C **G2015** Comprehensive (60 mins) home care plan oversight. For use only in a Medicare-approved CMMI model. (Services must be furnished within a beneficiary's home, domiciliary, rest home, assisted living and/ or nursing facility within 90 days following discharge from an inpatient facility.)　　B

BETOS: M4A　Home visit
Price established by carriers

CARE MANAGEMENT SERVICES (G2021-G2025)

C **G2021** Health care practitioners rendering treatment in place (TIP)　　E1

BETOS: M5D　Specialist - other
Service not separately priced by Part B

C **G2022** A model participant (ambulance supplier/ provider), the beneficiary refuses services covered under the model (transport to an alternate destination/treatment in place)   E1
BETOS: M5D Specialist - other
Service not separately priced by Part B

● C **G2023** Specimen collection for severe acute respiratory syndrome coronavirus 2 (sars-cov-2) (coronavirus disease [covid-19]), any specimen source   B
BETOS: T1H Lab tests - other (non-Medicare fee schedule)
Price subject to national limitation amount
Coding Clinic: 2020, Q2

● C **G2024** Specimen collection for severe acute respiratory syndrome coronavirus 2 (sars-cov-2) (coronavirus disease [covid-19]) from an individual in a SNF or by a laboratory on behalf of a HHA, any specimen source   B
BETOS: T1H Lab tests - other (non-Medicare fee schedule)
Price subject to national limitation amount
Coding Clinic: 2020, Q2

● C **G2025** Payment for a telehealth distant site service furnished by a rural health clinic (RHC) or federally qualified health center (FQHC) only   A
BETOS: M6 Consultations
Price established by carriers
Coding Clinic: 2020, Q2

ONLINE ASSESSMENT BY QUALIFIED NONPHYSICIAN HEALTHCARE PROFESSIONAL (G2061-G2063)

▲ C **G2061** Qualified nonphysician healthcare professional online assessment and management service, for an established patient, for up to seven days, cumulative time during the 7 days; 5-10 minutes   A
BETOS: M5D Specialist - other
Price established by carriers

▲ C **G2062** Qualified nonphysician healthcare professional online assessment and management service, for an established patient, for up to seven days, cumulative time during the 7 days; 11-20 minutes   A
BETOS: M5D Specialist - other
Price established by carriers

▲ C **G2063** Qualified nonphysician healthcare professional online assessment and management service, for an established patient, for up to seven days, cumulative time during the 7 days; 21 or more minutes   A
BETOS: M5D Specialist - other
Price established by carriers

COMPREHENSIVE CARE MANAGEMENT SERVICES (G2064-G2065)

C **G2064** Comprehensive care management services for a single high-risk disease, e.g., principal care management, at least 30 minutes of physician or other qualified health care professional time per calendar month with the following elements: one complex chronic condition lasting at least 3 months, which is the focus of the care plan, the condition is of sufficient severity to place patient at risk of hospitalization or have been the cause of a recent hospitalization, the condition requires development or revision of disease-specific care plan, the condition requires frequent adjustments in the medication regimen, and/or the management of the condition is unusually complex due to comorbidities   M
BETOS: M5D Specialist - other
Price established by carriers

C **G2065** Comprehensive care management for a single high-risk disease services, e.g. principal care management, at least 30 minutes of clinical staff time directed by a physician or other qualified health care professional, per calendar month with the following elements: one complex chronic condition lasting at least 3 months, which is the focus of the care plan, the condition is of sufficient severity to place patient at risk of hospitalization or have been cause of a recent hospitalization, the condition requires development or revision of disease-specific care plan, the condition requires frequent adjustments in the medication regimen, and/or the management of the condition is unusually complex due to comorbidities   S
BETOS: M5D Specialist - other
Price established by carriers

CARDIAC DEVICE EVALUATION (G2066)

C **G2066** Interrogation device evaluation(s), (remote) up to 30 days; implantable cardiovascular physiologic monitor system, implantable loop recorder system, or subcutaneous cardiac rhythm monitor system, remote data acquisition(s), receipt of transmissions and technician review, technical support and distribution of results   N
BETOS: M5D Specialist - other
Price established by carriers

MEDICATION ASSISTED TREATMENT PROGRAM (G2067-G2075)

C **G2067** Medication assisted treatment, methadone; weekly bundle including dispensing and/or administration, substance use counseling, individual and group therapy, and toxicology testing, if performed (provision of the services by a Medicare-enrolled opioid treatment program)   A
BETOS: M5D Specialist - other
Price established by carriers

● New code   ▲ Revised code   C Carrier judgment   D Special coverage instructions apply
I Not payable by Medicare   M Non-covered by Medicare   S Non-covered by Medicare statute   AHA Coding Clinic®

C **G2068** Medication assisted treatment, buprenorphine (oral); weekly bundle including dispensing and/or administration, substance use counseling, individual and group therapy, and toxicology testing if performed (provision of the services by a Medicare-enrolled opioid treatment program)   A
BETOS: M5D   Specialist - other
Price established by carriers

C **G2069** Medication assisted treatment, buprenorphine (injectable); weekly bundle including dispensing and/or administration, substance use counseling, individual and group therapy, and toxicology testing if performed (provision of the services by a Medicare-enrolled opioid treatment program)   A
BETOS: M5D   Specialist - other
Price established by carriers

C **G2070** Medication assisted treatment, buprenorphine (implant insertion); weekly bundle including dispensing and/or administration, substance use counseling, individual and group therapy, and toxicology testing if performed (provision of the services by a Medicare-enrolled opioid treatment program)   A
BETOS: M5D   Specialist - other
Price established by carriers

C **G2071** Medication assisted treatment, buprenorphine (implant removal); weekly bundle including dispensing and/or administration, substance use counseling, individual and group therapy, and toxicology testing if performed (provision of the services by a Medicare-enrolled opioid treatment program)   A
BETOS: M5D   Specialist - other
Price established by carriers

C **G2072** Medication assisted treatment, buprenorphine (implant insertion and removal); weekly bundle including dispensing and/or administration, substance use counseling, individual and group therapy, and toxicology testing if performed (provision of the services by a Medicare-enrolled opioid treatment program)   A
BETOS: M5D   Specialist - other
Price established by carriers

C **G2073** Medication assisted treatment, naltrexone; weekly bundle including dispensing and/or administration, substance use counseling, individual and group therapy, and toxicology testing if performed (provision of the services by a Medicare-enrolled opioid treatment program)   A
BETOS: M5D   Specialist - other
Price established by carriers

C **G2074** Medication assisted treatment, weekly bundle not including the drug, including substance use counseling, individual and group therapy, and toxicology testing if performed (provision of the services by a Medicare-enrolled opioid treatment program)   A
BETOS: M5D   Specialist - other
Price established by carriers

C **G2075** Medication assisted treatment, medication not otherwise specified; weekly bundle including dispensing and/or administration, substance use counseling, individual and group therapy, and toxicology testing, if performed (provision of the services by a Medicare-enrolled opioid treatment program)   A
BETOS: M5D   Specialist - other
Price established by carriers

OPIOID USE DISORDER - EVALUATION AND TREATMENT (G2076-G2081)

C **G2076** Intake activities, including initial medical examination that is a complete, fully documented physical evaluation and initial assessment by a program physician or a primary care physician, or an authorized healthcare professional under the supervision of a program physician qualified personnel that includes preparation of a treatment plan that includes the patient's short-term goals and the tasks the patient must perform to complete the short-term goals; the patient's requirements for education, vocational rehabilitation, and employment; and the medical, psycho-social, economic, legal, or other supportive services that a patient needs, conducted by qualified personnel (provision of the services by a Medicare-enrolled opioid treatment program); list separately in addition to code for primary procedure   A
BETOS: M5D   Specialist - other
Price established by carriers

C **G2077** Periodic assessment; assessing periodically by qualified personnel to determine the most appropriate combination of services and treatment (provision of the services by a Medicare-enrolled opioid treatment program); list separately in addition to code for primary procedure   A
BETOS: M5D   Specialist - other
Price established by carriers

C **G2078** Take-home supply of methadone; up to 7 additional day supply (provision of the services by a Medicare-enrolled opioid treatment program); list separately in addition to code for primary procedure   A
BETOS: M5D   Specialist - other
Price established by carriers

♂ Male only   ♀ Female only   🅐 Age   A2 - Z3 = ASC Payment indicator   A - Y = APC Status indicator
ASC = ASC Approved Procedure   **DME** Paid under the DME fee schedule   **MIPS** MIPS code

C **G2079** Take-home supply of buprenorphine (oral); up to 7 additional day supply (provision of the services by a Medicare-enrolled opioid treatment program); list separately in addition to code for primary procedure   A
BETOS: M5D   Specialist - other
Price established by carriers

C **G2080** Each additional 30 minutes of counseling in a week of medication assisted treatment, (provision of the services by a Medicare-enrolled opioid treatment program); list separately in addition to code for primary procedure   A
BETOS: M5D   Specialist - other
Price established by carriers

C **G2081** Patients age 66 and older in institutional special needs plans (SNP) or residing in long-term care with a POS code 32, 33, 34, 54 or 56 for more than 90 days during the measurement period   Ⓐ M MIPS
BETOS: Z2   Undefined codes
Service not separately priced by Part B

EVALUATION AND MANAGEMENT SERVICES (G2082-G2083)

C **G2082** Office or other outpatient visit for the evaluation and management of an established patient that requires the supervision of a physician or other qualified health care professional and provision of up to 56 mg of esketamine nasal self-administration, includes 2 hours post-administration observation   S
BETOS: M1B   Office visits - established
Price established by carriers

C **G2083** Office or other outpatient visit for the evaluation and management of an established patient that requires the supervision of a physician or other qualified health care professional and provision of greater than 56 mg esketamine nasal self-administration, includes 2 hours post-administration observation   S
BETOS: M1B   Office visits - established
Price established by carriers

OPIOID USE DISORDER - TREATMENT (OFFICE BASED) (G2086-G2088)

C **G2086** Office-based treatment for opioid use disorder, including development of the treatment plan, care coordination, individual therapy and group therapy and counseling; at least 70 minutes in the first calendar month   S
BETOS: M5D   Specialist - other
Price established by carriers
Coding Clinic: 2020, Q1

C **G2087** Office-based treatment for opioid use disorder, including care coordination, individual therapy and group therapy and counseling; at least 60 minutes in a subsequent calendar month   S
BETOS: M5D   Specialist - other
Price established by carriers
Coding Clinic: 2020, Q1

C **G2088** Office-based treatment for opioid use disorder, including care coordination, individual therapy and group therapy and counseling; each additional 30 minutes beyond the first 120 minutes (list separately in addition to code for primary procedure)   N
BETOS: M5D   Specialist - other
Price established by carriers
Coding Clinic: 2020, Q1

FUNCTIONAL STATUS (G2090-G2152)

C **G2090** Patients 66 years of age and older with at least one claim/encounter for frailty during the measurement period and a dispensed medication for dementia during the measurement period or the year prior to the measurement period   Ⓐ M MIPS
BETOS: Z2   Undefined codes
Service not separately priced by Part B

C **G2091** Patients 66 years of age and older with at least one claim/encounter for frailty during the measurement period and either one acute inpatient encounter with a diagnosis of advanced illness or two outpatient, observation, ED or nonacute inpatient encounters on different dates of service with an advanced illness diagnosis during the measurement period or the year prior to the measurement period   Ⓐ M MIPS
BETOS: Z2   Undefined codes
Service not separately priced by Part B

C **G2092** Angiotensin converting enzyme (ACE) inhibitor or angiotensin receptor blocker (ARB) or angiotensin receptor-neprilysin inhibitor (ARNI) therapy prescribed or currently being taken   M MIPS
BETOS: Z2   Undefined codes
Service not separately priced by Part B

C **G2093** Documentation of medical reason(s) for not prescribing ACE inhibitor or ARB or ARNI therapy (e.g., hypotensive patients who are at immediate risk of cardiogenic shock, hospitalized patients who have experienced marked azotemia, allergy, intolerance, other medical reasons)   M MIPS
BETOS: Z2   Undefined codes
Service not separately priced by Part B

C **G2094** Documentation of patient reason(s) for not prescribing ACE inhibitor or ARB or ARNI therapy (e.g., patient declined, other patient reasons)   M MIPS
BETOS: Z2   Undefined codes
Service not separately priced by Part B

● New code   ▲ Revised code   C Carrier judgment   D Special coverage instructions apply
Ⅰ Not payable by Medicare   M Non-covered by Medicare   S Non-covered by Medicare statute   AHA Coding Clinic®

C **G2095** Documentation of system reason(s) for not prescribing ACE inhibitor or ARB or ARNI therapy (e.g., other system reasons)   M MIPS
     BETOS: Z2   Undefined codes
     Service not separately priced by Part B

C **G2096** Angiotensin converting enzyme (ACE) inhibitor or angiotensin receptor blocker (ARB) or angiotensin receptor-neprilysin inhibitor (ARNI) therapy was not prescribed, reason not given   M MIPS
     BETOS: Z2   Undefined codes
     Service not separately priced by Part B

▲ C **G2097** Episodes where the patient had a competing diagnosis within three days after the episode date (e.g., intestinal infection, pertussis, bacterial infection, lyme disease, otitis media, acute sinusitis, chronic sinusitis, infection of the adenoids, prostatitis, cellulitis, mastoiditis, or bone infections, acute lymphadenitis, impetigo, skin staph infections, pneumonia/gonococcal infections, venereal disease (syphilis, chlamydia, inflammatory diseases [female reproductive organs]), infections of the kidney, cystitis or UTI)   M
     BETOS: Z2   Undefined codes
     Service not separately priced by Part B

C **G2098** Patients 66 years of age and older with at least one claim/encounter for frailty during the measurement period and a dispensed medication for dementia during the measurement period or the year prior to the measurement period   A M MIPS
     BETOS: Z2   Undefined codes
     Service not separately priced by Part B

C **G2099** Patients 66 years of age and older with at least one claim/encounter for frailty during the measurement period and either one acute inpatient encounter with a diagnosis of advanced illness or two outpatient, observation, ED or nonacute inpatient encounters on different dates of service with an advanced illness diagnosis during the measurement period or the year prior to the measurement period   A M MIPS
     BETOS: Z2   Undefined codes
     Service not separately priced by Part B

C **G2100** Patients 66 years of age and older with at least one claim/encounter for frailty during the measurement period and a dispensed medication for dementia during the measurement period or the year prior to the measurement period   A M MIPS
     BETOS: Z2   Undefined codes
     Service not separately priced by Part B

C **G2101** Patients 66 years of age and older with at least one claim/encounter for frailty during the measurement period and either one acute inpatient encounter with a diagnosis

of advanced illness or two outpatient, observation, ED or nonacute inpatient encounters on different dates of service with an advanced illness diagnosis during the measurement period or the year prior to the measurement period   A M MIPS
     BETOS: Z2   Undefined codes
     Service not separately priced by Part B

▲ C **G2105** Patient age 66 or older in institutional special needs plans (SNP) or residing in long-term care with pos code 32, 33, 34, 54 or 56 for more than 90 consecutive days during the measurement period   A M MIPS
     BETOS: Z2   Undefined codes
     Service not separately priced by Part B

C **G2106** Patients 66 years of age and older with at least one claim/encounter for frailty during the measurement period and a dispensed medication for dementia during the measurement period or the year prior to the measurement period   A M MIPS
     BETOS: Z2   Undefined codes
     Service not separately priced by Part B

C **G2107** Patients 66 years of age and older with at least one claim/encounter for frailty during the measurement period and either one acute inpatient encounter with a diagnosis of advanced illness or two outpatient, observation, ED or nonacute inpatient encounters on different dates of service with an advanced illness diagnosis during the measurement period or the year prior to the measurement period   A M MIPS
     BETOS: Z2   Undefined codes
     Service not separately priced by Part B

▲ C **G2108** Patient age 66 or older in institutional special needs plans (SNP) or residing in long-term care with pos code 32, 33, 34, 54 or 56 for more than 90 consecutive days during the measurement period   M MIPS
     BETOS: Z2   Undefined codes
     Service not separately priced by Part B

C **G2109** Patients 66 years of age and older with at least one claim/encounter for frailty during the measurement period and a dispensed medication for dementia during the measurement period or the year prior to the measurement period   A M MIPS
     BETOS: Z2   Undefined codes
     Service not separately priced by Part B

C **G2110** Patients 66 years of age and older with at least one claim/encounter for frailty during the measurement period and either one acute inpatient encounter with a diagnosis of advanced illness or two outpatient, observation, ED or nonacute inpatient encounters on different dates of service with an advanced illness diagnosis during the measurement period or the year prior to the measurement period   A M MIPS

BETOS: Z2   Undefined codes
Service not separately priced by Part B

C G2112 Patient receiving <=5 mg daily prednisone (or equivalent), or RA activity is worsening, or glucocorticoid use is for less than 6 months   M MIPS
BETOS: Z2   Undefined codes
Service not separately priced by Part B

C G2113 Patient receiving >5 mg daily prednisone (or equivalent) for longer than 6 months, and improvement or no change in disease activity   M MIPS
BETOS: Z2   Undefined codes
Service not separately priced by Part B

▲ **C G2115** Patients 66 - 80 years of age with at least one claim/encounter for frailty during the measurement period and a dispensed medication for dementia during the measurement period or the year prior to the measurement period   Ⓐ M MIPS
BETOS: Z2   Undefined codes
Service not separately priced by Part B

▲ **C G2116** Patients 66 - 80 years of age with at least one claim/encounter for frailty during the measurement period and either one acute inpatient encounter with a diagnosis of advanced illness or two outpatient, observation, ed or nonacute inpatient encounters on different dates of service with an advanced illness diagnosis during the measurement period or the year prior to the measurement period   Ⓐ M MIPS
BETOS: Z2   Undefined codes
Service not separately priced by Part B

▲ **C G2118** Patients 81 years of age and older with at least one claim/encounter for frailty during the measurement period   Ⓐ M
BETOS: Z2   Undefined codes
Service not separately priced by Part B

C G2121 Psychosis, depression, anxiety, apathy, and impulse control disorder assessed   M MIPS
BETOS: Z2   Undefined codes
Service not separately priced by Part B

C G2122 Psychosis, depression, anxiety, apathy, and impulse control disorder not assessed   M MIPS
BETOS: Z2   Undefined codes
Service not separately priced by Part B

▲ **C G2125** Patients 81 years of age and older with at least one claim/encounter for frailty during the six months prior to the measurement period through December 31 of the measurement period   Ⓐ M
BETOS: Z2   Undefined codes
Service not separately priced by Part B

▲ **C G2126** Patients 66 - 80 years of age with at least one claim/encounter for frailty during the measurement period and either one acute inpatient encounter with a diagnosis of advanced illness or two outpatient, observation, ed or nonacute inpatient encounters on different dates of service with an advanced illness diagnosis during the measurement period or the year prior to the measurement period   Ⓐ M MIPS
BETOS: Z2   Undefined codes
Service not separately priced by Part B

▲ **C G2127** Patients 66 - 80 years of age with at least one claim/encounter for frailty during the measurement period and a dispensed medication for dementia during the measurement period or the year prior to the measurement period   Ⓐ M MIPS
BETOS: Z2   Undefined codes
Service not separately priced by Part B

C G2128 Documentation of medical reason(s) for not on a daily aspirin or other antiplatelet (e.g. history of gastrointestinal bleed, intra-cranial bleed, blood disorders, idiopathic thrombocytopenic purpura (ITP), gastric bypass or documentation of active anticoagulant use during the measurement period)   M MIPS
BETOS: Z2   Undefined codes
Service not separately priced by Part B

C G2129 Procedure-related BP's not taken during an outpatient visit. Examples include same day surgery, ambulatory service center, G.I. lab, dialysis, infusion center, chemotherapy M MIPS
BETOS: Z2   Undefined codes
Service not separately priced by Part B

C G2136 Back pain measured by the visual analog scale (VAS) at three months (6 - 20 weeks) postoperatively was less than or equal to 3.0 or back pain measured by the visual analog scale (VAS) within three months preoperatively and at three months (6 - 20 weeks) postoperatively demonstrated an improvement of 5.0 points or greater   M MIPS
BETOS: Z2   Undefined codes
Service not separately priced by Part B

C G2137 Back pain measured by the visual analog scale (VAS) at three months (6 - 20 weeks) postoperatively was greater than 3.0 and back pain measured by the visual analog scale (VAS) within three months preoperatively and at three months (6 - 20 weeks) postoperatively demonstrated a change of less than an improvement of 5.0 points   M MIPS
BETOS: Z2   Undefined codes
Service not separately priced by Part B

● New code   ▲ Revised code   **C** Carrier judgment   **D** Special coverage instructions apply
I Not payable by Medicare   **M** Non-covered by Medicare   **S** Non-covered by Medicare statute   AHA Coding Clinic®

C **G2138** Back pain as measured by the visual analog scale (VAS) at one year (9 to 15 months) postoperatively was less than or equal to 3.0 or back pain measured by the visual analog scale (VAS) within three months preoperatively and at one year (9 to 15 months) postoperatively demonstrated a change of 5.0 points or greater M MIPS

BETOS: Z2   Undefined codes
Service not separately priced by Part B

C **G2139** Back pain measured by the visual analog scale (VAS) pain at one year (9 to 15 months) postoperatively was greater than 3.0 and back pain measured by the visual analog scale (VAS) within three months preoperatively and at one year (9 to 15 months) postoperatively demonstrated a change of less than 5.0 M MIPS

BETOS: Z2   Undefined codes
Service not separately priced by Part B

C **G2140** Leg pain measured by the visual analog scale (VAS) at three months (6 - 20 weeks) postoperatively was less than or equal to 3.0 or leg pain measured by the visual analog scale (VAS) within three months preoperatively and at three months (6 - 20 weeks) postoperatively demonstrated an improvement of 5.0 points or greater M MIPS

BETOS: Z2   Undefined codes
Service not separately priced by Part B

C **G2141** Leg pain measured by the visual analog scale (VAS) at three months (6 - 20 weeks) postoperatively was greater than 3.0 and leg pain measured by the visual analog scale (VAS) within three months preoperatively and at three months (6 - 20 weeks) postoperatively demonstrated less than an improvement of 5.0 points M MIPS

BETOS: Z2   Undefined codes
Service not separately priced by Part B

C **G2142** Functional status measured by the oswestry disability index (ODI version 2.1a) at one year (9 to 15 months) postoperatively was less than or equal to 22 or functional status measured by the ODI version 2.1a within three months preoperatively and at one year (9 to 15 months) postoperatively demonstrated a change of 30 points or greater M MIPS

BETOS: Z2   Undefined codes
Service not separately priced by Part B

C **G2143** Functional status measured by the oswestry disability index (ODI version 2.1a) at one year (9 to 15 months) postoperatively was greater than 22 and functional status measured by the ODI version 2.1a within three months preoperatively and at one year (9 to 15 months) postoperatively demonstrated a change of less than 30 points M MIPS

BETOS: Z2   Undefined codes
Service not separately priced by Part B

C **G2144** Functional status measured by the oswestry disability index (ODI version 2.1a) at three months (6 - 20 weeks) postoperatively was less than or equal to 22 or functional status measured by the ODI version 2.1a within three months preoperatively and at three months (6 - 20 weeks) postoperatively demonstrated a change of 30 points or greater M MIPS

BETOS: Z2   Undefined codes
Service not separately priced by Part B

C **G2145** Functional status measured by the oswestry disability index (ODI version 2.1a) at three months (6 - 20 weeks) postoperatively was greater than 22 and functional status measured by the ODI version 2.1a within three months preoperatively and at three months (6 - 20 weeks) postoperatively demonstrated a change of less than 30 points M MIPS

BETOS: Z2   Undefined codes
Service not separately priced by Part B

C **G2146** Leg pain as measured by the visual analog scale (VAS) at one year (9 to 15 months) postoperatively was less than or equal to 3.0 or leg pain measured by the visual analog scale (VAS) within three months preoperatively and at one year (9 to 15 months) postoperatively demonstrated an improvement of 5.0 points or greater M MIPS

BETOS: Z2   Undefined codes
Service not separately priced by Part B

C **G2147** Leg pain measured by the visual analog scale (VAS) at one year (9 to 15 months) postoperatively was greater than 3.0 and leg pain measured by the visual analog scale (VAS) within three months preoperatively and at one year (9 to 15 months) postoperatively demonstrated less than an improvement of 5.0 points M MIPS

BETOS: Z2   Undefined codes
Service not separately priced by Part B

C **G2148** Performance met: multimodal pain management was used M MIPS

BETOS: Z2   Undefined codes
Service not separately priced by Part B

C **G2149** Documentation of medical reason(s) for not using multimodal pain management (e.g., allergy to multiple classes of analgesics, intubated patient, hepatic failure, patient reports no pain during PACU stay, other medical reason(s)) M MIPS

BETOS: Z2   Undefined codes
Service not separately priced by Part B

G2138 - G2149

PROCEDURES / PROFESSIONAL SERVICES (G0008-G9987)

C G2150 Performance not met: multimodal pain management was not used   M MIPS

BETOS: Z2   Undefined codes

Service not separately priced by Part B

▲ **C G2151** Documentation stating patient has a diagnosis of a degenerative neurological condition such as ALS, MS, or parkinson's diagnosed at any time before or during the episode of care   M MIPS

BETOS: Z2   Undefined codes

Service not separately priced by Part B

▲ **C G2152** Risk-adjusted functional status change residual score for the neck impairment successfully calculated and the score was equal to zero (0) or greater than zero (> 0)   M MIPS

BETOS: Z2   Undefined codes

Service not separately priced by Part B

PERFORMANCE MEASURES (G2167-G2171)

▲ **C G2167** Risk-adjusted functional status change residual score for the neck impairment successfully calculated and the score was less than zero (< 0)   M MIPS

BETOS: Z2   Undefined codes

Service not separately priced by Part B

● **C G2168** Services performed by a physical therapist assistant in the home health setting in the delivery of a safe and effective physical therapy maintenance program, each 15 minutes   B

BETOS: Y1   Other - Medicare fee schedule

Service not separately priced by Part B

● **C G2169** Services performed by an occupational therapist assistant in the home health setting in the delivery of a safe and effective occupational therapy maintenance program, each 15 minutes   B

BETOS: Y1   Other - Medicare fee schedule

Service not separately priced by Part B

● **C G2170** Percutaneous arteriovenous fistula creation (AVF), direct, any site, by tissue approximation using thermal resistance energy, and secondary procedures to redirect blood flow (e.g., transluminal balloon angioplasty, coil embolization) when performed, and includes all imaging and radiologic guidance, supervision and interpretation, when performed   G2 ASC J1

BETOS: P1G   Major procedure - Other

Price established by carriers

Coding Clinic: 2020, Q2

● **C G2171** Percutaneous arteriovenous fistula creation (AVF), direct, any site, using magnetic-guided arterial and venous catheters and radiofrequency energy, including flow-directing procedures (e.g., vascular coil embolization with radiologic supervision and interpretation, wen performed) and fistulogram(s), angiography, enography, and/or ultrasound, with radiologic supervision and interpretation, when performed   J8 ASC J1

BETOS: P1G   Major procedure - Other

Price established by carriers

Coding Clinic: 2020, Q2

CLINICIAN DOCUMENTATION AND MANAGEMENT SERVICES (G2173-G2210)

● **C G2173** Uri episodes where the patient had a competing comorbid condition during the 12 months prior to or on the episode date (e.g., tuberculosis, neutropenia, cystic fibrosis, chronic bronchitis, pulmonary edema, respiratory failure, rheumatoid lung disease)   M

BETOS: Z2   Undefined codes

Service not separately priced by Part B

● **C G2174** Uri episodes when the patient had a new or refill prescription of antibiotics (table 1) in the 30 days prior to or on the episode date   M

BETOS: Z2   Undefined codes

Service not separately priced by Part B

● **C G2175** Episodes where the patient had a competing comorbid condition during the 12 months prior to or on the episode date (e.g., tuberculosis, neutropenia, cystic fibrosis, chronic bronchitis, pulmonary edema, respiratory failure, rheumatoid lung disease)   M

BETOS: Z2   Undefined codes

Service not separately priced by Part B

● **C G2176** Outpatient, ed, or observation visits that result in an inpatient admission   M

BETOS: Z2   Undefined codes

Service not separately priced by Part B

● **C G2177** Acute bronchitis/bronchiolitis episodes when the patient had a new or refill prescription of antibiotics (table 1) in the 30 days prior to or on the episode date   M

BETOS: Z2   Undefined codes

Service not separately priced by Part B

● **C G2178** Clinician documented that patient was not an eligible candidate for lower extremity neurological exam measure, for example patient bilateral amputee; patient has condition that would not allow them to accurately respond to a neurological exam (dementia, alzheimer's, etc.); patient has previously documented diabetic peripheral neuropathy with loss of protective sensation   M

BETOS: Z2   Undefined codes

Service not separately priced by Part B

● **C G2179** Clinician documented that patient had medical reason for not performing lower extremity neurological exam   M

BETOS: Z2   Undefined codes

Service not separately priced by Part B

● New code   ▲ Revised code   **C** Carrier judgment   **D** Special coverage instructions apply

I Not payable by Medicare   **M** Non-covered by Medicare   **S** Non-covered by Medicare statute   AHA Coding Clinic®

● C **G2180** Clinician documented that patient was not an eligible candidate for evaluation of footwear as patient is bilateral lower extremity amputee M
 BETOS: Z2 Undefined codes
 Service not separately priced by Part B

● C **G2181** BMI not documented due to medical reason or patient refusal of height or weight measurement M
 BETOS: Z2 Undefined codes
 Service not separately priced by Part B

● C **G2182** Patient receiving first-time biologic disease modifying anti-rheumatic drug therapy M
 BETOS: Z2 Undefined codes
 Service not separately priced by Part B

● C **G2183** Documentation patient unable to communicate and informant not available M
 BETOS: Z2 Undefined codes
 Service not separately priced by Part B

● C **G2184** Patient does not have a caregiver M
 BETOS: Z2 Undefined codes
 Service not separately priced by Part B

● C **G2185** Documentation caregiver is trained and certified in dementia care M
 BETOS: Z2 Undefined codes
 Service not separately priced by Part B

● C **G2186** Patient /caregiver dyad has been referred to appropriate resources and connection to those resources is confirmed M
 BETOS: Z2 Undefined codes
 Service not separately priced by Part B

● C **G2187** Patients with clinical indications for imaging of the head: head trauma M
 BETOS: Z2 Undefined codes
 Service not separately priced by Part B

● C **G2188** Patients with clinical indications for imaging of the head: new or change in headache above 50 years of age Ⓐ M
 BETOS: Z2 Undefined codes
 Service not separately priced by Part B

● C **G2189** Patients with clinical indications for imaging of the head: abnormal neurologic exam M
 BETOS: Z2 Undefined codes
 Service not separately priced by Part B

● C **G2190** Patients with clinical indications for imaging of the head: headache radiating to the neck M
 BETOS: Z2 Undefined codes
 Service not separately priced by Part B

● C **G2191** Patients with clinical indications for imaging of the head: positional headaches M
 BETOS: Z2 Undefined codes
 Service not separately priced by Part B

● C **G2192** Patients with clinical indications for imaging of the head: temporal headaches in patients over 55 years of age Ⓐ M

BETOS: Z2 Undefined codes
Service not separately priced by Part B

● C **G2193** Patients with clinical indications for imaging of the head: new onset headache in preschool children or younger (<6 years of age) Ⓐ M
 BETOS: Z2 Undefined codes
 Service not separately priced by Part B

● C **G2194** Patients with clinical indications for imaging of the head: new onset headache in pediatric patients with disabilities for which headache is a concern as inferred from behavior Ⓐ M
 BETOS: Z2 Undefined codes
 Service not separately priced by Part B

● C **G2195** Patients with clinical indications for imaging of the head: occipital headache in children Ⓐ M
 BETOS: Z2 Undefined codes
 Service not separately priced by Part B

● C **G2196** Patient identified as an unhealthy alcohol user when screened for unhealthy alcohol use using a systematic screening method M
 BETOS: Z2 Undefined codes
 Service not separately priced by Part B

● C **G2197** Patient screened for unhealthy alcohol use using a systematic screening method and not identified as an unhealthy alcohol user M
 BETOS: Z2 Undefined codes
 Service not separately priced by Part B

● C **G2198** Documentation of medical reason(s) for not screening for unhealthy alcohol use using a systematic screening method (e.g., limited life expectancy, other medical reasons) M
 BETOS: Z2 Undefined codes
 Service not separately priced by Part B

● C **G2199** Patient not screened for unhealthy alcohol use using a systematic screening method, reason not given M
 BETOS: Z2 Undefined codes
 Service not separately priced by Part B

● C **G2200** Patient identified as an unhealthy alcohol user received brief counseling M
 BETOS: Z2 Undefined codes
 Service not separately priced by Part B

● C **G2201** Documentation of medical reason(s) for not providing brief counseling (e.g., limited life expectancy, other medical reasons) M
 BETOS: Z2 Undefined codes
 Service not separately priced by Part B

● C **G2202** Patient did not receive brief counseling if identified as an unhealthy alcohol user, reason not given M
 BETOS: Z2 Undefined codes
 Service not separately priced by Part B

PROCEDURES / PROFESSIONAL SERVICES (G0008-G9987)

● C **G2203** Documentation of medical reason(s) for not providing brief counseling if identified as an unhealthy alcohol user (e.g., limited life expectancy, other medical reasons) M
BETOS: Z2 Undefined codes
Service not separately priced by Part B

● C **G2204** Patients between 50 and 85 years of age who received a screening colonoscopy during the performance period Ⓐ M
BETOS: Z2 Undefined codes
Service not separately priced by Part B

● C **G2205** Patients with pregnancy during adjuvant treatment course ♀ M
BETOS: Z2 Undefined codes
Service not separately priced by Part B

● C **G2206** Patient received adjuvant treatment course including both chemotherapy and her2-targeted therapy M
BETOS: Z2 Undefined codes
Service not separately priced by Part B

● C **G2207** Reason for not administering adjuvant treatment course including both chemotherapy and her2-targeted therapy (e.g. poor performance status (ecog 3-4; karnofsky =50), cardiac contraindications, insufficient renal function, insufficient hepatic function, other active or secondary cancer diagnoses, other medical contraindications, patients who died during initial treatment course or transferred during or after initial treatment course) M
BETOS: Z2 Undefined codes
Service not separately priced by Part B

● C **G2208** Patient did not receive adjuvant treatment course including both chemotherapy and her2-targeted therapy M
BETOS: Z2 Undefined codes
Service not separately priced by Part B

● C **G2209** Patient refused to participate M
BETOS: Z2 Undefined codes
Service not separately priced by Part B

● C **G2210** Risk-adjusted functional status change residual score for the neck impairment not measured because the patient did not complete the neck FS PROM at initial evaluation and/or near discharge, reason not given M
BETOS: Z2 Undefined codes
Service not separately priced by Part B

EVALUATION AND CARE MANAGEMENT SERVICES (G2211-G2214)

● C **G2211** Visit complexity inherent to evaluation and management associated with medical care services that serve as the continuing focal point for all needed health care services and/ or with medical care services that are part of ongoing care related to a patient's single, serious condition or a complex condition. (add-on code, list separately in addition to office/outpatient evaluation and management visit, new or established) N
BETOS: Z2 Undefined codes
Service not separately priced by Part B

● C **G2212** Prolonged office or other outpatient evaluation and management service(s) beyond the maximum required time of the primary procedure which has been selected using total time on the date of the primary service; each additional 15 minutes by the physician or qualified healthcare professional, with or without direct patient contact (list separately in addition to CPT® codes 99205, 99215 for office or other outpatient evaluation and management services) (do not report g2212 on the same date of service as 99354, 99355, 99358, 99359, 99415, 99416). (do not report g2212 for any time unit less than 15 minutes) N
BETOS: M5D Specialist - other
Price established using national RVUs

● C **G2213** Initiation of medication for the treatment of opioid use disorder in the emergency department setting, including assessment, referral to ongoing care, and arranging access to supportive services (list separately in addition to code for primary procedure) N
BETOS: Z2 Undefined codes
Price established using national RVUs

● C **G2214** Initial or subsequent psychiatric collaborative care management, first 30 minutes in a month of behavioral health care manager activities, in consultation with a psychiatric consultant, and directed by the treating physician or other qualified health care professional S
BETOS: M5D Specialist - other
Price established using national RVUs

TAKE HOME SUPPLIES (G2215-G2216)

● C **G2215** Take-home supply of nasal naloxone (provision of the services by a Medicare-enrolled opioid treatment program); list separately in addition to code for primary procedure A
BETOS: Z2 Undefined codes
Price established using national RVUs

● C **G2216** Take-home supply of injectable naloxone (provision of the services by a Medicare-enrolled opioid treatment program); list separately in addition to code for primary procedure A
BETOS: Z2 Undefined codes
Price established using national RVUs

| ● New code | ▲ Revised code | C Carrier judgment | D Special coverage instructions apply |
| I Not payable by Medicare | M Non-covered by Medicare | S Non-covered by Medicare statute | AHA Coding Clinic® |

DOCUMENTATION ASSESSMENT (REMOTE) (G2250)

- **C G2250** Remote assessment of recorded video and/or images submitted by an established patient (e.g., store and forward), including interpretation with follow-up with the patient within 24 business hours, not originating from a related service provided within the previous 7 days nor leading to a service or procedure within the next 24 hours or soonest available appointment A

  BETOS: M5D Specialist - other
  Price established by carriers

BRIEF COMMUNICATION TECHNOLOGY-BASED SERVICES (G2251-G2252)

- **C G2251** Brief communication technology-based service, e.g. virtual check-in, by a qualified health care professional who cannot report evaluation and management services, provided to an established patient, not originating from a related service provided within the previous 7 days nor leading to a service or procedure within the next 24 hours or soonest available appointment; 5-10 minutes of clinical discussion A

  BETOS: M5D Specialist - other
  Price established by carriers

- **C G2252** Brief communication technology-based service, e.g. virtual check-in, by a physician or other qualified health care professional who can report evaluation and management services, provided to an established patient, not originating from a related e/m service provided within the previous 7 days nor leading to an e/m service or procedure within the next 24 hours or soonest available appointment; 11-20 minutes of medical discussion A

  BETOS: M5D Specialist - other
  Price established by carriers

RADIATION THERAPY SERVICES (G6001-G6017)

- **D G6001** Ultrasonic guidance for placement of radiation therapy fields B

  CPT® Crosswalk: 76978, 76979, 77373, 77387, 77402, 77407, 77412

  BETOS: I3F Echography/ultrasonography - other
  Price established by carriers

- **C G6002** Stereoscopic X-ray guidance for localization of target volume for the delivery of radiation therapy B

  CPT® Crosswalk: 01922, 19294, 77373, 77387, 77402, 77407, 77412

  BETOS: I4B Imaging/procedure - other
  Price established by carriers

- **C G6003** Radiation treatment delivery, single treatment area, single port or parallel opposed ports, simple blocks or no blocks: up to 5 MeV B

  BETOS: P7A Oncology - radiation therapy
  Price established by carriers

- **C G6004** Radiation treatment delivery, single treatment area, single port or parallel opposed ports, simple blocks or no blocks: 6-10 MeV B

  BETOS: P7A Oncology - radiation therapy
  Price established by carriers

- **C G6005** Radiation treatment delivery, single treatment area, single port or parallel opposed ports, simple blocks or no blocks: 11-19 MeV B

  BETOS: P7A Oncology - radiation therapy
  Price established by carriers

- **C G6006** Radiation treatment delivery, single treatment area, single port or parallel opposed ports, simple blocks or no blocks: 20 MeV or greater B

  BETOS: P7A Oncology - radiation therapy
  Price established by carriers

- **C G6007** Radiation treatment delivery, 2 separate treatment areas, 3 or more ports on a single treatment area, use of multiple blocks: up to 5 MeV B

  BETOS: P7A Oncology - radiation therapy
  Price established by carriers

- **C G6008** Radiation treatment delivery, 2 separate treatment areas, 3 or more ports on a single treatment area, use of multiple blocks: 6-10 MeV B

  BETOS: P7A Oncology - radiation therapy
  Price established by carriers

- **C G6009** Radiation treatment delivery, 2 separate treatment areas, 3 or more ports on a single treatment area, use of multiple blocks: 11-19 MeV B

  BETOS: P7A Oncology - radiation therapy
  Price established by carriers

- **C G6010** Radiation treatment delivery, 2 separate treatment areas, 3 or more ports on a single treatment area, use of multiple blocks: 20 MeV or greater B

  BETOS: P7A Oncology - radiation therapy
  Price established by carriers

- **C G6011** Radiation treatment delivery, 3 or more separate treatment areas, custom blocking, tangential ports, wedges, rotational beam, compensators, electron beam; up to 5 MeV B

  BETOS: P7A Oncology - radiation therapy
  Price established by carriers

- **C G6012** Radiation treatment delivery, 3 or more separate treatment areas, custom blocking, tangential ports, wedges, rotational beam, compensators, electron beam; 6-10 MeV B

  BETOS: P7A Oncology - radiation therapy
  Price established by carriers

♂ Male only ♀ Female only Ⓐ Age A2 - Z3 = ASC Payment indicator A - Y = APC Status indicator
ASC = ASC Approved Procedure DME Paid under the DME fee schedule MIPS MIPS code

G6013 Radiation treatment delivery, 3 or more separate treatment areas, custom blocking, tangential ports, wedges, rotational beam, compensators, electron beam; 11-19 MeV   B
BETOS: P7A   Oncology - radiation therapy
Price established by carriers

G6014 Radiation treatment delivery, 3 or more separate treatment areas, custom blocking, tangential ports, wedges, rotational beam, compensators, electron beam; 20 MeV or greater   B
BETOS: P7A   Oncology - radiation therapy
Price established by carriers

G6015 Intensity modulated treatment delivery, single or multiple fields/arcs, via narrow spatially and temporally modulated beams, binary, dynamic MLC, per treatment session   B
BETOS: P7A   Oncology - radiation therapy
Price established by carriers

G6016 Compensator-based beam modulation treatment delivery of inverse planned treatment using 3 or more high resolution (milled or cast) compensator, convergent beam modulated fields, per treatment session   B
BETOS: P7A   Oncology - radiation therapy
Price established by carriers

G6017 Intra-fraction localization and tracking of target or patient motion during delivery of radiation therapy (e.g., 3D positional tracking, gating, 3D surface tracking), each fraction of treatment   B
BETOS: P6C   Minor procedures - other (Medicare fee schedule)
Price established by carriers

ADDITIONAL QUALITY MEASURES (G8395-G8635)

G8395 Left ventricular ejection fraction (LVEF) >= 40% or documentation as normal or mildly depressed left ventricular systolic function   M
BETOS: M5D   Specialist - other
Service not separately priced by Part B

G8396 Left ventricular ejection fraction (LVEF) not performed or documented   M
BETOS: M5D   Specialist - other
Service not separately priced by Part B

G8397 Dilated macular or fundus exam performed, including documentation of the presence or absence of macular edema and level of severity of retinopathy   M MIPS
BETOS: M5D   Specialist - other
Service not separately priced by Part B

G8399 Patient with documented results of a central dual-energy X-ray absorptiometry (DXA) ever being performed   M MIPS
BETOS: M5D   Specialist - other
Service not separately priced by Part B

G8400 Patient with central dual-energy X-ray absorptiometry (DXA) results not documented, reason not given   M MIPS
BETOS: M5D   Specialist - other
Service not separately priced by Part B

G8404 Lower extremity neurological exam performed and documented   M MIPS
BETOS: M5D   Specialist - other
Service not separately priced by Part B

G8405 Lower extremity neurological exam not performed   M MIPS
BETOS: M5D   Specialist - other
Service not separately priced by Part B

G8410 Footwear evaluation performed and documented   M MIPS
BETOS: M5D   Specialist - other
Service not separately priced by Part B

G8415 Footwear evaluation was not performed   M MIPS
BETOS: M5D   Specialist - other
Service not separately priced by Part B

G8416 Clinician documented that patient was not an eligible candidate for footwear evaluation measure   M MIPS
BETOS: M5D   Specialist - other
Service not separately priced by Part B

G8417 BMI is documented above normal parameters and a follow-up plan is documented   A M MIPS
BETOS: M5D   Specialist - other
Service not separately priced by Part B

G8418 BMI is documented below normal parameters and a follow-up plan is documented   A M MIPS
BETOS: M5D   Specialist - other
Service not separately priced by Part B

G8419 BMI documented outside normal parameters, no follow-up plan documented, no reason given   A M MIPS
BETOS: M5D   Specialist - other
Service not separately priced by Part B

G8420 BMI is documented within normal parameters and no follow-up plan is required   A M MIPS
BETOS: M5D   Specialist - other
Service not separately priced by Part B

G8421 BMI not documented and no reason is given   A M MIPS
BETOS: M5D   Specialist - other
Service not separately priced by Part B

G8422 BMI not documented, documentation the patient is not eligible for BMI calculation   A M MIPS
BETOS: M5D   Specialist - other
Service not separately priced by Part B

● New code   ▲ Revised code   C Carrier judgment   D Special coverage instructions apply
I Not payable by Medicare   M Non-covered by Medicare   S Non-covered by Medicare statute   AHA Coding Clinic®

C **G8427** Eligible clinician attests to documenting in the medical record they obtained, updated, or reviewed the patient's current medications M MIPS

BETOS: M5D   Specialist - other
Service not separately priced by Part B

C **G8428** Current list of medications not documented as obtained, updated, or reviewed by the eligible clinician, reason not given M MIPS

BETOS: M5D   Specialist - other
Service not separately priced by Part B

▲ C **G8430** Documentation of a medical reason(s) for not documenting, updating, or reviewing the patient's current medications list (e.g., patient is in an urgent or emergent medical situation) M MIPS

BETOS: M5D   Specialist - other
Service not separately priced by Part B

C **G8431** Screening for depression is documented as being positive and a follow-up plan is documented M MIPS

BETOS: M5D   Specialist - other
Service not separately priced by Part B

C **G8432** Depression screening not documented, reason not given M MIPS

BETOS: M5D   Specialist - other
Service not separately priced by Part B

C **G8433** Screening for depression not completed, documented reason M MIPS

BETOS: M5D   Specialist - other
Service not separately priced by Part B

C **G8450** Beta-blocker therapy prescribed M MIPS

BETOS: M5D   Specialist - other
Service not separately priced by Part B

C **G8451** Beta-blocker therapy for LVEF < 40% not prescribed for reasons documented by the clinician (e.g., low blood pressure, fluid overload, asthma, patients recently treated with an intravenous positive inotropic agent, allergy, intolerance, other medical reasons, patient declined, other patient reasons, or other reasons attributable to the healthcare system) M MIPS

BETOS: M5D   Specialist - other
Service not separately priced by Part B

C **G8452** Beta-blocker therapy not prescribed M MIPS

BETOS: M5D   Specialist - other
Service not separately priced by Part B

C **G8465** High or very high risk of recurrence of prostate cancer ♂ M MIPS

BETOS: M5D   Specialist - other
Service not separately priced by Part B

C **G8473** Angiotensin converting enzyme (ACE) inhibitor or angiotensin receptor blocker (ARB) therapy prescribed M MIPS

BETOS: M5D   Specialist - other
Service not separately priced by Part B

C **G8474** Angiotensin converting enzyme (ACE) inhibitor or angiotensin receptor blocker (ARB) therapy not prescribed for reasons documented by the clinician (e.g., allergy, intolerance, pregnancy, renal failure due to ACE inhibitor, diseases of the aortic or mitral valve, other medical reasons) or (e.g., patient declined, other patient reasons) or (e.g., lack of drug availability, other reasons attributable to the health care system) M MIPS

BETOS: M5D   Specialist - other
Service not separately priced by Part B

C **G8475** Angiotensin converting enzyme (ACE) inhibitor or angiotensin receptor blocker (ARB) therapy not prescribed, reason not given M MIPS

BETOS: M5D   Specialist - other
Service not separately priced by Part B

C **G8476** Most recent blood pressure has a systolic measurement of < 140 mmHg and a diastolic measurement of < 90 mmHg M

BETOS: M5D   Specialist - other
Service not separately priced by Part B

C **G8477** Most recent blood pressure has a systolic measurement of >=140 mmHg and/or a diastolic measurement of >=90 mmHg M

BETOS: M5D   Specialist - other
Service not separately priced by Part B

C **G8478** Blood pressure measurement not performed or documented, reason not given M

BETOS: M5D   Specialist - other
Service not separately priced by Part B

C **G8482** Influenza immunization administered or previously received M MIPS

BETOS: M5D   Specialist - other
Service not separately priced by Part B

C **G8483** Influenza immunization was not administered for reasons documented by clinician (e.g., patient allergy or other medical reasons, patient declined or other patient reasons, vaccine not available or other system reasons) M MIPS

BETOS: M5D   Specialist - other
Service not separately priced by Part B

C **G8484** Influenza immunization was not administered, reason not given M MIPS

BETOS: M5D   Specialist - other
Service not separately priced by Part B

C **G8506** Patient receiving angiotensin converting enzyme (ACE) inhibitor or angiotensin receptor blocker (ARB) therapy M MIPS

BETOS: M5D   Specialist - other
Service not separately priced by Part B
Coding Clinic: 2008, Q4

♂ Male only   ♀ Female only   Ⓐ Age   A2 - Z3 = ASC Payment indicator   A - Y = APC Status indicator
ASC = ASC Approved Procedure   DME Paid under the DME fee schedule   MIPS MIPS code

C G8510 Screening for depression is documented as negative, a follow-up plan is not required   M MIPS
BETOS: M5D   Specialist - other
Service not separately priced by Part B
Coding Clinic: 2008, Q4

C G8511 Screening for depression documented as positive, follow-up plan not documented, reason not given   M MIPS
BETOS: M5D   Specialist - other
Service not separately priced by Part B
Coding Clinic: 2008, Q4

C G8535 Elder maltreatment screen not documented; documentation that patient is not eligible for the elder maltreatment screen at the time of the encounter   A M MIPS
BETOS: M5D   Specialist - other
Service not separately priced by Part B
Coding Clinic: 2008, Q4

C G8536 No documentation of an elder maltreatment screen, reason not given   A M MIPS
BETOS: M5D   Specialist - other
Service not separately priced by Part B
Coding Clinic: 2008, Q4

C G8539 Functional outcome assessment documented as positive using a standardized tool and a care plan based on identified deficiencies on the date of functional outcome assessment, is documented   A M MIPS
BETOS: M5D   Specialist - other
Service not separately priced by Part B
Coding Clinic: 2008, Q4

C G8540 Functional outcome assessment not documented as being performed, documentation the patient is not eligible for a functional outcome assessment using a standardized tool at the time of the encounter   A M MIPS
BETOS: M5D   Specialist - other
Service not separately priced by Part B
Coding Clinic: 2008, Q4

C G8541 Functional outcome assessment using a standardized tool not documented, reason not given   M MIPS
BETOS: M5D   Specialist - other
Service not separately priced by Part B
Coding Clinic: 2008, Q4

C G8542 Functional outcome assessment using a standardized tool is documented; no functional deficiencies identified, care plan not required   A M MIPS
BETOS: M5D   Specialist - other
Service not separately priced by Part B
Coding Clinic: 2008, Q4

C G8543 Documentation of a positive functional outcome assessment using a standardized tool; care plan not documented, reason not given   A M MIPS
BETOS: M5D   Specialist - other
Service not separately priced by Part B
Coding Clinic: 2008, Q4

C G8559 Patient referred to a physician (preferably a physician with training in disorders of the ear) for an otologic evaluation   M
BETOS: M5D   Specialist - other
Service not separately priced by Part B

C G8560 Patient has a history of active drainage from the ear within the previous 90 days   M
BETOS: M5D   Specialist - other
Service not separately priced by Part B

C G8561 Patient is not eligible for the referral for otologic evaluation for patients with a history of active drainage measure   M
BETOS: M5D   Specialist - other
Service not separately priced by Part B

C G8562 Patient does not have a history of active drainage from the ear within the previous 90 days   M
BETOS: M5D   Specialist - other
Service not separately priced by Part B

C G8563 Patient not referred to a physician (preferably a physician with training in disorders of the ear) for an otologic evaluation, reason not given   M
BETOS: M5D   Specialist - other
Service not separately priced by Part B

C G8564 Patient was referred to a physician (preferably a physician with training in disorders of the ear) for an otologic evaluation, reason not specified)   M
BETOS: M5D   Specialist - other
Service not separately priced by Part B

C G8565 Verification and documentation of sudden or rapidly progressive hearing loss   M
BETOS: M5D   Specialist - other
Service not separately priced by Part B

C G8566 Patient is not eligible for the "referral for otologic evaluation for sudden or rapidly progressive hearing loss" measure   M
BETOS: M5D   Specialist - other
Service not separately priced by Part B

C G8567 Patient does not have verification and documentation of sudden or rapidly progressive hearing loss   M
BETOS: M5D   Specialist - other
Service not separately priced by Part B

C G8568 Patient was not referred to a physician (preferably a physician with training in disorders of the ear) for an otologic evaluation, reason not given   M
BETOS: M5D   Specialist - other
Service not separately priced by Part B

● New code   ▲ Revised code   **C** Carrier judgment   **D** Special coverage instructions apply
I Not payable by Medicare   **M** Non-covered by Medicare   **S** Non-covered by Medicare statute   AHA Coding Clinic®

C **G8569** Prolonged postoperative intubation (> 24 hrs) required **M** **MIPS**
BETOS: M5D　Specialist - other
Service not separately priced by Part B

C **G8570** Prolonged postoperative intubation (> 24 hrs) not required **M** **MIPS**
BETOS: M5D　Specialist - other
Service not separately priced by Part B

C **G8575** Developed postoperative renal failure or required dialysis **M** **MIPS**
BETOS: M5D　Specialist - other
Service not separately priced by Part B

C **G8576** No postoperative renal failure/dialysis not required **M** **MIPS**
BETOS: M5D　Specialist - other
Service not separately priced by Part B

C **G8577** Re-exploration required due to mediastinal bleeding with or without tamponade, graft occlusion, valve dysfunction or other cardiac reason **M** **MIPS**
BETOS: M5D　Specialist - other
Service not separately priced by Part B

C **G8578** Re-exploration not required due to mediastinal bleeding with or without tamponade, graft occlusion, valve dysfunction or other cardiac reason **M** **MIPS**
BETOS: M5D　Specialist - other
Service not separately priced by Part B

C **G8598** Aspirin or another antiplatelet therapy used **M**
BETOS: M5D　Specialist - other
Service not separately priced by Part B

C **G8599** Aspirin or another antiplatelet therapy not used, reason not given **M**
BETOS: M5D　Specialist - other
Service not separately priced by Part B

C **G8600** IV tPA initiated within three hours (<= 180 minutes) of time last known well **M** **MIPS**
BETOS: M5D　Specialist - other
Service not separately priced by Part B

▲ **C** **G8601** IV alteplase not initiated within three hours (<= 180 minutes) of time last known well for reasons documented by clinician (e.g. patient enrolled in clinical trial for stroke, patient admitted for elective carotid intervention, patient received tenecteplase (tnk)) **M** **MIPS**
BETOS: M5D　Specialist - other
Service not separately priced by Part B

C **G8602** IV tPA not initiated within three hours (<= 180 minutes) of time last known well, reason not given **M** **MIPS**
BETOS: M5D　Specialist - other
Service not separately priced by Part B

C **G8633** Pharmacologic therapy (other than minerals/vitamins) for osteoporosis prescribed **M** **MIPS**
BETOS: M5B　Specialist - psychiatry
Service not separately priced by Part B

C **G8635** Pharmacologic therapy for osteoporosis was not prescribed, reason not given **M** **MIPS**
BETOS: M5B　Specialist - psychiatry
Service not separately priced by Part B

QUALITY MEASURES RELATED FOR RISK-ADJUSTED FUNCTIONAL STATUS SCORING (G8647-G8670)

C **G8647** Risk-adjusted functional status change residual score for the knee impairment successfully calculated and the score was equal to zero (0) or greater than zero (> 0) **M** **MIPS**
BETOS: M5B　Specialist - psychiatry
Service not separately priced by Part B

C **G8648** Risk-adjusted functional status change residual score for the knee impairment successfully calculated and the score was less than zero (< 0) **M** **MIPS**
BETOS: M5B　Specialist - psychiatry
Service not separately priced by Part B

▲ **C** **G8650** Risk-adjusted functional status change residual score for the knee impairment not measured because the patient did not complete the LEPF PROM at initial evaluation and/or near discharge, reason not given **M** **MIPS**
BETOS: M5B　Specialist - psychiatry
Service not separately priced by Part B

C **G8651** Risk-adjusted functional status change residual score for the hip impairment successfully calculated and the score was equal to zero (0) or greater than zero (> 0) **M** **MIPS**
BETOS: M5B　Specialist - psychiatry
Service not separately priced by Part B

C **G8652** Risk-adjusted functional status change residual score for the hip impairment successfully calculated and the score was less than zero (< 0) **M** **MIPS**
BETOS: M5B　Specialist - psychiatry
Service not separately priced by Part B

▲ **C** **G8654** Risk-adjusted functional status change residual score for the hip impairment not measured because the patient did not complete the LEPF PROM at initial evaluation and/or near discharge, reason not given **M** **MIPS**
BETOS: M5B　Specialist - psychiatry
Service not separately priced by Part B

C **G8655** Risk-adjusted functional status change residual score for the lower leg, foot or ankle impairment successfully calculated and the score was equal to zero (0) or greater than zero (> 0) **M** **MIPS**
BETOS: M5B　Specialist - psychiatry
Service not separately priced by Part B

♂ Male only　♀ Female only　ⒶＡge　A2 - Z3 = ASC Payment indicator　A - Y = APC Status indicator
ASC = ASC Approved Procedure　**DME** Paid under the DME fee schedule　**MIPS** MIPS code

CPT® is a registered trademark of the American Medical Association. All rights reserved.　　　　　　　223

C **G8656** Risk-adjusted functional status change residual score for the lower leg, foot or ankle impairment successfully calculated and the score was less than zero (< 0) M MIPS
BETOS: M5B Specialist - psychiatry
Service not separately priced by Part B

▲ **C** **G8658** Risk-adjusted functional status change residual score for the lower leg, foot or ankle impairment not measured because the patient did not complete the LEPF PROM at initial evaluation and/or near discharge, reason not given M MIPS
BETOS: M5B Specialist - psychiatry
Service not separately priced by Part B

C **G8659** Risk-adjusted functional status change residual score for the low back impairment successfully calculated and the score was equal to zero (0) or greater than zero (> 0) M MIPS
BETOS: M5B Specialist - psychiatry
Service not separately priced by Part B

C **G8660** Risk-adjusted functional status change residual score for the low back impairment successfully calculated and the score was less than zero (< 0) M MIPS
BETOS: M5B Specialist - psychiatry
Service not separately priced by Part B

C **G8661** Risk-adjusted functional status change residual score for the low back impairment not measured because the patient did not complete the FS status survey near discharge, patient not appropriate M
BETOS: M5B Specialist - psychiatry
Service not separately priced by Part B

C **G8662** Risk-adjusted functional status change residual score for the low back impairment not measured because the patient did not complete the low back FS PROM at initial evaluation and/or near discharge, reason not given M MIPS
BETOS: M5B Specialist - psychiatry
Service not separately priced by Part B

C **G8663** Risk-adjusted functional status change residual score for the shoulder impairment successfully calculated and the score was equal to zero (0) or greater than zero (> 0) M MIPS
BETOS: M5B Specialist - psychiatry
Service not separately priced by Part B

C **G8664** Risk-adjusted functional status change residual score for the shoulder impairment successfully calculated and the score was less than zero (< 0) M MIPS
BETOS: M5B Specialist - psychiatry
Service not separately priced by Part B

C **G8666** Risk-adjusted functional status change residual score for the shoulder impairment not measured because the patient did not complete the shoulder FS PROM at initial evaluation and/or near discharge, reason not given M MIPS
BETOS: M5B Specialist - psychiatry
Service not separately priced by Part B

C **G8667** Risk-adjusted functional status change residual score for the elbow, wrist or hand impairment successfully calculated and the score was equal to zero (0) or greater than zero (> 0) M MIPS
BETOS: M5B Specialist - psychiatry
Service not separately priced by Part B

C **G8668** Risk-adjusted functional status change residual score for the elbow, wrist or hand impairment successfully calculated and the score was less than zero (< 0) M MIPS
BETOS: M5B Specialist - psychiatry
Service not separately priced by Part B

C **G8670** Risk-adjusted functional status change residual score for the elbow, wrist or hand impairment not measured because the patient did not complete the elbow/wrist/hand FS PROM at initial evaluation and/or near discharge, reason not given M MIPS
BETOS: M5B Specialist - psychiatry
Service not separately priced by Part B

ADDITIONAL QUALITY MEASURES (G8694-G8970)

▲ **C** **G8694** Left ventricular ejection fraction (LVEF) < 40% or documentation of moderate or severe LVSD M MIPS
BETOS: M5B Specialist - psychiatry
Service not separately priced by Part B

C **G8708** Patient not prescribed or dispensed antibiotic Ⓐ M MIPS
BETOS: M5B Specialist - psychiatry
Service not separately priced by Part B

▲ **C** **G8709** Uri episodes when the patient had competing diagnoses on or three days after the episode date (e.g., intestinal infection, pertussis, bacterial infection, lyme disease, otitis media, acute sinusitis, acute pharyngitis, acute tonsillitis, chronic sinusitis, infection of the pharynx/larynx/tonsils/adenoids, prostatitis, cellulitis, mastoiditis, or bone infections, acute lymphadenitis, impetigo, skin staph infections, pneumonia/gonococcal infections, venereal disease (syphilis, chlamydia, inflammatory diseases [female reproductive organs]), infections of the kidney, cystitis or UTI, and acne) Ⓐ M MIPS
BETOS: M5B Specialist - psychiatry
Service not separately priced by Part B

C **G8710** Patient prescribed or dispensed antibiotic Ⓐ M MIPS
BETOS: M5B Specialist - psychiatry
Service not separately priced by Part B

● New code   ▲ Revised code   **C** Carrier judgment   **D** Special coverage instructions apply
I Not payable by Medicare   **M** Non-covered by Medicare   **S** Non-covered by Medicare statute   AHA Coding Clinic®

CPT® is a registered trademark of the American Medical Association. All rights reserved.

C G8711 Prescribed or dispensed antibiotic　　M MIPS
BETOS: M5B　Specialist - psychiatry
Service not separately priced by Part B

C G8712 Antibiotic not prescribed or dispensed　　M
BETOS: M5B　Specialist - psychiatry
Service not separately priced by Part B

C G8721 pT category (primary tumor), pN category (regional lymph nodes), and histologic grade were documented in pathology report　　M
BETOS: M5B　Specialist - psychiatry
Service not separately priced by Part B

C G8722 Documentation of medical reason(s) for not including the PT category, the pN category or the histologic grade in the pathology report (e.g., re-excision without residual tumor; non-carcinomasanal canal)　　M
BETOS: M5B　Specialist - psychiatry
Service not separately priced by Part B

C G8723 Specimen site is other than anatomic location of primary tumor　　M
BETOS: M5B　Specialist - psychiatry
Service not separately priced by Part B

C G8724 pT category, pN category and histologic grade were not documented in the pathology report, reason not given　　M
BETOS: M5B　Specialist - psychiatry
Service not separately priced by Part B

C G8733 Elder maltreatment screen documented as positive and a follow-up plan is documented　　M MIPS
BETOS: M5B　Specialist - psychiatry
Service not separately priced by Part B

C G8734 Elder maltreatment screen documented as negative, no follow-up required　　M MIPS
BETOS: M5B　Specialist - psychiatry
Service not separately priced by Part B

C G8735 Elder maltreatment screen documented as positive, follow-up plan not documented, reason not given　　M MIPS
BETOS: M5B　Specialist - psychiatry
Service not separately priced by Part B

C G8749 Absence of signs of melanoma (tenderness, jaundice, localized neurologic signs such as weakness, or any other sign suggesting systemic spread) or absence of symptoms of melanoma (cough, dyspnea, pain, paresthesia, or any other symptom suggesting the possibility of systemic spread of melanoma)　　M
BETOS: M5B　Specialist - psychiatry
Service not separately priced by Part B

C G8752 Most recent systolic blood pressure < 140 mmHg　　M MIPS
BETOS: M5B　Specialist - psychiatry
Service not separately priced by Part B

C G8753 Most recent systolic blood pressure >= 140 mmHg　　M MIPS
BETOS: M5B　Specialist - psychiatry
Service not separately priced by Part B

C G8754 Most recent diastolic blood pressure < 90 mmHg　　M MIPS
BETOS: M5B　Specialist - psychiatry
Service not separately priced by Part B

C G8755 Most recent diastolic blood pressure >= 90 mmHg　　M MIPS
BETOS: M5B　Specialist - psychiatry
Service not separately priced by Part B

C G8756 No documentation of blood pressure measurement, reason not given　　M MIPS
BETOS: M5B　Specialist - psychiatry
Service not separately priced by Part B

C G8783 Normal blood pressure reading documented, follow-up not required　　M MIPS
BETOS: M5B　Specialist - psychiatry
Service not separately priced by Part B

C G8785 Blood pressure reading not documented, reason not given　　M MIPS
BETOS: M5B　Specialist - psychiatry
Service not separately priced by Part B

C G8797 Specimen site other than anatomic location of esophagus　　M MIPS
BETOS: M5B　Specialist - psychiatry
Service not separately priced by Part B

C G8798 Specimen site other than anatomic location of prostate　　♂ M MIPS
BETOS: M5B　Specialist - psychiatry
Service not separately priced by Part B

C G8806 Performance of trans-abdominal or trans-vaginal ultrasound and pregnancy location documented　　♀ Ⓐ M MIPS
BETOS: M5B　Specialist - psychiatry
Service not separately priced by Part B

C G8807 Trans-abdominal or trans-vaginal ultrasound not performed for reasons documented by clinician (e.g., patient has visited the ED multiple times within 72 hours, patient has a documented intrauterine pregnancy [IUP])　　♀ Ⓐ M MIPS
BETOS: M5B　Specialist - psychiatry
Service not separately priced by Part B

C G8808 Trans-abdominal or trans-vaginal ultrasound not performed, reason not given　　♀ M MIPS
BETOS: M5B　Specialist - psychiatry
Service not separately priced by Part B

C G8815 Documented reason in the medical records for why the statin therapy was not prescribed (i.e., lower extremity bypass was for a patient with non-artherosclerotic disease)　　M
BETOS: M5B　Specialist - psychiatry
Service not separately priced by Part B

♂ Male only　　♀ Female only　　Ⓐ Age　　A2 - Z3 = ASC Payment indicator　　A - Y = APC Status indicator
ASC = ASC Approved Procedure　　**DME** Paid under the DME fee schedule　　MIPS MIPS code

C **G8816** Statin medication prescribed at discharge   M
BETOS: M5B   Specialist - psychiatry
Service not separately priced by Part B

C **G8817** Statin therapy not prescribed at discharge, reason not given   M
BETOS: M5B   Specialist - psychiatry
Service not separately priced by Part B

C **G8818** Patient discharge to home no later than post-operative day #7   M MIPS
BETOS: M5B   Specialist - psychiatry
Service not separately priced by Part B

C **G8825** Patient not discharged to home by post-operative day #7   M MIPS
BETOS: M5B   Specialist - psychiatry
Service not separately priced by Part B

C **G8826** Patient discharge to home no later than post-operative day #2 following EVAR   M MIPS
BETOS: M5B   Specialist - psychiatry
Service not separately priced by Part B

C **G8833** Patient not discharged to home by post-operative day #2 following EVAR   M MIPS
BETOS: M5B   Specialist - psychiatry
Service not separately priced by Part B

C **G8834** Patient discharged to home no later than post-operative day #2 following CEA   M MIPS
BETOS: M5B   Specialist - psychiatry
Service not separately priced by Part B

C **G8838** Patient not discharged to home by post-operative day #2 following CEA   M MIPS
BETOS: M5B   Specialist - psychiatry
Service not separately priced by Part B

C **G8839** Sleep apnea symptoms assessed, including presence or absence of snoring and daytime sleepiness   M
BETOS: M5B   Specialist - psychiatry
Service not separately priced by Part B

C **G8840** Documentation of reason(s) for not documenting an assessment of sleep symptoms (e.g., patient didn't have initial daytime sleepiness, patient visited between initial testing and initiation of therapy)   M
BETOS: M5B   Specialist - psychiatry
Service not separately priced by Part B

C **G8841** Sleep apnea symptoms not assessed, reason not given   M
BETOS: M5B   Specialist - psychiatry
Service not separately priced by Part B

C **G8842** Apnea hypopnea index (AHI) or respiratory disturbance index (RDI) measured at the time of initial diagnosis   M MIPS
BETOS: M5B   Specialist - psychiatry
Service not separately priced by Part B

C **G8843** Documentation of reason(s) for not measuring an apnea hypopnea index (AHI) or a respiratory disturbance index (RDI) at the time of initial diagnosis (e.g., psychiatric disease, dementia, patient declined, financial, insurance coverage, test ordered but not yet completed)   M MIPS
BETOS: M5B   Specialist - psychiatry
Service not separately priced by Part B

C **G8844** Apnea hypopnea index (AHI) or respiratory disturbance index (RDI) not measured at the time of initial diagnosis, reason not given   M MIPS
BETOS: M5B   Specialist - psychiatry
Service not separately priced by Part B

C **G8845** Positive airway pressure therapy prescribed   M
BETOS: M5B   Specialist - psychiatry
Service not separately priced by Part B

C **G8846** Moderate or severe obstructive sleep apnea (apnea hypopnea index (AHI) or respiratory disturbance index (RDI) of 15 or greater)   M
BETOS: M5B   Specialist - psychiatry
Service not separately priced by Part B

C **G8849** Documentation of reason(s) for not prescribing positive airway pressure therapy (e.g., patient unable to tolerate, alternative therapies use, patient declined, financial, insurance coverage)   M
BETOS: M5B   Specialist - psychiatry
Service not separately priced by Part B

C **G8850** Positive airway pressure therapy not prescribed, reason not given   M
BETOS: M5B   Specialist - psychiatry
Service not separately priced by Part B

C **G8851** Objective measurement of adherence to positive airway pressure therapy, documented   M MIPS
BETOS: M5B   Specialist - psychiatry
Service not separately priced by Part B

C **G8852** Positive airway pressure therapy prescribed   M MIPS
BETOS: M5B   Specialist - psychiatry
Service not separately priced by Part B

C **G8854** Documentation of reason(s) for not objectively measuring adherence to positive airway pressure therapy (e.g., patient didn't bring data from continuous positive airway pressure [CPAP], therapy not yet initiated, not available on machine)   M MIPS
BETOS: M5B   Specialist - psychiatry
Service not separately priced by Part B

C **G8855** Objective measurement of adherence to positive airway pressure therapy not performed, reason not given   M MIPS
BETOS: M5B   Specialist - psychiatry
Service not separately priced by Part B

● New code   ▲ Revised code   **C** Carrier judgment   **D** Special coverage instructions apply
I Not payable by Medicare   **M** Non-covered by Medicare   **S** Non-covered by Medicare statute   AHA Coding Clinic®

C **G8856** Referral to a physician for an otologic evaluation performed　　M MIPS
BETOS: M5B　Specialist - psychiatry
Service not separately priced by Part B

C **G8857** Patient is not eligible for the referral for otologic evaluation measure (e.g., patients who are already under the care of a physician for acute or chronic dizziness)　　M MIPS
BETOS: M5B　Specialist - psychiatry
Service not separately priced by Part B

C **G8858** Referral to a physician for an otologic evaluation not performed, reason not given　　M MIPS
BETOS: M5B　Specialist - psychiatry
Service not separately priced by Part B

C **G8863** Patients not assessed for risk of bone loss, reason not given　　M
BETOS: M5B　Specialist - psychiatry
Service not separately priced by Part B

C **G8864** Pneumococcal vaccine administered or previously received　　M
BETOS: M5B　Specialist - psychiatry
Service not separately priced by Part B

C **G8865** Documentation of medical reason(s) for not administering or previously receiving pneumococcal vaccine (e.g., patient allergic reaction, potential adverse drug reaction)　　M
BETOS: M5B　Specialist - psychiatry
Service not separately priced by Part B

C **G8866** Documentation of patient reason(s) for not administering or previously receiving pneumococcal vaccine (e.g., patient refusal)　　M
BETOS: M5B　Specialist - psychiatry
Service not separately priced by Part B

C **G8867** Pneumococcal vaccine not administered or previously received, reason not given　　M
BETOS: M5B　Specialist - psychiatry
Service not separately priced by Part B

C **G8869** Patient has documented immunity to Hepatitis B and initiating anti-TNF therapy　　M MIPS
BETOS: M5B　Specialist - psychiatry
Service not separately priced by Part B

C **G8875** Clinician diagnosed breast cancer preoperatively by a minimally invasive biopsy method　　M
BETOS: M5B　Specialist - psychiatry
Service not separately priced by Part B

C **G8876** Documentation of reason(s) for not performing minimally invasive biopsy to diagnose breast cancer preoperatively (e.g., lesion too close to skin, implant, chest wall, etc., lesion could not be adequately visualized for needle biopsy, patient condition prevents needle biopsy [weight, breast thickness, etc.], duct excision without imaging abnormality, prophylactic mastectomy, reduction mammoplasty, excisional biopsy performed by another physician)　　M
BETOS: M5B　Specialist - psychiatry
Service not separately priced by Part B

C **G8877** Clinician did not attempt to achieve the diagnosis of breast cancer preoperatively by a minimally invasive biopsy method, reason not given　　M
BETOS: M5B　Specialist - psychiatry
Service not separately priced by Part B

C **G8878** Sentinel lymph node biopsy procedure performed　　M MIPS
BETOS: M5B　Specialist - psychiatry
Service not separately priced by Part B

C **G8880** Documentation of reason(s) sentinel lymph node biopsy not performed (e.g., reasons could include but not limited to; non-invasive cancer, incidental discovery of breast cancer on prophylactic mastectomy, incidental discovery of breast cancer on reduction mammoplasty, pre-operative biopsy proven lymph node (LN) metastases, inflammatory carcinoma, stage 3 locally advanced cancer, recurrent invasive breast cancer, clinically node positive after neoadjuvant systemic therapy, patient refusal after informed consent, patient with significant age, comorbidities, or limited life expectancy and favorable tumor; adjuvant systemic therapy unlikely to change)　　M MIPS
BETOS: M5B　Specialist - psychiatry
Service not separately priced by Part B

C **G8881** Stage of breast cancer is greater than T1N0M0 or T2N0M0　　M
BETOS: M5B　Specialist - psychiatry
Service not separately priced by Part B

C **G8882** Sentinel lymph node biopsy procedure not performed, reason not given　　M MIPS
BETOS: M5B　Specialist - psychiatry
Service not separately priced by Part B

C **G8883** Biopsy results reviewed, communicated, tracked and documented　　M MIPS
BETOS: M5B　Specialist - psychiatry
Service not separately priced by Part B

C **G8884** Clinician documented reason that patient's biopsy results were not reviewed　　M MIPS
BETOS: M5B　Specialist - psychiatry
Service not separately priced by Part B

C **G8885** Biopsy results not reviewed, communicated, tracked or documented　　M MIPS
BETOS: M5B　Specialist - psychiatry
Service not separately priced by Part B

♂ Male only　　♀ Female only　　Ⓐ Age　　A2 - Z3 = ASC Payment indicator　　A - Y = APC Status indicator
ASC = ASC Approved Procedure　　**DME** Paid under the DME fee schedule　　MIPS MIPS code

G8907 Patient documented not to have experienced any of the following events: a burn prior to discharge; a fall within the facility; wrong site/ side/patient/procedure/implant event; or a hospital transfer or hospital admission upon discharge from the facility M
BETOS: M5B Specialist - psychiatry
Service not separately priced by Part B

G8908 Patient documented to have received a burn prior to discharge M
BETOS: M5B Specialist - psychiatry
Service not separately priced by Part B

G8909 Patient documented not to have received a burn prior to discharge M
BETOS: M5B Specialist - psychiatry
Service not separately priced by Part B

G8910 Patient documented to have experienced a fall within ASC M
BETOS: M5B Specialist - psychiatry
Service not separately priced by Part B

G8911 Patient documented not to have experienced a fall within ambulatory surgical center M
BETOS: M5B Specialist - psychiatry
Service not separately priced by Part B

G8912 Patient documented to have experienced a wrong site, wrong side, wrong patient, wrong procedure or wrong implant event M
BETOS: M5B Specialist - psychiatry
Service not separately priced by Part B

G8913 Patient documented not to have experienced a wrong site, wrong side, wrong patient, wrong procedure or wrong implant event M
BETOS: M5B Specialist - psychiatry
Service not separately priced by Part B

G8914 Patient documented to have experienced a hospital transfer or hospital admission upon discharge from ASC M
BETOS: M5B Specialist - psychiatry
Service not separately priced by Part B

G8915 Patient documented not to have experienced a hospital transfer or hospital admission upon discharge from ASC M
BETOS: M5B Specialist - psychiatry
Service not separately priced by Part B

G8916 Patient with preoperative order for IV antibiotic surgical site infection (SSI) prophylaxis, antibiotic initiated on time M
BETOS: M5B Specialist - psychiatry
Service not separately priced by Part B

G8917 Patient with preoperative order for IV antibiotic surgical site infection (SSI) prophylaxis, antibiotic not initiated on time M
BETOS: M5B Specialist - psychiatry
Service not separately priced by Part B

G8918 Patient without preoperative order for IV antibiotic surgical site infection (SSI) prophylaxis M
BETOS: M5B Specialist - psychiatry
Service not separately priced by Part B

G8923 Left ventricular ejection fraction (LVEF) < 40% or documentation of moderately or severely depressed left ventricular systolic function M MIPS
BETOS: M5B Specialist - psychiatry
Service not separately priced by Part B

▲ **G8924** Spirometry test results demonstrate FEV1/ FVC < 70%, FEV1 < 60% predicted and patient has COPD symptoms (e.g., dyspnea, cough/sputum, wheezing) M MIPS
BETOS: M5B Specialist - psychiatry
Service not separately priced by Part B

G8925 Spirometry test results demonstrate fev1 >= 60% FEV1/FVC >= 70%, predicted or patient does not have COPD symptoms M
BETOS: M5B Specialist - psychiatry
Service not separately priced by Part B

G8926 Spirometry test not performed or documented, reason not given M
BETOS: M5B Specialist - psychiatry
Service not separately priced by Part B

G8934 Left ventricular ejection fraction (LVEF) <40% or documentation of moderately or severely depressed left ventricular systolic function M MIPS
BETOS: M5B Specialist - psychiatry
Service not separately priced by Part B

G8935 Clinician prescribed angiotensin converting enzyme (ACE) inhibitor or angiotensin receptor blocker (ARB) therapy M MIPS
BETOS: M5B Specialist - psychiatry
Service not separately priced by Part B

G8936 Clinician documented that patient was not an eligible candidate for angiotensin converting enzyme (ACE) inhibitor or angiotensin receptor blocker (ARB) therapy (e.g., allergy, intolerance, pregnancy, renal failure due to ACE inhibitor, diseases of the aortic or mitral valve, other medical reasons) or (e.g., patient declined, other patient reasons) or (e.g., lack of drug availability, other reasons attributable to the health care system) M MIPS
BETOS: M5B Specialist - psychiatry
Service not separately priced by Part B

G8937 Clinician did not prescribe angiotensin converting enzyme (ACE) inhibitor or angiotensin receptor blocker (ARB) therapy, reason not given Ⓞ M MIPS
BETOS: M5B Specialist - psychiatry
Service not separately priced by Part B

● New code ▲ Revised code C Carrier judgment D Special coverage instructions apply
I Not payable by Medicare M Non-covered by Medicare S Non-covered by Medicare statute AHA Coding Clinic®

▲ C **G8938** BMI is documented as being outside of normal parameters, follow-up plan is not documented, documentation the patient is not eligible Ⓐ M MIPS

BETOS: M5B   Specialist - psychiatry
Service not separately priced by Part B

C **G8941** Elder maltreatment screen documented as positive, follow-up plan not documented, documentation the patient is not eligible for follow-up plan at the time of the encounter Ⓐ M MIPS

BETOS: M5B   Specialist - psychiatry
Service not separately priced by Part B

C **G8942** Functional outcomes assessment using a standardized tool is documented within the previous 30 days and care plan, based on identified deficiencies on the date of the functional outcome assessment, is documented Ⓐ M MIPS

BETOS: M5B   Specialist - psychiatry
Service not separately priced by Part B

C **G8944** AJCC melanoma cancer Stage 0 through IIC melanoma M

BETOS: M5B   Specialist - psychiatry
Service not separately priced by Part B

C **G8946** Minimally invasive biopsy method attempted but not diagnostic of breast cancer (e.g., high risk lesion of breast such as atypical ductal hyperplasia, lobular neoplasia, atypical lobular hyperplasia, lobular carcinoma in situ, atypical columnar hyperplasia, flat epithelial atypia, radial scar, complex sclerosing lesion, papillary lesion, or any lesion with spindle cells) Ⓐ M

BETOS: M5B   Specialist - psychiatry
Service not separately priced by Part B

C **G8950** Pre-hypertensive or hypertensive blood pressure reading documented, and the indicated follow-up is documented M MIPS

BETOS: M5B   Specialist - psychiatry
Service not separately priced by Part B

C **G8952** Pre-hypertensive or hypertensive blood pressure reading documented, indicated follow-up not documented, reason not given M MIPS

BETOS: M5B   Specialist - psychiatry
Service not separately priced by Part B

C **G8955** Most recent assessment of adequacy of volume management documented Ⓐ M

BETOS: M5B   Specialist - psychiatry
Service not separately priced by Part B

C **G8956** Patient receiving maintenance hemodialysis in an outpatient dialysis facility Ⓐ M

BETOS: M5B   Specialist - psychiatry
Service not separately priced by Part B

C **G8958** Assessment of adequacy of volume management not documented, reason not given Ⓐ M

BETOS: M5B   Specialist - psychiatry
Service not separately priced by Part B

C **G8961** Cardiac stress imaging test primarily performed on low-risk surgery patient for preoperative evaluation within 30 days preceding this surgery Ⓐ M MIPS

BETOS: M5B   Specialist - psychiatry
Service not separately priced by Part B

C **G8962** Cardiac stress imaging test performed on patient for any reason including those who did not have low risk surgery or test that was performed more than 30 days preceding low risk surgery Ⓐ M MIPS

BETOS: M5B   Specialist - psychiatry
Service not separately priced by Part B

C **G8963** Cardiac stress imaging performed primarily for monitoring of asymptomatic patient who had PCI within 2 years Ⓐ M MIPS

BETOS: M5B   Specialist - psychiatry
Service not separately priced by Part B

C **G8964** Cardiac stress imaging test performed primarily for any other reason than monitoring of asymptomatic patient who had PCI within 2 years (e.g., symptomatic patient, patient greater than 2 years since PCI, initial evaluation, etc) Ⓐ M MIPS

BETOS: M5B   Specialist - psychiatry
Service not separately priced by Part B

C **G8965** Cardiac stress imaging test primarily performed on low CHD risk patient for initial detection and risk assessment Ⓐ M MIPS

BETOS: M5B   Specialist - psychiatry
Service not separately priced by Part B

C **G8966** Cardiac stress imaging test performed on symptomatic or higher than low CHD risk patient or for any reason other than initial detection and risk assessment Ⓐ M MIPS

BETOS: M5B   Specialist - psychiatry
Service not separately priced by Part B

C **G8967** Warfarin or another FDA-approved oral anticoagulant is prescribed Ⓐ M MIPS

BETOS: M5B   Specialist - psychiatry
Service not separately priced by Part B

C **G8968** Documentation of medical reason(s) for not prescribing warfarin or another FDA-approved anticoagulant (e.g., atrial appendage device in place) Ⓐ M MIPS

BETOS: M5B   Specialist - psychiatry
Service not separately priced by Part B

▲ C **G8969** Documentation of patient reason(s) for not prescribing warfarin or another oral anticoagulant that is FDA approved for the prevention of thromboembolism (e.g., patient choice of having atrial appendage device placed) Ⓐ M MIPS

BETOS: M5B   Specialist - psychiatry
Service not separately priced by Part B

♂ Male only   ♀ Female only   Ⓐ Age   A2 - Z3 = ASC Payment indicator   A - Y = APC Status indicator
ASC = ASC Approved Procedure   **DME** Paid under the DME fee schedule   **MIPS** MIPS code

229

C **G8970** No risk factors or one moderate risk factor for thromboembolism   Ⓐ M
BETOS: M5B   Specialist - psychiatry
Service not separately priced by Part B

MEDICARE COORDINATED CARE DEMONSTRATION (MCCD) SERVICES (G9001-G9012)

D **G9001** Coordinated care fee, initial rate   B
BETOS: Y2   Other - non-Medicare fee schedule
Service not separately priced by Part B

D **G9002** Coordinated care fee, maintenance rate   B
BETOS: Y2   Other - non-Medicare fee schedule
Service not separately priced by Part B

D **G9003** Coordinated care fee, risk adjusted high, initial   B
BETOS: Y2   Other - non-Medicare fee schedule
Service not separately priced by Part B

D **G9004** Coordinated care fee, risk adjusted low, initial   B
BETOS: Y2   Other - non-Medicare fee schedule
Service not separately priced by Part B

D **G9005** Coordinated care fee, risk adjusted maintenance   B
BETOS: Y2   Other - non-Medicare fee schedule
Service not separately priced by Part B

D **G9006** Coordinated care fee, home monitoring   B
BETOS: Y2   Other - non-Medicare fee schedule
Service not separately priced by Part B

D **G9007** Coordinated care fee, scheduled team conference   B
BETOS: Y2   Other - non-Medicare fee schedule
Service not separately priced by Part B

D **G9008** Coordinated care fee, physician coordinated care oversight services   B
BETOS: Y2   Other - non-Medicare fee schedule
Service not separately priced by Part B

D **G9009** Coordinated care fee, risk adjusted maintenance, level 3   B
BETOS: Y2   Other - non-Medicare fee schedule
Service not separately priced by Part B

D **G9010** Coordinated care fee, risk adjusted maintenance, level 4   B
BETOS: Y2   Other - non-Medicare fee schedule
Service not separately priced by Part B

D **G9011** Coordinated care fee, risk adjusted maintenance, level 5   B
BETOS: Y2   Other - non-Medicare fee schedule
Service not separately priced by Part B

D **G9012** Other specified case management service not elsewhere classified   B
BETOS: Y2   Other - non-Medicare fee schedule
Service not separately priced by Part B

MEDICARE DEMONSTRATION PROJECTS (G9013-G9140)

M **G9013** ESRD demo basic bundle level I   E1
BETOS: Y2   Other - non-Medicare fee schedule
Service not separately priced by Part B

M **G9014** ESRD demo expanded bundle including venous access and related services   E1
BETOS: Y2   Other - non-Medicare fee schedule
Service not separately priced by Part B

M **G9016** Smoking cessation counseling, individual, in the absence of or in addition to any other evaluation and management service, per session (6-10 minutes) [demo project code only]   E1
BETOS: Y2   Other - non-Medicare fee schedule
Service not separately priced by Part B

I **G9050** Oncology; primary focus of visit; work-up, evaluation, or staging at the time of cancer diagnosis or recurrence (for use in a Medicare-approved demonstration project)   E1
BETOS: P7B   Oncology - other
Service not separately priced by Part B

I **G9051** Oncology; primary focus of visit; treatment decision-making after disease is staged or restaged, discussion of treatment options, supervising/coordinating active cancer directed therapy or managing consequences of cancer directed therapy (for use in a Medicare-approved demonstration project)   E1
BETOS: P7B   Oncology - other
Service not separately priced by Part B

I **G9052** Oncology; primary focus of visit; surveillance for disease recurrence for patient who has completed definitive cancer-directed therapy and currently lacks evidence of recurrent disease; cancer directed therapy might be considered in the future (for use in a Medicare-approved demonstration project)   E1
BETOS: P7B   Oncology - other
Service not separately priced by Part B

● New code   ▲ Revised code   C Carrier judgment   D Special coverage instructions apply
I Not payable by Medicare   M Non-covered by Medicare   S Non-covered by Medicare statute   AHA Coding Clinic®

I **G9053** Oncology; primary focus of visit; expectant management of patient with evidence of cancer for whom no cancer directed therapy is being administered or arranged at present; cancer directed therapy might be considered in the future (for use in a Medicare-approved demonstration project)   E1

    BETOS: P7B   Oncology - other
    Service not separately priced by Part B

I **G9054** Oncology; primary focus of visit; supervising, coordinating or managing care of patient with terminal cancer or for whom other medical illness prevents further cancer treatment; includes symptom management, end-of-life care planning, management of palliative therapies (for use in a Medicare-approved demonstration project)   E1

    BETOS: P7B   Oncology - other
    Service not separately priced by Part B

I **G9055** Oncology; primary focus of visit; other, unspecified service not otherwise listed (for use in a Medicare-approved demonstration project)   E1

    BETOS: P7B   Oncology - other
    Service not separately priced by Part B

I **G9056** Oncology; practice guidelines; management adheres to guidelines (for use in a Medicare-approved demonstration project)   E1

    BETOS: P7B   Oncology - other
    Service not separately priced by Part B

I **G9057** Oncology; practice guidelines; management differs from guidelines as a result of patient enrollment in an institutional review board approved clinical trial (for use in a Medicare-approved demonstration project)   E1

    BETOS: P7B   Oncology - other
    Service not separately priced by Part B

I **G9058** Oncology; practice guidelines; management differs from guidelines because the treating physician disagrees with guideline recommendations (for use in a Medicare-approved demonstration project)   E1

    BETOS: P7B   Oncology - other
    Service not separately priced by Part B

I **G9059** Oncology; practice guidelines; management differs from guidelines because the patient, after being offered treatment consistent with guidelines, has opted for alternative treatment or management, including no treatment (for use in a Medicare-approved demonstration project)   E1

    BETOS: P7B   Oncology - other
    Service not separately priced by Part B

I **G9060** Oncology; practice guidelines; management differs from guidelines for reason(s) associated with patient comorbid illness or performance status not factored into guidelines (for use in a Medicare-approved demonstration project)   E1

    BETOS: P7B   Oncology - other
    Service not separately priced by Part B

I **G9061** Oncology; practice guidelines; patient's condition not addressed by available guidelines (for use in a Medicare-approved demonstration project)   E1

    BETOS: P7B   Oncology - other
    Service not separately priced by Part B

I **G9062** Oncology; practice guidelines; management differs from guidelines for other reason(s) not listed (for use in a Medicare-approved demonstration project)   E1

    BETOS: P7B   Oncology - other
    Service not separately priced by Part B

C **G9063** Oncology; disease status; limited to non-small cell lung cancer; extent of disease initially established as Stage I (prior to neo-adjuvant therapy, if any) with no evidence of disease progression, recurrence, or metastases (for use in a Medicare-approved demonstration project)   M

    BETOS: P7B   Oncology - other
    Service not separately priced by Part B

C **G9064** Oncology; disease status; limited to non-small cell lung cancer; extent of disease initially established as Stage II (prior to neo-adjuvant therapy, if any) with no evidence of disease progression, recurrence, or metastases (for use in a Medicare-approved demonstration project)   M

    BETOS: P7B   Oncology - other
    Service not separately priced by Part B

C **G9065** Oncology; disease status; limited to non-small cell lung cancer; extent of disease initially established as Stage III A (prior to neo-adjuvant therapy, if any) with no evidence of disease progression, recurrence, or metastases (for use in a Medicare-approved demonstration project)   M

    BETOS: P7B   Oncology - other
    Service not separately priced by Part B

C **G9066** Oncology; disease status; limited to non-small cell lung cancer; Stage III B- IV at diagnosis, metastatic, locally recurrent, or progressive (for use in a Medicare-approved demonstration project)   M

    BETOS: P7B   Oncology - other
    Service not separately priced by Part B

C **G9067** Oncology; disease status; limited to non-small cell lung cancer; extent of disease unknown, staging in progress, or not listed (for use in a Medicare-approved demonstration project)   M

    BETOS: P7B   Oncology - other
    Service not separately priced by Part B

♂ Male only   ♀ Female only   **A** Age   A2 - Z3 = ASC Payment indicator   A - Y = APC Status indicator
ASC = ASC Approved Procedure   **DME** Paid under the DME fee schedule   **MIPS** MIPS code

C **G9068** Oncology; disease status; limited to small cell and combined small cell/non-small cell; extent of disease initially established as limited with no evidence of disease progression, recurrence, or metastases (for use in a Medicare-approved demonstration project)   M

BETOS: P7B   Oncology - other
Service not separately priced by Part B

C **G9069** Oncology; disease status; small cell lung cancer, limited to small cell and combined small cell/non-small cell; extensive Stage at diagnosis, metastatic, locally recurrent, or progressive (for use in a Medicare-approved demonstration project)   M

BETOS: P7B   Oncology - other
Service not separately priced by Part B

C **G9070** Oncology; disease status; small cell lung cancer, limited to small cell and combined small cell/non-small; extent of disease unknown, staging in progress, or not listed (for use in a Medicare-approved demonstration project)   M

BETOS: P7B   Oncology - other
Service not separately priced by Part B

C **G9071** Oncology; disease status; invasive female breast cancer (does not include ductal carcinoma in situ); adenocarcinoma as predominant cell type; Stage I or Stage IIA-IIB; or T3, N1, M0; and ER and/or pr positive; with no evidence of disease progression, recurrence, or metastases (for use in a Medicare-approved demonstration project) M

BETOS: P7B   Oncology - other
Service not separately priced by Part B

C **G9072** Oncology; disease status; invasive female breast cancer (does not include ductal carcinoma in situ); adenocarcinoma as predominant cell type; Stage I, or Stage IIA-IIB; or T3, N1, M0; and ER and PR negative; with no evidence of disease progression, recurrence, or metastases (for use in a Medicare-approved demonstration project)   M

BETOS: P7B   Oncology - other
Service not separately priced by Part B

C **G9073** Oncology; disease status; invasive female breast cancer (does not include ductal carcinoma in situ); adenocarcinoma as predominant cell type; Stage IIIA-IIIB; and not T3, N1, M0; and ER and/or PR positive; with no evidence of disease progression, recurrence, or metastases (for use in a Medicare-approved demonstration project) M

BETOS: P7B   Oncology - other
Service not separately priced by Part B

C **G9074** Oncology; disease status; invasive female breast cancer (does not include ductal carcinoma in situ); adenocarcinoma as

predominant cell type; Stage IIIA-IIIB; and not T3, N1, M0; and ER and PR negative; with no evidence of disease progression, recurrence, or metastases (for use in a Medicare-approved demonstration project)   M

BETOS: P7B   Oncology - other
Service not separately priced by Part B

C **G9075** Oncology; disease status; invasive female breast cancer (does not include ductal carcinoma in situ); adenocarcinoma as predominant cell type; M1 at diagnosis, metastatic, locally recurrent, or progressive (for use in a Medicare-approved demonstration project)   M

BETOS: P7B   Oncology - other
Service not separately priced by Part B

C **G9077** Oncology; disease status; prostate cancer, limited to adenocarcinoma as predominant cell type; T1-T3C and gleason 2-7 and PSA < or equal to 20 at diagnosis with no evidence of disease progression, recurrence, or metastases (for use in a Medicare-approved demonstration project)   ♂ M

BETOS: P7B   Oncology - other
Service not separately priced by Part B

C **G9078** Oncology; disease status; prostate cancer, limited to adenocarcinoma as predominant cell type; T2 or T3A Gleason 8-10 or PSA > 20 at diagnosis with no evidence of disease progression, recurrence, or metastases (for use in a Medicare-approved demonstration project)   ♂ M

BETOS: P7B   Oncology - other
Service not separately priced by Part B

C **G9079** Oncology; disease status; prostate cancer, limited to adenocarcinoma as predominant cell type; T3B-T4, any N; any T, N1 at diagnosis with no evidence of disease progression, recurrence, or metastases (for use in a Medicare-approved demonstration project)   ♂ M

BETOS: P7B   Oncology - other
Service not separately priced by Part B

C **G9080** Oncology; disease status; prostate cancer, limited to adenocarcinoma; after initial treatment with rising PSA or failure of PSA decline (for use in a Medicare-approved demonstration project)   ♂ M

BETOS: P7B   Oncology - other
Service not separately priced by Part B

C **G9083** Oncology; disease status; prostate cancer, limited to adenocarcinoma; extent of disease unknown, staging in progress, or not listed (for use in a Medicare-approved demonstration project)   ♂ M

BETOS: P7B   Oncology - other
Service not separately priced by Part B

● New code   ▲ Revised code   **C** Carrier judgment   **D** Special coverage instructions apply
I Not payable by Medicare   **M** Non-covered by Medicare   **S** Non-covered by Medicare statute   AHA Coding Clinic®

C **G9084** Oncology; disease status; colon cancer, limited to invasive cancer, adenocarcinoma as predominant cell type; extent of disease initially established as T1-3, N0, M0 with no evidence of disease progression, recurrence, or metastases (for use in a Medicare-approved demonstration project) M
    BETOS: P7B   Oncology - other
    Service not separately priced by Part B

C **G9085** Oncology; disease status; colon cancer, limited to invasive cancer, adenocarcinoma as predominant cell type; extent of disease initially established as T4, N0, M0 with no evidence of disease progression, recurrence, or metastases (for use in a Medicare-approved demonstration project) M
    BETOS: P7B   Oncology - other
    Service not separately priced by Part B

C **G9086** Oncology; disease status; colon cancer, limited to invasive cancer, adenocarcinoma as predominant cell type; extent of disease initially established as T1-4, N1-2, M0 with no evidence of disease progression, recurrence, or metastases (for use in a Medicare-approved demonstration project) M
    BETOS: P7B   Oncology - other
    Service not separately priced by Part B

C **G9087** Oncology; disease status; colon cancer, limited to invasive cancer, adenocarcinoma as predominant cell type; M1 at diagnosis, metastatic, locally recurrent, or progressive with current clinical, radiologic, or biochemical evidence of disease (for use in a Medicare-approved demonstration project) M
    BETOS: P7B   Oncology - other
    Service not separately priced by Part B

C **G9088** Oncology; disease status; colon cancer, limited to invasive cancer, adenocarcinoma as predominant cell type; M1 at diagnosis, metastatic, locally recurrent, or progressive without current clinical, radiologic, or biochemical evidence of disease (for use in a Medicare-approved demonstration project) M
    BETOS: P7B   Oncology - other
    Service not separately priced by Part B

C **G9089** Oncology; disease status; colon cancer, limited to invasive cancer, adenocarcinoma as predominant cell type; extent of disease unknown, staging in progress, or not listed (for use in a Medicare-approved demonstration project) M
    BETOS: P7B   Oncology - other
    Service not separately priced by Part B

C **G9090** Oncology; disease status; rectal cancer, limited to invasive cancer, adenocarcinoma as predominant cell type; extent of disease initially established as T1-2, N0, M0 (prior to neo-adjuvant therapy, if any) with no evidence of disease progression, recurrence, or metastases (for use in a Medicare-approved demonstration project) M

    BETOS: P7B   Oncology - other
    Service not separately priced by Part B

C **G9091** Oncology; disease status; rectal cancer, limited to invasive cancer, adenocarcinoma as predominant cell type; extent of disease initially established as T3, N0, M0 (prior to neo-adjuvant therapy, if any) with no evidence of disease progression, recurrence, or metastases (for use in a Medicare-approved demonstration project) M
    BETOS: P7B   Oncology - other
    Service not separately priced by Part B

C **G9092** Oncology; disease status; rectal cancer, limited to invasive cancer, adenocarcinoma as predominant cell type; extent of disease initially established as T1-3, N1-2, M0 (prior to neo-adjuvant therapy, if any) with no evidence of disease progression, recurrence, or metastases (for use in a Medicare-approved demonstration project) M
    BETOS: P7B   Oncology - other
    Service not separately priced by Part B

C **G9093** Oncology; disease status; rectal cancer, limited to invasive cancer, adenocarcinoma as predominant cell type; extent of disease initially established as T4, any N, M0 (prior to neo-adjuvant therapy, if any) with no evidence of disease progression, recurrence, or metastases (for use in a Medicare-approved demonstration project) M
    BETOS: P7B   Oncology - other
    Service not separately priced by Part B

C **G9094** Oncology; disease status; rectal cancer, limited to invasive cancer, adenocarcinoma as predominant cell type; M1 at diagnosis, metastatic, locally recurrent, or progressive (for use in a Medicare-approved demonstration project) M
    BETOS: P7B   Oncology - other
    Service not separately priced by Part B

C **G9095** Oncology; disease status; rectal cancer, limited to invasive cancer, adenocarcinoma as predominant cell type; extent of disease unknown, staging in progress, or not listed (for use in a Medicare-approved demonstration project) M
    BETOS: P7B   Oncology - other
    Service not separately priced by Part B

C **G9096** Oncology; disease status; esophageal cancer, limited to adenocarcinoma or squamous cell carcinoma as predominant cell type; extent of disease initially established as T1-T3, N0-N1 or NX (prior to neo-adjuvant therapy, if any) with no evidence of disease progression, recurrence, or metastases (for use in a Medicare-approved demonstration project) M
    BETOS: P7B   Oncology - other
    Service not separately priced by Part B

♂ Male only   ♀ Female only   **A** Age   A2 - Z3 = ASC Payment indicator   A - Y = APC Status indicator
ASC = ASC Approved Procedure   **DME** Paid under the DME fee schedule   **MIPS** MIPS code

G9097-G9110

PROCEDURES / PROFESSIONAL SERVICES (G0008-G9987)

C **G9097** Oncology; disease status; esophageal cancer, limited to adenocarcinoma or squamous cell carcinoma as predominant cell type; extent of disease initially established as T4, any N, M0 (prior to neo-adjuvant therapy, if any) with no evidence of disease progression, recurrence, or metastases (for use in a Medicare-approved demonstration project)   M

BETOS: P7B   Oncology - other
Service not separately priced by Part B

C **G9098** Oncology; disease status; esophageal cancer, limited to adenocarcinoma or squamous cell carcinoma as predominant cell type; M1 at diagnosis, metastatic, locally recurrent, or progressive (for use in a Medicare-approved demonstration project)   M

BETOS: P7B   Oncology - other
Service not separately priced by Part B

C **G9099** Oncology; disease status; esophageal cancer, limited to adenocarcinoma or squamous cell carcinoma as predominant cell type; extent of disease unknown, staging in progress, or not listed (for use in a Medicare-approved demonstration project)   M

BETOS: P7B   Oncology - other
Service not separately priced by Part B

C **G9100** Oncology; disease status; gastric cancer, limited to adenocarcinoma as predominant cell type; post R0 resection (with or without neoadjuvant therapy) with no evidence of disease recurrence, progression, or metastases (for use in a Medicare-approved demonstration project)   M

BETOS: P7B   Oncology - other
Service not separately priced by Part B

C **G9101** Oncology; disease status; gastric cancer, limited to adenocarcinoma as predominant cell type; post R1 or R2 resection (with or without neoadjuvant therapy) with no evidence of disease progression, or metastases (for use in a Medicare-approved demonstration project)   M

BETOS: P7B   Oncology - other
Service not separately priced by Part B

C **G9102** Oncology; disease status; gastric cancer, limited to adenocarcinoma as predominant cell type; clinical or pathologic M0, unresectable with no evidence of disease progression, or metastases (for use in a Medicare-approved demonstration project) M

BETOS: P7B   Oncology - other
Service not separately priced by Part B

C **G9103** Oncology; disease status; gastric cancer, limited to adenocarcinoma as predominant cell type; clinical or pathologic M1 at diagnosis, metastatic, locally recurrent, or progressive (for use in a Medicare-approved demonstration project)   M

BETOS: P7B   Oncology - other
Service not separately priced by Part B

C **G9104** Oncology; disease status; gastric cancer, limited to adenocarcinoma as predominant cell type; extent of disease unknown, staging in progress, or not listed (for use in a Medicare-approved demonstration project) M

BETOS: P7B   Oncology - other
Service not separately priced by Part B

C **G9105** Oncology; disease status; pancreatic cancer, limited to adenocarcinoma as predominant cell type; post R0 resection without evidence of disease progression, recurrence, or metastases (for use in a Medicare-approved demonstration project)   M

BETOS: P7B   Oncology - other
Service not separately priced by Part B

C **G9106** Oncology; disease status; pancreatic cancer, limited to adenocarcinoma; post R1 or R2 resection with no evidence of disease progression, or metastases (for use in a Medicare-approved demonstration project) M

BETOS: P7B   Oncology - other
Service not separately priced by Part B

C **G9107** Oncology; disease status; pancreatic cancer, limited to adenocarcinoma; unresectable at diagnosis, M1 at diagnosis, metastatic, locally recurrent, or progressive (for use in a Medicare-approved demonstration project)   M

BETOS: P7B   Oncology - other
Service not separately priced by Part B

C **G9108** Oncology; disease status; pancreatic cancer, limited to adenocarcinoma; extent of disease unknown, staging in progress, or not listed (for use in a Medicare-approved demonstration project)   M

BETOS: P7B   Oncology - other
Service not separately priced by Part B

C **G9109** Oncology; disease status; head and neck cancer, limited to cancers of oral cavity, pharynx and larynx with squamous cell as predominant cell type; extent of disease initially established as T1-T2 and N0, M0 (prior to neo-adjuvant therapy, if any) with no evidence of disease progression, recurrence, or metastases (for use in a Medicare-approved demonstration project)   M

BETOS: P7B   Oncology - other
Service not separately priced by Part B

C **G9110** Oncology; disease status; head and neck cancer, limited to cancers of oral cavity, pharynx and larynx with squamous cell as predominant cell type; extent of disease initially established as T3-4 and/or N1-3, M0 (prior to neo-adjuvant therapy, if any) with no evidence of disease progression, recurrence, or metastases (for use in a Medicare-approved demonstration project)   M

BETOS: P7B   Oncology - other
Service not separately priced by Part B

● New code   ▲ Revised code   **C** Carrier judgment   **D** Special coverage instructions apply
I Not payable by Medicare   **M** Non-covered by Medicare   **S** Non-covered by Medicare statute   AHA Coding Clinic®

C **G9111** Oncology; disease status; head and neck cancer, limited to cancers of oral cavity, pharynx and larynx with squamous cell as predominant cell type; M1 at diagnosis, metastatic, locally recurrent, or progressive (for use in a Medicare-approved demonstration project) M
BETOS: P7B   Oncology - other
Service not separately priced by Part B

C **G9112** Oncology; disease status; head and neck cancer, limited to cancers of oral cavity, pharynx and larynx with squamous cell as predominant cell type; extent of disease unknown, staging in progress, or not listed (for use in a Medicare-approved demonstration project) M
BETOS: P7B   Oncology - other
Service not separately priced by Part B

C **G9113** Oncology; disease status; ovarian cancer, limited to epithelial cancer; pathologic Stage IA-B (Grade 1) without evidence of disease progression, recurrence, or metastases (for use in a Medicare-approved demonstration project) ♀ M
BETOS: P7B   Oncology - other
Service not separately priced by Part B

C **G9114** Oncology; disease status; ovarian cancer, limited to epithelial cancer; pathologic Stage IA-B (Grade 2-3); or Stage IC (all grades); or Stage II; without evidence of disease progression, recurrence, or metastases (for use in a Medicare-approved demonstration project) ♀ M
BETOS: P7B   Oncology - other
Service not separately priced by Part B

C **G9115** Oncology; disease status; ovarian cancer, limited to epithelial cancer; pathologic Stage III-IV; without evidence of progression, recurrence, or metastases (for use in a Medicare-approved demonstration project) ♀ M
BETOS: P7B   Oncology - other
Service not separately priced by Part B

C **G9116** Oncology; disease status; ovarian cancer, limited to epithelial cancer; evidence of disease progression, or recurrence, and/or platinum resistance (for use in a Medicare-approved demonstration project) ♀ M
BETOS: P7B   Oncology - other
Service not separately priced by Part B

C **G9117** Oncology; disease status; ovarian cancer, limited to epithelial cancer; extent of disease unknown, staging in progress, or not listed (for use in a Medicare-approved demonstration project) ♀ M
BETOS: P7B   Oncology - other
Service not separately priced by Part B

C **G9123** Oncology; disease status; chronic myelogenous leukemia, limited to Philadelphia chromosome positive and/or BCR-ABL positive; chronic phase not in hematologic, cytogenetic, or molecular remission (for use in a Medicare-approved demonstration project) M
BETOS: P7B   Oncology - other
Service not separately priced by Part B

C **G9124** Oncology; disease status; chronic myelogenous leukemia, limited to Philadelphia chromosome positive and/or BCR-ABL positive; accelerated phase not in hematologic cytogenetic, or molecular remission (for use in a Medicare-approved demonstration project) M
BETOS: P7B   Oncology - other
Service not separately priced by Part B

C **G9125** Oncology; disease status; chronic myelogenous leukemia, limited to Philadelphia chromosome positive and/or BCR-ABL positive; blast phase not in hematologic, cytogenetic, or molecular remission (for use in a Medicare-approved demonstration project) M
BETOS: P7B   Oncology - other
Service not separately priced by Part B

C **G9126** Oncology; disease status; chronic myelogenous leukemia, limited to Philadelphia chromosome positive and/or BCR-ABL positive; in hematologic, cytogenetic, or molecular remission (for use in a Medicare-approved demonstration project) M
BETOS: P7B   Oncology - other
Service not separately priced by Part B

C **G9128** Oncology; disease status; limited to multiple myeloma, systemic disease; smoldering, Stage I (for use in a Medicare-approved demonstration project) M
BETOS: P7B   Oncology - other
Service not separately priced by Part B

C **G9129** Oncology; disease status; limited to multiple myeloma, systemic disease; Stage II or higher (for use in a Medicare-approved demonstration project) M
BETOS: P7B   Oncology - other
Service not separately priced by Part B

C **G9130** Oncology; disease status; limited to multiple myeloma, systemic disease; extent of disease unknown, staging in progress, or not listed (for use in a Medicare-approved demonstration project) M
BETOS: P7B   Oncology - other
Service not separately priced by Part B

♂ Male only   ♀ Female only   Ⓐ Age   A2 - Z3 = ASC Payment indicator   A - Y = APC Status indicator
ASC = ASC Approved Procedure   **DME** Paid under the DME fee schedule   **MIPS** MIPS code

C G9131 Oncology; disease status; invasive female breast cancer (does not include ductal carcinoma in situ); adenocarcinoma as predominant cell type; extent of disease unknown, staging in progress, or not listed (for use in a Medicare-approved demonstration project) M
BETOS: P7B   Oncology - other
Service not separately priced by Part B

C G9132 Oncology; disease status; prostate cancer, limited to adenocarcinoma; hormone-refractory/androgen-independent (e.g., rising PSA on anti-androgen therapy or post-orchiectomy); clinical metastases (for use in a Medicare-approved demonstration project) ♂ M
BETOS: P7B   Oncology - other
Service not separately priced by Part B

C G9133 Oncology; disease status; prostate cancer, limited to adenocarcinoma; hormone-responsive; clinical metastases or M1 at diagnosis (for use in a Medicare-approved demonstration project) ♂ M
BETOS: P7B   Oncology - other
Service not separately priced by Part B

C G9134 Oncology; disease status; non-Hodgkin's lymphoma, any cellular classification; Stage I, II at diagnosis, not relapsed, not refractory (for use in a Medicare-approved demonstration project) M
BETOS: P7B   Oncology - other
Service not separately priced by Part B

C G9135 Oncology; disease status; non-Hodgkin's lymphoma, any cellular classification; Stage III, IV, not relapsed, not refractory (for use in a Medicare-approved demonstration project) M
BETOS: P7B   Oncology - other
Service not separately priced by Part B

C G9136 Oncology; disease status; non-Hodgkin's lymphoma, transformed from original cellular diagnosis to a second cellular classification (for use in a Medicare-approved demonstration project) M
BETOS: P7B   Oncology - other
Service not separately priced by Part B

C G9137 Oncology; disease status; non-Hodgkin's lymphoma, any cellular classification; relapsed/refractory (for use in a Medicare-approved demonstration project) M
BETOS: P7B   Oncology - other
Service not separately priced by Part B

C G9138 Oncology; disease status; non-Hodgkin's lymphoma, any cellular classification; diagnostic evaluation, stage not determined, evaluation of possible relapse or non-response to therapy, or not listed (for use in a Medicare-approved demonstration project) M

BETOS: P7B   Oncology - other
Service not separately priced by Part B

C G9139 Oncology; disease status; chronic myelogenous leukemia, limited to Philadelphia chromosome positive and/or BCR-ABL positive; extent of disease unknown, staging in progress, not listed (for use in a Medicare-approved demonstration project) M
BETOS: P7B   Oncology - other
Service not separately priced by Part B

C G9140 Frontier extended stay clinic demonstration; for a patient stay in a clinic approved for the CMS demonstration project; the following measures should be present: the stay must be equal to or greater than 4 hours; weather or other conditions must prevent transfer or the case falls into a category of monitoring and observation cases that are permitted by the rules of the demonstration; there is a maximum frontier extended stay clinic (FESC) visit of 48 hours, except in the case when weather or other conditions prevent transfer; payment is made on each period up to 4 hours, after the first 4 hours A
BETOS: Z2   Undefined codes
Service not separately priced by Part B

WARFARIN RESPONSIVENESS TESTING (G9143)

C G9143 Warfarin responsiveness testing by genetic technique using any method, any number of specimen(s) N
BETOS: M5D   Specialist - other
Price established by carriers
Coding Clinic: 2010, Q1
Pub: 100-4, Chapter-32, 250.1; 100-4, Chapter-32, 250.2

OUTPATIENT INTRAVENOUS INSULIN TREATMENT (G9147)

M G9147 Outpatient intravenous insulin treatment (OIVIT) either pulsatile or continuous, by any means, guided by the results of measurements for: respiratory quotient; and/or, urine urea nitrogen (UUN); and/or, arterial, venous or capillary glucose; and/or potassium concentration E1
BETOS: P5E   Ambulatory procedures - other
Service not separately priced by Part B
Coding Clinic: 2010, Q1
Pub: 100-4, Chapter-4, 320.2; 100-4, Chapter-4, 320.1

PRIMARY CARE QUALITY MEASURES (G9148-G9153)

C G9148 National Committee for Quality Assurance - Level 1 medical home M
BETOS: Z2   Undefined codes
Service not separately priced by Part B

● New code   ▲ Revised code   **C** Carrier judgment   **D** Special coverage instructions apply
I Not payable by Medicare   **M** Non-covered by Medicare   **S** Non-covered by Medicare statute   AHA Coding Clinic®

C **G9149** National Committee for Quality Assurance - Level 2 medical home   M
BETOS: Z2   Undefined codes
Service not separately priced by Part B

C **G9150** National Committee for Quality Assurance - Level 3 medical home   M
BETOS: Z2   Undefined codes
Service not separately priced by Part B

C **G9151** MAPCP Demonstration - state provided services   M
BETOS: Z2   Undefined codes
Service not separately priced by Part B

C **G9152** MAPCP Demonstration - Community Health Teams   M
BETOS: Z2   Undefined codes
Service not separately priced by Part B

C **G9153** MAPCP Demonstration - Physician Incentive Pool   M
BETOS: Z2   Undefined codes
Service not separately priced by Part B

PROVIDER ASSESSMENT FOR WHEELCHAIR (G9156)

C **G9156** Evaluation for wheelchair requiring face to face visit with physician   M
BETOS: Z2   Undefined codes
Service not separately priced by Part B

DIAGNOSTIC CARDIAC DOPPLER ULTRASOUND (G9157)

C **G9157** Transesophageal doppler measurement of cardiac output (including probe placement, image acquisition, and interpretation per course of treatment) for monitoring purposes   B
BETOS: T2C   Other tests - EKG monitoring
Service not separately priced by Part B
Pub: 100-4, Chapter-32, 300.2

BUNDLED PAYMENT CARE (G9187)

C **G9187** Bundled payments for care improvement initiative home visit for patient assessment performed by a qualified health care professional for individuals not considered homebound including, but not limited to, assessment of safety, falls, clinical status, fluid status, medication reconciliation/ management, patient compliance with orders/plan of care, performance of activities of daily living, appropriateness of care setting; (for use only in the Medicare-approved bundled payments for care improvement initiative); may not be billed for a 30-day period covered by a transitional care management code   E1
BETOS: M5D   Specialist - other
Price established by carriers

ADDITIONAL QUALITY MEASURES (G9188-G9893)

C **G9188** Beta-blocker therapy not prescribed, reason not given   M MIPS
BETOS: M5B   Specialist - psychiatry
Service not separately priced by Part B

C **G9189** Beta-blocker therapy prescribed or currently being taken   M MIPS
BETOS: M5B   Specialist - psychiatry
Service not separately priced by Part B

C **G9190** Documentation of medical reason(s) for not prescribing beta-blocker therapy (e.g., allergy, intolerance, other medical reasons)   M MIPS
BETOS: M5B   Specialist - psychiatry
Service not separately priced by Part B

C **G9191** Documentation of patient reason(s) for not prescribing beta-blocker therapy (e.g., patient declined, other patient reasons)   M MIPS
BETOS: M5B   Specialist - psychiatry
Service not separately priced by Part B

C **G9192** Documentation of system reason(s) for not prescribing beta-blocker therapy (e.g., other reasons attributable to the health care system)   M MIPS
BETOS: M5B   Specialist - psychiatry
Service not separately priced by Part B

C **G9196** Documentation of medical reason(s) for not ordering a first or second generation cephalosporin for antimicrobial prophylaxis (e.g., patients enrolled in clinical trials, patients with documented infection prior to surgical procedure of interest, patients who were receiving antibiotics more than 24 hours prior to surgery [except colon surgery patients taking oral prophylactic antibiotics], patients who were receiving antibiotics within 24 hours prior to arrival [except colon surgery patients taking oral prophylactic antibiotics], other medical reason(s))   M MIPS
BETOS: M5B   Specialist - psychiatry
Service not separately priced by Part B

C **G9197** Documentation of order for first or second generation cephalosporin for antimicrobial prophylaxis   M MIPS
BETOS: M5B   Specialist - psychiatry
Service not separately priced by Part B

C **G9198** Order for first or second generation cephalosporin for antimicrobial prophylaxis was not documented, reason not given   M MIPS
BETOS: M5B   Specialist - psychiatry
Service not separately priced by Part B

C **G9212** DSM-IVTM criteria for major depressive disorder documented at the initial evaluation   M
BETOS: M5B   Specialist - psychiatry
Service not separately priced by Part B

♂ Male only   ♀ Female only   Ⓐ Age   A2 - Z3 = ASC Payment indicator   A - Y = APC Status indicator
ASC = ASC Approved Procedure   **DME** Paid under the DME fee schedule   **MIPS** MIPS code

C **G9213** DSM-IV-TR criteria for major depressive disorder not documented at the initial evaluation, reason not otherwise specified M
BETOS: M5B   Specialist - psychiatry
Service not separately priced by Part B

C **G9223** Pneumocystis jiroveci pneumonia prophylaxis prescribed within 3 months of low CD4+ cell count below 500 cells/mm3 or a CD4 percentage below 15% M
BETOS: M5B   Specialist - psychiatry
Service not separately priced by Part B

C **G9225** Foot exam was not performed, reason not given M
BETOS: M5B   Specialist - psychiatry
Service not separately priced by Part B

C **G9226** Foot examination performed (includes examination through visual inspection, sensory exam with 10-g monofilament plus testing any one of the following: vibration using 128-Hz tuning fork, pinprick sensation, ankle reflexes, or vibration perception threshold, and pulse exam; report when all of the 3 components are completed) M
BETOS: M5B   Specialist - psychiatry
Service not separately priced by Part B

C **G9227** Functional outcome assessment documented, care plan not documented, documentation the patient is not eligible for a care plan at the time of the encounter M MIPS
BETOS: M5B   Specialist - psychiatry
Service not separately priced by Part B

C **G9228** Chlamydia, gonorrhea and syphilis screening results documented (report when results are present for all of the 3 screenings) M MIPS
BETOS: M5B   Specialist - psychiatry
Service not separately priced by Part B

C **G9229** Chlamydia, gonorrhea, and syphilis screening results not documented (patient refusal is the only allowed exception) M MIPS
BETOS: M5B   Specialist - psychiatry
Service not separately priced by Part B

C **G9230** Chlamydia, gonorrhea, and syphilis not screened, reason not given M MIPS
BETOS: M5B   Specialist - psychiatry
Service not separately priced by Part B

C **G9231** Documentation of end stage renal disease (ESRD), dialysis, renal transplant before or during the measurement period or pregnancy during the measurement period ♀ M MIPS
BETOS: M5B   Specialist - psychiatry
Service not separately priced by Part B

C **G9242** Documentation of viral load equal to or greater than 200 copies/ml or viral load not performed M MIPS
BETOS: M5B   Specialist - psychiatry
Service not separately priced by Part B

C **G9243** Documentation of viral load less than 200 copies/ml M MIPS
BETOS: M5B   Specialist - psychiatry
Service not separately priced by Part B

C **G9246** Patient did not have at least one medical visit in each 6 month period of the 24 month measurement period, with a minimum of 60 days between medical visits M MIPS
BETOS: M5B   Specialist - psychiatry
Service not separately priced by Part B

C **G9247** Patient had at least one medical visit in each 6 month period of the 24 month measurement period, with a minimum of 60 days between medical visits M MIPS
BETOS: M5B   Specialist - psychiatry
Service not separately priced by Part B

C **G9250** Documentation of patient pain brought to a comfortable level within 48 hours from initial assessment M MIPS
BETOS: M5B   Specialist - psychiatry
Service not separately priced by Part B

C **G9251** Documentation of patient with pain not brought to a comfortable level within 48 hours from initial assessment M MIPS
BETOS: M5B   Specialist - psychiatry
Service not separately priced by Part B

C **G9254** Documentation of patient discharged to home later than post-operative day 2 following CAS M MIPS
BETOS: M5B   Specialist - psychiatry
Service not separately priced by Part B

C **G9255** Documentation of patient discharged to home no later than post operative day 2 following CAS M MIPS
BETOS: M5B   Specialist - psychiatry
Service not separately priced by Part B

C **G9267** Documentation of patient with one or more complications or mortality within 30 days M MIPS
BETOS: M5B   Specialist - psychiatry
Service not separately priced by Part B

C **G9268** Documentation of patient with one or more complications within 90 days M MIPS
BETOS: M5B   Specialist - psychiatry
Service not separately priced by Part B

C **G9269** Documentation of patient without one or more complications and without mortality within 30 days M MIPS
BETOS: M5B   Specialist - psychiatry
Service not separately priced by Part B

C **G9270** Documentation of patient without one or more complications within 90 days M MIPS
BETOS: M5B   Specialist - psychiatry
Service not separately priced by Part B

● New code   ▲ Revised code   **C** Carrier judgment   **D** Special coverage instructions apply
I Not payable by Medicare   **M** Non-covered by Medicare   **S** Non-covered by Medicare statute   AHA Coding Clinic®

G9273 Blood pressure has a systolic value of < 140 and a diastolic value of < 90   M
BETOS: M5B   Specialist - psychiatry
Service not separately priced by Part B

G9274 Blood pressure has a systolic value of =140 and a diastolic value of = 90 or systolic value < 140 and diastolic value = 90 or systolic value = 140 and diastolic value < 90   M
BETOS: M5B   Specialist - psychiatry
Service not separately priced by Part B

G9275 Documentation that patient is a current non-tobacco user   Ⓐ M
BETOS: M5B   Specialist - psychiatry
Service not separately priced by Part B

G9276 Documentation that patient is a current tobacco user   Ⓐ M
BETOS: M5B   Specialist - psychiatry
Service not separately priced by Part B

G9277 Documentation that the patient is on daily aspirin or anti-platelet or has documentation of a valid contraindication or exception to aspirin/anti-platelet; contraindications/exceptions include anti-coagulant use, allergy to aspirin or anti-platelets, history of gastrointestinal bleed and bleeding disorder; additionally, the following exceptions documented by the physician as a reason for not taking daily aspirin or anti-platelet are acceptable (use of non-steroidal anti-inflammatory agents, documented risk for drug interaction, uncontrolled hypertension defined as >180 systolic or >110 diastolic or gastroesophageal reflux)   M
BETOS: M5B   Specialist - psychiatry
Service not separately priced by Part B

G9278 Documentation that the patient is not on daily aspirin or anti-platelet regimen   M
BETOS: M5B   Specialist - psychiatry
Service not separately priced by Part B

G9279 Pneumococcal screening performed and documentation of vaccination received prior to discharge   M
BETOS: M5B   Specialist - psychiatry
Service not separately priced by Part B

G9280 Pneumococcal vaccination not administered prior to discharge, reason not specified   M
BETOS: M5B   Specialist - psychiatry
Service not separately priced by Part B

G9281 Screening performed and documentation that vaccination not indicated/patient refusal   M
BETOS: M5B   Specialist - psychiatry
Service not separately priced by Part B

G9282 Documentation of medical reason(s) for not reporting the histological type or NSCLC-NOS classification with an explanation (e.g., biopsy taken for other purposes in a patient

with a history of non-small cell lung cancer or other documented medical reasons)   M
BETOS: M5B   Specialist - psychiatry
Service not separately priced by Part B

G9283 Non-small cell lung cancer biopsy and cytology specimen report documents classification into specific histologic type or classified as NSCLC-NOS with an explanation   M
BETOS: M5B   Specialist - psychiatry
Service not separately priced by Part B

G9284 Non-small cell lung cancer biopsy and cytology specimen report does not document classification into specific histologic type or classified as NSCLC-NOS with an explanation   M
BETOS: M5B   Specialist - psychiatry
Service not separately priced by Part B

G9285 Specimen site other than anatomic location of lung or is not classified as non-small cell lung cancer   M
BETOS: M5B   Specialist - psychiatry
Service not separately priced by Part B

G9286 Antibiotic regimen prescribed within 10 days after onset of symptoms   M MIPS
BETOS: M5B   Specialist - psychiatry
Service not separately priced by Part B

G9287 Antibiotic regimen not prescribed within 10 days after onset of symptoms   M MIPS
BETOS: M5B   Specialist - psychiatry
Service not separately priced by Part B

G9288 Documentation of medical reason(s) for not reporting the histological type or NSCLC-NOS classification with an explanation (e.g., a solitary fibrous tumor in a person with a history of non-small cell carcinoma or other documented medical reasons)   M
BETOS: M5B   Specialist - psychiatry
Service not separately priced by Part B

G9289 Non-small cell lung cancer biopsy and cytology specimen report documents classification into specific histologic type or classified as NSCLC-NOS with an explanation   M
BETOS: M5B   Specialist - psychiatry
Service not separately priced by Part B

G9290 Non-small cell lung cancer biopsy and cytology specimen report does not document classification into specific histologic type or classified as NSCLC-NOS with an explanation   M
BETOS: M5B   Specialist - psychiatry
Service not separately priced by Part B

G9291 Specimen site other than anatomic location of lung, is not classified as non-small cell lung cancer or classified as NSCLC-NOS   M
BETOS: M5B   Specialist - psychiatry
Service not separately priced by Part B

♂ Male only   ♀ Female only   Ⓐ Age   A2 - Z3 = ASC Payment indicator   A - Y = APC Status indicator
ASC = ASC Approved Procedure   **DME** Paid under the DME fee schedule   **MIPS** MIPS code

G9292 - G9316

PROCEDURES / PROFESSIONAL SERVICES (G0008-G9987)

C **G9292** Documentation of medical reason(s) for not reporting PT category and a statement on thickness and ulceration and for PT1, mitotic rate (e.g., negative skin biopsies in a patient with a history of melanoma or other documented medical reasons)   M
    BETOS: M5B   Specialist - psychiatry
    Service not separately priced by Part B

C **G9293** Pathology report does not include the PT category and a statement on thickness and ulceration and for PT1, mitotic rate   M
    BETOS: M5B   Specialist - psychiatry
    Service not separately priced by Part B

C **G9294** Pathology report includes the PT category and a statement on thickness and ulceration and for PT1, mitotic rate   M
    BETOS: M5B   Specialist - psychiatry
    Service not separately priced by Part B

C **G9295** Specimen site other than anatomic cutaneous location   M
    BETOS: M5B   Specialist - psychiatry
    Service not separately priced by Part B

C **G9296** Patients with documented shared decision-making including discussion of conservative (non-surgical) therapy (e.g., NSAIDS, analgesics, weight loss, exercise, injections) prior to the procedure   M MIPS
    BETOS: M5B   Specialist - psychiatry
    Service not separately priced by Part B

C **G9297** Shared decision-making including discussion of conservative (non-surgical) therapy (e.g., NSAIDS, analgesics, weight loss, exercise, injections) prior to the procedure, not documented, reason not given   M MIPS
    BETOS: M5B   Specialist - psychiatry
    Service not separately priced by Part B

C **G9298** Patients who are evaluated for venous thromboembolic and cardiovascular risk factors within 30 days prior to the procedure (e.g. history of DVT, PE, MI, arrhythmia and stroke)   M MIPS
    BETOS: M5B   Specialist - psychiatry
    Service not separately priced by Part B

▲ **C** **G9299** Patients who are not evaluated for venous thromboembolic and cardiovascular risk factors within 30 days prior to the procedure (e.g., history of DVT, PE, MI, arrhythmia and stroke, reason not given)   M MIPS
    BETOS: M5B   Specialist - psychiatry
    Service not separately priced by Part B

C **G9305** Intervention for presence of leak of endoluminal contents through an anastomosis not required   M MIPS
    BETOS: M5B   Specialist - psychiatry
    Service not separately priced by Part B

C **G9306** Intervention for presence of leak of endoluminal contents through an anastomosis required   M MIPS
    BETOS: M5B   Specialist - psychiatry
    Service not separately priced by Part B

C **G9307** No return to the operating room for a surgical procedure, for complications of the principal operative procedure, within 30 days of the principal operative procedure   M MIPS
    BETOS: M5B   Specialist - psychiatry
    Service not separately priced by Part B

C **G9308** Unplanned return to the operating room for a surgical procedure, for complications of the principal operative procedure, within 30 days of the principal operative procedure   M MIPS
    BETOS: M5B   Specialist - psychiatry
    Service not separately priced by Part B

C **G9309** No unplanned hospital readmission within 30 days of principal procedure   M MIPS
    BETOS: M5B   Specialist - psychiatry
    Service not separately priced by Part B

C **G9310** Unplanned hospital readmission within 30 days of principal procedure   M MIPS
    BETOS: M5B   Specialist - psychiatry
    Service not separately priced by Part B

C **G9311** No surgical site infection   M MIPS
    BETOS: M5B   Specialist - psychiatry
    Service not separately priced by Part B

C **G9312** Surgical site infection   M MIPS
    BETOS: M5B   Specialist - psychiatry
    Service not separately priced by Part B

C **G9313** Amoxicillin, with or without clavulanate, not prescribed as first line antibiotic at the time of diagnosis for documented reason   M MIPS
    BETOS: M5B   Specialist - psychiatry
    Service not separately priced by Part B

C **G9314** Amoxicillin, with or without clavulanate, not prescribed as first line antibiotic at the time of diagnosis, reason not given   M MIPS
    BETOS: M5B   Specialist - psychiatry
    Service not separately priced by Part B

C **G9315** Documentation amoxicillin, with or without clavulanate, prescribed as a first line antibiotic at the time of diagnosis   M MIPS
    BETOS: M5B   Specialist - psychiatry
    Service not separately priced by Part B

C **G9316** Documentation of patient-specific risk assessment with a risk calculator based on multi-institutional clinical data, the specific risk calculator used, and communication of risk assessment from risk calculator with the patient or family   M MIPS
    BETOS: M5B   Specialist - psychiatry
    Service not separately priced by Part B

● New code   ▲ Revised code   **C** Carrier judgment   **D** Special coverage instructions apply
I Not payable by Medicare   **M** Non-covered by Medicare   **S** Non-covered by Medicare statute   AHA Coding Clinic®

G9317 Documentation of patient-specific risk assessment with a risk calculator based on multi-institutional clinical data, the specific risk calculator used, and communication of risk assessment from risk calculator with the patient or family not completed   M MIPS

   BETOS: M5B   Specialist - psychiatry
   Service not separately priced by Part B

G9318 Imaging study named according to standardized nomenclature   M

   BETOS: M5B   Specialist - psychiatry
   Service not separately priced by Part B

G9319 Imaging study not named according to standardized nomenclature, reason not given   M

   BETOS: M5B   Specialist - psychiatry
   Service not separately priced by Part B

G9321 Count of previous CT (any type of CT) and cardiac nuclear medicine (myocardial perfusion) studies documented in the 12-month period prior to the current study   M MIPS

   BETOS: M5B   Specialist - psychiatry
   Service not separately priced by Part B

G9322 Count of previous CT and cardiac nuclear medicine (myocardial perfusion) studies not documented in the 12-month period prior to the current study, reason not given   M MIPS

   BETOS: M5B   Specialist - psychiatry
   Service not separately priced by Part B

G9341 Search conducted for prior patient CT studies completed at non-affiliated external healthcare facilities or entities within the past 12-months and are available through a secure, authorized, media-free, shared archive prior to an imaging study being performed   M

   BETOS: M5B   Specialist - psychiatry
   Service not separately priced by Part B

G9342 Search not conducted prior to an imaging study being performed for prior patient CT studies completed at non-affiliated external healthcare facilities or entities within the past 12-months and are available through a secure, authorized, media-free, shared archive, reason not given   M

   BETOS: M5B   Specialist - psychiatry
   Service not separately priced by Part B

G9344 Due to system reasons search not conducted for dicom format images for prior patient CT imaging studies completed at non-affiliated external healthcare facilities or entities within the past 12 months that are available through a secure, authorized, media-free, shared archive (e.g., non-affiliated external healthcare facilities or entities does not have archival abilities through a shared archival system)   M

   BETOS: M5B   Specialist - psychiatry
   Service not separately priced by Part B

G9345 Follow-up recommendations documented according to recommended guidelines for incidentally detected pulmonary nodules (e.g., follow-up CT imaging studies needed or that no follow-up is needed) based at a minimum on nodule size and patient risk factors   A M MIPS

   BETOS: M5B   Specialist - psychiatry
   Service not separately priced by Part B

G9347 Follow-up recommendations not documented according to recommended guidelines for incidentally detected pulmonary nodules, reason not given   A M MIPS

   BETOS: M5B   Specialist - psychiatry
   Service not separately priced by Part B

G9348 CT scan of the paranasal sinuses ordered at the time of diagnosis for documented reasons   M MIPS

   BETOS: M5B   Specialist - psychiatry
   Service not separately priced by Part B

G9349 CT scan of the paranasal sinuses ordered at the time of diagnosis or received within 28 days after date of diagnosis   M MIPS

   BETOS: M5B   Specialist - psychiatry
   Service not separately priced by Part B

G9350 CT scan of the paranasal sinuses not ordered at the time of diagnosis or received within 28 days after date of diagnosis   M MIPS

   BETOS: M5B   Specialist - psychiatry
   Service not separately priced by Part B

G9351 More than one CT scan of the paranasal sinuses ordered or received within 90 days after diagnosis   M

   BETOS: M5B   Specialist - psychiatry
   Service not separately priced by Part B

G9352 More than one CT scan of the paranasal sinuses ordered or received within 90 days after the date of diagnosis, reason not given   M

   BETOS: M5B   Specialist - psychiatry
   Service not separately priced by Part B

G9353 More than one CT scan of the paranasal sinuses ordered or received within 90 days after the date of diagnosis for documented reasons (e.g., patients with complications, second CT obtained prior to surgery, other medical reasons)   M

   BETOS: M5B   Specialist - psychiatry
   Service not separately priced by Part B

G9354 One CT scan or no CT scan of the paranasal sinuses ordered within 90 days after the date of diagnosis   M

   BETOS: M5B   Specialist - psychiatry
   Service not separately priced by Part B

♂ Male only   ♀ Female only   A Age   A2 - Z3 = ASC Payment indicator   A - Y = APC Status indicator
ASC = ASC Approved Procedure   DME Paid under the DME fee schedule   MIPS MIPS code

▲ **C** **G9355** Early elective delivery by c-section, or early elective induction, not performed (less than 39 weeks gestation) ♀ Ⓐ M **MIPS**
BETOS: M5B Specialist - psychiatry
Service not separately priced by Part B

▲ **C** **G9356** Early elective delivery by c-section, or early elective induction, performed (less than 39 week gestation) ♀ Ⓐ M **MIPS**
BETOS: M5B Specialist - psychiatry
Service not separately priced by Part B

C **G9357** Post-partum screenings, evaluations and education performed ♀ Ⓐ M **MIPS**
BETOS: M5B Specialist - psychiatry
Service not separately priced by Part B

C **G9358** Post-partum screenings, evaluations and education not performed ♀ Ⓐ M **MIPS**
BETOS: M5B Specialist - psychiatry
Service not separately priced by Part B

C **G9359** Documentation of negative or managed positive TB screen with further evidence that TB is not active prior to the treatment with a biologic immune response modifier M **MIPS**
BETOS: M5B Specialist - psychiatry
Service not separately priced by Part B

C **G9360** No documentation of negative or managed positive TB screen M **MIPS**
BETOS: M5B Specialist - psychiatry
Service not separately priced by Part B

C **G9361** Medical indication for induction [documentation of reason(s) for elective delivery (C-section) or early induction (e.g., hemorrhage and placental complications, hypertension, preeclampsia and eclampsia, rupture of membranes-premature or prolonged, maternal conditions complicating pregnancy/delivery, fetal conditions complicating pregnancy/delivery, late pregnancy, prior uterine surgery, or participation in clinical trial)] ♀ Ⓐ M **MIPS**
BETOS: Z2 Undefined codes
Service not separately priced by Part B

C **G9364** Sinusitis caused by, or presumed to be caused by, bacterial infection M **MIPS**
BETOS: Z2 Undefined codes
Service not separately priced by Part B

C **G9367** At least two orders for the same high-risk medication M **MIPS**
BETOS: Z2 Undefined codes
Service not separately priced by Part B

C **G9368** At least two orders for the same high-risk medications not ordered M **MIPS**
BETOS: Z2 Undefined codes
Service not separately priced by Part B

C **G9380** Patient offered assistance with end of life issues during the measurement period M **MIPS**
BETOS: Z2 Undefined codes
Service not separately priced by Part B

C **G9382** Patient not offered assistance with end of life issues during the measurement period M **MIPS**
BETOS: Z2 Undefined codes
Service not separately priced by Part B

C **G9383** Patient received screening for HCV infection within the 12 month reporting period M **MIPS**
BETOS: Z2 Undefined codes
Service not separately priced by Part B

C **G9384** Documentation of medical reason(s) for not receiving annual screening for HCV infection (e.g., decompensated cirrhosis indicating advanced disease [i.e., ascites, esophageal variceal bleeding, hepatic encephalopathy], hepatocellular carcinoma, waitlist for organ transplant, limited life expectancy, other medical reasons) M **MIPS**
BETOS: Z2 Undefined codes
Service not separately priced by Part B

C **G9385** Documentation of patient reason(s) for not receiving annual screening for HCV infection (e.g., patient declined, other patient reasons) M **MIPS**
BETOS: Z2 Undefined codes
Service not separately priced by Part B

C **G9386** Screening for HCV infection not received within the 12 month reporting period, reason not given M **MIPS**
BETOS: Z2 Undefined codes
Service not separately priced by Part B

C **G9393** Patient with an initial PHQ-9 score greater than nine who achieves remission at twelve months as demonstrated by a twelve month (+/- 30 days) PHQ-9 score of less than five M
BETOS: Z2 Undefined codes
Service not separately priced by Part B

C **G9394** Patient who had a diagnosis of bipolar disorder or personality disorder, death, permanent nursing home resident or receiving hospice or palliative care any time during the measurement or assessment period M
BETOS: Z2 Undefined codes
Service not separately priced by Part B

C **G9395** Patient with an initial PHQ-9 score greater than nine who did not achieve remission at twelve months as demonstrated by a twelve month (+/- 30 days) PHQ-9 score greater than or equal to five M
BETOS: Z2 Undefined codes
Service not separately priced by Part B

C **G9396** Patient with an initial PHQ-9 score greater than nine who was not assessed for remission at twelve months (+/- 30 days) M
BETOS: Z2 Undefined codes
Service not separately priced by Part B

● New code ▲ Revised code **C** Carrier judgment **D** Special coverage instructions apply
I Not payable by Medicare **M** Non-covered by Medicare **S** Non-covered by Medicare statute AHA Coding Clinic®

C **G9399** Documentation in the patient record of a discussion between the physician/clinician and the patient that includes all of the following: treatment choices appropriate to genotype, risks and benefits, evidence of effectiveness, and patient preferences toward the outcome of the treatment M MIPS

BETOS: Z2   Undefined codes
Service not separately priced by Part B

C **G9400** Documentation of medical or patient reason(s) for not discussing treatment options; medical reasons: patient is not a candidate for treatment due to advanced physical or mental health comorbidity (including active substance use); currently receiving antiviral treatment; successful antiviral treatment (with sustained virologic response) prior to reporting period; other documented medical reasons; patient reasons: patient unable or unwilling to participate in the discussion or other patient reasons M MIPS

BETOS: Z2   Undefined codes
Service not separately priced by Part B

▲ **C** **G9401** No documentation in the patient record of a discussion between the physician or other qualified healthcare professional and the patient that includes all of the following: treatment choices appropriate to genotype, risks and benefits, evidence of effectiveness, and patient preferences toward treatment M MIPS

BETOS: Z2   Undefined codes
Service not separately priced by Part B

▲ **C** **G9402** Patient received follow-up within 30 days after discharge M MIPS

BETOS: Z2   Undefined codes
Service not separately priced by Part B

C **G9403** Clinician documented reason patient was not able to complete 30 day follow-up from acute inpatient setting discharge (e.g., patient death prior to follow-up visit, patient non-compliant for visit follow-up) M MIPS

BETOS: Z2   Undefined codes
Service not separately priced by Part B

C **G9404** Patient did not receive follow-up on the date of discharge or within 30 days after discharge M MIPS

BETOS: Z2   Undefined codes
Service not separately priced by Part B

C **G9405** Patient received follow-up within 7 days after discharge M MIPS

BETOS: Z2   Undefined codes
Service not separately priced by Part B

C **G9406** Clinician documented reason patient was not able to complete 7 day follow-up from acute inpatient setting discharge (i.e patient

death prior to follow-up visit, patient non-compliance for visit follow-up) M MIPS

BETOS: Z2   Undefined codes
Service not separately priced by Part B

C **G9407** Patient did not receive follow-up on or within 7 days after discharge M MIPS

BETOS: Z2   Undefined codes
Service not separately priced by Part B

C **G9408** Patients with cardiac tamponade and/or pericardiocentesis occurring within 30 days M MIPS

BETOS: Z2   Undefined codes
Service not separately priced by Part B

C **G9409** Patients without cardiac tamponade and/or pericardiocentesis occurring within 30 days M MIPS

BETOS: Z2   Undefined codes
Service not separately priced by Part B

C **G9410** Patient admitted within 180 days, status post CIED implantation, replacement, or revision with an infection requiring device removal or surgical revision M MIPS

BETOS: Z2   Undefined codes
Service not separately priced by Part B

C **G9411** Patient not admitted within 180 days, status post CIED implantation, replacement, or revision with an infection requiring device removal or surgical revision M MIPS

BETOS: Z2   Undefined codes
Service not separately priced by Part B

C **G9412** Patient admitted within 180 days, status post CIED implantation, replacement, or revision with an infection requiring device removal or surgical revision M MIPS

BETOS: Z2   Undefined codes
Service not separately priced by Part B

C **G9413** Patient not admitted within 180 days, status post CIED implantation, replacement, or revision with an infection requiring device removal or surgical revision M MIPS

BETOS: Z2   Undefined codes
Service not separately priced by Part B

C **G9414** Patient had one dose of meningococcal vaccine (serogroups A, C, W, Y) on or between the patient's 11th and 13th birthdays Ⓐ M MIPS

BETOS: Z2   Undefined codes
Service not separately priced by Part B

▲ **C** **G9415** Patient did not have one dose of meningococcal vaccine (serogroups A, C, W, Y) on or between the patient's 11th and 13th birthdays Ⓐ M MIPS

BETOS: Z2   Undefined codes
Service not separately priced by Part B

G9416 Patient had one tetanus, diphtheria toxoids and acellular pertussis vaccine (TDAP) on or between the patient's 10th and 13th birthdays Ⓐ M MIPS
BETOS: Z2   Undefined codes
Service not separately priced by Part B

G9417 Patient did not have one tetanus, diphtheria toxoids and acellular pertussis vaccine (TDAP) on or between the patient's 10th and 13th birthdays Ⓐ M MIPS
BETOS: Z2   Undefined codes
Service not separately priced by Part B

G9418 Primary non-small cell lung cancer biopsy and cytology specimen report documents classification into specific histologic type or classified as NSCLC-NOS with an explanation M MIPS
BETOS: Z2   Undefined codes
Service not separately priced by Part B

G9419 Documentation of medical reason(s) for not including the histological type or NSCLC-NOS classification with an explanation (e.g., biopsy taken for other purposes in a patient with a history of primary non-small cell lung cancer or other documented medical reasons) M MIPS
BETOS: Z2   Undefined codes
Service not separately priced by Part B

G9420 Specimen site other than anatomic location of lung or is not classified as primary non-small cell lung cancer M MIPS
BETOS: Z2   Undefined codes
Service not separately priced by Part B

G9421 Primary non-small cell lung cancer biopsy and cytology specimen report does not document classification into specific histologic type or classified as NSCLC-NOS with an explanation M MIPS
BETOS: Z2   Undefined codes
Service not separately priced by Part B

G9422 Primary lung carcinoma resection report documents PT category, pN category and for non-small cell lung cancer, histologic type (squamous cell carcinoma, adenocarcinoma and not NSCLC-NOS) M MIPS
BETOS: Z2   Undefined codes
Service not separately priced by Part B

G9423 Documentation of medical reason for not including PT category, pN category and histologic type [for patient with appropriate exclusion criteria (e.g., metastatic disease, benign tumors, malignant tumors other than carcinomas, inadequate surgical specimens)] M MIPS
BETOS: Z2   Undefined codes
Service not separately priced by Part B

G9424 Specimen site other than anatomic location of lung, or classified as NSCLC-NOS M MIPS

BETOS: Z2   Undefined codes
Service not separately priced by Part B

G9425 Primary lung carcinoma resection report does not document PT category, pN category and for non-small cell lung cancer, histologic type (squamous cell carcinoma, adenocarcinoma) M MIPS
BETOS: Z2   Undefined codes
Service not separately priced by Part B

G9426 Improvement in median time from ED arrival to initial ED oral or parenteral pain medication administration performed for ED admitted patients M
BETOS: Z2   Undefined codes
Service not separately priced by Part B

G9427 Improvement in median time from ED arrival to initial ED oral or parenteral pain medication administration not performed for ED admitted patients M
BETOS: Z2   Undefined codes
Service not separately priced by Part B

G9428 Pathology report includes the PT category and a statement on thickness, ulceration and mitotic rate M MIPS
BETOS: Z2   Undefined codes
Service not separately priced by Part B

G9429 Documentation of medical reason(s) for not including PT category and a statement on thickness, ulceration and mitotic rate (e.g., negative skin biopsies in a patient with a history of melanoma or other documented medical reasons) M MIPS
BETOS: Z2   Undefined codes
Service not separately priced by Part B

G9430 Specimen site other than anatomic cutaneous location M MIPS
BETOS: Z2   Undefined codes
Service not separately priced by Part B

G9431 Pathology report does not include the PT category and a statement on thickness, ulceration and mitotic rate M MIPS
BETOS: Z2   Undefined codes
Service not separately priced by Part B

G9432 Asthma well-controlled based on the ACT, C-ACT, ACQ, or ATAQ score and results documented M MIPS
BETOS: Z2   Undefined codes
Service not separately priced by Part B

G9434 Asthma not well-controlled based on the ACT, C-ACT, ACQ, or ATAQ score, or specified asthma control tool not used, reason not given M MIPS
BETOS: Z2   Undefined codes
Service not separately priced by Part B

▲ **G9448** Patients who were born in the years 1945 to 1965 M MIPS
BETOS: Z2   Undefined codes
Service not separately priced by Part B

● New code   ▲ Revised code   Ⓒ Carrier judgment   Ⓓ Special coverage instructions apply
Ⓘ Not payable by Medicare   Ⓜ Non-covered by Medicare   Ⓢ Non-covered by Medicare statute   AHA Coding Clinic®

C **G9449** History of receiving blood transfusions prior to 1992   M MIPS

       BETOS: Z2   Undefined codes
       Service not separately priced by Part B

C **G9450** History of injection drug use   M MIPS

       BETOS: Z2   Undefined codes
       Service not separately priced by Part B

C **G9451** Patient received one-time screening for HCV infection   M MIPS

       BETOS: Z2   Undefined codes
       Service not separately priced by Part B

C **G9452** Documentation of medical reason(s) for not receiving one-time screening for HCV infection (e.g., decompensated cirrhosis indicating advanced disease [ie, ascites, esophageal variceal bleeding, hepatic encephalopathy], hepatocellular carcinoma, waitlist for organ transplant, limited life expectancy, other medical reasons)   M MIPS

       BETOS: Z2   Undefined codes
       Service not separately priced by Part B

C **G9453** Documentation of patient reason(s) for not receiving one-time screening for HCV infection (e.g., patient declined, other patient reasons)   M MIPS

       BETOS: Z2   Undefined codes
       Service not separately priced by Part B

C **G9454** One-time screening for HCV infection not received within 12-month reporting period and no documentation of prior screening for HCV infection, reason not given   M MIPS

       BETOS: Z2   Undefined codes
       Service not separately priced by Part B

C **G9455** Patient underwent abdominal imaging with ultrasound, contrast enhanced CT or contrast MRI for HCC   M MIPS

       BETOS: Z2   Undefined codes
       Service not separately priced by Part B

C **G9456** Documentation of medical or patient reason(s) for not ordering or performing screening for HCC. medical reason: comorbid medical conditions with expected survival < 5 years, hepatic decompensation and not a candidate for liver transplantation, or other medical reasons; patient reasons: patient declined or other patient reasons (e.g., cost of tests, time related to accessing testing equipment)   M MIPS

       BETOS: Z2   Undefined codes
       Service not separately priced by Part B

C **G9457** Patient did not undergo abdominal imaging and did not have a documented reason for not undergoing abdominal imaging in the submission period   M MIPS

       BETOS: Z2   Undefined codes
       Service not separately priced by Part B

C **G9458** Patient documented as tobacco user and received tobacco cessation intervention (must include at least one of the following: advice given to quit smoking or tobacco use, counseling on the benefits of quitting smoking or tobacco use, assistance with or referral to external smoking or tobacco cessation support programs, or current enrollment in smoking or tobacco use cessation program) if identified as a tobacco user   M MIPS

       BETOS: Z2   Undefined codes
       Service not separately priced by Part B

C **G9459** Currently a tobacco non-user   M MIPS

       BETOS: Z2   Undefined codes
       Service not separately priced by Part B

C **G9460** Tobacco assessment or tobacco cessation intervention not performed, reason not given   M MIPS

       BETOS: Z2   Undefined codes
       Service not separately priced by Part B

C **G9468** Patient not receiving corticosteroids greater than or equal to 10 mg/day of prednisone equivalents for 60 or greater consecutive days or a single prescription equating to 600 mg prednisone or greater for all fills   M

       BETOS: Z2   Undefined codes
       Service not separately priced by Part B

C **G9470** Patients not receiving corticosteroids greater than or equal to 10 mg/day of prednisone equivalents for 60 or greater consecutive days or a single prescription equating to 600 mg prednisone or greater for all fills   M

       BETOS: Z2   Undefined codes
       Service not separately priced by Part B

C **G9471** Within the past 2 years, central dual-energy X-ray absorptiometry (DXA) not ordered or documented   M

       BETOS: Z2   Undefined codes
       Service not separately priced by Part B

C **G9473** Services performed by chaplain in the hospice setting, each 15 minutes   B

       BETOS: M5D   Specialist - other
       Service not separately priced by Part B

C **G9474** Services performed by dietary counselor in the hospice setting, each 15 minutes   B

       BETOS: M5D   Specialist - other
       Service not separately priced by Part B

C **G9475** Services performed by other counselor in the hospice setting, each 15 minutes   B

       BETOS: M5D   Specialist - other
       Service not separately priced by Part B

C **G9476** Services performed by volunteer in the hospice setting, each 15 minutes   B

       BETOS: M5D   Specialist - other
       Service not separately priced by Part B

♂ Male only   ♀ Female only   **A** Age   A2 - Z3 = ASC Payment indicator   A - Y = APC Status indicator

ASC = ASC Approved Procedure   **DME** Paid under the DME fee schedule   MIPS MIPS code

C **G9477** Services performed by care coordinator in the hospice setting, each 15 minutes B
BETOS: M5D Specialist - other
Service not separately priced by Part B

C **G9478** Services performed by other qualified therapist in the hospice setting, each 15 minutes B
BETOS: M5D Specialist - other
Service not separately priced by Part B

C **G9479** Services performed by qualified pharmacist in the hospice setting, each 15 minutes B
BETOS: M5D Specialist - other
Service not separately priced by Part B

C **G9480** Admission to medicare care choice model program (MCCM) B
BETOS: M5D Specialist - other
Service not separately priced by Part B

C **G9481** Remote in-home visit for the evaluation and management of a new patient for use only in a Medicare-approved CMS innovation center demonstration project, which requires these 3 key components: a problem focused history; a problem focused examination; and straightforward medical decision making, furnished in real time using interactive audio and video technology. Counseling and coordination of care with other physicians, other qualified health care professionals or agencies are provided consistent with the nature of the problem(s) and the needs of the patient or the family or both. Usually, the presenting problem(s) are self-limited or minor. Typically, 10 minutes are spent with the patient or family or both via real time, audio and video intercommunications technology B
BETOS: Z2 Undefined codes
Service not separately priced by Part B
Coding Clinic: 2016, Q1

C **G9482** Remote in-home visit for the evaluation and management of a new patient for use only in a Medicare-approved CMS innovation center demonstration project, which requires these 3 key components: an expanded problem focused history; an expanded problem focused examination; straightforward medical decision making, furnished in real time using interactive audio and video technology. Counseling and coordination of care with other physicians, other qualified health care professionals or agencies are provided consistent with the nature of the problem(s) and the needs of the patient or the family or both. Usually, the presenting problem(s) are of low to moderate severity. Typically, 20 minutes are spent with the patient or family or both via real time, audio and video intercommunications technology B

BETOS: Z2 Undefined codes
Service not separately priced by Part B
Coding Clinic: 2016, Q1

C **G9483** Remote in-home visit for the evaluation and management of a new patient for use only in a Medicare-approved CMS innovation center demonstration project, which requires these 3 key components: a detailed history; a detailed examination; medical decision making of low complexity, furnished in real time using interactive audio and video technology. Counseling and coordination of care with other physicians, other qualified health care professionals or agencies are provided consistent with the nature of the problem(s) and the needs of the patient or the family or both. Usually, the presenting problem(s) are of moderate severity. Typically, 30 minutes are spent with the patient or family or both via real time, audio and video intercommunications technology B
BETOS: Z2 Undefined codes
Service not separately priced by Part B
Coding Clinic: 2016, Q1

C **G9484** Remote in-home visit for the evaluation and management of a new patient for use only in a Medicare-approved CMS innovation center demonstration project, which requires these 3 key components: a comprehensive history; a comprehensive examination; medical decision making of moderate complexity, furnished in real time using interactive audio and video technology. Counseling and coordination of care with other physicians, other qualified health care professionals or agencies are provided consistent with the nature of the problem(s) and the needs of the patient or the family or both. Usually, the presenting problem(s) are of moderate to high severity. Typically, 45 minutes are spent with the patient or family or both via real time, audio and video intercommunications technology B
BETOS: Z2 Undefined codes
Service not separately priced by Part B
Coding Clinic: 2016, Q1

C **G9485** Remote in-home visit for the evaluation and management of a new patient for use only in a Medicare-approved CMS innovation center demonstration project, which requires these 3 key components: a comprehensive history; a comprehensive examination; medical decision making of high complexity, furnished in real time using interactive audio and video technology. Counseling and coordination of care with other physicians, other qualified health care professionals or agencies are provided consistent with the nature of the problem(s) and the needs of the patient or the family or both. Usually, the presenting problem(s) are of moderate to high severity. Typically, 60 minutes are spent with the patient or family or both via real time, audio and video intercommunications technology　　　　　　　　　　　　　B

BETOS: Z2　Undefined codes
Service not separately priced by Part B
Coding Clinic: 2016, Q1

C **G9486** Remote in-home visit for the evaluation and management of an established patient for use only in a Medicare-approved CMS innovation center demonstration project, which requires at least 2 of the following 3 key components: a problem focused history; a problem focused examination; straightforward medical decision making, furnished in real time using interactive audio and video technology. Counseling and coordination of care with other physicians, other qualified health care professionals or agencies are provided consistent with the nature of the problem(s) and the needs of the patient or the family or both. Usually, the presenting problem(s) are self-limited or minor. Typically, 10 minutes are spent with the patient or family or both via real time, audio and video intercommunications technology　　　　　　　　　　　　　B

BETOS: Z2　Undefined codes
Service not separately priced by Part B
Coding Clinic: 2016, Q1

C **G9487** Remote in-home visit for the evaluation and management of an established patient for use only in a Medicare-approved CMS innovation center demonstration project, which requires at least 2 of the following 3 key components: an expanded problem focused history; an expanded problem focused examination; medical decision making of low complexity, furnished in real time using interactive audio and video technology. Counseling and coordination of care with other physicians, other qualified health care professionals or agencies are provided consistent with the nature of the problem(s) and the needs of the patient or the family or both. Usually, the presenting problem(s) are of low to moderate severity. Typically, 15 minutes are spent with the patient or family or both via real time, audio and video intercommunications technology　B

BETOS: Z2　Undefined codes
Service not separately priced by Part B
Coding Clinic: 2016, Q1

C **G9488** Remote in-home visit for the evaluation and management of an established patient for use only in a Medicare-approved CMS innovation center demonstration project, which requires at least 2 of the following 3 key components: a detailed history; a detailed examination; medical decision making of moderate complexity, furnished in

real time using interactive audio and video technology. Counseling and coordination of care with other physicians, other qualified health care professionals or agencies are provided consistent with the nature of the problem(s) and the needs of the patient or the family or both. Usually, the presenting problem(s) are of moderate to high severity. Typically, 25 minutes are spent with the patient or family or both via real time, audio and video intercommunications technology　B

BETOS: Z2　Undefined codes
Service not separately priced by Part B
Coding Clinic: 2016, Q1

C **G9489** Remote in-home visit for the evaluation and management of an established patient for use only in a Medicare-approved CMS innovation center demonstration project, which requires at least 2 of the following 3 key components: a comprehensive history; a comprehensive examination; medical decision making of high complexity, furnished in real time using interactive audio and video technology. Counseling and coordination of care with other physicians, other qualified health care professionals or agencies are provided consistent with the nature of the problem(s) and the needs of the patient or the family or both. Usually, the presenting problem(s) are of moderate to high severity. Typically, 40 minutes are spent with the patient or family or both via real time, audio and video intercommunications technology　B

BETOS: Z2　Undefined codes
Service not separately priced by Part B
Coding Clinic: 2016, Q1

C **G9490** CMS innovation center models, home visit for patient assessment performed by clinical staff for an individual not considered homebound, including, but not necessarily limited to patient assessment of clinical status, safety/fall prevention, functional status/ambulation, medication reconciliation/management, compliance with orders/plan of care, performance of activities of daily living, and ensuring beneficiary connections to community and other services. (for use only in Medicare-approved CMS innovation center models); may not be billed for a 30 day period covered by a transitional care management code　　　　　　　　　　　　　B

BETOS: Z2　Undefined codes
Service not separately priced by Part B
Coding Clinic: 2016, Q1

C **G9497** Received instruction from the anesthesiologist or proxy prior to the day of surgery to abstain from smoking on the day of surgery　　　　　　　　　　　M **MIPS**

BETOS: Z2　Undefined codes
Service not separately priced by Part B

♂ Male only　♀ Female only　**A** Age　A2 - Z3 = ASC Payment indicator　A - Y = APC Status indicator
ASC = ASC Approved Procedure　**DME** Paid under the DME fee schedule　**MIPS** MIPS code

CPT® is a registered trademark of the American Medical Association. All rights reserved.　　　　　　　**247**

C **G9498** Antibiotic regimen prescribed   M MIPS
BETOS: Z2   Undefined codes
Service not separately priced by Part B

C **G9500** Radiation exposure indices, or exposure time and number of fluorographic images in final report for procedures using fluoroscopy, documented   M MIPS
BETOS: Z2   Undefined codes
Service not separately priced by Part B

C **G9501** Radiation exposure indices, or exposure time and number of fluorographic images not documented in final report for procedure using fluoroscopy, reason not given   M MIPS
BETOS: Z2   Undefined codes
Service not separately priced by Part B

C **G9502** Documentation of medical reason for not performing foot exam (i.e., patients who have had either a bilateral amputation above or below the knee, or both a left and right amputation above or below the knee before or during the measurement period)   M
BETOS: Z2   Undefined codes
Service not separately priced by Part B

C **G9504** Documented reason for not assessing Hepatitis B virus (HBV) status (e.g., patient not initiating anti-TNF therapy, patient declined) prior to initiating anti-TNF therapy   M MIPS
BETOS: Z2   Undefined codes
Service not separately priced by Part B

C **G9505** Antibiotic regimen prescribed within 10 days after onset of symptoms for documented medical reason   M MIPS
BETOS: Z2   Undefined codes
Service not separately priced by Part B

C **G9506** Biologic immune response modifier prescribed   M MIPS
BETOS: Z2   Undefined codes
Service not separately priced by Part B

C **G9507** Documentation that the patient is on a statin medication or has documentation of a valid contraindication or exception to statin medications; contraindications/exceptions that can be defined by diagnosis codes include pregnancy during the measurement period, active liver disease, rhabdomyolysis, end stage renal disease on dialysis and heart failure; provider documented contraindications/exceptions include breastfeeding during the measurement period, woman of child-bearing age not actively taking birth control, allergy to statin, drug interaction (HIV protease inhibitors, nefazodone, cyclosporine, gemfibrozil, and danazol) and intolerance (with supporting documentation of trying a statin at least once within the last 5 years or diagnosis codes for myositis or toxic myopathy related to drugs)   M

BETOS: Z2   Undefined codes
Service not separately priced by Part B

C **G9508** Documentation that the patient is not on a statin medication   M
BETOS: Z2   Undefined codes
Service not separately priced by Part B

C **G9509** Adult patients 18 years of age or older with major depression or dysthymia who reached remission at twelve months as demonstrated by a twelve month (+/-60 days) PHQ-9 or PHQ-9M score of less than 5   M MIPS
BETOS: Z2   Undefined codes
Service not separately priced by Part B

C **G9510** Adult patients 18 years of age or older with major depression or dysthymia who did not reach remission at twelve months as demonstrated by a twelve month (+/-60 days) PHQ-9 or PHQ-9M score of less than 5. Either PHQ-9 or PHQ-9M score was not assessed or is greater than or equal to 5   M MIPS
BETOS: Z2   Undefined codes
Service not separately priced by Part B

C **G9511** Index event date PHQ-9 or PHQ-9M score greater than 9 documented during the twelve month denominator identification period   M MIPS
BETOS: Z2   Undefined codes
Service not separately priced by Part B

C **G9512** Individual had a PDC of 0.8 or greater M MIPS
BETOS: Z2   Undefined codes
Service not separately priced by Part B

C **G9513** Individual did not have a PDC of 0.8 or greater   M MIPS
BETOS: Z2   Undefined codes
Service not separately priced by Part B

C **G9514** Patient required a return to the operating room within 90 days of surgery   M MIPS
BETOS: Z2   Undefined codes
Service not separately priced by Part B

C **G9515** Patient did not require a return to the operating room within 90 days of surgery   M MIPS
BETOS: Z2   Undefined codes
Service not separately priced by Part B

C **G9516** Patient achieved an improvement in visual acuity, from their preoperative level, within 90 days of surgery   M MIPS
BETOS: Z2   Undefined codes
Service not separately priced by Part B

C **G9517** Patient did not achieve an improvement in visual acuity, from their preoperative level, within 90 days of surgery, reason not given   M MIPS
BETOS: Z2   Undefined codes
Service not separately priced by Part B

● New code   ▲ Revised code   C Carrier judgment   D Special coverage instructions apply
I Not payable by Medicare   M Non-covered by Medicare   S Non-covered by Medicare statute   AHA Coding Clinic®

C **G9518** Documentation of active injection drug use M MIPS
BETOS: Z2 Undefined codes
Service not separately priced by Part B

C **G9519** Patient achieves final refraction (spherical equivalent) +/- 1.0 diopters of their planned refraction within 90 days of surgery M MIPS
BETOS: Z2 Undefined codes
Service not separately priced by Part B

C **G9520** Patient does not achieve final refraction (spherical equivalent) +/- 1.0 diopters of their planned refraction within 90 days of surgery M MIPS
BETOS: Z2 Undefined codes
Service not separately priced by Part B

C **G9521** Total number of emergency department visits and inpatient hospitalizations less than two in the past 12 months M MIPS
BETOS: Z2 Undefined codes
Service not separately priced by Part B

C **G9522** Total number of emergency department visits and inpatient hospitalizations equal to or greater than two in the past 12 months or patient not screened, reason not given M MIPS
BETOS: Z2 Undefined codes
Service not separately priced by Part B

C **G9529** Patient with minor blunt head trauma had an appropriate indication(s) for a head CT M MIPS
BETOS: Z2 Undefined codes
Service not separately priced by Part B

C **G9530** Patient presented with a minor blunt head trauma and had a head CT ordered for trauma by an emergency care provider M MIPS
BETOS: Z2 Undefined codes
Service not separately priced by Part B

C **G9531** Patient has documentation of ventricular shunt, brain tumor, multisystem trauma, or is currently taking an antiplatelet medication including: abciximab, anagrelide, cangrelor, cilostazol, clopidogrel, dipyridamole, eptifibatide, prasugrel, ticlopidine, ticagrelor, tirofiban, or vorapaxar M MIPS
BETOS: Z2 Undefined codes
Service not separately priced by Part B

C **G9533** Patient with minor blunt head trauma did not have an appropriate indication(s) for a head CT M MIPS
BETOS: Z2 Undefined codes
Service not separately priced by Part B

▲ C **G9537** Imaging needed as part of a clinical trial; or other clinician ordered the study M MIPS
BETOS: Z2 Undefined codes
Service not separately priced by Part B

C **G9539** Intent for potential removal at time of placement M MIPS
BETOS: Z2 Undefined codes
Service not separately priced by Part B

C **G9540** Patient alive 3 months post procedure M MIPS
BETOS: Z2 Undefined codes
Service not separately priced by Part B

C **G9541** Filter removed within 3 months of placement M MIPS
BETOS: Z2 Undefined codes
Service not separately priced by Part B

C **G9542** Documented re-assessment for the appropriateness of filter removal within 3 months of placement M MIPS
BETOS: Z2 Undefined codes
Service not separately priced by Part B

C **G9543** Documentation of at least two attempts to reach the patient to arrange a clinical re-assessment for the appropriateness of filter removal within 3 months of placement M MIPS
BETOS: Z2 Undefined codes
Service not separately priced by Part B

C **G9544** Patients that do not have the filter removed, documented re-assessment for the appropriateness of filter removal, or documentation of at least two attempts to reach the patient to arrange a clinical re-assessment for the appropriateness of filter removal within 3 months of placement M MIPS
BETOS: Z2 Undefined codes
Service not separately priced by Part B

C **G9547** Cystic renal lesion that is simple appearing (Bosniak I or II), or adrenal lesion less than or equal to 1.0 cm or adrenal lesion greater than 1.0 cm but less than or equal to 4.0 cm classified as likely benign by unenhanced CT or washout protocol CT, or MRI with in- and opposed-phase sequences or other equivalent institutional imaging protocols M MIPS
BETOS: Z2 Undefined codes
Service not separately priced by Part B

C **G9548** Final reports for imaging studies stating no follow-up imaging is recommended M MIPS
BETOS: Z2 Undefined codes
Service not separately priced by Part B

C **G9549** Documentation of medical reason(s) that follow-up imaging is indicated (e.g., patient has lymphadenopathy, signs of metastasis or an active diagnosis or history of cancer, and other medical reason(s)) M MIPS
BETOS: Z2 Undefined codes
Service not separately priced by Part B

▲ C **G9550** Final reports for imaging studies with follow-up imaging recommended, or final reports that do not include a specific recommendation of no follow-up M MIPS
BETOS: Z2 Undefined codes
Service not separately priced by Part B

♂ Male only ♀ Female only Ⓐ Age A2 - Z3 = ASC Payment indicator A - Y = APC Status indicator
ASC = ASC Approved Procedure DME Paid under the DME fee schedule MIPS MIPS code

C **G9551** Final reports for imaging studies without an incidentally found lesion noted   M
BETOS: Z2   Undefined codes
Service not separately priced by Part B

C **G9552** Incidental thyroid nodule < 1.0 cm noted in report   M MIPS
BETOS: Z2   Undefined codes
Service not separately priced by Part B

C **G9553** Prior thyroid disease diagnosis   M
BETOS: Z2   Undefined codes
Service not separately priced by Part B

C **G9554** Final reports for CT, CTA, MRI or MRA of the chest or neck or ultrasound of the neck with follow-up imaging recommended   M MIPS
BETOS: Z2   Undefined codes
Service not separately priced by Part B

C **G9555** Documentation of medical reason(s) for recommending follow-up imaging (e.g., patient has multiple endocrine neoplasia, patient has cervical lymphadenopathy, other medical reason(s))   M MIPS
BETOS: Z2   Undefined codes
Service not separately priced by Part B

C **G9556** Final reports for CT, CTA, MRI or MRA of the chest or neck or ultrasound of the neck with follow-up imaging not recommended   M MIPS
BETOS: Z2   Undefined codes
Service not separately priced by Part B

C **G9557** Final reports for CT, CTA, MRI or MRA studies of the chest or neck or ultrasound of the neck without an incidentally found thyroid nodule < 1.0 cm noted or no nodule found   M
BETOS: Z2   Undefined codes
Service not separately priced by Part B

C **G9561** Patients prescribed opiates for longer than six weeks   M MIPS
BETOS: Z2   Undefined codes
Service not separately priced by Part B

C **G9562** Patients who had a follow-up evaluation conducted at least every three months during opioid therapy   M MIPS
BETOS: Z2   Undefined codes
Service not separately priced by Part B

C **G9563** Patients who did not have a follow-up evaluation conducted at least every three months during opioid therapy   M MIPS
BETOS: Z2   Undefined codes
Service not separately priced by Part B

C **G9577** Patients prescribed opiates for longer than six weeks   M MIPS
BETOS: Z2   Undefined codes
Service not separately priced by Part B

C **G9578** Documentation of signed opioid treatment agreement at least once during opioid therapy   M MIPS
BETOS: Z2   Undefined codes
Service not separately priced by Part B

C **G9579** No documentation of signed an opioid treatment agreement at least once during opioid therapy   M MIPS
BETOS: Z2   Undefined codes
Service not separately priced by Part B

C **G9580** Door to puncture time of less than 2 hours   M MIPS
BETOS: Z2   Undefined codes
Service not separately priced by Part B

C **G9582** Door to puncture time of greater than 2 hours, no reason given   M MIPS
BETOS: Z2   Undefined codes
Service not separately priced by Part B

C **G9583** Patients prescribed opiates for longer than six weeks   M MIPS
BETOS: Z2   Undefined codes
Service not separately priced by Part B

C **G9584** Patient evaluated for risk of misuse of opiates by using a brief validated instrument (e.g., opioid risk tool, SOAPP-R) or patient interviewed at least once during opioid therapy   M MIPS
BETOS: Z2   Undefined codes
Service not separately priced by Part B

C **G9585** Patient not evaluated for risk of misuse of opiates by using a brief validated instrument (e.g., opioid risk tool, SOAPP-R) or patient not interviewed at least once during opioid therapy   M MIPS
BETOS: Z2   Undefined codes
Service not separately priced by Part B

C **G9593** Pediatric patient with minor blunt head trauma classified as low risk according to the PECARN prediction rules   Ⓐ M MIPS
BETOS: Z2   Undefined codes
Service not separately priced by Part B

C **G9594** Patient presented with a minor blunt head trauma and had a head CT ordered for trauma by an emergency care provider   M MIPS
BETOS: Z2   Undefined codes
Service not separately priced by Part B

C **G9595** Patient has documentation of ventricular shunt, brain tumor, or coagulopathy   M MIPS
BETOS: Z2   Undefined codes
Service not separately priced by Part B

C **G9596** Pediatric patient had a head CT for trauma ordered by someone other than an emergency care provider or was ordered for a reason other than trauma   Ⓐ M
BETOS: Z2   Undefined codes
Service not separately priced by Part B

C **G9597** Pediatric patient with minor blunt head trauma not classified as low risk according to the PECARN prediction rules   Ⓐ M MIPS
BETOS: Z2   Undefined codes
Service not separately priced by Part B

● New code   ▲ Revised code   **C** Carrier judgment   **D** Special coverage instructions apply
I Not payable by Medicare   **M** Non-covered by Medicare   **S** Non-covered by Medicare statute   AHA Coding Clinic®

C **G9598** Aortic aneurysm 5.5 - 5.9 cm maximum diameter on centerline formatted CT or minor diameter on axial formatted CT M
BETOS: Z2 Undefined codes
Service not separately priced by Part B

C **G9599** Aortic aneurysm 6.0 cm or greater maximum diameter on centerline formatted CT or minor diameter on axial formatted CT M
BETOS: Z2 Undefined codes
Service not separately priced by Part B

C **G9603** Patient survey score improved from baseline following treatment M [MIPS]
BETOS: Z2 Undefined codes
Service not separately priced by Part B

C **G9604** Patient survey results not available M [MIPS]
BETOS: Z2 Undefined codes
Service not separately priced by Part B

C **G9605** Patient survey score did not improve from baseline following treatment M [MIPS]
BETOS: Z2 Undefined codes
Service not separately priced by Part B

C **G9606** Intraoperative cystoscopy performed to evaluate for lower tract injury M [MIPS]
BETOS: Z2 Undefined codes
Service not separately priced by Part B

C **G9607** Documented medical reasons for not performing intraoperative cystoscopy (e.g., urethral pathology precluding cystoscopy, any patient who has a congenital or acquired absence of the urethra) or in the case of patient death M [MIPS]
BETOS: Z2 Undefined codes
Service not separately priced by Part B

C **G9608** Intraoperative cystoscopy not performed to evaluate for lower tract injury M [MIPS]
BETOS: Z2 Undefined codes
Service not separately priced by Part B

C **G9609** Documentation of an order for anti-platelet agents M
BETOS: Z2 Undefined codes
Service not separately priced by Part B

C **G9610** Documentation of medical reason(s) in the patient's record for not ordering anti-platelet agents M
BETOS: Z2 Undefined codes
Service not separately priced by Part B

C **G9611** Order for anti-platelet agents was not documented in the patient's record, reason not given M
BETOS: Z2 Undefined codes
Service not separately priced by Part B

C **G9612** Photodocumentation of two or more cecal landmarks to establish a complete examination M [MIPS]
BETOS: Z2 Undefined codes
Service not separately priced by Part B

C **G9613** Documentation of post-surgical anatomy (e.g., right hemicolectomy, ileocecal resection, etc.) M [MIPS]
BETOS: Z2 Undefined codes
Service not separately priced by Part B

C **G9614** Photodocumentation of less than two cecal landmarks (i.e., no cecal landmarks or only one cecal landmark) to establish a complete examination M [MIPS]
BETOS: Z2 Undefined codes
Service not separately priced by Part B

C **G9618** Documentation of screening for uterine malignancy or those that had an ultrasound and/or endometrial sampling of any kind ♀ M [MIPS]
BETOS: Z2 Undefined codes
Service not separately priced by Part B

C **G9620** Patient not screened for uterine malignancy, or those that have not had an ultrasound and/or endometrial sampling of any kind, reason not given ♀ M [MIPS]
BETOS: Z2 Undefined codes
Service not separately priced by Part B

C **G9621** Patient identified as an unhealthy alcohol user when screened for unhealthy alcohol use using a systematic screening method and received brief counseling M [MIPS]
BETOS: Z2 Undefined codes
Service not separately priced by Part B

C **G9622** Patient not identified as an unhealthy alcohol user when screened for unhealthy alcohol use using a systematic screening method M [MIPS]
BETOS: Z2 Undefined codes
Service not separately priced by Part B

C **G9623** Documentation of medical reason(s) for not screening for unhealthy alcohol use (e.g., limited life expectancy, other medical reasons) M [MIPS]
BETOS: Z2 Undefined codes
Service not separately priced by Part B

C **G9624** Patient not screened for unhealthy alcohol use using a systematic screening method or patient did not receive brief counseling if identified as an unhealthy alcohol user, reason not given M [MIPS]
BETOS: Z2 Undefined codes
Service not separately priced by Part B

C **G9625** Patient sustained bladder injury at the time of surgery or discovered subsequently up to 30 days post-surgery M [MIPS]
BETOS: Z2 Undefined codes
Service not separately priced by Part B

C **G9626** Documented medical reason for not reporting bladder injury (e.g., gynecologic or other pelvic malignancy documented, concurrent surgery involving bladder

---

♂ Male only ♀ Female only **A** Age A2 - Z3 = ASC Payment indicator A - Y = APC Status indicator
ASC = ASC Approved Procedure **DME** Paid under the DME fee schedule [MIPS] MIPS code

pathology, injury that occurs during urinary incontinence procedure, patient death from non-medical causes not related to surgery, patient died during procedure without evidence of bladder injury) M MIPS

    BETOS: Z2 Undefined codes
    Service not separately priced by Part B

C G9627 Patient did not sustain bladder injury at the time of surgery nor discovered subsequently up to 30n days post-surgery M MIPS

    BETOS: Z2 Undefined codes
    Service not separately priced by Part B

C G9628 Patient sustained bowel injury at the time of surgery or discovered subsequently up to 30 days post-surgery M MIPS

    BETOS: Z2 Undefined codes
    Service not separately priced by Part B

C G9629 Documented medical reasons for not reporting bowel injury (e.g., gynecologic or other pelvic malignancy documented, planned (e.g., not due to an unexpected bowel injury) resection and/or re-anastomosis of bowel, or patient death from non-medical causes not related to surgery, patient died during procedure without evidence of bowel injury) M MIPS

    BETOS: Z2 Undefined codes
    Service not separately priced by Part B

C G9630 Patient did not sustain a bowel injury at the time of surgery nor discovered subsequently up to 30 days post-surgery M MIPS

    BETOS: Z2 Undefined codes
    Service not separately priced by Part B

C G9631 Patient sustained ureter injury at the time of surgery or discovered subsequently up to 30 days post-surgery M MIPS

    BETOS: Z2 Undefined codes
    Service not separately priced by Part B

C G9632 Documented medical reasons for not reporting ureter injury (e.g., gynecologic or other pelvic malignancy documented, concurrent surgery involving bladder pathology, injury that occurs during a urinary incontinence procedure, patient death from non-medical causes not related to surgery, patient died during procedure without evidence of ureter injury) M MIPS

    BETOS: Z2 Undefined codes
    Service not separately priced by Part B

C G9633 Patient did not sustain ureter injury at the time of surgery nor discovered subsequently up to 30 days post-surgery M MIPS

    BETOS: Z2 Undefined codes
    Service not separately priced by Part B

C G9634 Health-related quality of life assessed with tool during at least two visits and quality of life score remained the same or improved M MIPS

    BETOS: Z2 Undefined codes
    Service not separately priced by Part B

C G9635 Health-related quality of life not assessed with tool for documented reason(s) (e.g., patient has a cognitive or neuropsychiatric impairment that impairs his/her ability to complete the HRQOL survey, patient has the inability to read and/or write in order to complete the hrqol questionnaire) M MIPS

    BETOS: Z2 Undefined codes
    Service not separately priced by Part B

C G9636 Health-related quality of life not assessed with tool during at least two visits or quality of life score declined M MIPS

    BETOS: Z2 Undefined codes
    Service not separately priced by Part B

C G9637 Final reports with documentation of one or more dose reduction techniques (e.g., automated exposure control, adjustment of the ma and/or kv according to patient size, use of iterative reconstruction technique) Ⓐ M MIPS

    BETOS: Z2 Undefined codes
    Service not separately priced by Part B

C G9638 Final reports without documentation of one or more dose reduction techniques (e.g., automated exposure control, adjustment of the ma and/or kv according to patient size, use of iterative reconstruction technique) Ⓐ M MIPS

    BETOS: Z2 Undefined codes
    Service not separately priced by Part B

C G9639 Major amputation or open surgical bypass not required within 48 hours of the index endovascular lower extremity revascularization procedure M MIPS

    BETOS: Z2 Undefined codes
    Service not separately priced by Part B

C G9640 Documentation of planned hybrid or staged procedure M MIPS

    BETOS: Z2 Undefined codes
    Service not separately priced by Part B

C G9641 Major amputation or open surgical bypass required within 48 hours of the index endovascular lower extremity revascularization procedure M MIPS

    BETOS: Z2 Undefined codes
    Service not separately priced by Part B

▲ **C G9642** Current smoker (e.g., cigarette, cigar, pipe, e-cigarette or marijuana) Ⓐ M MIPS

    BETOS: Z2 Undefined codes
    Service not separately priced by Part B

C G9643 Elective surgery Ⓐ M MIPS

    BETOS: Z2 Undefined codes
    Service not separately priced by Part B

● New code   ▲ Revised code   **C** Carrier judgment   **D** Special coverage instructions apply
I Not payable by Medicare   **M** Non-covered by Medicare   **S** Non-covered by Medicare statute   AHA Coding Clinic®

C **G9644** Patients who abstained from smoking prior to anesthesia on the day of surgery or procedure M MIPS

BETOS: Z2 Undefined codes
Service not separately priced by Part B

C **G9645** Patients who did not abstain from smoking prior to anesthesia on the day of surgery or procedure M MIPS

BETOS: Z2 Undefined codes
Service not separately priced by Part B

C **G9646** Patients with 90 day MRS score of 0 to 2 M MIPS

BETOS: Z2 Undefined codes
Service not separately priced by Part B

C **G9647** Patients in whom MRS score could not be obtained at 90 day follow-up M MIPS

BETOS: Z2 Undefined codes
Service not separately priced by Part B

C **G9648** Patients with 90 day MRS score greater than 2 M MIPS

BETOS: Z2 Undefined codes
Service not separately priced by Part B

C **G9649** Psoriasis assessment tool documented meeting any one of the specified benchmarks (e.g., (PGA; 5-point or 6-point scale), body surface area (BSA), psoriasis area and severity index (PASI) and/or dermatology life quality index) (DLQI)) M MIPS

BETOS: Z2 Undefined codes
Service not separately priced by Part B

C **G9651** Psoriasis assessment tool documented not meeting any one of the specified benchmarks (e.g., (PGA; 5-point or 6-point scale), body surface area (BSA), psoriasis area and severity index (PASI) and/or dermatology life quality index) (DLQI)) or psoriasis assessment tool not documented M MIPS

BETOS: Z2 Undefined codes
Service not separately priced by Part B

C **G9654** Monitored anesthesia care (MAC) M MIPS

BETOS: Z2 Undefined codes
Service not separately priced by Part B

C **G9655** A transfer of care protocol or handoff tool/checklist that includes the required key handoff elements is used M

BETOS: Z2 Undefined codes
Service not separately priced by Part B

C **G9656** Patient transferred directly from anesthetizing location to PACU or other non-ICU location M

BETOS: Z2 Undefined codes
Service not separately priced by Part B

C **G9658** A transfer of care protocol or handoff tool/checklist that includes the required key handoff elements is not used M

BETOS: Z2 Undefined codes
Service not separately priced by Part B

▲ **C** **G9659** Patients greater than or equal to 86 years of age who underwent a screening colonoscopy and did not have a history of colorectal cancer or other valid medical reason for the colonoscopy, including: iron deficiency anemia, lower gastrointestinal bleeding, crohn's disease (i.e., regional enteritis), familial adenomatous polyposis, lynch syndrome (i.e., hereditary non-polyposis colorectal cancer), inflammatory bowel disease, ulcerative colitis, abnormal finding of gastrointestinal tract, or changes in bowel habits Ⓐ M MIPS

BETOS: Z2 Undefined codes
Service not separately priced by Part B

▲ **C** **G9660** Documentation of medical reason(s) for a colonoscopy performed on a patient greater than or equal to 86 years of age (e.g., iron deficiency anemia, lower gastrointestinal bleeding, crohn's disease (i.e., regional enteritis), familial history of adenomatous polyposis, lynch syndrome (i.e., hereditary non-polyposis colorectal cancer), inflammatory bowel disease, ulcerative colitis, abnormal finding of gastrointestinal tract, or changes in bowel habits) Ⓐ M MIPS

BETOS: Z2 Undefined codes
Service not separately priced by Part B

▲ **C** **G9661** Patients greater than or equal to 86 years of age who received a colonoscopy for an assessment of signs/symptoms of GI tract illness, and/or because the patient meets high risk criteria, and/or to follow-up on previously diagnosed advanced lesions Ⓐ M MIPS

BETOS: Z2 Undefined codes
Service not separately priced by Part B

C **G9662** Previously diagnosed or have an active diagnosis of clinical ASCVD Ⓐ M MIPS

BETOS: Z2 Undefined codes
Service not separately priced by Part B

▲ **C** **G9663** Any fasting or direct LDL-C laboratory test result >= 190 mg/dl Ⓐ M MIPS

BETOS: Z2 Undefined codes
Service not separately priced by Part B

C **G9664** Patients who are currently statin therapy users or received an order (prescription) for statin therapy M MIPS

BETOS: Z2 Undefined codes
Service not separately priced by Part B

C **G9665** Patients who are not currently statin therapy users or did not receive an order (prescription) for statin therapy M MIPS

BETOS: Z2 Undefined codes
Service not separately priced by Part B

▲ C **G9666** Patient's highest fasting or direct LDL-C laboratory test result in the measurement period or two years prior to the beginning of the measurement period is 70-189 mg/dl   Ⓐ M MIPS
BETOS: Z2 Undefined codes
Service not separately priced by Part B

C **G9674** Patients with clinical ASCVD diagnosis   M
BETOS: Z2 Undefined codes
Service not separately priced by Part B

C **G9675** Patients who have ever had a fasting or direct laboratory result of LDL-C = 190 mg/dl   M
BETOS: Z2 Undefined codes
Service not separately priced by Part B

C **G9676** Patients aged 40 to 75 years at the beginning of the measurement period with type 1 or type 2 diabetes and with an LDL-C result of 70-189 mg/dl recorded as the highest fasting or direct laboratory test result in the measurement year or during the two years prior to the beginning of the measurement period   Ⓐ M
BETOS: Z2 Undefined codes
Service not separately priced by Part B

C **G9678** Oncology care model (OCM) monthly enhanced oncology services (MEOS) payment for OCM enhanced services. G9678 payments may only be made to OCM practitioners for OCM beneficiaries for the furnishment of enhanced services as defined in the OCM participation agreement   B
BETOS: Z2 Undefined codes
Service not separately priced by Part B

C **G9679** This code is for onsite acute care treatment of a nursing facility resident with pneumonia; may only be billed once per day per beneficiary   B
BETOS: Z2 Undefined codes
Service not separately priced by Part B

C **G9680** This code is for onsite acute care treatment of a nursing facility resident with CHF; may only be billed once per day per beneficiary   B
BETOS: Z2 Undefined codes
Service not separately priced by Part B

C **G9681** This code is for onsite acute care treatment of a resident with COPD or asthma; may only be billed once per day per beneficiary   B
BETOS: Z2 Undefined codes
Service not separately priced by Part B

C **G9682** This code is for the onsite acute care treatment a nursing facility resident with a skin infection; may only be billed once per day per beneficiary   B
BETOS: Z2 Undefined codes
Service not separately priced by Part B

C **G9683** Facility service(s) for the onsite acute care treatment of a nursing facility resident with fluid or electrolyte disorder. (may only be billed once per day per beneficiary). This service is for a demonstration project   B
BETOS: Z2 Undefined codes
Service not separately priced by Part B

C **G9684** This code is for the onsite acute care treatment of a nursing facility resident for a UTI; may only be billed once per day per beneficiary   B
BETOS: Z2 Undefined codes
Service not separately priced by Part B

C **G9685** Physician service or other qualified health care professional for the evaluation and management of a beneficiary's acute change in condition in a nursing facility. This service is for a demonstration project   M
BETOS: Z2 Undefined codes
Service not separately priced by Part B

C **G9687** Hospice services provided to patient any time during the measurement period   M MIPS
BETOS: Z2 Undefined codes
Service not separately priced by Part B

C **G9688** Patients using hospice services any time during the measurement period   M MIPS
BETOS: Z2 Undefined codes
Service not separately priced by Part B

C **G9689** Patient admitted for performance of elective carotid intervention   M
BETOS: Z2 Undefined codes
Service not separately priced by Part B

C **G9690** Patient receiving hospice services any time during the measurement period   M MIPS
BETOS: Z2 Undefined codes
Service not separately priced by Part B

C **G9691** Patient had hospice services any time during the measurement period   M
BETOS: Z2 Undefined codes
Service not separately priced by Part B

C **G9692** Hospice services received by patient any time during the measurement period   M MIPS
BETOS: Z2 Undefined codes
Service not separately priced by Part B

C **G9693** Patient use of hospice services any time during the measurement period   M MIPS
BETOS: Z2 Undefined codes
Service not separately priced by Part B

C **G9694** Hospice services utilized by patient any time during the measurement period   M MIPS
BETOS: Z2 Undefined codes
Service not separately priced by Part B

C **G9695** Long-acting inhaled bronchodilator prescribed   M MIPS
BETOS: Z2 Undefined codes
Service not separately priced by Part B

● New code   ▲ Revised code   C Carrier judgment   D Special coverage instructions apply
I Not payable by Medicare   M Non-covered by Medicare   S Non-covered by Medicare statute   AHA Coding Clinic®

C **G9696** Documentation of medical reason(s) for not prescribing a long-acting inhaled bronchodilator M MIPS

BETOS: Z2   Undefined codes
Service not separately priced by Part B

C **G9697** Documentation of patient reason(s) for not prescribing a long-acting inhaled bronchodilator M MIPS

BETOS: Z2   Undefined codes
Service not separately priced by Part B

C **G9698** Documentation of system reason(s) for not prescribing a long-acting inhaled bronchodilator M MIPS

BETOS: Z2   Undefined codes
Service not separately priced by Part B

C **G9699** Long-acting inhaled bronchodilator not prescribed, reason not otherwise specified M MIPS

BETOS: Z2   Undefined codes
Service not separately priced by Part B

C **G9700** Patients who use hospice services any time during the measurement period M MIPS

BETOS: Z2   Undefined codes
Service not separately priced by Part B

C **G9702** Patients who use hospice services any time during the measurement period M MIPS

BETOS: Z2   Undefined codes
Service not separately priced by Part B

▲ **C** **G9703** Episodes where the patient is taking antibiotics (table 1) in the 30 days prior to the episode date Ⓐ M MIPS

BETOS: Z2   Undefined codes
Service not separately priced by Part B

C **G9704** AJCC breast cancer stage I: T1 mic or T1a documented M

BETOS: Z2   Undefined codes
Service not separately priced by Part B

C **G9705** AJCC breast cancer stage I: T1b (tumor > 0.5 cm but <= 1 cm in greatest dimension) documented M

BETOS: Z2   Undefined codes
Service not separately priced by Part B

C **G9706** Low (or very low) risk of recurrence, prostate cancer ♂ M MIPS

BETOS: Z2   Undefined codes
Service not separately priced by Part B

C **G9707** Patient received hospice services any time during the measurement period M MIPS

BETOS: Z2   Undefined codes
Service not separately priced by Part B

C **G9708** Women who had a bilateral mastectomy or who have a history of a bilateral mastectomy or for whom there is evidence of a right and a left unilateral mastectomy ♀ M MIPS

BETOS: Z2   Undefined codes
Service not separately priced by Part B

C **G9709** Hospice services used by patient any time during the measurement period M MIPS

BETOS: Z2   Undefined codes
Service not separately priced by Part B

C **G9710** Patient was provided hospice services any time during the measurement period M MIPS

BETOS: Z2   Undefined codes
Service not separately priced by Part B

C **G9711** Patients with a diagnosis or past history of total colectomy or colorectal cancer M MIPS

BETOS: Z2   Undefined codes
Service not separately priced by Part B

C **G9712** Documentation of medical reason(s) for prescribing or dispensing antibiotic (e.g., intestinal infection, pertussis, bacterial infection, lyme disease, otitis media, acute sinusitis, acute pharyngitis, acute tonsillitis, chronic sinusitis, infection of the pharynx/larynx/tonsils/adenoids, prostatitis, cellulitis/ mastoiditis/bone infections, acute lymphadenitis, impetigo, skin staph infections, pneumonia, gonococcal infections/ venereal disease (syphilis, chlamydia, inflammatory diseases [female reproductive organs]), infections of the kidney, cystitis/UTI, acne, HIV disease/asymptomatic HIV, cystic fibrosis, disorders of the immune system, malignancy neoplasms, chronic bronchitis, emphysema, bronchiectasis, extrinsic allergic alveolitis, chronic airway obstruction, chronic obstructive asthma, pneumoconiosis and other lung disease due to external agents, other diseases of the respiratory system, and tuberculosis M MIPS

BETOS: Z2   Undefined codes
Service not separately priced by Part B

C **G9713** Patients who use hospice services any time during the measurement period M MIPS

BETOS: Z2   Undefined codes
Service not separately priced by Part B

C **G9714** Patient is using hospice services any time during the measurement period M MIPS

BETOS: Z2   Undefined codes
Service not separately priced by Part B

C **G9715** Patients who use hospice services any time during the measurement period M MIPS

BETOS: Z2   Undefined codes
Service not separately priced by Part B

▲ **C** **G9716** BMI is documented as being outside of normal parameters, follow-up plan is not completed for documented reason M MIPS

BETOS: Z2   Undefined codes
Service not separately priced by Part B

▲ **C** **G9717** Documentation stating the patient has had a diagnosis of depression or has had a diagnosis of bipolar disorder M MIPS

BETOS: Z2   Undefined codes
Service not separately priced by Part B

♂ Male only   ♀ Female only   Ⓐ Age   A2 - Z3 = ASC Payment indicator   A - Y = APC Status indicator
ASC = ASC Approved Procedure   **DME** Paid under the DME fee schedule   **MIPS** MIPS code

C **G9718** Hospice services for patient provided any time during the measurement period M MIPS
  BETOS: Z2 Undefined codes
  Service not separately priced by Part B

C **G9719** Patient is not ambulatory, bed ridden, immobile, confined to chair, wheelchair bound, dependent on helper pushing wheelchair, independent in wheelchair or minimal help in wheelchair M
  BETOS: Z2 Undefined codes
  Service not separately priced by Part B

C **G9720** Hospice services for patient occurred any time during the measurement period M MIPS
  BETOS: Z2 Undefined codes
  Service not separately priced by Part B

C **G9721** Patient not ambulatory, bed ridden, immobile, confined to chair, wheelchair bound, dependent on helper pushing wheelchair, independent in wheelchair or minimal help in wheelchair M
  BETOS: Z2 Undefined codes
  Service not separately priced by Part B

▲ C **G9722** Documented history of renal failure or baseline serum creatinine >= 4.0 mg/dl; renal transplant recipients are not considered to have preoperative renal failure, unless, since transplantation the CR has been or is 4.0 or higher M MIPS
  BETOS: Z2 Undefined codes
  Service not separately priced by Part B

C **G9723** Hospice services for patient received any time during the measurement period M
  BETOS: Z2 Undefined codes
  Service not separately priced by Part B

C **G9724** Patients who had documentation of use of anticoagulant medications overlapping the measurement year M
  BETOS: Z2 Undefined codes
  Service not separately priced by Part B

C **G9725** Patients who use hospice services any time during the measurement period M MIPS
  BETOS: Z2 Undefined codes
  Service not separately priced by Part B

C **G9726** Patient refused to participate M MIPS
  BETOS: Z2 Undefined codes
  Service not separately priced by Part B

▲ C **G9727** Patient unable to complete the LEPF PROM at initial evaluation and/or discharge due to blindness, illiteracy, severe mental incapacity or language incompatibility and an adequate proxy is not available M MIPS
  BETOS: Z2 Undefined codes
  Service not separately priced by Part B

C **G9728** Patient refused to participate M MIPS
  BETOS: Z2 Undefined codes
  Service not separately priced by Part B

▲ C **G9729** Patient unable to complete the LEPF PROM at initial evaluation and/or discharge due to blindness, illiteracy, severe mental incapacity or language incompatibility and an adequate proxy is not available M MIPS
  BETOS: Z2 Undefined codes
  Service not separately priced by Part B

C **G9730** Patient refused to participate M MIPS
  BETOS: Z2 Undefined codes
  Service not separately priced by Part B

▲ C **G9731** Patient unable to complete the LEPF PROM at initial evaluation and/or discharge due to blindness, illiteracy, severe mental incapacity or language incompatibility and an adequate proxy is not available M MIPS
  BETOS: Z2 Undefined codes
  Service not separately priced by Part B

C **G9732** Patient refused to participate M MIPS
  BETOS: Z2 Undefined codes
  Service not separately priced by Part B

C **G9733** Patient unable to complete the low back FS PROM at initial evaluation and/or discharge due to blindness, illiteracy, severe mental incapacity or language incompatibility and an adequate proxy is not available M MIPS
  BETOS: Z2 Undefined codes
  Service not separately priced by Part B

C **G9734** Patient refused to participate M MIPS
  BETOS: Z2 Undefined codes
  Service not separately priced by Part B

C **G9735** Patient unable to complete the shoulder FS PROM at initial evaluation and/or discharge due to blindness, illiteracy, severe mental incapacity or language incompatibility and an adequate proxy is not available M MIPS
  BETOS: Z2 Undefined codes
  Service not separately priced by Part B

C **G9736** Patient refused to participate M MIPS
  BETOS: Z2 Undefined codes
  Service not separately priced by Part B

C **G9737** Patient unable to complete the elbow/wrist/hand FS PROM at initial evaluation and/or discharge due to blindness, illiteracy, severe mental incapacity or language incompatibility and an adequate proxy is not available M MIPS
  BETOS: Z2 Undefined codes
  Service not separately priced by Part B

C **G9740** Hospice services given to patient any time during the measurement period M MIPS
  BETOS: Z2 Undefined codes
  Service not separately priced by Part B

C **G9741** Patients who use hospice services any time during the measurement period M MIPS
  BETOS: Z2 Undefined codes
  Service not separately priced by Part B

● New code   ▲ Revised code   C Carrier judgment   D Special coverage instructions apply
I Not payable by Medicare   M Non-covered by Medicare   S Non-covered by Medicare statute   AHA Coding Clinic®

C **G9744** Patient not eligible due to active diagnosis of hypertension M MIPS
BETOS: Z2 Undefined codes
Service not separately priced by Part B

C **G9745** Documented reason for not screening or recommending a follow-up for high blood pressure M MIPS
BETOS: Z2 Undefined codes
Service not separately priced by Part B

C **G9746** Patient has mitral stenosis or prosthetic heart valves or patient has transient or reversible cause of AF (e.g., pneumonia, hyperthyroidism, pregnancy, cardiac surgery) M
BETOS: Z2 Undefined codes
Service not separately priced by Part B

C **G9751** Patient died at any time during the 24-month measurement period M MIPS
BETOS: Z2 Undefined codes
Service not separately priced by Part B

C **G9752** Emergency surgery M MIPS
BETOS: Z2 Undefined codes
Service not separately priced by Part B

C **G9753** Documentation of medical reason for not conducting a search for dicom format images for prior patient CT imaging studies completed at non-affiliated external healthcare facilities or entities within the past 12 months that are available through a secure, authorized, media-free, shared archive (e.g., trauma, acute myocardial infarction, stroke, aortic aneurysm where time is of the essence) M
BETOS: Z2 Undefined codes
Service not separately priced by Part B

C **G9754** A finding of an incidental pulmonary nodule M MIPS
BETOS: Z2 Undefined codes
Service not separately priced by Part B

C **G9755** Documentation of medical reason(s) for not including a recommended interval and modality for follow-up or for no follow-up, and source of recommendations (e.g., patients with unexplained fever, immunocompromised patients who are at risk for infection) M MIPS
BETOS: Z2 Undefined codes
Service not separately priced by Part B

C **G9756** Surgical procedures that included the use of silicone oil M MIPS
BETOS: Z2 Undefined codes
Service not separately priced by Part B

C **G9757** Surgical procedures that included the use of silicone oil M MIPS
BETOS: Z2 Undefined codes
Service not separately priced by Part B

C **G9758** Patient in hospice at any time during the measurement period M MIPS
BETOS: Z2 Undefined codes
Service not separately priced by Part B

C **G9760** Patients who use hospice services any time during the measurement period M MIPS
BETOS: Z2 Undefined codes
Service not separately priced by Part B

C **G9761** Patients who use hospice services any time during the measurement period M MIPS
BETOS: Z2 Undefined codes
Service not separately priced by Part B

C **G9762** Patient had at least two HPV vaccines (with at least 146 days between the two) or three HPV vaccines on or between the patient's 9th and 13th birthdays ♀ Ⓐ M MIPS
BETOS: Z2 Undefined codes
Service not separately priced by Part B

C **G9763** Patient did not have at least two HPV vaccines (with at least 146 days between the two) or three HPV vaccines on or between the patient's 9th and 13th birthdays ♀ Ⓐ M MIPS
BETOS: Z2 Undefined codes
Service not separately priced by Part B

C **G9764** Patient has been treated with a systemic medication for psoriasis vulgaris M MIPS
BETOS: Z2 Undefined codes
Service not separately priced by Part B

C **G9765** Documentation that the patient declined change in medication or alternative therapies were unavailable, has documented contraindications, or has not been treated with a systemic medication for at least six consecutive months (e.g., experienced adverse effects or lack of efficacy with all other therapy options) in order to achieve better disease control as measured by PGA, BSA, PASI, or DLQI M MIPS
BETOS: Z2 Undefined codes
Service not separately priced by Part B

C **G9766** Patients who are transferred from one institution to another with a known diagnosis of CVA for endovascular stroke treatment M MIPS
BETOS: Z2 Undefined codes
Service not separately priced by Part B

C **G9767** Hospitalized patients with newly diagnosed CVA considered for endovascular stroke treatment M MIPS
BETOS: Z2 Undefined codes
Service not separately priced by Part B

C **G9768** Patients who utilize hospice services any time during the measurement period M MIPS
BETOS: Z2 Undefined codes
Service not separately priced by Part B

♂ Male only   ♀ Female only   Ⓐ Age   A2 - Z3 = ASC Payment indicator   A - Y = APC Status indicator
ASC = ASC Approved Procedure   **DME** Paid under the DME fee schedule   MIPS MIPS code

C **G9769** Patient had a bone mineral density test in the past two years or received osteoporosis medication or therapy in the past 12 months   M MIPS
    BETOS: Z2   Undefined codes
    Service not separately priced by Part B

C **G9770** Peripheral nerve block (PNB)   M MIPS
    BETOS: Z2   Undefined codes
    Service not separately priced by Part B

C **G9771** At least 1 body temperature measurement equal to or greater than 35.5 degrees celsius (or 95.9 degrees fahrenheit) achieved within the 30 minutes immediately before or the 15 minutes immediately after anesthesia end time   M MIPS
    BETOS: Z2   Undefined codes
    Service not separately priced by Part B

C **G9772** Documentation of medical reason(s) for not achieving at least 1 body temperature measurement equal to or greater than 35.5 degrees celsius (or 95.9 degrees fahrenheit) within the 30 minutes immediately before or the 15 minutes immediately after anesthesia end time (e.g., emergency cases, intentional hypothermia, etc.)   M MIPS
    BETOS: Z2   Undefined codes
    Service not separately priced by Part B

C **G9773** At least 1 body temperature measurement equal to or greater than 35.5 degrees celsius (or 95.9 degrees Fahrenheit) not achieved within the 30 minutes immediately before or the 15 minutes immediately after anesthesia end time, reason not given   M MIPS
    BETOS: Z2   Undefined codes
    Service not separately priced by Part B

C **G9774** Patients who have had a hysterectomy   ♀ M MIPS
    BETOS: Z2   Undefined codes
    Service not separately priced by Part B

C **G9775** Patient received at least 2 prophylactic pharmacologic anti-emetic agents of different classes preoperatively and/or intraoperatively   M MIPS
    BETOS: Z2   Undefined codes
    Service not separately priced by Part B

C **G9776** Documentation of medical reason for not receiving at least 2 prophylactic pharmacologic anti-emetic agents of different classes preoperatively and/or intraoperatively (e.g., intolerance or other medical reason)   M MIPS
    BETOS: Z2   Undefined codes
    Service not separately priced by Part B

C **G9777** Patient did not receive at least 2 prophylactic pharmacologic anti-emetic agents of different classes preoperatively and/or intraoperatively   M MIPS
    BETOS: Z2   Undefined codes
    Service not separately priced by Part B

C **G9778** Patients who have a diagnosis of pregnancy   ♀ A M MIPS
    BETOS: Z2   Undefined codes
    Service not separately priced by Part B

C **G9779** Patients who are breastfeeding   ♀ A M MIPS
    BETOS: Z2   Undefined codes
    Service not separately priced by Part B

C **G9780** Patients who have a diagnosis of rhabdomyolysis   M MIPS
    BETOS: Z2   Undefined codes
    Service not separately priced by Part B

C **G9781** Documentation of medical reason(s) for not currently being a statin therapy user or receive an order (prescription) for statin therapy (e.g., patient with adverse effect, allergy or intolerance to statin medication therapy, patients who are receiving palliative or hospice care, patients with active liver disease or hepatic disease or insufficiency, and patients with end stage renal disease (ESRD))   M MIPS
    BETOS: Z2   Undefined codes
    Service not separately priced by Part B

C **G9782** History of or active diagnosis of familial or pure hypercholesterolemia   M MIPS
    BETOS: Z2   Undefined codes
    Service not separately priced by Part B

C **G9783** Documentation of patients with diabetes who have a most recent fasting or direct LDL-C laboratory test result < 70 mg/dl and are not taking statin therapy   M MIPS
    BETOS: Z2   Undefined codes
    Service not separately priced by Part B

C **G9784** Pathologists/dermatopathologists providing a second opinion on a biopsy   M MIPS
    BETOS: Z2   Undefined codes
    Service not separately priced by Part B

C **G9785** Pathology report diagnosing cutaneous basal cell carcinoma, squamous cell carcinoma, or melanoma (to include in situ disease) sent from the pathologist/ dermatopathologist to the biopsying clinician for review within 7 days from the time when the tissue specimen was received by the pathologist   M MIPS
    BETOS: Z2   Undefined codes
    Service not separately priced by Part B

C **G9786** Pathology report diagnosing cutaneous basal cell carcinoma, squamous cell carcinoma, or melanoma (to include in situ disease) was not sent from the pathologist/ dermatopathologist to the biopsying clinician for review within 7 days from the time when the tissue specimen was received by the pathologist   M MIPS
    BETOS: Z2   Undefined codes
    Service not separately priced by Part B

● New code   ▲ Revised code   **C** Carrier judgment   **D** Special coverage instructions apply
I Not payable by Medicare   **M** Non-covered by Medicare   **S** Non-covered by Medicare statute   AHA Coding Clinic®

C G9787 Patient alive as of the last day of the measurement year M MIPS
BETOS: Z2 Undefined codes
Service not separately priced by Part B

C G9788 Most recent BP is less than or equal to 140/90 mmHg M MIPS
BETOS: Z2 Undefined codes
Service not separately priced by Part B

C G9789 Blood pressure recorded during inpatient stays, emergency room visits, urgent care visits, and patient self-reported BP's (home and health fair BP results) M MIPS
BETOS: Z2 Undefined codes
Service not separately priced by Part B

C G9790 Most recent BP is greater than 140/90 mmHg, or blood pressure not documented M MIPS
BETOS: Z2 Undefined codes
Service not separately priced by Part B

C G9791 Most recent tobacco status is tobacco free M MIPS
BETOS: Z2 Undefined codes
Service not separately priced by Part B

C G9792 Most recent tobacco status is not tobacco free M MIPS
BETOS: Z2 Undefined codes
Service not separately priced by Part B

C G9793 Patient is currently on a daily aspirin or other antiplatelet M MIPS
BETOS: Z2 Undefined codes
Service not separately priced by Part B

C G9794 Documentation of medical reason(s) for not on a daily aspirin or other antiplatelet (e.g., history of gastrointestinal bleed, intra-cranial bleed, idiopathic thrombocytopenic purpura (ITP), gastric bypass or documentation of active anticoagulant use during the measurement period) M
BETOS: Z2 Undefined codes
Service not separately priced by Part B

C G9795 Patient is not currently on a daily aspirin or other antiplatelet M MIPS
BETOS: Z2 Undefined codes
Service not separately priced by Part B

C G9796 Patient is currently on a statin therapy M MIPS
BETOS: Z2 Undefined codes
Service not separately priced by Part B

C G9797 Patient is not on a statin therapy M MIPS
BETOS: Z2 Undefined codes
Service not separately priced by Part B

C G9805 Patients who use hospice services any time during the measurement period M MIPS
BETOS: Z2 Undefined codes
Service not separately priced by Part B

C G9806 Patients who received cervical cytology or an HPV test ♀ M MIPS
BETOS: Z2 Undefined codes
Service not separately priced by Part B

C G9807 Patients who did not receive cervical cytology or an HPV test ♀ M MIPS
BETOS: Z2 Undefined codes
Service not separately priced by Part B

C G9808 Any patients who had no asthma controller medications dispensed during the measurement year M MIPS
BETOS: Z2 Undefined codes
Service not separately priced by Part B

C G9809 Patients who use hospice services any time during the measurement period M MIPS
BETOS: Z2 Undefined codes
Service not separately priced by Part B

C G9810 Patient achieved a PDC of at least 75% for their asthma controller medication M MIPS
BETOS: Z2 Undefined codes
Service not separately priced by Part B

C G9811 Patient did not achieve a PDC of at least 75% for their asthma controller medication M MIPS
BETOS: Z2 Undefined codes
Service not separately priced by Part B

C G9812 Patient died including all deaths occurring during the hospitalization in which the operation was performed, even if after 30 days, and those deaths occurring after discharge from the hospital, but within 30 days of the procedure M MIPS
BETOS: Z2 Undefined codes
Service not separately priced by Part B

C G9813 Patient did not die within 30 days of the procedure or during the index hospitalization M MIPS
BETOS: Z2 Undefined codes
Service not separately priced by Part B

C G9818 Documentation of sexual activity M
BETOS: Z2 Undefined codes
Service not separately priced by Part B

C G9819 Patients who use hospice services any time during the measurement period M
BETOS: Z2 Undefined codes
Service not separately priced by Part B

C G9820 Documentation of a chlamydia screening test with proper follow-up M
BETOS: Z2 Undefined codes
Service not separately priced by Part B

C G9821 No documentation of a chlamydia screening test with proper follow-up M
BETOS: Z2 Undefined codes
Service not separately priced by Part B

♂ Male only   ♀ Female only   Ⓐ Age   A2 - Z3 = ASC Payment indicator   A - Y = APC Status indicator
ASC = ASC Approved Procedure   **DME** Paid under the DME fee schedule   **MIPS** MIPS code

C **G9822** Women who had an endometrial ablation procedure during the year prior to the index date (exclusive of the index date) ♀ M MIPS
BETOS: Z2   Undefined codes
Service not separately priced by Part B

C **G9823** Endometrial sampling or hysteroscopy with biopsy and results documented ♀ M MIPS
BETOS: Z2   Undefined codes
Service not separately priced by Part B

C **G9824** Endometrial sampling or hysteroscopy with biopsy and results not documented ♀ M MIPS
BETOS: Z2   Undefined codes
Service not separately priced by Part B

C **G9830** HER2/neu positive ♀ M MIPS
BETOS: Z2   Undefined codes
Service not separately priced by Part B

C **G9831** AJCC stage at breast cancer diagnosis = II or III M MIPS
BETOS: Z2   Undefined codes
Service not separately priced by Part B

C **G9832** AJCC stage at breast cancer diagnosis = I (Ia or Ib) and t-stage at breast cancer diagnosis does not equal = t1, t1a, t1b M MIPS
BETOS: Z2   Undefined codes
Service not separately priced by Part B

C **G9838** Patient has metastatic disease at diagnosis M MIPS
BETOS: Z2   Undefined codes
Service not separately priced by Part B

C **G9839** Anti-EGFR monoclonal antibody therapy M MIPS
BETOS: Z2   Undefined codes
Service not separately priced by Part B

C **G9840** RAS (KRAS and NRAS) gene mutation testing performed before initiation of anti-EGFR MoAb M MIPS
BETOS: Z2   Undefined codes
Service not separately priced by Part B

C **G9841** RAS (KRAS and NRAS) gene mutation testing not performed before initiation of anti-EGFR MoAb M MIPS
BETOS: Z2   Undefined codes
Service not separately priced by Part B

C **G9842** Patient has metastatic disease at diagnosis M MIPS
BETOS: Z2   Undefined codes
Service not separately priced by Part B

C **G9843** RAS (KRAS and NRAS) gene mutation M MIPS
BETOS: Z2   Undefined codes
Service not separately priced by Part B

C **G9844** Patient did not receive Anti-EGFR monoclonal antibody therapy M MIPS
BETOS: Z2   Undefined codes
Service not separately priced by Part B

C **G9845** Patient received Anti-EGFR monoclonal antibody therapy M MIPS
BETOS: Z2   Undefined codes
Service not separately priced by Part B

C **G9846** Patients who died from cancer M MIPS
BETOS: Z2   Undefined codes
Service not separately priced by Part B

C **G9847** Patient received chemotherapy in the last 14 days of life M MIPS
BETOS: Z2   Undefined codes
Service not separately priced by Part B

C **G9848** Patient did not receive chemotherapy in the last 14 days of life M MIPS
BETOS: Z2   Undefined codes
Service not separately priced by Part B

C **G9852** Patients who died from cancer M MIPS
BETOS: Z2   Undefined codes
Service not separately priced by Part B

C **G9853** Patient admitted to the ICU in the last 30 days of life M MIPS
BETOS: Z2   Undefined codes
Service not separately priced by Part B

C **G9854** Patient was not admitted to the ICU in the last 30 days of life M MIPS
BETOS: Z2   Undefined codes
Service not separately priced by Part B

C **G9858** Patient enrolled in hospice M MIPS
BETOS: Z2   Undefined codes
Service not separately priced by Part B

C **G9859** Patients who died from cancer M MIPS
BETOS: Z2   Undefined codes
Service not separately priced by Part B

C **G9860** Patient spent less than three days in hospice care M MIPS
BETOS: Z2   Undefined codes
Service not separately priced by Part B

C **G9861** Patient spent greater than or equal to three days in hospice care M MIPS
BETOS: Z2   Undefined codes
Service not separately priced by Part B

C **G9862** Documentation of medical reason(s) for not recommending at least a 10 year follow-up interval (e.g., inadequate prep, familial or personal history of colonic polyps, patient had no adenoma and age is = 66 years old, or life expectancy < 10 years old, other medical reasons) M
BETOS: Z2   Undefined codes
Service not separately priced by Part B

C **G9868** Receipt and analysis of remote, asynchronous images for dermatologic and/or ophthalmologic evaluation, for use under the Next Generation ACO model, less than 10 minutes B
BETOS: M5D   Specialist - other
Price established by carriers

● New code   ▲ Revised code   C Carrier judgment   D Special coverage instructions apply
I Not payable by Medicare   M Non-covered by Medicare   S Non-covered by Medicare statute   AHA Coding Clinic®

C **G9869** Receipt and analysis of remote, asynchronous images for dermatologic and/or ophthalmologic evaluation, for use under the Next Generation ACO model, 10-20 minutes B

BETOS: M5D Specialist - other
Price established by carriers

C **G9870** Receipt and analysis of remote, asynchronous images for dermatologic and/or ophthalmologic evaluation, for use under the Next Generation ACO model, 20 or more minutes B

BETOS: M5D Specialist - other
Price established by carriers

C **G9873** First Medicare diabetes prevention program (MDPP) core session was attended by an MDPP beneficiary under the MDPP expanded model (EM). A core session is an MDPP service that: (1) is furnished by an MDPP supplier during months 1 through 6 of the MDPP services period; (2) is approximately 1 hour in length; and (3) adheres to a CDC-approved DPP curriculum for core sessions M

BETOS: Y1 Other - Medicare fee schedule
Service not separately priced by Part B

C **G9874** Four total Medicare diabetes prevention program (MDPP) core sessions were attended by an MDPP beneficiary under the MDPP expanded model (EM). A core session is an MDPP service that: (1) is furnished by an MDPP supplier during months 1 through 6 of the MDPP services period; (2) is approximately 1 hour in length; and (3) adheres to a CDC-approved DPP curriculum for core sessions M

BETOS: Y1 Other - Medicare fee schedule
Service not separately priced by Part B

C **G9875** Nine total Medicare diabetes prevention program (MDPP) core sessions were attended by an MDPP beneficiary under the MDPP expanded model (EM). A core session is an MDPP service that: (1) is furnished by an MDPP supplier during months 1 through 6 of the MDPP services period; (2) is approximately 1 hour in length; and (3) adheres to a CDC-approved DPP curriculum for core sessions M

BETOS: Y1 Other - Medicare fee schedule
Service not separately priced by Part B

C **G9876** Two Medicare diabetes prevention program (MDPP) core maintenance sessions (MS) were attended by an MDPP beneficiary in months (MO) 7-9 under the MDPP expanded model (EM). A core maintenance session is an MDPP service that: (1) is furnished by an MDPP supplier during months 7 through 12 of the MDPP services period; (2) is approximately 1 hour in length; and (3) adheres to a CDC-approved DPP curriculum

for maintenance sessions. The beneficiary did not achieve at least 5% weight loss (WL) from his/her baseline weight, as measured by at least one in-person weight measurement at a core maintenance session in months 7-9 M

BETOS: Y1 Other - Medicare fee schedule
Service not separately priced by Part B

C **G9877** Two Medicare diabetes prevention program (MDPP) core maintenance sessions (MS) were attended by an MDPP beneficiary in months (MO) 10-12 under the MDPP expanded model (EM). A core maintenance session is an MDPP service that: (1) is furnished by an MDPP supplier during months 7 through 12 of the MDPP services period; (2) is approximately 1 hour in length; and (3) adheres to a CDC-approved DPP curriculum for maintenance sessions. The beneficiary did not achieve at least 5% weight loss (WL) from his/her baseline weight, as measured by at least one in-person weight measurement at a core maintenance session in months 10-12 M

BETOS: Y1 Other - Medicare fee schedule
Service not separately priced by Part B

C **G9878** Two Medicare diabetes prevention program (MDPP) core maintenance sessions (MS) were attended by an MDPP beneficiary in months (MO) 7-9 under the MDPP expanded model (EM). A core maintenance session is an MDPP service that: (1) is furnished by an MDPP supplier during months 7 through 12 of the MDPP services period; (2) is approximately 1 hour in length; and (3) adheres to a CDC-approved DPP curriculum for maintenance sessions. The beneficiary achieved at least 5% weight loss (WL) from his/her baseline weight, as measured by at least one in-person weight measurement at a core maintenance session in months 7-9 M

BETOS: Y1 Other - Medicare fee schedule
Service not separately priced by Part B

C **G9879** Two Medicare diabetes prevention program (MDPP) core maintenance sessions (MS) were attended by an MDPP beneficiary in months (MO) 10-12 under the MDPP expanded model (EM). A core maintenance session is an MDPP service that: (1) is furnished by an MDPP supplier during months 7 through 12 of the MDPP services period; (2) is approximately 1 hour in length; and (3) adheres to a CDC-approved DPP curriculum for maintenance sessions. The beneficiary achieved at least 5% weight loss (WL) from his/her baseline weight, as measured by at least one in-person weight measurement at a core maintenance session in months 10-12 M

BETOS: Y1 Other - Medicare fee schedule
Service not separately priced by Part B

♂ Male only ♀ Female only **A** Age A2 - Z3 = ASC Payment indicator A - Y = APC Status indicator
ASC = ASC Approved Procedure **DME** Paid under the DME fee schedule **MIPS** MIPS code

G9869 - G9879

PROCEDURES / PROFESSIONAL SERVICES (G0008-G9987)

G9880 — G9891

PROCEDURES / PROFESSIONAL SERVICES (G0008-G9987)

C **G9880** The MDPP beneficiary achieved at least 5% weight loss (WL) from his/her baseline weight in months 1-12 of the MDPP services period under the MDPP expanded model (EM). This is a one-time payment available when a beneficiary first achieves at least 5% weight loss from baseline as measured by an in-person weight measurement at a core session or core maintenance session   **M**
BETOS: Y1   Other - Medicare fee schedule
Service not separately priced by Part B

C **G9881** The MDPP beneficiary achieved at least 9% weight loss (WL) from his/her baseline weight in months 1-24 under the MDPP expanded model (EM). This is a one-time payment available when a beneficiary first achieves at least 9% weight loss from baseline as measured by an in-person weight measurement at a core session, core maintenance session, or ongoing maintenance session   **M**
BETOS: Y1   Other - Medicare fee schedule
Service not separately priced by Part B

C **G9882** Two Medicare diabetes prevention program (MDPP) ongoing maintenance sessions (MS) were attended by an MDPP beneficiary in months (MO) 13-15 under the MDPP expanded model (EM). An ongoing maintenance session is an MDPP service that: (1) is furnished by an MDPP supplier during months 13 through 24 of the MDPP services period; (2) is approximately 1 hour in length; and (3) adheres to a CDC-approved DPP curriculum for maintenance sessions. The beneficiary maintained at least 5% weight loss (WL) from his/her baseline weight, as measured by at least one in-person weight measurement at an ongoing maintenance session in months 13-15   **M**
BETOS: Y1   Other - Medicare fee schedule
Service not separately priced by Part B

C **G9883** Two Medicare diabetes prevention program (MDPP) ongoing maintenance sessions (MS) were attended by an MDPP beneficiary in months (MO) 16-18 under the MDPP expanded model (EM). An ongoing maintenance session is an MDPP service that: (1) is furnished by an MDPP supplier during months 13 through 24 of the MDPP services period; (2) is approximately 1 hour in length; and (3) adheres to a CDC-approved DPP curriculum for maintenance sessions. The beneficiary maintained at least 5% weight loss (WL) from his/her baseline weight, as measured by at least one in-person weight measurement at an ongoing maintenance session in months 16-18   **M**
BETOS: Y1   Other - Medicare fee schedule
Service not separately priced by Part B

C **G9884** Two Medicare diabetes prevention program (MDPP) ongoing maintenance sessions (MS) were attended by an MDPP beneficiary in months (MO) 19-21 under the MDPP expanded model (EM). An ongoing maintenance session is an MDPP service that: (1) is furnished by an MDPP supplier during months 13 through 24 of the MDPP services period; (2) is approximately 1 hour in length; and (3) adheres to a CDC-approved DPP curriculum for maintenance sessions. The beneficiary maintained at least 5% weight loss (WL) from his/her baseline weight, as measured by at least one in-person weight measurement at an ongoing maintenance session in months 19-21   **M**
BETOS: Y1   Other - Medicare fee schedule
Service not separately priced by Part B

C **G9885** Two Medicare diabetes prevention program (MDPP) ongoing maintenance sessions (MS) were attended by an MDPP beneficiary in months (MO) 22-24 under the MDPP expanded model (EM). An ongoing maintenance session is an MDPP service that: (1) is furnished by an MDPP supplier during months 13 through 24 of the MDPP services period; (2) is approximately 1 hour in length; and (3) adheres to a CDC-approved DPP curriculum for maintenance sessions. The beneficiary maintained at least 5% weight loss (WL) from his/her baseline weight, as measured by at least one in-person weight measurement at an ongoing maintenance session in months 22-24   **M**
BETOS: Y1   Other - Medicare fee schedule
Service not separately priced by Part B

C **G9890** Bridge payment: a one-time payment for the first Medicare diabetes prevention program (MDPP) core session, core maintenance session, or ongoing maintenance session furnished by an MDPP supplier to an MDPP beneficiary during months 1-24 of the MDPP expanded model (EM) who has previously received MDPP services from a different MDPP supplier under the MDPP expanded model. A supplier may only receive one bridge payment per MDPP beneficiary   **M**
BETOS: Y1   Other - Medicare fee schedule
Service not separately priced by Part B

C **G9891** MDPP session reported as a line-item on a claim for a payable MDPP expanded model (EM) HCPCS code for a session furnished by the billing supplier under the MDPP expanded model and counting toward achievement of the attendance performance goal for the payable MDPP expanded model HCPCS code (this code is for reporting purposes only)   **M**
BETOS: Y1   Other - Medicare fee schedule
Service not separately priced by Part B

● New code   ▲ Revised code   **C** Carrier judgment   **D** Special coverage instructions apply
I Not payable by Medicare   **M** Non-covered by Medicare   **S** Non-covered by Medicare statute   AHA Coding Clinic®

CPT® is a registered trademark of the American Medical Association. All rights reserved.

C **G9892** Documentation of patient reason(s) for not performing a dilated macular examination M MIPS

> **BETOS:** Z2 Undefined codes
> Service not separately priced by Part B

C **G9893** Dilated macular exam was not performed, reason not otherwise specified M MIPS

> **BETOS:** Z2 Undefined codes
> Service not separately priced by Part B

RADIOLOGY SERVICES PROSTATE (G9894-G9897)

C **G9894** Androgen deprivation therapy prescribed/administered in combination with external beam radiotherapy to the prostate ♂ M MIPS

> **BETOS:** Z2 Undefined codes
> Service not separately priced by Part B

C **G9895** Documentation of medical reason(s) for not prescribing/administering androgen deprivation therapy in combination with external beam radiotherapy to the prostate (e.g., salvage therapy) ♂ M MIPS

> **BETOS:** Z2 Undefined codes
> Service not separately priced by Part B

C **G9896** Documentation of patient reason(s) for not prescribing/administering androgen deprivation therapy in combination with external beam radiotherapy to the prostate ♂ M MIPS

> **BETOS:** Z2 Undefined codes
> Service not separately priced by Part B

C **G9897** Patients who were not prescribed/administered androgen deprivation therapy in combination with external beam radiotherapy to the prostate, reason not given ♂ M MIPS

> **BETOS:** Z2 Undefined codes
> Service not separately priced by Part B

GERIATRIC CARE MANAGEMENT (G9898)

▲ **C** **G9898** Patients age 66 or older in institutional special needs plans (SNP) or residing in long-term care with pos code 32, 33, 34, 54, or 56 for more than 90 consecutive days during the measurement period Ⓐ M MIPS

> **BETOS:** Z2 Undefined codes
> Service not separately priced by Part B

BREAST SCREENING/DIAGNOSTICS/THERAPEUTICS (G9899-G9900)

C **G9899** Screening, diagnostic, film, digital or digital breast tomosynthesis (3D) mammography results documented and reviewed M MIPS

> **BETOS:** Z2 Undefined codes
> Service not separately priced by Part B

C **G9900** Screening, diagnostic, film, digital or digital breast tomosynthesis (3D) mammography results were not documented and reviewed, reason not otherwise specified M MIPS

> **BETOS:** Z2 Undefined codes
> Service not separately priced by Part B

ADDITIONAL GERIATRIC CARE MANAGEMENT (G9901)

▲ **C** **G9901** Patient age 66 or older in institutional special needs plans (SNP) or residing in long-term care with pos code 32, 33, 34, 54, or 56 for more than 90 consecutive days during the measurement period Ⓐ M MIPS

> **BETOS:** Z2 Undefined codes
> Service not separately priced by Part B

TOBACCO SCREENING (G9902-G9909)

C **G9902** Patient screened for tobacco use and identified as a tobacco user M MIPS

> **BETOS:** Z2 Undefined codes
> Service not separately priced by Part B

C **G9903** Patient screened for tobacco use and identified as a tobacco non-user M MIPS

> **BETOS:** Z2 Undefined codes
> Service not separately priced by Part B

C **G9904** Documentation of medical reason(s) for not screening for tobacco use (e.g., limited life expectancy, other medical reason) M MIPS

> **BETOS:** Z2 Undefined codes
> Service not separately priced by Part B

C **G9905** Patient not screened for tobacco use, reason not given M MIPS

> **BETOS:** Z2 Undefined codes
> Service not separately priced by Part B

C **G9906** Patient identified as a tobacco user received tobacco cessation intervention (counseling and/or pharmacotherapy) M MIPS

> **BETOS:** Z2 Undefined codes
> Service not separately priced by Part B

C **G9907** Documentation of medical reason(s) for not providing tobacco cessation intervention (e.g., limited life expectancy, other medical reason) M MIPS

> **BETOS:** Z2 Undefined codes
> Service not separately priced by Part B

C **G9908** Patient identified as tobacco user did not receive tobacco cessation intervention (counseling and/or pharmacotherapy), reason not given M MIPS

> **BETOS:** Z2 Undefined codes
> Service not separately priced by Part B

C **G9909** Documentation of medical reason(s) for not providing tobacco cessation intervention if identified as a tobacco user (e.g., limited life expectancy, other medical reason) M MIPS

> **BETOS:** Z2 Undefined codes
> Service not separately priced by Part B

♂ Male only ♀ Female only Ⓐ Age A2 - Z3 = ASC Payment indicator A - Y = APC Status indicator
ASC = ASC Approved Procedure **DME** Paid under the DME fee schedule **MIPS** MIPS code

OTHER GERIATRIC CARE MANAGEMENT (G9910)

▲ [C] **G9910** Patients age 66 or older in institutional special needs plans (SNP) or residing in long-term care with pos code 32, 33, 34, 54 or 56 for more than 90 consecutive days during the measurement period ⒶM [MIPS]
BETOS: Z2 Undefined codes
Service not separately priced by Part B

BREAST CANCER CLASSIFICATION (G9911)

[C] **G9911** Clinically node negative (t1n0m0 or t2n0m0) invasive breast cancer before or after neoadjuvant systemic therapy M [MIPS]
BETOS: Z2 Undefined codes
Service not separately priced by Part B

ANTI-TNF DIAGNOSTICS FOR HBV STATUS (G9912-G9915)

[C] **G9912** Hepatitis B virus (HBV) status assessed and results interpreted prior to initiating anti-TNF (tumor necrosis factor) therapy M [MIPS]
BETOS: Z2 Undefined codes
Service not separately priced by Part B

[C] **G9913** Hepatitis B virus (HBV) status not assessed and results interpreted prior to initiating anti-TNF (tumor necrosis factor) therapy, reason not given M [MIPS]
BETOS: Z2 Undefined codes
Service not separately priced by Part B

[C] **G9914** Patient receiving an anti-TNF agent M [MIPS]
BETOS: Z2 Undefined codes
Service not separately priced by Part B

[C] **G9915** No record of HBV results documented M [MIPS]
BETOS: Z2 Undefined codes
Service not separately priced by Part B

FUNCTIONAL STATUS CODES (G9916-G9918)

[C] **G9916** Functional status performed once in the last 12 months M [MIPS]
BETOS: Z2 Undefined codes
Service not separately priced by Part B

[C] **G9917** Documentation of advanced stage dementia and caregiver knowledge is limited M
BETOS: Z2 Undefined codes
Service not separately priced by Part B

[C] **G9918** Functional status not performed, reason not otherwise specified M [MIPS]
BETOS: Z2 Undefined codes
Service not separately priced by Part B

SCREENING (G9919-G9932)

[C] **G9919** Screening performed and positive and provision of recommendations M [MIPS]
BETOS: Z2 Undefined codes
Service not separately priced by Part B

[C] **G9920** Screening performed and negative M [MIPS]
BETOS: Z2 Undefined codes
Service not separately priced by Part B

[C] **G9921** No screening performed, partial screening performed or positive screen without recommendations and reason is not given or otherwise specified M [MIPS]
BETOS: Z2 Undefined codes
Service not separately priced by Part B

[C] **G9922** Safety concerns screen provided and if positive then documented mitigation recommendations M [MIPS]
BETOS: Z2 Undefined codes
Service not separately priced by Part B

[C] **G9923** Safety concerns screen provided and negative M [MIPS]
BETOS: Z2 Undefined codes
Service not separately priced by Part B

[C] **G9925** Safety concerns screening not provided, reason not otherwise specified M [MIPS]
BETOS: Z2 Undefined codes
Service not separately priced by Part B

[C] **G9926** Safety concerns screening positive screen is without provision of mitigation recommendations, including but not limited to referral to other resources M [MIPS]
BETOS: Z2 Undefined codes
Service not separately priced by Part B

[C] **G9927** Documentation of system reason(s) for not prescribing warfarin or another FDA-approved anticoagulation due to patient being currently enrolled in a clinical trial related to AF/atrial flutter treatment M [MIPS]
BETOS: Z2 Undefined codes
Service not separately priced by Part B

[C] **G9928** Warfarin or another FDA-approved anticoagulant not prescribed, reason not given M [MIPS]
BETOS: Z2 Undefined codes
Service not separately priced by Part B

[C] **G9929** Patient with transient or reversible cause of AF (e.g., pneumonia, hyperthyroidism, pregnancy, cardiac surgery) M [MIPS]
BETOS: Z2 Undefined codes
Service not separately priced by Part B

[C] **G9930** Patients who are receiving comfort care only M [MIPS]
BETOS: Z2 Undefined codes
Service not separately priced by Part B

▲ [C] **G9931** Documentation of CHA2DS2-VASC risk score of 0 or 1 for men; or 0, 1, or 2 for women M [MIPS]
BETOS: Z2 Undefined codes
Service not separately priced by Part B

● New code ▲ Revised code [C] Carrier judgment [D] Special coverage instructions apply
[I] Not payable by Medicare [M] Non-covered by Medicare [S] Non-covered by Medicare statute AHA Coding Clinic®

C **G9932** Documentation of patient reason(s) for not having records of negative or managed positive TB screen (e.g., patient does not return for mantoux (PPD) skin test evaluation) M [MIPS]
BETOS: Z2 Undefined codes
Service not separately priced by Part B

GERIATRIC CARE MANAGEMENT AND OTHER SERVICES (G9938-G9940)

▲ C **G9938** Patients age 66 or older in institutional special needs plans (SNP) or residing in long-term care with pos code 32, 33, 34, 54, or 56 for more than 90 consecutive days during the six months prior to the measurement period through December 31 of the measurement period Ⓐ M [MIPS]
BETOS: Z2 Undefined codes
Service not separately priced by Part B

C **G9939** Pathologists/dermatopathologists is the same clinician who performed the biopsy M [MIPS]
BETOS: Z2 Undefined codes
Service not separately priced by Part B

C **G9940** Documentation of medical reason(s) for not on a statin (e.g., pregnancy, in vitro fertilization, clomiphene Rx, ESRD, cirrhosis, muscular pain and disease during the measurement period or prior year) M [MIPS]
BETOS: Z2 Undefined codes
Service not separately priced by Part B

PAIN ASSESSMENT (G9942-G9949)

C **G9942** Patient had any additional spine procedures performed on the same date as the lumbar discectomy/laminectomy M [MIPS]
BETOS: Z2 Undefined codes
Service not separately priced by Part B

C **G9943** Back pain was not measured by the visual analog scale (VAS) within three months preoperatively and at three months (6 - 20 weeks) postoperatively M [MIPS]
BETOS: Z2 Undefined codes
Service not separately priced by Part B

▲ C **G9945** Patient had cancer, acute fracture or infection related to the lumbar spine or patient had neuromuscular, idiopathic or congenital lumbar scoliosis M [MIPS]
BETOS: Z2 Undefined codes
Service not separately priced by Part B

C **G9946** Back pain was not measured by the visual analog scale (VAS) within three months preoperatively and at one year (9 to 15 months) postoperatively M [MIPS]
BETOS: Z2 Undefined codes
Service not separately priced by Part B

C **G9948** Patient had any additional spine procedures performed on the same date as the lumbar discectomy/laminectomy M [MIPS]
BETOS: Z2 Undefined codes
Service not separately priced by Part B

C **G9949** Leg pain was not measured by the visual analog scale (VAS) at three months (6 - 20 weeks) postoperatively M [MIPS]
BETOS: Z2 Undefined codes
Service not separately priced by Part B

MEDICATIONS (ANTIEMETICS AND ANTIMICROBIALS) (G9954-G9961)

C **G9954** Patient exhibits 2 or more risk factors for post-operative vomiting M [MIPS]
BETOS: Z2 Undefined codes
Service not separately priced by Part B

C **G9955** Cases in which an inhalational anesthetic is used only for induction M [MIPS]
BETOS: Z2 Undefined codes
Service not separately priced by Part B

C **G9956** Patient received combination therapy consisting of at least two prophylactic pharmacologic anti-emetic agents of different classes preoperatively and/or intraoperatively M [MIPS]
BETOS: Z2 Undefined codes
Service not separately priced by Part B

C **G9957** Documentation of medical reason for not receiving combination therapy consisting of at least two prophylactic pharmacologic anti-emetic agents of different classes preoperatively and/or intraoperatively (e.g., intolerance or other medical reason) M [MIPS]
BETOS: Z2 Undefined codes
Service not separately priced by Part B

C **G9958** Patient did not receive combination therapy consisting of at least two prophylactic pharmacologic anti-emetic agents of different classes preoperatively and/or intraoperatively M [MIPS]
BETOS: Z2 Undefined codes
Service not separately priced by Part B

C **G9959** Systemic antimicrobials not prescribed M [MIPS]
BETOS: Z2 Undefined codes
Service not separately priced by Part B

C **G9960** Documentation of medical reason(s) for prescribing systemic antimicrobials M [MIPS]
BETOS: Z2 Undefined codes
Service not separately priced by Part B

C **G9961** Systemic antimicrobials prescribed M [MIPS]
BETOS: Z2 Undefined codes
Service not separately priced by Part B

♂ Male only	♀ Female only	Ⓐ Age	A2 - Z3 = ASC Payment indicator	A - Y = APC Status indicator
ASC = ASC Approved Procedure		[DME] Paid under the DME fee schedule		[MIPS] MIPS code

G9962 - G9980

PROCEDURES / PROFESSIONAL SERVICES (G0008-G9987)

EMBOLIZATION (G9962-G9963)

C **G9962** Embolization endpoints are documented separately for each embolized vessel and ovarian artery angiography or embolization performed in the presence of variant uterine artery anatomy ♀ M MIPS

BETOS: Z2 Undefined codes
Service not separately priced by Part B

C **G9963** Embolization endpoints are not documented separately for each embolized vessel or ovarian artery angiography or embolization not performed in the presence of variant uterine artery anatomy ♀ M MIPS

BETOS: Z2 Undefined codes
Service not separately priced by Part B

SCREENING, WELLNESS AND PHYSICIAN VISITS (G9964-G9970)

C **G9964** Patient received at least one well-child visit with a PCP during the performance period ⒶM

BETOS: Z2 Undefined codes
Service not separately priced by Part B

C **G9965** Patient did not receive at least one well-child visit with a PCP during the performance period ⒶM

BETOS: Z2 Undefined codes
Service not separately priced by Part B

C **G9968** Patient was referred to another provider or specialist during the performance period M MIPS

BETOS: Z2 Undefined codes
Service not separately priced by Part B

C **G9969** Provider who referred the patient to another provider received a report from the provider to whom the patient was referred M MIPS

BETOS: Z2 Undefined codes
Service not separately priced by Part B

C **G9970** Provider who referred the patient to another provider did not receive a report from the provider to whom the patient was referred M MIPS

BETOS: Z2 Undefined codes
Service not separately priced by Part B

VISION ASSESSMENT (G9974-G9975)

C **G9974** Dilated macular exam performed, including documentation of the presence or absence of macular thickening or geographic atrophy or hemorrhage and the level of macular degeneration severity M MIPS

BETOS: Z2 Undefined codes
Service not separately priced by Part B

C **G9975** Documentation of medical reason(s) for not performing a dilated macular examination M MIPS

BETOS: Z2 Undefined codes
Service not separately priced by Part B

REMOTE IN-HOUSE EVALUATION AND MANAGEMENT ASSESSMENT (G9978-G9987)

C **G9978** Remote in-home visit for the evaluation and management of a new patient for use only in a Medicare-approved bundled payments for care improvement advanced (BPCI advanced) model episode of care, which requires these 3 key components: a problem focused history; a problem focused examination; and straightforward medical decision making, furnished in real time using interactive audio and video technology. Counseling and coordination of care with other physicians, other qualified health care professionals or agencies are provided consistent with the nature of the problem(s) and the needs of the patient or the family or both. Usually, the presenting problem(s) are self-limited or minor. Typically, 10 minutes are spent with the patient or family or both via real time, audio and video intercommunications technology B

BETOS: M1A Office visits - new
Price established by carriers

C **G9979** Remote in-home visit for the evaluation and management of a new patient for use only in a Medicare-approved bundled payments for care improvement advanced (BPCI advanced) model episode of care, which requires these 3 key components: an expanded problem focused history; an expanded problem focused examination; straightforward medical decision making, furnished in real time using interactive audio and video technology. Counseling and coordination of care with other physicians, other qualified health care professionals or agencies are provided consistent with the nature of the problem(s) and the needs of the patient or the family or both. Usually, the presenting problem(s) are of low to moderate severity. Typically, 20 minutes are spent with the patient or family or both via real time, audio and video intercommunications technology B

BETOS: M1A Office visits - new
Price established by carriers

C **G9980** Remote in-home visit for the evaluation and management of a new patient for use only in a Medicare-approved bundled payments for care improvement advanced (BPCI advanced) model episode of care, which requires these 3 key components: a detailed history; a detailed examination; medical decision making of low complexity, furnished in real time using interactive audio and video technology. Counseling and coordination of care with other physicians, other qualified health care professionals or agencies are provided consistent with the nature of the problem(s) and the needs of the patient or

---

● New code   ▲ Revised code   **C** Carrier judgment   **D** Special coverage instructions apply
I Not payable by Medicare   **M** Non-covered by Medicare   **S** Non-covered by Medicare statute   AHA Coding Clinic®

the family or both. Usually, the presenting problem(s) are of moderate severity. Typically, 30 minutes are spent with the patient or family or both via real time, audio and video intercommunications technology B

BETOS: M1A   Office visits - new
Price established by carriers

C G9981 Remote in-home visit for the evaluation and management of a new patient for use only in a Medicare-approved bundled payments for care improvement advanced (BPCI advanced) model episode of care, which requires these 3 key components: a comprehensive history; a comprehensive examination; medical decision making of moderate complexity, furnished in real time using interactive audio and video technology. Counseling and coordination of care with other physicians, other qualified health care professionals or agencies are provided consistent with the nature of the problem(s) and the needs of the patient or the family or both. Usually, the presenting problem(s) are of moderate to high severity. Typically, 45 minutes are spent with the patient or family or both via real time, audio and video intercommunications technology   B

BETOS: M1A   Office visits - new
Price established by carriers

C G9982 Remote in-home visit for the evaluation and management of a new patient for use only in a Medicare-approved bundled payments for care improvement advanced (BPCI advanced) model episode of care, which requires these 3 key components: a comprehensive history; a comprehensive examination; medical decision making of high complexity, furnished in real time using interactive audio and video technology. Counseling and coordination of care with other physicians, other qualified health care professionals or agencies are provided consistent with the nature of the problem(s) and the needs of the patient or the family or both. Usually, the presenting problem(s) are of moderate to high severity. Typically, 60 minutes are spent with the patient or family or both via real time, audio and video intercommunications technology   B

BETOS: M1A   Office visits - new
Price established by carriers

C G9983 Remote in-home visit for the evaluation and management of an established patient for use only in a Medicare-approved bundled payments for care improvement advanced (BPCI advanced) model episode of care, which requires at least 2 of the following 3 key components: a problem focused history; a problem focused examination; straightforward medical decision making, furnished in real time using interactive audio

and video technology. Counseling and coordination of care with other physicians, other qualified health care professionals or agencies are provided consistent with the nature of the problem(s) and the needs of the patient or the family or both. Usually, the presenting problem(s) are self-limited or minor. Typically, 10 minutes are spent with the patient or family or both via real time, audio and video intercommunications technology   B

BETOS: M1B   Office visits - established
Price established by carriers

C G9984 Remote in-home visit for the evaluation and management of an established patient for use only in a Medicare-approved bundled payments for care improvement advanced (BPCI advanced) model episode of care, which requires at least 2 of the following 3 key components: an expanded problem focused history; an expanded problem focused examination; medical decision making of low complexity, furnished in real time using interactive audio and video technology. Counseling and coordination of care with other physicians, other qualified health care professionals or agencies are provided consistent with the nature of the problem(s) and the needs of the patient or the family or both. Usually, the presenting problem(s) are of low to moderate severity. Typically, 15 minutes are spent with the patient or family or both via real time, audio and video intercommunications technology B

BETOS: M1B   Office visits - established
Price established by carriers

C G9985 Remote in-home visit for the evaluation and management of an established patient for use only in a Medicare-approved bundled payments for care improvement advanced (BPCI advanced) model episode of care, which requires at least 2 of the following 3 key components: a detailed history; a detailed examination; medical decision making of moderate complexity, furnished in real time using interactive audio and video technology. Counseling and coordination of care with other physicians, other qualified health care professionals or agencies are provided consistent with the nature of the problem(s) and the needs of the patient or the family or both. Usually, the presenting problem(s) are of moderate to high severity. Typically, 25 minutes are spent with the patient or family or both via real time, audio and video intercommunications technology B

BETOS: M1B   Office visits - established
Price established by carriers

♂ Male only   ♀ Female only   Ⓐ Age   A2 - Z3 = ASC Payment indicator   A - Y = APC Status indicator
ASC = ASC Approved Procedure   DME Paid under the DME fee schedule   MIPS MIPS code

CPT® is a registered trademark of the American Medical Association. All rights reserved.   **267**

C **G9986** Remote in-home visit for the evaluation and management of an established patient for use only in a Medicare-approved bundled payments for care improvement advanced (BPCI advanced) model episode of care, which requires at least 2 of the following 3 key components: a comprehensive history; a comprehensive examination; medical decision making of high complexity, furnished in real time using interactive audio and video technology. Counseling and coordination of care with other physicians, other qualified health care professionals or agencies are provided consistent with the nature of the problem(s) and the needs of the patient or the family or both. Usually, the presenting problem(s) are of moderate to high severity. Typically, 40 minutes are spent with the patient or family or both via real time, audio and video intercommunications technology B

BETOS: M1B   Office visits - established
Price established by carriers

C **G9987** Bundled payments for care improvement advanced (BPCI advanced) model home visit for patient assessment performed by clinical staff for an individual not considered homebound, including, but not necessarily limited to patient assessment of clinical status, safety/fall prevention, functional status/ambulation, medication reconciliation/ management, compliance with orders/plan of care, performance of activities of daily living, and ensuring beneficiary connections to community and other services; for use only for a BPCI advanced model episode of care; may not be billed for a 30-day period covered by a transitional care management code B

BETOS: M5D   Specialist - other
Price established by carriers

CPT® is a registered trademark of the American Medical Association. All rights reserved.

ALCOHOL AND DRUG ABUSE TREATMENT (H0001-H2037)

DRUG, ALCOHOL, AND BEHAVIORAL HEALTH SERVICES (H0001-H0030)

H0001 Alcohol and/or drug assessment
BETOS: Z2   Undefined codes
Service not separately priced by Part B
Coding Clinic: 2009, Q2

H0002 Behavioral health screening to determine eligibility for admission to treatment program   MIPS
BETOS: Z2   Undefined codes
Service not separately priced by Part B

H0003 Alcohol and/or drug screening; laboratory analysis of specimens for presence of alcohol and/or drugs
BETOS: Z2   Undefined codes
Service not separately priced by Part B

H0004 Behavioral health counseling and therapy, per 15 minutes   MIPS
BETOS: Z2   Undefined codes
Service not separately priced by Part B

H0005 Alcohol and/or drug services; group counseling by a clinician
BETOS: Z2   Undefined codes
Service not separately priced by Part B

H0006 Alcohol and/or drug services; case management
BETOS: Z2   Undefined codes
Service not separately priced by Part B

H0007 Alcohol and/or drug services; crisis intervention (outpatient)
BETOS: Z2   Undefined codes
Service not separately priced by Part B

H0008 Alcohol and/or drug services; sub-acute detoxification (hospital inpatient)
BETOS: Z2   Undefined codes
Service not separately priced by Part B

H0009 Alcohol and/or drug services; acute detoxification (hospital inpatient)
BETOS: Z2   Undefined codes
Service not separately priced by Part B

H0010 Alcohol and/or drug services; sub-acute detoxification (residential addiction program inpatient)
BETOS: Z2   Undefined codes
Service not separately priced by Part B

H0011 Alcohol and/or drug services; acute detoxification (residential addiction program inpatient)
BETOS: Z2   Undefined codes
Service not separately priced by Part B

H0012 Alcohol and/or drug services; sub-acute detoxification (residential addiction program outpatient)
BETOS: Z2   Undefined codes
Service not separately priced by Part B

H0013 Alcohol and/or drug services; acute detoxification (residential addiction program outpatient)
BETOS: Z2   Undefined codes
Service not separately priced by Part B

H0014 Alcohol and/or drug services; ambulatory detoxification
BETOS: Z2   Undefined codes
Service not separately priced by Part B

H0015 Alcohol and/or drug services; intensive outpatient (treatment program that operates at least 3 hours/day and at least 3 days/week and is based on an individualized treatment plan), including assessment, counseling; crisis intervention, and activity therapies or education
BETOS: Z2   Undefined codes
Service not separately priced by Part B

H0016 Alcohol and/or drug services; medical/somatic (medical intervention in ambulatory setting)
BETOS: Z2   Undefined codes
Service not separately priced by Part B

H0017 Behavioral health; residential (hospital residential treatment program), without room and board, per diem   MIPS
BETOS: Z2   Undefined codes
Service not separately priced by Part B

H0018 Behavioral health; short-term residential (non-hospital residential treatment program), without room and board, per diem   MIPS
BETOS: Z2   Undefined codes
Service not separately priced by Part B

H0019 Behavioral health; long-term residential (non-medical, non-acute care in a residential treatment program where stay is typically longer than 30 days), without room and board, per diem   MIPS
BETOS: Z2   Undefined codes
Service not separately priced by Part B

H0020 Alcohol and/or drug services; methadone administration and/or service (provision of the drug by a licensed program)
BETOS: Z2   Undefined codes
Service not separately priced by Part B

H0021 Alcohol and/or drug training service (for staff and personnel not employed by providers)
BETOS: Z2   Undefined codes
Service not separately priced by Part B

♂ Male only   ♀ Female only   Ⓐ Age   A2 - Z3 = ASC Payment indicator   A - Y = APC Status indicator
ASC = ASC Approved Procedure   DME Paid under the DME fee schedule   MIPS MIPS code

H0022 Alcohol and/or drug intervention service (planned facilitation)
BETOS: Z2   Undefined codes
Service not separately priced by Part B

H0023 Behavioral health outreach service (planned approach to reach a targeted population)
BETOS: Z2   Undefined codes
Service not separately priced by Part B

H0024 Behavioral health prevention information dissemination service (one-way direct or non-direct contact with service audiences to affect knowledge and attitude)
BETOS: Z2   Undefined codes
Service not separately priced by Part B

H0025 Behavioral health prevention education service (delivery of services with target population to affect knowledge, attitude and/or behavior)
BETOS: Z2   Undefined codes
Service not separately priced by Part B

H0026 Alcohol and/or drug prevention process service, community-based (delivery of services to develop skills of impactors)
BETOS: Z2   Undefined codes
Service not separately priced by Part B

H0027 Alcohol and/or drug prevention environmental service (broad range of external activities geared toward modifying systems in order to mainstream prevention through policy and law)
BETOS: Z2   Undefined codes
Service not separately priced by Part B

H0028 Alcohol and/or drug prevention problem identification and referral service (e.g., student assistance and employee assistance programs), does not include assessment
BETOS: Z2   Undefined codes
Service not separately priced by Part B

H0029 Alcohol and/or drug prevention alternatives service (services for populations that exclude alcohol and other drug use e.g., alcohol free social events)
BETOS: Z2   Undefined codes
Service not separately priced by Part B

H0030 Behavioral health hotline service
BETOS: Z2   Undefined codes
Service not separately priced by Part B

MENTAL HEALTH PROGRAMS AND MEDICATION ADMINISTRATION TRAINING (H0031-H0040)

H0031 Mental health assessment, by non-physician   MIPS
BETOS: Z2   Undefined codes
Service not separately priced by Part B

H0032 Mental health service plan development by non-physician
BETOS: Z2   Undefined codes
Service not separately priced by Part B

H0033 Oral medication administration, direct observation
BETOS: Z2   Undefined codes
Service not separately priced by Part B

H0034 Medication training and support, per 15 minutes   MIPS
BETOS: Z2   Undefined codes
Service not separately priced by Part B

H0035 Mental health partial hospitalization, treatment, less than 24 hours   MIPS
BETOS: Z2   Undefined codes
Service not separately priced by Part B

H0036 Community psychiatric supportive treatment, face-to-face, per 15 minutes   MIPS
BETOS: Z2   Undefined codes
Service not separately priced by Part B

H0037 Community psychiatric supportive treatment program, per diem   MIPS
BETOS: Z2   Undefined codes
Service not separately priced by Part B

H0038 Self-help/peer services, per 15 minutes
BETOS: Z2   Undefined codes
Service not separately priced by Part B

H0039 Assertive community treatment, face-to-face, per 15 minutes   MIPS
BETOS: Z2   Undefined codes
Service not separately priced by Part B

H0040 Assertive community treatment program, per diem   MIPS
BETOS: Z2   Undefined codes
Service not separately priced by Part B

FOSTER CARE (H0041, H0042)

H0041 Foster care, child, non-therapeutic, per diem   A
BETOS: Z2   Undefined codes
Service not separately priced by Part B

H0042 Foster care, child, non-therapeutic, per month   A
BETOS: Z2   Undefined codes
Service not separately priced by Part B

SUPPORTED HOUSING (H0043, H0044)

H0043 Supported housing, per diem
BETOS: Z2   Undefined codes
Service not separately priced by Part B

H0044 Supported housing, per month
BETOS: Z2   Undefined codes
Service not separately priced by Part B

● New code   ▲ Revised code   C Carrier judgment   D Special coverage instructions apply
I Not payable by Medicare   M Non-covered by Medicare   S Non-covered by Medicare statute   AHA Coding Clinic®

MISCELLANEOUS DRUG AND ALCOHOL SERVICES (H0045-H0050)

H0045 Respite care services, not in the home, per diem
BETOS: Z2   Undefined codes
Service not separately priced by Part B

H0046 Mental health services, not otherwise specified
BETOS: Z2   Undefined codes
Service not separately priced by Part B

H0047 Alcohol and/or other drug abuse services, not otherwise specified
BETOS: Z2   Undefined codes
Service not separately priced by Part B

H0048 Alcohol and/or other drug testing: collection and handling only, specimens other than blood
BETOS: Z2   Undefined codes
Service not separately priced by Part B

H0049 Alcohol and/or drug screening
BETOS: Z2   Undefined codes
Service not separately priced by Part B

H0050 Alcohol and/or drug services, brief intervention, per 15 minutes
BETOS: Z2   Undefined codes
Service not separately priced by Part B

PRENATAL CARE AND FAMILY PLANNING ASSESSMENT (H1000-H1011)

H1000 Prenatal care, at-risk assessment ♀ Ⓐ
BETOS: Z2   Undefined codes
Service not separately priced by Part B
Coding Clinic: 2002, Q1

H1001 Prenatal care, at-risk enhanced service; antepartum management ♀ Ⓐ
BETOS: Z2   Undefined codes
Service not separately priced by Part B
Coding Clinic: 2002, Q1

H1002 Prenatal care, at risk enhanced service; care coordination ♀ Ⓐ
BETOS: Z2   Undefined codes
Service not separately priced by Part B
Coding Clinic: 2002, Q1

H1003 Prenatal care, at-risk enhanced service; education ♀ Ⓐ
BETOS: Z2   Undefined codes
Service not separately priced by Part B
Coding Clinic: 2002, Q1

H1004 Prenatal care, at-risk enhanced service; follow-up home visit ♀ Ⓐ
BETOS: Z2   Undefined codes
Service not separately priced by Part B
Coding Clinic: 2002, Q1

H1005 Prenatal care, at-risk enhanced service package (includes H1001-H1004) ♀ Ⓐ
BETOS: Z2   Undefined codes
Service not separately priced by Part B
Coding Clinic: 2002, Q1

H1010 Non-medical family planning education, per session
BETOS: Z2   Undefined codes
Service not separately priced by Part B

H1011 Family assessment by licensed behavioral health professional for state defined purposes
BETOS: Z2   Undefined codes
Service not separately priced by Part B

OTHER MENTAL HEALTH AND COMMUNITY SUPPORT SERVICES (H2000-H2037)

H2000 Comprehensive multidisciplinary evaluation MIPS
BETOS: Z2   Undefined codes
Service not separately priced by Part B

H2001 Rehabilitation program, per 1/2 day MIPS
BETOS: Z2   Undefined codes
Service not separately priced by Part B

H2010 Comprehensive medication services, per 15 minutes MIPS
BETOS: Z2   Undefined codes
Service not separately priced by Part B

H2011 Crisis intervention service, per 15 minutes MIPS
BETOS: Z2   Undefined codes
Service not separately priced by Part B

H2012 Behavioral health day treatment, per hour MIPS
BETOS: Z2   Undefined codes
Service not separately priced by Part B

H2013 Psychiatric health facility service, per diem MIPS
BETOS: Z2   Undefined codes
Service not separately priced by Part B

H2014 Skills training and development, per 15 minutes MIPS
BETOS: Z2   Undefined codes
Service not separately priced by Part B

H2015 Comprehensive community support services, per 15 minutes MIPS
BETOS: Z2   Undefined codes
Service not separately priced by Part B

H2016 Comprehensive community support services, per diem MIPS
BETOS: Z2   Undefined codes
Service not separately priced by Part B

H2017 Psychosocial rehabilitation services, per 15 minutes MIPS
BETOS: Z2   Undefined codes
Service not separately priced by Part B

♂ Male only   ♀ Female only   Ⓐ Age   A2 - Z3 = ASC Payment indicator   A - Y = APC Status indicator
ASC = ASC Approved Procedure   **DME** Paid under the DME fee schedule   MIPS MIPS code

H2018 Psychosocial rehabilitation services,
per diem · MIPS
BETOS: Z2 Undefined codes
Service not separately priced by Part B

H2019 Therapeutic behavioral services,
per 15 minutes · MIPS
BETOS: Z2 Undefined codes
Service not separately priced by Part B

H2020 Therapeutic behavioral services,
per diem · MIPS
BETOS: Z2 Undefined codes
Service not separately priced by Part B

H2021 Community-based wrap-around services,
per 15 minutes
BETOS: Z2 Undefined codes
Service not separately priced by Part B

H2022 Community-based wrap-around services,
per diem
BETOS: Z2 Undefined codes
Service not separately priced by Part B

H2023 Supported employment, per 15 minutes
BETOS: Z2 Undefined codes
Service not separately priced by Part B

H2024 Supported employment, per diem
BETOS: Z2 Undefined codes
Service not separately priced by Part B

H2025 Ongoing support to maintain employment,
per 15 minutes
BETOS: Z2 Undefined codes
Service not separately priced by Part B

H2026 Ongoing support to maintain employment,
per diem
BETOS: Z2 Undefined codes
Service not separately priced by Part B

H2027 Psychoeducational service, per 15 minutes
BETOS: Z2 Undefined codes
Service not separately priced by Part B

H2028 Sexual offender treatment service,
per 15 minutes
BETOS: Z2 Undefined codes
Service not separately priced by Part B

H2029 Sexual offender treatment service, per diem
BETOS: Z2 Undefined codes
Service not separately priced by Part B

H2030 Mental health clubhouse services,
per 15 minutes
BETOS: Z2 Undefined codes
Service not separately priced by Part B

H2031 Mental health clubhouse services, per diem
BETOS: Z2 Undefined codes
Service not separately priced by Part B

H2032 Activity therapy, per 15 minutes
BETOS: Z2 Undefined codes
Service not separately priced by Part B

H2033 Multisystemic therapy for juveniles,
per 15 minutes · Ⓐ
BETOS: Z2 Undefined codes
Service not separately priced by Part B

H2034 Alcohol and/or drug abuse halfway house
services, per diem
BETOS: Z2 Undefined codes
Service not separately priced by Part B

H2035 Alcohol and/or other drug treatment program,
per hour
BETOS: Z2 Undefined codes
Service not separately priced by Part B

H2036 Alcohol and/or other drug treatment program,
per diem
BETOS: Z2 Undefined codes
Service not separately priced by Part B

H2037 Developmental delay prevention activities,
dependent child of client, per 15 minutes · Ⓐ
BETOS: Z2 Undefined codes
Service not separately priced by Part B
Coding Clinic: 2009, Q2

DRUGS ADMINISTERED OTHER THAN ORAL METHOD (J0120-J8999)

DRUGS, ADMINISTERED BY INJECTION (J0120-J7175)

D **J0120** Injection, tetracycline, up to 250 mg　　　　　　　　N1 ASC N
BETOS: O1E　Other drugs

C **J0121** Injection, omadacycline, 1 mg　　K2 ASC G
BETOS: O1E　Other drugs
Drugs: NUZYRA
Coding Clinic: 2019, Q4

C **J0122** Injection, eravacycline, 1 mg　　N1 ASC N
BETOS: O1E　Other drugs
Drugs: XERAVA
Coding Clinic: 2019, Q4

C **J0129** Injection, abatacept, 10 mg (code may be used for Medicare when drug administered under the direct supervision of a physician, not for use when drug is self administered)　　　　　　K2 ASC K
BETOS: O1E　Other drugs
Drugs: ABATACEPT, ORENCIA, ORENCIA CLICKJECT
Coding Clinic: 2006, Q4

D **J0130** Injection abciximab, 10 mg　　N1 ASC N
BETOS: O1E　Other drugs

C **J0131** Injection, acetaminophen, 10 mg　N1 ASC N
BETOS: O1E　Other drugs

C **J0132** Injection, acetylcysteine, 100 mg　N1 ASC N
BETOS: O1E　Other drugs
Drugs: ACETADOTE, ACETYLCYSTEINE, ACETYLCYSTEINE INJ, ACETYLCYSTEINE INJECTION

C **J0133** Injection, acyclovir, 5 mg　　N1 ASC N
BETOS: O1E　Other drugs
Drugs: ACYCLOVIR SODIUM

C **J0135** Injection, adalimumab, 20 mg　K2 ASC K MIPS
BETOS: O1E　Other drugs
Drugs: HUMIRA
Coding Clinic: 2005, Q3; 2005, Q2

D **J0153** Injection, adenosine, 1 mg (not to be used to report any adenosine phosphate compounds)　　　　　N1 ASC N
BETOS: O1E　Other drugs
Drugs: ADENOCARD, ADENOSCAN, ADENOSINE

D **J0171** Injection, adrenalin, epinephrine, 0.1 mg　　　　　　N1 ASC N
BETOS: O1E　Other drugs
Drugs: ADRENALIN, EPINEPHRINE HCL
Coding Clinic: 2011, Q1

C **J0178** Injection, aflibercept, 1 mg　　K2 ASC K
BETOS: O1E　Other drugs
Drugs: EYLEA

C **J0179** Injection, brolucizumab-dbll, 1 mg　K2 ASC G
BETOS: O1E　Other drugs
Drugs: BEOVU
Coding Clinic: 2020, Q1

C **J0180** Injection, agalsidase beta, 1 mg　　K2 ASC K
BETOS: O1E　Other drugs
Drugs: FABRAZYME
Coding Clinic: 2005, Q2

C **J0185** Injection, aprepitant, 1 mg　　K2 ASC K
BETOS: O1E　Other drugs
Drugs: CINVANTI
Coding Clinic: 2019, Q1

D **J0190** Injection, biperiden lactate, per 5 mg　　　　　　K5 ASC E2
BETOS: O1E　Other drugs

D **J0200** Injection, alatrofloxacin mesylate, 100 mg　　　　　K5 ASC E2
BETOS: O1E　Other drugs

C **J0202** Injection, alemtuzumab, 1 mg　　K2 ASC K
BETOS: O1E　Other drugs
Drugs: LEMTRADA
Coding Clinic: 2016, Q1

D **J0205** Injection, alglucerase, per 10 units K5 ASC E2
BETOS: O1E　Other drugs
Coding Clinic: 2005, Q2

D **J0207** Injection, amifostine, 500 mg　　K2 ASC K
BETOS: O1D　Chemotherapy
Drugs: ETHYOL

D **J0210** Injection, methyldopate HCl, up to 250 mg　　　　　K5 ASC E2
BETOS: O1E　Other drugs

C **J0215** Injection, alefacept, 0.5 mg　　K5 ASC E2
BETOS: O1E　Other drugs

C **J0220** Injection, alglucosidase alfa, 10 mg, not otherwise specified　　K2 ASC K
BETOS: O1E　Other drugs
Coding Clinic: 2008, Q1; 2012, Q1

C **J0221** Injection, alglucosidase alfa, (Lumizyme), 10 mg　　　　K2 ASC K
BETOS: O1E　Other drugs
Drugs: LUMIZYME

C **J0222** Injection, patisiran, 0.1 mg　　K2 ASC G
BETOS: O1E　Other drugs
Drugs: ONPATTRO
Coding Clinic: 2019, Q4

● **C** **J0223** Injection, givosiran, 0.5 mg　　K2 ASC G
BETOS: O1E　Other drugs
Drugs: GIVLAARI
Coding Clinic: 2020, Q2

D **J0256** Injection, alpha 1 proteinase inhibitor (human), not otherwise specified, 10 mg　　　　　　K2 ASC K
BETOS: O1E　Other drugs

♂ Male only　　♀ Female only　　Ⓐ Age　　A2 - Z3 = ASC Payment indicator　　A - Y = APC Status indicator
ASC = ASC Approved Procedure　　**DME** Paid under the DME fee schedule　　**MIPS** MIPS code

Drugs: ARALAST NP, PROLASTIN-C, ZEMAIRA
Coding Clinic: 2005, Q2; 2012, Q1

D J0257 Injection, alpha 1 proteinase inhibitor (human), (Glassia), 10 mg   K2 ASC K
BETOS: O1E   Other drugs
Drugs: GLASSIA
Coding Clinic: 2012, Q1

D J0270 Injection, alprostadil, 1.25 mcg (code may be used for Medicare when drug administered under the direct supervision of a physician, not for use when drug is self administered)   B
BETOS: O1E   Other drugs

D J0275 Alprostadil urethral suppository (code may be used for Medicare when drug administered under the direct supervision of a physician, not for use when drug is self administered)   B
BETOS: O1E   Other drugs

C J0278 Injection, amikacin sulfate, 100 mg   N1 ASC N
BETOS: O1E   Other drugs
Drugs: AMIKACIN SULFATE

D J0280 Injection, aminophyllin, up to 250 mg   N1 ASC N
BETOS: O1E   Other drugs
Drugs: AMINOPHYLLINE
Coding Clinic: 2005, Q4

D J0282 Injection, amiodarone hydrochloride, 30 mg   N1 ASC N
BETOS: O1E   Other drugs

D J0285 Injection, amphotericin B, 50 mg   N1 ASC N
BETOS: O1E   Other drugs
Drugs: AMPHOTERICIN B

D J0287 Injection, amphotericin B lipid complex, 10 mg   K2 ASC K
BETOS: O1E   Other drugs
Drugs: ABELCET

D J0288 Injection, amphotericin B cholesteryl sulfate complex, 10 mg   K5 ASC E2
BETOS: O1E   Other drugs

D J0289 Injection, amphotericin B liposome, 10 mg   K2 ASC K
BETOS: O1E   Other drugs
Drugs: AMBISOME

D J0290 Injection, ampicillin sodium, 500 mg   N1 ASC N
BETOS: O1E   Other drugs
Drugs: AMPICILLIN, AMPICILLIN FOR INJECTION, AMPICILLIN SODIUM

C J0291 Injection, plazomicin, 5 mg   K2 ASC G
BETOS: O1E   Other drugs
Drugs: ZEMDRI (PLAZOMICIN)
Coding Clinic: 2019, Q4

D J0295 Injection, ampicillin sodium/sulbactam sodium, per 1.5 gm   N1 ASC N

BETOS: O1E   Other drugs
Drugs: AMPICILLIN-SULBACTAM, UNASYN 1.5GM, UNASYN 15GM, UNASYN 3GM

D J0300 Injection, amobarbital, up to 125 mg   K2 ASC K
BETOS: O1E   Other drugs

D J0330 Injection, succinylcholine chloride, up to 20 mg   N1 ASC N
BETOS: O1E   Other drugs

C J0348 Injection, anidulafungin, 1 mg   N1 ASC N
BETOS: O1E   Other drugs
Drugs: ERAXIS

D J0350 Injection, anistreplase, per 30 units   K5 ASC E2
BETOS: O1E   Other drugs

D J0360 Injection, hydralazine HCl, up to 20 mg   N1 ASC N
BETOS: O1E   Other drugs
Drugs: HYDRALAZINE HCL

C J0364 Injection, apomorphine hydrochloride, 1 mg   K5 ASC E2
BETOS: O1E   Other drugs

D J0365 Injection, aprotinin, 10,000 kiu   K5 ASC E2
BETOS: O1E   Other drugs

D J0380 Injection, metaraminol bitartrate, per 10 mg   K5 ASC E2
BETOS: O1E   Other drugs

D J0390 Injection, chloroquine hydrochloride, up to 250 mg   K2 ASC K
BETOS: O1E   Other drugs

D J0395 Injection, arbutamine HCl, 1 mg   K5 ASC E2
BETOS: O1E   Other drugs

C J0400 Injection, aripiprazole, intramuscular, 0.25 mg   N1 ASC N
BETOS: O1E   Other drugs
Coding Clinic: 2008, Q1

C J0401 Injection, aripiprazole, extended release, 1 mg   K2 ASC K
BETOS: O1E   Other drugs
Drugs: ABILIFY MAINTENA
Coding Clinic: 2014, Q1

D J0456 Injection, azithromycin, 500 mg   N1 ASC N
BETOS: O1E   Other drugs
Drugs: AZITHROMYCIN, ZITHROMAX

D J0461 Injection, atropine sulfate, 0.01 mg   N1 ASC N
BETOS: O1E   Other drugs
Drugs: ATROPINE SULFATE

D J0470 Injection, dimercaprol, per 100 mg   N1 ASC N
BETOS: O1E   Other drugs

D J0475 Injection, baclofen, 10 mg   K2 ASC K
BETOS: O1E   Other drugs
Drugs: BACLOFEN, GABLOFEN, LIORESAL

● New code   ▲ Revised code   **C** Carrier judgment   **D** Special coverage instructions apply
I Not payable by Medicare   **M** Non-covered by Medicare   **S** Non-covered by Medicare statute   *AHA Coding Clinic®*

D J0476 Injection, baclofen, 50 mcg for intrathecal trial   N1 ASC N
BETOS: O1E   Other drugs
Drugs: GABLOFEN, LIORESAL

D J0480 Injection, basiliximab, 20 mg   K2 ASC K
BETOS: O1E   Other drugs
Drugs: SIMULECT

C J0485 Injection, belatacept, 1 mg   K2 ASC K
BETOS: O1E   Other drugs
Drugs: NULOJIX

C J0490 Injection, belimumab, 10 mg   K2 ASC K
BETOS: O1E   Other drugs
Drugs: BENLYSTA

D J0500 Injection, dicyclomine HCl, up to 20 mg   N1 ASC N
BETOS: O1E   Other drugs
Drugs: BENTYL, DICYCLOMINE HCl, DICYCLOMINE HCL

D J0515 Injection, benztropine mesylate, per 1 mg   N1 ASC N
BETOS: O1E   Other drugs
Drugs: BENZTROPINE, COGENTIN

C J0517 Injection, benralizumab, 1 mg   K2 ASC K
BETOS: O1E   Other drugs
Drugs: FASENRA
Coding Clinic: 2019, Q1

D J0520 Injection, bethanechol chloride, myotonachol or urecholine, up to 5 mg   K5 ASC E2
BETOS: O1E   Other drugs

C J0558 Injection, penicillin G benzathine and penicillin G procaine, 100,000 units   K2 ASC K
BETOS: O1E   Other drugs
Drugs: BICILLIN C-R, BICILLIN CR PEDIATRIC
Coding Clinic: 2011, Q1

D J0561 Injection, penicillin G benzathine, 100,000 units   K2 ASC K
BETOS: O1E   Other drugs
Drugs: BICILLIN L-A
Coding Clinic: 2011, Q1

C J0565 Injection, bezlotoxumab, 10 mg   K2 ASC K
BETOS: O1E   Other drugs
Drugs: ZINPLAVA

C J0567 Injection, cerliponase alfa, 1 mg   N1 Ⓐ ASC N
BETOS: O1E   Other drugs
Coding Clinic: 2019, Q1

C J0570 Buprenorphine implant, 74.2 mg   K2 ASC K
BETOS: O1E   Other drugs
Drugs: PROBUPHINE SYSTEM KIT
Coding Clinic: 2011, Q1; 2017, Q1

D J0571 Buprenorphine, oral, 1 mg   E1
BETOS: O1E   Other drugs
Service not separately priced by Part B
Coding Clinic: 2014, Q4; 2016, Q1

D J0572 Buprenorphine/naloxone, oral, less than or equal to 3 mg buprenorphine   E1
BETOS: O1E   Other drugs
Service not separately priced by Part B
Coding Clinic: 2014, Q4; 2016, Q1

D J0573 Buprenorphine/naloxone, oral, greater than 3 mg, but less than or equal to 6 mg buprenorphine   E1
BETOS: O1E   Other drugs
Service not separately priced by Part B
Coding Clinic: 2014, Q4; 2016, Q1

D J0574 Buprenorphine/naloxone, oral, greater than 6 mg, but less than or equal to 10 mg buprenorphine   E1
BETOS: O1E   Other drugs
Service not separately priced by Part B
Coding Clinic: 2014, Q4; 2016, Q1

D J0575 Buprenorphine/naloxone, oral, greater than 10 mg buprenorphine   E1
BETOS: O1E   Other drugs
Service not separately priced by Part B
Coding Clinic: 2014, Q4; 2016, Q1

C J0583 Injection, bivalirudin, 1 mg   N1 ASC N
BETOS: O1E   Other drugs
Drugs: ANGIOMAX, BIVALIRUDIN, BIVALIRUDIN RTU

C J0584 Injection, burosumab-twza 1 mg   K2 ASC K
BETOS: O1E   Other drugs
Drugs: CRYSVITA
Coding Clinic: 2019, Q1

D J0585 Injection, onabotulinumtoxinA, 1 unit   K2 ASC K
BETOS: O1E   Other drugs
Drugs: BOTOX, BOTOX COSMETIC

C J0586 Injection, abobotulinumtoxinA, 5 units   K2 ASC K
BETOS: O1E   Other drugs
Drugs: DYSPORT

D J0587 Injection, rimabotulinumtoxinB, 100 units   K2 ASC K
BETOS: O1E   Other drugs
Drugs: MYOBLOC
Coding Clinic: 2002, Q2; 2002, Q1

C J0588 Injection, incobotulinumtoxin A, 1 unit   K2 ASC K
BETOS: O1E   Other drugs
Drugs: XEOMIN

● **C J0591** Injection, deoxycholic acid, 1 mg   E1
BETOS: O1E   Other drugs
Coding Clinic: 2020, Q2

D J0592 Injection, buprenorphine hydrochloride, 0.1 mg   N1 ASC N
BETOS: O1E   Other drugs
Drugs: BUPRENEX, BUPRENORPHINE HCL, BUPRENORPHINE HCL INJECTION

♂ Male only   ♀ Female only   Ⓐ Age   A2 - Z3 = ASC Payment indicator   A - Y = APC Status indicator
ASC = ASC Approved Procedure   **DME** Paid under the DME fee schedule   **MIPS** MIPS code

C **J0593** Injection, lanadelumab-flyo, 1 mg (code may be used for Medicare when drug administered under direct supervision of a physician, not for use when drug is self-administered)   N1 ASC N
BETOS: O1E   Other drugs
Coding Clinic: 2019, Q4

C **J0594** Injection, Busulfan, 1 mg   K2 ASC K
BETOS: O1E   Other drugs
Drugs: BUSULFAN

C **J0595** Injection, butorphanol tartrate, 1 mg   N1 ASC N
BETOS: O1E   Other drugs
Drugs: BUTORPHANOL TARTRATE
Coding Clinic: 2005, Q2

C **J0596** Injection, C1 esterase inhibitor (recombinant), ruconest, 10 units   K2 ASC K
BETOS: O1E   Other drugs
Drugs: RUCONEST
Coding Clinic: 2016, Q1

C **J0597** Injection, C-1 esterase inhibitor (human), Berinert, 10 units   K2 ASC K
BETOS: O1E   Other drugs
Drugs: BERINERT
Coding Clinic: 2011, Q1

C **J0598** Injection, C-1 esterase inhibitor (human), Cinryze, 10 units   K2 ASC K
BETOS: O1E   Other drugs
Drugs: CINRYZE

C **J0599** Injection, C-1 esterase inhibitor (human), (HAEGARDA®), 10 units   K2 ASC K
BETOS: O1E   Other drugs
Coding Clinic: 2019, Q1

D **J0600** Injection, edetate calcium disodium, up to 1000 mg   K2 ASC K
BETOS: O1E   Other drugs
Drugs: CALCIUM DISODIUM VERSENATE

D **J0604** Cinacalcet, oral, 1 mg, (for ESRD on dialysis)   B
BETOS: O1E   Other drugs
Coding Clinic: 2018, Q1

D **J0606** Injection, etelcalcetide, 0.1 mg   N1 ASC N
BETOS: O1E   Other drugs
Coding Clinic: 2018, Q1; 2018, Q2

D **J0610** Injection, calcium gluconate, per 10 ml   N1 ASC N
BETOS: O1E   Other drugs
Drugs: CALCIUM GLUCONATE

D **J0620** Injection, calcium glycerophosphate and calcium lactate, per 10 ml   N1 ASC N
BETOS: O1E   Other drugs

D **J0630** Injection, calcitonin salmon, up to 400 units   K2 ASC K
BETOS: O1E   Other drugs

Drugs: MIACALCIN
Pub: 100-4, Chapter-10, 90.1

D **J0636** Injection, calcitriol, 0.1 mcg   N1 ASC N
BETOS: O1E   Other drugs
Drugs: CALCITRIOL

C **J0637** Injection, caspofungin acetate, 5 mg   N1 ASC N
BETOS: O1E   Other drugs
Drugs: CANCIDAS, CASPOFUNGIN, CASPOFUNGIN ACETATE

C **J0638** Injection, canakinumab, 1 mg   K2 ASC K
BETOS: O1E   Other drugs
Drugs: ILARIS
Coding Clinic: 2011, Q1; 2011, Q4

D **J0640** Injection, leucovorin calcium, per 50 mg   N1 ASC N
BETOS: O1E   Other drugs
Drugs: LEUCOVORIN CALCIUM
Coding Clinic: 2009, Q1

D **J0641** Injection, levoleucovorin, not otherwise specified, 0.5 mg   K2 ASC K
BETOS: O1E   Other drugs
Drugs: LEVOLEUCOVORIN CALCIUM
Coding Clinic: 2009, Q1; 2008, Q4; 2019, Q4

C **J0642** Injection, levoleucovorin (KHAPZORYTM), 0.5 mg   K2 ASC G
BETOS: O1E   Other drugs
Drugs: KHAPZORY
Coding Clinic: 2019, Q4; 2020, Q1

D **J0670** Injection, mepivacaine hydrochloride, per 10 ml   N1 ASC N
BETOS: O1E   Other drugs
Drugs: POLOCAINE, POLOCAINE-MPF

D **J0690** Injection, cefazolin sodium, 500 mg N1 ASC N
BETOS: O1E   Other drugs
Drugs: CEFAZOLIN SODIUM, CEFAZOLIN SODIUM IN DEXTROSE

● **C** **J0691** Injection, lefamulin, 1 mg   K2 ASC G
BETOS: O1E   Other drugs
Drugs: XENLETA
Coding Clinic: 2020, Q2

C **J0692** Injection, cefepime hydrochloride, 500 mg   N1 ASC N
BETOS: O1E   Other drugs
Drugs: CEFEPIME, CEFEPIME HCL, CEFEPIME HCL IN DEXTROSE, MAXIPIME
Coding Clinic: 2002, Q1

● **C** **J0693** Injection, cefiderocol, 5 mg   K2 Ⓐ ASC G
BETOS: O1E   Other drugs
Drugs: FETROJA

D **J0694** Injection, cefoxitin sodium, 1 gm   N1 ASC N
BETOS: O1E   Other drugs
Drugs: CEFOXITIN SODIUM, PREMIERPRO RX CEFOXITIN SODIUM

● New code   ▲ Revised code   **C** Carrier judgment   **D** Special coverage instructions apply
I Not payable by Medicare   **M** Non-covered by Medicare   **S** Non-covered by Medicare statute   AHA Coding Clinic®

C **J0695** Injection, ceftolozane 50 mg and tazobactam 25 mg   K2 ASC K
BETOS: O1E   Other drugs
Drugs: ZERBAXA
Coding Clinic: 2016, Q1

D **J0696** Injection, ceftriaxone sodium, per 250 mg   N1 ASC N
BETOS: O1E   Other drugs
Drugs: CEFTRIAXONE, CEFTRIAXONE IN D5W, CEFTRIAXONE SODIUM

D **J0697** Injection, sterile cefuroxime sodium, per 750 mg   N1 ASC N
BETOS: O1E   Other drugs
Drugs: CEFUROXIME SODIUM, ZINACEF

D **J0698** Injection, cefotaxime sodium, per gm   N1 ASC N
BETOS: O1E   Other drugs
Drugs: CEFOTAXIME SODIUM

D **J0702** Injection, betamethasone acetate 3 mg and betamethasone sodium phosphate 3 mg   N1 ASC N
BETOS: O1E   Other drugs
Drugs: BETAMETHASONE SODIUM PHOSPHATE AND BETAMETHASONE ACETATE, CELESTONE SOLUSPAN
Coding Clinic: 2018, Q4

C **J0706** Injection, caffeine citrate, 5 mg   N1 ASC N
BETOS: O1E   Other drugs
Coding Clinic: 2002, Q2; 2002, Q1

D **J0710** Injection, cephapirin sodium, up to 1 gm   K5 ASC E2
BETOS: O1E   Other drugs

C **J0712** Injection, ceftaroline fosamil, 10 mg   K2 ASC K
BETOS: O1E   Other drugs
Drugs: TEFLARO

D **J0713** Injection, ceftazidime, per 500 mg   N1 ASC N
BETOS: O1E   Other drugs
Drugs: CEFTAZIDIME, FORTAZ, FORTAZ (ADD-V), FORTAZ ADD-V, TAZICEF

C **J0714** Injection, ceftazidime and avibactam, 0.5 g/0.125 g   K2 ASC K
BETOS: O1E   Other drugs
Drugs: AVYCAZ
Coding Clinic: 2016, Q1

D **J0715** Injection, ceftizoxime sodium, per 500 mg   N1 ASC N
BETOS: O1E   Other drugs

C **J0716** Injection, centruroides immune f(ab)2, up to 120 milligrams   K2 ASC K
BETOS: O1E   Other drugs
Drugs: ANASCORP

C **J0717** Injection, certolizumab pegol, 1 mg (code may be used for Medicare when drug administered under the direct supervision of a physician, not for use when drug is self administered)   K2 ASC K MIPS

BETOS: O1E   Other drugs
Drugs: CIMZIA
Coding Clinic: 2014, Q1

D **J0720** Injection, chloramphenicol sodium succinate, up to 1 gm   N1 ASC N
BETOS: O1E   Other drugs
Drugs: CHLORAMPHENICOL SOD SUCCINATE

D **J0725** Injection, chorionic gonadotropin, per 1,000 USP units   N1 ♀ Ⓐ ASC N
BETOS: O1E   Other drugs
Drugs: CHORIONIC GONADOTROPIN, NOVAREL

D **J0735** Injection, clonidine hydrochloride, 1 mg   N1 ASC N
BETOS: O1E   Other drugs
Drugs: CLONIDINE HYDROCHLORIDE, CLONIDINE HYDROCHLORIDE INJECTION, DURACLON

D **J0740** Injection, cidofovir, 375 mg   K2 ASC K
BETOS: O1E   Other drugs
Drugs: CIDOFOVIR

● **C** **J0742** Injection, imipenem 4 mg, cilastatin 4 mg and relebactam 2 mg   K2 ASC G
BETOS: O1E   Other drugs
Drugs: RECARBRIO
Coding Clinic: 2020, Q2

D **J0743** Injection, cilastatin sodium; imipenem, per 250 mg   N1 ASC N
BETOS: O1E   Other drugs
Drugs: IMIPENEM AND CILASTATIN, PRIMAXIN IV

C **J0744** Injection, ciprofloxacin for intravenous infusion, 200 mg   N1 ASC N
BETOS: O1E   Other drugs
Drugs: CIPRO, CIPROFLOXACIN
Coding Clinic: 2002, Q1

D **J0745** Injection, codeine phosphate, per 30 mg   K2 ASC K
BETOS: O1E   Other drugs

D **J0770** Injection, colistimethate sodium, up to 150 mg   N1 ASC N
BETOS: O1E   Other drugs
Drugs: COLISTIMETHATE SODIUM, COLY-MYCIN M PARENTERAL

C **J0775** Injection, collagenase, clostridium histolyticum, 0.01 mg   K2 ASC K
BETOS: O1E   Other drugs
Drugs: XIAFLEX (COLLAGENASE CLOSTRIDIUM HISTOLYTICUM)
Coding Clinic: 2011, Q1

D **J0780** Injection, prochlorperazine, up to 10 mg   N1 ASC N
BETOS: O1E   Other drugs
Drugs: PROCHLORPERAZINE EDISYLATE

♂ Male only   ♀ Female only   Ⓐ Age   A2 - Z3 = ASC Payment indicator   A - Y = APC Status indicator
ASC = ASC Approved Procedure   DME Paid under the DME fee schedule   MIPS MIPS code

● **C** **J0791** Injection, crizanlizumab-tmca,
5 mg   K2 ASC G
BETOS: O1E   Other drugs
Drugs: ADAKVEO
Coding Clinic: 2020, Q2

D **J0795** Injection, corticorelin ovine triflutate,
1 microgram   K2 ASC K
BETOS: O1E   Other drugs
Drugs: ACTHREL

D **J0800** Injection, corticotropin, up to
40 units   N1 ASC N
BETOS: O1E   Other drugs
Drugs: H.P. ACTHAR

C **J0834** Injection, cosyntropin, 0.25 mg   N1 ASC N
BETOS: O1E   Other drugs
Drugs: CORTROSYN, COSYNTROPIN,
COSYNTROPIN (CORTROSYN GENERIC)

C **J0840** Injection, crotalidae polyvalent immune FAB
(Ovine), up to 1 gram   K2 ASC K
BETOS: O1E   Other drugs
Drugs: CROFAB POWDER FOR
SOLUTION

C **J0841** Injection, crotalidae immune F(ab')2
(equine), 120 mg   K2 ASC K
BETOS: O1E   Other drugs
Drugs: ANAVIP
Coding Clinic: 2019, Q1

D **J0850** Injection, cytomegalovirus immune globulin
intravenous (human), per vial   K2 ASC K
BETOS: O1E   Other drugs
Drugs: CYTOGAM

C **J0875** Injection, dalbavancin, 5 mg   K2 ASC K
BETOS: O1E   Other drugs
Drugs: DALVANCE
Coding Clinic: 2016, Q1

C **J0878** Injection, daptomycin, 1 mg   N1 ASC N
BETOS: O1E   Other drugs
Drugs: CUBICIN, DAPTOMYCIN
Coding Clinic: 2005, Q2

D **J0881** Injection, darbepoetin alfa, 1 microgram
(non-ESRD use)   K2 ASC K
BETOS: O1E   Other drugs
Drugs: ARANESP

D **J0882** Injection, darbepoetin alfa, 1 microgram
(for ESRD on dialysis)   K2 ASC K
BETOS: O1E   Other drugs
Other carrier priced
Drugs: ARANESP

D **J0883** Injection, argatroban, 1 mg
(for non-ESRD use)   K2 Ⓐ ASC K
BETOS: O1E   Other drugs
Drugs: ARGATROBAN

D **J0884** Injection, argatroban, 1 mg (for ESRD on
dialysis)   K2 Ⓐ ASC K
BETOS: O1E   Other drugs
Drugs: ARGATROBAN

D **J0885** Injection, epoetin alfa, (for non-ESRD use),
1000 units   K2 ASC K
BETOS: O1E   Other drugs
Drugs: EPOGEN, PROCRIT
Coding Clinic: 2006, Q2; 2006, Q2

D **J0887** Injection, epoetin beta, 1 microgram,
(for ESRD on dialysis)   N1 ASC N
BETOS: O1E   Other drugs
Other carrier priced
Drugs: MIRCERA

D **J0888** Injection, epoetin beta, 1 microgram,
(for Non ESRD use)   K2 ASC K
BETOS: O1E   Other drugs
Other carrier priced
Drugs: MIRCERA

C **J0890** Injection, peginesatide, 0.1 mg (for ESRD on
dialysis)   E1
BETOS: O1E   Other drugs

C **J0894** Injection, decitabine, 1 mg   K2 ASC K
BETOS: O1E   Other drugs
Drugs: DACOGEN, DECITABINE

D **J0895** Injection, deferoxamine mesylate,
500 mg   N1 ASC N
BETOS: O1E   Other drugs
Drugs: DEFEROXAMINE MESYLATE,
DESFERAL

● **C** **J0896** Injection, luspatercept-aamt,
0.25 mg   K2 ASC G
BETOS: O1E   Other drugs
Drugs: REBLOZYL
Coding Clinic: 2020, Q2

C **J0897** Injection, denosumab, 1 mg   K2 ASC K
BETOS: O1E   Other drugs
Drugs: PROLIA, XGEVA
Coding Clinic: 2013, Q1; 2016, Q1

D **J0945** Injection, brompheniramine maleate, per
10 mg   N1 ASC N
BETOS: O1E   Other drugs

D **J1000** Injection, depo-estradiol cypionate, up to
5 mg   N1 ASC N
BETOS: O1E   Other drugs
Drugs: DEPO-ESTRADIOL

D **J1020** Injection, methylprednisolone acetate,
20 mg   N1 ASC N
BETOS: O1E   Other drugs
Drugs: DEPO-MEDROL,
METHYLPREDNISOLONE ACETATE USP
Coding Clinic: 2005, Q3; 2009, Q2; 2018,
Q4; 2019, Q3

D **J1030** Injection, methylprednisolone acetate,
40 mg   N1 ASC N
BETOS: O1E   Other drugs
Drugs: DEPO-MEDROL,
METHYLPREDNISOLONE ACETATE,
METHYLPREDNISOLONE ACETATE USP
Coding Clinic: 2005, Q3; 2009, Q2; 2018,
Q4; 2019, Q3

● New code   ▲ Revised code   **C** Carrier judgment   **D** Special coverage instructions apply
I Not payable by Medicare   **M** Non-covered by Medicare   **S** Non-covered by Medicare statute   AHA Coding Clinic®

D **J1040** Injection, methylprednisolone acetate,
80 mg   N1 ASC N
BETOS: O1E   Other drugs
Drugs: DEPO-MEDROL,
METHYLPREDNISOLONE ACETATE
Coding Clinic: 2009, Q2; 2018, Q4

C **J1050** Injection, medroxyprogesterone acetate,
1 mg   N1 ♀ ASC N
BETOS: O1E   Other drugs
Drugs: DEPO-PROVERA

D **J1071** Injection, testosterone cypionate,
1 mg   N1 ♂ ASC N
BETOS: O1E   Other drugs
Drugs: DEPO-TESTOSTERONE,
TESTOSTERONE CYPIONATE

D **J1094** Injection, dexamethasone acetate,
1 mg   N1 ASC N
BETOS: O1E   Other drugs

D **J1095** Injection, dexamethasone 9 percent,
intraocular, 1 microgram   K2 ASC G
BETOS: O1E   Other drugs
Statute: 1833T
Drugs: DEXYCU (INTRAOCULAR
SUSPENSION)
Coding Clinic: 2019, Q1

C **J1096** Dexamethasone, lacrimal ophthalmic insert,
0.1 mg   K2 ASC G
BETOS: O1E   Other drugs
Drugs: DEXTENZA
Coding Clinic: 2019, Q4

C **J1097** Phenylephrine 10.16 mg/ml and ketorolac
2.88 mg/ml ophthalmic irrigation solution,
1 ml   K2 ASC N
BETOS: O1E   Other drugs
Drugs: OMIDRIA (PHENYLEPHRINE 1% +
KETOROLAC 0.3% IRRIGATION)
Coding Clinic: 2019, Q4

D **J1100** Injection, dexamethasone sodium
phosphate, 1 mg   N1 ASC N
BETOS: O1E   Other drugs
Drugs: DEXAMETHASONE SODIUM
PHOSPHATE

D **J1110** Injection, dihydroergotamine mesylate, per
1 mg   N1 ASC N
BETOS: O1E   Other drugs
Drugs: D.H.E. 45, DIHYDROERGOTAMINE
MESYLATE

D **J1120** Injection, acetazolamide sodium, up to
500 mg   N1 ASC N
BETOS: O1E   Other drugs
Drugs: ACETAZOLAMIDE SODIUM
Coding Clinic: 2005, Q4

C **J1130** Injection, diclofenac sodium,
0.5 mg   N1 Ⓐ ASC N
BETOS: O1E   Other drugs
Coding Clinic: 2017, Q1

D **J1160** Injection, digoxin, up to 0.5 mg   N1 ASC N
BETOS: O1E   Other drugs
Drugs: DIGOXIN, LANOXIN

D **J1162** Injection, digoxin immune FAB (Ovine), per
vial   K2 ASC K
BETOS: O1E   Other drugs
Drugs: DIGIFAB

D **J1165** Injection, phenytoin sodium,
per 50 mg   N1 ASC N
BETOS: O1E   Other drugs
Drugs: PHENYTOIN SODIUM

D **J1170** Injection, hydromorphone, up to
4 mg   N1 ASC N
BETOS: O1E   Other drugs
Drugs: DILAUDID, DILAUDID (PFSYR),
HYDROMORPHONE, HYDROMORPHONE
HCL, HYDROMORPHONE
HYDROCHLORIDE

D **J1180** Injection, dyphylline, up to 500 mg   K5 ASC E2
BETOS: O1E   Other drugs

D **J1190** Injection, dexrazoxane hydrochloride, per
250 mg   K2 ASC K
BETOS: O1E   Other drugs
Drugs: DEXRAZOXANE, TOTECT,
ZINECARD

D **J1200** Injection, diphenhydramine HCl,
up to 50 mg   N1 ASC N
BETOS: O1E   Other drugs
Drugs: BENADRYL, DIPHENHYDRAMINE
HCL
Coding Clinic: 2002, Q1

● **C** **J1201** Injection, cetirizine hydrochloride,
0.5 mg   K2 ASC G
BETOS: O1E   Other drugs
Drugs: QUZYTTIR
Coding Clinic: 2020, Q2

D **J1205** Injection, chlorothiazide sodium,
per 500 mg   N1 ASC N
BETOS: O1E   Other drugs
Drugs: CHLOROTHIAZIDE SODIUM,
DIURIL IV

D **J1212** Injection, DMSO, dimethyl sulfoxide,
50%, 50 ml   K2 ASC K
BETOS: O1E   Other drugs
Drugs: RIMSO-50

D **J1230** Injection, methadone HCl, up to
10 mg   N1 ASC N
BETOS: O1E   Other drugs
Drugs: METHADONE HCL

D **J1240** Injection, dimenhydrinate, up to
50 mg   N1 ASC N
BETOS: O1E   Other drugs
Drugs: DIMENHYDRINATE

D **J1245** Injection, dipyridamole, per 10 mg   N1 ASC N
BETOS: O1E   Other drugs
Drugs: DIPYRIDAMOLE

♂ Male only   ♀ Female only   Ⓐ Age   A2 - Z3 = ASC Payment indicator   A - Y = APC Status indicator
ASC = ASC Approved Procedure   **DME** Paid under the DME fee schedule   **MIPS** MIPS code

D J1250 Injection, Dobutamine hydrochloride, per 250 mg   N1 ASC N
BETOS: O1E   Other drugs
Drugs: DOBUTAMINE HCL

D J1260 Injection, dolasetron mesylate, 10 mg   N1 ASC N
BETOS: O1D   Chemotherapy

C J1265 Injection, dopamine HCl, 40 mg   N1 ASC N
BETOS: O1E   Other drugs
Drugs: DOPAMINE, DOPAMINE 200MG/5ML, DOPAMINE HCL 400MGIN 5% DEXTROSE   LIFECARE 250ML, DOPAMINE HCL 800MGIN 5% DEXTROSE LIFECARE 250ML, DOPAMINE IN D5W
Coding Clinic: 2005, Q4

C J1267 Injection, doripenem, 10 mg   N1 ASC N
BETOS: O1E   Other drugs
Coding Clinic: 2008, Q4

C J1270 Injection, doxercalciferol, 1 mcg   N1 ASC N
BETOS: O1E   Other drugs
Drugs: DOXERCALCIFEROL, HECTOROL
Coding Clinic: 2002, Q1

C J1290 Injection, ecallantide, 1 mg   K2 ASC K
BETOS: O1E   Other drugs
Drugs: KALBITOR®
Coding Clinic: 2011, Q1

C J1300 Injection, eculizumab, 10 mg   K2 ASC K
BETOS: O1E   Other drugs
Drugs: SOLIRIS
Coding Clinic: 2008, Q1

C J1301 Injection, edaravone, 1 mg   K2 ASC K
BETOS: O1E   Other drugs
Drugs: RADICAVA
Coding Clinic: 2019, Q1

C J1303 Injection, ravulizumab-cwvz, 10 mg   K2 ASC G
BETOS: O1E   Other drugs
Drugs: ULTOMIRIS
Coding Clinic: 2019, Q4

D J1320 Injection, amitriptyline HCl, up to 20 mg   N1 ASC N
BETOS: O1E   Other drugs

C J1322 Injection, elosulfase alfa, 1 mg   K2 ASC K
BETOS: O1E   Other drugs
Drugs: VIMIZIM

C J1324 Injection, enfuvirtide, 1 mg   K5 ASC E2
BETOS: O1E   Other drugs

D J1325 Injection, epoprostenol, 0.5 mg   N1 ASC N
BETOS: O1E   Other drugs
Drugs: EPOPROSTENOL, EPOPROSTENOL (VELETRI), FLOLAN

D J1327 Injection, eptifibatide, 5 mg   N1 ASC N
BETOS: O1E   Other drugs

D J1330 Injection, ergonovine maleate, up to 0.2 mg   K5 ♀ ASC E2
BETOS: O1E   Other drugs

C J1335 Injection, ertapenem sodium, 500 mg   N1 ASC N
BETOS: O1E   Other drugs
Drugs: ERTAPENEM, INVANZ

D J1364 Injection, erythromycin lactobionate, per 500 mg   K2 ASC K
BETOS: O1E   Other drugs
Drugs: ERYTHROMYCIN, ERYTHROMYCIN LACTOBIONATE

D J1380 Injection, estradiol valerate, up to 10 mg   N1 ASC N
BETOS: O1E   Other drugs
Drugs: DELESTROGEN, ESTRADIOL VALERATE
Coding Clinic: 2011, Q1

D J1410 Injection, estrogen conjugated, per 25 mg   K2 ASC K
BETOS: O1E   Other drugs
Drugs: PREMARIN

C J1428 Injection, eteplirsen, 10 mg   N1 ASC N
BETOS: O1E   Other drugs

● **C J1429** Injection, golodirsen, 10 mg   K2 ASC G
BETOS: O1E   Other drugs
Drugs: VYONDYS 53
Coding Clinic: 2020, Q2

D J1430 Injection, ethanolamine oleate, 100 mg   K2 ASC K
BETOS: O1E   Other drugs
Drugs: ETHANOLAMINE OLEATE

D J1435 Injection, estrone, per 1 mg   K5 ♀ ASC E2
BETOS: O1E   Other drugs

D J1436 Injection, etidronate disodium, per 300 mg   E1
BETOS: O1E   Other drugs

● **C J1437** Injection, ferric derisomaltose, 10 mg   K2 ASC G
BETOS: O1E   Other drugs
Drugs: MONOFERRIC

D J1438 Injection, etanercept, 25 mg (code may be used for Medicare when drug administered under the direct supervision of a physician, not for use when drug is self administered)   K2 ASC K
BETOS: O1E   Other drugs
Drugs: ENBREL, ENBREL (ETANERCEPT)

C J1439 Injection, ferric carboxymaltose, 1 mg   K2 ASC K
BETOS: O1E   Other drugs
Drugs: INJECTAFER

D J1442 Injection, filgrastim (G-CSF), excludes biosimilars, 1 microgram   K2 ASC K
BETOS: O1E   Other drugs
Drugs: NEUPOGEN
Coding Clinic: 2014, Q1

C J1443 Injection, ferric pyrophosphate citrate solution, 0.1 mg of iron   K5 ASC E2

● New code   ▲ Revised code   **C** Carrier judgment   **D** Special coverage instructions apply
I Not payable by Medicare   **M** Non-covered by Medicare   **S** Non-covered by Medicare statute   *AHA Coding Clinic®*

BETOS: O1E   Other drugs
Coding Clinic: 2016, Q1

C **J1444** Injection, ferric pyrophosphate citrate powder, 0.1 mg of iron   K5 ASC E2
BETOS: O1E   Other drugs
Coding Clinic: 2019, Q3

D **J1447** Injection, TBO-filgrastim, 1 microgram   K2 ASC K
BETOS: O1E   Other drugs
Drugs: GRANIX
Coding Clinic: 2016, Q1

D **J1450** Injection fluconazole, 200 mg   N1 ASC N
BETOS: O1E   Other drugs
Drugs: FLUCONAZOLE IN SODIUM CHLORIDE, FLUCONAZOLE INJECTION

D **J1451** Injection, fomepizole, 15 mg   K2 ASC K
BETOS: O1E   Other drugs
Drugs: FOMEPIZOLE

D **J1452** Injection, fomivirsen sodium, intraocular, 1.65 mg   K5 ASC E2
BETOS: O1E   Other drugs

C **J1453** Injection, fosaprepitant, 1 mg   K2 ASC K
BETOS: O1E   Other drugs
Drugs: EMEND FOR INJECTION 150MG, FOSAPREPITANT FOR INJECTION 150 MG
Coding Clinic: 2008, Q4

D **J1454** Injection, fosnetupitant 235 mg and palonosetron 0.25 mg   K2 ASC K
BETOS: O1E   Other drugs
Drugs: AKYNZEO (IV INJECTION)
Coding Clinic: 2018, Q4; 2019, Q1

D **J1455** Injection, foscarnet sodium, per 1000 mg   K2 ASC K
BETOS: O1E   Other drugs
Drugs: FOSCAVIR

C **J1457** Injection, gallium nitrate, 1 mg   K5 ASC E2
BETOS: O1E   Other drugs
Coding Clinic: 2005, Q2

C **J1458** Injection, galsulfase, 1 mg   K2 ASC K
BETOS: O1E   Other drugs
Drugs: NAGLAZYME

C **J1459** Injection, immune globulin (Privigen), intravenous, non-lyophilized (e.g., liquid), 500 mg   K2 ASC K
BETOS: O1E   Other drugs
Drugs: PRIVIGEN
Coding Clinic: 2008, Q4

D **J1460** Injection, gamma globulin, intramuscular, 1 cc   K2 ASC K
BETOS: O1E   Other drugs
Drugs: GAMASTAN, GAMASTAN S/D
Coding Clinic: 2011, Q1

C **J1555** Injection, immune globulin (Cuvitru), 100 mg   K2 ASC K

BETOS: D1G   Drugs Administered through DME
Drugs: CUVITRU
Coding Clinic: 2018, Q1

C **J1556** Injection, immune globulin (bivigam), 500 mg   K2 ASC K
BETOS: O1E   Other drugs
Drugs: BIVIGAM
Coding Clinic: 2013, Q4

C **J1557** Injection, immune globulin, (Gammaplex), intravenous, non-lyophilized (e.g., liquid), 500 mg   K2 ASC K
BETOS: O1E   Other drugs
Drugs: GAMMAPLEX

● **C** **J1558** Injection, immune globulin (xembify), 100 mg   K2 ASC K
BETOS: O1E   Other drugs
Drugs: XEMBIFY
Coding Clinic: 2020, Q2

C **J1559** Injection, immune globulin (Hizentra), 100 mg   K2 ASC K
BETOS: O1E   Other drugs
Drugs: HIZENTRA
Coding Clinic: 2011, Q1

D **J1560** Injection, gamma globulin, intramuscular, over 10 cc   K2 ASC K
BETOS: O1E   Other drugs
Drugs: GAMASTAN, GAMASTAN S/D

D **J1561** Injection, immune globulin, (Gamunex-C/Gammaked), non-lyophilized (e.g., liquid), 500 mg   K2 ASC K
BETOS: O1E   Other drugs
Drugs: GAMMAKED, GAMUNEX-C
Coding Clinic: 2002, Q2; 2007, Q4; 2008, Q1; 2012, Q1

C **J1562** Injection, immune globulin (Vivaglobin), 100 mg   K5 ASC E2
BETOS: O1E   Other drugs

D **J1566** Injection, immune globulin, intravenous, lyophilized (e.g., powder), not otherwise specified, 500 mg   K2 ASC K
BETOS: O1E   Other drugs
Drugs: CARIMUNE NF, GAMMAGARD S/D
Coding Clinic: 2006, Q1

C **J1568** Injection, immune globulin, (Octagam), intravenous, non-lyophilized (e.g., liquid), 500 mg   K2 ASC K
BETOS: O1E   Other drugs
Drugs: OCTAGAM
Coding Clinic: 2007, Q4; 2008, Q1

D **J1569** Injection, immune globulin, (Gammagard liquid), non-lyophilized, (e.g., liquid), 500 mg   K2 ASC K
BETOS: O1E   Other drugs
Drugs: GAMMAGARD LIQUID
Coding Clinic: 2007, Q4; 2008, Q1

♂ Male only   ♀ Female only   **A** Age   A2 - Z3 = ASC Payment indicator   A - Y = APC Status indicator
ASC = ASC Approved Procedure   **DME** Paid under the DME fee schedule   **MIPS** MIPS code

D J1570 Injection, ganciclovir sodium, 500 mg   N1 ASC N
BETOS: O1E   Other drugs
Drugs: CYTOVENE, GANCICLOVIR

D J1571 Injection, Hepatitis B immune globulin (HepaGam B), intramuscular, 0.5 ml   K2 ASC K
BETOS: O1E   Other drugs
Drugs: CBI HEPAGAM B 1 ML, CBI HEPAGAM B 5 ML, HEPAGAM B
Coding Clinic: 2007, Q4; 2008, Q1; 2008, Q3

D J1572 Injection, immune globulin, (Flebogamma/Flebogamma Dif), intravenous, non-lyophilized (e.g., liquid), 500 mg   K2 ASC K
BETOS: O1E   Other drugs
Drugs: FLEBOGAMMA 10% DIF, FLEBOGAMMA DIF
Coding Clinic: 2007, Q4; 2008, Q1

C J1573 Injection, Hepatitis B immune globulin (HepaGam B), intravenous, 0.5 ml K2 ASC K
BETOS: O1E   Other drugs
Drugs: CBI HEPAGAM B 1 ML, CBI HEPAGAM B 5 ML, HEPAGAM B
Coding Clinic: 2008, Q1; 2008, Q3

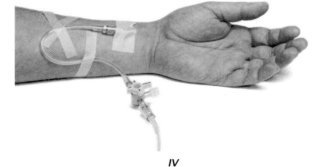

IV

C J1575 Injection, immune globulin/hyaluronidase, (HYQVIA), 100 mg immuneglobulin K2 ASC K
BETOS: O1E   Other drugs
Drugs: HYQVIA
Coding Clinic: 2016, Q1

D J1580 Injection, garamycin, gentamicin, up to 80 mg   N1 ASC N
BETOS: O1E   Other drugs
Drugs: GENTAMICIN SULFATE

D J1595 Injection, glatiramer acetate, 20 mg K2 ASC K
BETOS: O1E   Other drugs
Drugs: COPAXONE

C J1599 Injection, immune globulin, intravenous, non-lyophilized (e.g., liquid), not otherwise specified, 500 mg   N1 ASC N
BETOS: O1E   Other drugs
Coding Clinic: 2011, Q1

D J1600 Injection, gold sodium thiomalate, up to 50 mg   K5 ASC E2
BETOS: O1E   Other drugs

C J1602 Injection, golimumab, 1 mg, for intravenous use   K2 ASC K
BETOS: O1E   Other drugs
Drugs: SIMPONI ARIA
Coding Clinic: 2014, Q1

D J1610 Injection, glucagon hydrochloride, per 1 mg   K2 ASC K
BETOS: O1E   Other drugs
Drugs: GLUCAGEN DIAGNOSTIC KIT, GLUCAGEN(R), GLUCAGON EMERGENCY, GLUCAGON HYDROCHLORIDE, GLUCAGON HYDROCHLORIDE KIT

D J1620 Injection, gonadorelin hydrochloride, per 100 mcg   K5 ASC E2
BETOS: O1E   Other drugs

D J1626 Injection, granisetron hydrochloride, 100 mcg   N1 ASC N
BETOS: O1E   Other drugs
Drugs: GRANISETRON HCL

C J1627 Injection, granisetron, extended-release, 0.1 mg   N1 ASC N
BETOS: O1E   Other drugs
Drugs: SUSTOL

C J1628 Injection, guselkumab, 1 mg   K2 ASC K
BETOS: O1E   Other drugs
Drugs: TREMFYA
Coding Clinic: 2019, Q1

D J1630 Injection, haloperidol, up to 5 mg   N1 ASC N
BETOS: O1E   Other drugs
Drugs: HALDOL, HALOPERIDOL LACTATE

D J1631 Injection, haloperidol decanoate, per 50 mg   N1 ASC N
BETOS: O1E   Other drugs
Drugs: HALDOL DECANOATE, HALOPERIDOL DECANOATE

● **C J1632** Injection, brexanolone, 1 mg   K2 ASC G
BETOS: O1E   Other drugs
Drugs: ZULRESSO

D J1640 Injection, hemin, 1 mg   K2 ASC K
BETOS: O1E   Other drugs
Drugs: PANHEMATIN

D J1642 Injection, heparin sodium, (heparin lock flush), per 10 units   N1 ASC N
BETOS: O1E   Other drugs
Drugs: HEPARIN (PORCINE) LOCK FLUSH, HEPARIN LOCK FLUSH
Coding Clinic: 2005, Q4

D J1644 Injection, heparin sodium, per 1000 units   N1 ASC N
BETOS: O1E   Other drugs
Drugs: HEPARIN (PORCINE) IN 0.45% NACL, HEPARIN (PORCINE) IN D5W, HEPARIN (PORCINE) IN NACL, HEPARIN SODIUM, HEPARIN SODIUM (PORCINE), HEPARIN SODIUM IN NACL, HEPARIN SODIUM/SODIUM CHL

● New code   ▲ Revised code   **C** Carrier judgment   **D** Special coverage instructions apply
I Not payable by Medicare   **M** Non-covered by Medicare   **S** Non-covered by Medicare statute   AHA Coding Clinic®

D **J1645** Injection, dalteparin sodium, per
2500 IU   N1 ASC N
BETOS: O1E   Other drugs
Drugs: FRAGMIN

C **J1650** Injection, enoxaparin sodium,
10 mg   N1 ASC N
BETOS: O1E   Other drugs
Drugs: ENOXAPARIN SODIUM, LOVENOX

D **J1652** Injection, fondaparinux sodium,
0.5 mg   N1 ASC N
BETOS: O1E   Other drugs
Drugs: ARIXTRA, FONDAPARINUX
SODIUM

C **J1655** Injection, tinzaparin sodium,
1000 IU   N1 ASC N
BETOS: O1E   Other drugs
Coding Clinic: 2002, Q1

D **J1670** Injection, tetanus immune globulin, human,
up to 250 units   K2 ASC K
BETOS: O1E   Other drugs
Drugs: HYPERTET S/D

D **J1675** Injection, histrelin acetate, 10 micrograms   B
BETOS: O1E   Other drugs

D **J1700** Injection, hydrocortisone acetate, up to
25 mg   N1 ASC N
BETOS: O1E   Other drugs

D **J1710** Injection, hydrocortisone sodium phosphate,
up to 50 mg   N1 ASC N
BETOS: O1E   Other drugs

D **J1720** Injection, hydrocortisone sodium succinate,
up to 100 mg   N1 ASC N
BETOS: O1E   Other drugs
Drugs: SOLU-CORTEF, SOLU-CORTEF
500MG 4ML

C **J1726** Injection, hydroxyprogesterone caproate,
(makena), 10 mg   K2 ♀ ASC K
BETOS: O1E   Other drugs
Drugs: HYDROXYPROGESTERONE
CAPROATE, MAKENA, MAKENA AUTO
INJECTOR

C **J1729** Injection, hydroxyprogesterone caproate, not
otherwise specified, 10 mg   K2 ♀ ASC K
BETOS: O1E   Other drugs

D **J1730** Injection, diazoxide, up to 300 mg K5 ASC E2
BETOS: O1E   Other drugs

● **C** **J1738** Injection, meloxicam, 1 mg   K2 ASC G
BETOS: O1E   Other drugs
Drugs: ANJESO

C **J1740** Injection, ibandronate sodium,
1 mg   K2 ASC K
BETOS: O1E   Other drugs
Drugs: BONIVA, IBANDRONATE SODIUM
Coding Clinic: 2006, Q4

C **J1741** Injection, ibuprofen, 100 mg   N1 ASC N
BETOS: O1E   Other drugs

D **J1742** Injection, ibutilide fumarate, 1 mg K2 ASC K
BETOS: O1E   Other drugs
Drugs: CORVERT, IBUTILIDE FUMARATE

C **J1743** Injection, idursulfase, 1 mg   N1 ASC N
BETOS: O1E   Other drugs
Drugs: ELAPRASE
Coding Clinic: 2008, Q1

C **J1744** Injection, icatibant, 1 mg   K2 ASC K
BETOS: O1E   Other drugs
Drugs: ICATIBANT

D **J1745** Injection, infliximab, excludes biosimilar,
10 mg   K2 ASC K MIPS
BETOS: O1E   Other drugs
Drugs: REMICADE

C **J1746** Injection, ibalizumab-uiyk, 10 mg   K2 ASC K
BETOS: O1E   Other drugs
Drugs: TROGARZO
Coding Clinic: 2019, Q1

D **J1750** Injection, iron dextran, 50 mg   K2 ASC K
BETOS: O1E   Other drugs
Drugs: INFED

C **J1756** Injection, iron sucrose, 1 mg   N1 ASC N
BETOS: O1E   Other drugs
Drugs: VENOFER

D **J1786** Injection, imiglucerase, 10 units   K2 ASC K
BETOS: O1E   Other drugs
Drugs: CEREZYME
Coding Clinic: 2011, Q1

D **J1790** Injection, droperidol, up to 5 mg   N1 ASC N
BETOS: O1E   Other drugs

D **J1800** Injection, propranolol HCl, up to
1 mg   N1 ASC N
BETOS: O1E   Other drugs
Drugs: PROPRANOLOL, PROPRANOLOL
HCL
Coding Clinic: 2005, Q4

D **J1810** Injection, droperidol and fentanyl citrate, up
to 2 ml ampule   E1
BETOS: O1E   Other drugs
Coding Clinic: 2002, Q2

D **J1815** Injection, insulin, per 5 units   N1 ASC N
BETOS: O1E   Other drugs
Drugs: FIASP, HUMALOG, HUMALOG
JUNIOR KWIKPEN, HUMALOG KWIKPEN,
HUMALOG MIX 50/50, HUMALOG MIX
75/25, HUMULIN 70/30, HUMULIN 70/30
KWIKPEN, HUMULIN N, HUMULIN N
(NPH), HUMULIN N KWIKPEN, HUMULIN
R, HUMULIN R U-500, INSULIN ASPART,
INSULIN ASPART FLEXPEN, INSULIN
ASPART PENFILL, INSULIN ASPART
PROTAMINE-INSULIN ASPART, INSULIN
ASPART PROTAMINE-INSULIN ASPART
FLEXPEN, INSULIN LISPRO, INSULIN
LISPRO JUNIOR KWIKPEN, INSULIN
LISPRO KWIKPEN, INSULIN LISPRO
PROTAMINE/INS LISPRO 75/25 KWIKPEN,

NOVOLIN 70/30, NOVOLIN N, NOVOLIN
N (NPH), NOVOLIN R, NOVOLOG,
NOVOLOG FLEXPEN, NOVOLOG MIX
70/30, NOVOLOG MIX 70/30 FLEXPEN,
NOVOLOG PENFILL
Coding Clinic: 2005, Q4

C J1817 Insulin for administration through DME
(i.e., insulin pump) per 50 units   N1 ASC N
BETOS: D1G   Drugs Administered through
DME
Drugs: HUMALOG, HUMALOG KWIKPEN,
HUMULIN R, INSULIN LISPRO,
INSULIN LISPRO JUNIOR KWIKPEN,
INSULIN LISPRO KWIKPEN, NOVOLIN
R, NOVOLOG, NOVOLOG FLEXPEN,
NOVOLOG PENFILL
Coding Clinic: 2005, Q4

● **C J1823** Injection, inebilizumab-cdon,
1 mg   K2 Ⓐ ASC K
BETOS: O1E   Other drugs
Drugs: UPLIZNA

C J1826 Injection, interferon beta-1a,
30 mcg   K2 ASC K
BETOS: O1E   Other drugs
Service not separately priced by Part B
Coding Clinic: 2011, Q2; 2011, Q2; 2011,
Q1; 2014, Q4

D J1830 Injection' interferon beta-1b, 0.25 mg (code
may be used for Medicare when drug
administered under the direct supervision
of a physician, not for use when drug is self
administered)   K2 ASC K
BETOS: O1E   Other drugs
Drugs: BETASERON

C J1833 Injection, isavuconazonium, 1 mg   K2 ASC K
BETOS: O1E   Other drugs
Drugs: CRESEMBA INJECTION
Coding Clinic: 2016, Q1

C J1835 Injection, itraconazole, 50 mg   K5 ASC E2
BETOS: O1E   Other drugs
Coding Clinic: 2002, Q1

D J1840 Injection, kanamycin sulfate,
up to 500 mg   N1 ASC N
BETOS: O1E   Other drugs

D J1850 Injection, kanamycin sulfate,
up to 75 mg   K5 ASC E2
BETOS: O1E   Other drugs

D J1885 Injection, ketorolac tromethamine,
per 15 mg   N1 ASC N
BETOS: O1E   Other drugs
Drugs: KETOROLAC TROMETHAMINE

D J1890 Injection, cephalothin sodium,
up to 1 gram   N1 ASC N
BETOS: O1E   Other drugs

C J1930 Injection, lanreotide, 1 mg   K2 ASC K
BETOS: O1E   Other drugs
Drugs: SOMATULINE DEPOT
Coding Clinic: 2008, Q4

C J1931 Injection, laronidase, 0.1 mg   K2 ASC K
BETOS: O1E   Other drugs
Drugs: ALDURAZYME
Coding Clinic: 2005, Q2; 2005, Q1

D J1940 Injection, furosemide, up to 20 mg N1 ASC N
BETOS: O1E   Other drugs
Drugs: FUROSEMIDE
Coding Clinic: 2005, Q4

C J1943 Injection, aripiprazole lauroxil, (ARISTADA
INITIO®), 1 mg   K2 ASC G
BETOS: O1E   Other drugs
Drugs: ARISTADA INITIO
Coding Clinic: 2019, Q4

C J1944 Injection, aripiprazole lauroxil,
(ARISTADA®), 1 mg   K2 ASC K
BETOS: O1E   Other drugs
Drugs: ARISTADA
Coding Clinic: 2019, Q4

D J1945 Injection, lepirudin, 50 mg   K5 ASC E2
BETOS: O1E   Other drugs

D J1950 Injection, leuprolide acetate (for depot
suspension), per 3.75 mg   K2 ASC K
BETOS: O1E   Other drugs
Drugs: LUPRON DEPOT 3-MONTH,
11.25MG, LUPRON DEPOT 3.75MG,
LUPRON DEPOT-PED 3-MONTH, 30 MG,
LUPRON DEPOT-PED 11.25MG, LUPRON
DEPOT-PED 3-MONTH, 11.25MG
Coding Clinic: 2019, Q2

C J1953 Injection, levetiracetam, 10 mg   N1 ASC N
BETOS: O1E   Other drugs
Drugs: LEVETIRACETAM,
LEVETIRACETAM (KEPPRA)
Coding Clinic: 2008, Q4

D J1955 Injection, levocarnitine, per 1 gm   B
BETOS: O1E   Other drugs
Drugs: CARNITOR

D J1956 Injection, levofloxacin, 250 mg   N1 ASC N
BETOS: O1E   Other drugs
Drugs: LEVOFLOXACIN

D J1960 Injection, levorphanol tartrate, up
to 2 mg   N1 ASC N
BETOS: O1E   Other drugs

D J1980 Injection, hyoscyamine sulfate,
up to 0.25 mg   N1 ASC N
BETOS: O1E   Other drugs
Drugs: LEVSIN

D J1990 Injection, chlordiazepoxide HCl, up to
100 mg   N1 ASC N
BETOS: O1E   Other drugs

D J2001 Injection, lidocaine HCl for intravenous
infusion, 10 mg   N1 ASC N
BETOS: O1E   Other drugs
Drugs: LIDOCAINE IN D5W

● New code   ▲ Revised code   **C** Carrier judgment   **D** Special coverage instructions apply
I Not payable by Medicare   **M** Non-covered by Medicare   **S** Non-covered by Medicare statute   AHA Coding Clinic®

[D] **J2010** Injection, lincomycin HCl, up to
300 mg　　　　　　　　N1 ASC N
BETOS: O1E　Other drugs
Drugs: LINCOCIN, LINCOMYCIN

[C] **J2020** Injection, linezolid, 200 mg　　N1 ASC N
BETOS: O1E　Other drugs
Drugs: LINEZOLID, ZYVOX
Coding Clinic: 2002, Q2; 2002, Q1

[D] **J2060** Injection, lorazepam, 2 mg　　N1 ASC N
BETOS: O1E　Other drugs
Drugs: ATIVAN, LORAZEPAM

[C] **J2062** Loxapine for inhalation, 1 mg　　K5 ASC E2
Coding Clinic: 2019, Q1

[D] **J2150** Injection, mannitol, 25% in 50 ml　N1 ASC N
BETOS: O1E　Other drugs
Drugs: MANNITOL

[C] **J2170** Injection, mecasermin, 1 mg　　N1 ASC N
BETOS: O1E　Other drugs

[D] **J2175** Injection, meperidine hydrochloride, per
100 mg　　　　　　　　N1 ASC N
BETOS: O1E　Other drugs
Drugs: DEMEROL, MEPERIDINE HCL

[D] **J2180** Injection, meperidine and promethazine HCl,
up to 50 mg　　　　　　N1 ASC N
BETOS: O1E　Other drugs

[C] **J2182** Injection, mepolizumab, 1 mg　　K2 [A] ASC K
BETOS: O1E　Other drugs
Drugs: NUCALA

[C] **J2185** Injection, meropenem, 100 mg　N1 ASC N
BETOS: O1E　Other drugs
Drugs: MEROPENEM, MERREM
Coding Clinic: 2005, Q2

[C] **J2186** Injection, meropenem and vaborbactam,
10mg/10mg (20mg)　　　K2 ASC K
BETOS: O1E　Other drugs
Drugs: VABOMERE (MEROPENEM-
VABORBACTAM)
Coding Clinic: 2019, Q1

[D] **J2210** Injection, methylergonovine maleate, up to
0.2 mg　　　　　　　　N1 ASC N
BETOS: O1E　Other drugs
Drugs: METHYLERGONOVINE MALEATE

[C] **J2212** Injection, methylnaltrexone, 0.1 mg　N1 ASC N
BETOS: O1E　Other drugs

[C] **J2248** Injection, micafungin sodium, 1 mg　K2 ASC K
BETOS: O1E　Other drugs
Drugs: MICAFUNGIN SODIUM
(MYCAMINE)
Coding Clinic: 2006, Q4

[D] **J2250** Injection, midazolam hydrochloride,
per 1 mg　　　　　　　N1 ASC N
BETOS: O1E　Other drugs
Drugs: MIDAZOLAM HCL

[D] **J2260** Injection, milrinone lactate, 5 mg　N1 ASC N
BETOS: O1E　Other drugs
Drugs: MILRINONE IN DEXTROSE,
MILRINONE LACTATE

[C] **J2265** Injection, minocycline hydrochloride,
1 mg　　　　　　　　　K2 ASC K
BETOS: O1E　Other drugs
Drugs: MINOCIN

[D] **J2270** Injection, morphine sulfate, up
to 10 mg　　　　　　　N1 ASC N
BETOS: O1E　Other drugs
Drugs: MORPHINE SULFATE
Coding Clinic: 2005, Q4

[D] **J2274** Injection, morphine sulfate, preservative-free
for epidural or intrathecal use,
10 mg　　　　　　　　N1 ASC N
BETOS: O1E　Other drugs
Drugs: DURAMORPH, INFUMORPH 200,
INFUMORPH 500, MITIGO, MORPHINE
SULFATE

[D] **J2278** Injection, ziconotide, 1 microgram　K2 ASC K
BETOS: O1E　Other drugs
Drugs: PRIALT

[C] **J2280** Injection, moxifloxacin, 100 mg　N1 ASC N
BETOS: O1E　Other drugs
Drugs: MOXIFLOXACIN HCL
Coding Clinic: 2005, Q2

[D] **J2300** Injection, nalbuphine hydrochloride, per
10 mg　　　　　　　　N1 ASC N
BETOS: O1E　Other drugs
Drugs: NALBUPHINE HCL

[D] **J2310** Injection, naloxone hydrochloride,
per 1 mg　　　　　　　N1 ASC N
BETOS: O1E　Other drugs
Drugs: NALOXONE HCL, NALOXONE
HYDROCHLORIDE

[C] **J2315** Injection, naltrexone, depot form,
1 mg　　　　　　　　　K2 ASC K
BETOS: O1E　Other drugs
Drugs: VIVITROL

[D] **J2320** Injection, nandrolone decanoate, up to
50 mg　　　　　　　　N1 ASC N
BETOS: O1E　Other drugs
Coding Clinic: 2011, Q1

[C] **J2323** Injection, natalizumab, 1 mg　　K2 ASC K
BETOS: O1E　Other drugs
Drugs: TYSABRI
Coding Clinic: 2008, Q1

[D] **J2325** Injection, nesiritide, 0.1 mg　　　　E1
BETOS: O1E　Other drugs

[C] **J2326** Injection, nusinersen, 0.1 mg　　K2 ASC K
BETOS: O1E　Other drugs
Drugs: SPINRAZA
Coding Clinic: 2020, Q1

♂ Male only　　♀ Female only　　[A] Age　　A2 - Z3 = ASC Payment indicator　　A - Y = APC Status indicator
ASC = ASC Approved Procedure　　**DME** Paid under the DME fee schedule　　**MIPS** MIPS code

C J2350 Injection, ocrelizumab, 1 mg   K2 ASC K
BETOS: O1E   Other drugs
Drugs: OCREVUS

C J2353 Injection, octreotide, depot form for intramuscular injection, 1 mg   K2 ASC K
BETOS: O1E   Other drugs
Drugs: SANDOSTATIN LAR DEPOT

C J2354 Injection, octreotide, non-depot form for subcutaneous or intravenous injection, 25 mcg   N1 ASC N
BETOS: O1E   Other drugs
Drugs: OCTREOTIDE ACETATE, SANDOSTATIN

D J2355 Injection, oprelvekin, 5 mg   N1 ASC N
BETOS: O1E   Other drugs
Coding Clinic: 2005, Q2

C J2357 Injection, omalizumab, 5 mg   K2 ASC K
BETOS: O1E   Other drugs
Drugs: XOLAIR
Coding Clinic: 2005, Q2

C J2358 Injection, olanzapine, long-acting, 1 mg   K2 ASC K
BETOS: O1E   Other drugs
Drugs: ZYPREXA RELPREVV
Coding Clinic: 2011, Q1

D J2360 Injection, orphenadrine citrate, up to 60 mg   N1 ASC N
BETOS: O1E   Other drugs
Drugs: ORPHENADRINE CITRATE, ORPHENADRINE CITRATE INJECTION

D J2370 Injection, phenylephrine HCl, up to 1 ml   N1 ASC N
BETOS: O1E   Other drugs

D J2400 Injection, chloroprocaine hydrochloride, per 30 ml   N1 ASC N
BETOS: O1E   Other drugs
Drugs: CHLOROPROCAINE HCL, CLOROTEKAL, NESACAINE, NESACAINE-MPF

D J2405 Injection, ondansetron hydrochloride, per 1 mg   N1 ASC N
BETOS: O1E   Other drugs
Drugs: ONDANSETRON HCL, ZOFRAN

D J2407 Injection, oritavancin, 10 mg   K2 ASC K
BETOS: O1E   Other drugs
Drugs: ORBACTIV
Coding Clinic: 2016, Q1

D J2410 Injection, oxymorphone HCl, up to 1 mg   N1 ASC N
BETOS: O1E   Other drugs

C J2425 Injection, palifermin, 50 micrograms   K2 ASC K
BETOS: O1E   Other drugs
Drugs: KEPIVANCE, KEPIVANCE/PALIFERMIN

C J2426 Injection, paliperidone palmitate extended release, 1 mg   K2 ASC K
BETOS: O1E   Other drugs
Drugs: INVEGA SUSTENNA
Coding Clinic: 2011, Q1

D J2430 Injection, pamidronate disodium, per 30 mg   N1 ASC N
BETOS: O1E   Other drugs
Drugs: PAMIDRONATE DISODIUM

D J2440 Injection, papaverine HCl, up to 60 mg   N1 ASC N
BETOS: O1E   Other drugs

D J2460 Injection, oxytetracycline HCl, up to 50 mg   K5 ASC E2
BETOS: O1E   Other drugs

C J2469 Injection, palonosetron HCl, 25 mcg   N1 ASC N
BETOS: O1E   Other drugs
Drugs: ALOXI, PALONOSETRON
Coding Clinic: 2005, Q2; 2005, Q1

D J2501 Injection, paricalcitol, 1 mcg   N1 ASC N
BETOS: O1E   Other drugs
Drugs: PARICALCITOL, ZEMPLAR

C J2502 Injection, pasireotide long acting, 1 mg   K2 ASC K
BETOS: O1E   Other drugs
Drugs: SIGNIFOR LAR
Coding Clinic: 2016, Q1

C J2503 Injection, pegaptanib sodium, 0.3 mg   N1 ASC N
BETOS: O1E   Other drugs
Drugs: MACUGEN

D J2504 Injection, pegademase bovine, 25 IU   K2 ASC K
BETOS: O1E   Other drugs
Drugs: ADAGEN

C J2505 Injection, pegfilgrastim, 6 mg   K2 ASC K
BETOS: O1E   Other drugs
Drugs: NEULASTA, NEULASTA DELIVERY KIT
Coding Clinic: 2009, Q3

C J2507 Injection, pegloticase, 1 mg   K2 ASC K
BETOS: O1E   Other drugs
Drugs: KRYSTEXXA

D J2510 Injection, penicillin G procaine, aqueous, up to 600,000 units   N1 ASC N
BETOS: O1E   Other drugs
Drugs: PENICILLIN G PROCAINE

D J2513 Injection, pentastarch, 10% solution, 100 ml   K5 ASC E2
BETOS: O1E   Other drugs

D J2515 Injection, pentobarbital sodium, per 50 mg   K2 ASC K
BETOS: O1E   Other drugs
Drugs: NEMBUTAL, PENTOBARBITAL

D J2540 Injection, penicillin G potassium, up to 600,000 units N1 ASC N
BETOS: O1E Other drugs
Drugs: PENICILLIN G POT IN DEXTROSE, PENICILLIN G POTASSIUM, PFIZERPEN, PFIZERPEN-G

D J2543 Injection, piperacillin sodium/tazobactam sodium, 1 gram/0.125 grams (1.125 grams) N1 ASC N
BETOS: O1E Other drugs
Drugs: PIPERACILLIN AND TAZOBACTAM, PIPERACILLIN SODIUM-TAZOBACTAM SODIUM, PIPERACILLIN SODIUM/ TAZO, PIPERACILLIN SODIUM/ TAZO (ADD-VANTAGE)

D J2545 Pentamidine isethionate, inhalation solution, FDA-approved final product, non-compounded, administered through DME, unit dose form, per 300 mg B
BETOS: D1G Drugs Administered through DME
Drugs: NEBUPENT

C J2547 Injection, peramivir, 1 mg K2 ASC K
BETOS: O1E Other drugs
Drugs: RAPIVAB
Coding Clinic: 2016, Q1

D J2550 Injection, promethazine HCl, up to 50 mg N1 ASC N
BETOS: O1E Other drugs
Drugs: PHENERGAN, PROMETHAZINE, PROMETHAZINE HCL

D J2560 Injection, phenobarbital sodium, up to 120 mg K2 ASC K
BETOS: O1E Other drugs
Drugs: PHENOBARBITAL SODIUM

C J2562 Injection, plerixafor, 1 mg K2 ASC K
BETOS: O1E Other drugs
Drugs: MOZOBIL (PLERIXAFOR)

D J2590 Injection, oxytocin, up to 10 units N1 ♀ ASC N
BETOS: O1E Other drugs

D J2597 Injection, desmopressin acetate, per 1 mcg K2 ASC K
BETOS: O1E Other drugs
Drugs: DDAVP, DESMOPRESSIN ACETATE

D J2650 Injection, prednisolone acetate, up to 1 ml N1 ASC N
BETOS: O1E Other drugs

D J2670 Injection, tolazoline HCl, up to 25 mg K5 ASC E2
BETOS: O1E Other drugs

D J2675 Injection, progesterone, per 50 mg N1 ♀ ASC N
BETOS: O1E Other drugs
Drugs: PROGESTERONE

D J2680 Injection, fluphenazine decanoate, up to 25 mg N1 ASC N
BETOS: O1E Other drugs
Drugs: FLUPHENAZINE DECANOATE

D J2690 Injection, procainamide HCl, up to 1 gm N1 ASC N
BETOS: O1E Other drugs
Drugs: PROCAINAMIDE HCL

D J2700 Injection, oxacillin sodium, up to 250 mg N1 ASC N
BETOS: O1E Other drugs
Drugs: BACTOCILL IN DEXTROSE, OXACILLIN, OXACILLIN SODIUM

C J2704 Injection, propofol, 10 mg N1 ASC N
BETOS: O1E Other drugs
Drugs: DIPRIVAN, PROPOFOL
Coding Clinic: 2014, Q4

D J2710 Injection, neostigmine methylsulfate, up to 0.5 mg N1 ASC N
BETOS: O1E Other drugs

D J2720 Injection, protamine sulfate, per 10 mg N1 ASC N
BETOS: O1E Other drugs
Drugs: PROTAMINE SULFATE

C J2724 Injection, protein C concentrate, intravenous, human, 10 IU K2 ASC K
BETOS: O1E Other drugs
Drugs: CEPROTIN
Coding Clinic: 2008, Q1

D J2725 Injection, protirelin, per 250 mcg K5 ASC E2
BETOS: O1E Other drugs

D J2730 Injection, pralidoxime chloride, up to 1 gm N1 ASC N
BETOS: O1E Other drugs

D J2760 Injection, phentolamine mesylate, up to 5 mg K2 ASC K
BETOS: O1E Other drugs
Drugs: PHENTOLAMINE MESYLATE

D J2765 Injection, metoclopramide HCl, up to 10 mg N1 ASC N
BETOS: O1E Other drugs
Drugs: METOCLOPRAMIDE HCL

D J2770 Injection, quinupristin/dalfopristin, 500 mg (150/350) K2 ASC K
BETOS: O1E Other drugs
Drugs: SYNERCID

C J2778 Injection, ranibizumab, 0.1 mg K2 ASC K
BETOS: O1E Other drugs
Drugs: LUCENTIS, LUCENTIS PFS
Coding Clinic: 2008, Q1

D J2780 Injection, ranitidine hydrochloride, 25 mg N1 ASC N
BETOS: O1E Other drugs
Drugs: RANITIDINE, ZANTAC

♂ Male only   ♀ Female only   **A** Age   A2 - Z3 = ASC Payment indicator   A - Y = APC Status indicator
ASC = ASC Approved Procedure   **DME** Paid under the DME fee schedule   **MIPS** MIPS code

C **J2783** Injection, rasburicase, 0.5 mg   K2 ASC K
BETOS: O1E   Other drugs
Drugs: ELITEK
Coding Clinic: 2004, Q2; 2005, Q2

C **J2785** Injection, regadenoson, 0.1 mg   N1 ASC N
BETOS: O1E   Other drugs
Drugs: REGADENOSON
Coding Clinic: 2008, Q4

C **J2786** Injection, reslizumab, 1 mg   K2 Ⓐ ASC K
BETOS: O1E   Other drugs
Drugs: CINQAIR

C **J2787** Riboflavin 5'-phosphate, ophthalmic solution, up to 3 ml   N
BETOS: O1E   Other drugs
Coding Clinic: 2019, Q1

D **J2788** Injection, Rho D immune globulin, human, minidose, 50 micrograms (250 IU)   N1 ASC N
BETOS: O1E   Other drugs
Drugs: HYPERRHO S/D, MICRHOGAM, MICRHOGAM UF PLUS

D **J2790** Injection, Rho D immune globulin, human, full dose, 300 micrograms (1500 IU)   N1 ASC N
BETOS: O1E   Other drugs
Drugs: HYPERRHO S/D, RHOGAM ULTRA-FILTERED PLUS

D **J2791** Injection, Rho D immune globulin (human), (Rhophylac), intramuscular or intravenous, 100 IU   N1 ASC N
BETOS: O1E   Other drugs
Drugs: RHOPHYLAC
Coding Clinic: 2007, Q4; 2008, Q1

D **J2792** Injection, Rho D immune globulin, intravenous, human, solvent detergent, 100 IU   K2 ASC K
BETOS: O1E   Other drugs
Drugs: WINRHO SDF

D **J2793** Injection, rilonacept, 1 mg   K5 ASC E2
BETOS: O1E   Other drugs

C **J2794** Injection, risperidone (risperdal consta), 0.5 mg   K2 ASC K
BETOS: O1E   Other drugs
Drugs: RISPERDAL CONSTA
Coding Clinic: 2005, Q2; 2005, Q1

C **J2795** Injection, ropivacaine hydrochloride, 1 mg   N1 ASC N
BETOS: O1E   Other drugs
Drugs: NAROPIN, ROPIVACAINE, ROPIVACAINE HYDROCHLORIDE

C **J2796** Injection, romiplostim, 10 micrograms   K2 ASC K
BETOS: O1E   Other drugs
Drugs: NPLATE

D **J2797** Injection, rolapitant, 0.5 mg   E1
BETOS: O1E   Other drugs
Coding Clinic: 2019, Q1

C **J2798** Injection, risperidone, (Perseris), 0.5 mg   K2 ASC G
BETOS: O1E   Other drugs
Drugs: PERSERIS
Coding Clinic: 2019, Q4

D **J2800** Injection, methocarbamol, up to 10 ml   N1 ASC N
BETOS: O1E   Other drugs
Drugs: METHOCARBAMOL, ROBAXIN

C **J2805** Injection, sincalide, 5 micrograms   N1 ASC N
BETOS: O1E   Other drugs
Drugs: SINCALIDE INJ
Coding Clinic: 2005, Q4

D **J2810** Injection, theophylline, per 40 mg   N1 ASC N
BETOS: O1E   Other drugs

D **J2820** Injection, sargramostim (GM-CSF), 50 mcg   K2 ASC K
BETOS: O1E   Other drugs
Drugs: LEUKINE (LYO PWD)

C **J2840** Injection, sebelipase alfa, 1 mg   K2 ASC K
BETOS: O1E   Other drugs
Drugs: KANUMA

D **J2850** Injection, secretin, synthetic, human, 1 microgram   K2 ASC K
BETOS: O1E   Other drugs
Drugs: CHIRHOSTIM

C **J2860** Injection, siltuximab, 10 mg   K2 ASC K
BETOS: O1E   Other drugs
Drugs: SYLVANT
Coding Clinic: 2016, Q1

D **J2910** Injection, aurothioglucose, up to 50 mg   K5 ASC E2
BETOS: O1E   Other drugs

D **J2916** Injection, sodium ferric gluconate complex in sucrose injection, 12.5 mg   N1 ASC N
BETOS: O1E   Other drugs
Drugs: FERRLECIT, SODIUM FERRIC GLUCONATE, SODIUM FERRIC GLUCONATE COMPLEX IN SUCROSE

D **J2920** Injection, methylprednisolone sodium succinate, up to 40 mg   N1 ASC N
BETOS: O1E   Other drugs
Drugs: METHYLPREDNISOLONE SODIUM SUCC, SOLU-MEDROL

D **J2930** Injection, methylprednisolone sodium succinate, up to 125 mg   N1 ASC N
BETOS: O1E   Other drugs
Drugs: METHYLPREDNISOLONE SODIUM SUCC, SOLU-MEDROL

D **J2940** Injection, somatrem, 1 mg   K5 ASC E2
BETOS: O1E   Other drugs
Statute: 1861s2b
Coding Clinic: 2002, Q2; 2002, Q1

D **J2941** Injection, somatropin, 1 mg   K2 ASC K
BETOS: O1E   Other drugs

● New code   ▲ Revised code   **C** Carrier judgment   **D** Special coverage instructions apply
I Not payable by Medicare   **M** Non-covered by Medicare   **S** Non-covered by Medicare statute   AHA Coding Clinic®

Statute: 1861s2b
Coding Clinic: 2002, Q2; 2002, Q1

D J2950 Injection, promazine HCl, up to
25 mg   N1 ASC N
BETOS: O1E   Other drugs

D J2993 Injection, reteplase, 18.1 mg   K2 ASC K
BETOS: O1E   Other drugs
Drugs: RETAVASE KIT

D J2995 Injection, streptokinase, per
250,000 IU   K5 ASC E2
BETOS: O1E   Other drugs

D J2997 Injection, alteplase recombinant,
1 mg   K2 ASC K
BETOS: O1E   Other drugs
Drugs: ACTIVASE, CATHFLO ACTIVASE

D J3000 Injection, streptomycin, up to 1 gm N1 ASC N
BETOS: O1E   Other drugs
Drugs: STREPTOMYCIN SULFATE

D J3010 Injection, fentanyl citrate, 0.1 mg   N1 ASC N
BETOS: O1E   Other drugs
Drugs: FENTANYL CITRATE, SUBLIMAZE

D J3030 Injection, sumatriptan succinate, 6 mg
(code may be used for Medicare when drug
administered under the direct supervision
of a physician, not for use when drug is self
administered)   N1 ASC N
BETOS: O1E   Other drugs

C J3031 Injection, fremanezumab-vfrm, 1 mg (code
may be used for Medicare when drug
administered under the direct supervision of
a physician, not for use when drug is self-
administered)   K2 ASC G
BETOS: O1E   Other drugs
Drugs: AJOVY
Coding Clinic: 2019, Q4

● **C J3032** Injection, eptinezumab-jjmr, 1 mg   K2 ASC G
BETOS: O1E   Other drugs
Drugs: VYEPTI

C J3060 Injection, taliglucerase alfa,
10 units   K2 ASC K
BETOS: O1E   Other drugs
Drugs: ELELYSO
Coding Clinic: 2013, Q4

D J3070 Injection, pentazocine, 30 mg   N1 ASC N
BETOS: O1E   Other drugs

C J3090 Injection, tedizolid phosphate, 1 mg K2 ASC K
BETOS: O1E   Other drugs
Drugs: SIVEXTRO
Coding Clinic: 2016, Q1

C J3095 Injection, telavancin, 10 mg   K2 ASC K
BETOS: O1E   Other drugs
Drugs: VIBATIV
Coding Clinic: 2011, Q1

C J3101 Injection, tenecteplase, 1 mg   K2 ASC K
BETOS: O1E   Other drugs
Drugs: TNKASE
Coding Clinic: 2008, Q4; 2020, Q3

D J3105 Injection, terbutaline sulfate, up
to 1 mg   N1 ASC N
BETOS: O1E   Other drugs
Drugs: TERBUTALINE, TERBUTALINE
SULFATE

D J3110 Injection, teriparatide, 10 mcg   B
BETOS: O1E   Other drugs
Pub: 100-4, Chapter-10, 90.1

C J3111 Injection, romosozumab-aqqg,
1 mg   K2 ASC G
BETOS: O1E   Other drugs
Drugs: EVENITY

D J3121 Injection, testosterone enanthate,
1 mg   N1 ♂ ASC N
BETOS: O1E   Other drugs
Drugs: TESTOSTERONE ENANTHATE

D J3145 Injection, testosterone undecanoate,
1 mg   K2 ♂ ASC K
BETOS: O1E   Other drugs
Drugs: AVEED

D J3230 Injection, chlorpromazine HCl, up
to 50 mg   N1 ASC N
BETOS: O1E   Other drugs
Drugs: CHLORPROMAZINE HCL

D J3240 Injection, thyrotropin alpha, 0.9 mg, provided
in 1.1 mg vial   K2 ASC K
BETOS: O1E   Other drugs
Drugs: THYROGEN
Coding Clinic: 2005, Q4; 2005, Q2

● **C J3241** Injection, teprotumumab-trbw,
10 mg   K2 ASC G
BETOS: O1E   Other drugs
Drugs: TEPEZZA

C J3243 Injection, tigecycline, 1 mg   K2 ASC K
BETOS: O1E   Other drugs
Drugs: TIGECYCLINE
Coding Clinic: 2006, Q4

C J3245 Injection, tildrakizumab, 1 mg   K2 ASC G
BETOS: O1E   Other drugs
Drugs: ILUMYA
Coding Clinic: 2005, Q1

C J3246 Injection, tirofiban HCl, 0.25 mg   K2 ASC K
BETOS: O1E   Other drugs
Drugs: AGGRASTAT
Coding Clinic: 2005, Q1

D J3250 Injection, trimethobenzamide HCl, up to
200 mg   N1 ASC N
BETOS: O1E   Other drugs
Drugs: TIGAN

♂ Male only   ♀ Female only   **A** Age   A2 - Z3 = ASC Payment indicator   A - Y = APC Status indicator
ASC = ASC Approved Procedure   **DME** Paid under the DME fee schedule   **MIPS** MIPS code

J3260 - J3398

D **J3260** Injection, tobramycin sulfate, up to 80 mg   N1 ASC N
BETOS: O1E   Other drugs
Drugs: TOBRAMYCIN SULFATE

C **J3262** Injection, tocilizumab, 1 mg   K2 ASC K
BETOS: O1E   Other drugs
Drugs: ACTEMRA
Coding Clinic: 2011, Q1

D **J3265** Injection, torsemide, 10 mg/ml   N1 ASC N
BETOS: O1E   Other drugs

D **J3280** Injection, thiethylperazine maleate, up to 10 mg   K5 ASC E2
BETOS: O1E   Other drugs

C **J3285** Injection, treprostinil, 1 mg   K2 ASC K
BETOS: O1E   Other drugs
Drugs: REMODULIN, TREPROSTINIL INJECTION

D **J3300** Injection, triamcinolone acetonide, preservative free, 1 mg   N1 ASC N
BETOS: O1E   Other drugs
Drugs: TRIAMCINOLONE ACETONIDE, PRESERVATIVE FREE
Coding Clinic: 2009, Q1; 2008, Q4

D **J3301** Injection, triamcinolone acetonide, not otherwise specified, 10 mg   N1 ASC N
BETOS: O1E   Other drugs
Drugs: KENALOG, KENALOG-10, KENALOG-40, KENALOG-80, TRIAMCINOLONE ACETONIDE
Coding Clinic: 2017, Q3; 2018, Q4

D **J3302** Injection, triamcinolone diacetate, per 5 mg   N1 ASC N
BETOS: O1E   Other drugs

D **J3303** Injection, triamcinolone hexacetonide, per 5 mg   N1 ASC N
BETOS: O1E   Other drugs

D **J3304** Injection, triamcinolone acetonide, preservative-free, extended-release, microsphere formulation, 1 mg   K2 ASC K
BETOS: O1E   Other drugs
Drugs: ZILRETTA
Coding Clinic: 2019, Q1

D **J3305** Injection, trimetrexate glucuronate, per 25 mg   K5 ASC E2
BETOS: O1E   Other drugs

D **J3310** Injection, perphenazine, up to 5 mg N1 ASC N
BETOS: O1E   Other drugs

D **J3315** Injection, triptorelin pamoate, 3.75 mg   K2 ♂ ASC K
BETOS: O1E   Other drugs
Drugs: TRELSTAR

D **J3316** Injection, triptorelin, extended-release, 3.75 mg   K2 ASC K
BETOS: O1E   Other drugs
Drugs: TRIPTODUR
Coding Clinic: 2019, Q1

D **J3320** Injection, spectinomycin dihydrochloride, up to 2 gm   K5 ASC E2
BETOS: O1E   Other drugs

D **J3350** Injection, urea, up to 40 gm   K5 ♀ ASC E2
BETOS: O1E   Other drugs

D **J3355** Injection, urofollitropin, 75 IU   K5 ♀ ASC E2
BETOS: O1E   Other drugs

C **J3357** Ustekinumab, for subcutaneous injection, 1 mg   K2 ASC K
BETOS: O1E   Other drugs
Drugs: STELARA
Coding Clinic: 2011, Q1; 2016, Q4; 2017, Q1

C **J3358** Ustekinumab, for intravenous injection, 1 mg   K2 ASC K
BETOS: O1E   Other drugs
Drugs: STELARA (IV INFUSION)

D **J3360** Injection, diazepam, up to 5 mg   N1 ASC N
BETOS: O1E   Other drugs
Drugs: DIAZEPAM
Coding Clinic: 2007, Q2

D **J3364** Injection, urokinase, 5000 IU vial   N1 ASC N
BETOS: O1E   Other drugs

D **J3365** Injection, IV, urokinase, 250,000 IU vial   K5 ASC E2
BETOS: O1E   Other drugs

D **J3370** Injection, vancomycin HCl, 500 mg N1 ASC N
BETOS: O1E   Other drugs
Drugs: VANCOCIN HCL, VANCOMYCIN, VANCOMYCIN HCL, VANCOMYCIN HYDROCHLORIDE

D **J3380** Injection, vedolizumab, 1 mg   K2 ASC K
BETOS: O1E   Other drugs
Drugs: ENTYVIO
Coding Clinic: 2016, Q1

C **J3385** Injection, velaglucerase alfa, 100 units   K2 ASC K
BETOS: O1E   Other drugs
Drugs: VPRIV
Coding Clinic: 2011, Q1

D **J3396** Injection, verteporfin, 0.1 mg   K2 ASC K
BETOS: O1E   Other drugs
Drugs: VISUDYNE
Coding Clinic: 2005, Q1; 2020, Q1
Pub: 100-4, Chapter-32, 300.1; 100-4, Chapter-32, 300.2

C **J3397** Injection, vestronidase alfa-vjbk, 1 mg   N1 ASC N
BETOS: O1E   Other drugs
Coding Clinic: 2019, Q1

C **J3398** Injection, voretigene neparvovec-rzyl, 1 billion vector genomes   K2 ASC K
BETOS: O1E   Other drugs
Drugs: LUXTURNA
Coding Clinic: 2019, Q1

● New code   ▲ Revised code   **C** Carrier judgment   **D** Special coverage instructions apply
I Not payable by Medicare   **M** Non-covered by Medicare   **S** Non-covered by Medicare statute   AHA Coding Clinic®

● **C** **J3399** Injection, onasemnogene abeparvovec-xioi, per treatment, up to 5x10^15 vector genomes   K

BETOS: O1E   Other drugs

Drugs: ZOLGENSMA 1X5.5 ML VIAL AND 2X8.3 ML VIAL KIT, ZOLGENSMA 1X5.5 ML VIAL AND 3X8.3 ML VIAL KIT, ZOLGENSMA 1X5.5 ML VIAL AND 4X8.3 ML VIAL KIT, ZOLGENSMA 1X5.5 ML VIAL AND 5X8.3 ML VIAL KIT, ZOLGENSMA 1X5.5 ML VIAL AND 6X8.3 ML VIAL KIT, ZOLGENSMA 1X5.5 ML VIAL AND 7X8.3 ML VIAL KIT, ZOLGENSMA 2X5.5 ML VIAL AND 1X8.3 ML VIAL KIT, ZOLGENSMA 2X5.5 ML VIAL AND 2X8.3 ML VIAL KIT, ZOLGENSMA 2X5.5 ML VIAL AND 3X8.3 ML VIAL KIT, ZOLGENSMA 2X5.5 ML VIAL AND 4X8.3 ML VIAL KIT, ZOLGENSMA 2X5.5 ML VIAL AND 5X8.3 ML VIAL KIT, ZOLGENSMA 2X5.5 ML VIAL AND 6X8.3 ML VIAL KIT, ZOLGENSMA 2X5.5 ML VIAL AND 7X8.3 ML VIAL KIT, ZOLGENSMA 2X8.3 ML VIAL KIT, ZOLGENSMA 3X8.3 ML VIAL KIT, ZOLGENSMA 4X8.3 ML VIAL KIT, ZOLGENSMA 5X8.3 ML VIAL KIT, ZOLGENSMA 6X8.3 ML VIAL KIT, ZOLGENSMA 7X8.3 ML VIAL KIT, ZOLGENSMA 8X8.3 ML VIAL KIT, ZOLGENSMA 9X8.3 ML VIAL KIT

Coding Clinic: 2020, Q2

D **J3400** Injection, triflupromazine HCl, up to 20 mg   K5 ASC E2

BETOS: O1E   Other drugs

D **J3410** Injection, hydroxyzine HCl, up to 25 mg   N1 ASC N

BETOS: O1E   Other drugs
Drugs: HYDROXYZINE HCL

C **J3411** Injection, thiamine HCl, 100 mg   N1 ASC N

BETOS: O1E   Other drugs
Drugs: THIAMINE HCL
Coding Clinic: 2005, Q2

C **J3415** Injection, pyridoxine HCl, 100 mg   N1 ASC N

BETOS: O1E   Other drugs
Drugs: PYRIDOXINE HCL
Coding Clinic: 2005, Q2

D **J3420** Injection, vitamin B-12 cyanocobalamin, up to 1000 mcg   N1 ASC N

BETOS: O1E   Other drugs
Drugs: CYANOCOBALAMIN

D **J3430** Injection, phytonadione (vitamin K), per 1 mg   N1 ASC N

BETOS: O1E   Other drugs
Drugs: PHYTONADIONE, VITAMIN K1

D **J3465** Injection, voriconazole, 10 mg   N1 ASC N

BETOS: O1E   Other drugs
Drugs: VFEND IV, VORICONAZOLE
Coding Clinic: 2005, Q2

D **J3470** Injection, hyaluronidase, up to 150 units   N1 ASC N

BETOS: O1E   Other drugs

D **J3471** Injection, hyaluronidase, ovine, preservative free, per 1 USP unit (up to 999 USP units)   N1 ASC N

BETOS: O1E   Other drugs
Drugs: VITRASE

D **J3472** Injection, hyaluronidase, ovine, preservative free, per 1000 USP units   N1 ASC N

BETOS: O1E   Other drugs

D **J3473** Injection, hyaluronidase, recombinant, 1 USP unit   N1 ASC N

BETOS: O1E   Other drugs
Drugs: HYLENEX

D **J3475** Injection, magnesium sulfate, per 500 mg   N1 ASC N

BETOS: O1E   Other drugs
Drugs: MAGNESIUM SULFATE, MAGNESIUM SULFATE IN 5% DEXTROSE

D **J3480** Injection, potassium chloride, per 2 mEq   N1 ASC N

BETOS: O1E   Other drugs
Drugs: POTASSIUM CHLORIDE, POTASSIUM CHLORIDE/DEXTROSE, POTASSIUM CHLORIDE/SODIUM CHLORIDE

D **J3485** Injection, zidovudine, 10 mg   N1 ASC N

BETOS: O1E   Other drugs
Drugs: RETROVIR

C **J3486** Injection, ziprasidone mesylate, 10 mg   N1 ASC N

BETOS: O1E   Other drugs
Drugs: GEODON, ZIPRASIDONE MESYLATE
Coding Clinic: 2005, Q2

C **J3489** Injection, zoledronic acid, 1 mg   N1 ASC N

BETOS: O1E   Other drugs
Drugs: RECLAST, ZOLEDRONIC ACID, ZOMETA
Coding Clinic: 2013, Q4

D **J3490** Unclassified drugs   N1 ASC N

BETOS: O1E   Other drugs
Coding Clinic: 2005, Q4; 2008, Q1; 2009, Q2; 2013, Q1; 2010, Q3; 2014, Q2; 2012, Q4; 2014, Q4; 2017, Q1; 2017, Q1
Pub: 100-4, Chapter-8, 60.2.1.1; 100-4, Chapter-10, 90.1; 100-4, Chapter-32, 280.2

M **J3520** Edetate disodium, per 150 mg   E1

BETOS: O1E   Other drugs
Service not separately priced by Part B

D **J3530** Nasal vaccine inhalation   N1 ASC N

BETOS: O1E   Other drugs

M **J3535** Drug administered through a metered dose inhaler   E1

BETOS: O1E   Other drugs
Service not separately priced by Part B

M **J3570** Laetrile, amygdalin, vitamin B17   E1

BETOS: O1E   Other drugs
Service not separately priced by Part B

C **J3590** Unclassified biologics   N1 ASC N
BETOS: O1E   Other drugs
Coding Clinic: 2012, Q4; 2016, Q4; 2017, Q1
Pub: 100-4, Chapter-32, 280.2

C **J3591** Unclassified drug or biological used for ESRD on dialysis   B
BETOS: O1E   Other drugs
Coding Clinic: 2019, Q1

D **J7030** Infusion, normal saline solution, 1000 cc   N1 ASC N
BETOS: O1E   Other drugs
Drugs: SODIUM CHLORIDE, SODIUM CHLORIDE

D **J7040** Infusion, normal saline solution, sterile (500 ml = 1 unit)   N1 ASC N
BETOS: O1E   Other drugs
Drugs: SODIUM CHLORIDE, SODIUM CHLORIDE

D **J7042** 5% dextrose/normal saline (500 ml = 1 unit)   N1 ASC N
BETOS: O1E   Other drugs
Drugs: DEXTROSE-NACL

D **J7050** Infusion, normal saline solution, 250 cc   N1 ASC N
BETOS: O1E   Other drugs
Drugs: SODIUM CHLORIDE, SODIUM CHLORIDE

D **J7060** 5% dextrose/water (500 ml = 1 unit)   N1 ASC N
BETOS: O1E   Other drugs
Drugs: DEXTROSE, DEXTROSE 5%

D **J7070** Infusion, D5W, 1000 cc   N1 ASC N
BETOS: O1E   Other drugs
Drugs: DEXTROSE, DEXTROSE 5%

D **J7100** Infusion, dextran 40, 500 ml   N1 ASC N
BETOS: O1E   Other drugs

D **J7110** Infusion, dextran 75, 500 ml   N1 ASC N
BETOS: O1E   Other drugs

D **J7120** Ringers lactate infusion, up to 1000 cc   N1 ASC N
BETOS: O1E   Other drugs
Drugs: LACTATED RINGERS

D **J7121** 5% Dextrose in lactated ringers infusion, up to 1000 cc   N1 ASC N
BETOS: O1E   Other drugs
Coding Clinic: 2016, Q1

D **J7131** Hypertonic saline solution, 1 ml   N1 ASC N
BETOS: O1E   Other drugs

● **C** **J7169** Injection, coagulation Factor XA (recombinant), inactivated-zhzo (andexxa), 10 mg   K2 ASC G
BETOS: O1E   Other drugs
Drugs: ANDEXXA
Coding Clinic: 2020, Q2

C **J7170** Injection, emicizumab-kxwh, 0.5 mg   K2 ASC K
BETOS: O1E   Other drugs
Drugs: HEMLIBRA
Coding Clinic: 2019, Q1

C **J7175** Injection, Factor X, (human), 1 IU   K2 ASC K
BETOS: O1E   Other drugs
Drugs: COAGADEX
Coding Clinic: 2017, Q1

CLOTTING FACTORS (J7177-J7212)

C **J7177** Injection, Human fibrinogen concentrate (Fibryga®), 1 mg   N1 ASC N
BETOS: O1E   Other drugs
Drugs: FIBRYGA
Coding Clinic: 2019, Q1

C **J7178** Injection, Human fibrinogen concentrate, not otherwise specified, 1 mg   K2 ASC K
BETOS: O1E   Other drugs
Drugs: RIASTAP

D **J7179** Injection, Von Willebrand Factor (recombinant), (Vonvendi), 1 IU VWF:RCo   K2 ASC K
BETOS: O1E   Other drugs
Drugs: VONVENDI
Coding Clinic: 2017, Q1

C **J7180** Injection, Factor XIII (Antihemophilic factor, human), 1 IU   K2 ASC K
BETOS: O1E   Other drugs
Drugs: CORIFACT
Coding Clinic: 2012, Q1

C **J7181** Injection, Factor XIII a-subunit, (recombinant), per IU   K2 ASC K
BETOS: O1E   Other drugs
Drugs: TRETTEN

C **J7182** Injection, Factor VIII, (Antihemophilic factor, recombinant), (Novoeight), per IU   K2 ASC K
BETOS: O1E   Other drugs
Drugs: NOVOEIGHT
Coding Clinic: 2014, Q4

D **J7183** Injection, Von Willebrand Factor complex (human), wilate, 1 IU VWF:RCo   K2 ASC K
BETOS: O1E   Other drugs
Drugs: WILATE

C **J7185** Injection, Factor VIII (Antihemophilic factor, recombinant) (XYNTHA), per IU   K2 ASC K
BETOS: O1E   Other drugs
Drugs: XYNTHA

D **J7186** Injection, Antihemophilic Factor VIII/Von Willebrand Factor complex (human), per Factor VIII IU   K2 ASC K
BETOS: O1E   Other drugs
Drugs: ALPHANATE / VON WILLEBRAND FACTOR COMPLEX
Coding Clinic: 2008, Q4

● New code   ▲ Revised code   **C** Carrier judgment   **D** Special coverage instructions apply
I Not payable by Medicare   **M** Non-covered by Medicare   **S** Non-covered by Medicare statute   AHA Coding Clinic®

D J7187 Injection, Von Willebrand Factor complex (Humate-P), per IU VWF:RCo　K2 ASC K
BETOS: O1E　Other drugs
Drugs: HUMATE-P LOW DILUENT

D J7188 Injection, Factor VIII (Antihemophilic factor, recombinant), (OBIZUR), per IU　K2 ASC K
BETOS: O1E　Other drugs
Drugs: OBIZUR
Coding Clinic: 2016, Q1

▲ **D J7189** Factor VIIA (Antihemophilic factor, recombinant), (novoseven rt), 1 microgram　K2 ASC K
BETOS: O1E　Other drugs
Drugs: NOVOSEVEN RT
Pub: 100-4, Chapter-3, 20.7.3; 100-4, Chapter-3, 20.7.3

D J7190 Factor VIII (Antihemophilic factor, human) per IU　K2 ASC K
BETOS: O1E　Other drugs
Drugs: ALPHANATE / VON WILLEBRAND FACTOR COMPLEX, HEMOFIL M, KOATE, KOATE-DVI

D J7191 Factor VIII (Antihemophilic factor (porcine)), per IU　K5 ASC E2
BETOS: O1E　Other drugs

D J7192 Factor VIII (Antihemophilic factor, recombinant) per IU, not otherwise specified　K2 ASC K
BETOS: O1E　Other drugs
Drugs: ADVATE, HELIXATE FS, HELIXATE FS 3000, KOGENATE FS, RECOMBINATE

D J7193 Factor IX (Antihemophilic factor, purified, non-recombinant) per IU　K2 ASC K
BETOS: O1E　Other drugs
Drugs: ALPHANINE® SD VF 1000 IU M2V USA, ALPHANINE® SD VF 1500 IU M2V USA, ALPHANINE® SD VF 500 IU M2V USA, MONONINE
Coding Clinic: 2002, Q2

D J7194 Factor IX, complex, per IU　K2 ASC K
BETOS: O1E　Other drugs
Drugs: PROFILNINE® SD FIX SD M2V(1000), PROFILNINE® SD FIX SD M2V(1500), PROFILNINE® SD FIX SD M2V(500)

D J7195 Injection, Factor IX (Antihemophilic factor, recombinant) per IU, not otherwise specified　K2 ASC K
BETOS: O1E　Other drugs
Drugs: BENEFIX
Coding Clinic: 2002, Q2; 2002, Q1

C J7196 Injection, Antithrombin recombinant, 50 IU　N1 ASC N
BETOS: O1E　Other drugs
Coding Clinic: 2011, Q1

D J7197 Antithrombin III (human), per IU　K2 ASC K
BETOS: O1E　Other drugs
Drugs: THROMBATE III

D J7198 Anti-inhibitor, per IU　K2 ASC K
BETOS: O1E　Other drugs
Drugs: FEIBA NF

D J7199 Hemophilia clotting factor, not otherwise classified　B
BETOS: O1E　Other drugs

D J7200 Injection, Factor IX, (Antihemophilic factor, recombinant), Rixubis, per IU　K2 ASC K
BETOS: O1E　Other drugs
Drugs: RIXUBIS

D J7201 Injection, Factor IX, Fc fusion protein, (recombinant), ALPROLIX, 1 IU　K2 ASC K
BETOS: O1E　Other drugs
Drugs: ALPROLIX

D J7202 Injection, Factor IX, albumin fusion protein, (recombinant), IDELVION, 1 IU　K2 ASC K
BETOS: O1E　Other drugs
Drugs: IDELVION

D J7203 Injection Factor IX, (Antihemophilic factor, recombinant), glycopegylated, (Rebinyn®), 1 IU　K2 ASC K
BETOS: O1E　Other drugs
Drugs: REBINYN
Coding Clinic: 2019, Q1

● **C J7204** Injection, Factor VIII, Antihemophilic factor (recombinant), (esperoct), glycopegylated-exei, per IU　K2 ASC G
BETOS: O1E　Other drugs
Drugs: ESPEROCT
Coding Clinic: 2020, Q2

D J7205 Injection, Factor VIII Fc fusion protein (recombinant), per IU　K2 ASC K
BETOS: O1E　Other drugs
Drugs: ELOCTATE
Coding Clinic: 2016, Q1

D J7207 Injection, Factor VIII, (Antihemophilic factor, recombinant), PEGYLATED, 1 IU　K2 ASC K
BETOS: O1E　Other drugs
Drugs: ADYNOVATE

D J7208 Injection, Factor VIII, (Antihemophilic factor, recombinant),PEGylated-aucl, (JIVI®), 1 I.U.　K2 ASC G
BETOS: O1E　Other drugs
Drugs: JIVI
Coding Clinic: 2019, Q3

C J7209 Injection, Factor VIII, (Antihemophilic factor, recombinant), (NUWIQ), 1 IU　K2 ASC K
BETOS: O1E　Other drugs
Drugs: NUWIQ

C J7210 Injection, Factor VIII, (Antihemophilic factor, recombinant), (AFSTYLA), 1 IU　K2 ASC K
BETOS: O1E　Other drugs
Drugs: AFSTYLA

♂ Male only　♀ Female only　Ⓐ Age　A2 - Z3 = ASC Payment indicator　A - Y = APC Status indicator
ASC = ASC Approved Procedure　**DME** Paid under the DME fee schedule　**MIPS** MIPS code

J7211 - J7316

DRUGS ADMINISTERED OTHER THAN ORAL METHOD (J0120-J8999)

C **J7211** Injection, Factor VIII, (Antihemophilic factor, recombinant), (KOVALTRY), 1 IU   K2 ASC K
BETOS: O1E   Other drugs
Drugs: KOVALTRY
Coding Clinic: 2018, Q1

● **C** **J7212** Factor viia (Antihemophilic factor, recombinant)-jncw (sevenfact), 1 microgram   K2 Ⓐ ASC K
BETOS: O1E   Other drugs
Drugs: SEVENFACT

CONTRACEPTIVE SYSTEMS (J7296-J7307)

S **J7296** Levonorgestrel-releasing intrauterine contraceptive system, (Kyleena), 19.5 mg   ♀ E1
BETOS: P6C   Minor procedures - other (Medicare fee schedule)
Service not separately priced by Part B
Statute: 1862(a)(1)

S **J7297** Levonorgestrel-releasing intrauterine contraceptive system (Liletta), 52 mg   ♀ Ⓐ E1
BETOS: P6C   Minor procedures - other (Medicare fee schedule)
Service not separately priced by Part B
Statute: 1862(a)(1)
Coding Clinic: 2016, Q1

S **J7298** Levonorgestrel-releasing intrauterine contraceptive system (Mirena), 52 mg ♀ Ⓐ E1
BETOS: P6C   Minor procedures - other (Medicare fee schedule)
Service not separately priced by Part B
Statute: 1862(a)(1)
Coding Clinic: 2016, Q1

S **J7300** Intrauterine copper contraceptive   ♀ Ⓐ E1
BETOS: P6C   Minor procedures - other (Medicare fee schedule)
Service not separately priced by Part B
Statute: 1862A1

S **J7301** Levonorgestrel-releasing intrauterine contraceptive system (Skyla), 13.5 mg   ♀ E1
BETOS: P6C   Minor procedures - other (Medicare fee schedule)
Service not separately priced by Part B
Statute: 1862(a)(1)
Coding Clinic: 2014, Q4

S **J7303** Contraceptive supply, hormone containing vaginal ring, each   ♀ Ⓐ E1
BETOS: Z2   Undefined codes
Service not separately priced by Part B
Statute: 1862.1

S **J7304** Contraceptive supply, hormone containing patch, each   ♀ Ⓐ E1
BETOS: Z2   Undefined codes
Service not separately priced by Part B
Statute: 1862.1

I **J7306** Levonorgestrel (contraceptive) implant system, including implants and supplies   E1
BETOS: P6C   Minor procedures - other (Medicare fee schedule)
Service not separately priced by Part B

I **J7307** Etonogestrel (contraceptive) implant system, including implant and supplies   E1
BETOS: Z2   Undefined codes
Service not separately priced by Part B

MISCELLANEOUS DRUGS (J7308-J7401)

C **J7308** Aminolevulinic acid HCl for topical administration, 20%, single unit dosage form (354 mg)   K2 ASC K
BETOS: O1E   Other drugs
Drugs: LEVULAN KERASTICK
Coding Clinic: 2002, Q1; 2005, Q2; 2020, Q1

D **J7309** Methyl aminolevulinate (MAL) for topical administration, 16.8%, 1 gram   K5 ASC E2
BETOS: O1E   Other drugs
Coding Clinic: 2011, Q1; 2020, Q1

D **J7310** Ganciclovir, 4.5 mg, long-acting implant   K5 ASC E2
BETOS: O1E   Other drugs

C **J7311** Injection, fluocinolone acetonide, intravitreal implant (Retisert), 0.01 mg   K2 ASC K
BETOS: O1E   Other drugs
Drugs: FLUOCINOLONE ACETONIDE IMPLT (RETISERT)

C **J7312** Injection, Dexamethasone, intravitreal implant, 0.1 mg   K2 ASC K
BETOS: O1E   Other drugs
Drugs: OZURDEX
Coding Clinic: 2011, Q1

C **J7313** Injection, fluocinolone acetonide, intravitreal implant (Iluvien), 0.01 mg   K2 ASC K
BETOS: O1E   Other drugs
Drugs: ILUVIEN
Coding Clinic: 2016, Q1

C **J7314** Injection, fluocinolone acetonide, intravitreal implant (YUTIQTM), 0.01 mg   K2 ASC K
BETOS: O1E   Other drugs
Drugs: YUTIQ
Coding Clinic: 2019, Q4

C **J7315** Mitomycin, ophthalmic, 0.2 mg   N1 ASC N
BETOS: O1E   Other drugs
Coding Clinic: 2002, Q2; 2014, Q2; 2016, Q4

C **J7316** Injection, Ocriplasmin, 0.125 mg   K2 ASC K
BETOS: O1E   Other drugs
Drugs: JETREA
Coding Clinic: 2002, Q2; 2002, Q1; 2013, Q4

● New code   ▲ Revised code   **C** Carrier judgment   **D** Special coverage instructions apply
I Not payable by Medicare   **M** Non-covered by Medicare   **S** Non-covered by Medicare statute   AHA Coding Clinic®

C **J7318** Hyaluronan or derivative, durolane, for intra-articular injection, 1 mg   K2 ASC K
BETOS: O1E   Other drugs
Drugs: DUROLANE
Coding Clinic: 2019, Q1

C **J7320** Hyaluronan or derivitive, Genvisc 850, for intra-articular injection, 1 mg   K2 ASC K
BETOS: O1E   Other drugs
Drugs: GENVISC 850
Coding Clinic: 2006, Q1

▲ C **J7321** Hyaluronan or derivative, hyalgan or supartz, for intra-articular injection, per dose   N1 ASC N
BETOS: O1E   Other drugs
Drugs: SUPARTZ FX
Coding Clinic: 2008, Q1; 2012, Q4; 2020, Q2

C **J7322** Hyaluronan or derivative, Hymovis, for intra-articular injection, 1 mg   K2 ASC K
BETOS: O1E   Other drugs
Drugs: HYMOVIS
Coding Clinic: 2008, Q1

C **J7323** Hyaluronan or derivative, Euflexxa, for intra-articular injection, per dose   K2 ASC K
BETOS: O1E   Other drugs
Drugs: EUFLEXXA
Coding Clinic: 2008, Q1; 2012, Q4

C **J7324** Hyaluronan or derivative, Orthovisc, for intra-articular injection, per dose   K2 ASC K
BETOS: O1E   Other drugs
Drugs: ORTHOVISC
Coding Clinic: 2008, Q1; 2012, Q4

C **J7325** Hyaluronan or derivative, Synvisc or Synvisc-One, for intra-articular injection, 1 mg   K2 ASC K
BETOS: O1E   Other drugs
Drugs: SYNVISC, SYNVISCONE
Coding Clinic: 2012, Q4

C **J7326** Hyaluronan or derivative, Gel-One, for intra-articular injection, per dose   K2 ASC K
BETOS: O1E   Other drugs
Drugs: GEL-ONE
Coding Clinic: 2012, Q1; 2012, Q4

C **J7327** Hyaluronan or derivative, Monovisc, for intra-articular injection, per dose   K2 ASC K
BETOS: O1E   Other drugs
Drugs: MONOVISC
Coding Clinic: 2014, Q4

C **J7328** Hyaluronan or derivative, Gel-Syn, for intra-articular injection, 0.1 mg   K2 ASC K
BETOS: O1E   Other drugs
Drugs: GELSYN-3
Coding Clinic: 2016, Q1

C **J7329** Hyaluronan or derivative, TriVisc®, for intra-articular injection, 1 mg   K2 ASC K

BETOS: O1E   Other drugs
Drugs: TRIVISC
Coding Clinic: 2019, Q1

C **J7330** Autologous cultured chondrocytes, implant   B
BETOS: O1E   Other drugs
Other carrier priced
Coding Clinic: 2010, Q4

C **J7331** Hyaluronan or derivative, SYNOJOYNTTM, for intra-articular injection, 1 mg   K2 ASC G
BETOS: O1E   Other drugs
Drugs: SYNOJOYNT
Coding Clinic: 2019, Q4

C **J7332** Hyaluronan or derivative, TRILURON™, for intra-articular injection, 1 mg   N
BETOS: O1E   Other drugs
Coding Clinic: 2019, Q4

● C **J7333** Hyaluronan or derivative, visco-3, for intra-articular injection, per dose   N1 ASC N
BETOS: O1E   Other drugs
Coding Clinic: 2020, Q2

C **J7336** Capsaicin 8% patch, per square centimeter   K2 ASC K
BETOS: O1E   Other drugs
Drugs: QUTENZA

C **J7340** Carbidopa 5 mg/Levodopa 20 mg enteral suspension, 100 ml   K2 ASC K
BETOS: O1E   Other drugs
Drugs: DUOPA
Coding Clinic: 2002, Q1; 2006, Q4; 2008, Q4; 2016, Q1

C **J7342** Instillation, Ciprofloxacin otic suspension, 6 mg   K2 ASC K
BETOS: O1E   Other drugs
Drugs: OTIPRIO
Coding Clinic: 2008, Q4

D **J7345** Aminolevulinic acid HCL for topical administration, 10% gel, 10 mg   K2 ASC K
BETOS: O1E   Other drugs
Drugs: AMELUZ GEL
Coding Clinic: 2008, Q1; 2017, Q4; 2018, Q1; 2020, Q1

● C **J7351** Injection, Bimatoprost, intracameral implant, 1 microgram   K2 ASC G
BETOS: O1E   Other drugs
Drugs: DURYSTA

● C **J7352** Afamelanotide implant, 1 mg   K2 Ⓐ ASC K
BETOS: O1E   Other drugs
Drugs: SCENESSE

C **J7401** Mometasone furoate sinus implant, 10 micrograms   N
BETOS: O1E   Other drugs
Coding Clinic: 2019, Q4

J7318 - J7401

DRUGS ADMINISTERED OTHER THAN ORAL METHOD (J0120-J8999)

IMMUNOSUPPRESSIVE DRUGS (J7500-J7599)

D **J7500** Azathioprine, oral, 50 mg　　　N1 ASC N
　　BETOS: O1E　Other drugs
　　Drugs: AZASAN, AZATHIOPRINE

D **J7501** Azathioprine, parenteral, 100 mg　K2 ASC K
　　BETOS: O1E　Other drugs
　　Drugs: AZATHIOPRINE INJECTION

D **J7502** Cyclosporine, oral, 100 mg　　N1 ASC N
　　BETOS: O1E　Other drugs
　　Other carrier priced
　　Drugs: CYCLOSPORINE, CYCLOSPORINE
　　MODIFIED, GENGRAF, NEORAL,
　　SANDIMMUNE

D **J7503** Tacrolimus, extended release, (Envarsus
　　XR), oral, 0.25 mg　　　N1 ASC N
　　BETOS: O1E　Other drugs
　　Drugs: ENVARSUS XR
　　Coding Clinic: 2016, Q1

D **J7504** Lymphocyte immune globulin, antithymocyte
　　globulin, equine, parenteral,
　　250 mg　　　　　　　　K2 ASC K
　　BETOS: O1E　Other drugs
　　Drugs: ATGAM

D **J7505** Muromonab-CD3, parenteral, 5 mg N1 ASC N
　　BETOS: O1E　Other drugs

D **J7507** Tacrolimus, immediate release, oral,
　　1 mg　　　　　　　　　N1 ASC N
　　BETOS: O1E　Other drugs
　　Drugs: PROGRAF, PROGRAF GRANULES,
　　TACROLIMUS

D **J7508** Tacrolimus, extended release, (Astagraf XL),
　　oral, 0.1 mg　　　　　N1 ASC N
　　BETOS: O1E　Other drugs
　　Drugs: ASTAGRAF XL
　　Coding Clinic: 2014, Q1; 2016, Q1

D **J7509** Methylprednisolone oral, per 4 mg　N1 ASC N
　　BETOS: O1E　Other drugs
　　Drugs: MEDROL, MEDROL
　　(PAK), METHYLPREDNISOLONE,
　　METHYLPREDNISOLONE (PAK)

D **J7510** Prednisolone oral, per 5 mg　　N1 ASC N
　　BETOS: O1E　Other drugs
　　Drugs: PREDNISOLONE

C **J7511** Lymphocyte immune globulin, antithymocyte
　　globulin, rabbit, parenteral, 25 mg　K2 ASC K
　　BETOS: O1E　Other drugs
　　Drugs: THYMOGLOBULIN
　　Coding Clinic: 2002, Q2; 2002, Q1

D **J7512** Prednisone, immediate release or delayed
　　release, oral, 1 mg　　　N1 ASC N
　　BETOS: O1E　Other drugs
　　Drugs: PREDNISONE, PREDNISONE
　　INTENSOL
　　Coding Clinic: 2016, Q1

D **J7513** Daclizumab, parenteral, 25 mg　K5 ASC E2
　　BETOS: O1E　Other drugs
　　Coding Clinic: 2005, Q2

C **J7515** Cyclosporine, oral, 25 mg　　N1 ASC N
　　BETOS: O1E　Other drugs
　　Drugs: CYCLOSPORINE, CYCLOSPORINE
　　MODIFIED, GENGRAF, NEORAL,
　　SANDIMMUNE

C **J7516** Cyclosporin, parenteral, 250 mg　N1 ASC N
　　BETOS: O1E　Other drugs
　　Drugs: CYCLOSPORINE, SANDIMMUNE

C **J7517** Mycophenolate mofetil, oral,
　　250 mg　　　　　　　　N1 ASC N
　　BETOS: O1E　Other drugs
　　Drugs: CELLCEPT, MYCOPHENOLATE
　　MOFETIL

D **J7518** Mycophenolic acid, oral, 180 mg　N1 ASC N
　　BETOS: O1E　Other drugs
　　Drugs: MYCOPHENOLIC ACID,
　　MYCOPHENOLIC ACID DR, MYFORTIC
　　Coding Clinic: 2005, Q2

D **J7520** Sirolimus, oral, 1 mg　　　N1 ASC N
　　BETOS: O1E　Other drugs
　　Drugs: RAPAMUNE, SIROLIMUS

D **J7525** Tacrolimus, parenteral, 5 mg　K2 ASC K
　　BETOS: O1E　Other drugs
　　Drugs: PROGRAF

D **J7527** Everolimus, oral, 0.25 mg　　N1 ASC N
　　BETOS: O1G　Immunizations/Vaccinations
　　Drugs: EVEROLIMUS, ZORTRESS

D **J7599** Immunosuppressive drug, not otherwise
　　classified　　　　　　N1 ASC N
　　BETOS: O1E　Other drugs

INHALATION SOLUTIONS (J7604-J7686)

C **J7604** Acetylcysteine, inhalation solution,
　　compounded product, administered through
　　DME, unit dose form, per gram　　M
　　BETOS: D1G　Drugs Administered through
　　DME

C **J7605** Arformoterol, inhalation solution, FDA-
　　approved final product, non-compounded,
　　administered through DME, unit dose form,
　　15 micrograms　　　　　　M
　　BETOS: D1G　Drugs Administered through
　　DME
　　Drugs: ARFORMOTEROL

C **J7606** Formoterol fumarate, inhalation solution,
　　FDA-approved final product, non-
　　compounded, administered through DME,
　　unit dose form, 20 micrograms　　M
　　BETOS: D1G　Drugs Administered through
　　DME
　　Drugs: PERFOROMIST
　　Coding Clinic: 2008, Q4

● New code　　▲ Revised code　　**C** Carrier judgment　　**D** Special coverage instructions apply
I Not payable by Medicare　　**M** Non-covered by Medicare　　**S** Non-covered by Medicare statute　　AHA Coding Clinic®

C **J7607** Levalbuterol, inhalation solution, compounded product, administered through DME, concentrated form, 0.5 mg   M

    BETOS: D1G   Drugs Administered through DME

D **J7608** Acetylcysteine, inhalation solution, FDA-approved final product, non-compounded, administered through DME, unit dose form, per gram   M

    BETOS: D1G   Drugs Administered through DME

    Drugs: ACETYLCYSTEINE

C **J7609** Albuterol, inhalation solution, compounded product, administered through DME, unit dose, 1 mg   M

    BETOS: D1G   Drugs Administered through DME

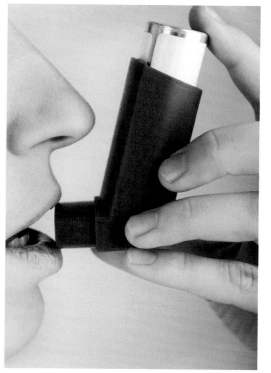

Inhaler

C **J7610** Albuterol, inhalation solution, compounded product, administered through DME, concentrated form, 1 mg   M

    BETOS: D1G   Drugs Administered through DME

D **J7611** Albuterol, inhalation solution, FDA-approved final product, non-compounded, administered through DME, concentrated form, 1 mg   M

    BETOS: D1G   Drugs Administered through DME

    Service not separately priced by Part B

    Drugs: ALBUTEROL SULFATE

    Coding Clinic: 2007, Q2; 2008, Q2; 2009, Q3

D **J7612** Levalbuterol, inhalation solution, FDA-approved final product, non-compounded, administered through DME, concentrated form, 0.5 mg   M

    BETOS: D1G   Drugs Administered through DME

    Service not separately priced by Part B

    Drugs: LEVALBUTEROL, LEVALBUTEROL INHALATION SOLUTION CONCENTRATED, XOPENEX

    Coding Clinic: 2007, Q2; 2008, Q2; 2009, Q3

D **J7613** Albuterol, inhalation solution, FDA-approved final product, non-compounded, administered through DME, unit dose, 1 mg   M

    BETOS: D1G   Drugs Administered through DME

    Service not separately priced by Part B

    Drugs: ALBUTEROL SULFATE

    Coding Clinic: 2007, Q2; 2008, Q2; 2009, Q3

D **J7614** Levalbuterol, inhalation solution, FDA-approved final product, non-compounded, administered through DME, unit dose, 0.5 mg   M

    BETOS: D1G   Drugs Administered through DME

    Service not separately priced by Part B

    Drugs: LEVALBUTEROL, XOPENEX

    Coding Clinic: 2007, Q2; 2008, Q2; 2009, Q3

C **J7615** Levalbuterol, inhalation solution, compounded product, administered through DME, unit dose, 0.5 mg   M

    BETOS: D1G   Drugs Administered through DME

D **J7620** Albuterol, up to 2.5 mg and ipratropium bromide, up to 0.5 mg, FDA-approved final product, non-compounded, administered through DME   M

    BETOS: D1G   Drugs Administered through DME

    Drugs: ALBUTEROL IPRATROPIUM

C **J7622** Beclomethasone, inhalation solution, compounded product, administered through DME, unit dose form, per milligram   M

    BETOS: D1G   Drugs Administered through DME

    Coding Clinic: 2002, Q1

C **J7624** Betamethasone, inhalation solution, compounded product, administered through DME, unit dose form, per milligram   M

    BETOS: D1G   Drugs Administered through DME

    Coding Clinic: 2002, Q1

♂ Male only   ♀ Female only   🅐 Age   A2 - Z3 = ASC Payment indicator   A - Y = APC Status indicator

ASC = ASC Approved Procedure   **DME** Paid under the DME fee schedule   **MIPS** MIPS code

C **J7626** Budesonide, inhalation solution, FDA-approved final product, non-compounded, administered through DME, unit dose form, up to 0.5 mg   M
BETOS: D1G   Drugs Administered through DME
Drugs: BUDESONIDE, PULMICORT
Coding Clinic: 2002, Q1

C **J7627** Budesonide, inhalation solution, compounded product, administered through DME, unit dose form, up to 0.5 mg   M
BETOS: D1G   Drugs Administered through DME

D **J7628** Bitolterol mesylate, inhalation solution, compounded product, administered through DME, concentrated form, per milligram   M
BETOS: D1G   Drugs Administered through DME

D **J7629** Bitolterol mesylate, inhalation solution, compounded product, administered through DME, unit dose form, per milligram   M
BETOS: D1G   Drugs Administered through DME

D **J7631** Cromolyn sodium, inhalation solution, FDA-approved final product, non-compounded, administered through DME, unit dose form, per 10 milligrams   M
BETOS: D1G   Drugs Administered through DME
Drugs: CROMOLYN SODIUM

C **J7632** Cromolyn sodium, inhalation solution, compounded product, administered through DME, unit dose form, per 10 milligrams   M
BETOS: D1G   Drugs Administered through DME

C **J7633** Budesonide, inhalation solution, FDA-approved final product, non-compounded, administered through DME, concentrated form, per 0.25 milligram   M
BETOS: D1G   Drugs Administered through DME

C **J7634** Budesonide, inhalation solution, compounded product, administered through DME, concentrated form, per 0.25 milligram   M
BETOS: D1G   Drugs Administered through DME

D **J7635** Atropine, inhalation solution, compounded product, administered through DME, concentrated form, per milligram   M
BETOS: D1G   Drugs Administered through DME

D **J7636** Atropine, inhalation solution, compounded product, administered through DME, unit dose form, per milligram   M
BETOS: D1G   Drugs Administered through DME

D **J7637** Dexamethasone, inhalation solution, compounded product, administered through DME, concentrated form, per milligram   M
BETOS: D1G   Drugs Administered through DME

D **J7638** Dexamethasone, inhalation solution, compounded product, administered through DME, unit dose form, per milligram   M
BETOS: D1G   Drugs Administered through DME

D **J7639** Dornase alfa, inhalation solution, FDA-approved final product, non-compounded, administered through DME, unit dose form, per milligram   M
BETOS: D1G   Drugs Administered through DME
Drugs: PULMOZYME

C **J7640** Formoterol, inhalation solution, compounded product, administered through DME, unit dose form, 12 micrograms   E1
BETOS: D1G   Drugs Administered through DME
Service not separately priced by Part B
Coding Clinic: 2006, Q1

C **J7641** Flunisolide, inhalation solution, compounded product, administered through DME, unit dose, per milligram   M
BETOS: D1G   Drugs Administered through DME
Coding Clinic: 2002, Q1

D **J7642** Glycopyrrolate, inhalation solution, compounded product, administered through DME, concentrated form, per milligram   M
BETOS: D1G   Drugs Administered through DME

D **J7643** Glycopyrrolate, inhalation solution, compounded product, administered through DME, unit dose form, per milligram   M
BETOS: D1G   Drugs Administered through DME

D **J7644** Ipratropium bromide, inhalation solution, FDA-approved final product, non-compounded, administered through DME, unit dose form, per milligram   M
BETOS: D1G   Drugs Administered through DME
Drugs: IPRATROPIUM BROMIDE

C **J7645** Ipratropium bromide, inhalation solution, compounded product, administered through DME, unit dose form, per milligram   M
BETOS: D1G   Drugs Administered through DME

C **J7647** Isoetharine HCl, inhalation solution, compounded product, administered through DME, concentrated form, per milligram   M
BETOS: D1G   Drugs Administered through DME

D **J7648** Isoetharine HCl, inhalation solution, FDA-approved final product, non-compounded, administered through DME, concentrated form, per milligram M

BETOS: D1G Drugs Administered through DME

D **J7649** Isoetharine HCl, inhalation solution, FDA-approved final product, non-compounded, administered through DME, unit dose form, per milligram M

BETOS: D1G Drugs Administered through DME

C **J7650** Isoetharine HCl, inhalation solution, compounded product, administered through DME, unit dose form, per milligram M

BETOS: D1G Drugs Administered through DME

C **J7657** Isoproterenol HCl, inhalation solution, compounded product, administered through DME, concentrated form, per milligram M

BETOS: D1G Drugs Administered through DME

D **J7658** Isoproterenol HCl, inhalation solution, FDA-approved final product, non-compounded, administered through DME, concentrated form, per milligram M

BETOS: D1G Drugs Administered through DME

D **J7659** Isoproterenol HCl, inhalation solution, FDA-approved final product, non-compounded, administered through DME, unit dose form, per milligram M

BETOS: D1G Drugs Administered through DME

C **J7660** Isoproterenol HCl, inhalation solution, compounded product, administered through DME, unit dose form, per milligram M

BETOS: D1G Drugs Administered through DME

C **J7665** Mannitol, administered through an inhaler, 5 mg N1 ASC N

BETOS: O1E Other drugs

C **J7667** Metaproterenol sulfate, inhalation solution, compounded product, concentrated form, per 10 milligrams M

BETOS: D1G Drugs Administered through DME

D **J7668** Metaproterenol sulfate, inhalation solution, FDA-approved final product, non-compounded, administered through DME, concentrated form, per 10 milligrams M

BETOS: D1G Drugs Administered through DME

D **J7669** Metaproterenol sulfate, inhalation solution, FDA-approved final product, non-compounded, administered through DME, unit dose form, per 10 milligrams M

BETOS: D1G Drugs Administered through DME

C **J7670** Metaproterenol sulfate, inhalation solution, compounded product, administered through DME, unit dose form, per 10 milligrams M

BETOS: D1G Drugs Administered through DME

C **J7674** Methacholine chloride administered as inhalation solution through a nebulizer, per 1 mg N1 ASC N

BETOS: O1E Other drugs
Drugs: PROVOCHOLINE
Coding Clinic: 2005, Q2

C **J7676** Pentamidine isethionate, inhalation solution, compounded product, administered through DME, unit dose form, per 300 mg M

BETOS: D1G Drugs Administered through DME

C **J7677** Revefenacin inhalation solution, FDA-approved final product, non-compounded, administered through DME, 1 microgram M

BETOS: D1G Drugs Administered through DME
Drugs: YUPELRI

D **J7680** Terbutaline sulfate, inhalation solution, compounded product, administered through DME, concentrated form, per milligram M

BETOS: D1G Drugs Administered through DME

D **J7681** Terbutaline sulfate, inhalation solution, compounded product, administered through DME, unit dose form, per milligram M

BETOS: D1G Drugs Administered through DME

D **J7682** Tobramycin, inhalation solution, FDA-approved final product, non-compounded, unit dose form, administered through DME, per 300 milligrams M

BETOS: D1G Drugs Administered through DME
Drugs: BETHKIS, KITABIS PAK, TOBI, TOBRAMYCIN, TOBRAMYCIN INHALATION

D **J7683** Triamcinolone, inhalation solution, compounded product, administered through DME, concentrated form, per milligram M

BETOS: D1G Drugs Administered through DME

D **J7684** Triamcinolone, inhalation solution, compounded product, administered through DME, unit dose form, per milligram M

BETOS: D1G Drugs Administered through DME

C **J7685** Tobramycin, inhalation solution, compounded product, administered through DME, unit dose form, per 300 milligrams M

BETOS: D1G Drugs Administered through DME

C **J7686** Treprostinil, inhalation solution, FDA-approved final product, non-compounded, administered through DME, unit dose form, 1.74 mg M
  BETOS: D1G Drugs Administered through DME
  Drugs: TYVASO, TYVASO (REFILL KIT), TYVASO (STARTER KIT)

DRUGS, NOT OTHERWISE CLASSIFIED (J7699-J8499)

D **J7699** Noc drugs, inhalation solution administered through DME M
  BETOS: D1G Drugs Administered through DME

D **J7799** Noc drugs, other than inhalation drugs, administered through DME N1 ASC N
  BETOS: D1G Drugs Administered through DME

D **J7999** Compounded drug, not otherwise classified N1 ASC N
  BETOS: O1E Other drugs
  Coding Clinic: 2016, Q1; 2016, Q4; 2017, Q1

D **J8498** Antiemetic drug, rectal/suppository, not otherwise specified B
  BETOS: O1D Chemotherapy
  Statute: 1861s2T

M **J8499** Prescription drug, oral, non chemotherapeutic, NOS E1
  BETOS: O1E Other drugs
  Service not separately priced by Part B

CHEMOTHERAPY DRUGS, ORAL ADMINISTRATION (J8501-J8999), SEE ALSO CHEMOTHERAPY DRUGS, ADMINISTERED BY INJECTION (J9000-J9999)

D **J8501** Aprepitant, oral, 5 mg N1 ASC N
  BETOS: O1E Other drugs
  Drugs: APREPITANT, APREPITANT (BI FOLD), APREPITANT (TRI-FOLD), APREPITANT 3-DAY PACK, EMEND, EMEND BI-PACK, EMEND TRI-FOLD
  Coding Clinic: 2005, Q3

D **J8510** Busulfan; oral, 2 mg N1 ASC N
  BETOS: O1D Chemotherapy

M **J8515** Cabergoline, oral, 0.25 mg E1
  BETOS: O1E Other drugs
  Service not separately priced by Part B

D **J8520** Capecitabine, oral, 150 mg N1 ASC N
  BETOS: O1D Chemotherapy
  Drugs: CAPECITABINE, XELODA

D **J8521** Capecitabine, oral, 500 mg N1 ASC N
  BETOS: O1D Chemotherapy
  Drugs: CAPECITABINE, XELODA

D **J8530** Cyclophosphamide; oral, 25 mg N1 ASC N
  BETOS: O1D Chemotherapy

  Drugs: CYCLOPHOSPHAMIDE
  Coding Clinic: 2002, Q1

D **J8540** Dexamethasone, oral, 0.25 mg N1 ASC N
  BETOS: O1E Other drugs
  Statute: 1861(s)2T
  Drugs: DEXAMETHASONE

D **J8560** Etoposide; oral, 50 mg K2 ASC K
  BETOS: O1D Chemotherapy
  Drugs: ETOPOSIDE

C **J8562** Fludarabine phosphate, oral, 10 mg K5 ASC E2
  BETOS: O1D Chemotherapy
  Coding Clinic: 2011, Q1

D **J8565** Gefitinib, oral, 250 mg K5 ASC E2
  BETOS: O1E Other drugs
  Service not separately priced by Part B
  Coding Clinic: 2014, Q4

D **J8597** Antiemetic drug, oral, not otherwise specified N1 ASC N
  BETOS: O1D Chemotherapy
  Statute: 1861s2T

D **J8600** Melphalan; oral, 2 mg N1 ASC N
  BETOS: O1D Chemotherapy

D **J8610** Methotrexate; oral, 2.5 mg N1 ASC N
  BETOS: O1D Chemotherapy
  Drugs: METHOTREXATE, TREXALL

C **J8650** Nabilone, oral, 1 mg K5 ASC E2
  BETOS: O1E Other drugs

D **J8655** Netupitant 300 mg and palonosetron 0.5 mg, oral K2 ASC K
  BETOS: O1E Other drugs
  Drugs: AKYNZEO
  Coding Clinic: 2016, Q1

D **J8670** Rolapitant, oral, 1 mg K2 ASC K
  BETOS: O1E Other drugs
  Drugs: VARUBI ORAL (ROLAPITANT)

D **J8700** Temozolomide, oral, 5 mg N1 ASC N
  BETOS: O1D Chemotherapy
  Drugs: TEMODAR, TEMOZOLOMIDE

C **J8705** Topotecan, oral, 0.25 mg N1 ASC N
  BETOS: O1D Chemotherapy
  Drugs: HYCAMTIN, ORAL
  Coding Clinic: 2009, Q1; 2008, Q4

D **J8999** Prescription drug, oral, chemotherapeutic, NOS B
  BETOS: O1D Chemotherapy

CHEMOTHERAPY DRUGS (J9000-J9999)

CHEMOTHERAPY DRUGS, ADMINISTERED BY INJECTION (J9000-J9999), SEE ALSO CHEMOTHERAPY DRUGS, ORAL ADMINISTRATION (J8501-J8999)

D J9000 Injection, doxorubicin hydrochloride,
10 mg   N1 ASC N
BETOS: O1D   Chemotherapy
Drugs: ADRIAMYCIN, DOXORUBICIN HCL, DOXORUBICIN HCL (LYO)
Coding Clinic: 2007, Q4

D J9015 Injection, aldesleukin, per single
use vial   K2 ASC K
BETOS: O1D   Chemotherapy
Coding Clinic: 2005, Q2

C J9017 Injection, arsenic trioxide, 1 mg   K2 ASC K
BETOS: O1D   Chemotherapy
Drugs: ARSENIC TRIOXIDE, TRISENOX
Coding Clinic: 2002, Q2; 2002, Q1; 2005, Q2

D J9019 Injection, asparaginase (Erwinaze),
1,000 IU   K2 ASC K
BETOS: O1D   Chemotherapy
Drugs: ERWINAZE

D J9020 Injection, asparaginase, not otherwise
specified, 10,000 units   K5 ASC E2
BETOS: O1D   Chemotherapy

C J9022 Injection, atezolizumab, 10 mg   K2 ASC K
BETOS: O1D   Chemotherapy
Drugs: TECENTRIQ, TECENTRIQ (ATEZOLIZUMAB)

C J9023 Injection, avelumab, 10 mg   K2 ASC K
BETOS: O1E   Other drugs
Drugs: BAVENCIO

C J9025 Injection, azacitidine, 1 mg   K2 ASC K
BETOS: O1D   Chemotherapy
Drugs: AZACITIDINE, AZACITIDINE (VIDAZA)

C J9027 Injection, clofarabine, 1 mg   K2 ASC K
BETOS: O1E   Other drugs
Drugs: CLOFARABINE, CLOLAR

D J9030 BCG live intravesical instillation,
1 mg   N1 ASC N
BETOS: O1D   Chemotherapy
Drugs: TICE BCG
Coding Clinic: 2019, Q3

C J9032 Injection, belinostat, 10 mg   K2 ASC K
BETOS: O1D   Chemotherapy
Drugs: BELEODAQ
Coding Clinic: 2016, Q1

C J9033 Injection, bendamustine HCL (treanda),
1 mg   K2 ASC K
BETOS: O1D   Chemotherapy
Drugs: TREANDA
Coding Clinic: 2008, Q4

C J9034 Injection, bendamustine HCL (bendeka),
1 mg   K2 ASC K
BETOS: O1D   Chemotherapy
Drugs: BENDEKA
Coding Clinic: 2017, Q1

C J9035 Injection, bevacizumab, 10 mg   K2 ASC K
BETOS: O1E   Other drugs
Drugs: AVASTIN
Coding Clinic: 2005, Q2; 2013, Q1; 2013, Q3

C J9036 Injection, bendamustine hydrochloride,
(BELRAPZO™/Bendamustine),
1 mg   K2 ASC G
BETOS: O1D   Chemotherapy
Drugs: BELRAPZO, BENDAMUSTINE
Coding Clinic: 2019, Q3

C J9039 Injection, blinatumomab,
1 microgram   K2 ASC K
BETOS: O1D   Chemotherapy
Drugs: BLINCYTO
Coding Clinic: 2016, Q1

D J9040 Injection, bleomycin sulfate,
15 units   N1 ASC N
BETOS: O1D   Chemotherapy
Drugs: BLEOMYCIN, BLEOMYCIN SULFATE

C J9041 Injection, bortezomib (velcade),
0.1 mg   K2 ASC K
BETOS: O1E   Other drugs
Drugs: VELCADE
Coding Clinic: 2005, Q2; 2005, Q1

C J9042 Injection, brentuximab vedotin,
1 mg   K2 ASC K
BETOS: O1D   Chemotherapy
Drugs: ADCETRIS

C J9043 Injection, cabazitaxel, 1 mg   K2 ASC K
BETOS: O1D   Chemotherapy
Drugs: JEVTANA

C J9044 Injection, bortezomib, not otherwise
specified, 0.1 mg   K2 ASC K
BETOS: O1E   Other drugs
Drugs: BORTEZOMIB
Coding Clinic: 2019, Q1

D J9045 Injection, carboplatin, 50 mg   N1 ASC N
BETOS: O1D   Chemotherapy
Drugs: CARBOPLATIN, PARAPLATIN

C J9047 Injection, carfilzomib, 1 mg   K2 ASC K
BETOS: O1D   Chemotherapy
Drugs: KYPROLIS
Coding Clinic: 2013, Q4

D J9050 Injection, carmustine, 100 mg   K2 ASC K
BETOS: O1D   Chemotherapy
Drugs: BICNU, CARMUSTINE

♂ Male only   ♀ Female only   **A** Age   A2 - Z3 = ASC Payment indicator   A - Y = APC Status indicator
ASC = ASC Approved Procedure   **DME** Paid under the DME fee schedule   **MIPS** MIPS code

J9055 - J9190 (left vertical margin)

CHEMOTHERAPY DRUGS (J9000-J9999) (left vertical margin)

| C | **J9055** | Injection, cetuximab, 10 mg | K2 ASC K |

BETOS: O1E   Other drugs
Drugs: ERBITUX
Coding Clinic: 2005, Q2

| C | **J9057** | Injection, copanlisib, 1 mg | K2 ASC K |

BETOS: O1D   Chemotherapy
Drugs: ALIQOPA
Coding Clinic: 2019, Q1

| D | **J9060** | Injection, cisplatin, powder or solution, 10 mg | N1 ASC N |

BETOS: O1D   Chemotherapy
Drugs: CISPLATIN
Coding Clinic: 2011, Q1

| D | **J9065** | Injection, cladribine, per 1 mg | K2 ASC K |

BETOS: O1D   Chemotherapy
Drugs: CLADRIBINE

| D | **J9070** | Cyclophosphamide, 100 mg | K2 ASC K |

BETOS: O1D   Chemotherapy
Drugs: CYCLOPHOSPHAMIDE
Coding Clinic: 2011, Q1

| C | **J9098** | Injection, cytarabine liposome, 10 mg | N1 ASC N |

BETOS: O1E   Other drugs

| D | **J9100** | Injection, cytarabine, 100 mg | N1 ASC N |

BETOS: O1D   Chemotherapy
Drugs: CYTARABINE
Coding Clinic: 2011, Q1

| C | **J9118** | Injection, calaspargase pegol-mknl, 10 units | K5 ASC E2 |

BETOS: O1D   Chemotherapy
Coding Clinic: 2019, Q4

| C | **J9119** | Injection, cemiplimab-rwlc, 1 mg | K2 ASC G |

BETOS: O1D   Chemotherapy
Drugs: LIBTAYO
Coding Clinic: 2019, Q4

| D | **J9120** | Injection, dactinomycin, 0.5 mg | K2 ASC K |

BETOS: O1D   Chemotherapy
Drugs: COSMEGEN, DACTINOMYCIN

| D | **J9130** | Dacarbazine, 100 mg | N1 ASC N |

BETOS: O1D   Chemotherapy
Drugs: DACARBAZINE
Coding Clinic: 2008, Q1; 2011, Q1

● | C | **J9144** | Injection, daratumumab, 10 mg and hyaluronidase-fihj | K2 ▲ ASC G |

BETOS: O1D   Chemotherapy
Drugs: DARZALEX

| D | **J9145** | Injection, daratumumab, 10 mg | K2 ASC K |

BETOS: O1D   Chemotherapy
Drugs: DARZALEX

| D | **J9150** | Injection, daunorubicin, 10 mg | K2 ASC K |

BETOS: O1D   Chemotherapy
Drugs: DAUNORUBICIN HCL

| D | **J9151** | Injection, daunorubicin citrate, liposomal formulation, 10 mg | K5 ASC E2 |

BETOS: O1D   Chemotherapy

| C | **J9153** | Injection, liposomal, 1 mg daunorubicin and 2.27 mg cytarabine | K2 ASC K |

BETOS: O1D   Chemotherapy
Drugs: VYXEOS
Coding Clinic: 2019, Q1

| C | **J9155** | Injection, degarelix, 1 mg | K2 ASC K |

BETOS: O1E   Other drugs
Drugs: FIRMAGON

| C | **J9160** | Injection, denileukin diftitox, 300 micrograms | K5 ASC E2 |

BETOS: O1E   Other drugs
Coding Clinic: 2005, Q2

| D | **J9165** | Injection, diethylstilbestrol diphosphate, 250 mg | K5 ♂ ASC E2 |

BETOS: O1D   Chemotherapy

| D | **J9171** | Injection, docetaxel, 1 mg | N1 ASC N |

BETOS: O1E   Other drugs
Drugs: DOCETAXEL, TAXOTERE

| C | **J9173** | Injection, durvalumab, 10 mg | K2 ASC K |

BETOS: O1E   Other drugs
Drugs: IMFINZI
Coding Clinic: 2019, Q1

| D | **J9175** | Injection, Elliotts' B solution, 1 ml | N1 ASC N |

BETOS: O1E   Other drugs

| C | **J9176** | Injection, elotuzumab, 1 mg | K2 ASC K |

BETOS: O1E   Other drugs
Drugs: EMPLICITI

● | C | **J9177** | Injection, enfortumab vedotin-ejfv, 0.25 mg | K2 ASC G |

BETOS: O1E   Other drugs
Drugs: PADCEV
Coding Clinic: 2020, Q2

| C | **J9178** | Injection, epirubicin HCl, 2 mg | N1 ASC N |

BETOS: O1E   Other drugs
Drugs: ELLENCE, EPIRUBICIN

| C | **J9179** | Injection, eribulin mesylate, 0.1 mg | K2 ASC K |

BETOS: O1D   Chemotherapy
Drugs: HALAVEN

| D | **J9181** | Injection, etoposide, 10 mg | N1 ASC N |

BETOS: O1D   Chemotherapy
Drugs: ETOPOPHOS, ETOPOSIDE

| D | **J9185** | Injection, fludarabine phosphate, 50 mg | N1 ASC N |

BETOS: O1D   Chemotherapy
Drugs: FLUDARABINE PHOSPHATE

| D | **J9190** | Injection, fluorouracil, 500 mg | N1 ASC N |

BETOS: O1D   Chemotherapy
Drugs: ADRUCIL, FLUOROURACIL

● New code   ▲ Revised code   C Carrier judgment   D Special coverage instructions apply
I Not payable by Medicare   M Non-covered by Medicare   S Non-covered by Medicare statute   *AHA Coding Clinic®*

● C **J9198** Injection, gemcitabine hydrochloride, (infugem), 100 mg   K2 ASC G
     BETOS: O1D   Chemotherapy
     Drugs: INFUGEM
     Coding Clinic: 2020, Q2; 2020, Q2

D **J9200** Injection, floxuridine, 500 mg   N1 ASC N
     BETOS: O1D   Chemotherapy
     Drugs: FLOXURIDINE

D **J9201** Injection, gemcitabine hydrochloride, not otherwise specified, 200 mg   N1 ASC N
     BETOS: O1D   Chemotherapy
     Drugs: GEMCITABINE, GEMCITABINE HYDROCHLORIDE, GEMZAR

D **J9202** Goserelin acetate implant, per 3.6 mg   K2 ASC K
     BETOS: O1D   Chemotherapy
     Drugs: ZOLADEX

C **J9203** Injection, gemtuzumab ozogamicin, 0.1 mg   K2 ASC K
     BETOS: O1D   Chemotherapy
     Drugs: MYLOTARG
     Coding Clinic: 2017, Q4; 2018, Q1

C **J9204** Injection, mogamulizumab-kpkc, 1 mg   K2 ASC G
     BETOS: O1D   Chemotherapy
     Drugs: POTELIGEO
     Coding Clinic: 2019, Q4

D **J9205** Injection, irinotecan liposome, 1 mg   K2 ASC K
     BETOS: O1D   Chemotherapy
     Drugs: ONIVYDE

D **J9206** Injection, irinotecan, 20 mg   N1 ASC N
     BETOS: O1D   Chemotherapy
     Drugs: CAMPTOSAR, IRINOTECAN HCL, IRINOTECAN HYDROCHLORIDE

C **J9207** Injection, ixabepilone, 1 mg   K2 ASC K
     BETOS: O1D   Chemotherapy
     Drugs: IXEMPRA KIT
     Coding Clinic: 2008, Q4

D **J9208** Injection, ifosfamide, 1 gram   N1 ASC N
     BETOS: O1D   Chemotherapy
     Drugs: IFEX, IFOSFAMIDE

D **J9209** Injection, mesna, 200 mg   N1 ASC N
     BETOS: O1D   Chemotherapy
     Drugs: MESNA, MESNEX

C **J9210** Injection, emapalumab-lzsg, 1 mg   K2 ASC G
     BETOS: O1D   Chemotherapy
     Drugs: GAMIFANT
     Coding Clinic: 2019, Q4

D **J9211** Injection, idarubicin hydrochloride, 5 mg   N1 ASC N
     BETOS: O1D   Chemotherapy
     Drugs: IDAMYCIN PFS, IDARUBICIN

D **J9212** Injection, interferon alfacon-1, recombinant, 1 microgram   K5 ASC E2
     BETOS: O1E   Other drugs

D **J9213** Injection, interferon, alfa-2a, recombinant, 3 million units   N1 ASC N
     BETOS: O1D   Chemotherapy

D **J9214** Injection, interferon, alfa-2b, recombinant, 1 million units   K2 ASC K
     BETOS: O1D   Chemotherapy
     Drugs: INTRON-A

D **J9215** Injection, interferon, alfa-N3, (human leukocyte derived), 250,000 IU   K5 ASC E2
     BETOS: O1D   Chemotherapy

D **J9216** Injection, interferon, gamma 1-b, 3 million units   K5 ASC E2
     BETOS: O1D   Chemotherapy
     Coding Clinic: 2005, Q2

D **J9217** Leuprolide acetate (for depot suspension), 7.5 mg   K2 ASC K
     BETOS: O1D   Chemotherapy
     Drugs: ELIGARD, LUPRON DEPOT 4-MONTH, 30MG , LUPRON DEPOT 6-MONTH, 45MG , LUPRON DEPOT 7.5 MG KIT, LUPRON DEPOT-3 MONTH 22.5MG KIT, LUPRON DEPOT-PED 15MG, LUPRON DEPOT-PED 7.5MG
     Coding Clinic: 2019, Q2

D **J9218** Leuprolide acetate, per 1 mg   N1 ASC N
     BETOS: O1D   Chemotherapy
     Drugs: LEUPROLIDE ACETATE
     Coding Clinic: 2019, Q2

D **J9219** Leuprolide acetate implant, 65 mg   K5 ASC E2
     BETOS: O1D   Chemotherapy
     Coding Clinic: 2001, Q4

● C **J9223** Injection, lurbinectedin, 0.1 mg   K2 Ⓐ ASC G
     BETOS: O1D   Chemotherapy
     Drugs: ZEPZELCA

D **J9225** Histrelin implant (Vantas), 50 mg   K2 ASC K
     BETOS: O1D   Chemotherapy
     Drugs: VANTAS IMPLANT

D **J9226** Histrelin implant (Supprelin LA), 50 mg   K2 ASC K
     BETOS: O1D   Chemotherapy
     Drugs: SUPPRELIN LA IMPLANT
     Coding Clinic: 2008, Q1

● C **J9227** Injection, isatuximab-irfc, 10 mg   K2 ASC G
     BETOS: O1D   Chemotherapy
     Drugs: SARCLISA

C **J9228** Injection, ipilimumab, 1 mg   K2 ASC K
     BETOS: O1D   Chemotherapy
     Drugs: YERVOY

C **J9229** Injection, inotuzumab ozogamicin, 0.1 mg   K2 ASC K
     BETOS: O1E   Other drugs
     Drugs: BESPONSA
     Coding Clinic: 2019, Q1

♂ Male only   ♀ Female only   Ⓐ Age   A2 - Z3 = ASC Payment indicator   A - Y = APC Status indicator
ASC = ASC Approved Procedure   **DME** Paid under the DME fee schedule   **MIPS** MIPS code

D **J9230** Injection, mechlorethamine hydrochloride, (nitrogen mustard), 10 mg K2 ASC K
BETOS: O1D   Chemotherapy
Drugs: MUSTARGEN

▲ **D** **J9245** Injection, melphalan hydrochloride, not otherwise specified, 50 mg K2 ASC K
BETOS: O1D   Chemotherapy
Drugs: ALKERAN, MELPHALAN
Coding Clinic: 2020, Q2

● **C** **J9246** Injection, melphalan (evomela), 1 mg K2 ASC K
BETOS: O1D   Chemotherapy
Drugs: EVOMELA
Coding Clinic: 2020, Q2

D **J9250** Methotrexate sodium, 5 mg N1 ASC N
BETOS: O1D   Chemotherapy
Drugs: METHOTREXATE, METHOTREXATE POWDER 1GM IN 50ML SD VIAL (P.F.), METHOTREXATE SODIUM

D **J9260** Methotrexate sodium, 50 mg N1 ASC N
BETOS: O1D   Chemotherapy
Drugs: METHOTREXATE, METHOTREXATE POWDER 1GM IN 50ML SD VIAL (P.F.), METHOTREXATE SODIUM

C **J9261** Injection, nelarabine, 50 mg K2 ASC K
BETOS: O1E   Other drugs
Drugs: ARRANON

C **J9262** Injection, omacetaxine mepesuccinate, 0.01 mg K2 ASC K
BETOS: O1D   Chemotherapy
Drugs: SYNRIBO
Coding Clinic: 2013, Q4

C **J9263** Injection, oxaliplatin, 0.5 mg N1 ASC N
BETOS: O1D   Chemotherapy
Drugs: OXALIPLATIN
Coding Clinic: 2009, Q1

C **J9264** Injection, paclitaxel protein-bound particles, 1 mg K2 ASC K
BETOS: O1E   Other drugs
Drugs: ABRAXANE

D **J9266** Injection, pegaspargase, per single dose vial K2 ASC K
BETOS: O1D   Chemotherapy
Drugs: ONCASPAR
Coding Clinic: 2002, Q2

D **J9267** Injection, paclitaxel, 1 mg N1 ASC N
BETOS: O1D   Chemotherapy
Drugs: PACLITAXEL

D **J9268** Injection, pentostatin, 10 mg K2 ASC K
BETOS: O1D   Chemotherapy
Drugs: NIPENT

C **J9269** Injection, tagraxofusp-erzs, 10 micrograms K2 ASC G
BETOS: O1D   Chemotherapy
Drugs: ELZONRIS
Coding Clinic: 2019, Q4

D **J9270** Injection, plicamycin, 2.5 mg K2 ASC K
BETOS: O1D   Chemotherapy

C **J9271** Injection, pembrolizumab, 1 mg K2 ASC K
BETOS: O1D   Chemotherapy
Drugs: KEYTRUDA
Coding Clinic: 2016, Q1

D **J9280** Injection, mitomycin, 5 mg K2 ASC K
BETOS: O1D   Chemotherapy
Drugs: MITOMYCIN, MUTAMYCIN
Coding Clinic: 2011, Q1; 2014, Q2; 2016, Q4; 2017, Q4

● **C** **J9281** Mitomycin pyelocalyceal instillation, 1 mg K2 Ⓐ ASC G
BETOS: O1D   Chemotherapy
Drugs: JELMYTO

C **J9285** Injection, olaratumab, 10 mg K2 ASC K
BETOS: O1D   Chemotherapy
Drugs: LARTRUVO

D **J9293** Injection, mitoxantrone hydrochloride, per 5 mg K2 ASC K
BETOS: O1D   Chemotherapy
Drugs: MITOXANTRONE HYDROCHLORIDE

C **J9295** Injection, necitumumab, 1 mg K2 ASC K
BETOS: O1D   Chemotherapy
Drugs: PORTRAZZA

D **J9299** Injection, nivolumab, 1 mg K2 ASC K
BETOS: O1D   Chemotherapy
Drugs: OPDIVO
Coding Clinic: 2016, Q1

C **J9301** Injection, obinutuzumab, 10 mg K2 ASC K
BETOS: O1D   Chemotherapy
Drugs: GAZYVA

C **J9302** Injection, ofatumumab, 10 mg K2 ASC K
BETOS: O1D   Chemotherapy
Drugs: ARZERRA
Coding Clinic: 2011, Q1

C **J9303** Injection, panitumumab, 10 mg K2 ASC K
BETOS: O1D   Chemotherapy
Drugs: PANITUMUMAB
Coding Clinic: 2008, Q1

● **C** **J9304** Injection, pemetrexed (pemfexy), 10 mg K5 ASC E2
BETOS: O1E   Other drugs

▲ **C** **J9305** Injection, pemetrexed, not otherwise specified, 10 mg K2 ASC K
BETOS: O1E   Other drugs
Drugs: ALIMTA
Coding Clinic: 2005, Q2

C **J9306** Injection, pertuzumab, 1 mg K2 ASC K
BETOS: O1D   Chemotherapy
Drugs: PERJETA
Coding Clinic: 2013, Q4

● New code   ▲ Revised code   **C** Carrier judgment   **D** Special coverage instructions apply
I Not payable by Medicare   **M** Non-covered by Medicare   **S** Non-covered by Medicare statute   AHA Coding Clinic®

CPT® is a registered trademark of the American Medical Association. All rights reserved.

C **J9307** Injection, pralatrexate, 1 mg   K2 ASC K
    BETOS: O1E   Other drugs
    Drugs: FOLOTYN
    Coding Clinic: 2011, Q1

C **J9308** Injection, ramucirumab, 5 mg   K2 ASC K
    BETOS: O1D   Chemotherapy
    Drugs: CYRAMZA
    Coding Clinic: 2016, Q1

C **J9309** Injection, polatuzumab vedotin-piiq, 1 mg   K2 ASC G
    BETOS: O1D   Chemotherapy
    Drugs: POLIVY

D **J9311** Injection, rituximab 10 mg and hyaluronidase   K2 ASC K
    BETOS: O1D   Chemotherapy
    Drugs: RITUXAN HYCELA
    Coding Clinic: 2019, Q1

D **J9312** Injection, rituximab, 10 mg   K2 ASC K
    BETOS: O1D   Chemotherapy
    Drugs: RITUXAN
    Coding Clinic: 2019, Q1

C **J9313** Injection, moxetumomab pasudotox-tdfk, 0.01 mg   K2 ASC G
    BETOS: O1D   Chemotherapy
    Drugs: LUMOXITI
    Coding Clinic: 2019, Q4

C **J9315** Injection, romidepsin, 1 mg   K2 ASC K
    BETOS: O1D   Chemotherapy
    Drugs: ISTODAX (ROMIDEPSIN), ROMIDEPSIN
    Coding Clinic: 2011, Q1

● C **J9316** Injection, pertuzumab, trastuzumab, and hyaluronidase-zzxf, per 10 mg   K2 Ⓐ ASC G
    BETOS: O1D   Chemotherapy
    Drugs: PHESGO

● C **J9317** Injection, sacituzumab govitecan-hziy, 2.5 mg   K2 Ⓐ ASC G
    BETOS: O1D   Chemotherapy
    Drugs: TRODELVY

D **J9320** Injection, streptozocin, 1 gram   K2 ASC K
    BETOS: O1D   Chemotherapy
    Drugs: ZANOSAR

C **J9325** Injection, talimogene laherparepvec, per 1 million plaque forming units   K2 ASC K
    BETOS: O1E   Other drugs
    Drugs: IMLYGIC
    Coding Clinic: 2019, Q2

C **J9328** Injection, temozolomide, 1 mg   K2 ASC K
    BETOS: O1D   Chemotherapy
    Drugs: TEMODAR IV

C **J9330** Injection, temsirolimus, 1 mg   K2 ASC K
    BETOS: O1D   Chemotherapy
    Drugs: TEMSIROLIMUS
    Coding Clinic: 2008, Q4

D **J9340** Injection, thiotepa, 15 mg   K2 ASC K
    BETOS: O1D   Chemotherapy
    Drugs: THIOTEPA

C **J9351** Injection, topotecan, 0.1 mg   N1 ASC N
    BETOS: O1D   Chemotherapy
    Drugs: HYCAMTIN, TOPOTECAN
    Coding Clinic: 2011, Q1

C **J9352** Injection, trabectedin, 0.1 mg   K2 ASC K
    BETOS: O1D   Chemotherapy
    Drugs: YONDELIS

C **J9354** Injection, ado-trastuzumab emtansine, 1 mg   K2 ASC K
    BETOS: O1D   Chemotherapy
    Drugs: KADCYLA
    Coding Clinic: 2013, Q4

C **J9355** Injection, trastuzumab, excludes biosimilar, 10 mg   K2 ASC K
    BETOS: O1E   Other drugs
    Drugs: HERCEPTIN
    Coding Clinic: 2006, Q2; 2019, Q3
    Pub: 100-4, Chapter-3, 20.7.3; 100-4, Chapter-3, 20.7.3

C **J9356** Injection, trastuzumab, 10 mg and hyaluronidase-oysk   K2 ASC G
    BETOS: O1E   Other drugs
    Drugs: HERCEPTIN HYLECTA
    Coding Clinic: 2019, Q3

D **J9357** Injection, valrubicin, intravesical, 200 mg   K2 ASC K
    BETOS: O1E   Other drugs
    Drugs: VALRUBICIN, VALSTAR

● C **J9358** Injection, fam-trastuzumab deruxtecan-nxki, 1 mg   K2 ASC G
    BETOS: O1E   Other drugs
    Drugs: ENHERTU
    Coding Clinic: 2020, Q2

D **J9360** Injection, vinblastine sulfate, 1 mg   N1 ASC N
    BETOS: O1D   Chemotherapy
    Drugs: VINBLASTINE SULFATE

D **J9370** Vincristine sulfate, 1 mg   N1 ASC N
    BETOS: O1D   Chemotherapy
    Drugs: VINCRISTINE SULFATE
    Coding Clinic: 2011, Q1

C **J9371** Injection, vincristine sulfate liposome, 1 mg   K2 ASC K
    BETOS: O1D   Chemotherapy
    Drugs: VINCRISTINE SULFATE
    Coding Clinic: 2014, Q1

D **J9390** Injection, vinorelbine tartrate, 10 mg   N1 ASC N
    BETOS: O1D   Chemotherapy
    Drugs: NAVELBINE, VINORELBINE TARTRATE
    Coding Clinic: 2005, Q2

♂ Male only   ♀ Female only   Ⓐ Age   A2 - Z3 = ASC Payment indicator   A - Y = APC Status indicator
ASC = ASC Approved Procedure   **DME** Paid under the DME fee schedule   **MIPS** MIPS code

C **J9395** Injection, fulvestrant, 25 mg   K2 ASC K
BETOS: O1E   Other drugs
Drugs: FASLODEX, FULVESTRANT

C **J9400** Injection, ziv-aflibercept, 1 mg   K2 ASC K
BETOS: O1E   Other drugs
Drugs: ZALTRAP
Coding Clinic: 2013, Q4

D **J9600** Injection, porfimer sodium, 75 mg   K2 ASC K
BETOS: O1D   Chemotherapy
Drugs: PHOTOFRIN
Coding Clinic: 2020, Q1

D **J9999** Not otherwise classified, antineoplastic
drugs   N1 ASC N
BETOS: O1D   Chemotherapy
Coding Clinic: 2002, Q1; 2008, Q1; 2009,
Q2; 2013, Q1; 2010, Q3; 2012, Q4; 2017, Q1

● New code   ▲ Revised code   **C** Carrier judgment   **D** Special coverage instructions apply
I Not payable by Medicare   **M** Non-covered by Medicare   **S** Non-covered by Medicare statute   AHA Coding Clinic®

DURABLE MEDICAL EQUIPMENT (DME) (K0001-K1012)

WHEELCHAIRS, COMPONENTS, AND ACCESSORIES (K0001-K0195)

C **K0001** Standard wheelchair   DME Y
   BETOS: D1D   Wheelchairs
   DME Modifier: RR

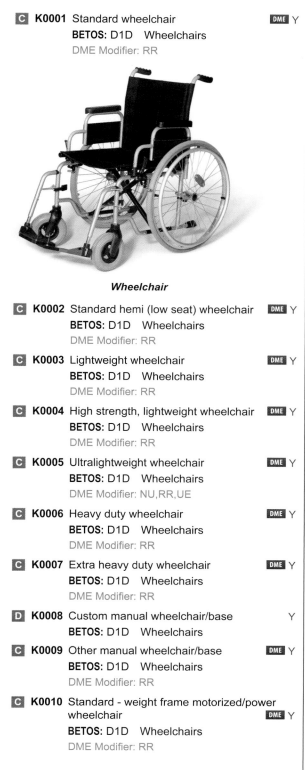

Wheelchair

C **K0002** Standard hemi (low seat) wheelchair   DME Y
   BETOS: D1D   Wheelchairs
   DME Modifier: RR

C **K0003** Lightweight wheelchair   DME Y
   BETOS: D1D   Wheelchairs
   DME Modifier: RR

C **K0004** High strength, lightweight wheelchair   DME Y
   BETOS: D1D   Wheelchairs
   DME Modifier: RR

C **K0005** Ultralightweight wheelchair   DME Y
   BETOS: D1D   Wheelchairs
   DME Modifier: NU,RR,UE

C **K0006** Heavy duty wheelchair   DME Y
   BETOS: D1D   Wheelchairs
   DME Modifier: RR

C **K0007** Extra heavy duty wheelchair   DME Y
   BETOS: D1D   Wheelchairs
   DME Modifier: RR

D **K0008** Custom manual wheelchair/base   Y
   BETOS: D1D   Wheelchairs

C **K0009** Other manual wheelchair/base   DME Y
   BETOS: D1D   Wheelchairs
   DME Modifier: RR

C **K0010** Standard - weight frame motorized/power wheelchair   DME Y
   BETOS: D1D   Wheelchairs
   DME Modifier: RR

C **K0011** Standard - weight frame motorized/power wheelchair with programmable control parameters for speed adjustment, tremor dampening, acceleration control and braking   DME Y
   BETOS: D1D   Wheelchairs
   DME Modifier: KF,RR

C **K0012** Lightweight portable motorized/power wheelchair   DME Y
   BETOS: D1D   Wheelchairs
   DME Modifier: RR

D **K0013** Custom motorized/power wheelchair base   Y
   BETOS: D1D   Wheelchairs

C **K0014** Other motorized/power wheelchair base   Y
   BETOS: D1D   Wheelchairs

C **K0015** Detachable, non-adjustable height armrest, replacement only, each   DME Y
   BETOS: D1D   Wheelchairs
   DME Modifier: KE,KU,RR

C **K0017** Detachable, adjustable height armrest, base, replacement only, each   DME Y
   BETOS: D1D   Wheelchairs
   DME Modifier: KE,KU,NU,RR,UE

C **K0018** Detachable, adjustable height armrest, upper portion, replacement only, each   DME Y
   BETOS: D1D   Wheelchairs
   DME Modifier: KE,KU,NU,RR,UE

C **K0019** Arm pad, replacement only, each   DME Y
   BETOS: D1D   Wheelchairs
   DME Modifier: KE,KU,NU,RR,UE

C **K0020** Fixed, adjustable height armrest, pair   DME Y
   BETOS: D1D   Wheelchairs
   DME Modifier: KE,KU,NU,RR,UE

C **K0037** High mount flip-up foot rest, each   DME Y
   BETOS: D1D   Wheelchairs
   DME Modifier: KE,KU,NU,RR,UE

C **K0038** Leg strap, each   DME Y
   BETOS: D1D   Wheelchairs
   DME Modifier: KE,KU,NU,RR,UE

C **K0039** Leg strap, H style, each   DME Y
   BETOS: D1D   Wheelchairs
   DME Modifier: KE,KU,NU,RR,UE

C **K0040** Adjustable angle footplate, each   DME Y
   BETOS: D1D   Wheelchairs
   DME Modifier: KE,KU,NU,RR,UE

C **K0041** Large size footplate, each   DME Y
   BETOS: D1D   Wheelchairs
   DME Modifier: KE,KU,NU,RR,UE

C **K0042** Standard size footplate, replacement only, each   DME Y
   BETOS: D1D   Wheelchairs
   DME Modifier: KE,KU,NU,RR,UE

C K0043 Foot rest, lower extension tube, replacement only, each DME Y
BETOS: D1D Wheelchairs
DME Modifier: KE,KU,NU,RR,UE

C K0044 Foot rest, upper hanger bracket, replacement only, each DME Y
BETOS: D1D Wheelchairs
DME Modifier: KE,KU,NU,RR,UE

C K0045 Foot rest, complete assembly, replacement only, each DME Y
BETOS: D1D Wheelchairs
DME Modifier: KE,KU,NU,RR,UE

C K0046 Elevating leg rest, lower extension tube, replacement only, each DME Y
BETOS: D1D Wheelchairs
DME Modifier: KE,KU,NU,RR,UE

C K0047 Elevating leg rest, upper hanger bracket, replacement only, each DME Y
BETOS: D1D Wheelchairs
DME Modifier: KE,KU,NU,RR,UE

C K0050 Ratchet assembly, replacement only DME Y
BETOS: D1D Wheelchairs
DME Modifier: KE,KU,NU,RR,UE

C K0051 Cam release assembly, foot rest or leg rest, replacement only, each DME Y
BETOS: D1D Wheelchairs
DME Modifier: KE,KU,NU,RR,UE

C K0052 Swingaway, detachable foot rests, replacement only, each DME Y
BETOS: D1D Wheelchairs
DME Modifier: KE,KU,NU,RR,UE

C K0053 Elevating foot rests, articulating (telescoping), each DME Y
BETOS: D1D Wheelchairs
DME Modifier: KE,KU,NU,RR,UE

C K0056 Seat height less than 17" or equal to or greater than 21" for a high strength, lightweight, or ultralightweight wheelchair DME Y
BETOS: D1D Wheelchairs
DME Modifier: KU,NU,RR,UE

C K0065 Spoke protectors, each DME Y
BETOS: D1D Wheelchairs
DME Modifier: KU,NU,RR,UE

C K0069 Rear wheel assembly, complete, with solid tire, spokes or molded, replacement only, each DME Y
BETOS: D1D Wheelchairs
DME Modifier: KU,NU,RR,UE

C K0070 Rear wheel assembly, complete, with pneumatic tire, spokes or molded, replacement only, each DME Y
BETOS: D1D Wheelchairs
DME Modifier: KU,RR

C K0071 Front caster assembly, complete, with pneumatic tire, replacement only, each DME Y
BETOS: D1D Wheelchairs
DME Modifier: KU,NU,RR,UE

C K0072 Front caster assembly, complete, with semi-pneumatic tire, replacement only, each DME Y
BETOS: D1D Wheelchairs
DME Modifier: KU,NU,RR,UE

C K0073 Caster pin lock, each DME Y
BETOS: D1D Wheelchairs
DME Modifier: KU,NU,RR,UE

C K0077 Front caster assembly, complete, with solid tire, replacement only, each DME Y
BETOS: D1D Wheelchairs
DME Modifier: KU,NU,RR,UE

C K0098 Drive belt for power wheelchair, replacement only DME Y
BETOS: D1D Wheelchairs
DME Modifier: KE,KU,NU,RR,UE

C K0105 IV hanger, each DME Y
BETOS: D1D Wheelchairs
DME Modifier: KU,NU,RR,UE

C K0108 Wheelchair component or accessory, not otherwise specified Y
BETOS: D1D Wheelchairs

D K0195 Elevating leg rests, pair (for use with capped rental wheelchair base) DME Y
BETOS: D1D Wheelchairs
DME Modifier: KE,KU,RR

INFUSION PUMPS AND SUPPLIES (K0455-K0605)

D K0455 Infusion pump used for uninterrupted parenteral administration of medication, (e.g., epoprostenol or treprostinol) DME Y
BETOS: D1E Other DME
DME Modifier: RR

Infusion pump

D **K0462** Temporary replacement for patient owned equipment being repaired, any type   Y
BETOS: D1E   Other DME

D **K0552** Supplies for external non-insulin drug infusion pump, syringe type cartridge, sterile, each   DME Y
BETOS: D1E   Other DME

D **K0553** Supply allowance for therapeutic continuous glucose monitor (CGM), includes all supplies and accessories, 1 month supply = 1 Unit Of Service   DME Y
BETOS: D1E   Other DME
DME Modifier: KF
Coding Clinic: 2017, Q2

D **K0554** Receiver (monitor), dedicated, for use with therapeutic glucose continuous monitor system   DME Y
BETOS: D1E   Other DME
DME Modifier: KF,NU,RR,UE
Coding Clinic: 2017, Q2

C **K0601** Replacement battery for external infusion pump owned by patient, silver oxide, 1.5 volt, each   DME Y
BETOS: D1E   Other DME
DME Modifier: NU
Coding Clinic: 2003, Q2

C **K0602** Replacement battery for external infusion pump owned by patient, silver oxide, 3 volt, each   DME Y
BETOS: D1E   Other DME
DME Modifier: NU
Coding Clinic: 2003, Q2

C **K0603** Replacement battery for external infusion pump owned by patient, alkaline, 1.5 volt, each   DME Y
BETOS: D1E   Other DME
DME Modifier: NU
Coding Clinic: 2003, Q2

C **K0604** Replacement battery for external infusion pump owned by patient, lithium, 3.6 volt, each   DME Y
BETOS: D1E   Other DME
DME Modifier: NU
Coding Clinic: 2003, Q2

C **K0605** Replacement battery for external infusion pump owned by patient, lithium, 4.5 volt, each   DME Y
BETOS: D1E   Other DME
DME Modifier: NU
Coding Clinic: 2003, Q2

AUTOMATED EXTERNAL DEFIBRILLATOR AND SUPPLIES (K0606-K0609)

C **K0606** Automatic external defibrillator, with integrated electrocardiogram analysis, garment type   DME Y
BETOS: D1E   Other DME
DME Modifier: KF,RR

C **K0607** Replacement battery for automated external defibrillator, garment type only, each   DME Y
BETOS: D1E   Other DME
DME Modifier: KF,RR

C **K0608** Replacement garment for use with automated external defibrillator, each   DME Y
BETOS: D1E   Other DME
DME Modifier: KF,NU,RR,UE

C **K0609** Replacement electrodes for use with automated external defibrillator, garment type only, each   DME Y
BETOS: D1E   Other DME
DME Modifier: KF

MISCELLANEOUS DME AND ACCESSORIES (K0669-K0746)

C **K0669** Wheelchair accessory, wheelchair seat or back cushion, does not meet specific code criteria or no written coding verification from DME PDAC   Y
BETOS: D1D   Wheelchairs

C **K0672** Addition to lower extremity orthosis, removable soft interface, all components, replacement only, each   DME A
BETOS: D1F   Prosthetic/Orthotic devices

C **K0730** Controlled dose inhalation drug delivery system   DME Y
BETOS: D1E   Other DME
DME Modifier: RR

C **K0733** Power wheelchair accessory, 12 to 24 amp hour sealed lead acid battery, each (e.g., gel cell, absorbed glassmat)   DME Y
BETOS: D1D   Wheelchairs
DME Modifier: KE,KU,NU,RR,UE

C **K0738** Portable gaseous oxygen system, rental; home compressor used to fill portable oxygen cylinders; includes portable containers, regulator, flowmeter, humidifier, cannula or mask, and tubing   DME Y
BETOS: D1C   Oxygen and supplies
DME Modifier: QB,QF,RR

C **K0739** Repair or nonroutine service for durable medical equipment other than oxygen equipment requiring the skill of a technician, labor component, per 15 minutes   Y
BETOS: D1E   Other DME

♂ Male only   ♀ Female only   **A** Age   A2 - Z3 = ASC Payment indicator   A - Y = APC Status indicator
ASC = ASC Approved Procedure   **DME** Paid under the DME fee schedule   **MIPS** MIPS code

M **K0740** Repair or nonroutine service for oxygen equipment requiring the skill of a technician, labor component, per 15 minutes   E1
   BETOS: D1C   Oxygen and supplies
   Service not separately priced by Part B

C **K0743** Suction pump, home model, portable, for use on wounds   Y
   BETOS: D1E   Other DME

C **K0744** Absorptive wound dressing for use with suction pump, home model, portable, pad size 16 square inches or less   A
   BETOS: D1E   Other DME

C **K0745** Absorptive wound dressing for use with suction pump, home model, portable, pad size more than 16 square inches but less than or equal to 48 square inches   A
   BETOS: D1E   Other DME

C **K0746** Absorptive wound dressing for use with suction pump, home model, portable, pad size greater than 48 square inches   A
   BETOS: D1E   Other DME

POWER OPERATED VEHICLES (K0800-K0812)

C **K0800** Power operated vehicle, group 1 standard, patient weight capacity up to and including 300 pounds   DME Y
   BETOS: D1D   Wheelchairs
   DME Modifier: NU,RR,UE

C **K0801** Power operated vehicle, group 1 heavy duty, patient weight capacity 301 to 450 pounds   DME Y
   BETOS: D1D   Wheelchairs
   DME Modifier: NU,RR,UE

C **K0802** Power operated vehicle, group 1 very heavy duty, patient weight capacity 451 to 600 pounds   DME Y
   BETOS: D1D   Wheelchairs
   DME Modifier: NU,RR,UE

C **K0806** Power operated vehicle, group 2 standard, patient weight capacity up to and including 300 pounds   DME Y
   BETOS: D1D   Wheelchairs
   DME Modifier: NU,RR,UE

C **K0807** Power operated vehicle, group 2 heavy duty, patient weight capacity 301 to 450 pounds   DME Y
   BETOS: D1D   Wheelchairs
   DME Modifier: NU,RR,UE

C **K0808** Power operated vehicle, group 2 very heavy duty, patient weight capacity 451 to 600 pounds   DME Y
   BETOS: D1D   Wheelchairs
   DME Modifier: NU,RR,UE

C **K0812** Power operated vehicle, not otherwise classified   Y
   BETOS: D1D   Wheelchairs

WHEELCHAIRS, POWER OPERATED (K0813-K0899)

C **K0813** Power wheelchair, group 1 standard, portable, sling/solid seat and back, patient weight capacity up to and including 300 pounds   DME Y
   BETOS: D1D   Wheelchairs
   DME Modifier: RR

C **K0814** Power wheelchair, group 1 standard, portable, captains chair, patient weight capacity up to and including 300 pounds   DME Y
   BETOS: D1D   Wheelchairs
   DME Modifier: RR

C **K0815** Power wheelchair, group 1 standard, sling/solid seat and back, patient weight capacity up to and including 300 pounds   DME Y
   BETOS: D1D   Wheelchairs
   DME Modifier: RR

C **K0816** Power wheelchair, group 1 standard, captains chair, patient weight capacity up to and including 300 pounds   DME Y
   BETOS: D1D   Wheelchairs
   DME Modifier: RR

C **K0820** Power wheelchair, group 2 standard, portable, sling/solid seat/back, patient weight capacity up to and including 300 pounds   DME Y
   BETOS: D1D   Wheelchairs
   DME Modifier: RR

C **K0821** Power wheelchair, group 2 standard, portable, captains chair, patient weight capacity up to and including 300 pounds   DME Y
   BETOS: D1D   Wheelchairs
   DME Modifier: RR

C **K0822** Power wheelchair, group 2 standard, sling/solid seat/back, patient weight capacity up to and including 300 pounds   DME Y
   BETOS: D1D   Wheelchairs
   DME Modifier: RR

C **K0823** Power wheelchair, group 2 standard, captains chair, patient weight capacity up to and including 300 pounds   DME Y
   BETOS: D1D   Wheelchairs
   DME Modifier: RR

C **K0824** Power wheelchair, group 2 heavy duty, sling/solid seat/back, patient weight capacity 301 to 450 pounds   DME Y
   BETOS: D1D   Wheelchairs
   DME Modifier: RR

● New code   ▲ Revised code   **C** Carrier judgment   **D** Special coverage instructions apply
I Not payable by Medicare   **M** Non-covered by Medicare   **S** Non-covered by Medicare statute   AHA Coding Clinic®

C **K0825** Power wheelchair, group 2 heavy duty, captains chair, patient weight capacity 301 to 450 pounds   DME Y
     BETOS: D1D   Wheelchairs
     DME Modifier: RR

C **K0826** Power wheelchair, group 2 very heavy duty, sling/solid seat/back, patient weight capacity 451 to 600 pounds   DME Y
     BETOS: D1D   Wheelchairs
     DME Modifier: RR

C **K0827** Power wheelchair, group 2 very heavy duty, captains chair, patient weight capacity 451 to 600 pounds   DME Y
     BETOS: D1D   Wheelchairs
     DME Modifier: RR

C **K0828** Power wheelchair, group 2 extra heavy duty, sling/solid seat/back, patient weight capacity 601 pounds or more   DME Y
     BETOS: D1D   Wheelchairs
     DME Modifier: RR

C **K0829** Power wheelchair, group 2 extra heavy duty, captains chair, patient weight 601 pounds or more   DME Y
     BETOS: D1D   Wheelchairs
     DME Modifier: RR

C **K0830** Power wheelchair, group 2 standard, seat elevator, sling/solid seat/back, patient weight capacity up to and including 300 pounds   Y
     BETOS: D1D   Wheelchairs

C **K0831** Power wheelchair, group 2 standard, seat elevator, captains chair, patient weight capacity up to and including 300 pounds   Y
     BETOS: D1D   Wheelchairs

C **K0835** Power wheelchair, group 2 standard, single power option, sling/solid seat/back, patient weight capacity up to and including 300 pounds   DME Y
     BETOS: D1D   Wheelchairs
     DME Modifier: RR

C **K0836** Power wheelchair, group 2 standard, single power option, captains chair, patient weight capacity up to and including 300 pounds   DME Y
     BETOS: D1D   Wheelchairs
     DME Modifier: RR

C **K0837** Power wheelchair, group 2 heavy duty, single power option, sling/solid seat/back, patient weight capacity 301 to 450 pounds   DME Y
     BETOS: D1D   Wheelchairs
     DME Modifier: RR

C **K0838** Power wheelchair, group 2 heavy duty, single power option, captains chair, patient weight capacity 301 to 450 pounds   DME Y
     BETOS: D1D   Wheelchairs
     DME Modifier: RR

C **K0839** Power wheelchair, group 2 very heavy duty, single power option, sling/solid seat/back, patient weight capacity 451 to 600 pounds   DME Y
     BETOS: D1D   Wheelchairs
     DME Modifier: RR

C **K0840** Power wheelchair, group 2 extra heavy duty, single power option, sling/solid seat/back, patient weight capacity 601 pounds or more   DME Y
     BETOS: D1D   Wheelchairs
     DME Modifier: RR

C **K0841** Power wheelchair, group 2 standard, multiple power option, sling/solid seat/back, patient weight capacity up to and including 300 pounds   DME Y
     BETOS: D1D   Wheelchairs
     DME Modifier: RR

C **K0842** Power wheelchair, group 2 standard, multiple power option, captains chair, patient weight capacity up to and including 300 pounds   DME Y
     BETOS: D1D   Wheelchairs
     DME Modifier: RR

C **K0843** Power wheelchair, group 2 heavy duty, multiple power option, sling/solid seat/back, patient weight capacity 301 to 450 pounds   DME Y
     BETOS: D1D   Wheelchairs
     DME Modifier: RR

C **K0848** Power wheelchair, group 3 standard, sling/solid seat/back, patient weight capacity up to and including 300 pounds   DME Y
     BETOS: D1D   Wheelchairs
     DME Modifier: RR

C **K0849** Power wheelchair, group 3 standard, captains chair, patient weight capacity up to and including 300 pounds   DME Y
     BETOS: D1D   Wheelchairs
     DME Modifier: RR

C **K0850** Power wheelchair, group 3 heavy duty, sling/solid seat/back, patient weight capacity 301 to 450 pounds   DME Y
     BETOS: D1D   Wheelchairs
     DME Modifier: RR

C **K0851** Power wheelchair, group 3 heavy duty, captains chair, patient weight capacity 301 to 450 pounds   DME Y
     BETOS: D1D   Wheelchairs
     DME Modifier: RR

C **K0852** Power wheelchair, group 3 very heavy duty, sling/solid seat/back, patient weight capacity 451 to 600 pounds   DME Y
     BETOS: D1D   Wheelchairs
     DME Modifier: RR

♂ Male only   ♀ Female only   A Age   A2 - Z3 = ASC Payment indicator   A - Y = APC Status indicator
ASC = ASC Approved Procedure   DME Paid under the DME fee schedule   MIPS MIPS code

C **K0853** Power wheelchair, group 3 very heavy duty, captains chair, patient weight capacity 451 to 600 pounds   **DME** Y

     BETOS: D1D   Wheelchairs

     DME Modifier: RR

C **K0854** Power wheelchair, group 3 extra heavy duty, sling/solid seat/back, patient weight capacity 601 pounds or more   **DME** Y

     BETOS: D1D   Wheelchairs

     DME Modifier: RR

C **K0855** Power wheelchair, group 3 extra heavy duty, captains chair, patient weight capacity 601 pounds or more   **DME** Y

     BETOS: D1D   Wheelchairs

     DME Modifier: RR

C **K0856** Power wheelchair, group 3 standard, single power option, sling/solid seat/back, patient weight capacity up to and including 300 pounds   **DME** Y

     BETOS: D1D   Wheelchairs

     DME Modifier: RR

C **K0857** Power wheelchair, group 3 standard, single power option, captains chair, patient weight capacity up to and including 300 pounds   **DME** Y

     BETOS: D1D   Wheelchairs

     DME Modifier: RR

C **K0858** Power wheelchair, group 3 heavy duty, single power option, sling/solid seat/back, patient weight 301 to 450 pounds   **DME** Y

     BETOS: D1D   Wheelchairs

     DME Modifier: RR

C **K0859** Power wheelchair, group 3 heavy duty, single power option, captains chair, patient weight capacity 301 to 450 pounds   **DME** Y

     BETOS: D1D   Wheelchairs

     DME Modifier: RR

C **K0860** Power wheelchair, group 3 very heavy duty, single power option, sling/solid seat/back, patient weight capacity 451 to 600 pounds   **DME** Y

     BETOS: D1D   Wheelchairs

     DME Modifier: RR

C **K0861** Power wheelchair, group 3 standard, multiple power option, sling/solid seat/back, patient weight capacity up to and including 300 pounds   **DME** Y

     BETOS: D1D   Wheelchairs

     DME Modifier: RR

C **K0862** Power wheelchair, group 3 heavy duty, multiple power option, sling/solid seat/back, patient weight capacity 301 to 450 pounds   **DME** Y

     BETOS: D1D   Wheelchairs

     DME Modifier: RR

C **K0863** Power wheelchair, group 3 very heavy duty, multiple power option, sling/solid seat/back, patient weight capacity 451 to 600 pounds   **DME** Y

     BETOS: D1D   Wheelchairs

     DME Modifier: RR

C **K0864** Power wheelchair, group 3 extra heavy duty, multiple power option, sling/solid seat/back, patient weight capacity 601 pounds or more   **DME** Y

     BETOS: D1D   Wheelchairs

     DME Modifier: RR

C **K0868** Power wheelchair, group 4 standard, sling/solid seat/back, patient weight capacity up to and including 300 pounds   Y

     BETOS: D1D   Wheelchairs

C **K0869** Power wheelchair, group 4 standard, captains chair, patient weight capacity up to and including 300 pounds   Y

     BETOS: D1D   Wheelchairs

C **K0870** Power wheelchair, group 4 heavy duty, sling/solid seat/back, patient weight capacity 301 to 450 pounds   Y

     BETOS: D1D   Wheelchairs

C **K0871** Power wheelchair, group 4 very heavy duty, sling/solid seat/back, patient weight capacity 451 to 600 pounds   Y

     BETOS: D1D   Wheelchairs

C **K0877** Power wheelchair, group 4 standard, single power option, sling/solid seat/back, patient weight capacity up to and including 300 pounds   Y

     BETOS: D1D   Wheelchairs

C **K0878** Power wheelchair, group 4 standard, single power option, captains chair, patient weight capacity up to and including 300 pounds   Y

     BETOS: D1D   Wheelchairs

C **K0879** Power wheelchair, group 4 heavy duty, single power option, sling/solid seat/back, patient weight capacity 301 to 450 pounds   Y

     BETOS: D1D   Wheelchairs

C **K0880** Power wheelchair, group 4 very heavy duty, single power option, sling/solid seat/back, patient weight 451 to 600 pounds   Y

     BETOS: D1D   Wheelchairs

C **K0884** Power wheelchair, group 4 standard, multiple power option, sling/solid seat/back, patient weight capacity up to and including 300 pounds   Y

     BETOS: D1D   Wheelchairs

C **K0885** Power wheelchair, group 4 standard, multiple power option, captains chair, patient weight capacity up to and including 300 pounds   Y

     BETOS: D1D   Wheelchairs

● New code   ▲ Revised code   **C** Carrier judgment   **D** Special coverage instructions apply

I Not payable by Medicare   **M** Non-covered by Medicare   **S** Non-covered by Medicare statute   AHA Coding Clinic®

C **K0886** Power wheelchair, group 4 heavy duty, multiple power option, sling/solid seat/back, patient weight capacity 301 to 450 pounds Y
BETOS: D1D Wheelchairs

C **K0890** Power wheelchair, group 5 pediatric, single power option, sling/solid seat/back, patient weight capacity up to and including 125 pounds Ⓐ Y
BETOS: D1D Wheelchairs

C **K0891** Power wheelchair, group 5 pediatric, multiple power option, sling/solid seat/back, patient weight capacity up to and including 125 pounds Ⓐ Y
BETOS: D1D Wheelchairs

C **K0898** Power wheelchair, not otherwise classified Y
BETOS: D1D Wheelchairs

C **K0899** Power mobility device, not coded by DME PDAC or does not meet criteria Y
BETOS: D1D Wheelchairs
Service not separately priced by Part B

CUSTOMIZED DME, OTHER THAN WHEELCHAIR (K0900)

D **K0900** Customized durable medical equipment, other than wheelchair Y
BETOS: D1E Other DME

COMPONENTS, ACCESSORIES AND SUPPLIES (K1001-K1012)

C **K1001** Electronic positional obstructive sleep apnea treatment, with sensor, includes all components and accessories, any type Y
BETOS: Z2 Undefined codes
Value not established

M **K1002** Cranial electrotherapy stimulation (CES) system, includes all supplies and accessories, any type E1
BETOS: Z2 Undefined codes
Service not separately priced by Part B

C **K1003** Whirlpool tub, walk-in, portable Y
BETOS: Z2 Undefined codes
Value not established

C **K1004** Low frequency ultrasonic diathermy treatment device for home use, includes all components and accessories Y
BETOS: Z2 Undefined codes
Value not established

C **K1005** Disposable collection and storage bag for breast milk, any size, any type, each Y
BETOS: Z2 Undefined codes
Value not established

● C **K1006** Suction pump, home model, portable or stationary, electric, any type, for use with external urine management system Y
BETOS: Z2 Undefined codes
Value not established

● C **K1007** Bilateral hip, knee, ankle, foot device, powered, includes pelvic component, single or double upright(s), knee joints any type, with or without ankle joints any type, includes all components and accessories, motors, microprocessors, sensors Y
BETOS: Z2 Undefined codes
Value not established

● C **K1009** Speech volume modulation system, any type, including all components and accessories Y
BETOS: Z2 Undefined codes
Value not established

● C **K1010** Indwelling intraurethral drainage device with valve, patient inserted, replacement only, each Y
BETOS: Z2 Undefined codes
Value not established

● C **K1011** Activation device for intraurethral drainage device with valve, replacement only, each Y
BETOS: Z2 Undefined codes
Value not established

● C **K1012** Charger and base station for intraurethral activation device, replacement only Y
BETOS: Z2 Undefined codes
Value not established

♂ Male only   ♀ Female only   Ⓐ Age   A2 - Z3 = ASC Payment indicator   A - Y = APC Status indicator
ASC = ASC Approved Procedure   **DME** Paid under the DME fee schedule   **MIPS** MIPS code

NOTES

ORTHOTIC PROCEDURES AND SERVICES (L0112-L4631)

CERVICAL ORTHOTICS (L0112-L0174)

C **L0112** Cranial-cervical orthosis (CCO), congenital torticollis type, with or without soft interface material, adjustable range of motion joint, custom fabricated　**DME** A
BETOS: D1F　Prosthetic/Orthotic devices

C **L0113** Cranial-cervical orthosis (CCO), torticollis type, with or without joint, with or without soft interface material, prefabricated, includes fitting and adjustment　**DME** A
BETOS: D1F　Prosthetic/Orthotic devices
Coding Clinic: 2008, Q4

C **L0120** Cervical, flexible, non-adjustable, prefabricated, off-the-shelf (foam collar)　**DME** A
BETOS: D1F　Prosthetic/Orthotic devices

C **L0130** Cervical, flexible, thermoplastic collar, molded to patient　**DME** A
BETOS: D1F　Prosthetic/Orthotic devices

C **L0140** Cervical, semi-rigid, adjustable (plastic collar)　**DME** A
BETOS: D1F　Prosthetic/Orthotic devices

C **L0150** Cervical, semi-rigid, adjustable molded chin cup (plastic collar with mandibular/occipital piece)　**DME** A
BETOS: D1F　Prosthetic/Orthotic devices

C **L0160** Cervical, semi-rigid, wire frame occipital/mandibular support, prefabricated, off-the-shelf　**DME** A
BETOS: D1F　Prosthetic/Orthotic devices

C **L0170** Cervical, collar, molded to patient model　**DME** A
BETOS: D1F　Prosthetic/Orthotic devices

C **L0172** Cervical, collar, semi-rigid thermoplastic foam, two-piece, prefabricated, off-the-shelf　**DME** A
BETOS: D1F　Prosthetic/Orthotic devices

C **L0174** Cervical, collar, semi-rigid, thermoplastic foam, two piece with thoracic extension, prefabricated, off-the-shelf　**DME** A
BETOS: D1F　Prosthetic/Orthotic devices

CERVICAL ORTHOTICS MULTI-POST COLLAR (L0180-L0200)

C **L0180** Cervical, multiple post collar, occipital/mandibular supports, adjustable　**DME** A
BETOS: D1F　Prosthetic/Orthotic devices

C **L0190** Cervical, multiple post collar, occipital/mandibular supports, adjustable cervical bars (SOMI, Guilford, Taylor types)　**DME** A
BETOS: D1F　Prosthetic/Orthotic devices

C **L0200** Cervical, multiple post collar, occipital/mandibular supports, adjustable cervical bars, and thoracic extension　**DME** A
BETOS: D1F　Prosthetic/Orthotic devices

THORACIC RIB BELTS (L0220)

C **L0220** Thoracic, rib belt, custom fabricated　**DME** A
BETOS: D1F　Prosthetic/Orthotic devices

THORACIC-LUMBAR-SACRAL ORTHOTICS (TLSO) (L0450-L0492), SEE ALSO LOW-PROFILE ADDITIONS, THORACIC-LUMBAR-SACRAL ORTHOTICS (L1200-L1290)

C **L0450** Thoracic-lumbar-sacral orthosis (TLSO), flexible, provides trunk support, upper thoracic region, produces intracavitary pressure to reduce load on the intervertebral disks with rigid stays or panel(s), includes shoulder straps and closures, prefabricated, off-the-shelf　**DME** A
BETOS: D1F　Prosthetic/Orthotic devices

Thoracic-lumbar-sacral orthosis

L0452 - L0466

ORTHOTIC PROCEDURES AND SERVICES (L0112-L4631)

[C] **L0452** Thoracic-lumbar-sacral orthosis (TLSO), flexible, provides trunk support, upper thoracic region, produces intracavitary pressure to reduce load on the intervertebral disks with rigid stays or panel(s), includes shoulder straps and closures, custom fabricated [DME] A

BETOS: D1F   Prosthetic/Orthotic devices

[C] **L0454** Thoracic-lumbar-sacral orthosis (TLSO), flexible, provides trunk support, extends from sacrococcygeal junction to above T-9 vertebra, restricts gross trunk motion in the sagittal plane, produces intracavitary pressure to reduce load on the intervertebral disks with rigid stays or panel(s), includes shoulder straps and closures, prefabricated item that has been trimmed, bent, molded, assembled, or otherwise customized to fit a specific patient by an individual with expertise [DME] A

BETOS: D1F   Prosthetic/Orthotic devices

[C] **L0455** Thoracic-lumbar-sacral orthosis (TLSO), flexible, provides trunk support, extends from sacrococcygeal junction to above T-9 vertebra, restricts gross trunk motion in the sagittal plane, produces intracavitary pressure to reduce load on the intervertebral disks with rigid stays or panel(s), includes shoulder straps and closures, prefabricated, off-the-shelf [DME] A

BETOS: D1F   Prosthetic/Orthotic devices

[C] **L0456** Thoracic-lumbar-sacral orthosis (TLSO), flexible, provides trunk support, thoracic region, rigid posterior panel and soft anterior apron, extends from the sacrococcygeal junction and terminates just inferior to the scapular spine, restricts gross trunk motion in the sagittal plane, produces intracavitary pressure to reduce load on the intervertebral disks, includes straps and closures, prefabricated item that has been trimmed, bent, molded, assembled, or otherwise customized to fit a specific patient by an individual with expertise [DME] A

BETOS: D1F   Prosthetic/Orthotic devices

[C] **L0457** Thoracic-lumbar-sacral orthosis (TLSO), flexible, provides trunk support, thoracic region, rigid posterior panel and soft anterior apron, extends from the sacrococcygeal junction and terminates just inferior to the scapular spine, restricts gross trunk motion in the sagittal plane, produces intracavitary pressure to reduce load on the intervertebral disks, includes straps and closures, prefabricated, off-the-shelf [DME] A

BETOS: D1F   Prosthetic/Orthotic devices

[C] **L0458** Thoracic-lumbar-sacral orthosis (TLSO), triplanar control, modular segmented spinal system, two rigid plastic shells, posterior extends from the sacrococcygeal junction and

terminates just inferior to the scapular spine, anterior extends from the symphysis pubis to the xiphoid, soft liner, restricts gross trunk motion in the sagittal, coronal, and transverse planes, lateral strength is provided by overlapping plastic and stabilizing closures, includes straps and closures, prefabricated, includes fitting and adjustment [DME] A

BETOS: D1F   Prosthetic/Orthotic devices

[C] **L0460** Thoracic-lumbar-sacral orthosis (TLSO), triplanar control, modular segmented spinal system, two rigid plastic shells, posterior extends from the sacrococcygeal junction and terminates just inferior to the scapular spine, anterior extends from the symphysis pubis to the sternal notch, soft liner, restricts gross trunk motion in the sagittal, coronal, and transverse planes, lateral strength is provided by overlapping plastic and stabilizing closures, includes straps and closures, prefabricated item that has been trimmed, bent, molded, assembled, or otherwise customized to fit a specific patient by an individual with expertise [DME] A

BETOS: D1F   Prosthetic/Orthotic devices

[C] **L0462** Thoracic-lumbar-sacral orthosis (TLSO), triplanar control, modular segmented spinal system, three rigid plastic shells, posterior extends from the sacrococcygeal junction and terminates just inferior to the scapular spine, anterior extends from the symphysis pubis to the sternal notch, soft liner, restricts gross trunk motion in the sagittal, coronal, and transverse planes, lateral strength is provided by overlapping plastic and stabilizing closures, includes straps and closures, prefabricated, includes fitting and adjustment [DME] A

BETOS: D1F   Prosthetic/Orthotic devices

[C] **L0464** Thoracic-lumbar-sacral orthosis (TLSO), triplanar control, modular segmented spinal system, four rigid plastic shells, posterior extends from sacrococcygeal junction and terminates just inferior to scapular spine, anterior extends from symphysis pubis to the sternal notch, soft liner, restricts gross trunk motion in sagittal, coronal, and transverse planes, lateral strength is provided by overlapping plastic and stabilizing closures, includes straps and closures, prefabricated, includes fitting and adjustment [DME] A

BETOS: D1F   Prosthetic/Orthotic devices

[C] **L0466** Thoracic-lumbar-sacral orthosis (TLSO), sagittal control, rigid posterior frame and flexible soft anterior apron with straps, closures and padding, restricts gross trunk motion in sagittal plane, produces intracavitary pressure to reduce load on intervertebral disks, prefabricated item that has been trimmed, bent, molded, assembled, or otherwise customized to fit a specific patient by an individual with expertise **DME** A

BETOS: D1F   Prosthetic/Orthotic devices

C **L0467** Thoracic-lumbar-sacral orthosis (TLSO), sagittal control, rigid posterior frame and flexible soft anterior apron with straps, closures and padding, restricts gross trunk motion in sagittal plane, produces intracavitary pressure to reduce load on intervertebral disks, prefabricated, off-the-shelf **DME** A

BETOS: D1F   Prosthetic/Orthotic devices

C **L0468** Thoracic-lumbar-sacral orthosis (TLSO), sagittal-coronal control, rigid posterior frame and flexible soft anterior apron with straps, closures and padding, extends from sacrococcygeal junction over scapulae, lateral strength provided by pelvic, thoracic, and lateral frame pieces, restricts gross trunk motion in sagittal, and coronal planes, produces intracavitary pressure to reduce load on intervertebral disks, prefabricated item that has been trimmed, bent, molded, assembled, or otherwise customized to fit a specific patient by an individual with expertise **DME** A

BETOS: D1F   Prosthetic/Orthotic devices

C **L0469** Thoracic-lumbar-sacral orthosis (TLSO), sagittal-coronal control, rigid posterior frame and flexible soft anterior apron with straps, closures and padding, extends from sacrococcygeal junction over scapulae, lateral strength provided by pelvic, thoracic, and lateral frame pieces, restricts gross trunk motion in sagittal and coronal planes, produces intracavitary pressure to reduce load on intervertebral disks, prefabricated, off-the-shelf **DME** A

BETOS: D1F   Prosthetic/Orthotic devices

C **L0470** Thoracic-lumbar-sacral orthosis (TLSO), triplanar control, rigid posterior frame and flexible soft anterior apron with straps, closures and padding, extends from sacrococcygeal junction to scapula, lateral strength provided by pelvic, thoracic, and lateral frame pieces, rotational strength provided by subclavicular extensions, restricts gross trunk motion in sagittal, coronal, and transverse planes, provides intracavitary pressure to reduce load on the intervertebral disks, includes fitting and shaping the frame, prefabricated, includes fitting and adjustment **DME** A

BETOS: D1F   Prosthetic/Orthotic devices

C **L0472** Thoracic-lumbar-sacral orthosis (TLSO), triplanar control, hyperextension, rigid anterior and lateral frame extends from symphysis pubis to sternal notch with two anterior components (one pubic and one sternal), posterior and lateral pads with

straps and closures, limits spinal flexion, restricts gross trunk motion in sagittal, coronal, and transverse planes, includes fitting and shaping the frame, prefabricated, includes fitting and adjustment **DME** A

BETOS: D1F   Prosthetic/Orthotic devices

C **L0480** Thoracic-lumbar-sacral orthosis (TLSO), triplanar control, one piece rigid plastic shell without interface liner, with multiple straps and closures, posterior extends from sacrococcygeal junction and terminates just inferior to scapular spine, anterior extends from symphysis pubis to sternal notch, anterior or posterior opening, restricts gross trunk motion in sagittal, coronal, and transverse planes, includes a carved plaster or CAD-CAM model, custom fabricated **DME** A

BETOS: D1F   Prosthetic/Orthotic devices

C **L0482** Thoracic-lumbar-sacral orthosis (TLSO), triplanar control, one piece rigid plastic shell with interface liner, multiple straps and closures, posterior extends from sacrococcygeal junction and terminates just inferior to scapular spine, anterior extends from symphysis pubis to sternal notch, anterior or posterior opening, restricts gross trunk motion in sagittal, coronal, and transverse planes, includes a carved plaster or CAD-CAM model, custom fabricated **DME** A

BETOS: D1F   Prosthetic/Orthotic devices

C **L0484** Thoracic-lumbar-sacral orthosis (TLSO), triplanar control, two piece rigid plastic shell without interface liner, with multiple straps and closures, posterior extends from sacrococcygeal junction and terminates just inferior to scapular spine, anterior extends from symphysis pubis to sternal notch, lateral strength is enhanced by overlapping plastic, restricts gross trunk motion in the sagittal, coronal, and transverse planes, includes a carved plaster or CAD-CAM model, custom fabricated **DME** A

BETOS: D1F   Prosthetic/Orthotic devices

C **L0486** Thoracic-lumbar-sacral orthosis (TLSO), triplanar control, two piece rigid plastic shell with interface liner, multiple straps and closures, posterior extends from sacrococcygeal junction and terminates just inferior to scapular spine, anterior extends from symphysis pubis to sternal notch, lateral strength is enhanced by overlapping plastic, restricts gross trunk motion in the sagittal, coronal, and transverse planes, includes a carved plaster or CAD-CAM model, custom fabricated **DME** A

BETOS: D1F   Prosthetic/Orthotic devices

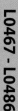

ORTHOTIC PROCEDURES AND SERVICES (L0112-L4631)

C **L0488** Thoracic-lumbar-sacral orthosis (TLSO), triplanar control, one piece rigid plastic shell with interface liner, multiple straps and closures, posterior extends from sacrococcygeal junction and terminates just inferior to scapular spine, anterior extends from symphysis pubis to sternal notch, anterior or posterior opening, restricts gross trunk motion in sagittal, coronal, and transverse planes, prefabricated, includes fitting and adjustment   DME A

BETOS: D1F   Prosthetic/Orthotic devices

C **L0490** Thoracic-lumbar-sacral orthosis (TLSO), sagittal-coronal control, one piece rigid plastic shell, with overlapping reinforced anterior, with multiple straps and closures, posterior extends from sacrococcygeal junction and terminates at or before the T-9 vertebra, anterior extends from symphysis pubis to xiphoid, anterior opening, restricts gross trunk motion in sagittal and coronal planes, prefabricated, includes fitting and adjustment   DME A

BETOS: D1F   Prosthetic/Orthotic devices

C **L0491** Thoracic-lumbar-sacral orthosis (TLSO), sagittal-coronal control, modular segmented spinal system, two rigid plastic shells, posterior extends from the sacrococcygeal junction and terminates just inferior to the scapular spine, anterior extends from the symphysis pubis to the xiphoid, soft liner, restricts gross trunk motion in the sagittal and coronal planes, lateral strength is provided by overlapping plastic and stabilizing closures, includes straps and closures, prefabricated, includes fitting and adjustment   DME A

BETOS: D1F   Prosthetic/Orthotic devices

C **L0492** Thoracic-lumbar-sacral orthosis (TLSO), sagittal-coronal control, modular segmented spinal system, three rigid plastic shells, posterior extends from the sacrococcygeal junction and terminates just inferior to the scapular spine, anterior extends from the symphysis pubis to the xiphoid, soft liner, restricts gross trunk motion in the sagittal and coronal planes, lateral strength is provided by overlapping plastic and stabilizing closures, includes straps and closures, prefabricated, includes fitting and adjustment   DME A

BETOS: D1F   Prosthetic/Orthotic devices

SACRAL ORTHOTICS (L0621-L0624)

C **L0621** Sacroiliac orthosis (SO), flexible, provides pelvic-sacral support, reduces motion about the sacroiliac joint, includes straps, closures, may include pendulous abdomen design, prefabricated, off-the-shelf   DME A

BETOS: D1F   Prosthetic/Orthotic devices

C **L0622** Sacroiliac orthosis (SO), flexible, provides pelvic-sacral support, reduces motion about the sacroiliac joint, includes straps, closures, may include pendulous abdomen design, custom fabricated   DME A

BETOS: D1F   Prosthetic/Orthotic devices

C **L0623** Sacroiliac orthosis (SO), provides pelvic-sacral support, with rigid or semi-rigid panels over the sacrum and abdomen, reduces motion about the sacroiliac joint, includes straps, closures, may include pendulous abdomen design, prefabricated, off-the-shelf   DME A

BETOS: D1F   Prosthetic/Orthotic devices

C **L0624** Sacroiliac orthosis (SO), provides pelvic-sacral support, with rigid or semi-rigid panels placed over the sacrum and abdomen, reduces motion about the sacroiliac joint, includes straps, closures, may include pendulous abdomen design, custom fabricated   DME A

BETOS: D1F   Prosthetic/Orthotic devices

LUMBAR ORTHOTICS (L0625-L0627), SEE ALSO LUMBAR ORTHOTICS SAGITTAL CONTROL (L0641, L0642)

C **L0625** Lumbar orthosis (LO), flexible, provides lumbar support, posterior extends from L-1 to below L-5 vertebra, produces intracavitary pressure to reduce load on the intervertebral discs, includes straps, closures, may include pendulous abdomen design, shoulder straps, stays, prefabricated, off-the-shelf   DME A

BETOS: D1F   Prosthetic/Orthotic devices

C **L0626** Lumbar orthosis (LO), sagittal control, with rigid posterior panel(s), posterior extends from L-1 to below L-5 vertebra, produces intracavitary pressure to reduce load on the intervertebral discs, includes straps, closures, may include padding, stays, shoulder straps, pendulous abdomen design, prefabricated item that has been trimmed, bent, molded, assembled, or otherwise customized to fit a specific patient by an individual with expertise   DME A

BETOS: D1F   Prosthetic/Orthotic devices

C **L0627** Lumbar orthosis (LO), sagittal control, with rigid anterior and posterior panels, posterior extends from L-1 to below L-5 vertebra, produces intracavitary pressure to reduce load on the intervertebral discs, includes straps, closures, may include padding, shoulder straps, pendulous abdomen design, prefabricated item that has been trimmed, bent, molded, assembled, or otherwise customized to fit a specific patient by an individual with expertise   DME A

BETOS: D1F   Prosthetic/Orthotic devices

LUMBAR-SACRAL ORTHOTICS (L0628-L0640), SEE ALSO
LUMBAR-SACRAL ORTHOTICS SAGITTAL CONTROL
(L0643-L0651)

C **L0628** Lumbar-sacral orthosis (LSO), flexible, provides lumbo-sacral support, posterior extends from sacrococcygeal junction to T-9 vertebra, produces intracavitary pressure to reduce load on the intervertebral discs, includes straps, closures, may include stays, shoulder straps, pendulous abdomen design, prefabricated, off-the-shelf **DME** A

BETOS: D1F   Prosthetic/Orthotic devices

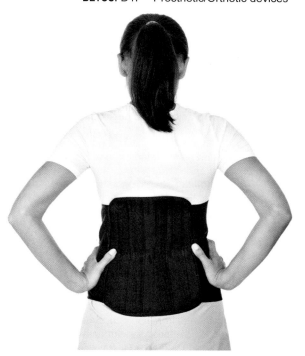

Lumbar-sacral orthosis

C **L0629** Lumbar-sacral orthosis (LSO), flexible, provides lumbo-sacral support, posterior extends from sacrococcygeal junction to T-9 vertebra, produces intracavitary pressure to reduce load on the intervertebral discs, includes straps, closures, may include stays, shoulder straps, pendulous abdomen design, custom fabricated **DME** A

BETOS: D1F   Prosthetic/Orthotic devices

C **L0630** Lumbar-sacral orthosis (LSO), sagittal control, with rigid posterior panel(s), posterior extends from sacrococcygeal junction to T-9 vertebra, produces intracavitary pressure to reduce load on the intervertebral discs, includes straps, closures, may include padding, stays, shoulder straps, pendulous abdomen design, prefabricated item that has been trimmed, bent, molded, assembled, or otherwise customized to fit a specific patient by an individual with expertise **DME** A

BETOS: D1F   Prosthetic/Orthotic devices

C **L0631** Lumbar-sacral orthosis (LSO), sagittal control, with rigid anterior and posterior panels, posterior extends from sacrococcygeal junction to T-9 vertebra, produces intracavitary pressure to reduce load on the intervertebral discs, includes straps, closures, may include padding, shoulder straps, pendulous abdomen design, prefabricated item that has been trimmed, bent, molded, assembled, or otherwise customized to fit a specific patient by an individual with expertise **DME** A

BETOS: D1F   Prosthetic/Orthotic devices

C **L0632** Lumbar-sacral orthosis (LSO), sagittal control, with rigid anterior and posterior panels, posterior extends from sacrococcygeal junction to T-9 vertebra, produces intracavitary pressure to reduce load on the intervertebral discs, includes straps, closures, may include padding, shoulder straps, pendulous abdomen design, custom fabricated **DME** A

BETOS: D1F   Prosthetic/Orthotic devices

C **L0633** Lumbar-sacral orthosis (LSO), sagittal-coronal control, with rigid posterior frame/panel(s), posterior extends from sacrococcygeal junction to T-9 vertebra, lateral strength provided by rigid lateral frame/panels, produces intracavitary pressure to reduce load on intervertebral discs, includes straps, closures, may include padding, stays, shoulder straps, pendulous abdomen design, prefabricated item that has been trimmed, bent, molded, assembled, or otherwise customized to fit a specific patient by an individual with expertise **DME** A

BETOS: D1F   Prosthetic/Orthotic devices

C **L0634** Lumbar-sacral orthosis (LSO), sagittal-coronal control, with rigid posterior frame/panel(s), posterior extends from sacrococcygeal junction to T-9 vertebra, lateral strength provided by rigid lateral frame/panel(s), produces intracavitary pressure to reduce load on intervertebral discs, includes straps, closures, may include padding, stays, shoulder straps, pendulous abdomen design, custom fabricated **DME** A

BETOS: D1F   Prosthetic/Orthotic devices

C **L0635** Lumbar-sacral orthosis (LSO), sagittal-coronal control, lumbar flexion, rigid posterior frame/panel(s), lateral articulating design to flex the lumbar spine, posterior extends from sacrococcygeal junction to T-9 vertebra, lateral strength provided by rigid lateral frame/panel(s), produces intracavitary pressure to reduce load on intervertebral discs, includes straps, closures, may include padding, anterior panel, pendulous abdomen design, prefabricated, includes fitting and adjustment **DME** A

BETOS: D1F   Prosthetic/Orthotic devices

C **L0636** Lumbar-sacral orthosis (LSO), sagittal-coronal control, lumbar flexion, rigid posterior frame/panels, lateral articulating design to flex the lumbar spine, posterior extends from sacrococcygeal junction to T-9 vertebra, lateral strength provided by rigid lateral frame/panels, produces intracavitary pressure to reduce load on intervertebral discs, includes straps, closures, may include padding, anterior panel, pendulous abdomen design, custom fabricated ▪DME▪ A
BETOS: D1F   Prosthetic/Orthotic devices

C **L0637** Lumbar-sacral orthosis (LSO), sagittal-coronal control, with rigid anterior and posterior frame/panels, posterior extends from sacrococcygeal junction to T-9 vertebra, lateral strength provided by rigid lateral frame/panels, produces intracavitary pressure to reduce load on intervertebral discs, includes straps, closures, may include padding, shoulder straps, pendulous abdomen design, prefabricated item that has been trimmed, bent, molded, assembled, or otherwise customized to fit a specific patient by an individual with expertise ▪DME▪ A
BETOS: D1F   Prosthetic/Orthotic devices

C **L0638** Lumbar-sacral orthosis (LSO), sagittal-coronal control, with rigid anterior and posterior frame/panels, posterior extends from sacrococcygeal junction to T-9 vertebra, lateral strength provided by rigid lateral frame/panels, produces intracavitary pressure to reduce load on intervertebral discs, includes straps, closures, may include padding, shoulder straps, pendulous abdomen design, custom fabricated ▪DME▪ A
BETOS: D1F   Prosthetic/Orthotic devices

C **L0639** Lumbar-sacral orthosis (LSO), sagittal-coronal control, rigid shell(s)/panel(s), posterior extends from sacrococcygeal junction to T-9 vertebra, anterior extends from symphysis pubis to xyphoid, produces intracavitary pressure to reduce load on the intervertebral discs, overall strength is provided by overlapping rigid material and stabilizing closures, includes straps, closures, may include soft interface, pendulous abdomen design, prefabricated item that has been trimmed, bent, molded, assembled, or otherwise customized to fit a specific patient by an individual with expertise ▪DME▪ A
BETOS: D1F   Prosthetic/Orthotic devices

C **L0640** Lumbar-sacral orthosis (LSO), sagittal-coronal control, rigid shell(s)/panel(s), posterior extends from sacrococcygeal junction to T-9 vertebra, anterior extends from symphysis pubis to xiphoid, produces intracavitary pressure to reduce load on the intervertebral discs, overall strength

is provided by overlapping rigid material and stabilizing closures, includes straps, closures, may include soft interface, pendulous abdomen design, custom fabricated ▪DME▪ A
BETOS: D1F   Prosthetic/Orthotic devices

LUMBAR ORTHOTICS SAGITTAL CONTROL (L0641, L0642), SEE ALSO LUMBAR ORTHOTICS (L0625-L0627)

C **L0641** Lumbar orthosis (LO), sagittal control, with rigid posterior panel(s), posterior extends from L-1 to below L-5 vertebra, produces intracavitary pressure to reduce load on the intervertebral discs, includes straps, closures, may include padding, stays, shoulder straps, pendulous abdomen design, prefabricated, off-the-shelf ▪DME▪ A
BETOS: D1F   Prosthetic/Orthotic devices

C **L0642** Lumbar orthosis (LO), sagittal control, with rigid anterior and posterior panels, posterior extends from L-1 to below L-5 vertebra, produces intracavitary pressure to reduce load on the intervertebral discs, includes straps, closures, may include padding, shoulder straps, pendulous abdomen design, prefabricated, off-the-shelf ▪DME▪ A
BETOS: D1F   Prosthetic/Orthotic devices

LUMBAR-SACRAL ORTHOTICS SAGITTAL CONTROL (L0643-L0651), SEE ALSO LUMBAR-SACRAL ORTHOTICS (L0628-L0640)

C **L0643** Lumbar-sacral orthosis (LSO), sagittal control, with rigid posterior panel(s), posterior extends from sacrococcygeal junction to T-9 vertebra, produces intracavitary pressure to reduce load on the intervertebral discs, includes straps, closures, may include padding, stays, shoulder straps, pendulous abdomen design, prefabricated, off-the-shelf ▪DME▪ A
BETOS: D1F   Prosthetic/Orthotic devices

C **L0648** Lumbar-sacral orthosis (LSO), sagittal control, with rigid anterior and posterior panels, posterior extends from sacrococcygeal junction to T-9 vertebra, produces intracavitary pressure to reduce load on the intervertebral discs, includes straps, closures, may include padding, shoulder straps, pendulous abdomen design, prefabricated, off-the-shelf ▪DME▪ A
BETOS: D1F   Prosthetic/Orthotic devices

C **L0649** Lumbar-sacral orthosis (LSO), sagittal-coronal control, with rigid posterior frame/panel(s), posterior extends from sacrococcygeal junction to T-9 vertebra, lateral strength provided by rigid lateral frame/panels, produces intracavitary pressure to reduce load on intervertebral discs, includes straps, closures, may include padding, stays, shoulder straps, pendulous abdomen design, prefabricated, off-the-shelf `DME` A

BETOS: D1F　Prosthetic/Orthotic devices

C L0650 Lumbar-sacral orthosis (LSO), sagittal-coronal control, with rigid anterior and posterior frame/panel(s), posterior extends from sacrococcygeal junction to T-9 vertebra, lateral strength provided by rigid lateral frame/panel(s), produces intracavitary pressure to reduce load on intervertebral discs, includes straps, closures, may include padding, shoulder straps, pendulous abdomen design, prefabricated, off-the-shelf `DME` A

BETOS: D1F　Prosthetic/Orthotic devices

C L0651 Lumbar-sacral orthosis (LSO), sagittal-coronal control, rigid shell(s)/panel(s), posterior extends from sacrococcygeal junction to T-9 vertebra, anterior extends from symphysis pubis to xyphoid, produces intracavitary pressure to reduce load on the intervertebral discs, overall strength is provided by overlapping rigid material and stabilizing closures, includes straps, closures, may include soft interface, pendulous abdomen design, prefabricated, off-the-shelf `DME` A

BETOS: D1F　Prosthetic/Orthotic devices

CERVICAL-THORACIC-LUMBAR-SACRAL ORTHOTICS (L0700, L0710)

C L0700 Cervical-thoracic-lumbar-sacral orthosis (CTLSO), anterior-posterior-lateral control, molded to patient model (Minerva type) `DME` A

BETOS: D1F　Prosthetic/Orthotic devices

C L0710 Cervical-thoracic-lumbar-sacral orthosis (CTLSO), anterior-posterior-lateral-control, molded to patient model, with interface material (Minerva type) `DME` A

BETOS: D1F　Prosthetic/Orthotic devices

CERVICAL HALO PROCEDURES (L0810-L0861)

C L0810 Halo procedure, cervical halo incorporated into jacket vest `DME` A

BETOS: D1F　Prosthetic/Orthotic devices

C L0820 Halo procedure, cervical halo incorporated into plaster body jacket `DME` A

BETOS: D1F　Prosthetic/Orthotic devices

C L0830 Halo procedure, cervical halo incorporated into Milwaukee type orthosis `DME` A

BETOS: D1F　Prosthetic/Orthotic devices

C L0859 Addition to halo procedure, magnetic resonance image compatible systems, rings and pins, any material `DME` A

BETOS: D1F　Prosthetic/Orthotic devices

C L0861 Addition to halo procedure, replacement liner/interface material `DME` A

BETOS: D1F　Prosthetic/Orthotic devices

ACCESSORIES FOR SPINAL ORTHOTICS INCLUDING THORACIC-LUMBAR-SACRAL ORTHOSES (TLSO) (L0970-L0999)

C L0970 Thoracic-lumbar-sacral orthosis (TLSO), corset front `DME` A

BETOS: D1F　Prosthetic/Orthotic devices

C L0972 Lumbar-sacral orthosis (LSO), corset front `DME` A

BETOS: D1F　Prosthetic/Orthotic devices

C L0974 Thoracic-lumbar-sacral orthosis (TLSO), full corset `DME` A

BETOS: D1F　Prosthetic/Orthotic devices

C L0976 Lumbar-sacral orthotic (LSO), full corset `DME` A

BETOS: D1F　Prosthetic/Orthotic devices

C L0978 Axillary crutch extension `DME` A

BETOS: D1F　Prosthetic/Orthotic devices

C L0980 Peroneal straps, prefabricated, off-the-shelf, pair `DME` A

BETOS: D1F　Prosthetic/Orthotic devices

C L0982 Stocking supporter grips, prefabricated, off-the-shelf, set of four (4) `DME` A

BETOS: D1F　Prosthetic/Orthotic devices

C L0984 Protective body sock, prefabricated, off-the-shelf, each `DME` A

BETOS: D1F　Prosthetic/Orthotic devices

C L0999 Addition to spinal orthosis, not otherwise specified A

BETOS: D1F　Prosthetic/Orthotic devices

SCOLIOSIS ORTHOTIC DEVICES INCLUDING CERVICAL-THORACIC-LUMBAR-SACRAL ORTHOSES (CTLSO) (L1000-L1120)

C L1000 Cervical-thoracic-lumbar-sacral orthosis (CTLSO) (Milwaukee), inclusive of furnishing initial orthosis, including model `DME` A

BETOS: D1F　Prosthetic/Orthotic devices

C L1001 Cervical-thoracic-lumbar-sacral orthosis (CTLSO), immobilizer, infant size, prefabricated, includes fitting and adjustment `DME` A

BETOS: D1F　Prosthetic/Orthotic devices

C L1005 Tension based scoliosis orthosis and accessory pads, includes fitting and adjustment `DME` A

BETOS: D1F　Prosthetic/Orthotic devices
Coding Clinic: 2002, Q1

C L1010 Addition to Cervical-thoracic-lumbar-sacral orthosis (CTLSO) or scoliosis orthosis, axilla sling `DME` A

BETOS: D1F　Prosthetic/Orthotic devices

♂ Male only　　♀ Female only　　Ⓐ Age　　A2 - Z3 = ASC Payment indicator　　A - Y = APC Status indicator
ASC = ASC Approved Procedure　　`DME` Paid under the DME fee schedule　　`MIPS` MIPS code

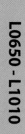

L1020 - L1499

ORTHOTIC PROCEDURES AND SERVICES (L0112-L4631)

C L1020 Addition to Cervical-thoracic-lumbar-sacral orthosis (CTLSO) or scoliosis orthosis, kyphosis pad   DME A
BETOS: D1F   Prosthetic/Orthotic devices

C L1025 Addition to Cervical-thoracic-lumbar-sacral orthosis (CTLSO) or scoliosis orthosis, kyphosis pad, floating   DME A
BETOS: D1F   Prosthetic/Orthotic devices

C L1030 Addition to Cervical-thoracic-lumbar-sacral orthosis (CTLSO) or scoliosis orthosis, lumbar bolster pad   DME A
BETOS: D1F   Prosthetic/Orthotic devices

C L1040 Addition to Cervical-thoracic-lumbar-sacral orthosis (CTLSO) or scoliosis orthosis, lumbar or lumbar rib pad   DME A
BETOS: D1F   Prosthetic/Orthotic devices

C L1050 Addition to Cervical-thoracic-lumbar-sacral orthosis (CTLSO) or scoliosis orthosis, sternal pad   DME A
BETOS: D1F   Prosthetic/Orthotic devices

C L1060 Addition to Cervical-thoracic-lumbar-sacral orthosis (CTLSO) or scoliosis orthosis, thoracic pad   DME A
BETOS: D1F   Prosthetic/Orthotic devices

C L1070 Addition to Cervical-thoracic-lumbar-sacral orthosis (CTLSO) or scoliosis orthosis, trapezius sling   DME A
BETOS: D1F   Prosthetic/Orthotic devices

C L1080 Addition to Cervical-thoracic-lumbar-sacral orthosis (CTLSO) or scoliosis orthosis, outrigger   DME A
BETOS: D1F   Prosthetic/Orthotic devices

C L1085 Addition to Cervical-thoracic-lumbar-sacral orthosis (CTLSO) or scoliosis orthosis, outrigger, bilateral with vertical extensions   DME A
BETOS: D1F   Prosthetic/Orthotic devices

C L1090 Addition to Cervical-thoracic-lumbar-sacral orthosis (CTLSO) or scoliosis orthosis, lumbar sling   DME A
BETOS: D1F   Prosthetic/Orthotic devices

C L1100 Addition to Cervical-thoracic-lumbar-sacral orthosis (CTLSO) or scoliosis orthosis, ring flange, plastic or leather   DME A
BETOS: D1F   Prosthetic/Orthotic devices

C L1110 Addition to Cervical-thoracic-lumbar-sacral orthosis (CTLSO) or scoliosis orthosis, ring flange, plastic or leather, molded to patient model   DME A
BETOS: D1F   Prosthetic/Orthotic devices

C L1120 Addition to Cervical-thoracic-lumbar-sacral orthosis (CTLSO), scoliosis orthosis, cover for upright, each   DME A
BETOS: D1F   Prosthetic/Orthotic devices

LOW-PROFILE ADDITIONS, THORACIC-LUMBAR-SACRAL ORTHOTICS (L1200-L1290), SEE ALSO THORACIC-LUMBAR-SACRAL (TLSO) ORTHOTICS (L0450-L0492)

C L1200 Thoracic-lumbar-sacral-orthosis (TLSO), inclusive of furnishing initial orthosis only   DME A
BETOS: D1F   Prosthetic/Orthotic devices

C L1210 Addition to Thoracic-lumbar-sacral-orthosis (TLSO), (low profile), lateral thoracic extension   DME A
BETOS: D1F   Prosthetic/Orthotic devices

C L1220 Addition to Thoracic-lumbar-sacral orthosis (TLSO), (low profile), anterior thoracic extension   DME A
BETOS: D1F   Prosthetic/Orthotic devices

C L1230 Addition to Thoracic-lumbar-sacral orthosis (TLSO), (low profile), Milwaukee type superstructure   DME A
BETOS: D1F   Prosthetic/Orthotic devices

C L1240 Addition to Thoracic-lumbar-sacral orthosis (TLSO), (low profile), lumbar derotation pad   DME A
BETOS: D1F   Prosthetic/Orthotic devices

C L1250 Addition to Thoracic-lumbar-sacral orthosis (TLSO), (low profile), anterior ASIS pad   DME A
BETOS: D1F   Prosthetic/Orthotic devices

C L1260 Addition to Thoracic-lumbar-sacral orthosis (TLSO), (low profile), anterior thoracic derotation pad   DME A
BETOS: D1F   Prosthetic/Orthotic devices

C L1270 Addition to Thoracic-lumbar-sacral orthosis (TLSO), (low profile), abdominal pad   DME A
BETOS: D1F   Prosthetic/Orthotic devices

C L1280 Addition to Thoracic-lumbar-sacral orthosis (TLSO), (low profile), rib gusset (elastic), each   DME A
BETOS: D1F   Prosthetic/Orthotic devices

C L1290 Addition to Thoracic-lumbar-sacral orthosis (TLSO), (low profile), lateral trochanteric pad   DME A
BETOS: D1F   Prosthetic/Orthotic devices

OTHER SCOLIOSIS AND SPINAL ORTHOTICS AND PROCEDURES (L1300-L1499)

C L1300 Other scoliosis procedure, body jacket molded to patient model   DME A
BETOS: D1F   Prosthetic/Orthotic devices

C L1310 Other scoliosis procedure, post-operative body jacket   DME A
BETOS: D1F   Prosthetic/Orthotic devices

C L1499 Spinal orthosis, not otherwise specified   A
BETOS: D1F   Prosthetic/Orthotic devices

● New code   ▲ Revised code   C Carrier judgment   D Special coverage instructions apply
I Not payable by Medicare   M Non-covered by Medicare   S Non-covered by Medicare statute   AHA Coding Clinic®

HIP ORTHOTICS (L1600-L1690)

C **L1600** Hip orthosis (HO), abduction control of hip joints, flexible, Frejka type with cover, prefabricated item that has been trimmed, bent, molded, assembled, or otherwise customized to fit a specific patient by an individual with expertise `DME` A
BETOS: D1F   Prosthetic/Orthotic devices

C **L1610** Hip orthosis (HO), abduction control of hip joints, flexible, (Frejka cover only), prefabricated item that has been trimmed, bent, molded, assembled, or otherwise customized to fit a specific patient by an individual with expertise `DME` A
BETOS: D1F   Prosthetic/Orthotic devices

C **L1620** Hip orthosis (HO), abduction control of hip joints, flexible, (Pavlik harness), prefabricated item that has been trimmed, bent, molded, assembled, or otherwise customized to fit a specific patient by an individual with expertise `DME` A
BETOS: D1F   Prosthetic/Orthotic devices

C **L1630** Hip orthosis (HO), abduction control of hip joints, semi-flexible (Von Rosen type), custom-fabricated `DME` A
BETOS: D1F   Prosthetic/Orthotic devices

C **L1640** Hip orthosis (HO), abduction control of hip joints, static, pelvic band or spreader bar, thigh cuffs, custom-fabricated `DME` A
BETOS: D1F   Prosthetic/Orthotic devices

C **L1650** Hip orthosis (HO), abduction control of hip joints, static, adjustable, (Ilfled type), prefabricated, includes fitting and adjustment `DME` A
BETOS: D1F   Prosthetic/Orthotic devices

C **L1652** Hip orthosis (HO), bilateral thigh cuffs with adjustable abductor spreader bar, adult size, prefabricated, includes fitting and adjustment, any type `DME` **A** A
BETOS: D1F   Prosthetic/Orthotic devices

C **L1660** Hip orthosis (HO), abduction control of hip joints, static, plastic, prefabricated, includes fitting and adjustment `DME` A
BETOS: D1F   Prosthetic/Orthotic devices

C **L1680** Hip orthosis (HO), abduction control of hip joints, dynamic, pelvic control, adjustable hip motion control, thigh cuffs (Rancho hip action type), custom fabricated `DME` A
BETOS: D1F   Prosthetic/Orthotic devices

C **L1685** Hip orthosis (HO), abduction control of hip joint, postoperative hip abduction type, custom fabricated `DME` A
BETOS: D1F   Prosthetic/Orthotic devices

C **L1686** Hip orthosis (HO), abduction control of hip joint, postoperative hip abduction type, prefabricated, includes fitting and adjustment `DME` A
BETOS: D1F   Prosthetic/Orthotic devices

C **L1690** Combination, bilateral, lumbar-sacral-hip-femur orthosis (LSHFO) providing adduction and internal rotation control, prefabricated, includes fitting and adjustment `DME` A
BETOS: D1F   Prosthetic/Orthotic devices

LEGG PERTHES ORTHOTICS (L1700-L1755)

C **L1700** Legg Perthes orthosis, (Toronto type), custom fabricated `DME` A
BETOS: D1F   Prosthetic/Orthotic devices

C **L1710** Legg Perthes orthosis, (Newington type), custom fabricated `DME` A
BETOS: D1F   Prosthetic/Orthotic devices

C **L1720** Legg Perthes orthosis, trilateral, (Tachdijan type), custom fabricated `DME` A
BETOS: D1F   Prosthetic/Orthotic devices

C **L1730** Legg Perthes orthosis, (Scottish Rite type), custom fabricated `DME` A
BETOS: D1F   Prosthetic/Orthotic devices

C **L1755** Legg Perthes orthosis, (Patten bottom type), custom fabricated `DME` A
BETOS: D1F   Prosthetic/Orthotic devices

KNEE ORTHOTICS (L1810-L1860)

C **L1810** Knee orthosis (KO), elastic with joints, prefabricated item that has been trimmed, bent, molded, assembled, or otherwise customized to fit a specific patient by an individual with expertise `DME` A
BETOS: D1F   Prosthetic/Orthotic devices

C **L1812** Knee orthosis (KO), elastic with joints, prefabricated, off-the-shelf `DME` A
BETOS: D1F   Prosthetic/Orthotic devices

C **L1820** Knee orthosis (KO), elastic with condylar pads and joints, with or without patellar control, prefabricated, includes fitting and adjustment `DME` A
BETOS: D1F   Prosthetic/Orthotic devices

C **L1830** Knee orthosis (KO), immobilizer, canvas longitudinal, prefabricated, off-the-shelf `DME` A
BETOS: D1F   Prosthetic/Orthotic devices

♂ Male only   ♀ Female only   **A** Age   A2 - Z3 = ASC Payment indicator   A - Y = APC Status indicator
ASC = ASC Approved Procedure   `DME` Paid under the DME fee schedule   `MIPS` MIPS code

L1831 - L1860

ORTHOTIC PROCEDURES AND SERVICES (L0112-L4631)

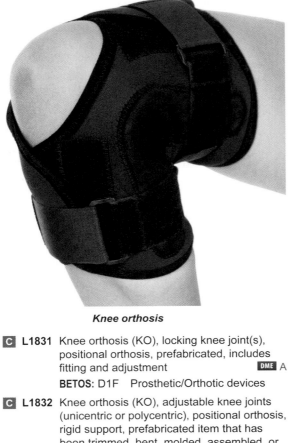

Knee orthosis

C **L1831** Knee orthosis (KO), locking knee joint(s), positional orthosis, prefabricated, includes fitting and adjustment **DME** A
    BETOS: D1F Prosthetic/Orthotic devices

C **L1832** Knee orthosis (KO), adjustable knee joints (unicentric or polycentric), positional orthosis, rigid support, prefabricated item that has been trimmed, bent, molded, assembled, or otherwise customized to fit a specific patient by an individual with expertise **DME** A
    BETOS: D1F Prosthetic/Orthotic devices

C **L1833** Knee orthosis (KO), adjustable knee joints (unicentric or polycentric), positional orthosis, rigid support, prefabricated, off-the-shelf **DME** A
    BETOS: D1F Prosthetic/Orthotic devices

C **L1834** Knee orthosis (KO), without knee joint, rigid, custom fabricated **DME** A
    BETOS: D1F Prosthetic/Orthotic devices

C **L1836** Knee orthosis (KO), rigid, without joint(s), includes soft interface material, prefabricated, off-the-shelf **DME** A
    BETOS: D1F Prosthetic/Orthotic devices

C **L1840** Knee orthosis (KO), derotation, medial-lateral, anterior cruciate ligament, custom fabricated **DME** A
    BETOS: D1F Prosthetic/Orthotic devices

C **L1843** Knee orthosis (KO), single upright, thigh and calf, with adjustable flexion and extension joint (unicentric or polycentric), medial-lateral and rotation control, with or without varus/valgus adjustment, prefabricated item that has been trimmed, bent, molded, assembled, or otherwise customized to fit a specific patient by an individual with expertise **DME** A
    BETOS: D1F Prosthetic/Orthotic devices

C **L1844** Knee orthosis (KO), single upright, thigh and calf, with adjustable flexion and extension joint (unicentric or polycentric), medial-lateral and rotation control, with or without varus/valgus adjustment, custom fabricated **DME** A
    BETOS: D1F Prosthetic/Orthotic devices

C **L1845** Knee orthosis (KO), double upright, thigh and calf, with adjustable flexion and extension joint (unicentric or polycentric), medial-lateral and rotation control, with or without varus/valgus adjustment, prefabricated item that has been trimmed, bent, molded, assembled, or otherwise customized to fit a specific patient by an individual with expertise **DME** A
    BETOS: D1F Prosthetic/Orthotic devices

C **L1846** Knee orthosis (KO), double upright, thigh and calf, with adjustable flexion and extension joint (unicentric or polycentric), medial-lateral and rotation control, with or without varus/valgus adjustment, custom fabricated **DME** A
    BETOS: D1F Prosthetic/Orthotic devices

C **L1847** Knee orthosis (KO), double upright with adjustable joint, with inflatable air support chamber(s), prefabricated item that has been trimmed, bent, molded, assembled, or otherwise customized to fit a specific patient by an individual with expertise **DME** A
    BETOS: D1F Prosthetic/Orthotic devices

C **L1848** Knee orthosis (KO), double upright with adjustable joint, with inflatable air support chamber(s), prefabricated, off-the-shelf **DME** A
    BETOS: D1F Prosthetic/Orthotic devices

C **L1850** Knee orthosis (KO), swedish type, prefabricated, off-the-shelf **DME** A
    BETOS: D1F Prosthetic/Orthotic devices

C **L1851** Knee orthosis (KO), single upright, thigh and calf, with adjustable flexion and extension joint (unicentric or polycentric), medial-lateral and rotation control, with or without varus/valgus adjustment, prefabricated, off-the-shelf **DME** A
    BETOS: D1F Prosthetic/Orthotic devices

C **L1852** Knee orthosis (KO), double upright, thigh and calf, with adjustable flexion and extension joint (unicentric or polycentric), medial-lateral and rotation control, with or without varus/valgus adjustment, prefabricated, off-the-shelf **DME** A
    BETOS: D1F Prosthetic/Orthotic devices

C **L1860** Knee orthosis (KO), modification of supracondylar prosthetic socket, custom fabricated (SK) **DME** A
    BETOS: D1F Prosthetic/Orthotic devices

● New code   ▲ Revised code   **C** Carrier judgment   **D** Special coverage instructions apply
I Not payable by Medicare   **M** Non-covered by Medicare   **S** Non-covered by Medicare statute   *AHA Coding Clinic®*

ANKLE-FOOT ORTHOTICS (L1900-L1990), SEE ALSO ANKLE-FOOT ORTHOTICS (L2106-L2116)

C L1900 Ankle-foot orthosis (AFO), spring wire, dorsiflexion assist calf band, custom fabricated **DME** A
BETOS: D1F Prosthetic/Orthotic devices

C L1902 Ankle orthosis (AO), ankle gauntlet or similar, with or without joints, prefabricated, off-the-shelf **DME** A
BETOS: D1F Prosthetic/Orthotic devices

C L1904 Ankle orthosis (AO), ankle gauntlet or similar, with or without joints, custom fabricated **DME** A
BETOS: D1F Prosthetic/Orthotic devices

C L1906 Ankle-foot orthosis (AFO), multiligamentous ankle support, prefabricated, off-the-shelf **DME** A
BETOS: D1F Prosthetic/Orthotic devices

C L1907 Ankle orthosis (AO), supramalleolar with straps, with or without interface/pads, custom fabricated **DME** A
BETOS: D1F Prosthetic/Orthotic devices

C L1910 Ankle-foot orthosis (AFO), posterior, single bar, clasp attachment to shoe counter, prefabricated, includes fitting and adjustment **DME** A
BETOS: D1F Prosthetic/Orthotic devices

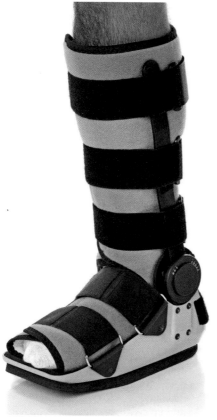

Ankle-foot orthosis

C L1920 Ankle-foot orthosis (AFO), single upright with static or adjustable stop (phelps or perlstein type), custom fabricated **DME** A
BETOS: D1F Prosthetic/Orthotic devices

C L1930 Ankle-foot orthosis (AFO), plastic or other material, prefabricated, includes fitting and adjustment **DME** A
BETOS: D1F Prosthetic/Orthotic devices

C L1932 Ankle-foot orthosis (AFO), rigid anterior tibial section, total carbon fiber or equal material, prefabricated, includes fitting and adjustment **DME** A
BETOS: D1F Prosthetic/Orthotic devices

C L1940 Ankle-foot orthosis (AFO), plastic or other material, custom fabricated **DME** A
BETOS: D1F Prosthetic/Orthotic devices

C L1945 Ankle-foot orthosis (AFO), plastic, rigid anterior tibial section (floor reaction), custom fabricated **DME** A
BETOS: D1F Prosthetic/Orthotic devices

C L1950 Ankle-foot orthosis (AFO), spiral, (institute of rehabilitative medicine type), plastic, custom fabricated **DME** A
BETOS: D1F Prosthetic/Orthotic devices

C L1951 Ankle-foot orthosis (AFO), spiral, (institute of rehabilitative medicine type), plastic or other material, prefabricated, includes fitting and adjustment **DME** A
BETOS: D1F Prosthetic/Orthotic devices

C L1960 Ankle-foot orthosis (AFO), posterior solid ankle, plastic, custom fabricated **DME** A
BETOS: D1F Prosthetic/Orthotic devices

C L1970 Ankle-foot orthosis (AFO), plastic with ankle joint, custom fabricated **DME** A
BETOS: D1F Prosthetic/Orthotic devices

C L1971 Ankle-foot orthosis (AFO), plastic or other material with ankle joint, prefabricated, includes fitting and adjustment **DME** A
BETOS: D1F Prosthetic/Orthotic devices

C L1980 Ankle-foot orthosis (AFO), single upright free plantar dorsiflexion, solid stirrup, calf band/cuff (single bar 'BK' orthosis), custom-fabricated **DME** A
BETOS: D1F Prosthetic/Orthotic devices

C L1990 Ankle-foot orthosis (AFO), double upright free plantar dorsiflexion, solid stirrup, calf band/cuff (double bar 'BK' orthosis), custom fabricated **DME** A
BETOS: D1F Prosthetic/Orthotic devices

L2000 - L2114 — ORTHOTIC PROCEDURES AND SERVICES (L0112-L4631)

KNEE-ANKLE-FOOT ORTHOTICS (L2000-L2038), SEE ALSO KNEE-ANKLE-FOOT ORTHOTICS (L2126-L2136)

C L2000 Knee-ankle-foot orthosis (KAFO), single upright, free knee, free ankle, solid stirrup, thigh and calf bands/cuffs (single bar 'AK' orthosis), custom fabricated **DME** A
BETOS: D1F   Prosthetic/Orthotic devices

C L2005 Knee-ankle-foot orthosis (KAFO), any material, single or double upright, stance control, automatic lock and swing phase release, any type activation, includes ankle joint, any type, custom fabricated **DME** A
BETOS: D1F   Prosthetic/Orthotic devices

C L2006 Knee-ankle-foot device, any material, single or double upright, swing and/or stance phase microprocessor control with adjustability, includes all components (e.g., sensors, batteries, charger), any type activation, with or without ankle joint(s), custom fabricated A
BETOS: Z2   Undefined codes
Value not established

C L2010 Knee-ankle-foot orthosis (KAFO), single upright, free ankle, solid stirrup, thigh and calf bands/cuffs (single bar 'AK' orthosis), without knee joint, custom-fabricated **DME** A
BETOS: D1F   Prosthetic/Orthotic devices

C L2020 Knee-ankle-foot orthosis (KAFO), double upright, free ankle, solid stirrup, thigh and calf bands/cuffs (double bar 'AK' orthosis), custom-fabricated **DME** A
BETOS: D1F   Prosthetic/Orthotic devices

C L2030 Knee-ankle-foot orthosis (KAFO), double upright, free ankle, solid stirrup, thigh and calf bands/cuffs, (double bar 'AK' orthosis), without knee joint, custom fabricated **DME** A
BETOS: D1F   Prosthetic/Orthotic devices

C L2034 Knee-ankle-foot orthosis (KAFO), full plastic, single upright, with or without free motion knee, medial lateral rotation control, with or without free motion ankle, custom fabricated **DME** A
BETOS: D1F   Prosthetic/Orthotic devices

C L2035 Knee-ankle-foot orthosis (KAFO), full plastic, static (pediatric size), without free motion ankle, prefabricated, includes fitting and adjustment **DME** Ⓐ A
BETOS: D1F   Prosthetic/Orthotic devices

C L2036 Knee-ankle-foot orthosis (KAFO), full plastic, double upright, with or without free motion knee, with or without free motion ankle, custom fabricated **DME** A
BETOS: D1F   Prosthetic/Orthotic devices

C L2037 Knee-ankle-foot orthosis (KAFO), full plastic, single upright, with or without free motion knee, with or without free motion ankle, custom fabricated **DME** A
BETOS: D1F   Prosthetic/Orthotic devices

C L2038 Knee-ankle-foot orthosis (KAFO), full plastic, with or without free motion knee, multi-axis ankle, custom fabricated **DME** A
BETOS: D1F   Prosthetic/Orthotic devices

HIP-KNEE-ANKLE-FOOT ORTHOTICS (L2040-L2090)

C L2040 Hip-knee-ankle-foot orthosis (HKAFO), torsion control, bilateral rotation straps, pelvic band/belt, custom fabricated **DME** A
BETOS: D1F   Prosthetic/Orthotic devices

C L2050 Hip-knee-ankle-foot orthosis (HKAFO), torsion control, bilateral torsion cables, hip joint, pelvic band/belt, custom fabricated **DME** A
BETOS: D1F   Prosthetic/Orthotic devices

C L2060 Hip-knee-ankle-foot orthosis (HKAFO), torsion control, bilateral torsion cables, ball bearing hip joint, pelvic band/ belt, custom fabricated **DME** A
BETOS: D1F   Prosthetic/Orthotic devices

C L2070 Hip-knee-ankle-foot orthosis (HKAFO), torsion control, unilateral rotation straps, pelvic band/belt, custom fabricated **DME** A
BETOS: D1F   Prosthetic/Orthotic devices

C L2080 Hip-knee-ankle-foot orthosis (HKAFO), torsion control, unilateral torsion cable, hip joint, pelvic band/belt, custom fabricated **DME** A
BETOS: D1F   Prosthetic/Orthotic devices

C L2090 Hip-knee-ankle-foot orthosis (HKAFO), torsion control, unilateral torsion cable, ball bearing hip joint, pelvic band/ belt, custom fabricated **DME** A
BETOS: D1F   Prosthetic/Orthotic devices

ANKLE-FOOT ORTHOTICS (L2106-L2116), SEE ALSO ANKLE-FOOT ORTHOTICS (L1900-L1990)

C L2106 Ankle-foot orthosis (AFO), fracture orthosis, tibial fracture cast orthosis, thermoplastic type casting material, custom fabricated **DME** A
BETOS: D1F   Prosthetic/Orthotic devices

C L2108 Ankle-foot orthosis (AFO), fracture orthosis, tibial fracture cast orthosis, custom fabricated **DME** A
BETOS: D1F   Prosthetic/Orthotic devices

C L2112 Ankle-foot orthosis (AFO), fracture orthosis, tibial fracture orthosis, soft, prefabricated, includes fitting and adjustment **DME** A
BETOS: D1F   Prosthetic/Orthotic devices

C L2114 Ankle-foot orthosis (AFO), fracture orthosis, tibial fracture orthosis, semi-rigid, prefabricated, includes fitting and adjustment **DME** A
BETOS: D1F   Prosthetic/Orthotic devices

● New code   ▲ Revised code   **C** Carrier judgment   **D** Special coverage instructions apply
I Not payable by Medicare   **M** Non-covered by Medicare   **S** Non-covered by Medicare statute   AHA Coding Clinic®

C **L2116** Ankle-foot orthosis (AFO), fracture orthosis, tibial fracture orthosis, rigid, prefabricated, includes fitting and adjustment DME A
  BETOS: D1F   Prosthetic/Orthotic devices

KNEE-ANKLE-FOOT ORTHOTICS (L2126-L2136), SEE ALSO KNEE-ANKLE-FOOT ORTHOTICS (L2000-L2038)

C **L2126** Knee-ankle-foot orthosis (KAFO), fracture orthosis, femoral fracture cast orthosis, thermoplastic type casting material, custom fabricated DME A
  BETOS: D1F   Prosthetic/Orthotic devices

C **L2128** Knee-ankle-foot orthosis(KAFO), fracture orthosis, femoral fracture cast orthosis, custom fabricated DME A
  BETOS: D1F   Prosthetic/Orthotic devices

C **L2132** Knee-ankle-foot orthosis(KAFO), fracture orthosis, femoral fracture cast orthosis, soft, prefabricated, includes fitting and adjustment DME A
  BETOS: D1F   Prosthetic/Orthotic devices

C **L2134** Knee-ankle-foot orthosis(KAFO), fracture orthosis, femoral fracture cast orthosis, semi-rigid, prefabricated, includes fitting and adjustment DME A
  BETOS: D1F   Prosthetic/Orthotic devices

C **L2136** Knee-ankle-foot orthosis(KAFO), fracture orthosis, femoral fracture cast orthosis, rigid, prefabricated, includes fitting and adjustment DME A
  BETOS: D1F   Prosthetic/Orthotic devices

ADDITIONS, LOWER EXTREMITY, FRACTURE ORTHOTICS (L2180-L2192)

C **L2180** Addition to lower extremity fracture orthosis, plastic shoe insert with ankle joints DME A
  BETOS: D1F   Prosthetic/Orthotic devices

C **L2182** Addition to lower extremity fracture orthosis, drop lock knee joint DME A
  BETOS: D1F   Prosthetic/Orthotic devices

C **L2184** Addition to lower extremity fracture orthosis, limited motion knee joint DME A
  BETOS: D1F   Prosthetic/Orthotic devices

C **L2186** Addition to lower extremity fracture orthosis, adjustable motion knee joint, lerman type DME A
  BETOS: D1F   Prosthetic/Orthotic devices

C **L2188** Addition to lower extremity fracture orthosis, quadrilateral brim DME A
  BETOS: D1F   Prosthetic/Orthotic devices

C **L2190** Addition to lower extremity fracture orthosis, waist belt DME A
  BETOS: D1F   Prosthetic/Orthotic devices

C **L2192** Addition to lower extremity fracture orthosis, hip joint, pelvic band, thigh flange, and pelvic belt DME A
  BETOS: D1F   Prosthetic/Orthotic devices

ADDITIONS, LOWER EXTREMITY ORTHOTICS (L2200-L2397)

C **L2200** Addition to lower extremity, limited ankle motion, each joint DME A
  BETOS: D1F   Prosthetic/Orthotic devices

C **L2210** Addition to lower extremity, dorsiflexion assist (plantar flexion resist), each joint DME A
  BETOS: D1F   Prosthetic/Orthotic devices

C **L2220** Addition to lower extremity, dorsiflexion and plantar flexion assist/resist, each joint DME A
  BETOS: D1F   Prosthetic/Orthotic devices

C **L2230** Addition to lower extremity, split flat caliper stirrups and plate attachment DME A
  BETOS: D1F   Prosthetic/Orthotic devices

C **L2232** Addition to lower extremity orthosis, rocker bottom for total contact ankle-foot orthosis (AFO), for custom fabricated orthosis only DME A
  BETOS: D1F   Prosthetic/Orthotic devices

C **L2240** Addition to lower extremity, round caliper and plate attachment DME A
  BETOS: D1F   Prosthetic/Orthotic devices

C **L2250** Addition to lower extremity, foot plate, molded to patient model, stirrup attachment DME A
  BETOS: D1F   Prosthetic/Orthotic devices

C **L2260** Addition to lower extremity, reinforced solid stirrup (Scott-Craig type) DME A
  BETOS: D1F   Prosthetic/Orthotic devices

C **L2265** Addition to lower extremity, long tongue stirrup DME A
  BETOS: D1F   Prosthetic/Orthotic devices

C **L2270** Addition to lower extremity, varus/valgus correction ('T') strap, padded/lined or malleolus pad DME A
  BETOS: D1F   Prosthetic/Orthotic devices

C **L2275** Addition to lower extremity, varus/valgus correction, plastic modification, padded/lined DME A
  BETOS: D1F   Prosthetic/Orthotic devices

C **L2280** Addition to lower extremity, molded inner boot DME A
  BETOS: D1F   Prosthetic/Orthotic devices

C **L2300** Addition to lower extremity, abduction bar (bilateral hip involvement), jointed, adjustable DME A
  BETOS: D1F   Prosthetic/Orthotic devices

C **L2310** Addition to lower extremity, abduction bar-straight DME A
  BETOS: D1F   Prosthetic/Orthotic devices

♂ Male only   ♀ Female only   Ⓐ Age   A2 - Z3 = ASC Payment indicator   A - Y = APC Status indicator
ASC = ASC Approved Procedure   DME Paid under the DME fee schedule   MIPS MIPS code

L2320 Addition to lower extremity, non-molded lacer, for custom fabricated orthosis only   DME A

BETOS: D1F   Prosthetic/Orthotic devices

L2330 Addition to lower extremity, lacer molded to patient model, for custom fabricated orthosis only   DME A

BETOS: D1F   Prosthetic/Orthotic devices

L2335 Addition to lower extremity, anterior swing band   DME A

BETOS: D1F   Prosthetic/Orthotic devices

L2340 Addition to lower extremity, pre-tibial shell, molded to patient model   DME A

BETOS: D1F   Prosthetic/Orthotic devices

L2350 Addition to lower extremity, prosthetic type, (BK) socket, molded to patient model, (used for 'PTB' 'AFO' orthosis)   DME A

BETOS: D1F   Prosthetic/Orthotic devices

L2360 Addition to lower extremity, extended steel shank   DME A

BETOS: D1F   Prosthetic/Orthotic devices

L2370 Addition to lower extremity, Patten bottom   DME A

BETOS: D1F   Prosthetic/Orthotic devices

L2375 Addition to lower extremity, torsion control, ankle joint and half solid stirrup   DME A

BETOS: D1F   Prosthetic/Orthotic devices

L2380 Addition to lower extremity, torsion control, straight knee joint, each joint   DME A

BETOS: D1F   Prosthetic/Orthotic devices

L2385 Addition to lower extremity, straight knee joint, heavy duty, each joint   DME A

BETOS: D1F   Prosthetic/Orthotic devices

L2387 Addition to lower extremity, polycentric knee joint, for custom fabricated knee-ankle-foot orthosis (KAFO), each joint   DME A

BETOS: D1F   Prosthetic/Orthotic devices

L2390 Addition to lower extremity, offset knee joint, each joint   DME A

BETOS: D1F   Prosthetic/Orthotic devices

L2395 Addition to lower extremity, offset knee joint, heavy duty, each joint   DME A

BETOS: D1F   Prosthetic/Orthotic devices

L2397 Addition to lower extremity orthosis, suspension sleeve   DME A

BETOS: D1F   Prosthetic/Orthotic devices

ORTHOTIC ADDITIONS TO KNEE JOINTS (L2405-L2492)

L2405 Addition to knee joint, drop lock, each   DME A

BETOS: D1F   Prosthetic/Orthotic devices

L2415 Addition to knee lock with integrated release mechanism (bail, cable, or equal), any material, each joint   DME A

BETOS: D1F   Prosthetic/Orthotic devices

L2425 Addition to knee joint, disc or dial lock for adjustable knee flexion, each joint   DME A

BETOS: D1F   Prosthetic/Orthotic devices

L2430 Addition to knee joint, ratchet lock for active and progressive knee extension, each joint   DME A

BETOS: D1F   Prosthetic/Orthotic devices

L2492 Addition to knee joint, lift loop for drop lock ring   DME A

BETOS: D1F   Prosthetic/Orthotic devices

ADDITIONS, WEIGHT-BEARING, LOWER EXTREMITIES (L2500-L2550)

L2500 Addition to lower extremity, thigh/weight bearing, gluteal/ ischial weight bearing, ring   DME A

BETOS: D1F   Prosthetic/Orthotic devices

L2510 Addition to lower extremity, thigh/weight bearing, quadri- lateral brim, molded to patient model   DME A

BETOS: D1F   Prosthetic/Orthotic devices

L2520 Addition to lower extremity, thigh/weight bearing, quadri- lateral brim, custom fitted   DME A

BETOS: D1F   Prosthetic/Orthotic devices

L2525 Addition to lower extremity, thigh/weight bearing, ischial containment/narrow M-L brim molded to patient model   DME A

BETOS: D1F   Prosthetic/Orthotic devices

L2526 Addition to lower extremity, thigh/weight bearing, ischial containment/narrow M-L brim, custom fitted   DME A

BETOS: D1F   Prosthetic/Orthotic devices

L2530 Addition to lower extremity, thigh-weight bearing, lacer, non-molded   DME A

BETOS: D1F   Prosthetic/Orthotic devices

L2540 Addition to lower extremity, thigh/weight bearing, lacer, molded to patient model   DME A

BETOS: D1F   Prosthetic/Orthotic devices

L2550 Addition to lower extremity, thigh/weight bearing, high roll cuff   DME A

BETOS: D1F   Prosthetic/Orthotic devices

ADDITIONS, PELVIC AND/OR THORACIC CONTROL, LOWER EXTREMITIES (L2570-L2680)

L2570 Addition to lower extremity, pelvic control, hip joint, Clevis-type two position joint, each   DME A

BETOS: D1F   Prosthetic/Orthotic devices

L2580 Addition to lower extremity, pelvic control, pelvic sling   DME A

BETOS: D1F   Prosthetic/Orthotic devices

● New code   ▲ Revised code   C Carrier judgment   D Special coverage instructions apply

I Not payable by Medicare   M Non-covered by Medicare   S Non-covered by Medicare statute   AHA Coding Clinic®

C **L2600** Addition to lower extremity, pelvic control, hip joint, Clevis-type, or thrust bearing, free, each DME A

  BETOS: D1F   Prosthetic/Orthotic devices

C **L2610** Addition to lower extremity, pelvic control, hip joint, Clevis-type or thrust bearing, lock, each DME A

  BETOS: D1F   Prosthetic/Orthotic devices

C **L2620** Addition to lower extremity, pelvic control, hip joint, heavy duty, each DME A

  BETOS: D1F   Prosthetic/Orthotic devices

C **L2622** Addition to lower extremity, pelvic control, hip joint, adjustable flexion, each DME A

  BETOS: D1F   Prosthetic/Orthotic devices

C **L2624** Addition to lower extremity, pelvic control, hip joint, adjustable flexion, extension, abduction control, each DME A

  BETOS: D1F   Prosthetic/Orthotic devices

C **L2627** Addition to lower extremity, pelvic control, plastic, molded to patient model, reciprocating hip joint and cables DME A

  BETOS: D1F   Prosthetic/Orthotic devices

C **L2628** Addition to lower extremity, pelvic control, metal frame, reciprocating hip joint and cables DME A

  BETOS: D1F   Prosthetic/Orthotic devices

C **L2630** Addition to lower extremity, pelvic control, band and belt, unilateral DME A

  BETOS: D1F   Prosthetic/Orthotic devices

C **L2640** Addition to lower extremity, pelvic control, band and belt, bilateral DME A

  BETOS: D1F   Prosthetic/Orthotic devices

C **L2650** Addition to lower extremity, pelvic and thoracic control, gluteal pad, each DME A

  BETOS: D1F   Prosthetic/Orthotic devices

C **L2660** Addition to lower extremity, thoracic control, thoracic band DME A

  BETOS: D1F   Prosthetic/Orthotic devices

C **L2670** Addition to lower extremity, thoracic control, paraspinal uprights DME A

  BETOS: D1F   Prosthetic/Orthotic devices

C **L2680** Addition to lower extremity, thoracic control, lateral support uprights DME A

  BETOS: D1F   Prosthetic/Orthotic devices

OTHER LOWER EXTREMITY ADDITIONS (L2750-L2999)

C **L2750** Addition to lower extremity orthosis, plating chrome or nickel, per bar DME A

  BETOS: D1F   Prosthetic/Orthotic devices

C **L2755** Addition to lower extremity orthosis, high strength, lightweight material, all hybrid lamination/prepreg composite, per segment, for custom fabricated orthosis only DME A

  BETOS: D1F   Prosthetic/Orthotic devices

C **L2760** Addition to lower extremity orthosis, extension, per extension, per bar (for lineal adjustment for growth) DME A

  BETOS: D1F   Prosthetic/Orthotic devices

C **L2768** Orthotic side bar disconnect device, per bar DME A

  BETOS: D1F   Prosthetic/Orthotic devices
  Coding Clinic: 2002, Q1

C **L2780** Addition to lower extremity orthosis, non-corrosive finish, per bar DME A

  BETOS: D1F   Prosthetic/Orthotic devices

C **L2785** Addition to lower extremity orthosis, drop lock retainer, each DME A

  BETOS: D1F   Prosthetic/Orthotic devices

C **L2795** Addition to lower extremity orthosis, knee control, full kneecap DME A

  BETOS: D1F   Prosthetic/Orthotic devices

C **L2800** Addition to lower extremity orthosis, knee control, knee cap, medial or lateral pull, for use with custom fabricated orthosis only DME A

  BETOS: D1F   Prosthetic/Orthotic devices

C **L2810** Addition to lower extremity orthosis, knee control, condylar pad DME A

  BETOS: D1F   Prosthetic/Orthotic devices

C **L2820** Addition to lower extremity orthosis, soft interface for molded plastic, below knee section DME A

  BETOS: D1F   Prosthetic/Orthotic devices

C **L2830** Addition to lower extremity orthosis, soft interface for molded plastic, above knee section DME A

  BETOS: D1F   Prosthetic/Orthotic devices

C **L2840** Addition to lower extremity orthosis, tibial length sock, fracture or equal, each DME A

  BETOS: D1F   Prosthetic/Orthotic devices

C **L2850** Addition to lower extremity orthosis, femoral length sock, fracture or equal, each DME A

  BETOS: D1F   Prosthetic/Orthotic devices

I **L2861** Addition to lower extremity joint, knee or ankle, concentric adjustable torsion style mechanism for custom fabricated orthotics only, each E1

  BETOS: D1F   Prosthetic/Orthotic devices
  Service not separately priced by Part B

C **L2999** Lower extremity orthoses, not otherwise specified A

  BETOS: D1F   Prosthetic/Orthotic devices

FOOT INSERTS, REMOVABLE (L3000-L3031)

D **L3000** Foot, insert, removable, molded to patient model, 'UCB' type, Berkeley Shell, each DME A

  BETOS: D1F   Prosthetic/Orthotic devices
  Service not separately priced by Part B

♂ Male only   ♀ Female only   Ⓐ Age   A2 - Z3 = ASC Payment indicator   A - Y = APC Status indicator
ASC = ASC Approved Procedure   DME Paid under the DME fee schedule   MIPS MIPS code

L3001 - L3160

ORTHOTIC PROCEDURES AND SERVICES (L0112-L4631)

D L3001 Foot, insert, removable, molded to patient model, Spenco, each DME A
BETOS: D1F Prosthetic/Orthotic devices
Service not separately priced by Part B

D L3002 Foot, insert, removable, molded to patient model, Plastazote or equal, each DME A
BETOS: D1F Prosthetic/Orthotic devices
Service not separately priced by Part B

D L3003 Foot, insert, removable, molded to patient model, silicone gel, each DME A
BETOS: D1F Prosthetic/Orthotic devices
Service not separately priced by Part B

D L3010 Foot, insert, removable, molded to patient model, longitudinal arch support, each DME A
BETOS: D1F Prosthetic/Orthotic devices
Service not separately priced by Part B

D L3020 Foot, insert, removable, molded to patient model, longitudinal/ metatarsal support, each DME A
BETOS: D1F Prosthetic/Orthotic devices
Service not separately priced by Part B

D L3030 Foot, insert, removable, formed to patient foot, each DME A
BETOS: D1F Prosthetic/Orthotic devices
Service not separately priced by Part B

C L3031 Foot, insert/plate, removable, addition to lower extremity orthosis, high strength, lightweight material, all hybrid lamination/ prepreg composite, each DME A
BETOS: D1F Prosthetic/Orthotic devices
Service not separately priced by Part B

FOOT ARCH SUPPORTS (L3040-L3090)

D L3040 Foot, arch support, removable, premolded, longitudinal, each DME A
BETOS: D1F Prosthetic/Orthotic devices
Service not separately priced by Part B

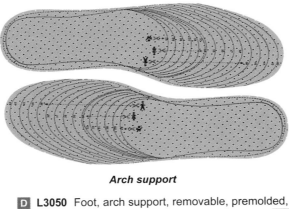

Arch support

D L3050 Foot, arch support, removable, premolded, metatarsal, each DME A
BETOS: D1F Prosthetic/Orthotic devices
Service not separately priced by Part B

D L3060 Foot, arch support, removable, premolded, longitudinal/ metatarsal, each DME A
BETOS: D1F Prosthetic/Orthotic devices
Service not separately priced by Part B

D L3070 Foot, arch support, non-removable attached to shoe, longitudinal, each DME A
BETOS: D1F Prosthetic/Orthotic devices
Service not separately priced by Part B

D L3080 Foot, arch support, non-removable attached to shoe, metatarsal, each DME A
BETOS: D1F Prosthetic/Orthotic devices
Service not separately priced by Part B

D L3090 Foot, arch support, non-removable attached to shoe, longitudinal/metatarsal, each DME A
BETOS: D1F Prosthetic/Orthotic devices
Service not separately priced by Part B

REPOSITIONING FOOT ORTHOTICS (L3100-L3170)

D L3100 Hallus-valgus night dynamic splint, prefabricated, off-the-shelf DME A
BETOS: D1F Prosthetic/Orthotic devices
Service not separately priced by Part B

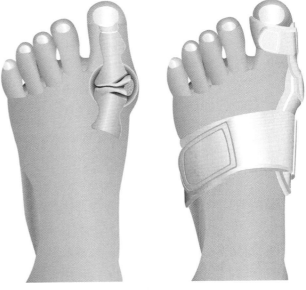

Hallux valgus splint

D L3140 Foot, abduction rotation bar, including shoes DME A
BETOS: D1F Prosthetic/Orthotic devices
Service not separately priced by Part B

D L3150 Foot, abduction rotation bar, without shoes DME A
BETOS: D1F Prosthetic/Orthotic devices
Service not separately priced by Part B

C L3160 Foot, adjustable shoe-styled positioning device A
BETOS: D1F Prosthetic/Orthotic devices
Service not separately priced by Part B

● New code ▲ Revised code **C** Carrier judgment **D** Special coverage instructions apply
I Not payable by Medicare **M** Non-covered by Medicare **S** Non-covered by Medicare statute AHA Coding Clinic®

D **L3170** Foot, plastic, silicone or equal, heel stabilizer, prefabricated, off-the-shelf, each **DME** A
BETOS: D1F   Prosthetic/Orthotic devices
Service not separately priced by Part B

ORTHOPEDIC SHOES (L3201-L3207)

D **L3201** Orthopedic shoe, Oxford with supinator or pronator, infant A
BETOS: D1F   Prosthetic/Orthotic devices
Service not separately priced by Part B

D **L3202** Orthopedic shoe, Oxford with supinator or pronator, child **A** A
BETOS: D1F   Prosthetic/Orthotic devices
Service not separately priced by Part B

D **L3203** Orthopedic shoe, Oxford with supinator or pronator, junior A
BETOS: D1F   Prosthetic/Orthotic devices
Service not separately priced by Part B

D **L3204** Orthopedic shoe, hightop with supinator or pronator, infant A
BETOS: D1F   Prosthetic/Orthotic devices
Service not separately priced by Part B

D **L3206** Orthopedic shoe, hightop with supinator or pronator, child **A** A
BETOS: D1F   Prosthetic/Orthotic devices
Service not separately priced by Part B

D **L3207** Orthopedic shoe, hightop with supinator or pronator, junior A
BETOS: D1F   Prosthetic/Orthotic devices
Service not separately priced by Part B

SURGICAL BOOTS (L3208-L3211)

D **L3208** Surgical boot, each, infant **A** A
BETOS: D1F   Prosthetic/Orthotic devices
Service not separately priced by Part B

D **L3209** Surgical boot, each, child **A** A
BETOS: D1F   Prosthetic/Orthotic devices
Service not separately priced by Part B

D **L3211** Surgical boot, each, junior A
BETOS: D1F   Prosthetic/Orthotic devices
Service not separately priced by Part B

BENESCH BOOTS (L3212-L3214)

D **L3212** Benesch boot, pair, infant A
BETOS: D1F   Prosthetic/Orthotic devices
Service not separately priced by Part B

D **L3213** Benesch boot, pair, child **A** A
BETOS: D1F   Prosthetic/Orthotic devices
Service not separately priced by Part B

D **L3214** Benesch boot, pair, junior A
BETOS: D1F   Prosthetic/Orthotic devices
Service not separately priced by Part B

OTHER ORTHOPEDIC FOOTWEAR (L3215-L3265)

S **L3215** Orthopedic footwear, ladies shoe, Oxford, each ♀ E1
BETOS: D1F   Prosthetic/Orthotic devices
Service not separately priced by Part B
Statute: 1862A8

S **L3216** Orthopedic footwear, ladies shoe, depth inlay, each ♀ E1
BETOS: D1F   Prosthetic/Orthotic devices
Service not separately priced by Part B
Statute: 1862A8

S **L3217** Orthopedic footwear, ladies shoe, hightop, depth inlay, each ♀ E1
BETOS: D1F   Prosthetic/Orthotic devices
Service not separately priced by Part B
Statute: 1862A8

S **L3219** Orthopedic footwear, mens shoe, Oxford, each ♂ E1
BETOS: D1F   Prosthetic/Orthotic devices
Service not separately priced by Part B
Statute: 1862A8

S **L3221** Orthopedic footwear, mens shoe, depth inlay, each ♂ E1
BETOS: D1F   Prosthetic/Orthotic devices
Service not separately priced by Part B
Statute: 1862A8

S **L3222** Orthopedic footwear, mens shoe, hightop, depth inlay, each E1
BETOS: D1F   Prosthetic/Orthotic devices
Service not separately priced by Part B
Statute: 1862A8

D **L3224** Orthopedic footwear, woman's shoe, Oxford, used as an integral part of a brace (orthosis) ♀ **DME** A
BETOS: D1F   Prosthetic/Orthotic devices

D **L3225** Orthopedic footwear, man's shoe, Oxford, used as an integral part of a brace (orthosis) ♂ **DME** A
BETOS: D1F   Prosthetic/Orthotic devices

D **L3230** Orthopedic footwear, custom shoe, depth inlay, each A
BETOS: D1F   Prosthetic/Orthotic devices
Service not separately priced by Part B

D **L3250** Orthopedic footwear, custom molded shoe, removable inner mold, prosthetic shoe, each A
BETOS: D1F   Prosthetic/Orthotic devices
Service not separately priced by Part B

D **L3251** Foot, shoe molded to patient model, silicone shoe, each A
BETOS: D1F   Prosthetic/Orthotic devices
Service not separately priced by Part B

D **L3252** Foot, shoe molded to patient model, Plastazote (or similar), custom fabricated, each A

♂ Male only   ♀ Female only   **A** Age   A2 - Z3 = ASC Payment indicator   A - Y = APC Status indicator
ASC = ASC Approved Procedure   **DME** Paid under the DME fee schedule   **MIPS** MIPS code

BETOS: D1F   Prosthetic/Orthotic devices
Service not separately priced by Part B

D L3253 Foot, molded shoe Plastazote (or similar) custom fitted, each   A
BETOS: D1F   Prosthetic/Orthotic devices
Service not separately priced by Part B

D L3254 Non-standard size or width   A
BETOS: D1F   Prosthetic/Orthotic devices
Service not separately priced by Part B

D L3255 Non-standard size or length   A
BETOS: D1F   Prosthetic/Orthotic devices
Service not separately priced by Part B

D L3257 Orthopedic footwear, additional charge for split size   A
BETOS: D1F   Prosthetic/Orthotic devices
Service not separately priced by Part B

D L3260 Surgical boot/shoe, each   E1
BETOS: D1F   Prosthetic/Orthotic devices
Service not separately priced by Part B

C L3265 Plastazote sandal, each   A
BETOS: D1F   Prosthetic/Orthotic devices
Service not separately priced by Part B

SHOE LIFTS (L3300-L3334)

D L3300 Lift, elevation, heel, tapered to metatarsals, per inch   DME A
BETOS: D1F   Prosthetic/Orthotic devices
Service not separately priced by Part B

D L3310 Lift, elevation, heel and sole, neoprene, per inch   DME A
BETOS: D1F   Prosthetic/Orthotic devices
Service not separately priced by Part B

D L3320 Lift, elevation, heel and sole, cork, per inch   A
BETOS: D1F   Prosthetic/Orthotic devices
Service not separately priced by Part B

D L3330 Lift, elevation, metal extension (skate) DME A
BETOS: D1F   Prosthetic/Orthotic devices
Service not separately priced by Part B

D L3332 Lift, elevation, inside shoe, tapered, up to one-half inch   DME A
BETOS: D1F   Prosthetic/Orthotic devices
Service not separately priced by Part B

D L3334 Lift, elevation, heel, per inch   DME A
BETOS: D1F   Prosthetic/Orthotic devices
Service not separately priced by Part B

SHOE WEDGES (L3340-L3420)

D L3340 Heel wedge, SACH   DME A
BETOS: D1F   Prosthetic/Orthotic devices
Service not separately priced by Part B

D L3350 Heel wedge   DME A
BETOS: D1F   Prosthetic/Orthotic devices
Service not separately priced by Part B

D L3360 Sole wedge, outside sole   DME A
BETOS: D1F   Prosthetic/Orthotic devices
Service not separately priced by Part B

D L3370 Sole wedge, between sole   DME A
BETOS: D1F   Prosthetic/Orthotic devices
Service not separately priced by Part B

D L3380 Clubfoot wedge   DME A
BETOS: D1F   Prosthetic/Orthotic devices
Service not separately priced by Part B

D L3390 Outflare wedge   DME A
BETOS: D1F   Prosthetic/Orthotic devices
Service not separately priced by Part B

D L3400 Metatarsal bar wedge, rocker   DME A
BETOS: D1F   Prosthetic/Orthotic devices
Service not separately priced by Part B

D L3410 Metatarsal bar wedge, between sole   DME A
BETOS: D1F   Prosthetic/Orthotic devices
Service not separately priced by Part B

D L3420 Full sole and heel wedge, between sole   DME A
BETOS: D1F   Prosthetic/Orthotic devices
Service not separately priced by Part B

SHOE HEELS (L3430-L3485)

D L3430 Heel, counter, plastic reinforced   DME A
BETOS: D1F   Prosthetic/Orthotic devices
Service not separately priced by Part B

D L3440 Heel, counter, leather reinforced   DME A
BETOS: D1F   Prosthetic/Orthotic devices
Service not separately priced by Part B

D L3450 Heel, SACH cushion type   DME A
BETOS: D1F   Prosthetic/Orthotic devices
Service not separately priced by Part B

D L3455 Heel, new leather, standard   DME A
BETOS: D1F   Prosthetic/Orthotic devices
Service not separately priced by Part B

D L3460 Heel, new rubber, standard   DME A
BETOS: D1F   Prosthetic/Orthotic devices
Service not separately priced by Part B

D L3465 Heel, Thomas with wedge   DME A
BETOS: D1F   Prosthetic/Orthotic devices
Service not separately priced by Part B

D L3470 Heel, Thomas extended to ball   DME A
BETOS: D1F   Prosthetic/Orthotic devices
Service not separately priced by Part B

D L3480 Heel, pad and depression for spur   DME A
BETOS: D1F   Prosthetic/Orthotic devices
Service not separately priced by Part B

D L3485 Heel, pad, removable for spur   A
BETOS: D1F   Prosthetic/Orthotic devices
Service not separately priced by Part B

● New code   ▲ Revised code   **C** Carrier judgment   **D** Special coverage instructions apply
I Not payable by Medicare   **M** Non-covered by Medicare   **S** Non-covered by Medicare statute   AHA Coding Clinic®

OTHER ORTHOPEDIC SHOE ADDITIONS (L3500-L3595)

D **L3500** Orthopedic shoe addition, insole, leather **DME** A
   BETOS: D1F   Prosthetic/Orthotic devices
   Service not separately priced by Part B

D **L3510** Orthopedic shoe addition, insole, rubber **DME** A
   BETOS: D1F   Prosthetic/Orthotic devices
   Service not separately priced by Part B

D **L3520** Orthopedic shoe addition, insole, felt covered with leather **DME** A
   BETOS: D1F   Prosthetic/Orthotic devices
   Service not separately priced by Part B

D **L3530** Orthopedic shoe addition, sole, half **DME** A
   BETOS: D1F   Prosthetic/Orthotic devices
   Service not separately priced by Part B

D **L3540** Orthopedic shoe addition, sole, full **DME** A
   BETOS: D1F   Prosthetic/Orthotic devices
   Service not separately priced by Part B

D **L3550** Orthopedic shoe addition, toe tap standard **DME** A
   BETOS: D1F   Prosthetic/Orthotic devices
   Service not separately priced by Part B

D **L3560** Orthopedic shoe addition, toe tap, horseshoe **DME** A
   BETOS: D1F   Prosthetic/Orthotic devices
   Service not separately priced by Part B

D **L3570** Orthopedic shoe addition, special extension to instep (leather with eyelets) **DME** A
   BETOS: D1F   Prosthetic/Orthotic devices
   Service not separately priced by Part B

D **L3580** Orthopedic shoe addition, convert instep to velcro closure **DME** A
   BETOS: D1F   Prosthetic/Orthotic devices
   Service not separately priced by Part B

D **L3590** Orthopedic shoe addition, convert firm shoe counter to soft counter **DME** A
   BETOS: D1F   Prosthetic/Orthotic devices
   Service not separately priced by Part B

D **L3595** Orthopedic shoe addition, March bar **DME** A
   BETOS: D1F   Prosthetic/Orthotic devices
   Service not separately priced by Part B

ORTHOSIS TRANSFERS (L3600-L3649)

D **L3600** Transfer of an orthosis from one shoe to another, caliper plate, existing **DME** A
   BETOS: D1F   Prosthetic/Orthotic devices
   Service not separately priced by Part B

D **L3610** Transfer of an orthosis from one shoe to another, caliper plate, new **DME** A
   BETOS: D1F   Prosthetic/Orthotic devices
   Service not separately priced by Part B

D **L3620** Transfer of an orthosis from one shoe to another, solid stirrup, existing **DME** A
   BETOS: D1F   Prosthetic/Orthotic devices
   Service not separately priced by Part B

D **L3630** Transfer of an orthosis from one shoe to another, solid stirrup, new **DME** A
   BETOS: D1F   Prosthetic/Orthotic devices
   Service not separately priced by Part B

D **L3640** Transfer of an orthosis from one shoe to another, dennis browne splint (Riveton), both shoes **DME** A
   BETOS: D1F   Prosthetic/Orthotic devices
   Service not separately priced by Part B

D **L3649** Orthopedic shoe, modification, addition or transfer, not otherwise specified A
   BETOS: D1F   Prosthetic/Orthotic devices
   Service not separately priced by Part B

SHOULDER ORTHOTICS (L3650-L3678)

C **L3650** Shoulder orthosis (SO), figure of eight design abduction restrainer, prefabricated, off-the-shelf **DME** A
   BETOS: D1F   Prosthetic/Orthotic devices

C **L3660** Shoulder orthosis (SO), figure of eight design abduction restrainer, canvas and webbing, prefabricated, off-the-shelf **DME** A
   BETOS: D1F   Prosthetic/Orthotic devices

C **L3670** Shoulder orthosis (SO), acromio/clavicular (canvas and webbing type), prefabricated, off-the-shelf **DME** A
   BETOS: D1F   Prosthetic/Orthotic devices

C **L3671** Shoulder orthosis (SO), shoulder joint design, without joints, may include soft interface, straps, custom fabricated, includes fitting and adjustment **DME** A
   BETOS: D1F   Prosthetic/Orthotic devices

C **L3674** Shoulder orthosis (SO), abduction positioning (airplane design), thoracic component and support bar, with or without nontorsion joint/turnbuckle, may include soft interface, straps, custom fabricated, includes fitting and adjustment **DME** A
   BETOS: D1F   Prosthetic/Orthotic devices

C **L3675** Shoulder orthosis (SO), vest type abduction restrainer, canvas webbing type or equal, prefabricated, off-the-shelf **DME** A
   BETOS: D1F   Prosthetic/Orthotic devices

D **L3677** Shoulder orthosis (SO), shoulder joint design, without joints, may include soft interface, straps, prefabricated item that has been trimmed, bent, molded, assembled, or otherwise customized to fit a specific patient by an individual with expertise A
   BETOS: Z2   Undefined codes
   Service not separately priced by Part B
   Coding Clinic: 2002, Q1

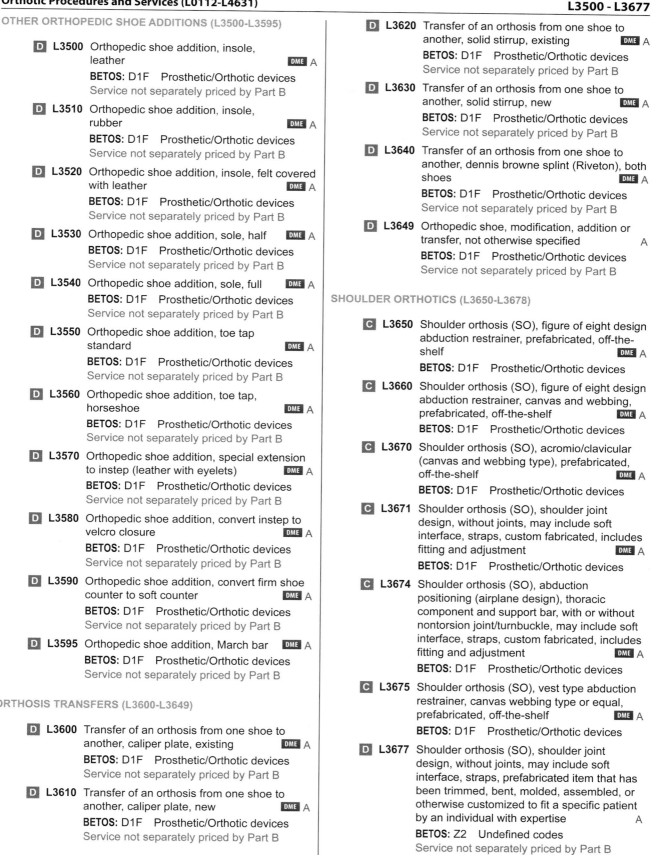

♂ Male only   ♀ Female only   **A** Age   A2 - Z3 = ASC Payment indicator   A - Y = APC Status indicator
ASC = ASC Approved Procedure   **DME** Paid under the DME fee schedule   **MIPS** MIPS code

L3678 Shoulder orthosis (SO), shoulder joint design, without joints, may include soft interface, straps, prefabricated, off-the-shelf A
BETOS: D1F   Prosthetic/Orthotic devices

ELBOW ORTHOTICS (L3702-L3762)

L3702 Elbow orthosis (EO), without joints, may include soft interface, straps, custom fabricated, includes fitting and adjustment DME A
BETOS: D1F   Prosthetic/Orthotic devices

L3710 Elbow orthosis (EO), elastic with metal joints, prefabricated, off-the-shelf DME A
BETOS: D1F   Prosthetic/Orthotic devices

L3720 Elbow orthosis (EO), double upright with forearm/arm cuffs, free motion, custom fabricated DME A
BETOS: D1F   Prosthetic/Orthotic devices

L3730 Elbow orthosis (EO), double upright with forearm/arm cuffs, extension/ flexion assist, custom fabricated DME A
BETOS: D1F   Prosthetic/Orthotic devices

L3740 Elbow orthosis (EO), double upright with forearm/arm cuffs, adjustable position lock with active control, custom fabricated DME A
BETOS: D1F   Prosthetic/Orthotic devices

L3760 Elbow orthosis (EO), with adjustable position locking joint(s), prefabricated, item that has been trimmed, bent, molded, assembled, or otherwise customized to fit a specific patient by an individual with expertise DME A
BETOS: D1F   Prosthetic/Orthotic devices

L3761 Elbow orthosis (EO), with adjustable position locking joint(s), prefabricated, off-the-shelf DME A
BETOS: D1F   Prosthetic/Orthotic devices

L3762 Elbow orthosis (EO), rigid, without joints, includes soft interface material, prefabricated, off-the-shelf DME A
BETOS: D1F   Prosthetic/Orthotic devices

ELBOW-WRIST-HAND-FINGER ORTHOTICS (L3763-L3766)

L3763 Elbow-wrist-hand orthosis (EWHO), rigid, without joints, may include soft interface, straps, custom fabricated, includes fitting and adjustment DME A
BETOS: D1F   Prosthetic/Orthotic devices

L3764 Elbow-wrist-hand orthosis (EWHO), includes one or more nontorsion joints, elastic bands, turnbuckles, may include soft interface, straps, custom fabricated, includes fitting and adjustment DME A
BETOS: D1F   Prosthetic/Orthotic devices

L3765 Elbow-wrist-hand-finger orthosis (EWHFO), rigid, without joints, may include soft interface, straps, custom fabricated, includes fitting and adjustment DME A
BETOS: D1F   Prosthetic/Orthotic devices

L3766 Elbow-wrist-hand-finger orthosis (EWHFO), includes one or more nontorsion joints, elastic bands, turnbuckles, may include soft interface, straps, custom fabricated, includes fitting and adjustment DME A
BETOS: D1F   Prosthetic/Orthotic devices

WRIST-HAND-FINGER ORTHOTICS (L3806-L3904)

L3806 Wrist-hand-finger orthosis (WHFO), includes one or more nontorsion joint(s), turnbuckles, elastic bands/springs, may include soft interface material, straps, custom fabricated, includes fitting and adjustment DME A
BETOS: D1F   Prosthetic/Orthotic devices

L3807 Wrist-hand-finger orthosis (WHFO), without joint(s), prefabricated item that has been trimmed, bent, molded, assembled, or otherwise customized to fit a specific patient by an individual with expertise DME A
BETOS: D1F   Prosthetic/Orthotic devices

L3808 Wrist-hand-finger orthosis (WHFO), rigid without joints, may include soft interface material; straps, custom fabricated, includes fitting and adjustment DME A
BETOS: D1F   Prosthetic/Orthotic devices

L3809 Wrist-hand-finger orthosis (WHFO), without joint(s), prefabricated, off-the-shelf, any type DME A
BETOS: D1F   Prosthetic/Orthotic devices

L3891 Addition to upper extremity joint, wrist or elbow, concentric adjustable torsion style mechanism for custom fabricated orthotics only, each E1
BETOS: D1F   Prosthetic/Orthotic devices
Service not separately priced by Part B

L3900 Wrist-hand-finger orthosis (WHFO), dynamic flexor hinge, reciprocal wrist extension/ flexion, finger flexion/extension, wrist or finger driven, custom fabricated DME A
BETOS: D1F   Prosthetic/Orthotic devices

L3901 Wrist-hand-finger orthosis (WHFO), dynamic flexor hinge, reciprocal wrist extension/ flexion, finger flexion/extension, cable driven, custom fabricated DME A
BETOS: D1F   Prosthetic/Orthotic devices

L3904 Wrist-hand-finger orthosis (WHFO), external powered, electric, custom fabricated DME A
BETOS: D1F   Prosthetic/Orthotic devices

● New code ▲ Revised code **C** Carrier judgment **D** Special coverage instructions apply
I Not payable by Medicare **M** Non-covered by Medicare **S** Non-covered by Medicare statute   AHA Coding Clinic®

WRIST-HAND ORTHOTICS (L3905-L3908)

C **L3905** Wrist-hand orthosis (WHO), includes one or more nontorsion joints, elastic bands, turnbuckles, may include soft interface, straps, custom fabricated, includes fitting and adjustment **DME** A

BETOS: D1F   Prosthetic/Orthotic devices

C **L3906** Wrist-hand orthosis (WHO), without joints, may include soft interface, straps, custom fabricated, includes fitting and adjustment **DME** A

BETOS: D1F   Prosthetic/Orthotic devices

C **L3908** Wrist-hand orthosis (WHO), wrist extension control cock-up, non molded, prefabricated, off-the-shelf **DME** A

BETOS: D1F   Prosthetic/Orthotic devices

ADDITIONAL MISCELLANEOUS ORTHOTICS, UPPER EXTREMITIES (L3912-L3956)

C **L3912** Hand-finger orthosis (HFO), flexion glove with elastic finger control, prefabricated, off-the-shelf **DME** A

BETOS: D1F   Prosthetic/Orthotic devices

C **L3913** Hand-finger orthosis (HFO), without joints, may include soft interface, straps, custom fabricated, includes fitting and adjustment **DME** A

BETOS: D1F   Prosthetic/Orthotic devices

C **L3915** Wrist-hand orthosis (WHO), includes one or more nontorsion joint(s), elastic bands, turnbuckles, may include soft interface, straps, prefabricated item that has been trimmed, bent, molded, assembled, or otherwise customized to fit a specific patient by an individual with expertise **DME** A

BETOS: D1F   Prosthetic/Orthotic devices

C **L3916** Wrist-hand orthosis (WHO), includes one or more nontorsion joint(s), elastic bands, turnbuckles, may include soft interface, straps, prefabricated, off-the-shelf **DME** A

BETOS: D1F   Prosthetic/Orthotic devices

C **L3917** Hand orthosis (HO), metacarpal fracture orthosis, prefabricated item that has been trimmed, bent, molded, assembled, or otherwise customized to fit a specific patient by an individual with expertise **DME** A

BETOS: D1F   Prosthetic/Orthotic devices

C **L3918** Hand orthosis (HO), metacarpal fracture orthosis, prefabricated, off-the-shelf **DME** A

BETOS: D1F   Prosthetic/Orthotic devices

C **L3919** Hand orthosis (HO), without joints, may include soft interface, straps, custom fabricated, includes fitting and adjustment **DME** A

BETOS: D1F   Prosthetic/Orthotic devices

C **L3921** Hand-finger orthosis (HFO), includes one or more nontorsion joints, elastic bands, turnbuckles, may include soft interface, straps, custom fabricated, includes fitting and adjustment **DME** A

BETOS: D1F   Prosthetic/Orthotic devices

C **L3923** Hand-finger orthosis (HFO), without joints, may include soft interface, straps, prefabricated item that has been trimmed, bent, molded, assembled, or otherwise customized to fit a specific patient by an individual with expertise **DME** A

BETOS: D1F   Prosthetic/Orthotic devices

C **L3924** Hand-finger orthosis (HFO), without joints, may include soft interface, straps, prefabricated, off-the-shelf **DME** A

BETOS: D1F   Prosthetic/Orthotic devices

C **L3925** Finger orthosis (FO), proximal interphalangeal (PIP)/distal interphalangeal (DIP), non torsion joint/spring, extension/flexion, may include soft interface material, prefabricated, off-the-shelf **DME** A

BETOS: D1F   Prosthetic/Orthotic devices

C **L3927** Finger orthosis (FO), proximal interphalangeal (PIP)/distal interphalangeal (DIP), without joint/spring, extension/flexion (e.g., static or ring type), may include soft interface material, prefabricated, off-the-shelf **DME** A

BETOS: D1F   Prosthetic/Orthotic devices

C **L3929** Hand-finger orthosis (HFO), includes one or more nontorsion joint(s), turnbuckles, elastic bands/springs, may include soft interface material, straps, prefabricated item that has been trimmed, bent, molded, assembled, or otherwise customized to fit a specific patient by an individual with expertise **DME** A

BETOS: D1F   Prosthetic/Orthotic devices

C **L3930** Hand-finger orthosis (HFO), includes one or more nontorsion joint(s), turnbuckles, elastic bands/springs, may include soft interface material, straps, prefabricated, off-the-shelf **DME** A

BETOS: D1F   Prosthetic/Orthotic devices

C **L3931** Wrist-hand-finger orthosis (WHFO), includes one or more nontorsion joint(s), turnbuckles, elastic bands/springs, may include soft interface material, straps, prefabricated, includes fitting and adjustment **DME** A

BETOS: D1F   Prosthetic/Orthotic devices

C **L3933** Finger orthosis (FO), without joints, may include soft interface, custom fabricated, includes fitting and adjustment **DME** A

BETOS: D1F   Prosthetic/Orthotic devices

C **L3935** Finger orthosis (FO), nontorsion joint, may include soft interface, custom fabricated, includes fitting and adjustment **DME** A

BETOS: D1F   Prosthetic/Orthotic devices

♂ Male only   ♀ Female only   **A** Age   A2 - Z3 = ASC Payment indicator   A - Y = APC Status indicator

ASC = ASC Approved Procedure   **DME** Paid under the DME fee schedule   **MIPS** MIPS code

C L3956 Addition of joint to upper extremity orthosis, any material; per joint `DME` A
BETOS: D1F   Prosthetic/Orthotic devices

SHOULDER-ELBOW-WRIST-HAND ORTHOTICS (L3960-L3973)

C L3960 Shoulder-elbow-wrist-hand orthosis (SEWHO), abduction positioning, airplane design, prefabricated, includes fitting and adjustment `DME` A
BETOS: D1F   Prosthetic/Orthotic devices

C L3961 Shoulder-elbow-wrist-hand orthosis (SEWHO), shoulder cap design, without joints, may include soft interface, straps, custom fabricated, includes fitting and adjustment `DME` A
BETOS: D1F   Prosthetic/Orthotic devices

C L3962 Shoulder-elbow-wrist-hand orthosis (SEWHO), abduction positioning, erbs palsey design, prefabricated, includes fitting and adjustment `DME` A
BETOS: D1F   Prosthetic/Orthotic devices

C L3967 Shoulder-elbow-wrist-hand orthosis (SEWHO), abduction positioning (airplane design), thoracic component and support bar, without joints, may include soft interface, straps, custom fabricated, includes fitting and adjustment `DME` A
BETOS: D1F   Prosthetic/Orthotic devices

C L3971 Shoulder-elbow-wrist-hand orthosis (SEWHO), shoulder cap design, includes one or more nontorsion joints, elastic bands, turnbuckles, may include soft interface, straps, custom fabricated, includes fitting and adjustment `DME` A
BETOS: D1F   Prosthetic/Orthotic devices

C L3973 Shoulder-elbow-wrist-hand orthosis (SEWHO), abduction positioning (airplane design), thoracic component and support bar, includes one or more nontorsion joints, elastic bands, turnbuckles, may include soft interface, straps, custom fabricated, includes fitting and adjustment `DME` A
BETOS: D1F   Prosthetic/Orthotic devices

SHOULDER-ELBOW-WRIST-HAND-FINGER ORTHOTICS (L3975-L3978)

C L3975 Shoulder-elbow-wrist-hand-finger orthosis (SEWHFO), shoulder cap design, without joints, may include soft interface, straps, custom fabricated, includes fitting and adjustment `DME` A
BETOS: D1F   Prosthetic/Orthotic devices

C L3976 Shoulder-elbow-wrist-hand-finger orthosis (SEWHFO), abduction positioning (airplane design), thoracic component and support bar, without joints, may include soft interface, straps, custom fabricated, includes fitting and adjustment `DME` A
BETOS: D1F   Prosthetic/Orthotic devices

C L3977 Shoulder-elbow-wrist-hand-finger orthosis (SEWHFO), shoulder cap design, includes one or more nontorsion joints, elastic bands, turnbuckles, may include soft interface, straps, custom fabricated, includes fitting and adjustment `DME` A
BETOS: D1F   Prosthetic/Orthotic devices

C L3978 Shoulder-elbow-wrist-hand-finger orthosis (SEWHFO), abduction positioning (airplane design), thoracic component and support bar, includes one or more nontorsion joints, elastic bands, turnbuckles, may include soft interface, straps, custom fabricated, includes fitting and adjustment `DME` A
BETOS: D1F   Prosthetic/Orthotic devices

FRACTURE, ADDITION, AND UNSPECIFIED ORTHOTICS, UPPER EXTREMITIES (L3980-L3999)

C L3980 Upper extremity fracture orthosis, humeral, prefabricated, includes fitting and adjustment `DME` A
BETOS: D1F   Prosthetic/Orthotic devices

C L3981 Upper extremity fracture orthosis, humeral, prefabricated, includes shoulder cap design, with or without joints, forearm section, may include soft interface, straps, includes fitting and adjustments `DME` A
BETOS: D1F   Prosthetic/Orthotic devices

C L3982 Upper extremity fracture orthosis, radius/ulnar, prefabricated, includes fitting and adjustment `DME` A
BETOS: D1F   Prosthetic/Orthotic devices

C L3984 Upper extremity fracture orthosis, wrist, prefabricated, includes fitting and adjustment `DME` A
BETOS: D1F   Prosthetic/Orthotic devices

C L3995 Addition to upper extremity orthosis, sock, fracture or equal, each `DME` A
BETOS: D1F   Prosthetic/Orthotic devices

C L3999 Upper limb orthosis, not otherwise specified A
BETOS: D1F   Prosthetic/Orthotic devices

ORTHOTIC REPLACEMENT PARTS OR REPAIR (L4000-L4210)

C L4000 Replace girdle for spinal orthosis (Cervical-thoracic-lumbar-sacral orthosis (CTLSO) or Shoulder orthosis (SO)) `DME` A
BETOS: D1F   Prosthetic/Orthotic devices

C L4002 Replacement strap, any orthosis, includes all components, any length, any type `DME` A
BETOS: D1F   Prosthetic/Orthotic devices

C L4010 Replace trilateral socket brim `DME` A
BETOS: D1F   Prosthetic/Orthotic devices

C L4020 Replace quadrilateral socket brim, molded to patient model `DME` A
BETOS: D1F   Prosthetic/Orthotic devices

C **L4030** Replace quadrilateral socket brim, custom fitted DME A
   BETOS: D1F   Prosthetic/Orthotic devices

C **L4040** Replace molded thigh lacer, for custom fabricated orthosis only DME A
   BETOS: D1F   Prosthetic/Orthotic devices

C **L4045** Replace non-molded thigh lacer, for custom fabricated orthosis only DME A
   BETOS: D1F   Prosthetic/Orthotic devices

C **L4050** Replace molded calf lacer, for custom fabricated orthosis only DME A
   BETOS: D1F   Prosthetic/Orthotic devices

C **L4055** Replace non-molded calf lacer, for custom fabricated orthosis only DME A
   BETOS: D1F   Prosthetic/Orthotic devices

C **L4060** Replace high roll cuff DME A
   BETOS: D1F   Prosthetic/Orthotic devices

C **L4070** Replace proximal and distal upright for KAFO DME A
   BETOS: D1F   Prosthetic/Orthotic devices

C **L4080** Replace metal bands KAFO, proximal thigh DME A
   BETOS: D1F   Prosthetic/Orthotic devices

C **L4090** Replace metal bands KAFO-AFO, calf or distal thigh DME A
   BETOS: D1F   Prosthetic/Orthotic devices

C **L4100** Replace leather cuff KAFO, proximal thigh DME A
   BETOS: D1F   Prosthetic/Orthotic devices

C **L4110** Replace leather cuff KAFO-AFO, calf or distal thigh DME A
   BETOS: D1F   Prosthetic/Orthotic devices

C **L4130** Replace pretibial shell DME A
   BETOS: D1F   Prosthetic/Orthotic devices

D **L4205** Repair of orthotic device, labor component, per 15 minutes A
   BETOS: D1F   Prosthetic/Orthotic devices

D **L4210** Repair of orthotic device, repair or replace minor parts A
   BETOS: D1F   Prosthetic/Orthotic devices

OTHER LOWER EXTREMITY ORTHOTICS (L4350-L4631)

C **L4350** Ankle control orthosis, stirrup style, rigid, includes any type interface (e.g., pneumatic, gel), prefabricated, off-the-shelf DME A
   BETOS: D1F   Prosthetic/Orthotic devices

C **L4360** Walking boot, pneumatic and/or vacuum, with or without joints, with or without interface material, prefabricated item that has been trimmed, bent, molded, assembled, or otherwise customized to fit a specific patient by an individual with expertise DME A
   BETOS: D1F   Prosthetic/Orthotic devices

C **L4361** Walking boot, pneumatic and/or vacuum, with or without joints, with or without interface material, prefabricated, off-the-shelf DME A
   BETOS: D1F   Prosthetic/Orthotic devices

C **L4370** Pneumatic full leg splint, prefabricated, off-the-shelf DME A
   BETOS: D1F   Prosthetic/Orthotic devices

C **L4386** Walking boot, non-pneumatic, with or without joints, with or without interface material, prefabricated item that has been trimmed, bent, molded, assembled, or otherwise customized to fit a specific patient by an individual with expertise DME A
   BETOS: D1F   Prosthetic/Orthotic devices

C **L4387** Walking boot, non-pneumatic, with or without joints, with or without interface material, prefabricated, off-the-shelf DME A
   BETOS: D1F   Prosthetic/Orthotic devices

C **L4392** Replacement, soft interface material, static AFO DME A
   BETOS: D1F   Prosthetic/Orthotic devices

C **L4394** Replace soft interface material, foot drop splint DME A
   BETOS: D1F   Prosthetic/Orthotic devices

C **L4396** Static or dynamic ankle-foot orthosis, including soft interface material, adjustable for fit, for positioning, may be used for minimal ambulation, prefabricated item that has been trimmed, bent, molded, assembled, or otherwise customized to fit a specific patient by an individual with expertise DME A
   BETOS: D1F   Prosthetic/Orthotic devices

C **L4397** Static or dynamic ankle-foot orthosis, including soft interface material, adjustable for fit, for positioning, may be used for minimal ambulation, prefabricated, off-the-shelf DME A
   BETOS: D1F   Prosthetic/Orthotic devices

C **L4398** Foot drop splint, recumbent positioning device, prefabricated, off-the-shelf DME A
   BETOS: D1F   Prosthetic/Orthotic devices

C **L4631** Ankle-foot orthosis (AFO), walking boot type, varus/valgus correction, rocker bottom, anterior tibial shell, soft interface, custom arch support, plastic or other material, includes straps and closures, custom fabricated DME A
   BETOS: D1F   Prosthetic/Orthotic devices

NOTES

PROSTHETIC PROCEDURES (L5000-L9900)

PARTIAL FOOT PROSTHETICS (L5000-L5020)

[D] L5000 Partial foot, shoe insert with longitudinal arch, toe filler **DME** A
BETOS: D1F Prosthetic/Orthotic devices

[D] L5010 Partial foot, molded socket, ankle height, with toe filler **DME** A
BETOS: D1F Prosthetic/Orthotic devices

[D] L5020 Partial foot, molded socket, tibial tubercle height, with toe filler **DME** A
BETOS: D1F Prosthetic/Orthotic devices

ANKLE PROSTHETICS (L5050, L5060)

[C] L5050 Ankle, Symes, molded socket, SACH foot **DME** A
BETOS: D1F Prosthetic/Orthotic devices

[C] L5060 Ankle, Symes, metal frame, molded leather socket, articulated ankle/foot **DME** A
BETOS: D1F Prosthetic/Orthotic devices

BELOW THE KNEE PROSTHETICS (L5100, L5105)

[C] L5100 Below knee, molded socket, shin, SACH foot **DME** A
BETOS: D1F Prosthetic/Orthotic devices

[C] L5105 Below knee, plastic socket, joints and thigh lacer, SACH foot **DME** A
BETOS: D1F Prosthetic/Orthotic devices

KNEE DISARTICULATION PROSTHETICS (L5150, L5160)

[C] L5150 Knee disarticulation (or through knee), molded socket, external knee joints, shin, SACH foot **DME** A
BETOS: D1F Prosthetic/Orthotic devices

[C] L5160 Knee disarticulation (or through knee), molded socket, bent knee configuration, external knee joints, shin, SACH foot **DME** A
BETOS: D1F Prosthetic/Orthotic devices

ABOVE THE KNEE PROSTHETICS (L5200-L5230)

[C] L5200 Above knee, molded socket, single axis constant friction knee, shin, SACH foot **DME** A
BETOS: D1F Prosthetic/Orthotic devices

[C] L5210 Above knee, short prosthesis, no knee joint ('stubbies'), with foot blocks, no ankle joints, each **DME** A
BETOS: D1F Prosthetic/Orthotic devices

[C] L5220 Above knee, short prosthesis, no knee joint ('stubbies'), with articulated ankle/foot, dynamically aligned, each **DME** A
BETOS: D1F Prosthetic/Orthotic devices

[C] L5230 Above knee, for proximal femoral focal deficiency, constant friction knee, shin, SACH foot **DME** A
BETOS: D1F Prosthetic/Orthotic devices

HIP DISARTICULATION PROSTHETICS (L5250, L5270)

[C] L5250 Hip disarticulation, Canadian type; molded socket, hip joint, single axis constant friction knee, shin, SACH foot **DME** A
BETOS: D1F Prosthetic/Orthotic devices

[C] L5270 Hip disarticulation, tilt table type; molded socket, locking hip joint, single axis constant friction knee, shin, SACH foot **DME** A
BETOS: D1F Prosthetic/Orthotic devices

ENDOSKELETAL PROSTHETICS, LOWER LIMBS (L5280-L5341)

[C] L5280 Hemipelvectomy, Canadian type; molded socket, hip joint, single axis constant friction knee, shin, SACH foot **DME** A
BETOS: D1F Prosthetic/Orthotic devices

[C] L5301 Below knee, molded socket, shin, SACH foot, endoskeletal system **DME** A
BETOS: D1F Prosthetic/Orthotic devices
Coding Clinic: 2002, Q1

[C] L5312 Knee disarticulation (or through knee), molded socket, single axis knee, pylon, SACH foot, endoskeletal system **DME** A
BETOS: D1F Prosthetic/Orthotic devices

[C] L5321 Above knee, molded socket, open end, SACH foot, endoskeletal system, single axis knee **DME** A
BETOS: D1F Prosthetic/Orthotic devices
Coding Clinic: 2002, Q1

[C] L5331 Hip disarticulation, Canadian type, molded socket, endoskeletal system, hip joint, single axis knee, SACH foot **DME** A
BETOS: D1F Prosthetic/Orthotic devices
Coding Clinic: 2002, Q1

[C] L5341 Hemipelvectomy, Canadian type, molded socket, endoskeletal system, hip joint, single axis knee, SACH foot **DME** A
BETOS: D1F Prosthetic/Orthotic devices
Coding Clinic: 2002, Q1

PROSTHETIC FITTING, IMMEDIATE POSTSURGICAL OR EARLY, LOWER LIMBS (L5400-L5460)

[C] L5400 Immediate post surgical or early fitting, application of initial rigid dressing, including fitting, alignment, suspension, and one cast change, below knee **DME** A
BETOS: D1F Prosthetic/Orthotic devices

C **L5410** Immediate post surgical or early fitting, application of initial rigid dressing, including fitting, alignment and suspension, below knee, each additional cast change and realignment `DME` A

BETOS: D1F   Prosthetic/Orthotic devices

C **L5420** Immediate post surgical or early fitting, application of initial rigid dressing, including fitting, alignment and suspension and one cast change 'AK' or knee disarticulation `DME` A

BETOS: D1F   Prosthetic/Orthotic devices

C **L5430** Immediate post surgical or early fitting, application of initial rigid dressing, incl. fitting, alignment and suspension, 'AK' or knee disarticulation, each additional cast change and realignment `DME` A

BETOS: D1F   Prosthetic/Orthotic devices

C **L5450** Immediate post surgical or early fitting, application of non-weight bearing rigid dressing, below knee `DME` A

BETOS: D1F   Prosthetic/Orthotic devices

C **L5460** Immediate post surgical or early fitting, application of non-weight bearing rigid dressing, above knee `DME` A

BETOS: D1F   Prosthetic/Orthotic devices

SUPPLY, INITIAL PROSTHESIS (L5500-L5505)

C **L5500** Initial, below knee 'PTB' type socket, non-alignable system, pylon, no cover, SACH foot, plaster socket, direct formed `DME` A

BETOS: D1F   Prosthetic/Orthotic devices

C **L5505** Initial, above knee - knee disarticulation, ischial level socket, non-alignable system, pylon, no cover, SACH foot, plaster socket, direct formed `DME` A

BETOS: D1F   Prosthetic/Orthotic devices

SUPPLY, PREPARATORY PROSTHESIS (L5510-L5600)

C **L5510** Preparatory, below knee 'PTB' type socket, non-alignable system, pylon, no cover, SACH foot, plaster socket, molded to model `DME` A

BETOS: D1F   Prosthetic/Orthotic devices

C **L5520** Preparatory, below knee 'PTB' type socket, non-alignable system, pylon, no cover, SACH foot, thermoplastic or equal, direct formed `DME` A

BETOS: D1F   Prosthetic/Orthotic devices

C **L5530** Preparatory, below knee 'PTB' type socket, non-alignable system, pylon, no cover, SACH foot, thermoplastic or equal, molded to model `DME` A

BETOS: D1F   Prosthetic/Orthotic devices

C **L5535** Preparatory, below knee 'PTB' type socket, non-alignable system, no cover, SACH foot, prefabricated, adjustable open end socket `DME` A

BETOS: D1F   Prosthetic/Orthotic devices

C **L5540** Preparatory, below knee 'PTB' type socket, non-alignable system, pylon, no cover, SACH foot, laminated socket, molded to model `DME` A

BETOS: D1F   Prosthetic/Orthotic devices

C **L5560** Preparatory, above knee- knee disarticulation, ischial level socket, non-alignable system, pylon, no cover, SACH foot, plaster socket, molded to model `DME` A

BETOS: D1F   Prosthetic/Orthotic devices

C **L5570** Preparatory, above knee - knee disarticulation, ischial level socket, non-alignable system, pylon, no cover, SACH foot, thermoplastic or equal, direct formed `DME` A

BETOS: D1F   Prosthetic/Orthotic devices

C **L5580** Preparatory, above knee - knee disarticulation ischial level socket, non-alignable system, pylon, no cover, SACH foot, thermoplastic or equal, molded to model `DME` A

BETOS: D1F   Prosthetic/Orthotic devices

C **L5585** Preparatory, above knee - knee disarticulation, ischial level socket, non-alignable system, pylon, no cover, SACH foot, prefabricated adjustable open end socket `DME` A

BETOS: D1F   Prosthetic/Orthotic devices

C **L5590** Preparatory, above knee - knee disarticulation ischial level socket, non-alignable system, pylon no cover, SACH foot, laminated socket, molded to model `DME` A

BETOS: D1F   Prosthetic/Orthotic devices

C **L5595** Preparatory, hip disarticulation-hemipelvectomy, pylon, no cover, SACH foot, thermoplastic or equal, molded to patient model `DME` A

BETOS: D1F   Prosthetic/Orthotic devices

C **L5600** Preparatory, hip disarticulation-hemipelvectomy, pylon, no cover, SACH foot, laminated socket, molded to patient model `DME` A

BETOS: D1F   Prosthetic/Orthotic devices

ENDOSKELETAL PROSTHETIC ADDITIONS, LOWER EXTREMITIES (L5610-L5617)

C **L5610** Addition to lower extremity, endoskeletal system, above knee, hydracadence system `DME` A

BETOS: D1F   Prosthetic/Orthotic devices

● New code   ▲ Revised code   **C** Carrier judgment   **D** Special coverage instructions apply

I Not payable by Medicare   **M** Non-covered by Medicare   **S** Non-covered by Medicare statute   AHA Coding Clinic®

C **L5611** Addition to lower extremity, endoskeletal system, above knee-knee disarticulation, 4 bar linkage, with friction swing phase control **DME** A
BETOS: D1F Prosthetic/Orthotic devices

C **L5613** Addition to lower extremity, endoskeletal system, above knee-knee disarticulation, 4 bar linkage, with hydraulic swing phase control **DME** A
BETOS: D1F Prosthetic/Orthotic devices

C **L5614** Addition to lower extremity, exoskeletal system, above knee-knee disarticulation, 4 bar linkage, with pneumatic swing phase control **DME** A
BETOS: D1F Prosthetic/Orthotic devices

C **L5616** Addition to lower extremity, endoskeletal system, above knee, universal multiplex system, friction swing phase control **DME** A
BETOS: D1F Prosthetic/Orthotic devices

C **L5617** Addition to lower extremity, quick change self-aligning unit, above knee or below knee, each **DME** A
BETOS: D1F Prosthetic/Orthotic devices

TEST SOCKET PROSTHETIC ADDITIONS, LOWER EXTREMITIES (L5618-L5628)

C **L5618** Addition to lower extremity, test socket, Symes **DME** A
BETOS: D1F Prosthetic/Orthotic devices

C **L5620** Addition to lower extremity, test socket, below knee **DME** A
BETOS: D1F Prosthetic/Orthotic devices

C **L5622** Addition to lower extremity, test socket, knee disarticulation **DME** A
BETOS: D1F Prosthetic/Orthotic devices

C **L5624** Addition to lower extremity, test socket, above knee **DME** A
BETOS: D1F Prosthetic/Orthotic devices

C **L5626** Addition to lower extremity, test socket, hip disarticulation **DME** A
BETOS: D1F Prosthetic/Orthotic devices

C **L5628** Addition to lower extremity, test socket, hemipelvectomy **DME** A
BETOS: D1F Prosthetic/Orthotic devices

VARIOUS PROSTHETIC SOCKETS (L5629-L5653)

C **L5629** Addition to lower extremity, below knee, acrylic socket **DME** A
BETOS: D1F Prosthetic/Orthotic devices

C **L5630** Addition to lower extremity, Symes type, expandable wall socket **DME** A
BETOS: D1F Prosthetic/Orthotic devices

C **L5631** Addition to lower extremity, above knee or knee disarticulation, acrylic socket **DME** A
BETOS: D1F Prosthetic/Orthotic devices

C **L5632** Addition to lower extremity, Symes type, 'PTB' brim design socket **DME** A
BETOS: D1F Prosthetic/Orthotic devices

C **L5634** Addition to lower extremity, Symes type, posterior opening (Canadian) socket **DME** A
BETOS: D1F Prosthetic/Orthotic devices

C **L5636** Addition to lower extremity, Symes type, medial opening socket **DME** A
BETOS: D1F Prosthetic/Orthotic devices

C **L5637** Addition to lower extremity, below knee, total contact **DME** A
BETOS: D1F Prosthetic/Orthotic devices

C **L5638** Addition to lower extremity, below knee, leather socket **DME** A
BETOS: D1F Prosthetic/Orthotic devices

C **L5639** Addition to lower extremity, below knee, wood socket **DME** A
BETOS: D1F Prosthetic/Orthotic devices

C **L5640** Addition to lower extremity, knee disarticulation, leather socket **DME** A
BETOS: D1F Prosthetic/Orthotic devices

C **L5642** Addition to lower extremity, above knee, leather socket **DME** A
BETOS: D1F Prosthetic/Orthotic devices

C **L5643** Addition to lower extremity, hip disarticulation, flexible inner socket, external frame **DME** A
BETOS: D1F Prosthetic/Orthotic devices

C **L5644** Addition to lower extremity, above knee, wood socket **DME** A
BETOS: D1F Prosthetic/Orthotic devices

C **L5645** Addition to lower extremity, below knee, flexible inner socket, external frame **DME** A
BETOS: D1F Prosthetic/Orthotic devices

C **L5646** Addition to lower extremity, below knee, air, fluid, gel or equal, cushion socket **DME** A
BETOS: D1F Prosthetic/Orthotic devices

C **L5647** Addition to lower extremity, below knee suction socket **DME** A
BETOS: D1F Prosthetic/Orthotic devices

C **L5648** Addition to lower extremity, above knee, air, fluid, gel or equal, cushion socket **DME** A
BETOS: D1F Prosthetic/Orthotic devices

C **L5649** Addition to lower extremity, ischial containment/narrow M-L socket **DME** A
BETOS: D1F Prosthetic/Orthotic devices

C **L5650** Additions to lower extremity, total contact, above knee or knee disarticulation socket **DME** A
BETOS: D1F Prosthetic/Orthotic devices

C **L5651** Addition to lower extremity, above knee, flexible inner socket, external frame **DME** A
BETOS: D1F Prosthetic/Orthotic devices

♂ Male only ♀ Female only Ⓐ Age A2 - Z3 = ASC Payment indicator A - Y = APC Status indicator
ASC = ASC Approved Procedure **DME** Paid under the DME fee schedule **MIPS** MIPS code

C L5652 Addition to lower extremity, suction suspension, above knee or knee disarticulation socket **DME** A
 BETOS: D1F   Prosthetic/Orthotic devices

C L5653 Addition to lower extremity, knee disarticulation, expandable wall socket **DME** A
 BETOS: D1F   Prosthetic/Orthotic devices

SOCKET INSERT, SUSPENSIONS, AND OTHER PROSTHETIC ADDITIONS (L5654-L5699)

C L5654 Addition to lower extremity, socket insert, Symes, (Kemblo, Pelite, Aliplast, Plastazote or equal) **DME** A
 BETOS: D1F   Prosthetic/Orthotic devices

C L5655 Addition to lower extremity, socket insert, below knee (Kemblo, Pelite, Aliplast, Plastazote or equal) **DME** A
 BETOS: D1F   Prosthetic/Orthotic devices

C L5656 Addition to lower extremity, socket insert, knee disarticulation (Kemblo, Pelite, Aliplast, Plastazote or equal) **DME** A
 BETOS: D1F   Prosthetic/Orthotic devices

C L5658 Addition to lower extremity, socket insert, above knee (Kemblo, Pelite, Aliplast, Plastazote or equal) **DME** A
 BETOS: D1F   Prosthetic/Orthotic devices

C L5661 Addition to lower extremity, socket insert, multi-durometer Symes **DME** A
 BETOS: D1F   Prosthetic/Orthotic devices

C L5665 Addition to lower extremity, socket insert, multi-durometer, below knee **DME** A
 BETOS: D1F   Prosthetic/Orthotic devices

C L5666 Addition to lower extremity, below knee, cuff suspension **DME** A
 BETOS: D1F   Prosthetic/Orthotic devices

C L5668 Addition to lower extremity, below knee, molded distal cushion **DME** A
 BETOS: D1F   Prosthetic/Orthotic devices

C L5670 Addition to lower extremity, below knee, molded supracondylar suspension ('PTS' or similar) **DME** A
 BETOS: D1F   Prosthetic/Orthotic devices

C L5671 Addition to lower extremity, below knee/above knee suspension locking mechanism (shuttle, lanyard or equal), excludes socket insert **DME** A
 BETOS: D1F   Prosthetic/Orthotic devices
 Coding Clinic: 2002, Q1

C L5672 Addition to lower extremity, below knee, removable medial brim suspension **DME** A
 BETOS: D1F   Prosthetic/Orthotic devices

C L5673 Addition to lower extremity, below knee/above knee, custom fabricated from existing mold or prefabricated, socket insert,

silicone gel, elastomeric or equal, for use with locking mechanism **DME** A
 BETOS: D1F   Prosthetic/Orthotic devices

C L5676 Additions to lower extremity, below knee, knee joints, single axis, pair **DME** A
 BETOS: D1F   Prosthetic/Orthotic devices

C L5677 Additions to lower extremity, below knee, knee joints, polycentric, pair **DME** A
 BETOS: D1F   Prosthetic/Orthotic devices

C L5678 Additions to lower extremity, below knee, joint covers, pair **DME** A
 BETOS: D1F   Prosthetic/Orthotic devices

C L5679 Addition to lower extremity, below knee/above knee, custom fabricated from existing mold or prefabricated, socket insert, silicone gel, elastomeric or equal, not for use with locking mechanism **DME** A
 BETOS: D1F   Prosthetic/Orthotic devices

C L5680 Addition to lower extremity, below knee, thigh lacer, nonmolded **DME** A
 BETOS: D1F   Prosthetic/Orthotic devices

C L5681 Addition to lower extremity, below knee/above knee, custom fabricated socket insert for congenital or atypical traumatic amputee, silicone gel, elastomeric or equal, for use with or without locking mechanism, initial only (for other than initial, use code L5673 or L5679) **DME** A
 BETOS: D1F   Prosthetic/Orthotic devices

C L5682 Addition to lower extremity, below knee, thigh lacer, gluteal/ischial, molded **DME** A
 BETOS: D1F   Prosthetic/Orthotic devices

C L5683 Addition to lower extremity, below knee/above knee, custom fabricated socket insert for other than congenital or atypical traumatic amputee, silicone gel, elastomeric or equal, for use with or without locking mechanism, initial only (for other than initial, use code L5673 or L5679) **DME** A
 BETOS: D1F   Prosthetic/Orthotic devices

C L5684 Addition to lower extremity, below knee, fork strap **DME** A
 BETOS: D1F   Prosthetic/Orthotic devices

C L5685 Addition to lower extremity prosthesis, below knee, suspension/sealing sleeve, with or without valve, any material, each **DME** A
 BETOS: D1F   Prosthetic/Orthotic devices

C L5686 Addition to lower extremity, below knee, back check (extension control) **DME** A
 BETOS: D1F   Prosthetic/Orthotic devices

C L5688 Addition to lower extremity, below knee, waist belt, webbing **DME** A
 BETOS: D1F   Prosthetic/Orthotic devices

C L5690 Addition to lower extremity, below knee, waist belt, padded and lined **DME** A
 BETOS: D1F   Prosthetic/Orthotic devices

C **L5692** Addition to lower extremity, above knee, pelvic control belt, light DME A

BETOS: D1F   Prosthetic/Orthotic devices

C **L5694** Addition to lower extremity, above knee, pelvic control belt, padded and lined DME A

BETOS: D1F   Prosthetic/Orthotic devices

C **L5695** Addition to lower extremity, above knee, pelvic control, sleeve suspension, neoprene or equal, each DME A

BETOS: D1F   Prosthetic/Orthotic devices

C **L5696** Addition to lower extremity, above knee or knee disarticulation, pelvic joint DME A

BETOS: D1F   Prosthetic/Orthotic devices

C **L5697** Addition to lower extremity, above knee or knee disarticulation, pelvic band DME A

BETOS: D1F   Prosthetic/Orthotic devices

C **L5698** Addition to lower extremity, above knee or knee disarticulation, Silesian bandage DME A

BETOS: D1F   Prosthetic/Orthotic devices

C **L5699** All lower extremity prostheses, shoulder harness DME A

BETOS: D1F   Prosthetic/Orthotic devices

REPLACEMENT SOCKETS (L5700-L5703)

C **L5700** Replacement, socket, below knee, molded to patient model DME A

BETOS: D1F   Prosthetic/Orthotic devices

C **L5701** Replacement, socket, above knee/knee disarticulation, including attachment plate, molded to patient model DME A

BETOS: D1F   Prosthetic/Orthotic devices

C **L5702** Replacement, socket, hip disarticulation, including hip joint, molded to patient model DME A

BETOS: D1F   Prosthetic/Orthotic devices

C **L5703** Ankle, Symes, molded to patient model, socket without solid ankle cushion heel (SACH) foot, replacement only DME A

BETOS: D1F   Prosthetic/Orthotic devices

CUSTOM-SHAPED PROTECTIVE COVERS (L5704-L5707)

C **L5704** Custom shaped protective cover, below knee DME A

BETOS: D1F   Prosthetic/Orthotic devices

C **L5705** Custom shaped protective cover, above knee DME A

BETOS: D1F   Prosthetic/Orthotic devices

C **L5706** Custom shaped protective cover, knee disarticulation DME A

BETOS: D1F   Prosthetic/Orthotic devices

C **L5707** Custom shaped protective cover, hip disarticulation DME A

BETOS: D1F   Prosthetic/Orthotic devices

EXOSKELETAL KNEE-SHIN SYSTEM ADDITIONS (L5710-L5780)

C **L5710** Addition, exoskeletal knee-shin system, single axis, manual lock DME A

BETOS: D1F   Prosthetic/Orthotic devices

C **L5711** Additions exoskeletal knee-shin system, single axis, manual lock, ultra-light material DME A

BETOS: D1F   Prosthetic/Orthotic devices

C **L5712** Addition, exoskeletal knee-shin system, single axis, friction swing and stance phase control (safety knee) DME A

BETOS: D1F   Prosthetic/Orthotic devices

C **L5714** Addition, exoskeletal knee-shin system, single axis, variable friction swing phase control DME A

BETOS: D1F   Prosthetic/Orthotic devices

C **L5716** Addition, exoskeletal knee-shin system, polycentric, mechanical stance phase lock DME A

BETOS: D1F   Prosthetic/Orthotic devices

C **L5718** Addition, exoskeletal knee-shin system, polycentric, friction swing and stance phase control DME A

BETOS: D1F   Prosthetic/Orthotic devices

C **L5722** Addition, exoskeletal knee-shin system, single axis, pneumatic swing, friction stance phase control DME A

BETOS: D1F   Prosthetic/Orthotic devices

C **L5724** Addition, exoskeletal knee-shin system, single axis, fluid swing phase control DME A

BETOS: D1F   Prosthetic/Orthotic devices

C **L5726** Addition, exoskeletal knee-shin system, single axis, external joints fluid swing phase control DME A

BETOS: D1F   Prosthetic/Orthotic devices

C **L5728** Addition, exoskeletal knee-shin system, single axis, fluid swing and stance phase control DME A

BETOS: D1F   Prosthetic/Orthotic devices

C **L5780** Addition, exoskeletal knee-shin system, single axis, pneumatic/hydra pneumatic swing phase control DME A

BETOS: D1F   Prosthetic/Orthotic devices

VACUUM PUMPS, LOWER LIMB PROSTHETIC ADDITIONS (L5781, L5782)

C **L5781** Addition to lower limb prosthesis, vacuum pump, residual limb volume management and moisture evacuation system DME A

BETOS: D1F   Prosthetic/Orthotic devices

♂ Male only   ♀ Female only   A Age   A2 - Z3 = ASC Payment indicator   A - Y = APC Status indicator

ASC = ASC Approved Procedure   DME Paid under the DME fee schedule   MIPS MIPS code

C **L5782** Addition to lower limb prosthesis, vacuum pump, residual limb volume management and moisture evacuation system, heavy duty   DME A
BETOS: D1F   Prosthetic/Orthotic devices

OTHER EXOSKELETAL ADDITIONS (L5785-L5795)

C **L5785** Addition, exoskeletal system, below knee, ultra-light material (titanium, carbon fiber or equal)   DME A
BETOS: D1F   Prosthetic/Orthotic devices

C **L5790** Addition, exoskeletal system, above knee, ultra-light material (titanium, carbon fiber or equal)   DME A
BETOS: D1F   Prosthetic/Orthotic devices

C **L5795** Addition, exoskeletal system, hip disarticulation, ultra-light material (titanium, carbon fiber or equal)   DME A
BETOS: D1F   Prosthetic/Orthotic devices

ENDOSKELETAL KNEE OR HIP SYSTEM ADDITIONS (L5810-L5966)

C **L5810** Addition, endoskeletal knee-shin system, single axis, manual lock   DME A
BETOS: D1F   Prosthetic/Orthotic devices

C **L5811** Addition, endoskeletal knee-shin system, single axis, manual lock, ultra-light material   DME A
BETOS: D1F   Prosthetic/Orthotic devices

C **L5812** Addition, endoskeletal knee-shin system, single axis, friction swing and stance phase control (safety knee)   DME A
BETOS: D1F   Prosthetic/Orthotic devices

C **L5814** Addition, endoskeletal knee-shin system, polycentric, hydraulic swing phase control, mechanical stance phase lock   DME A
BETOS: D1F   Prosthetic/Orthotic devices

C **L5816** Addition, endoskeletal knee-shin system, polycentric, mechanical stance phase lock   DME A
BETOS: D1F   Prosthetic/Orthotic devices

C **L5818** Addition, endoskeletal knee-shin system, polycentric, friction swing, and stance phase control   DME A
BETOS: D1F   Prosthetic/Orthotic devices

C **L5822** Addition, endoskeletal knee-shin system, single axis, pneumatic swing, friction stance phase control   DME A
BETOS: D1F   Prosthetic/Orthotic devices

C **L5824** Addition, endoskeletal knee-shin system, single axis, fluid swing phase control   DME A
BETOS: D1F   Prosthetic/Orthotic devices

C **L5826** Addition, endoskeletal knee-shin system, single axis, hydraulic swing phase control, with miniature high activity frame   DME A
BETOS: D1F   Prosthetic/Orthotic devices

C **L5828** Addition, endoskeletal knee-shin system, single axis, fluid swing and stance phase control   DME A
BETOS: D1F   Prosthetic/Orthotic devices

C **L5830** Addition, endoskeletal knee-shin system, single axis, pneumatic/ swing phase control   DME A
BETOS: D1F   Prosthetic/Orthotic devices

C **L5840** Addition, endoskeletal knee/shin system, 4-bar linkage or multiaxial, pneumatic swing phase control   DME A
BETOS: D1F   Prosthetic/Orthotic devices

C **L5845** Addition, endoskeletal, knee-shin system, stance flexion feature, adjustable   DME A
BETOS: D1F   Prosthetic/Orthotic devices

C **L5848** Addition to endoskeletal knee-shin system, fluid stance extension, dampening feature, with or without adjustability   DME A
BETOS: D1F   Prosthetic/Orthotic devices

C **L5850** Addition, endoskeletal system, above knee or hip disarticulation, knee extension assist   DME A
BETOS: D1F   Prosthetic/Orthotic devices

C **L5855** Addition, endoskeletal system, hip disarticulation, mechanical hip extension assist   DME A
BETOS: D1F   Prosthetic/Orthotic devices

C **L5856** Addition to lower extremity prosthesis, endoskeletal knee-shin system, microprocessor control feature, swing and stance phase, includes electronic sensor(s), any type   DME A
BETOS: D1F   Prosthetic/Orthotic devices

C **L5857** Addition to lower extremity prosthesis, endoskeletal knee-shin system, microprocessor control feature, swing phase only, includes electronic sensor(s), any type   DME A
BETOS: D1F   Prosthetic/Orthotic devices

C **L5858** Addition to lower extremity prosthesis, endoskeletal knee shin system, microprocessor control feature, stance phase only, includes electronic sensor(s), any type   DME A
BETOS: D1F   Prosthetic/Orthotic devices

C **L5859** Addition to lower extremity prosthesis, endoskeletal knee-shin system, powered and programmable flexion/extension assist control, includes any type motor(s)   DME A
BETOS: D1F   Prosthetic/Orthotic devices

● New code   ▲ Revised code   C Carrier judgment   D Special coverage instructions apply
I Not payable by Medicare   M Non-covered by Medicare   S Non-covered by Medicare statute   *AHA Coding Clinic®*

Leg prosthesis

C L5910 Addition, endoskeletal system, below knee, alignable system **DME** A
    BETOS: D1F   Prosthetic/Orthotic devices

C L5920 Addition, endoskeletal system, above knee or hip disarticulation, alignable system **DME** A
    BETOS: D1F   Prosthetic/Orthotic devices

C L5925 Addition, endoskeletal system, above knee, knee disarticulation or hip disarticulation, manual lock **DME** A
    BETOS: D1F   Prosthetic/Orthotic devices

C L5930 Addition, endoskeletal system, high activity knee control frame **DME** A
    BETOS: D1F   Prosthetic/Orthotic devices

C L5940 Addition, endoskeletal system, below knee, ultra-light material (titanium, carbon fiber or equal) **DME** A
    BETOS: D1F   Prosthetic/Orthotic devices

C L5950 Addition, endoskeletal system, above knee, ultra-light material (titanium, carbon fiber or equal) **DME** A
    BETOS: D1F   Prosthetic/Orthotic devices

C L5960 Addition, endoskeletal system, hip disarticulation, ultra-light material (titanium, carbon fiber or equal) **DME** A
    BETOS: D1F   Prosthetic/Orthotic devices

C L5961 Addition, endoskeletal system, polycentric hip joint, pneumatic or hydraulic control, rotation control, with or without flexion and/or extension control **DME** A
    BETOS: D1F   Prosthetic/Orthotic devices

C L5962 Addition, endoskeletal system, below knee, flexible protective outer surface covering system **DME** A
    BETOS: D1F   Prosthetic/Orthotic devices

C L5964 Addition, endoskeletal system, above knee, flexible protective outer surface covering system **DME** A
    BETOS: D1F   Prosthetic/Orthotic devices

C L5966 Addition, endoskeletal system, hip disarticulation, flexible protective outer surface covering system **DME** A
    BETOS: D1F   Prosthetic/Orthotic devices

ANKLE AND/OR FOOT PROSTHETICS AND ADDITIONS (L5968-L5999)

C L5968 Addition to lower limb prosthesis, multiaxial ankle with swing phase active dorsiflexion feature **DME** A
    BETOS: D1F   Prosthetic/Orthotic devices

C L5969 Addition, endoskeletal ankle-foot or ankle system, power assist, includes any type motor(s) A
    BETOS: D1F   Prosthetic/Orthotic devices

C L5970 All lower extremity prostheses, foot, external keel, solid ankle cushion heel (SACH) foot **DME** A
    BETOS: D1F   Prosthetic/Orthotic devices

C L5971 All lower extremity prosthesis, solid ankle cushion heel (SACH) foot, replacement only **DME** A
    BETOS: D1F   Prosthetic/Orthotic devices

C L5972 All lower extremity prostheses, foot, flexible keel **DME** A
    BETOS: D1F   Prosthetic/Orthotic devices

C L5973 Endoskeletal ankle-foot system, microprocessor controlled feature, dorsiflexion and/or plantar flexion control, includes power source **DME** A
    BETOS: D1F   Prosthetic/Orthotic devices

C L5974 All lower extremity prostheses, foot, single axis ankle/foot **DME** A
    BETOS: D1F   Prosthetic/Orthotic devices

C L5975 All lower extremity prosthesis, combination single axis ankle and flexible keel foot **DME** A
    BETOS: D1F   Prosthetic/Orthotic devices

C L5976 All lower extremity prostheses, energy storing foot (seattle carbon copy II or equal) **DME** A
    BETOS: D1F   Prosthetic/Orthotic devices

C L5978 All lower extremity prostheses, foot, multiaxial ankle/foot **DME** A
    BETOS: D1F   Prosthetic/Orthotic devices

C L5979 All lower extremity prosthesis, multi-axial ankle, dynamic response foot, one piece system **DME** A
    BETOS: D1F   Prosthetic/Orthotic devices

C L5980 All lower extremity prostheses, flex foot system **DME** A
    BETOS: D1F   Prosthetic/Orthotic devices

♂ Male only   ♀ Female only   **A** Age   A2 - Z3 = ASC Payment indicator   A - Y = APC Status indicator
ASC = ASC Approved Procedure   **DME** Paid under the DME fee schedule   **MIPS** MIPS code

C **L5981** All lower extremity prostheses, flex-walk system or equal   DME A
BETOS: D1F   Prosthetic/Orthotic devices

C **L5982** All exoskeletal lower extremity prostheses, axial rotation unit   DME A
BETOS: D1F   Prosthetic/Orthotic devices

C **L5984** All endoskeletal lower extremity prosthesis, axial rotation unit, with or without adjustability   DME A
BETOS: D1F   Prosthetic/Orthotic devices

C **L5985** All endoskeletal lower extremity prostheses, dynamic prosthetic pylon   DME A
BETOS: D1F   Prosthetic/Orthotic devices

C **L5986** All lower extremity prostheses, multi-axial rotation unit ('MCP' or equal)   DME A
BETOS: D1F   Prosthetic/Orthotic devices

C **L5987** All lower extremity prosthesis, shank foot system with vertical loading pylon   DME A
BETOS: D1F   Prosthetic/Orthotic devices

C **L5988** Addition to lower limb prosthesis, vertical shock reducing pylon feature   DME A
BETOS: D1F   Prosthetic/Orthotic devices

C **L5990** Addition to lower extremity prosthesis, user adjustable heel height   DME A
BETOS: D1F   Prosthetic/Orthotic devices
Coding Clinic: 2002, Q1

C **L5999** Lower extremity prosthesis, not otherwise specified   A
BETOS: D1F   Prosthetic/Orthotic devices

PARTIAL HAND PROSTHETICS (L6000-L6026)

C **L6000** Partial hand, thumb remaining   DME A
BETOS: D1F   Prosthetic/Orthotic devices

C **L6010** Partial hand, little and/or ring finger remaining   DME A
BETOS: D1F   Prosthetic/Orthotic devices

C **L6020** Partial hand, no finger remaining   DME A
BETOS: D1F   Prosthetic/Orthotic devices

C **L6026** Transcarpal/metacarpal or partial hand disarticulation prosthesis, external power, self-suspended, inner socket with removable forearm section, electrodes and cables, two batteries, charger, myoelectric control of terminal device, excludes terminal device(s)   DME A
BETOS: D1F   Prosthetic/Orthotic devices

WRIST DISARTICULATION, HAND PROSTHETICS (L6050-L6055)

C **L6050** Wrist disarticulation, molded socket, flexible elbow hinges, triceps pad   DME A
BETOS: D1F   Prosthetic/Orthotic devices

C **L6055** Wrist disarticulation, molded socket with expandable interface, flexible elbow hinges, triceps pad   DME A
BETOS: D1F   Prosthetic/Orthotic devices

BELOW ELBOW, FOREARM AND HAND PROSTHETICS (L6100-L6130)

C **L6100** Below elbow, molded socket, flexible elbow hinge, triceps pad   DME A
BETOS: D1F   Prosthetic/Orthotic devices

C **L6110** Below elbow, molded socket, (Muenster or Northwestern suspension types)   DME A
BETOS: D1F   Prosthetic/Orthotic devices

C **L6120** Below elbow, molded double wall split socket, step-up hinges, half cuff   DME A
BETOS: D1F   Prosthetic/Orthotic devices

C **L6130** Below elbow, molded double wall split socket, stump activated locking hinge, half cuff   DME A
BETOS: D1F   Prosthetic/Orthotic devices

ELBOW DISARTICULATION, FOREARM AND HAND PROSTHETICS (L6200-L6205)

C **L6200** Elbow disarticulation, molded socket, outside locking hinge, forearm   DME A
BETOS: D1F   Prosthetic/Orthotic devices

C **L6205** Elbow disarticulation, molded socket with expandable interface, outside locking hinges, forearm   DME A
BETOS: D1F   Prosthetic/Orthotic devices

ABOVE ELBOW, FOREARM AND HAND PROSTHETICS (L6250)

C **L6250** Above elbow, molded double wall socket, internal locking elbow, forearm   DME A
BETOS: D1F   Prosthetic/Orthotic devices

SHOULDER DISARTICULATION, ARM AND HAND PROSTHETICS (L6300-L6320)

C **L6300** Shoulder disarticulation, molded socket, shoulder bulkhead, humeral section, internal locking elbow, forearm   DME A
BETOS: D1F   Prosthetic/Orthotic devices

C **L6310** Shoulder disarticulation, passive restoration (complete prosthesis)   DME A
BETOS: D1F   Prosthetic/Orthotic devices

C **L6320** Shoulder disarticulation, passive restoration (shoulder cap only)   DME A
BETOS: D1F   Prosthetic/Orthotic devices

INTERSCAPULAR THORACIC, ARM, AND HAND PROSTHETICS (L6350-L6370)

C L6350 Interscapular thoracic, molded socket, shoulder bulkhead, humeral section, internal locking elbow, forearm **DME** A
BETOS: D1F   Prosthetic/Orthotic devices

C L6360 Interscapular thoracic, passive restoration (complete prosthesis) **DME** A
BETOS: D1F   Prosthetic/Orthotic devices

C L6370 Interscapular thoracic, passive restoration (shoulder cap only) **DME** A
BETOS: D1F   Prosthetic/Orthotic devices

PROSTHETIC FITTING, IMMEDIATE POSTSURGICAL OR EARLY, UPPER LIMBS (L6380-L6388)

C L6380 Immediate post surgical or early fitting, application of initial rigid dressing, including fitting alignment and suspension of components, and one cast change, wrist disarticulation or below elbow **DME** A
BETOS: D1F   Prosthetic/Orthotic devices

C L6382 Immediate post surgical or early fitting, application of initial rigid dressing including fitting alignment and suspension of components, and one cast change, elbow disarticulation or above elbow **DME** A
BETOS: D1F   Prosthetic/Orthotic devices

C L6384 Immediate post surgical or early fitting, application of initial rigid dressing including fitting alignment and suspension of components, and one cast change, shoulder disarticulation or interscapular thoracic **DME** A
BETOS: D1F   Prosthetic/Orthotic devices

C L6386 Immediate post surgical or early fitting, each additional cast change and realignment **DME** A
BETOS: D1F   Prosthetic/Orthotic devices

C L6388 Immediate post surgical or early fitting, application of rigid dressing only **DME** A
BETOS: D1F   Prosthetic/Orthotic devices

MOLDED SOCKET ENDOSKELETAL PROSTHETIC SYSTEM, UPPER LIMBS (L6400-L6570)

C L6400 Below elbow, molded socket, endoskeletal system, including soft prosthetic tissue shaping **DME** A
BETOS: D1F   Prosthetic/Orthotic devices

C L6450 Elbow disarticulation, molded socket, endoskeletal system, including soft prosthetic tissue shaping **DME** A
BETOS: D1F   Prosthetic/Orthotic devices

C L6500 Above elbow, molded socket, endoskeletal system, including soft prosthetic tissue shaping **DME** A
BETOS: D1F   Prosthetic/Orthotic devices

C L6550 Shoulder disarticulation, molded socket, endoskeletal system, including soft prosthetic tissue shaping **DME** A
BETOS: D1F   Prosthetic/Orthotic devices

C L6570 Interscapular thoracic, molded socket, endoskeletal system, including soft prosthetic tissue shaping **DME** A
BETOS: D1F   Prosthetic/Orthotic devices

PREPARATORY PROSTHETIC, UPPER LIMBS (L6580-L6590)

C L6580 Preparatory, wrist disarticulation or below elbow, single wall plastic socket, friction wrist, flexible elbow hinges, figure of eight harness, humeral cuff, Bowden cable control, USMC or equal pylon, no cover, molded to patient model **DME** A
BETOS: D1F   Prosthetic/Orthotic devices

C L6582 Preparatory, wrist disarticulation or below elbow, single wall socket, friction wrist, flexible elbow hinges, figure of eight harness, humeral cuff, Bowden cable control, USMC or equal pylon, no cover, direct formed **DME** A
BETOS: D1F   Prosthetic/Orthotic devices

C L6584 Preparatory, elbow disarticulation or above elbow, single wall plastic socket, friction wrist, locking elbow, figure of eight harness, fair lead cable control, USMC or equal pylon, no cover, molded to patient model **DME** A
BETOS: D1F   Prosthetic/Orthotic devices

C L6586 Preparatory, elbow disarticulation or above elbow, single wall socket, friction wrist, locking elbow, figure of eight harness, fair lead cable control, USMC or equal pylon, no cover, direct formed **DME** A
BETOS: D1F   Prosthetic/Orthotic devices

C L6588 Preparatory, shoulder disarticulation or interscapular thoracic, single wall plastic socket, shoulder joint, locking elbow, friction wrist, chest strap, fair lead cable control, USMC or equal pylon, no cover, molded to patient model **DME** A
BETOS: D1F   Prosthetic/Orthotic devices

C L6590 Preparatory, shoulder disarticulation or interscapular thoracic, single wall socket, shoulder joint, locking elbow, friction wrist, chest strap, fair lead cable control, USMC or equal pylon, no cover, direct formed **DME** A
BETOS: D1F   Prosthetic/Orthotic devices

UPPER EXTREMITY PROSTHETIC ADDITIONS (L6600-L6698)

C L6600 Upper extremity additions, polycentric hinge, pair **DME** A
BETOS: D1F   Prosthetic/Orthotic devices

C L6605 Upper extremity additions, single pivot hinge, pair **DME** A
BETOS: D1F   Prosthetic/Orthotic devices

♂ Male only   ♀ Female only   **A** Age   A2 - Z3 = ASC Payment indicator   A - Y = APC Status indicator
ASC = ASC Approved Procedure   **DME** Paid under the DME fee schedule   **MIPS** MIPS code

CPT® is a registered trademark of the American Medical Association. All rights reserved.   **347**

C **L6610** Upper extremity additions, flexible metal hinge, pair DME A
BETOS: D1F   Prosthetic/Orthotic devices

C **L6611** Addition to upper extremity prosthesis, external powered, additional switch, any type DME A
BETOS: D1F   Prosthetic/Orthotic devices

C **L6615** Upper extremity addition, disconnect locking wrist unit DME A
BETOS: D1F   Prosthetic/Orthotic devices

C **L6616** Upper extremity addition, additional disconnect insert for locking wrist unit, each DME A
BETOS: D1F   Prosthetic/Orthotic devices

C **L6620** Upper extremity addition, flexion/extension wrist unit, with or without friction DME A
BETOS: D1F   Prosthetic/Orthotic devices

C **L6621** Upper extremity prosthesis addition, flexion/extension wrist with or without friction, for use with external powered terminal device DME A
BETOS: D1F   Prosthetic/Orthotic devices

C **L6623** Upper extremity addition, spring assisted rotational wrist unit with latch release DME A
BETOS: D1F   Prosthetic/Orthotic devices

C **L6624** Upper extremity addition, flexion/extension and rotation wrist unit DME A
BETOS: D1F   Prosthetic/Orthotic devices

C **L6625** Upper extremity addition, rotation wrist unit with cable lock DME A
BETOS: D1F   Prosthetic/Orthotic devices

C **L6628** Upper extremity addition, quick disconnect hook adapter, Otto Bock or equal DME A
BETOS: D1F   Prosthetic/Orthotic devices

C **L6629** Upper extremity addition, quick disconnect lamination collar with coupling piece, Otto Bock or equal DME A
BETOS: D1F   Prosthetic/Orthotic devices

C **L6630** Upper extremity addition, stainless steel, any wrist DME A
BETOS: D1F   Prosthetic/Orthotic devices

C **L6632** Upper extremity addition, latex suspension sleeve, each DME A
BETOS: D1F   Prosthetic/Orthotic devices

C **L6635** Upper extremity addition, lift assist for elbow DME A
BETOS: D1F   Prosthetic/Orthotic devices

C **L6637** Upper extremity addition, nudge control elbow lock DME A
BETOS: D1F   Prosthetic/Orthotic devices

C **L6638** Upper extremity addition to prosthesis, electric locking feature, only for use with manually powered elbow DME A
BETOS: D1F   Prosthetic/Orthotic devices

C **L6640** Upper extremity additions, shoulder abduction joint, pair DME A
BETOS: D1F   Prosthetic/Orthotic devices

C **L6641** Upper extremity addition, excursion amplifier, pulley type DME A
BETOS: D1F   Prosthetic/Orthotic devices

C **L6642** Upper extremity addition, excursion amplifier, lever type DME A
BETOS: D1F   Prosthetic/Orthotic devices

C **L6645** Upper extremity addition, shoulder flexion-abduction joint, each DME A
BETOS: D1F   Prosthetic/Orthotic devices

C **L6646** Upper extremity addition, shoulder joint, multipositional locking, flexion, adjustable abduction friction control, for use with body powered or external powered system DME A
BETOS: D1F   Prosthetic/Orthotic devices

C **L6647** Upper extremity addition, shoulder lock mechanism, body powered actuator DME A
BETOS: D1F   Prosthetic/Orthotic devices

C **L6648** Upper extremity addition, shoulder lock mechanism, external powered actuator DME A
BETOS: D1F   Prosthetic/Orthotic devices

C **L6650** Upper extremity addition, shoulder universal joint, each DME A
BETOS: D1F   Prosthetic/Orthotic devices

C **L6655** Upper extremity addition, standard control cable, extra DME A
BETOS: D1F   Prosthetic/Orthotic devices

C **L6660** Upper extremity addition, heavy duty control cable DME A
BETOS: D1F   Prosthetic/Orthotic devices

C **L6665** Upper extremity addition, Teflon, or equal, cable lining DME A
BETOS: D1F   Prosthetic/Orthotic devices

C **L6670** Upper extremity addition, hook to hand, cable adapter DME A
BETOS: D1F   Prosthetic/Orthotic devices

C **L6672** Upper extremity addition, harness, chest or shoulder, saddle type DME A
BETOS: D1F   Prosthetic/Orthotic devices

C **L6675** Upper extremity addition, harness, (e.g., figure of eight type), single cable design DME A
BETOS: D1F   Prosthetic/Orthotic devices

C **L6676** Upper extremity addition, harness, (e.g., figure of eight type), dual cable design DME A
BETOS: D1F   Prosthetic/Orthotic devices

C **L6677** Upper extremity addition, harness, triple control, simultaneous operation of terminal device and elbow DME A
BETOS: D1F   Prosthetic/Orthotic devices

● New code   ▲ Revised code   C Carrier judgment   D Special coverage instructions apply
I Not payable by Medicare   M Non-covered by Medicare   S Non-covered by Medicare statute   AHA Coding Clinic®

C **L6680** Upper extremity addition, test socket, wrist disarticulation or below elbow **DME** A
    BETOS: D1F   Prosthetic/Orthotic devices

C **L6682** Upper extremity addition, test socket, elbow disarticulation or above elbow **DME** A
    BETOS: D1F   Prosthetic/Orthotic devices

C **L6684** Upper extremity addition, test socket, shoulder disarticulation or interscapular thoracic **DME** A
    BETOS: D1F   Prosthetic/Orthotic devices

C **L6686** Upper extremity addition, suction socket **DME** A
    BETOS: D1F   Prosthetic/Orthotic devices

C **L6687** Upper extremity addition, frame type socket, below elbow or wrist disarticulation **DME** A
    BETOS: D1F   Prosthetic/Orthotic devices

C **L6688** Upper extremity addition, frame type socket, above elbow or elbow disarticulation **DME** A
    BETOS: D1F   Prosthetic/Orthotic devices

C **L6689** Upper extremity addition, frame type socket, shoulder disarticulation **DME** A
    BETOS: D1F   Prosthetic/Orthotic devices

C **L6690** Upper extremity addition, frame type socket, interscapular-thoracic **DME** A
    BETOS: D1F   Prosthetic/Orthotic devices

C **L6691** Upper extremity addition, removable insert, each **DME** A
    BETOS: D1F   Prosthetic/Orthotic devices

C **L6692** Upper extremity addition, silicone gel insert or equal, each **DME** A
    BETOS: D1F   Prosthetic/Orthotic devices

C **L6693** Upper extremity addition, locking elbow, forearm counterbalance **DME** A
    BETOS: D1F   Prosthetic/Orthotic devices

C **L6694** Addition to upper extremity prosthesis, below elbow/above elbow, custom fabricated from existing mold or prefabricated, socket insert, silicone gel, elastomeric or equal, for use with locking mechanism **DME** A
    BETOS: D1F   Prosthetic/Orthotic devices

C **L6695** Addition to upper extremity prosthesis, below elbow/above elbow, custom fabricated from existing mold or prefabricated, socket insert, silicone gel, elastomeric or equal, not for use with locking mechanism **DME** A
    BETOS: D1F   Prosthetic/Orthotic devices

C **L6696** Addition to upper extremity prosthesis, below elbow/above elbow, custom fabricated socket insert for congenital or atypical traumatic amputee, silicone gel, elastomeric or equal, for use with or without locking mechanism, initial only (for other than initial, use code L6694 or L6695) **DME** A
    BETOS: D1F   Prosthetic/Orthotic devices

C **L6697** Addition to upper extremity prosthesis, below elbow/above elbow, custom fabricated socket insert for other than congenital or atypical traumatic amputee, silicone gel, elastomeric or equal, for use with or without locking mechanism, initial only (for other than initial, use code L6694 or L6695) **DME** A
    BETOS: D1F   Prosthetic/Orthotic devices

C **L6698** Addition to upper extremity prosthesis, below elbow/above elbow, lock mechanism, excludes socket insert **DME** A
    BETOS: D1F   Prosthetic/Orthotic devices

TERMINAL DEVICES AND ADDITIONS (L6703-L6882)

C **L6703** Terminal device, passive hand/mitt, any material, any size **DME** A
    BETOS: D1F   Prosthetic/Orthotic devices

C **L6704** Terminal device, sport/recreational/work attachment, any material, any size **DME** A
    BETOS: D1F   Prosthetic/Orthotic devices

C **L6706** Terminal device, hook, mechanical, voluntary opening, any material, any size, lined or unlined **DME** A
    BETOS: D1F   Prosthetic/Orthotic devices

C **L6707** Terminal device, hook, mechanical, voluntary closing, any material, any size, lined or unlined **DME** A
    BETOS: D1F   Prosthetic/Orthotic devices

C **L6708** Terminal device, hand, mechanical, voluntary opening, any material, any size **DME** A
    BETOS: D1F   Prosthetic/Orthotic devices

C **L6709** Terminal device, hand, mechanical, voluntary closing, any material, any size **DME** A
    BETOS: D1F   Prosthetic/Orthotic devices

C **L6711** Terminal device, hook, mechanical, voluntary opening, any material, any size, lined or unlined, pediatric **DME** Ⓐ A
    BETOS: D1F   Prosthetic/Orthotic devices
    Coding Clinic: 2008, Q4

C **L6712** Terminal device, hook, mechanical, voluntary closing, any material, any size, lined or unlined, pediatric **DME** Ⓐ A
    BETOS: D1F   Prosthetic/Orthotic devices
    Coding Clinic: 2008, Q4

C **L6713** Terminal device, hand, mechanical, voluntary opening, any material, any size, pediatric **DME** Ⓐ A
    BETOS: D1F   Prosthetic/Orthotic devices
    Coding Clinic: 2008, Q4

C **L6714** Terminal device, hand, mechanical, voluntary closing, any material, any size, pediatric **DME** Ⓐ A
    BETOS: D1F   Prosthetic/Orthotic devices
    Coding Clinic: 2008, Q4

C **L6715** Terminal device, multiple articulating digit, includes motor(s), initial issue or replacement **DME** A

    BETOS: D1F   Prosthetic/Orthotic devices

C **L6721** Terminal device, hook or hand, heavy duty, mechanical, voluntary opening, any material, any size, lined or unlined **DME** A

    BETOS: D1F   Prosthetic/Orthotic devices
    Coding Clinic: 2008, Q4

C **L6722** Terminal device, hook or hand, heavy duty, mechanical, voluntary closing, any material, any size, lined or unlined **DME** A

    BETOS: D1F   Prosthetic/Orthotic devices
    Coding Clinic: 2008, Q4

D **L6805** Addition to terminal device, modifier wrist unit **DME** A

    BETOS: D1F   Prosthetic/Orthotic devices

D **L6810** Addition to terminal device, precision pinch device **DME** A

    BETOS: D1F   Prosthetic/Orthotic devices

C **L6880** Electric hand, switch or myoelectric controlled, independently articulating digits, any grasp pattern or combination of grasp patterns, includes motor(s) **DME** A

    BETOS: D1F   Prosthetic/Orthotic devices

C **L6881** Automatic grasp feature, addition to upper limb electric prosthetic terminal device **DME** A

    BETOS: D1F   Prosthetic/Orthotic devices
    Coding Clinic: 2002, Q1

D **L6882** Microprocessor control feature, addition to upper limb prosthetic terminal device **DME** A

    BETOS: D1F   Prosthetic/Orthotic devices
    Coding Clinic: 2002, Q1

REPLACEMENT SOCKETS, UPPER LIMBS (L6883-L6885)

C **L6883** Replacement socket, below elbow/wrist disarticulation, molded to patient model, for use with or without external power **DME** A

    BETOS: D1F   Prosthetic/Orthotic devices

C **L6884** Replacement socket, above elbow/elbow disarticulation, molded to patient model, for use with or without external power **DME** A

    BETOS: D1F   Prosthetic/Orthotic devices

C **L6885** Replacement socket, shoulder disarticulation/interscapular thoracic, molded to patient model, for use with or without external power **DME** A

    BETOS: D1F   Prosthetic/Orthotic devices

HAND RESTORATION PROSTHETICS AND ADDITIONS (L6890-L6915)

C **L6890** Addition to upper extremity prosthesis, glove for terminal device, any material, prefabricated, includes fitting and adjustment **DME** A

    BETOS: D1F   Prosthetic/Orthotic devices

C **L6895** Addition to upper extremity prosthesis, glove for terminal device, any material, custom fabricated **DME** A

    BETOS: D1F   Prosthetic/Orthotic devices

C **L6900** Hand restoration (casts, shading and measurements included), partial hand, with glove, thumb or one finger remaining **DME** A

    BETOS: D1F   Prosthetic/Orthotic devices

C **L6905** Hand restoration (casts, shading and measurements included), partial hand, with glove, multiple fingers remaining **DME** A

    BETOS: D1F   Prosthetic/Orthotic devices

C **L6910** Hand restoration (casts, shading and measurements included), partial hand, with glove, no fingers remaining **DME** A

    BETOS: D1F   Prosthetic/Orthotic devices

C **L6915** Hand restoration (shading, and measurements included), replacement glove for above **DME** A

    BETOS: D1F   Prosthetic/Orthotic devices

EXTERNAL POWER UPPER LIMB PROSTHETICS (L6920-L6975)

C **L6920** Wrist disarticulation, external power, self-suspended inner socket, removable forearm shell, Otto Bock or equal, switch, cables, two batteries and one charger, switch control of terminal device **DME** A

    BETOS: D1F   Prosthetic/Orthotic devices

C **L6925** Wrist disarticulation, external power, self-suspended inner socket, removable forearm shell, Otto Bock or equal electrodes, cables, two batteries and one charger, myoelectric control of terminal device **DME** A

    BETOS: D1F   Prosthetic/Orthotic devices

C **L6930** Below elbow, external power, self-suspended inner socket, removable forearm shell, Otto Bock or equal switch, cables, two batteries and one charger, switch control of terminal device **DME** A

    BETOS: D1F   Prosthetic/Orthotic devices

C **L6935** Below elbow, external power, self-suspended inner socket, removable forearm shell, Otto Bock or equal electrodes, cables, two batteries and one charger, myoelectric control of terminal device **DME** A

    BETOS: D1F   Prosthetic/Orthotic devices

C **L6940** Elbow disarticulation, external power, molded inner socket, removable humeral shell, outside locking hinges, forearm, Otto Bock or equal switch, cables, two batteries and one charger, switch control of terminal device **DME** A

    BETOS: D1F   Prosthetic/Orthotic devices

● New code   ▲ Revised code   **C** Carrier judgment   **D** Special coverage instructions apply
I Not payable by Medicare   **M** Non-covered by Medicare   **S** Non-covered by Medicare statute   AHA Coding Clinic®

C **L6945** Elbow disarticulation, external power, molded inner socket, removable humeral shell, outside locking hinges, forearm, Otto Bock or equal electrodes, cables, two batteries and one charger, myoelectronic control of terminal device `DME` A

BETOS: D1F   Prosthetic/Orthotic devices

C **L6950** Above elbow, external power, molded inner socket, removable humeral shell, internal locking elbow, forearm, Otto Bock or equal switch, cables, two batteries and one charger, switch control of terminal device `DME` A

BETOS: D1F   Prosthetic/Orthotic devices

C **L6955** Above elbow, external power, molded inner socket, removable humeral shell, internal locking elbow, forearm, Otto Bock or equal electrodes, cables, two batteries and one charger, myoelectronic control of terminal device `DME` A

BETOS: D1F   Prosthetic/Orthotic devices

C **L6960** Shoulder disarticulation, external power, molded inner socket, removable shoulder shell, shoulder bulkhead, humeral section, mechanical elbow, forearm, Otto Bock or equal switch, cables, two batteries and one charger, switch control of terminal device `DME` A

BETOS: D1F   Prosthetic/Orthotic devices

C **L6965** Shoulder disarticulation, external power, molded inner socket, removable shoulder shell, shoulder bulkhead, humeral section, mechanical elbow, forearm, Otto Bock or equal electrodes, cables, two batteries and one charger, myoelectronic control of terminal device `DME` A

BETOS: D1F   Prosthetic/Orthotic devices

C **L6970** Interscapular-thoracic, external power, molded inner socket, removable shoulder shell, shoulder bulkhead, humeral section, mechanical elbow, forearm, Otto Bock or equal switch, cables, two batteries and one charger, switch control of terminal device `DME` A

BETOS: D1F   Prosthetic/Orthotic devices

C **L6975** Interscapular-thoracic, external power, molded inner socket, removable shoulder shell, shoulder bulkhead, humeral section, mechanical elbow, forearm, Otto Bock or equal electrodes, cables, two batteries and one charger, myoelectronic control of terminal device `DME` A

BETOS: D1F   Prosthetic/Orthotic devices

ELECTRIC HAND OR HOOK AND ADDITIONS (L7007-L7045)

C **L7007** Electric hand, switch or myoelectric controlled, adult `DME` Ⓐ A

BETOS: D1F   Prosthetic/Orthotic devices

C **L7008** Electric hand, switch or myoelectric, controlled, pediatric `DME` Ⓐ A

BETOS: D1F   Prosthetic/Orthotic devices

C **L7009** Electric hook, switch or myoelectric controlled, adult `DME` Ⓐ A

BETOS: D1F   Prosthetic/Orthotic devices

C **L7040** Prehensile actuator, switch controlled `DME` A

BETOS: D1F   Prosthetic/Orthotic devices

C **L7045** Electric hook, switch or myoelectric controlled, pediatric `DME` Ⓐ A

BETOS: D1F   Prosthetic/Orthotic devices

ELECTRONIC ELBOW AND ADDITIONS (L7170-L7259)

C **L7170** Electronic elbow, Hosmer or equal, switch controlled `DME` A

BETOS: D1F   Prosthetic/Orthotic devices

C **L7180** Electronic elbow, microprocessor sequential control of elbow and terminal device `DME` A

BETOS: D1F   Prosthetic/Orthotic devices

C **L7181** Electronic elbow, microprocessor simultaneous control of elbow and terminal device `DME` A

BETOS: D1F   Prosthetic/Orthotic devices

C **L7185** Electronic elbow, adolescent, Variety Village or equal, switch controlled `DME` A

BETOS: D1F   Prosthetic/Orthotic devices

C **L7186** Electronic elbow, child, Variety Village or equal, switch controlled `DME` Ⓐ A

BETOS: D1F   Prosthetic/Orthotic devices

C **L7190** Electronic elbow, adolescent, Variety Village or equal, myoelectronically controlled `DME` A

BETOS: D1F   Prosthetic/Orthotic devices

C **L7191** Electronic elbow, child, Variety Village or equal, myoelectronically controlled `DME` Ⓐ A

BETOS: D1F   Prosthetic/Orthotic devices

C **L7259** Electronic wrist rotator, any type `DME` A

BETOS: D1F   Prosthetic/Orthotic devices

BATTERIES AND ACCESSORIES (L7360-L7368)

C **L7360** Six volt battery, each `DME` A

BETOS: D1F   Prosthetic/Orthotic devices

C **L7362** Battery charger, six volt, each `DME` A

BETOS: D1F   Prosthetic/Orthotic devices

C **L7364** Twelve volt battery, each `DME` A

BETOS: D1F   Prosthetic/Orthotic devices

C **L7366** Battery charger, twelve volt, each `DME` A

BETOS: D1F   Prosthetic/Orthotic devices

C **L7367** Lithium ion battery, rechargeable, replacement `DME` A

BETOS: D1F   Prosthetic/Orthotic devices

C **L7368** Lithium ion battery charger, replacement only `DME` A

BETOS: D1F   Prosthetic/Orthotic devices

♂ Male only   ♀ Female only   Ⓐ Age   A2 - Z3 = ASC Payment indicator   A - Y = APC Status indicator
ASC = ASC Approved Procedure   `DME` Paid under the DME fee schedule   `MIPS` MIPS code

ADDITIONS FOR UPPER EXTREMITY PROSTHETICS (L7400-L7405)

C **L7400** Addition to upper extremity prosthesis, below elbow/wrist disarticulation, ultralight material (titanium, carbon fiber or equal) **DME** A
BETOS: D1F   Prosthetic/Orthotic devices

Arm prosthesis

C **L7401** Addition to upper extremity prosthesis, above elbow disarticulation, ultralight material (titanium, carbon fiber or equal) **DME** A
BETOS: D1F   Prosthetic/Orthotic devices

C **L7402** Addition to upper extremity prosthesis, shoulder disarticulation/interscapular thoracic, ultralight material (titanium, carbon fiber or equal) **DME** A
BETOS: D1F   Prosthetic/Orthotic devices

C **L7403** Addition to upper extremity prosthesis, below elbow/wrist disarticulation, acrylic material **DME** A
BETOS: D1F   Prosthetic/Orthotic devices

C **L7404** Addition to upper extremity prosthesis, above elbow disarticulation, acrylic material **DME** A
BETOS: D1F   Prosthetic/Orthotic devices

C **L7405** Addition to upper extremity prosthesis, shoulder disarticulation/interscapular thoracic, acrylic material **DME** A
BETOS: D1F   Prosthetic/Orthotic devices

UPPER EXTREMITY PROSTHETICS, NOT OTHERWISE SPECIFIED (NOS) (L7499)

C **L7499** Upper extremity prosthesis, not otherwise specified A
BETOS: D1F   Prosthetic/Orthotic devices

PROSTHETIC REPAIR (L7510, L7520)

D **L7510** Repair of prosthetic device, repair or replace minor parts A
BETOS: D1F   Prosthetic/Orthotic devices

C **L7520** Repair prosthetic device, labor component, per 15 minutes A
BETOS: D1F   Prosthetic/Orthotic devices

PROSTHETIC DONNING SLEEVE (L7600)

S **L7600** Prosthetic donning sleeve, any material, each E1
BETOS: D1F   Prosthetic/Orthotic devices
Service not separately priced by Part B
Statute: 1862(1)(a)

GASKET OR SEAL WITH PROSTHETIC (L7700)

C **L7700** Gasket or seal, for use with prosthetic socket insert, any type, each **DME** A
BETOS: D1F   Prosthetic/Orthotic devices

PENILE PROSTHETICS (L7900, L7902)

S **L7900** Male vacuum erection system ♂ E1
BETOS: D1F   Prosthetic/Orthotic devices
Service not separately priced by Part B
Statute: 1834a

S **L7902** Tension ring, for vacuum erection device, any type, replacement only, each ♂ E1
BETOS: D1F   Prosthetic/Orthotic devices
Service not separately priced by Part B
Statute: 1834a

BREAST PROSTHETICS AND ACCESSORIES (L8000-L8039), SEE ALSO PROSTHETIC BREAST IMPLANT (L8600)

D **L8000** Breast prosthesis, mastectomy bra, without integrated breast prosthesis form, any size, any type **DME** A
BETOS: D1F   Prosthetic/Orthotic devices

D **L8001** Breast prosthesis, mastectomy bra, with integrated breast prosthesis form, unilateral, any size, any type **DME** A
BETOS: D1F   Prosthetic/Orthotic devices
Coding Clinic: 2002, Q1

D **L8002** Breast prosthesis, mastectomy bra, with integrated breast prosthesis form, bilateral, any size, any type **DME** A
BETOS: D1F   Prosthetic/Orthotic devices
Coding Clinic: 2002, Q1

D **L8010** Breast prosthesis, mastectomy sleeve A
BETOS: D1F   Prosthetic/Orthotic devices
Service not separately priced by Part B

D **L8015** External breast prosthesis garment, with mastectomy form, post mastectomy **DME** A
BETOS: D1F   Prosthetic/Orthotic devices

D **L8020** Breast prosthesis, mastectomy form **DME** A
BETOS: D1F   Prosthetic/Orthotic devices

D **L8030** Breast prosthesis, silicone or equal, without integral adhesive **DME** A
BETOS: D1F   Prosthetic/Orthotic devices

D **L8031** Breast prosthesis, silicone or equal, with integral adhesive **DME** A
BETOS: D1F   Prosthetic/Orthotic devices

● New code   ▲ Revised code   **C** Carrier judgment   **D** Special coverage instructions apply
I Not payable by Medicare   **M** Non-covered by Medicare   **S** Non-covered by Medicare statute   AHA Coding Clinic®

| C | **L8032** | Nipple prosthesis, prefabricated, reusable, any type, each   **DME** A |

L8032 Nipple prosthesis, prefabricated, reusable, any type, each   **DME** A
     BETOS: D1F   Prosthetic/Orthotic devices

L8033 Nipple prosthesis, custom fabricated, reusable, any material, any type, each   A
     BETOS: D1F   Prosthetic/Orthotic devices

L8035 Custom breast prosthesis, post mastectomy, molded to patient model   **DME** A
     BETOS: D1F   Prosthetic/Orthotic devices

L8039 Breast prosthesis, not otherwise specified   A
     BETOS: D1F   Prosthetic/Orthotic devices

FACIAL AND EXTERNAL EAR PROSTHETICS (L8040-L8049)

L8040 Nasal prosthesis, provided by a non-physician   **DME** A
     BETOS: D1F   Prosthetic/Orthotic devices
     DME Modifier: KM,KN

L8041 Midfacial prosthesis, provided by a non-physician   **DME** A
     BETOS: D1F   Prosthetic/Orthotic devices
     DME Modifier: KM,KN

L8042 Orbital prosthesis, provided by a non-physician   **DME** A
     BETOS: D1F   Prosthetic/Orthotic devices
     DME Modifier: KM,KN

L8043 Upper facial prosthesis, provided by a non-physician   **DME** A
     BETOS: D1F   Prosthetic/Orthotic devices
     DME Modifier: KM,KN

L8044 Hemi-facial prosthesis, provided by a non-physician   **DME** A
     BETOS: D1F   Prosthetic/Orthotic devices
     DME Modifier: KM,KN

L8045 Auricular prosthesis, provided by a non-physician   **DME** A
     BETOS: D1F   Prosthetic/Orthotic devices
     DME Modifier: KM,KN

L8046 Partial facial prosthesis, provided by a non-physician   **DME** A
     BETOS: D1F   Prosthetic/Orthotic devices
     DME Modifier: KM,KN

L8047 Nasal septal prosthesis, provided by a non-physician   **DME** A
     BETOS: D1F   Prosthetic/Orthotic devices
     DME Modifier: KM,KN

L8048 Unspecified maxillofacial prosthesis, by report, provided by a non-physician   A
     BETOS: D1F   Prosthetic/Orthotic devices

L8049 Repair or modification of maxillofacial prosthesis, labor component, 15 minute increments, provided by a non-physician   A
     BETOS: D1F   Prosthetic/Orthotic devices

HERNIA TRUSSES (L8300-L8330)

L8300 Truss, single with standard pad   **DME** A
     BETOS: D1F   Prosthetic/Orthotic devices

L8310 Truss, double with standard pads   **DME** A
     BETOS: D1F   Prosthetic/Orthotic devices

L8320 Truss, addition to standard pad, water pad   **DME** A
     BETOS: D1F   Prosthetic/Orthotic devices

L8330 Truss, addition to standard pad, scrotal pad   ♂ **DME** A
     BETOS: D1F   Prosthetic/Orthotic devices

PROSTHETIC SHEATHS, SOCKS, AND SHRINKERS (L8400-L8485)

L8400 Prosthetic sheath, below knee, each   **DME** A
     BETOS: D1F   Prosthetic/Orthotic devices

L8410 Prosthetic sheath, above knee, each   **DME** A
     BETOS: D1F   Prosthetic/Orthotic devices

L8415 Prosthetic sheath, upper limb, each   **DME** A
     BETOS: D1F   Prosthetic/Orthotic devices

L8417 Prosthetic sheath/sock, including a gel cushion layer, below knee or above knee, each   **DME** A
     BETOS: D1F   Prosthetic/Orthotic devices

L8420 Prosthetic sock, multiple ply, below knee, each   **DME** A
     BETOS: D1F   Prosthetic/Orthotic devices

L8430 Prosthetic sock, multiple ply, above knee, each   **DME** A
     BETOS: D1F   Prosthetic/Orthotic devices

L8435 Prosthetic sock, multiple ply, upper limb, each   **DME** A
     BETOS: D1F   Prosthetic/Orthotic devices

L8440 Prosthetic shrinker, below knee, each   **DME** A
     BETOS: D1F   Prosthetic/Orthotic devices

L8460 Prosthetic shrinker, above knee, each   **DME** A
     BETOS: D1F   Prosthetic/Orthotic devices

L8465 Prosthetic shrinker, upper limb, each   **DME** A
     BETOS: D1F   Prosthetic/Orthotic devices

L8470 Prosthetic sock, single ply, fitting, below knee, each   **DME** A
     BETOS: D1F   Prosthetic/Orthotic devices

L8480 Prosthetic sock, single ply, fitting, above knee, each   **DME** A
     BETOS: D1F   Prosthetic/Orthotic devices

L8485 Prosthetic sock, single ply, fitting, upper limb, each   **DME** A
     BETOS: D1F   Prosthetic/Orthotic devices

♂ Male only   ♀ Female only   Ⓐ Age   A2 - Z3 = ASC Payment indicator   A - Y = APC Status indicator
ASC = ASC Approved Procedure   **DME** Paid under the DME fee schedule   **MIPS** MIPS code

UNLISTED PROSTHETIC PROCEDURES (L8499)

C L8499 Unlisted procedure for miscellaneous prosthetic services   A
BETOS: D1F   Prosthetic/Orthotic devices

VOICE PROSTHETICS AND ACCESSORIES (L8500-L8515)

D L8500 Artificial larynx, any type   DME A
BETOS: D1F   Prosthetic/Orthotic devices

D L8501 Tracheostomy speaking valve   DME A
BETOS: D1F   Prosthetic/Orthotic devices

C L8505 Artificial larynx replacement battery/accessory, any type   A
BETOS: D1F   Prosthetic/Orthotic devices
Coding Clinic: 2002, Q1

C L8507 Tracheo-esophageal voice prosthesis, patient inserted, any type, each   DME A
BETOS: D1F   Prosthetic/Orthotic devices
Coding Clinic: 2002, Q1

C L8509 Tracheo-esophageal voice prosthesis, inserted by a licensed health care provider, any type   DME A
BETOS: D1F   Prosthetic/Orthotic devices
Coding Clinic: 2002, Q1

D L8510 Voice amplifier   DME A
BETOS: D1F   Prosthetic/Orthotic devices
Coding Clinic: 2002, Q1

C L8511 Insert for indwelling tracheoesophageal prosthesis, with or without valve, replacement only, each   DME A
BETOS: D1F   Prosthetic/Orthotic devices

C L8512 Gelatin capsules or equivalent, for use with tracheoesophageal voice prosthesis, replacement only, per 10   DME A
BETOS: D1F   Prosthetic/Orthotic devices

C L8513 Cleaning device used with tracheoesophageal voice prosthesis, pipet, brush, or equal, replacement only, each   DME A
BETOS: D1F   Prosthetic/Orthotic devices

C L8514 Tracheoesophageal puncture dilator, replacement only, each   DME A
BETOS: D1F   Prosthetic/Orthotic devices

C L8515 Gelatin capsule, application device for use with tracheoesophageal voice prosthesis, each   DME A
BETOS: D1F   Prosthetic/Orthotic devices

PROSTHETIC BREAST IMPLANT (L8600), SEE ALSO BREAST PROSTHETICS AND ACCESSORIES (L8000-L8039)

D L8600 Implantable breast prosthesis, silicone or equal   N1 DME ASC N
BETOS: D1F   Prosthetic/Orthotic devices

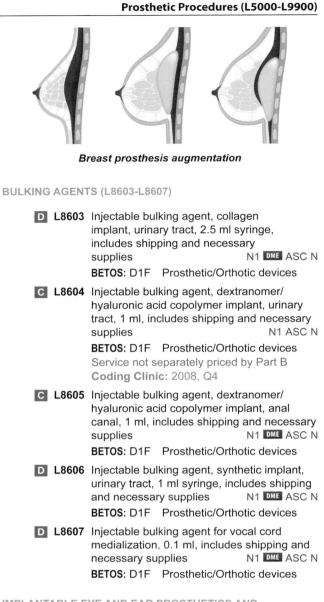

Breast prosthesis augmentation

BULKING AGENTS (L8603-L8607)

D L8603 Injectable bulking agent, collagen implant, urinary tract, 2.5 ml syringe, includes shipping and necessary supplies   N1 DME ASC N
BETOS: D1F   Prosthetic/Orthotic devices

C L8604 Injectable bulking agent, dextranomer/hyaluronic acid copolymer implant, urinary tract, 1 ml, includes shipping and necessary supplies   N1 ASC N
BETOS: D1F   Prosthetic/Orthotic devices
Service not separately priced by Part B
Coding Clinic: 2008, Q4

C L8605 Injectable bulking agent, dextranomer/hyaluronic acid copolymer implant, anal canal, 1 ml, includes shipping and necessary supplies   N1 DME ASC N
BETOS: D1F   Prosthetic/Orthotic devices

D L8606 Injectable bulking agent, synthetic implant, urinary tract, 1 ml syringe, includes shipping and necessary supplies   N1 DME ASC N
BETOS: D1F   Prosthetic/Orthotic devices

D L8607 Injectable bulking agent for vocal cord medialization, 0.1 ml, includes shipping and necessary supplies   N1 DME ASC N
BETOS: D1F   Prosthetic/Orthotic devices

IMPLANTABLE EYE AND EAR PROSTHETICS AND ACCESSORIES (L8608-L8629)

C L8608 Miscellaneous external component, supply or accessory for use with the argus II retinal prosthesis system   N
BETOS: D1F   Prosthetic/Orthotic devices

C L8609 Artificial cornea   N1 DME ASC N
BETOS: D1F   Prosthetic/Orthotic devices

D L8610 Ocular implant   N1 DME ASC N
BETOS: D1F   Prosthetic/Orthotic devices

D L8612 Aqueous shunt   N1 DME ASC N
BETOS: D1F   Prosthetic/Orthotic devices

D L8613 Ossicula implant   N1 DME ASC N
BETOS: D1F   Prosthetic/Orthotic devices

● New code   ▲ Revised code   **C** Carrier judgment   **D** Special coverage instructions apply
I Not payable by Medicare   **M** Non-covered by Medicare   **S** Non-covered by Medicare statute   AHA Coding Clinic®

D **L8614** Cochlear device, includes all internal and external components   N1 **DME** ASC N

     BETOS: D1F   Prosthetic/Orthotic devices

     Coding Clinic: 2001, Q1; 2002, Q3; 2003, Q4; 2016, Q3

D **L8615** Headset/headpiece for use with cochlear implant device, replacement   **DME** A

     BETOS: D1F   Prosthetic/Orthotic devices

D **L8616** Microphone for use with cochlear implant device, replacement   **DME** A

     BETOS: D1F   Prosthetic/Orthotic devices

D **L8617** Transmitting coil for use with cochlear implant device, replacement   **DME** A

     BETOS: D1F   Prosthetic/Orthotic devices

D **L8618** Transmitter cable for use with cochlear implant device or auditory osseointegrated device, replacement   **DME** A

     BETOS: D1F   Prosthetic/Orthotic devices

D **L8619** Cochlear implant, external speech processor and controller, integrated system, replacement   **DME** A

     BETOS: D1F   Prosthetic/Orthotic devices

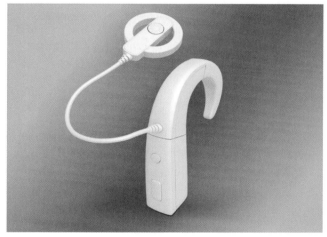

Cochlear device

C **L8621** Zinc air battery for use with cochlear implant device and auditory osseointegrated sound processors, replacement, each   **DME** A

     BETOS: D1F   Prosthetic/Orthotic devices

C **L8622** Alkaline battery for use with cochlear implant device, any size, replacement, each   **DME** A

     BETOS: D1F   Prosthetic/Orthotic devices

C **L8623** Lithium ion battery for use with cochlear implant device speech processor, other than ear level, replacement, each   **DME** A

     BETOS: D1F   Prosthetic/Orthotic devices

C **L8624** Lithium ion battery for use with cochlear implant or auditory osseointegrated device speech processor, ear level, replacement, each   **DME** A

     BETOS: D1F   Prosthetic/Orthotic devices

D **L8625** External recharging system for battery for use with cochlear implant or auditory osseointegrated device, replacement only, each   **DME** A

     BETOS: D1F   Prosthetic/Orthotic devices

D **L8627** Cochlear implant, external speech processor, component, replacement   **DME** A

     BETOS: D1F   Prosthetic/Orthotic devices

D **L8628** Cochlear implant, external controller component, replacement   **DME** A

     BETOS: D1F   Prosthetic/Orthotic devices

D **L8629** Transmitting coil and cable, integrated, for use with cochlear implant device, replacement   **DME** A

     BETOS: D1F   Prosthetic/Orthotic devices

IMPLANTABLE HAND AND FEET PROSTHETICS (L8630-L8659)

D **L8630** Metacarpophalangeal joint implant   N1 **DME** ASC N

     BETOS: D1F   Prosthetic/Orthotic devices

D **L8631** Metacarpal phalangeal joint replacement, two or more pieces, metal (e.g., stainless steel or cobalt chrome), ceramic-like material (e.g., pyrocarbon), for surgical implantation (all sizes, includes entire system)   N1 **DME** ASC N

     BETOS: D1F   Prosthetic/Orthotic devices

D **L8641** Metatarsal joint implant   N1 **DME** ASC N

     BETOS: D1F   Prosthetic/Orthotic devices

D **L8642** Hallux implant   N1 **DME** ASC N

     BETOS: D1F   Prosthetic/Orthotic devices

D **L8658** Interphalangeal joint spacer, silicone or equal, each   N1 **DME** ASC N

     BETOS: D1F   Prosthetic/Orthotic devices

D **L8659** Interphalangeal finger joint replacement, 2 or more pieces, metal (e.g., stainless steel or cobalt chrome), ceramic-like material (e.g., pyrocarbon) for surgical implantation, any size   N1 **DME** ASC N

     BETOS: D1F   Prosthetic/Orthotic devices

VASCULAR IMPLANTS (L8670)

D **L8670** Vascular graft material, synthetic, implant   N1 **DME** ASC N

     BETOS: D1F   Prosthetic/Orthotic devices

IMPLANTABLE NEUROSTIMULATORS AND COMPONENTS (L8679-L8689)

D **L8679** Implantable neurostimulator, pulse generator, any type   N1 **DME** ASC N

     BETOS: D1F   Prosthetic/Orthotic devices

♂ Male only   ♀ Female only   **A** Age   A2 - Z3 = ASC Payment indicator   A - Y = APC Status indicator

ASC = ASC Approved Procedure   **DME** Paid under the DME fee schedule   **MIPS** MIPS code

L8680 - L9900

I L8680 Implantable neurostimulator electrode, each   E1
    BETOS: D1F Prosthetic/Orthotic devices
    Service not separately priced by Part B

D L8681 Patient programmer (external) for use with implantable programmable neurostimulator pulse generator, replacement only **DME** A
    BETOS: D1F Prosthetic/Orthotic devices

D L8682 Implantable neurostimulator radiofrequency receiver   N1 **DME** ASC N
    BETOS: D1F Prosthetic/Orthotic devices

D L8683 Radiofrequency transmitter (external) for use with implantable neurostimulator radiofrequency receiver **DME** A
    BETOS: D1F Prosthetic/Orthotic devices

D L8684 Radiofrequency transmitter (external) for use with implantable sacral root neurostimulator receiver for bowel and bladder management, replacement **DME** A
    BETOS: D1F Prosthetic/Orthotic devices

I L8685 Implantable neurostimulator pulse generator, single array, rechargeable, includes extension   E1
    BETOS: D1F Prosthetic/Orthotic devices
    Service not separately priced by Part B

I L8686 Implantable neurostimulator pulse generator, single array, non-rechargeable, includes extension   E1
    BETOS: D1F Prosthetic/Orthotic devices
    Service not separately priced by Part B

I L8687 Implantable neurostimulator pulse generator, dual array, rechargeable, includes extension   E1
    BETOS: D1F Prosthetic/Orthotic devices
    Service not separately priced by Part B

I L8688 Implantable neurostimulator pulse generator, dual array, non-rechargeable, includes extension   E1
    BETOS: D1F Prosthetic/Orthotic devices
    Service not separately priced by Part B

D L8689 External recharging system for battery (internal) for use with implantable neurostimulator, replacement only **DME** A
    BETOS: D1F Prosthetic/Orthotic devices

MISCELLANEOUS ORTHOTIC AND PROSTHETIC SERVICES AND SUPPLIES (L8690-L9900)

C L8690 Auditory osseointegrated device, includes all internal and external components   N1 **DME** ASC N
    BETOS: D1F Prosthetic/Orthotic devices
    Coding Clinic: 2007, Q1; 2016, Q3

C L8691 Auditory osseointegrated device, external sound processor, excludes transducer/actuator, replacement only, each **DME** A
    BETOS: D1F Prosthetic/Orthotic devices

S L8692 Auditory osseointegrated device, external sound processor, used without osseointegration, body worn, includes headband or other means of external attachment   E1
    BETOS: D1F Prosthetic/Orthotic devices
    Service not separately priced by Part B
    Statute: 1862(a)(7)

C L8693 Auditory osseointegrated device abutment, any length, replacement only **DME** A
    BETOS: D1F Prosthetic/Orthotic devices

C L8694 Auditory osseointegrated device, transducer/actuator, replacement only, each **DME** A
    BETOS: D1F Prosthetic/Orthotic devices

D L8695 External recharging system for battery (external) for use with implantable neurostimulator, replacement only **DME** A
    BETOS: D1F Prosthetic/Orthotic devices

D L8696 Antenna (external) for use with implantable diaphragmatic/phrenic nerve stimulation device, replacement, each **DME** A
    BETOS: D1F Prosthetic/Orthotic devices

D L8698 Miscellaneous component, supply or accessory for use with total artificial heart system   A
    BETOS: D1F Prosthetic/Orthotic devices

C L8699 Prosthetic implant, not otherwise specified   N1 ASC N
    BETOS: D1F Prosthetic/Orthotic devices

▲ C L8701 Elbow, wrist, hand device, powered, with single or double upright(s), any type joint(s), includes microprocessor, sensors, all components and accessories   A
    BETOS: D1E Other DME

▲ C L8702 Elbow, wrist, hand, finger device, powered, with single or double upright(s), any type joint(s), includes microprocessor, sensors, all components and accessories   A
    BETOS: D1E Other DME

C L9900 Orthotic and prosthetic supply, accessory, and/or service component of another HCPCS "L" code   N1 ASC N
    BETOS: D1F Prosthetic/Orthotic devices

● New code ▲ Revised code C Carrier judgment D Special coverage instructions apply I Not payable by Medicare M Non-covered by Medicare S Non-covered by Medicare statute AHA Coding Clinic®

MEDICAL SERVICES (M0075-M1149)

MISCELLANEOUS MEDICAL SERVICES (M0075-M0301)

M **M0075** Cellular therapy E1
BETOS: Y2 Other - non-Medicare fee schedule
Service not separately priced by Part B

M **M0076** Prolotherapy E1
BETOS: Y2 Other - non-Medicare fee schedule
Service not separately priced by Part B

M **M0100** Intragastric hypothermia using gastric freezing E1
BETOS: P1G Major procedure - Other
Service not separately priced by Part B
Pub: 100-4, Chapter-10, 40.2

● **C** **M0239** Intravenous infusion, bamlanivimab-xxxx, includes infusion and post administration monitoring S
BETOS: O1G Immunizations/Vaccinations

● **C** **M0243** Intravenous infusion, casirivimab and imdevimab includes infusion and post administration monitoring S
BETOS: O1G Immunizations/Vaccinations

M **M0300** IV chelation therapy (chemical endarterectomy) E1
BETOS: Y2 Other - non-Medicare fee schedule
Service not separately priced by Part B

M **M0301** Fabric wrapping of abdominal aneurysm E1
BETOS: P1G Major procedure - Other
Service not separately priced by Part B
Coding Clinic: 2009, Q2

TB SCREENING (M1003-M1005)

▲ **C** **M1003** Tb screening performed and results interpreted within twelve months prior to initiation of first-time biologic disease modifying anti-rheumatic drug therapy M MIPS
BETOS: Z2 Undefined codes
Service not separately priced by Part B

C **M1004** Documentation of medical reason for not screening for TB or interpreting results (i.e., patient positive for TB and documentation of past treatment; patient who has recently completed a course of anti-TB therapy) M MIPS
BETOS: Z2 Undefined codes
Service not separately priced by Part B

C **M1005** TB screening not performed or results not interpreted, reason not given M MIPS
BETOS: Z2 Undefined codes
Service not separately priced by Part B

EVALUATION AND ASSESSMENT (M1006-M1014)

C **M1006** Disease activity not assessed, reason not given M MIPS
BETOS: Z2 Undefined codes
Service not separately priced by Part B

C **M1007** >=50% of total number of a patient's outpatient RA encounters assessed M MIPS
BETOS: Z2 Undefined codes
Service not separately priced by Part B

C **M1008** <50% of total number of a patient's outpatient RA encounters assessed M MIPS
BETOS: Z2 Undefined codes
Service not separately priced by Part B

C **M1009***Discharge/discontinuation of the episode of care documented in the medical record M MIPS
BETOS: Z2 Undefined codes
Service not separately priced by Part B

C **M1010***Discharge/discontinuation of the episode of care documented in the medical record M MIPS
BETOS: Z2 Undefined codes
Service not separately priced by Part B

C **M1011***Discharge/discontinuation of the episode of care documented in the medical record M MIPS
BETOS: Z2 Undefined codes
Service not separately priced by Part B

C **M1012***Discharge/discontinuation of the episode of care documented in the medical record M MIPS
BETOS: Z2 Undefined codes
Service not separately priced by Part B

C **M1013***Discharge/discontinuation of the episode of care documented in the medical record M MIPS
BETOS: Z2 Undefined codes
Service not separately priced by Part B

C **M1014***Discharge/discontinuation of the episode of care documented in the medical record M MIPS
BETOS: Z2 Undefined codes
Service not separately priced by Part B

PATIENT STATUS (M1016-M1018)

C **M1016** Female patients unable to bear children ♀ M MIPS
BETOS: Z2 Undefined codes
Service not separately priced by Part B

C **M1017** Patient admitted to palliative care services M MIPS
BETOS: Z2 Undefined codes
Service not separately priced by Part B

*This code has the same descriptor as another code. At press time, CMS did not provide any further explanation.

♂ Male only   ♀ Female only   Ⓐ Age   A2 - Z3 = ASC Payment indicator   A - Y = APC Status indicator
ASC = ASC Approved Procedure   **DME** Paid under the DME fee schedule   **MIPS** MIPS code

C M1018 Patients with an active diagnosis or history of cancer (except basal cell and squamous cell skin carcinoma), patients who are heavy tobacco smokers, lung cancer screening patients   M MIPS
BETOS: Z2   Undefined codes
Service not separately priced by Part B

ADOLESCENT DEPRESSION, REMISSION AND MANAGEMENT (M1019-M1026)

C M1019 Adolescent patients 12 to 17 years of age with major depression or dysthymia who reached remission at twelve months as demonstrated by a twelve month (+/-60 days) PHQ-9 or PHQ-9M score of less than 5   Ⓐ M MIPS
BETOS: Z2   Undefined codes
Service not separately priced by Part B

C M1020 Adolescent patients 12 to 17 years of age with major depression or dysthymia who did not reach remission at twelve months as demonstrated by a twelve month (+/-60 days) PHQ-9 or PHQ-9M score of less than 5. Either PHQ-9 or PHQ-9M score was not assessed or is greater than or equal to 5   Ⓐ M MIPS
BETOS: Z2   Undefined codes
Service not separately priced by Part B
Pub: 100-4, Chapter-10, 40.2

C M1021 Patient had only urgent care visits during the performance period   M MIPS
BETOS: Z2   Undefined codes
Service not separately priced by Part B

C M1022 Patients who were in hospice at any time during the performance period   M MIPS
BETOS: Z2   Undefined codes
Service not separately priced by Part B
Pub: 100-4, Chapter-10, 40.2

C M1025 Patients who were in hospice at any time during the performance period   M MIPS
BETOS: Z2   Undefined codes
Service not separately priced by Part B

C M1026 Patients who were in hospice at any time during the performance period   M MIPS
BETOS: Z2   Undefined codes
Service not separately priced by Part B

HEAD IMAGING (M1027-M1031)

C M1027 Imaging of the head (CT or MRI) was obtained   M MIPS
BETOS: Z2   Undefined codes
Service not separately priced by Part B

C M1028 Documentation of patients with primary headache diagnosis and imaging other than CT or MRI obtained   M MIPS
BETOS: Z2   Undefined codes
Service not separately priced by Part B

C M1029 Imaging of the head (CT or MRI) was not obtained, reason not given   M MIPS
BETOS: Z2   Undefined codes
Service not separately priced by Part B

C M1031 Patients with no clinical indications for imaging of the head   M MIPS
BETOS: Z2   Undefined codes
Service not separately priced by Part B

PHARMACOTHERAPY FOR OUD (M1032-M1036)

C M1032 Adults currently taking pharmacotherapy for OUD   Ⓐ M MIPS
BETOS: Z2   Undefined codes
Service not separately priced by Part B

C M1034 Adults who have at least 180 days of continuous pharmacotherapy with a medication prescribed for OUD without a gap of more than seven days   Ⓐ M MIPS
BETOS: Z2   Undefined codes
Service not separately priced by Part B

C M1035 Adults who are deliberately phased out of medication assisted treatment (MAT) prior to 180 days of continuous treatment   Ⓐ M MIPS
BETOS: Z2   Undefined codes
Service not separately priced by Part B

C M1036 Adults who have not had at least 180 days of continuous pharmacotherapy with a medication prescribed for OUD without a gap of more than seven days   Ⓐ M MIPS
BETOS: Z2   Undefined codes
Service not separately priced by Part B

LUMBAR SPINE ASSOCIATED CONDITIONS (M1037-M1041)

C M1037 Patients with a diagnosis of lumbar spine region cancer at the time of the procedure   M
BETOS: Z2   Undefined codes
Service not separately priced by Part B

C M1038 Patients with a diagnosis of lumbar spine region fracture at the time of the procedure   M
BETOS: Z2   Undefined codes
Service not separately priced by Part B

C M1039 Patients with a diagnosis of lumbar spine region infection at the time of the procedure   M
BETOS: Z2   Undefined codes
Service not separately priced by Part B

C M1040 Patients with a diagnosis of lumbar idiopathic or congenital scoliosis   M
BETOS: Z2   Undefined codes
Service not separately priced by Part B

▲ C M1041 Patient had cancer, acute fracture or infection related to the lumbar spine or patient had neuromuscular, idiopathic or congenital lumbar scoliosis   M MIPS
BETOS: Z2   Undefined codes
Service not separately priced by Part B

● New code   ▲ Revised code   **C** Carrier judgment   **D** Special coverage instructions apply
I Not payable by Medicare   **M** Non-covered by Medicare   **S** Non-covered by Medicare statute   AHA Coding Clinic®

FUNCTIONAL STATUS MEASUREMENT (M1043-M1049)

C **M1043** Functional status was not measured by the oswestry disability index (ODI version 2.1a) at one year (9 to 15 months) postoperatively M MIPS

BETOS: Z2 Undefined codes
Service not separately priced by Part B

▲ C **M1045** Functional status measured by the oxford knee score (OKS) at one year (9 to 15 months) postoperatively was greater than or equal to 37 or knee injury and osteoarthritis outcome score joint replacement (koos, jr.) was greater than or equal to 71 M MIPS

BETOS: Z2 Undefined codes
Service not separately priced by Part B

▲ C **M1046** Functional status measured by the oxford knee score (OKS) at one year (9 to 15 months) postoperatively was less than 37 or the knee injury and osteoarthritis outcome score joint replacement (koos, jr.) was less than 71 postoperatively M MIPS

BETOS: Z2 Undefined codes
Service not separately priced by Part B

C **M1049** Functional status was not measured by the oswestry disability index (ODI version 2.1a) at three months (6 - 20 weeks) postoperatively M MIPS

BETOS: Z2 Undefined codes
Service not separately priced by Part B

LUMBAR SPINE CONDITIONS (M1051)

▲ C **M1051** Patient had cancer, acute fracture or infection related to the lumbar spine or patient had neuromuscular, idiopathic or congenital lumbar scoliosis M MIPS

BETOS: Z2 Undefined codes
Service not separately priced by Part B

LIMB PAIN ASSESSMENT (M1052)

C **M1052** Leg pain was not measured by the visual analog scale (VAS) at one year (9 to 15 months) postoperatively M MIPS

BETOS: Z2 Undefined codes
Service not separately priced by Part B

URGENT CARE VISIT (M1054)

C **M1054** Patient had only urgent care visits during the performance period M

BETOS: Z2 Undefined codes
Service not separately priced by Part B

ANTICOAGULATION MANAGEMENT (M1055-M1057)

C **M1055** Aspirin or another antiplatelet therapy used M

BETOS: Z2 Undefined codes
Service not separately priced by Part B

C **M1056** Prescribed anticoagulant medication during the performance period, history of GI bleeding, history of intracranial bleeding, bleeding disorder and specific provider documented reasons: allergy to aspirin or anti-platelets, use of non-steroidal anti-inflammatory agents, drug-drug interaction, uncontrolled hypertension > 180/110 mmHg or gastroesophageal reflux disease M

BETOS: Z2 Undefined codes
Service not separately priced by Part B

C **M1057** Aspirin or another antiplatelet therapy not used, reason not given M

BETOS: Z2 Undefined codes
Service not separately priced by Part B

PERFORMANCE ASSESSMENT (M1058-M1060)

C **M1058** Patient was a permanent nursing home resident at any time during the performance period M

BETOS: Z2 Undefined codes
Service not separately priced by Part B

C **M1059** Patient was in hospice or receiving palliative care at any time during the performance period M

BETOS: Z2 Undefined codes
Service not separately priced by Part B

C **M1060** Patient died prior to the end of the performance period M

BETOS: Z2 Undefined codes
Service not separately priced by Part B

HOSPICE SERVICES (M1067)

C **M1067** Hospice services for patient provided any time during the measurement period M

BETOS: Z2 Undefined codes
Service not separately priced by Part B

MOBILITY STATUS (M1068)

C **M1068** Adults who are not ambulatory Ⓐ M

BETOS: Z2 Undefined codes
Service not separately priced by Part B

FALL RISK ASSESSMENT (M1069-M1070)

C **M1069** Patient screened for future fall risk M

BETOS: Z2 Undefined codes
Service not separately priced by Part B

C **M1070** Patient not screened for future fall risk, reason not given M

BETOS: Z2 Undefined codes
Service not separately priced by Part B

♂ Male only   ♀ Female only   Ⓐ Age   A2 - Z3 = ASC Payment indicator   A - Y = APC Status indicator
ASC = ASC Approved Procedure   **DME** Paid under the DME fee schedule   **MIPS** MIPS code

M1043 - M1070

MEDICAL SERVICES (M0075-M1149)

SPINAL PROCEDURES (M1071)

C M1071 Patient had any additional spine procedures performed on the same date as the lumbar discectomy/laminotomy   M MIPS
BETOS: Z2   Undefined codes
Service not separately priced by Part B

EPISODE OF CARE (M1106-M1143)

C M1106 The start of an episode of care documented in the medical record   M MIPS
BETOS: Z2   Undefined codes
Service not separately priced by Part B

C M1107 Documentation stating patient has a diagnosis of a degenerative neurological condition such as ALS, MS, or Parkinson's diagnosed at any time before or during the episode of care   M MIPS
BETOS: Z2   Undefined codes
Service not separately priced by Part B

▲ **C M1108** Ongoing care not clinically indicated because the patient needed a home program only, referral to another provider or facility, or consultation only, as documented in the medical record   M MIPS
BETOS: Z2   Undefined codes
Service not separately priced by Part B

▲ **C M1109** Ongoing care not medically possible because the patient was discharged early due to specific medical events, documented in the medical record, such as the patient became hospitalized or scheduled for surgery   M MIPS
BETOS: Z2   Undefined codes
Service not separately priced by Part B

▲ **C M1110** Ongoing care not possible because the patient self-discharged early (e.g., financial or insurance reasons, transportation problems, or reason unknown)   M MIPS
BETOS: Z2   Undefined codes
Service not separately priced by Part B

C M1111 The start of an episode of care documented in the medical record   M MIPS
BETOS: Z2   Undefined codes
Service not separately priced by Part B

C M1112 Documentation stating patient has a diagnosis of a degenerative neurological condition such as ALS, MS, or Parkinson's diagnosed at any time before or during the episode of care   M MIPS
BETOS: Z2   Undefined codes
Service not separately priced by Part B

▲ **C M1113** Ongoing care not clinically indicated because the patient needed a home program only, referral to another provider or facility, or consultation only, as documented in the medical record   M MIPS
BETOS: Z2   Undefined codes
Service not separately priced by Part B

▲ **C M1114** Ongoing care not medically possible because the patient was discharged early due to specific medical events, documented in the medical record, such as the patient became hospitalized or scheduled for surgery   M MIPS
BETOS: Z2   Undefined codes
Service not separately priced by Part B

▲ **C M1115** Ongoing care not possible because the patient self-discharged early (e.g., financial or insurance reasons, transportation problems, or reason unknown)   M MIPS
BETOS: Z2   Undefined codes
Service not separately priced by Part B

C M1116 The start of an episode of care documented in the medical record   M MIPS
BETOS: Z2   Undefined codes
Service not separately priced by Part B

C M1117 Documentation stating patient has a diagnosis of a degenerative neurological condition such as ALS, MS, or Parkinson's diagnosed at any time before or during the episode of care   M MIPS
BETOS: Z2   Undefined codes
Service not separately priced by Part B

▲ **C M1118** Ongoing care not clinically indicated because the patient needed a home program only, referral to another provider or facility, or consultation only, as documented in the medical record   M MIPS
BETOS: Z2   Undefined codes
Service not separately priced by Part B

▲ **C M1119** Ongoing care not medically possible because the patient was discharged early due to specific medical events, documented in the medical record, such as the patient became hospitalized or scheduled for surgery   M MIPS
BETOS: Z2   Undefined codes
Service not separately priced by Part B

▲ **C M1120** Ongoing care not possible because the patient self-discharged early (e.g., financial or insurance reasons, transportation problems, or reason unknown)   M MIPS
BETOS: Z2   Undefined codes
Service not separately priced by Part B

C M1121 The start of an episode of care documented in the medical record   M MIPS
BETOS: Z2   Undefined codes
Service not separately priced by Part B

C M1122 Documentation stating patient has a diagnosis of a degenerative neurological condition such as ALS, MS, or Parkinson's diagnosed at any time before or during the episode of care   M MIPS
BETOS: Z2   Undefined codes
Service not separately priced by Part B

● New code   ▲ Revised code   **C** Carrier judgment   **D** Special coverage instructions apply
I Not payable by Medicare   **M** Non-covered by Medicare   **S** Non-covered by Medicare statute   AHA Coding Clinic®

▲ C **M1123** Ongoing care not clinically indicated because the patient needed a home program only, referral to another provider or facility, or consultation only, as documented in the medical record M MIPS

    BETOS: Z2 Undefined codes

    Service not separately priced by Part B

▲ C **M1124** Ongoing care not medically possible because the patient was discharged early due to specific medical events, documented in the medical record, such as the patient became hospitalized or scheduled for surgery M MIPS

    BETOS: Z2 Undefined codes

    Service not separately priced by Part B

▲ C **M1125** Ongoing care not possible because the patient self-discharged early (e.g., financial or insurance reasons, transportation problems, or reason unknown) M MIPS

    BETOS: Z2 Undefined codes

    Service not separately priced by Part B

C **M1126** The start of an episode of care documented in the medical record M MIPS

    BETOS: Z2 Undefined codes

    Service not separately priced by Part B

C **M1127** Documentation stating patient has a diagnosis of a degenerative neurological condition such as ALS, MS, or Parkinson's diagnosed at any time before or during the episode of care M MIPS

    BETOS: Z2 Undefined codes

    Service not separately priced by Part B

▲ C **M1128** Ongoing care not clinically indicated because the patient needed a home program only, referral to another provider or facility, or consultation only, as documented in the medical record M MIPS

    BETOS: Z2 Undefined codes

    Service not separately priced by Part B

▲ C **M1129** Ongoing care not medically possible because the patient was discharged early due to specific medical events, documented in the medical record, such as the patient became hospitalized or scheduled for surgery M MIPS

    BETOS: Z2 Undefined codes

    Service not separately priced by Part B

▲ C **M1130** Ongoing care not possible because the patient self-discharged early (e.g., financial or insurance reasons, transportation problems, or reason unknown) M MIPS

    BETOS: Z2 Undefined codes

    Service not separately priced by Part B

C **M1131** Documentation stating patient has a diagnosis of a degenerative neurological condition such as ALS, MS, or Parkinson's diagnosed at any time before or during the episode of care M MIPS

BETOS: Z2 Undefined codes

Service not separately priced by Part B

▲ C **M1132** Ongoing care not clinically indicated because the patient needed a home program only, referral to another provider or facility, or consultation only, as documented in the medical record M MIPS

    BETOS: Z2 Undefined codes

    Service not separately priced by Part B

▲ C **M1133** Ongoing care not medically possible because the patient was discharged early due to specific medical events, documented in the medical record, such as the patient became hospitalized or scheduled for surgery M MIPS

    BETOS: Z2 Undefined codes

    Service not separately priced by Part B

▲ C **M1134** Ongoing care not possible because the patient self-discharged early (e.g., financial or insurance reasons, transportation problems, or reason unknown) M MIPS

    BETOS: Z2 Undefined codes

    Service not separately priced by Part B

C **M1135** The start of an episode of care documented in the medical record M MIPS

    BETOS: Z2 Undefined codes

    Service not separately priced by Part B

▲ C **M1141** Functional status was not measured by the oxford knee score (oks) or the knee injury and osteoarthritis outcome score joint replacement (koos, jr.) at one year (9 to 15 months) postoperatively M MIPS

    BETOS: Z2 Undefined codes

    Service not separately priced by Part B

C **M1142** Emergent cases M MIPS

    BETOS: Z2 Undefined codes

    Service not separately priced by Part B

C **M1143** Initiated episode of rehabilitation therapy, medical, or chiropractic care for neck impairment M MIPS

    BETOS: Z2 Undefined codes

    Service not separately priced by Part B

OTHER SERVICES (M1145-M1149)

● C **M1145** Most favored nation (MFN) model drug add-on amount, per dose, (do not bill with line items that have the JW modifier) K

    BETOS: Z2 Undefined codes

    Service not separately priced by Part B

● C **M1146** Ongoing care not clinically indicated because the patient needed a home program only, referral to another provider or facility, or consultation only, as documented in the medical record M

    BETOS: Z2 Undefined codes

    Service not separately priced by Part B

♂ Male only   ♀ Female only   A Age   A2 - Z3 = ASC Payment indicator   A - Y = APC Status indicator

ASC = ASC Approved Procedure   DME Paid under the DME fee schedule   MIPS MIPS code

● **C** **M1147** Ongoing care not medically possible because the patient was discharged early due to specific medical events, documented in the medical record, such as the patient became hospitalized or scheduled for surgery   M
    BETOS: Z2   Undefined codes
    Service not separately priced by Part B

● **C** **M1148** Ongoing care not possible because the patient self-discharged early (e.g., financial or insurance reasons, transportation problems, or reason unknown)   M
    BETOS: Z2   Undefined codes
    Service not separately priced by Part B

● **C** **M1149** Patient unable to complete the neck FS PROM at initial evaluation and/or discharge due to blindness, illiteracy, severe mental incapacity or language incompatibility, and an adequate proxy is not available   M
    BETOS: Z2   Undefined codes
    Service not separately priced by Part B

PATHOLOGY AND LABORATORY SERVICES (P2028-P9615)

LABORATORY TESTS OF BLOOD AND HAIR (P2028-P2038)

D **P2028** Cephalin flocculation, blood   A
BETOS: T1H   Lab tests - other (non-Medicare fee schedule)
Other carrier priced

D **P2029** Congo red, blood   A
BETOS: T1H   Lab tests - other (non-Medicare fee schedule)
Other carrier priced

M **P2031** Hair analysis (excluding arsenic)   E1
BETOS: T1H   Lab tests - other (non-Medicare fee schedule)
Service not separately priced by Part B

D **P2033** Thymol turbidity, blood   A
BETOS: T1H   Lab tests - other (non-Medicare fee schedule)
Other carrier priced

D **P2038** Mucoprotein, blood (seromucoid) (medical necessity procedure)   A
BETOS: T1H   Lab tests - other (non-Medicare fee schedule)
Price subject to national limitation amount

PAP SMEARS (P3000, P3001)

D **P3000** Screening Papanicolaou smear, cervical or vaginal, up to three smears, by technician under physician supervision   ♀ A
BETOS: T1H   Lab tests - other (non-Medicare fee schedule)
Price subject to national limitation amount

D **P3001** Screening Papanicolaou smear, cervical or vaginal, up to three smears, requiring interpretation by physician   ♀ B
BETOS: T1G   Lab tests - other (Medicare fee schedule)
Price established using national RVUs

URINE BACTERIAL CULTURE AND SENSITIVITY STUDIES (P7001)

I **P7001** Culture, bacterial, urine; quantitative, sensitivity study   E1
BETOS: T1H   Lab tests - other (non-Medicare fee schedule)
Service not separately priced by Part B

BLOOD AND BLOOD PRODUCTS, WITH ASSOCIATED PROCEDURES (P9010-P9100)

D **P9010** Blood (whole), for transfusion, per unit   R
BETOS: T1H   Lab tests - other (non-Medicare fee schedule)
Reasonable charge
Coding Clinic: 2004, Q3

D **P9011** Blood, split unit   R
BETOS: T1H   Lab tests - other (non-Medicare fee schedule)
Reasonable charge
Coding Clinic: 2004, Q3; 2005, Q2
Pub: 1100-4, Chapter-4, 231.4

D **P9012** Cryoprecipitate, each unit   R
BETOS: T1H   Lab tests - other (non-Medicare fee schedule)
Reasonable charge
Coding Clinic: 2004, Q3

D **P9016** Red blood cells, leukocytes reduced, each unit   R
BETOS: T1H   Lab tests - other (non-Medicare fee schedule)
Reasonable charge
Coding Clinic: 2004, Q4; 2004, Q3

D **P9017** Fresh frozen plasma (single donor), frozen within 8 hours of collection, each unit   R
BETOS: T1H   Lab tests - other (non-Medicare fee schedule)
Reasonable charge
Coding Clinic: 2004, Q3

D **P9019** Platelets, each unit   R
BETOS: T1H   Lab tests - other (non-Medicare fee schedule)
Reasonable charge
Coding Clinic: 2004, Q3

D **P9020** Platelet rich plasma, each unit   R
BETOS: T1H   Lab tests - other (non-Medicare fee schedule)
Reasonable charge
Coding Clinic: 2004, Q3

D **P9021** Red blood cells, each unit   R
BETOS: T1H   Lab tests - other (non-Medicare fee schedule)
Reasonable charge
Coding Clinic: 2004, Q4; 2004, Q3

D **P9022** Red blood cells, washed, each unit   R
BETOS: T1H   Lab tests - other (non-Medicare fee schedule)
Reasonable charge
Coding Clinic: 2004, Q3

D **P9023** Plasma, pooled multiple donor, solvent/detergent treated, frozen, each unit   R
BETOS: T1H   Lab tests - other (non-Medicare fee schedule)
Reasonable charge
Coding Clinic: 2004, Q3

D **P9031** Platelets, leukocytes reduced, each unit   R
BETOS: T1H   Lab tests - other (non-Medicare fee schedule)
Reasonable charge
Coding Clinic: 2004, Q3

♂ Male only   ♀ Female only   **A** Age   A2 - Z3 = ASC Payment indicator   A - Y = APC Status indicator
ASC = ASC Approved Procedure   **DME** Paid under the DME fee schedule   **MIPS** MIPS code

D P9032 Platelets, irradiated, each unit R
BETOS: T1H   Lab tests - other
(non-Medicare fee schedule)
Reasonable charge
Coding Clinic: 2004, Q3; 2005, Q2

D P9033 Platelets, leukocytes reduced, irradiated,
each unit R
BETOS: T1H   Lab tests - other
(non-Medicare fee schedule)
Reasonable charge
Coding Clinic: 2004, Q3; 2005, Q2

D P9034 Platelets, pheresis, each unit R
BETOS: T1H   Lab tests - other
(non-Medicare fee schedule)
Reasonable charge
Coding Clinic: 2004, Q3

D P9035 Platelets, pheresis, leukocytes reduced,
each unit R
BETOS: T1H   Lab tests - other
(non-Medicare fee schedule)
Reasonable charge
Coding Clinic: 2004, Q3

D P9036 Platelets, pheresis, irradiated, each unit R
BETOS: T1H   Lab tests - other
(non-Medicare fee schedule)
Reasonable charge
Coding Clinic: 2004, Q3; 2005, Q2

D P9037 Platelets, pheresis, leukocytes reduced,
irradiated, each unit R
BETOS: T1H   Lab tests - other
(non-Medicare fee schedule)
Reasonable charge
Coding Clinic: 2004, Q3; 2005, Q2

D P9038 Red blood cells, irradiated, each unit R
BETOS: T1H   Lab tests - other
(non-Medicare fee schedule)
Reasonable charge
Coding Clinic: 2004, Q3; 2005, Q2

D P9039 Red blood cells, deglycerolized, each unit R
BETOS: T1H   Lab tests - other
(non-Medicare fee schedule)
Reasonable charge
Coding Clinic: 2004, Q3

D P9040 Red blood cells, leukocytes reduced,
irradiated, each unit R
BETOS: T1H   Lab tests - other
(non-Medicare fee schedule)
Reasonable charge
Coding Clinic: 2004, Q3; 2005, Q2

C P9041 Infusion, albumin (human), 5%,
50 ml K2 ASC K
BETOS: T1H   Lab tests - other
(non-Medicare fee schedule)
Reasonable charge
Drugs: ALBUMIN (HUMAN), ALBUMINAR-5,
ALBUMINEX 5%, ALBURX, ALBUTEIN 5%,

ALBUTEIN®, ALBUTEIN® 5% ALBUMIN 500
ML, BUMINATE, PLASBUMIN-5
Coding Clinic: 2004, Q3

D P9043 Infusion, plasma protein fraction (human),
5%, 50 ml R
BETOS: T1H   Lab tests - other
(non-Medicare fee schedule)
Reasonable charge
Coding Clinic: 2004, Q3

D P9044 Plasma, cryoprecipitate reduced, each unit R
BETOS: T1H   Lab tests - other
(non-Medicare fee schedule)
Reasonable charge
Coding Clinic: 2004, Q3

C P9045 Infusion, albumin (human), 5%,
250 ml K2 ASC K
BETOS: Y2   Other - non-Medicare fee
schedule
Reasonable charge
Drugs: ALBUKED 5, ALBUMIN (HUMAN),
ALBUMINAR-5, ALBUMINEX 5%, ALBURX,
ALBUTEIN® 5% ALBUMIN 500 ML,
ALBUTEIN® 5%, BUMINATE, PLASBUMIN-5
Coding Clinic: 2002, Q1; 2004, Q3

C P9046 Infusion, albumin (human), 25%,
20 ml K2 ASC K
BETOS: Y2   Other - non-Medicare fee
schedule
Reasonable charge
Drugs: ALBUKED 25, ALBUMIN (HUMAN),
ALBUMINAR-25, ALBUMINEX 25%,
ALBURX, ALBUTEIN 25%, ALBUTEIN®,
ALBUTEIN® 25% ALBUMIN 100 ML,
BUMINATE, FLEXBUMIN, KEDBUMIN,
PLASBUMIN-25
Coding Clinic: 2002, Q1; 2004, Q3

C P9047 Infusion, albumin (human), 25%,
50 ml K2 ASC K
BETOS: Y2   Other - non-Medicare fee
schedule
Reasonable charge
Drugs: ALBUKED 25, ALBUMIN (HUMAN),
ALBUMINAR-25, ALBUMINEX 25%,
ALBURX, ALBUTEIN® 25%, ALBUTEIN®
25% ALBUMIN 100 ML, BUMINATE,
FLEXBUMIN, HUMAN ALBUMIN GRIFOLS,
KEDBUMIN, PLASBUMIN-25
Coding Clinic: 2002, Q1; 2004, Q3

C P9048 Infusion, plasma protein fraction (human),
5%, 250 ml R
BETOS: Y2   Other - non-Medicare fee
schedule
Reasonable charge
Coding Clinic: 2002, Q1; 2004, Q3

C P9050 Granulocytes, pheresis,
each unit K5 ASC E2
BETOS: Z2   Undefined codes
Reasonable charge
Coding Clinic: 2002, Q1; 2004, Q3

● New code   ▲ Revised code   **C** Carrier judgment   **D** Special coverage instructions apply
I Not payable by Medicare   **M** Non-covered by Medicare   **S** Non-covered by Medicare statute   AHA Coding Clinic®

D **P9051** Whole blood or red blood cells, leukocytes reduced, CMV-negative, each unit R
BETOS: T1H   Lab tests - other (non-Medicare fee schedule)
Reasonable charge
Statute: 1833T
Coding Clinic: 2004, Q3

D **P9052** Platelets, HLA-matched leukocytes reduced, apheresis/pheresis, each unit R
BETOS: T1H   Lab tests - other (non-Medicare fee schedule)
Reasonable charge
Statute: 1833T
Coding Clinic: 2004, Q3

D **P9053** Platelets, pheresis, leukocytes reduced, CMV-negative, irradiated, each unit R
BETOS: T1H   Lab tests - other (non-Medicare fee schedule)
Reasonable charge
Statute: 1833T
Coding Clinic: 2004, Q3; 2005, Q2

D **P9054** Whole blood or red blood cells, leukocytes reduced, frozen, deglycerol, washed, each unit R
BETOS: T1H   Lab tests - other (non-Medicare fee schedule)
Reasonable charge
Statute: 1833T
Coding Clinic: 2004, Q3

D **P9055** Platelets, leukocytes reduced, CMV-negative, apheresis/pheresis, each unit R
BETOS: T1H   Lab tests - other (non-Medicare fee schedule)
Reasonable charge
Statute: 1833T
Coding Clinic: 2004, Q3

D **P9056** Whole blood, leukocytes reduced, irradiated, each unit R
BETOS: T1H   Lab tests - other (non-Medicare fee schedule)
Reasonable charge
Statute: 1833T
Coding Clinic: 2004, Q3; 2005, Q2

D **P9057** Red blood cells, frozen/deglycerolized/ washed, leukocytes reduced, irradiated, each unit R
BETOS: T1H   Lab tests - other (non-Medicare fee schedule)
Reasonable charge
Statute: 1833T
Coding Clinic: 2004, Q3; 2005, Q2

D **P9058** Red blood cells, leukocytes reduced, CMV-negative, irradiated, each unit R
BETOS: T1H   Lab tests - other (non-Medicare fee schedule)
Reasonable charge
Statute: 1833T
Coding Clinic: 2004, Q3; 2005, Q2

D **P9059** Fresh frozen plasma between 8-24 hours of collection, each unit R
BETOS: T1H   Lab tests - other (non-Medicare fee schedule)
Reasonable charge
Statute: 1833T
Coding Clinic: 2004, Q3

D **P9060** Fresh frozen plasma, donor retested, each unit R
BETOS: T1H   Lab tests - other (non-Medicare fee schedule)
Reasonable charge
Statute: 1833T
Coding Clinic: 2004, Q3

D **P9070** Plasma, pooled multiple donor, pathogen reduced, frozen, each unit R
BETOS: T1H   Lab tests - other (non-Medicare fee schedule)
Reasonable charge
Statute: 1833T
Coding Clinic: 2016, Q1

D **P9071** Plasma (single donor), pathogen reduced, frozen, each unit R
BETOS: T1H   Lab tests - other (non-Medicare fee schedule)
Reasonable charge
Statute: 1833T
Coding Clinic: 2016, Q1

D **P9073** Platelets, pheresis, pathogen-reduced, each unit R
BETOS: T1H   Lab tests - other (non-Medicare fee schedule)
Reasonable charge
Statute: 1833T
Coding Clinic: 2018, Q1

C **P9099** Blood component or product not otherwise classified R
BETOS: T1H   Lab tests - other (non-Medicare fee schedule)
Reasonable charge

D **P9100** Pathogen(s) test for platelets S
BETOS: T1H   Lab tests - other (non-Medicare fee schedule)
Other carrier priced
Coding Clinic: 2018, Q1

SPECIMEN COLLECTION, TRAVEL ALLOWANCE (P9603, P9604)

D **P9603** Travel allowance one-way in connection with medically necessary laboratory specimen collection drawn from home bound or nursing home bound patient; prorated miles actually travelled A
BETOS: Y2   Other - non-Medicare fee schedule
Price established by carriers
Pub: 100-4, Chapter-16, 60.2

D **P9604** Travel allowance one-way in connection with medically necessary laboratory specimen collection drawn from home bound or nursing home bound patient; prorated trip charge   A

BETOS: Y2   Other - non-Medicare fee schedule

Price established by carriers

Pub: 100-4, Chapter-16, 60.2

SPECIMEN COLLECTION, CATHETERIZATION (P9612, P9615)

D **P9612** Catheterization for collection of specimen, single patient, all places of service   A

BETOS: T1H   Lab tests - other (non-Medicare fee schedule)

Other carrier priced

Coding Clinic: 2007, Q3; 2009, Q2

D **P9615** Catheterization for collection of specimen(s) (multiple patients)   N

BETOS: T1H   Lab tests - other (non-Medicare fee schedule)

Other carrier priced

TEMPORARY CODES (Q0035-Q9992)

MISCELLANEOUS DRUGS AND TESTS (Q0035-Q0144)

D **Q0035** Cardiokymography N
BETOS: T2D Other tests - other
Price established using national RVUs

D **Q0081** Infusion therapy, using other than chemotherapeutic drugs, per visit B
BETOS: P6C Minor procedures - other (Medicare fee schedule)
Service not separately priced by Part B
Coding Clinic: 2002, Q4; 2002, Q2; 2002, Q2; 2002, Q1; 2004, Q4; 2004, Q2; 2004, Q1; 2005, Q1; 2006, Q4

C **Q0083** Chemotherapy administration by other than infusion technique only (e.g., subcutaneous, intramuscular, push), per visit B
BETOS: O1D Chemotherapy
Service not separately priced by Part B
Coding Clinic: 2002, Q1; 2002, Q1; 2004, Q4; 2004, Q1; 2005, Q1; 2006, Q4

D **Q0084** Chemotherapy administration by infusion technique only, per visit B
BETOS: O1D Chemotherapy
Service not separately priced by Part B
Coding Clinic: 2002, Q1; 2002, Q1; 2004, Q4; 2004, Q2; 2004, Q1; 2005, Q1; 2006, Q4

C **Q0085** Chemotherapy administration by both infusion technique and other technique(s) (e.g., subcutaneous, intramuscular, push), per visit B
BETOS: O1D Chemotherapy
Service not separately priced by Part B
Coding Clinic: 2002, Q1; 2002, Q1; 2004, Q4; 2004, Q1; 2006, Q4

D **Q0091** Screening Papanicolaou smear; obtaining, preparing and conveyance of cervical or vaginal smear to laboratory ♀ S
BETOS: P6C Minor procedures - other (Medicare fee schedule)
Price established using national RVUs
Coding Clinic: 2002, Q4; 2008, Q4

D **Q0092** Set-up portable X-ray equipment N
BETOS: I1F Standard imaging - other
Price established using national RVUs

C **Q0111** Wet mounts, including preparations of vaginal, cervical or skin specimens ♀ A
BETOS: T1H Lab tests - other (non-Medicare fee schedule)
Price subject to national limitation amount

C **Q0112** All potassium hydroxide (KOH) preparations A
BETOS: T1H Lab tests - other (non-Medicare fee schedule)
Price subject to national limitation amount

C **Q0113** Pinworm examinations A
BETOS: T1H Lab tests - other (non-Medicare fee schedule)
Price subject to national limitation amount

C **Q0114** Fern test ♀ Ⓐ A
BETOS: T1H Lab tests - other (non-Medicare fee schedule)
Price subject to national limitation amount

C **Q0115** Post-coital direct, qualitative examinations of vaginal or cervical mucous ♀ A
BETOS: T1H Lab tests - other (non-Medicare fee schedule)
Price subject to national limitation amount

C **Q0138** Injection, ferumoxytol, for treatment of iron deficiency anemia, 1 mg (non-ESRD use) K2 ASC K
BETOS: O1E Other drugs
Drugs: FERAHEME

C **Q0139** Injection, ferumoxytol, for treatment of iron deficiency anemia, 1 mg (for ESRD on dialysis) K2 ASC K
BETOS: O1E Other drugs
Drugs: FERAHEME

M **Q0144** Azithromycin dihydrate, oral, capsules/powder, 1 gram E1
BETOS: O1E Other drugs
Service not separately priced by Part B

CHEMOTHERAPY ANTI-EMETIC MEDICATIONS (Q0161-Q0181), SEE ALSO CHEMOTHERAPY MEDICATIONS (Q5101-Q5106)

C **Q0161** Chlorpromazine hydrochloride, 5 mg, oral, FDA-approved prescription anti-emetic, for use as a complete therapeutic substitute for an IV anti-emetic at the time of chemotherapy treatment, not to exceed a 48-hour dosage regimen N1 ASC N
BETOS: O1D Chemotherapy
Coding Clinic: 2002, Q2; 2014, Q1

D **Q0162** Ondansetron 1 mg, oral, FDA-approved prescription anti-emetic, for use as a complete therapeutic substitute for an IV anti-emetic at the time of chemotherapy treatment, not to exceed a 48-hour dosage regimen N1 ASC N
BETOS: O1D Chemotherapy
Statute: 4557
Drugs: ONDANSETRON, ONDANSETRON HCL, ONDANSETRON ODT, ZOFRAN

D **Q0163** Diphenhydramine hydrochloride, 50 mg, oral, FDA-approved prescription anti-emetic, for use as a complete therapeutic substitute for an IV anti-emetic at time of chemotherapy treatment not to exceed a 48-hour dosage regimen N1 ASC N
BETOS: O1D Chemotherapy
Statute: 4557
Coding Clinic: 2002, Q1; 2008, Q1; 2009, Q2; 2012, Q2; 2019, Q4; 2020, Q1

♂ Male only ♀ Female only Ⓐ Age A2 - Z3 = ASC Payment indicator A - Y = APC Status indicator
ASC = ASC Approved Procedure **DME** Paid under the DME fee schedule **MIPS** MIPS code

Q0164 **D** Prochlorperazine maleate, 5 mg, oral, FDA-approved prescription anti-emetic, for use as a complete therapeutic substitute for an IV anti-emetic at the time of chemotherapy treatment, not to exceed a 48-hour dosage regimen   N1 ASC N
BETOS: O1D   Chemotherapy
Statute: 4557
Drugs: PROCHLORPERAZINE MALEATE

Q0166 **D** Granisetron hydrochloride, 1 mg, oral, FDA-approved prescription anti-emetic, for use as a complete therapeutic substitute for an IV anti-emetic at the time of chemotherapy treatment, not to exceed a 24-hour dosage regimen   N1 ASC N
BETOS: O1D   Chemotherapy
Statute: 4557
Drugs: GRANISETRON HCL

Q0167 **D** Dronabinol, 2.5 mg, oral, FDA-approved prescription anti-emetic, for use as a complete therapeutic substitute for an IV anti-emetic at the time of chemotherapy treatment, not to exceed a 48-hour dosage regimen   N1 ASC N
BETOS: O1D   Chemotherapy
Statute: 4557
Drugs: DRONABINOL, MARINOL

Q0169 **D** Promethazine hydrochloride, 12.5 mg, oral, FDA-approved prescription anti-emetic, for use as a complete therapeutic substitute for an IV anti-emetic at the time of chemotherapy treatment, not to exceed a 48-hour dosage regimen   N1 ASC N
BETOS: O1D   Chemotherapy
Statute: 4557

Q0173 **D** Trimethobenzamide hydrochloride, 250 mg, oral, FDA-approved prescription anti-emetic, for use as a complete therapeutic substitute for an IV anti-emetic at the time of chemotherapy treatment, not to exceed a 48-hour dosage regimen   N1 ASC N
BETOS: O1D   Chemotherapy
Statute: 4557

Q0174 **D** Thiethylperazine maleate, 10 mg, oral, FDA-approved prescription anti-emetic, for use as a complete therapeutic substitute for an IV anti-emetic at the time of chemotherapy treatment, not to exceed a 48-hour dosage regimen   K5 ASC E2
BETOS: O1D   Chemotherapy
Statute: 4557

Q0175 **D** Perphenazine, 4 mg, oral, FDA-approved prescription anti-emetic, for use as a complete therapeutic substitute for an IV anti-emetic at the time of chemotherapy treatment, not to exceed a 48-hour dosage regimen   N1 ASC N
BETOS: O1D   Chemotherapy
Statute: 4557

Q0177 **D** Hydroxyzine pamoate, 25 mg, oral, FDA-approved prescription anti-emetic, for use as a complete therapeutic substitute for an IV anti-emetic at the time of chemotherapy treatment, not to exceed a 48-hour dosage regimen   N1 ASC N
BETOS: O1D   Chemotherapy
Statute: 4557

Q0180 **D** Dolasetron mesylate, 100 mg, oral, FDA-approved prescription anti-emetic, for use as a complete therapeutic substitute for an IV anti-emetic at the time of chemotherapy treatment, not to exceed a 24-hour dosage regimen   N1 ASC N
BETOS: O1D   Chemotherapy
Statute: 4557

Q0181 **D** Unspecified oral dosage form, FDA-approved prescription anti-emetic, for use as a complete therapeutic substitute for a IV anti-emetic at the time of chemotherapy treatment, not to exceed a 48-hour dosage regimen   N1 ASC N
BETOS: O1D   Chemotherapy
Statute: 4557
Coding Clinic: 2006, Q1; 2008, Q1; 2009, Q2; 2012, Q2; 2019, Q4; 2020, Q1

MONOCLONAL ANTIBODIES (Q0239-Q0243)

● **C** **Q0239** Injection, bamlanivimab-xxxx, 700 mg   L1 ASC L
BETOS: O1G   Immunizations/Vaccinations

● **C** **Q0243** Injection, casirivimab and imdevimab, 2400 mg   L
BETOS: O1G   Immunizations/Vaccinations

VENTRICULAR ASSIST DEVICES (Q0477-Q0509)

Q0477 **D** Power module patient cable for use with electric or electric/pneumatic ventricular assist device, replacement only   DME A
BETOS: D1F   Prosthetic/Orthotic devices

Q0478 **D** Power adapter for use with electric or electric/pneumatic ventricular assist device, vehicle type   DME A
BETOS: D1F   Prosthetic/Orthotic devices

Q0479 **D** Power module for use with electric or electric/pneumatic ventricular assist device, replacement only   DME A
BETOS: D1F   Prosthetic/Orthotic devices

Q0480 **D** Driver for use with pneumatic ventricular assist device, replacement only   DME A
BETOS: D1F   Prosthetic/Orthotic devices
Coding Clinic: 2005, Q3

Q0481 **D** Microprocessor control unit for use with electric ventricular assist device, replacement only   DME A
BETOS: D1F   Prosthetic/Orthotic devices
Coding Clinic: 2005, Q3

● New code   ▲ Revised code   **C** Carrier judgment   **D** Special coverage instructions apply
I Not payable by Medicare   **M** Non-covered by Medicare   **S** Non-covered by Medicare statute   AHA Coding Clinic®

D **Q0482** Microprocessor control unit for use with electric/pneumatic combination ventricular assist device, replacement only **DME** A
BETOS: D1F   Prosthetic/Orthotic devices
Coding Clinic: 2005, Q3

D **Q0483** Monitor/display module for use with electric ventricular assist device, replacement only **DME** A
BETOS: D1F   Prosthetic/Orthotic devices
Coding Clinic: 2005, Q3

D **Q0484** Monitor/display module for use with electric or electric/pneumatic ventricular assist device, replacement only **DME** A
BETOS: D1F   Prosthetic/Orthotic devices
Coding Clinic: 2005, Q3

D **Q0485** Monitor control cable for use with electric ventricular assist device, replacement only **DME** A
BETOS: D1F   Prosthetic/Orthotic devices
Coding Clinic: 2005, Q3

D **Q0486** Monitor control cable for use with electric/pneumatic ventricular assist device, replacement only **DME** A
BETOS: D1F   Prosthetic/Orthotic devices
Coding Clinic: 2005, Q3

D **Q0487** Leads (pneumatic/electrical) for use with any type electric/pneumatic ventricular assist device, replacement only **DME** A
BETOS: D1F   Prosthetic/Orthotic devices
Coding Clinic: 2005, Q3

D **Q0488** Power pack base for use with electric ventricular assist device, replacement only A
BETOS: D1F   Prosthetic/Orthotic devices
Coding Clinic: 2005, Q3

D **Q0489** Power pack base for use with electric/pneumatic ventricular assist device, replacement only **DME** A
BETOS: D1F   Prosthetic/Orthotic devices
Coding Clinic: 2005, Q3

D **Q0490** Emergency power source for use with electric ventricular assist device, replacement only **DME** A
BETOS: D1F   Prosthetic/Orthotic devices
Coding Clinic: 2005, Q3

D **Q0491** Emergency power source for use with electric/pneumatic ventricular assist device, replacement only **DME** A
BETOS: D1F   Prosthetic/Orthotic devices
Coding Clinic: 2005, Q3

D **Q0492** Emergency power supply cable for use with electric ventricular assist device, replacement only **DME** A
BETOS: D1F   Prosthetic/Orthotic devices
Coding Clinic: 2005, Q3

D **Q0493** Emergency power supply cable for use with electric/pneumatic ventricular assist device, replacement only **DME** A
BETOS: D1F   Prosthetic/Orthotic devices
Coding Clinic: 2005, Q3

D **Q0494** Emergency hand pump for use with electric or electric/pneumatic ventricular assist device, replacement only **DME** A
BETOS: D1F   Prosthetic/Orthotic devices
Coding Clinic: 2005, Q3

D **Q0495** Battery/power pack charger for use with electric or electric/pneumatic ventricular assist device, replacement only **DME** A
BETOS: D1F   Prosthetic/Orthotic devices
Coding Clinic: 2005, Q3

D **Q0496** Battery, other than lithium-ion, for use with electric or electric/pneumatic ventricular assist device, replacement only **DME** A
BETOS: D1F   Prosthetic/Orthotic devices
Coding Clinic: 2005, Q3

D **Q0497** Battery clips for use with electric or electric/pneumatic ventricular assist device, replacement only **DME** A
BETOS: D1F   Prosthetic/Orthotic devices
Coding Clinic: 2005, Q3

D **Q0498** Holster for use with electric or electric/pneumatic ventricular assist device, replacement only **DME** A
BETOS: D1F   Prosthetic/Orthotic devices
Coding Clinic: 2005, Q3

D **Q0499** Belt/vest/bag for use to carry external peripheral components of any type ventricular assist device, replacement only **DME** A
BETOS: D1F   Prosthetic/Orthotic devices
Coding Clinic: 2005, Q3

D **Q0500** Filters for use with electric or electric/pneumatic ventricular assist device, replacement only **DME** A
BETOS: D1F   Prosthetic/Orthotic devices
Coding Clinic: 2005, Q3

D **Q0501** Shower cover for use with electric or electric/pneumatic ventricular assist device, replacement only **DME** A
BETOS: D1F   Prosthetic/Orthotic devices
Coding Clinic: 2005, Q3

D **Q0502** Mobility cart for pneumatic ventricular assist device, replacement only **DME** A
BETOS: D1F   Prosthetic/Orthotic devices
Coding Clinic: 2005, Q3

D **Q0503** Battery for pneumatic ventricular assist device, replacement only, each **DME** A
BETOS: D1F   Prosthetic/Orthotic devices
Coding Clinic: 2005, Q3

TEMPORARY CODES (Q0035-Q9992)

D **Q0504** Power adapter for pneumatic ventricular assist device, replacement only, vehicle type **DME** A
    BETOS: D1F   Prosthetic/Orthotic devices
    Coding Clinic: 2005, Q3

D **Q0506** Battery, lithium-ion, for use with electric or electric/pneumatic ventricular assist device, replacement only **DME** A
    BETOS: D1F   Prosthetic/Orthotic devices

D **Q0507** Miscellaneous supply or accessory for use with an external ventricular assist device A
    BETOS: D1F   Prosthetic/Orthotic devices

D **Q0508** Miscellaneous supply or accessory for use with an implanted ventricular assist device A
    BETOS: D1F   Prosthetic/Orthotic devices

D **Q0509** Miscellaneous supply or accessory for use with any implanted ventricular assist device for which payment was not made under Medicare Part A A
    BETOS: D1F   Prosthetic/Orthotic devices

PHARMACY SUPPLY AND DISPENSING FEES (Q0510-Q0514)

D **Q0510** Pharmacy supply fee for initial immunosuppressive drug(s), first month following transplant B
    BETOS: O1E   Other drugs

D **Q0511** Pharmacy supply fee for oral anti-cancer, oral anti-emetic or immunosuppressive drug(s); for the first prescription in a 30-day period B
    BETOS: O1E   Other drugs

D **Q0512** Pharmacy supply fee for oral anti-cancer, oral anti-emetic or immunosuppressive drug(s); for a subsequent prescription in a 30-day period B
    BETOS: O1E   Other drugs

D **Q0513** Pharmacy dispensing fee for inhalation drug(s); per 30 days B
    BETOS: O1E   Other drugs

D **Q0514** Pharmacy dispensing fee for inhalation drug(s); per 90 days B
    BETOS: O1E   Other drugs

MISCELLANEOUS DRUG AND NEW TECHNOLOGY CODES (Q0515-Q2028)

D **Q0515** Injection, sermorelin acetate, 1 microgram K5 ASC E2
    BETOS: O1E   Other drugs

D **Q1004** New technology intraocular lens category 4 as defined in Federal Register notice E1
    BETOS: D1F   Prosthetic/Orthotic devices
    Other carrier priced

D **Q1005** New technology intraocular lens category 5 as defined in Federal Register notice E1

BETOS: D1F   Prosthetic/Orthotic devices
Other carrier priced

D **Q2004** Irrigation solution for treatment of bladder calculi, for example renacidin, per 500 ml N1 ASC N
    BETOS: O1E   Other drugs
    Statute: 1861S2B

D **Q2009** Injection, fosphenytoin, 50 mg phenytoin equivalent N1 ASC N
    BETOS: O1E   Other drugs
    Statute: 1861S2B

D **Q2017** Injection, teniposide, 50 mg K2 ASC K
    BETOS: O1D   Chemotherapy
    Statute: 1861S2B
    Drugs: TENIPOSIDE

D **Q2026** Injection, Radiesse, 0.1 ml K2 ASC K
    BETOS: O1E   Other drugs
    Coding Clinic: 2010, Q3
    Pub: 100-4, Chapter-32, 260.2.1; 100-4, Chapter-32, 260.2.2

D **Q2028** Injection, sculptra, 0.5 mg K2 ASC K
    BETOS: O1E   Other drugs
    Coding Clinic: 2014, Q1

INFLUENZA VIRUS VACCINES (Q2034-Q2039)

D **Q2034** Influenza virus vaccine, split-virus, for intramuscular use (Agriflu) L1 ASC L
    BETOS: O1G   Immunizations/Vaccinations
    Coding Clinic: 2012, Q3

D **Q2035** Influenza virus vaccine, split-virus, when administered to individuals 3 years of age and older, for intramuscular use (Afluria) L1 Ⓐ ASC L
    BETOS: O1G   Immunizations/Vaccinations
    Drugs: AFLURIA (2018/2019)
    Coding Clinic: 2011, Q1; 2010, Q4

D **Q2036** Influenza virus vaccine, split-virus, when administered to individuals 3 years of age and older, for intramuscular use (Flulaval) L1 Ⓐ ASC L
    BETOS: O1G   Immunizations/Vaccinations
    Coding Clinic: 2011, Q1; 2010, Q4

D **Q2037** Influenza virus vaccine, split-virus, when administered to individuals 3 years of age and older, for intramuscular use (Fluvirin) L1 Ⓐ ASC L
    BETOS: O1G   Immunizations/Vaccinations
    Coding Clinic: 2011, Q1; 2010, Q4

D **Q2038** Influenza virus vaccine, split-virus, when administered to individuals 3 years of age and older, for intramuscular use (Fluzone) L1 Ⓐ ASC L
    BETOS: O1G   Immunizations/Vaccinations
    Coding Clinic: 2011, Q1; 2010, Q4

● New code   ▲ Revised code   **C** Carrier judgment   **D** Special coverage instructions apply
I Not payable by Medicare   **M** Non-covered by Medicare   **S** Non-covered by Medicare statute   AHA Coding Clinic®

D **Q2039** Influenza virus vaccine, not otherwise specified   L1 ASC L

    BETOS: O1G   Immunizations/Vaccinations

    Coding Clinic: 2011, Q1; 2010, Q4; 2017, Q4

OTHER DRUGS AND SERVICE FEES (Q2041-Q3031)

C **Q2041** Axicabtagene ciloleucel, up to 200 million autologous anti-CD19 car positive viable T cells, including leukapheresis and dose preparation procedures, per therapeutic dose   K

    BETOS: O1E   Other drugs

    Drugs: YESCARTA

    Coding Clinic: 2012, Q1; 2018, Q1; 2018, Q2; 2019, Q2

C **Q2042** Tisagenlecleucel, up to 600 million car-positive viable t cells, including leukapheresis and dose preparation procedures, per therapeutic dose   K

    BETOS: O1E   Other drugs

    Drugs: KYMRIAH (ADULT DOSE), KYMRIAH (PEDIATRIC DOSE)

    Coding Clinic: 2012, Q1; 2019, Q1; 2019, Q2

D **Q2043** Sipuleucel-T, minimum of 50 million autologous CD54+ cells activated with PAP-GM-CSF, including leukapheresis and all other preparatory procedures, per infusion   K2 ♂ ASC K

    BETOS: P1G   Major procedure - Other

    Drugs: PROVENGE®

    Coding Clinic: 2012, Q1; 2012, Q2

    Pub: 100-4, Chapter-32, 280.5; 100-4, Chapter-32, 280.4; 100-4, Chapter-32, 280.2

C **Q2049** Injection, doxorubicin hydrochloride, liposomal, imported Lipodox, 10 mg   K2 ASC K

    BETOS: O1D   Chemotherapy

    Coding Clinic: 2012, Q3

D **Q2050** Injection, doxorubicin hydrochloride, liposomal, not otherwise specified, 10 mg   K2 ASC K

    BETOS: O1D   Chemotherapy

    Drugs: DOXIL, DOXORUBICIN HCL, LIPOSOMAL,

    Coding Clinic: 2013, Q3; 2013, Q4

D **Q2052** Services, supplies and accessories used in the home under the Medicare intravenous immune globulin (IVIG) demonstration   E1

    BETOS: O1E   Other drugs

    Other carrier priced

    Coding Clinic: 2014, Q2

D **Q3001** Radioelements for brachytherapy, any type, each   N

    BETOS: P7A   Oncology - radiation therapy

    Other carrier priced

C **Q3014** Telehealth originating site facility fee   A

    BETOS: Y2   Other - non-Medicare fee schedule

    Coding Clinic: 2019, Q3

    Pub: 100-4, Chapter-12, 190.5

D **Q3027** Injection, interferon beta-1a, 1 mcg for intramuscular use   K2 ASC K

    BETOS: O1E   Other drugs

    Drugs: AVONEX, AVONEX PEN

    Coding Clinic: 2014, Q1

I **Q3028** Injection, interferon beta-1a, 1 mcg for subcutaneous use   E1

    BETOS: O1E   Other drugs

    Service not separately priced by Part B

D **Q3031** Collagen skin test   N1 ASC N

    BETOS: D1A   Medical/surgical supplies

    Price established using national RVUs

CAST AND SPLINT SUPPLIES (Q4001-Q4051)

C **Q4001** Casting supplies, body cast adult, with or without head, plaster   DME Ⓐ B

    BETOS: D1A   Medical/surgical supplies

    Coding Clinic: 2002, Q2

C **Q4002** Cast supplies, body cast adult, with or without head, fiberglass   DME Ⓐ B

    BETOS: D1A   Medical/surgical supplies

C **Q4003** Cast supplies, shoulder cast, adult (11 years +), plaster   DME Ⓐ B

    BETOS: D1A   Medical/surgical supplies

C **Q4004** Cast supplies, shoulder cast, adult (11 years +), fiberglass   DME Ⓐ B

    BETOS: D1A   Medical/surgical supplies

C **Q4005** Cast supplies, long arm cast, adult (11 years +), plaster   DME Ⓐ B

    BETOS: D1A   Medical/surgical supplies

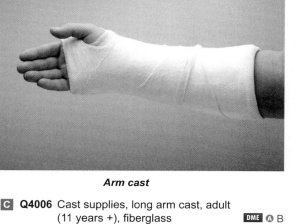

Arm cast

C **Q4006** Cast supplies, long arm cast, adult (11 years +), fiberglass   DME Ⓐ B

    BETOS: D1A   Medical/surgical supplies

♂ Male only   ♀ Female only   Ⓐ Age   A2 - Z3 = ASC Payment indicator   A - Y = APC Status indicator

ASC = ASC Approved Procedure   **DME** Paid under the DME fee schedule   **MIPS** MIPS code

C Q4007 Cast supplies, long arm cast, pediatric (0-10 years), plaster   DME A B
    BETOS: D1A   Medical/surgical supplies

C Q4008 Cast supplies, long arm cast, pediatric (0-10 years), fiberglass   DME A B
    BETOS: D1A   Medical/surgical supplies

C Q4009 Cast supplies, short arm cast, adult (11 years +), plaster   DME A B
    BETOS: D1A   Medical/surgical supplies

C Q4010 Cast supplies, short arm cast, adult (11 years +), fiberglass   DME A B
    BETOS: D1A   Medical/surgical supplies

C Q4011 Cast supplies, short arm cast, pediatric (0-10 years), plaster   DME A B
    BETOS: D1A   Medical/surgical supplies

C Q4012 Cast supplies, short arm cast, pediatric (0-10 years), fiberglass   DME A B
    BETOS: D1A   Medical/surgical supplies

C Q4013 Cast supplies, gauntlet cast (includes lower forearm and hand), adult (11 years +), plaster   DME A B
    BETOS: D1A   Medical/surgical supplies

C Q4014 Cast supplies, gauntlet cast (includes lower forearm and hand), adult (11 years +), fiberglass   DME A B
    BETOS: D1A   Medical/surgical supplies

C Q4015 Cast supplies, gauntlet cast (includes lower forearm and hand), pediatric (0-10 years), plaster   DME A B
    BETOS: D1A   Medical/surgical supplies

C Q4016 Cast supplies, gauntlet cast (includes lower forearm and hand), pediatric (0-10 years), fiberglass   DME A B
    BETOS: D1A   Medical/surgical supplies

C Q4017 Cast supplies, long arm splint, adult (11 years +), plaster   DME A B
    BETOS: D1A   Medical/surgical supplies

C Q4018 Cast supplies, long arm splint, adult (11 years +), fiberglass   DME A B
    BETOS: D1A   Medical/surgical supplies

C Q4019 Cast supplies, long arm splint, pediatric (0-10 years), plaster   DME A B
    BETOS: D1A   Medical/surgical supplies

C Q4020 Cast supplies, long arm splint, pediatric (0-10 years), fiberglass   DME A B
    BETOS: D1A   Medical/surgical supplies

C Q4021 Cast supplies, short arm splint, adult (11 years +), plaster   DME A B
    BETOS: D1A   Medical/surgical supplies

C Q4022 Cast supplies, short arm splint, adult (11 years +), fiberglass   DME A B
    BETOS: D1A   Medical/surgical supplies

C Q4023 Cast supplies, short arm splint, pediatric (0-10 years), plaster   DME A B
    BETOS: D1A   Medical/surgical supplies

C Q4024 Cast supplies, short arm splint, pediatric (0-10 years), fiberglass   DME A B
    BETOS: D1A   Medical/surgical supplies

C Q4025 Cast supplies, hip spica (one or both legs), adult (11 years +), plaster   DME A B
    BETOS: D1A   Medical/surgical supplies

C Q4026 Cast supplies, hip spica (one or both legs), adult (11 years +), fiberglass   DME A B
    BETOS: D1A   Medical/surgical supplies

C Q4027 Cast supplies, hip spica (one or both legs), pediatric (0-10 years), plaster   DME A B
    BETOS: D1A   Medical/surgical supplies

C Q4028 Cast supplies, hip spica (one or both legs), pediatric (0-10 years), fiberglass   DME A B
    BETOS: D1A   Medical/surgical supplies

C Q4029 Cast supplies, long leg cast, adult (11 years +), plaster   DME A B
    BETOS: D1A   Medical/surgical supplies

C Q4030 Cast supplies, long leg cast, adult (11 years +), fiberglass   DME A B
    BETOS: D1A   Medical/surgical supplies

C Q4031 Cast supplies, long leg cast, pediatric (0-10 years), plaster   DME A B
    BETOS: D1A   Medical/surgical supplies

C Q4032 Cast supplies, long leg cast, pediatric (0-10 years), fiberglass   DME A B
    BETOS: D1A   Medical/surgical supplies

C Q4033 Cast supplies, long leg cylinder cast, adult (11 years +), plaster   DME A B
    BETOS: D1A   Medical/surgical supplies

C Q4034 Cast supplies, long leg cylinder cast, adult (11 years +), fiberglass   DME A B
    BETOS: D1A   Medical/surgical supplies

C Q4035 Cast supplies, long leg cylinder cast, pediatric (0-10 years), plaster   DME A B
    BETOS: D1A   Medical/surgical supplies

C Q4036 Cast supplies, long leg cylinder cast, pediatric (0-10 years), fiberglass   DME A B
    BETOS: D1A   Medical/surgical supplies

C Q4037 Cast supplies, short leg cast, adult (11 years +), plaster   DME A B
    BETOS: D1A   Medical/surgical supplies

C Q4038 Cast supplies, short leg cast, adult (11 years +), fiberglass   DME A B
    BETOS: D1A   Medical/surgical supplies

C Q4039 Cast supplies, short leg cast, pediatric (0-10 years), plaster   DME A B
    BETOS: D1A   Medical/surgical supplies

C Q4040 Cast supplies, short leg cast, pediatric (0-10 years), fiberglass   DME A B
    BETOS: D1A   Medical/surgical supplies

● New code   ▲ Revised code   **C** Carrier judgment   **D** Special coverage instructions apply
I Not payable by Medicare   **M** Non-covered by Medicare   **S** Non-covered by Medicare statute   AHA Coding Clinic®

C **Q4041** Cast supplies, long leg splint, adult (11 years +), plaster `DME` Ⓐ B
BETOS: D1A   Medical/surgical supplies

C **Q4042** Cast supplies, long leg splint, adult (11 years +), fiberglass `DME` Ⓐ B
BETOS: D1A   Medical/surgical supplies

C **Q4043** Cast supplies, long leg splint, pediatric (0-10 years), plaster `DME` Ⓐ B
BETOS: D1A   Medical/surgical supplies

C **Q4044** Cast supplies, long leg splint, pediatric (0-10 years), fiberglass `DME` Ⓐ B
BETOS: D1A   Medical/surgical supplies

C **Q4045** Cast supplies, short leg splint, adult (11 years +), plaster `DME` Ⓐ B
BETOS: D1A   Medical/surgical supplies

C **Q4046** Cast supplies, short leg splint, adult (11 years +), fiberglass `DME` Ⓐ B
BETOS: D1A   Medical/surgical supplies

C **Q4047** Cast supplies, short leg splint, pediatric (0-10 years), plaster `DME` Ⓐ B
BETOS: D1A   Medical/surgical supplies

C **Q4048** Cast supplies, short leg splint, pediatric (0-10 years), fiberglass `DME` Ⓐ B
BETOS: D1A   Medical/surgical supplies

C **Q4049** Finger splint, static `DME` B
BETOS: D1A   Medical/surgical supplies
Coding Clinic: 2007, Q2

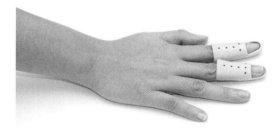

Finger splint

C **Q4050** Cast supplies, for unlisted types and materials of casts B
BETOS: D1A   Medical/surgical supplies
Other carrier priced

C **Q4051** Splint supplies, miscellaneous (includes thermoplastics, strapping, fasteners, padding and other supplies) B
BETOS: D1A   Medical/surgical supplies
Other carrier priced
Coding Clinic: 2002, Q2

MISCELLANEOUS DRUGS (Q4074-Q4082)

C **Q4074** Iloprost, inhalation solution, FDA-approved final product, non-compounded, administered through DME, unit dose form, up to 20 micrograms Y
BETOS: D1G   Drugs Administered through DME
Drugs: VENTAVIS

D **Q4081** Injection, epoetin alfa, 100 units (for ESRD on dialysis) N
BETOS: O1E   Other drugs
Other carrier priced
Drugs: EPOGEN, PROCRIT

C **Q4082** Drug or biological, not otherwise classified, Part B drug competitive acquisition program (CAP) B
BETOS: D1E   Other DME

SKIN SUBSTITUTES AND BIOLOGICALS (Q4100-Q4255)

C **Q4100** Skin substitute, not otherwise specified N1 ASC N
BETOS: O1E   Other drugs
Coding Clinic: 2009, Q1; 2008, Q4; 2012, Q2; 2010, Q1; 2018, Q2

C **Q4101** Apligraf, per square centimeter N1 ASC N
BETOS: O1E   Other drugs
Drugs: APLIGRAF
Coding Clinic: 2008, Q4; 2011, Q1; 2012, Q2; 2010, Q1

C **Q4102** Oasis wound matrix, per square centimeter N1 ASC N
BETOS: O1E   Other drugs
Drugs: OASIS WOUND MATRIX
Coding Clinic: 2008, Q4; 2011, Q1; 2012, Q2; 2012, Q3; 2010, Q1

C **Q4103** Oasis burn matrix, per square centimeter N1 ASC N
BETOS: O1E   Other drugs
Coding Clinic: 2008, Q4; 2011, Q1; 2012, Q2; 2010, Q1

C **Q4104** Integra bilayer matrix wound dressing (BMWD), per square centimeter N1 ASC N
BETOS: O1E   Other drugs
Coding Clinic: 2008, Q4; 2011, Q1; 2012, Q2; 2010, Q1; 2010, Q1; 2014, Q3

C **Q4105** Integra dermal regeneration template (DRT) or integra omnigraft dermal regeneration matrix, per square centimeter N1 ASC N
BETOS: O1E   Other drugs
Coding Clinic: 2008, Q4; 2011, Q1; 2012, Q2; 2010, Q1; 2010, Q1

C **Q4106** Dermagraft, per square centimeter N1 ASC N
BETOS: O1E   Other drugs
Drugs: DERMAGRAFT
Coding Clinic: 2008, Q4; 2011, Q1; 2012, Q2; 2010, Q1

♂ Male only   ♀ Female only   Ⓐ Age   A2 - Z3 = ASC Payment indicator   A - Y = APC Status indicator
ASC = ASC Approved Procedure   `DME` Paid under the DME fee schedule   `MIPS` MIPS code

C **Q4107** GRAFTJACKET, per square centimeter   N1 ASC N
BETOS: O1E   Other drugs
Coding Clinic: 2008, Q4; 2011, Q1; 2012, Q2; 2010, Q1

C **Q4108** Integra matrix, per square centimeter   N1 ASC N
BETOS: O1E   Other drugs
Coding Clinic: 2008, Q4; 2011, Q1; 2012, Q2; 2010, Q1; 2010, Q1

C **Q4110** PriMatrix, per square centimeter   N1 ASC N
BETOS: O1E   Other drugs
Drugs: PRIMATRIX, PRIMATRIX AG
Coding Clinic: 2008, Q4; 2011, Q1; 2012, Q2; 2010, Q1

C **Q4111** GammaGraft, per square centimeter   N1 ASC N
BETOS: O1E   Other drugs
Drugs: GAMMAGRAFT
Coding Clinic: 2009, Q1; 2008, Q4; 2011, Q1; 2012, Q2; 2010, Q1

C **Q4112** Cymetra, injectable, 1 cc   N1 ASC N
BETOS: O1E   Other drugs
Coding Clinic: 2008, Q4; 2011, Q1; 2012, Q2; 2010, Q1

C **Q4113** GRAFTJACKET XPRESS, injectable, 1 cc   N1 ASC N
BETOS: O1E   Other drugs
Coding Clinic: 2008, Q4; 2011, Q1; 2012, Q2; 2010, Q1

C **Q4114** Integra flowable wound matrix, injectable, 1 cc   N1 ASC N
BETOS: O1E   Other drugs
Coding Clinic: 2008, Q4; 2012, Q2; 2010, Q1; 2010, Q1

C **Q4115** AlloSkin, per square centimeter   N1 ASC N
BETOS: O1E   Other drugs
Coding Clinic: 2009, Q3; 2011, Q1; 2012, Q2; 2010, Q1

C **Q4116** AlloDerm, per square centimeter   N1 ASC N
BETOS: O1E   Other drugs
Coding Clinic: 2009, Q3; 2011, Q1; 2012, Q2; 2010, Q1

C **Q4117** HYALOMATRIX, per square centimeter   N1 ASC N
BETOS: O1E   Other drugs

C **Q4118** MatriStem micromatrix, 1 mg   N1 ASC N
BETOS: O1E   Other drugs
Coding Clinic: 2011, Q1; 2012, Q2; 2013, Q4

C **Q4121** TheraSkin, per square centimeter   N1 ASC N
BETOS: O1E   Other drugs
Drugs: THERASKIN
Coding Clinic: 2011, Q1; 2012, Q2

C **Q4122** DermACELL dermACELL AWM® or dermACELL AWM® porous, per square centimeter   N1 ASC N
BETOS: O1E   Other drugs
Coding Clinic: 2012, Q1; 2012, Q2

C **Q4123** AlloSkin RT, per square centimeter   N1 ASC N
BETOS: O1E   Other drugs

C **Q4124** OASIS ultra tri-layer wound matrix, per square centimeter   N1 ASC N
BETOS: O1E   Other drugs
Coding Clinic: 2012, Q2

C **Q4125** Arthroflex, per square centimeter   N1 ASC N
BETOS: O1E   Other drugs

C **Q4126** MemoDerm, DermaSpan, TranZgraft or InteguPly, per square centimeter   N1 ASC N
BETOS: O1E   Other drugs

C **Q4127** Talymed, per square centimeter   N1 ASC N
BETOS: O1E   Other drugs

C **Q4128** FlexHD, AllopatchHD, or MatrixHD, per square centimeter   N1 ASC N
BETOS: O1E   Other drugs

C **Q4130** Strattice TM, per square centimeter N1 ASC N
BETOS: O1E   Other drugs
Coding Clinic: 2012, Q2

C **Q4132** Grafix CORE and GrafixPL CORE, per square centimeter   N1 ASC N
BETOS: O1E   Other drugs
Drugs: GRAFIX CORE

C **Q4133** Grafix prime, GrafixPL PRIME™, Stravix® and StravixPL, per square centimeter   N1 ASC N
BETOS: O1E   Other drugs
Drugs: GRAFIX PRIME, GRAFIX XC, GRAFIXPL PRIME, STRAVIX

C **Q4134** Hmatrix, per square centimeter   N1 ASC N
BETOS: O1E   Other drugs

C **Q4135** Mediskin, per square centimeter   N1 ASC N
BETOS: O1E   Other drugs

C **Q4136** E-Z Derm, per square centimeter   N1 ASC N
BETOS: O1E   Other drugs

C **Q4137** Amnioexcel®, Aminoexcel Plus® or BioDExCel™, per square centimeter N1 ASC N
BETOS: O1E   Other drugs
Drugs: AMNIOEXCEL, AMNIOEXCEL PLUS

C **Q4138** BioDFence dryflex, per square centimeter   N1 ASC N
BETOS: O1E   Other drugs
Coding Clinic: 2014, Q1

C **Q4139** AmnioMatrix or biodmatrix, injectable, 1 cc   N1 ASC N
BETOS: O1E   Other drugs
Coding Clinic: 2014, Q1

C **Q4140** Biodfence, per square centimeter   N1 ASC N
BETOS: O1E   Other drugs
Coding Clinic: 2014, Q1

C **Q4141** AlloSkin AC, per square centimeter N1 ASC N
BETOS: O1E   Other drugs
Coding Clinic: 2014, Q1

● New code   ▲ Revised code   **C** Carrier judgment   **D** Special coverage instructions apply
I Not payable by Medicare   **M** Non-covered by Medicare   **S** Non-covered by Medicare statute   AHA Coding Clinic®

C Q4142 XCM BIOLOGIC tissue matrix, per square centimeter   N1 ASC N
BETOS: O1E   Other drugs
Coding Clinic: 2014, Q1

C Q4143 Repriza, per square centimeter   N1 ASC N
BETOS: O1E   Other drugs
Coding Clinic: 2014, Q1

C Q4145 EpiFix, injectable, 1 mg   N1 ASC N
BETOS: O1E   Other drugs
Drugs: EPIFIX MICRONIZED AMNIOTIC MEMBRANE ALLOGRAFT
Coding Clinic: 2014, Q1

C Q4146 Tensix, per square centimeter   N1 ASC N
BETOS: O1E   Other drugs
Coding Clinic: 2014, Q1

C Q4147 Architect, Architect PX, or Architect FX, extracellular matrix, per square centimeter   N1 ASC N
BETOS: O1E   Other drugs
Coding Clinic: 2014, Q1

C Q4148 NEOX CORD 1K, NEOX CORD RT, or CLARIX CORD 1K, per square centimeter   N1 ASC N
BETOS: O1E   Other drugs
Coding Clinic: 2014, Q1

C Q4149 Excellagen, 0.1 cc   N1 ASC N
BETOS: O1E   Other drugs
Coding Clinic: 2014, Q1

C Q4150 Allowrap DS or Dry, per square centimeter   N1 ASC N
BETOS: O1E   Other drugs
Coding Clinic: 2014, Q4

C Q4151 AmnioBand or Guardian, per square centimeter   N1 ASC N
BETOS: O1E   Other drugs
Drugs: AMNIOBAND MEMBRANE, AMNIOBAND VIABLE, WC AMNIOBAND
Coding Clinic: 2014, Q4

C Q4152 DermaPure, per square centimeter N1 ASC N
BETOS: O1E   Other drugs
Coding Clinic: 2014, Q4

C Q4153 Dermavest and plurivest, per square centimeter   N1 ASC N
BETOS: O1E   Other drugs
Coding Clinic: 2014, Q4; 2016, Q1

C Q4154 Biovance, per square centimeter   N1 ASC N
BETOS: O1E   Other drugs
Drugs: BIOVANCE
Coding Clinic: 2014, Q4

C Q4155 NeoxFlo or clarixFlo, 1 mg   N1 ASC N
BETOS: O1E   Other drugs
Coding Clinic: 2014, Q4

C Q4156 NEOX 100 or CLARIX 100, per square centimeter   N1 ASC N
BETOS: O1E   Other drugs
Coding Clinic: 2014, Q4

C Q4157 Revitalon, per square centimeter   N1 ASC N
BETOS: O1E   Other drugs
Coding Clinic: 2014, Q4

C Q4158 Kerecis Omega3, per square centimeter   N1 ASC N
BETOS: O1E   Other drugs
Coding Clinic: 2014, Q4

C Q4159 Affinity, per square centimeter   N1 ASC N
BETOS: O1E   Other drugs
Coding Clinic: 2014, Q4

C Q4160 NuShield, per square centimeter   N1 ASC N
BETOS: O1E   Other drugs
Drugs: NUSHIELD
Coding Clinic: 2014, Q4

C Q4161 Bio-ConneKt wound matrix, per square centimeter   N1 ASC N
BETOS: O1E   Other drugs
Coding Clinic: 2016, Q1

C Q4162 WoundEx Flow, BioSkin Flow, 0.5 cc   N1 ASC N
BETOS: O1E   Other drugs
Coding Clinic: 2016, Q1

C Q4163 WoundEx, BioSkin, per square centimeter   N1 ASC N
BETOS: O1E   Other drugs
Coding Clinic: 2016, Q1

C Q4164 Helicoll, per square centimeter   N1 ASC N
BETOS: O1E   Other drugs
Coding Clinic: 2016, Q1

C Q4165 Keramatrix or kerasorb, per square centimeter   N1 ASC N
BETOS: O1E   Other drugs
Coding Clinic: 2016, Q1

C Q4166 Cytal, per square centimeter   N1 ASC N
BETOS: O1E   Other drugs
Coding Clinic: 2017, Q1

C Q4167 Truskin, per square centimeter   N1 ASC N
BETOS: O1E   Other drugs
Coding Clinic: 2017, Q1

C Q4168 Amnioband, 1 mg   N1 ASC N
BETOS: O1E   Other drugs
Coding Clinic: 2017, Q1

C Q4169 Artacent wound, per square centimeter   N1 ASC N
BETOS: O1E   Other drugs
Coding Clinic: 2017, Q1

C Q4170 Cygnus, per square centimeter   N1 ASC N
BETOS: O1E   Other drugs
Coding Clinic: 2017, Q1

C Q4171 Interfyl, 1 mg   N1 ASC N
BETOS: O1E   Other drugs
Coding Clinic: 2017, Q1

♂ Male only   ♀ Female only   **A** Age   A2 - Z3 = ASC Payment indicator   A - Y = APC Status indicator
ASC = ASC Approved Procedure   **DME** Paid under the DME fee schedule   **MIPS** MIPS code

C Q4173 Palingen or palingen xplus, per square centimeter   N1 ASC N
BETOS: O1E   Other drugs
Coding Clinic: 2017, Q1

C Q4174 Palingen or promatrx, 0.36 mg per 0.25 cc   N1 ASC N
BETOS: O1E   Other drugs
Coding Clinic: 2017, Q1

C Q4175 Miroderm, per square centimeter   N1 ASC N
BETOS: O1E   Other drugs
Coding Clinic: 2017, Q1

▲ **C Q4176** Neopatch or therion, per square centimeter   N1 ASC N
BETOS: O1E   Other drugs
Coding Clinic: 2018, Q1; 2020, Q2

C Q4177 Floweramnioflo, 0.1 cc   N1 ASC N
BETOS: O1E   Other drugs
Coding Clinic: 2018, Q1

C Q4178 Floweramniopatch, per square centimeter   N1 ASC N
BETOS: O1E   Other drugs
Coding Clinic: 2018, Q1

C Q4179 Flowerderm, per square centimeter N1 ASC N
BETOS: O1E   Other drugs
Coding Clinic: 2018, Q1

C Q4180 Revita, per square centimeter   N1 ASC N
BETOS: O1E   Other drugs
Coding Clinic: 2018, Q1

C Q4181 Amnio wound, per square centimeter   N1 ASC N
BETOS: O1E   Other drugs
Coding Clinic: 2018, Q1

C Q4182 Transcyte, per square centimeter   N1 ASC N
BETOS: O1E   Other drugs
Coding Clinic: 2018, Q1

C Q4183 Surgigraft, per square centimeter   N1 ASC N
BETOS: O1E   Other drugs
Coding Clinic: 2019, Q1

C Q4184 Cellesta or cellesta duo, per square centimeter   N1 ASC N
BETOS: O1E   Other drugs
Coding Clinic: 2019, Q1

C Q4185 Cellesta flowable amnion (25 mg per cc); per 0.5 cc   N1 ASC N
BETOS: O1E   Other drugs
Coding Clinic: 2019, Q1

C Q4186 EpiFix®, per square centimeter   N1 ASC N
BETOS: O1E   Other drugs
Drugs: EPIFIX, EPIFIX AMNIOTIC MEMBRANE ALLOGRAFT
Coding Clinic: 2019, Q1

C Q4187 EpiCord®, per square centimeter   N1 ASC N
BETOS: O1E   Other drugs
Coding Clinic: 2019, Q1

C Q4188 Amnioarmor, per square centimeter   N1 ASC N
BETOS: O1E   Other drugs
Coding Clinic: 2019, Q1

C Q4189 Artacent AC, 1 mg   N1 ASC N
BETOS: O1E   Other drugs
Coding Clinic: 2019, Q1

C Q4190 Artacent AC, per square centimeter   N1 ASC N
BETOS: O1E   Other drugs
Coding Clinic: 2019, Q1

C Q4191 Restorigin™, per square centimeter N1 ASC N
BETOS: O1E   Other drugs
Coding Clinic: 2019, Q1

C Q4192 Restorigin™, 1 cc   N1 ASC N
BETOS: O1E   Other drugs
Coding Clinic: 2019, Q1

C Q4193 Coll-e-derm™, per square centimeter   N1 ASC N
BETOS: O1E   Other drugs
Coding Clinic: 2019, Q1

C Q4194 Novachor, per square centimeter N1 ASC N
BETOS: O1E   Other drugs
Coding Clinic: 2019, Q1

C Q4195 PuraPly®, per square centimeter   N1 ASC N
BETOS: O1E   Other drugs
Drugs: PURAPLY
Coding Clinic: 2019, Q1

C Q4196 PuraPly® AM, per square centimeter   N1 ASC N
BETOS: O1E   Other drugs
Drugs: PURAPLY AM
Coding Clinic: 2019, Q1

C Q4197 PuraPly® XT, per square centimeter   N1 ASC N
BETOS: O1E   Other drugs
Coding Clinic: 2019, Q1

C Q4198 Genesis amniotic membrane, per square centimeter   N1 ASC N
BETOS: O1E   Other drugs
Coding Clinic: 2019, Q1

C Q4200 Skin TE, per square centimeter   N1 ASC N
BETOS: O1E   Other drugs
Coding Clinic: 2019, Q1

C Q4201 Matrion, per square centimeter   N1 ASC N
BETOS: O1E   Other drugs
Coding Clinic: 2019, Q1

C Q4202 Keroxx (2.5g/cc), 1cc   N1 ASC N
BETOS: O1E   Other drugs
Coding Clinic: 2019, Q1

C Q4203 Derma-gide, per square centimeter   N1 ASC N
BETOS: O1E   Other drugs
Coding Clinic: 2019, Q1

● New code   ▲ Revised code   **C** Carrier judgment   **D** Special coverage instructions apply
I Not payable by Medicare   **M** Non-covered by Medicare   **S** Non-covered by Medicare statute   AHA Coding Clinic®

C Q4204 X-wrap, per square centimeter   N1 ASC N
BETOS: O1E   Other drugs
Coding Clinic: 2019, Q1

C Q4205 Membrane graft or membrane wrap, per square centimeter   N
BETOS: O1E   Other drugs
Coding Clinic: 2019, Q4

C Q4206 Fluid flow or fluid gf, 1 cc   N
BETOS: O1E   Other drugs
Coding Clinic: 2019, Q4

C Q4208 Novafix, per square centimeter   N
BETOS: O1E   Other drugs
Coding Clinic: 2019, Q4

C Q4209 Surgraft, per square centimeter   N
BETOS: O1E   Other drugs
Coding Clinic: 2019, Q4

C Q4210 Axolotl graft or Axolotl Dualgraft™, per square centimeter   N
BETOS: O1E   Other drugs
Coding Clinic: 2019, Q4

C Q4211 Amnion bio or axobiomembrane, per square centimeter   N
BETOS: O1E   Other drugs
Coding Clinic: 2019, Q4

C Q4212 AlloGen®, per cc   N
BETOS: O1E   Other drugs
Coding Clinic: 2019, Q4

C Q4213 Ascent, 0.5 mg   N
BETOS: O1E   Other drugs
Coding Clinic: 2019, Q4

C Q4214 Cellesta cord, per square centimeter   N
BETOS: O1E   Other drugs
Coding Clinic: 2019, Q4

C Q4215 Axolotl AmbientTM or Axolotl Cryo™, 0.1 mg   N
BETOS: O1E   Other drugs
Coding Clinic: 2019, Q4

C Q4216 Artacent cord, per square centimeter   N
BETOS: O1E   Other drugs
Coding Clinic: 2019, Q4

C Q4217 Woundfix, biowound, woundfix plus, biowound plus, woundfix xplus or biowound xplus, per square centimeter   N
BETOS: O1E   Other drugs
Coding Clinic: 2019, Q4

C Q4218 Surgicord, per square centimeter   N
BETOS: O1E   Other drugs
Coding Clinic: 2019, Q4

C Q4219 Surgigraft-dual, per square centimeter   N
BETOS: O1E   Other drugs
Coding Clinic: 2019, Q4

C Q4220 BellaCell HD or SureDerm®, per square centimeter   N
BETOS: O1E   Other drugs
Coding Clinic: 2019, Q4

C Q4221 AmnioWrap2™, per square centimeter   N
BETOS: O1E   Other drugs
Coding Clinic: 2019, Q4

C Q4222 ProgenaMatrix™, per square centimeter   N
BETOS: O1E   Other drugs
Coding Clinic: 2019, Q4

C Q4226 MyOwn Skin™, includes harvesting and preparation procedures, per square centimeter   N
BETOS: O1E   Other drugs
Coding Clinic: 2019, Q4

● C Q4227 Amniocore, per square centimeter N1 ASC N
BETOS: O1E   Other drugs
Coding Clinic: 2020, Q2

● C Q4228 Bionextpatch, per square centimeter   N1 ASC N
BETOS: O1E   Other drugs
Coding Clinic: 2020, Q2

● C Q4229 Cogenex amniotic membrane, per square centimeter   N1 ASC N
BETOS: O1E   Other drugs
Coding Clinic: 2020, Q2

● C Q4230 Cogenex flowable amnion, per 0.5 cc   N1 ASC N
BETOS: O1E   Other drugs
Coding Clinic: 2020, Q2

● C Q4231 Corplex p, per cc   N1 ASC N
BETOS: O1E   Other drugs
Coding Clinic: 2020, Q2

● C Q4232 Corplex, per square centimeter   N1 ASC N
BETOS: O1E   Other drugs
Coding Clinic: 2020, Q2

● C Q4233 Surfactor or nudyn, per 0.5 cc   N1 ASC N
BETOS: O1E   Other drugs
Coding Clinic: 2020, Q2

● C Q4234 Xcellerate, per square centimeter N1 ASC N
BETOS: O1E   Other drugs
Coding Clinic: 2020, Q2

● C Q4235 Amniorepair or altiply, per square centimeter   N1 ASC N
BETOS: O1E   Other drugs
Coding Clinic: 2020, Q2

● C Q4236 Carepatch, per square centimeter N1 ASC N
BETOS: O1E   Other drugs
Coding Clinic: 2020, Q2

● C Q4237 Cryo-cord, per square centimeter N1 ASC N
BETOS: O1E   Other drugs
Coding Clinic: 2020, Q2

♂ Male only   ♀ Female only   Ⓐ Age   A2 - Z3 = ASC Payment indicator   A - Y = APC Status indicator
ASC = ASC Approved Procedure   DME Paid under the DME fee schedule   MIPS MIPS code

● **C** **Q4238** Derm-maxx, per square
centimeter   N1 ASC N
BETOS: O1E   Other drugs
Coding Clinic: 2020, Q2

● **C** **Q4239** Amnio-maxx or amnio-maxx lite,
per square centimeter   N1 ASC N
BETOS: O1E   Other drugs
Coding Clinic: 2020, Q2

● **C** **Q4240** Corecyte, for topical use only,
per 0.5 cc   N1 ASC N
BETOS: O1E   Other drugs
Coding Clinic: 2020, Q2

● **C** **Q4241** Polycyte, for topical use only,
per 0.5 cc   N1 ASC N
BETOS: O1E   Other drugs
Coding Clinic: 2020, Q2

● **C** **Q4242** Amniocyte plus, per 0.5 cc   N1 ASC N
BETOS: O1E   Other drugs
Coding Clinic: 2020, Q2

● **C** **Q4244** Procenta, per 200 mg   N1 ASC N
BETOS: O1E   Other drugs
Coding Clinic: 2020, Q2

● **C** **Q4245** Amniotext, per cc   N1 ASC N
BETOS: O1E   Other drugs
Coding Clinic: 2020, Q2

● **C** **Q4246** Coretext or protext, per cc   N1 ASC N
BETOS: O1E   Other drugs
Coding Clinic: 2020, Q2

● **C** **Q4247** Amniotext patch, per square
centimeter   N1 ASC N
BETOS: O1E   Other drugs
Coding Clinic: 2020, Q2

● **C** **Q4248** Dermacyte amniotic membrane allograft,
per square centimeter   N1 ASC N
BETOS: O1E   Other drugs
Coding Clinic: 2020, Q2

● **C** **Q4249** Amniply, for topical use only, per square
centimeter   N
BETOS: O1E   Other drugs

● **C** **Q4250** Amnioamp-mp, per square centimeter   N
BETOS: O1E   Other drugs

● **C** **Q4254** Novafix dl, per square centimeter   N
BETOS: O1E   Other drugs

● **C** **Q4255** Reguard, for topical use only, per square
centimeter   N
BETOS: O1E   Other drugs

HOSPICE AND HOME HEALTH CARE (Q5001-Q5010)

D **Q5001** Hospice or home health care provided in
patient's home/residence   B
BETOS: Y2   Other - non-Medicare fee
schedule
Service not separately priced by Part B

Pub: 100-4, Chapter-10, 40.2; 100-4,
Chapter-11, 30.3

D **Q5002** Hospice or home health care provided in
assisted living facility   B
BETOS: Y2   Other - non-Medicare fee
schedule
Service not separately priced by Part B
Pub: 100-4, Chapter-11, 30.3; 100-4,
Chapter-10, 40.2

D **Q5003** Hospice care provided in nursing long term
care facility (LTC) or non-skilled nursing
facility (NF)   B
BETOS: Y2   Other - non-Medicare fee
schedule
Service not separately priced by Part B
Pub: 100-4, Chapter-11, 30.3

D **Q5004** Hospice care provided in skilled nursing
facility (SNF)   B
BETOS: Y2   Other - non-Medicare fee
schedule
Service not separately priced by Part B
Pub: 100-4, Chapter-11, 30.3

D **Q5005** Hospice care provided in inpatient hospital B
BETOS: Y2   Other - non-Medicare fee
schedule
Service not separately priced by Part B
Pub: 100-4, Chapter-11, 30.3

D **Q5006** Hospice care provided in inpatient hospice
facility   B
BETOS: Y2   Other - non-Medicare fee
schedule
Service not separately priced by Part B
Pub: 100-4, Chapter-11, 30.3

D **Q5007** Hospice care provided in long term care
facility   B
BETOS: Y2   Other - non-Medicare fee
schedule
Service not separately priced by Part B
Pub: 100-4, Chapter-11, 30.3

D **Q5008** Hospice care provided in inpatient
psychiatric facility   B
BETOS: Y2   Other - non-Medicare fee
schedule
Service not separately priced by Part B
Pub: 100-4, Chapter-11, 30.3

D **Q5009** Hospice or home health care provided in
place not otherwise specified (NOS)   B
BETOS: Y2   Other - non-Medicare fee
schedule
Service not separately priced by Part B
Pub: 100-4, Chapter-11, 30.3; 100-4,
Chapter-10, 40.2

D **Q5010** Hospice home care provided in a hospice
facility   B
BETOS: Y2   Other - non-Medicare fee
schedule
Service not separately priced by Part B
Pub: 100-4, Chapter-11, 30.3

● New code   ▲ Revised code   **C** Carrier judgment   **D** Special coverage instructions apply
I Not payable by Medicare   **M** Non-covered by Medicare   **S** Non-covered by Medicare statute   AHA Coding Clinic®

CHEMOTHERAPY MEDICATIONS (Q5101-Q5106), SEE ALSO
CHEMOTHERAPY ANTI-EMETIC MEDICATIONS (Q0161-Q0181)

D Q5101 Injection, filgrastim-sndz, biosimilar, (Zarxio),
1 microgram   K2 ASC K
BETOS: O1E   Other drugs
Drugs: ZARXIO® (FILGRASTIM-SNDZ)
Coding Clinic: 2016, Q2; 2018, Q1; 2018,
Q2

D Q5103 Injection, infliximab-dyyb, biosimilar,
(Inflectra), 10 mg   K2 ASC K
BETOS: O1E   Other drugs
Drugs: INFLECTRA
Coding Clinic: 2018, Q1; 2018, Q2; 2018,
Q2

D Q5104 Injection, infliximab-abda, biosimilar,
(Renflexis), 10 mg   K2 ASC K
BETOS: O1E   Other drugs
Drugs: RENFLEXIS
Coding Clinic: 2018, Q1; 2018, Q2; 2018,
Q2; 2018, Q2

D Q5105 Injection, epoetin alfa-epbx, biosimilar,
(Retacrit) (for ESRD on dialysis),
100 units   N1 ASC N
BETOS: O1E   Other drugs
Other carrier priced
Drugs: RETACRIT
Coding Clinic: 2018, Q2

D Q5106 Injection, epoetin alfa-epbx, biosimilar,
(Retacrit) (for non-ESRD use),
1000 units   K2 ASC K
BETOS: O1E   Other drugs
Drugs: RETACRIT
Coding Clinic: 2018, Q2

ANTI-INFLAMMATORY MEDICATION (Q5107-Q5111)

D Q5107 Injection, bevacizumab-awwb, biosimilar,
(MVASI), 10 mg   K2 ASC G
BETOS: O1E   Other drugs
Drugs: MVASI
Coding Clinic: 2019, Q1; 2019, Q4

C Q5108 Injection, pegfilgrastim-jmdb, biosimilar,
(Fulphila), 0.5 mg   K2 ASC G
BETOS: O1E   Other drugs
Drugs: FULPHILA (PEGFILGRASTIM-
JMDB)
Coding Clinic: 2018, Q3; 2018, Q4; 2019,
Q1

D Q5109 Injection, infliximab-qbtx, biosimilar, (IXIFI),
10 mg   K5 ASC E2
BETOS: O1E   Other drugs
Coding Clinic: 2019, Q1

D Q5110 Injection, filgrastim-aafi, biosimilar,
(Nivestym), 1 microgram   K2 ASC G
BETOS: O1E   Other drugs
Drugs: NIVESTYM
Coding Clinic: 2018, Q3; 2019, Q1

C Q5111 Injection, pegfilgrastim-cbqv, biosimilar,
(udenyca), 0.5 mg   K2 ASC G
BETOS: O1E   Other drugs
Drugs: UDENYCA (PEGFILGRASTIM-
CBQV)
Coding Clinic: 2019, Q1

CANCER TREATMENT DRUGS (Q5112-Q5122)

C Q5112 Injection, trastuzumab-dttb, biosimilar,
(Ontruzant), 10 mg   K2 ASC G
BETOS: O1E   Other drugs
Drugs: ONTRUZANT
Coding Clinic: 2019, Q3

C Q5113 Injection, trastuzumab-pkrb, biosimilar,
(HERZUMA®), 10 mg   K2 ASC G
BETOS: O1E   Other drugs
Drugs: HERZUMA
Coding Clinic: 2019, Q3

C Q5114 Injection, trastuzumab-dkst, biosimilar,
(Ogivri), 10 mg   K2 ASC G
BETOS: O1E   Other drugs
Drugs: OGIVRI
Coding Clinic: 2019, Q3

D Q5115 Injection, rituximab-abbs, biosimilar,
(Truxima), 10 mg   K2 ASC G
BETOS: O1D   Chemotherapy
Drugs: TRUXIMA
Coding Clinic: 2019, Q3

C Q5116 Injection, trastuzumab-qyyp, biosimilar,
(Trazimera), 10 mg   K2 ASC G
BETOS: O1E   Other drugs
Drugs: TRAZIMERA
Coding Clinic: 2019, Q4

C Q5117 Injection, trastuzumab-anns, biosimilar,
(KANJINTI™), 10 mg   K2 ASC G
BETOS: O1E   Other drugs
Drugs: KANJINTI
Coding Clinic: 2019, Q4

C Q5118 Injection, bevacizumab-bvzr, biosimilar,
(ZIRABEVTM), 10 mg   K2 ASC G
BETOS: O1E   Other drugs
Drugs: ZIRABEV
Coding Clinic: 2019, Q4

● **C Q5119** Injection, rituximab-pvvr, biosimilar,
(ruxience), 10 mg   K2 ASC G
BETOS: O1D   Chemotherapy
Drugs: RUXIENCE
Coding Clinic: 2020, Q2

● **C Q5120** Injection, pegfilgrastim-bmez, biosimilar,
(ziextenzo), 0.5 mg   K2 ASC G
BETOS: O1E   Other drugs
Drugs: ZIEXTENZO
Coding Clinic: 2020, Q2

♂ Male only   ♀ Female only   **A** Age   A2 - Z3 = ASC Payment indicator   A - Y = APC Status indicator
ASC = ASC Approved Procedure   **DME** Paid under the DME fee schedule   **MIPS** MIPS code

● [C] **Q5121** Injection, infliximab-axxq, biosimilar, (avsola), 10 mg　　　　　　　　　　　　K2 ASC G
BETOS: O1E　Other drugs
Drugs: AVSOLA
Coding Clinic: 2020, Q2

● [C] **Q5122** Injection, pegfilgrastim-apgf, biosimilar, (nyvepria), 0.5 mg　　　　　K5 ASC E2
BETOS: O1E　Other drugs

ASSESSMENT AND COUSELING-DEPARTMENT OF VETERANS AFFAIRS CHAPLAIN SERVICES (Q9001-Q9003)

● [C] **Q9001** Assessment by department of veterans affairs chaplain services　　　　　E1
BETOS: Z2　Undefined codes
Value not established

● [C] **Q9002** Counseling, individual, by department of veterans affairs chaplain services　　E1
BETOS: Z2　Undefined codes
Value not established

● [C] **Q9003** Counseling, group, by department of veterans affairs chaplain services　　　E1
BETOS: Z2　Undefined codes
Value not established

CONTRAST AGENTS/DIAGNOSTIC IMAGING (Q9950-Q9992), SEE ALSO IMAGING STUDIES (S8030-S8092)

[C] **Q9950** Injection, sulfur hexafluoride lipid microspheres, per ml　　　　N1 ASC N
BETOS: I1F　Standard imaging - other
Other carrier priced
Drugs: LUMASON
Coding Clinic: 2006, Q1; 2008, Q1; 2016, Q1; 2016, Q4

[D] **Q9951** Low osmolar contrast material, 400 or greater mg/ml iodine concentration, per ml　　　　　　　　　　　N1 ASC N
BETOS: I1E　Standard imaging - nuclear medicine
Coding Clinic: 2006, Q1; 2012, Q3

[D] **Q9953** Injection, iron-based magnetic resonance contrast agent, per ml　　N1 ASC N
BETOS: I1F　Standard imaging - other
Other carrier priced
Coding Clinic: 2006, Q1; 2012, Q3

[D] **Q9954** Oral magnetic resonance contrast agent, per 100 ml　　　　　N1 ASC N
BETOS: I1F　Standard imaging - other
Other carrier priced
Coding Clinic: 2006, Q1; 2012, Q3
Pub: 100-4, Chapter-13, 40

[C] **Q9955** Injection, perflexane lipid microspheres, per ml　　　　　　　N1 ASC N
BETOS: I1F　Standard imaging - other
Other carrier priced
Coding Clinic: 2012, Q3

[C] **Q9956** Injection, octafluoropropane microspheres, per ml　　　　　N1 ASC N
BETOS: I1F　Standard imaging - other
Other carrier priced
Drugs: OPTISON
Coding Clinic: 2012, Q3

[C] **Q9957** Injection, perflutren lipid microspheres, per ml　　　　　N1 ASC N
BETOS: I1F　Standard imaging - other
Other carrier priced
Drugs: DEFINITY
Coding Clinic: 2012, Q3

[D] **Q9958** High osmolar contrast material, up to 149 mg/ml iodine concentration, per ml　　　　　　　　　　N1 ASC N
BETOS: I1E　Standard imaging - nuclear medicine
Drugs: CONRAY 30, CYSTO-CONRAY II, CYSTOGRAFIN, CYSTOGRAFIN-DILUTE
Coding Clinic: 2005, Q3; 2007, Q1; 2011, Q4; 2012, Q3
Pub: 100-4, Chapter-13, 40

[D] **Q9959** High osmolar contrast material, 150-199 mg/ml iodine concentration, per ml　　　　　　　　　　N1 ASC N
BETOS: I1E　Standard imaging - nuclear medicine
Coding Clinic: 2005, Q3; 2007, Q1; 2012, Q3

[D] **Q9960** High osmolar contrast material, 200-249 mg/ml iodine concentration, per ml　　　　　　　　　　N1 ASC N
BETOS: I1E　Standard imaging - nuclear medicine
Drugs: CONRAY 43
Coding Clinic: 2005, Q3; 2007, Q1; 2012, Q3

[D] **Q9961** High osmolar contrast material, 250-299 mg/ml iodine concentration, per ml　　　　　　　　　　N1 ASC N
BETOS: I1E　Standard imaging - nuclear medicine
Drugs: CONRAY
Coding Clinic: 2005, Q3; 2007, Q1; 2012, Q3

[D] **Q9962** High osmolar contrast material, 300-349 mg/ml iodine concentration, per ml　　　　　　　　　　N1 ASC N
BETOS: I1E　Standard imaging - nuclear medicine
Coding Clinic: 2005, Q3; 2007, Q1; 2012, Q3

[D] **Q9963** High osmolar contrast material, 350-399 mg/ml iodine concentration, per ml　　　　　　　　　　N1 ASC N
BETOS: I1E　Standard imaging - nuclear medicine
Drugs: GASTROGRAFIN, MD GASTROVIEW, MD-76R
Coding Clinic: 2005, Q3; 2007, Q1; 2012, Q3

● New code　　▲ Revised code　　[C] Carrier judgment　　[D] Special coverage instructions apply
[I] Not payable by Medicare　　[M] Non-covered by Medicare　　[S] Non-covered by Medicare statute　　AHA Coding Clinic®

D Q9964 High osmolar contrast material, 400 or greater mg/ml iodine concentration, per ml   N1 ASC N
BETOS: I1E   Standard imaging - nuclear medicine
Coding Clinic: 2005, Q3; 2007, Q1; 2011, Q4; 2012, Q3
Pub: 100-4, Chapter-13, 40

D Q9965 Low osmolar contrast material, 100-199 mg/ml iodine concentration, per ml   N1 ASC N
BETOS: I1E   Standard imaging - nuclear medicine
Drugs: OMNIPAQUE 140, OMNIPAQUE 180
Coding Clinic: 2008, Q1; 2011, Q4; 2012, Q3

D Q9966 Low osmolar contrast material, 200-299 mg/ml iodine concentration, per ml   N1 ASC N
BETOS: I1E   Standard imaging - nuclear medicine
Drugs: ISOVUE-200, ISOVUE-250, ISOVUE-250 MULTIPACK, ISOVUE-M-200, OMNIPAQUE 240, OPTIRAY 240, ULTRAVIST 240, VISIPAQUE 270
Coding Clinic: 2008, Q1; 2012, Q3

D Q9967 Low osmolar contrast material, 300-399 mg/ml iodine concentration, per ml   N1 ASC N
BETOS: I1E   Standard imaging - nuclear medicine
Drugs: ISOVUE-300, ISOVUE-300 MULTI PACK, ISOVUE-370, ISOVUE-370 MULTI PACK, ISOVUE-M-300, OMNIPAQUE 300, OMNIPAQUE 300 (NOVAPLUS), OMNIPAQUE 350, OMNIPAQUE 350 (NOVAPLUS), OPTIRAY 300, OPTIRAY 320, OPTIRAY 350, OXILAN 350, ULTRAVIST 300, ULTRAVIST 370, VISIPAQUE 320
Coding Clinic: 2008, Q1; 2011, Q4; 2012, Q3

C Q9968 Injection, non-radioactive, non-contrast, visualization adjunct (e.g., methylene blue, isosulfan blue), 1 mg   K2 ASC K
BETOS: I1E   Standard imaging - nuclear medicine
Drugs: ISOSULFAN BLUE INJECTION, METHYLENE BLUE, PROVAYBLUE

D Q9969 Tc-99m from non-highly enriched uranium source, full cost recovery add-on, per study dose   K
BETOS: Y1   Other - Medicare fee schedule

D Q9982 Flutemetamol f18, diagnostic, per study dose, up to 5 millicuries   N1 ASC N
BETOS: I1E   Standard imaging - nuclear medicine
Service not separately priced by Part B
Coding Clinic: 2016, Q2; 2016, Q2

D Q9983 Florbetaben f18, diagnostic, per study dose, up to 8.1 millicuries   N1 ASC N
BETOS: I1E   Standard imaging - nuclear medicine
Service not separately priced by Part B
Coding Clinic: 2016, Q2; 2016, Q2

C Q9991 Injection, buprenorphine extended-release (Sublocade), less than or equal to 100 mg   K2 ASC K
BETOS: O1E   Other drugs
Drugs: SUBLOCADE
Coding Clinic: 2018, Q2

C Q9992 Injection, buprenorphine extended-release (Sublocade), greater than 100 mg   K2 ASC K
BETOS: O1E   Other drugs
Drugs: SUBLOCADE
Coding Clinic: 2018, Q2

NOTES

DIAGNOSTIC RADIOLOGY SERVICES
(R0070-R0076)

TRANSPORTATION, PORTABLE RADIOLOGY EQUIPMENT
(R0070-R0076)

D **R0070** Transportation of portable X-ray equipment and personnel to home or nursing home, per trip to facility or location, one patient seen   B
BETOS: I1F   Standard imaging - other
Price established by carriers

D **R0075** Transportation of portable X-ray equipment and personnel to home or nursing home, per trip to facility or location, more than one patient seen   B
BETOS: I1F   Standard imaging - other
Price established by carriers

D **R0076** Transportation of portable EKG to facility or location, per patient   B
BETOS: I1F   Standard imaging - other
Price established by carriers

♂ Male only   ♀ Female only   🅐 Age   A2 - Z3 = ASC Payment indicator   A - Y = APC Status indicator
ASC = ASC Approved Procedure   **DME** Paid under the DME fee schedule   **MIPS** MIPS code

383

NOTES

TEMPORARY NATIONAL CODES (NON-MEDICARE) (S0012-S9999)

NON-MEDICARE DRUG CODES (S0012-S0197)

S0012 Butorphanol tartrate, nasal spray, 25 mg
BETOS: Z2 Undefined codes
Service not separately priced by Part B

● **S0013** Esketamine, nasal spray, 1 mg Ⓐ
BETOS: Z2 Undefined codes
Service not separately priced by Part B

S0014 Tacrine hydrochloride, 10 mg
BETOS: Z2 Undefined codes
Service not separately priced by Part B

S0017 Injection, aminocaproic acid, 5 grams
BETOS: Z2 Undefined codes
Service not separately priced by Part B

S0020 Injection, bupivacaine hydrochloride, 30 ml
BETOS: Z2 Undefined codes
Service not separately priced by Part B

S0021 Injection, cefoperazone sodium, 1 gram
BETOS: Z2 Undefined codes
Service not separately priced by Part B

S0023 Injection, cimetidine hydrochloride, 300 mg
BETOS: Z2 Undefined codes
Service not separately priced by Part B

S0028 Injection, famotidine, 20 mg
BETOS: Z2 Undefined codes
Service not separately priced by Part B

S0030 Injection, metronidazole, 500 mg
BETOS: Z2 Undefined codes
Service not separately priced by Part B

S0032 Injection, nafcillin sodium, 2 grams
BETOS: Z2 Undefined codes
Service not separately priced by Part B

S0034 Injection, ofloxacin, 400 mg
BETOS: Z2 Undefined codes
Service not separately priced by Part B

S0039 Injection, sulfamethoxazole and trimethoprim, 10 ml
BETOS: Z2 Undefined codes
Service not separately priced by Part B

S0040 Injection, ticarcillin disodium and clavulanate potassium, 3.1 grams
BETOS: Z2 Undefined codes
Service not separately priced by Part B

S0073 Injection, aztreonam, 500 mg
BETOS: Z2 Undefined codes
Service not separately priced by Part B

S0074 Injection, cefotetan disodium, 500 mg
BETOS: Z2 Undefined codes
Service not separately priced by Part B

S0077 Injection, clindamycin phosphate, 300 mg
BETOS: Z2 Undefined codes
Service not separately priced by Part B

S0078 Injection, fosphenytoin sodium, 750 mg
BETOS: Z2 Undefined codes
Service not separately priced by Part B

S0080 Injection, pentamidine isethionate, 300 mg
BETOS: Z2 Undefined codes
Service not separately priced by Part B

S0081 Injection, piperacillin sodium, 500 mg
BETOS: Z2 Undefined codes
Service not separately priced by Part B

S0088 Imatinib, 100 mg
BETOS: Z2 Undefined codes
Service not separately priced by Part B

S0090 Sildenafil citrate, 25 mg
BETOS: Z2 Undefined codes
Service not separately priced by Part B

S0091 Granisetron hydrochloride, 1 mg (for circumstances falling under the Medicare statute, use Q0166)
BETOS: Z2 Undefined codes
Service not separately priced by Part B

S0092 Injection, hydromorphone hydrochloride, 250 mg (loading dose for infusion pump)
BETOS: Z2 Undefined codes
Service not separately priced by Part B

S0093 Injection, morphine sulfate, 500 mg (loading dose for infusion pump)
BETOS: Z2 Undefined codes
Service not separately priced by Part B

S0104 Zidovudine, oral, 100 mg
BETOS: Z2 Undefined codes
Service not separately priced by Part B

S0106 Bupropion HCL sustained release tablet, 150 mg, per bottle of 60 tablets
BETOS: Z2 Undefined codes
Service not separately priced by Part B

S0108 Mercaptopurine, oral, 50 mg
BETOS: Z2 Undefined codes
Service not separately priced by Part B

S0109 Methadone, oral, 5 mg
BETOS: Z2 Undefined codes
Service not separately priced by Part B

S0117 Tretinoin, topical, 5 grams
BETOS: Z2 Undefined codes
Service not separately priced by Part B

S0119 Ondansetron, oral, 4 mg (for circumstances falling under the Medicare statute, use HCPCS Q code)
BETOS: Z2 Undefined codes
Service not separately priced by Part B

♂ Male only   ♀ Female only   Ⓐ Age   A2 - Z3 = ASC Payment indicator   A - Y = APC Status indicator
ASC = ASC Approved Procedure   **DME** Paid under the DME fee schedule   **MIPS** MIPS code

S0122 Injection, menotropins, 75 IU
BETOS: Z2   Undefined codes
Service not separately priced by Part B

S0126 Injection, follitropin alfa, 75 IU
BETOS: Z2   Undefined codes
Service not separately priced by Part B

S0128 Injection, follitropin beta, 75 IU
BETOS: Z2   Undefined codes
Service not separately priced by Part B

S0132 Injection, ganirelix acetate, 250 mcg
BETOS: Z2   Undefined codes
Service not separately priced by Part B

S0136 Clozapine, 25 mg
BETOS: Z2   Undefined codes
Service not separately priced by Part B

S0137 Didanosine (ddi), 25 mg
BETOS: Z2   Undefined codes
Service not separately priced by Part B

S0138 Finasteride, 5 mg
BETOS: Z2   Undefined codes
Service not separately priced by Part B

S0139 Minoxidil, 10 mg
BETOS: Z2   Undefined codes
Service not separately priced by Part B

S0140 Saquinavir, 200 mg
BETOS: Z2   Undefined codes
Service not separately priced by Part B

S0142 Colistimethate sodium, inhalation solution administered through DME, concentrated form, per mg
BETOS: Z2   Undefined codes
Service not separately priced by Part B

S0145 Injection, pegylated interferon alfa-2a, 180 mcg per ml
BETOS: Z2   Undefined codes
Service not separately priced by Part B

S0148 Injection, pegylated interferon alfa-2b, 10 mcg
BETOS: Z2   Undefined codes
Service not separately priced by Part B

S0155 Sterile dilutant for epoprostenol, 50ml
BETOS: Z2   Undefined codes
Service not separately priced by Part B

S0156 Exemestane, 25 mg
BETOS: Z2   Undefined codes
Service not separately priced by Part B

S0157 Becaplermin gel 0.01%, 0.5 gm
BETOS: Z2   Undefined codes
Service not separately priced by Part B

S0160 Dextroamphetamine sulfate, 5 mg
BETOS: Z2   Undefined codes
Service not separately priced by Part B

S0164 Injection, pantoprazole sodium, 40 mg
BETOS: Z2   Undefined codes
Service not separately priced by Part B

S0166 Injection, olanzapine, 2.5 mg
BETOS: Z2   Undefined codes
Service not separately priced by Part B

S0169 Calcitrol, 0.25 microgram
BETOS: Z2   Undefined codes
Service not separately priced by Part B

S0170 Anastrozole, oral, 1 mg
BETOS: Z2   Undefined codes
Service not separately priced by Part B

S0171 Injection, bumetanide, 0.5 mg
BETOS: Z2   Undefined codes
Service not separately priced by Part B

S0172 Chlorambucil, oral, 2 mg
BETOS: Z2   Undefined codes
Service not separately priced by Part B

S0174 Dolasetron mesylate, oral 50 mg (for circumstances falling under the Medicare statute, use Q0180)
BETOS: Z2   Undefined codes
Service not separately priced by Part B

S0175 Flutamide, oral, 125 mg
BETOS: Z2   Undefined codes
Service not separately priced by Part B

S0176 Hydroxyurea, oral, 500 mg
BETOS: Z2   Undefined codes
Service not separately priced by Part B

S0177 Levamisole hydrochloride, oral, 50 mg
BETOS: Z2   Undefined codes
Service not separately priced by Part B

S0178 Lomustine, oral, 10 mg
BETOS: Z2   Undefined codes
Service not separately priced by Part B

S0179 Megestrol acetate, oral, 20 mg
BETOS: Z2   Undefined codes
Service not separately priced by Part B

S0182 Procarbazine hydrochloride, oral, 50 mg
BETOS: Z2   Undefined codes
Service not separately priced by Part B

S0183 Prochlorperazine maleate, oral, 5 mg (for circumstances falling under the Medicare statute, use Q0164)
BETOS: Z2   Undefined codes
Service not separately priced by Part B

S0187 Tamoxifen citrate, oral, 10 mg
BETOS: Z2   Undefined codes
Service not separately priced by Part B

S0189 Testosterone pellet, 75 mg
BETOS: Z2   Undefined codes
Service not separately priced by Part B

● New code   ▲ Revised code   **C** Carrier judgment   **D** Special coverage instructions apply
I Not payable by Medicare   **M** Non-covered by Medicare   **S** Non-covered by Medicare statute   *AHA Coding Clinic®*

■ S0190 Mifepristone, oral, 200 mg ♀
BETOS: Z2 Undefined codes
Service not separately priced by Part B

■ S0191 Misoprostol, oral, 200 mcg ♀ Ⓐ
BETOS: Z2 Undefined codes
Service not separately priced by Part B

■ S0194 Dialysis/stress vitamin supplement, oral, 100 capsules
BETOS: Z2 Undefined codes
Service not separately priced by Part B

■ S0197 Prenatal vitamins, 30-day supply ♀ Ⓐ
BETOS: Z2 Undefined codes
Service not separately priced by Part B

MISCELLANEOUS PROVIDER SERVICES (S0199-S0400), SEE ALSO MISCELLANEOUS PROVIDER SERVICES AND SUPPLIES (S0630-S3722)

■ S0199 Medically-induced abortion by oral ingestion of medication including all associated services and supplies (e.g., patient counseling, office visits, confirmation of pregnancy by HCG, ultrasound to confirm duration of pregnancy, ultrasound to confirm completion of abortion) except drugs ♀ Ⓐ
BETOS: Z2 Undefined codes
Service not separately priced by Part B

■ S0201 Partial hospitalization services, less than 24 hours, per diem [MIPS]
BETOS: Z2 Undefined codes
Service not separately priced by Part B

■ S0207 Paramedic intercept, non-hospital-based ALS service (non-voluntary), non-transport
BETOS: Z2 Undefined codes
Service not separately priced by Part B

■ S0208 Paramedic intercept, hospital-based ALS service (non-voluntary), non-transport
BETOS: Z2 Undefined codes
Service not separately priced by Part B

■ S0209 Wheelchair van, mileage, per mile
BETOS: Z2 Undefined codes
Service not separately priced by Part B

■ S0215 Non-emergency transportation; mileage, per mile
BETOS: Z2 Undefined codes
Service not separately priced by Part B

■ S0220 Medical conference by a physician with interdisciplinary team of health professionals or representatives of community agencies to coordinate activities of patient care (patient is present); approximately 30 minutes
BETOS: Z2 Undefined codes
Service not separately priced by Part B

■ S0221 Medical conference by a physician with interdisciplinary team of health professionals or representatives of community agencies to coordinate activities of patient care (patient is present); approximately 60 minutes
BETOS: Z2 Undefined codes
Service not separately priced by Part B

■ S0250 Comprehensive geriatric assessment and treatment planning performed by assessment team
BETOS: Z2 Undefined codes
Service not separately priced by Part B

■ S0255 Hospice referral visit (advising patient and family of care options) performed by nurse, social worker, or other designated staff
BETOS: Z2 Undefined codes
Service not separately priced by Part B

■ S0257 Counseling and discussion regarding advance directives or end of life care planning and decisions, with patient and/or surrogate (list separately in addition to code for appropriate evaluation and management service)
BETOS: Z2 Undefined codes
Service not separately priced by Part B

■ S0260 History and physical (outpatient or office) related to surgical procedure (list separately in addition to code for appropriate evaluation and management service)
BETOS: Z2 Undefined codes
Service not separately priced by Part B

■ S0265 Genetic counseling, under physician supervision, each 15 minutes
BETOS: Z2 Undefined codes
Service not separately priced by Part B

■ S0270 Physician management of patient home care, standard monthly case rate (per 30 days)
BETOS: Z2 Undefined codes
Service not separately priced by Part B

■ S0271 Physician management of patient home care, hospice monthly case rate (per 30 days)
BETOS: Z2 Undefined codes
Service not separately priced by Part B

■ S0272 Physician management of patient home care, episodic care monthly case rate (per 30 days)
BETOS: Z2 Undefined codes
Service not separately priced by Part B

■ S0273 Physician visit at member's home, outside of a capitation arrangement
BETOS: Z2 Undefined codes
Service not separately priced by Part B

■ S0274 Nurse practitioner visit at member's home, outside of a capitation arrangement
BETOS: Z2 Undefined codes
Service not separately priced by Part B

♂ Male only   ♀ Female only   Ⓐ Age   A2 - Z3 = ASC Payment indicator   A - Y = APC Status indicator
ASC = ASC Approved Procedure   **DME** Paid under the DME fee schedule   **MIPS** MIPS code

TEMPORARY NATIONAL CODES (NON-MEDICARE) (S0012-S9999)

S0280 - S0510

I **S0280** Medical home program, comprehensive care coordination and planning, initial plan
BETOS: Z2   Undefined codes
Service not separately priced by Part B

I **S0281** Medical home program, comprehensive care coordination and planning, maintenance of plan
BETOS: Z2   Undefined codes
Service not separately priced by Part B

I **S0285** Colonoscopy consultation performed prior to a screening colonoscopy procedure
BETOS: Z2   Undefined codes
Service not separately priced by Part B
Coding Clinic: 2016, Q2

I **S0302** Completed early periodic screening diagnosis and treatment (EPSDT) service (list in addition to code for appropriate evaluation and management service) Ⓐ
BETOS: Z2   Undefined codes
Service not separately priced by Part B

I **S0310** Hospitalist services (list separately in addition to code for appropriate evaluation and management service)
BETOS: Z2   Undefined codes
Service not separately priced by Part B

I **S0311** Comprehensive management and care coordination for advanced illness, per calendar month
BETOS: Z2   Undefined codes
Service not separately priced by Part B
Coding Clinic: 2016, Q2

I **S0315** Disease management program; initial assessment and initiation of the program
BETOS: Z2   Undefined codes
Service not separately priced by Part B

I **S0316** Disease management program, follow-up/reassessment
BETOS: Z2   Undefined codes
Service not separately priced by Part B

I **S0317** Disease management program; per diem
BETOS: Z2   Undefined codes
Service not separately priced by Part B

I **S0320** Telephone calls by a registered nurse to a disease management program member for monitoring purposes; per month
BETOS: Z2   Undefined codes
Service not separately priced by Part B

I **S0340** Lifestyle modification program for management of coronary artery disease, including all supportive services; first quarter / stage
BETOS: Z2   Undefined codes
Service not separately priced by Part B

I **S0341** Lifestyle modification program for management of coronary artery disease,

including all supportive services; second or third quarter / stage
BETOS: Z2   Undefined codes
Service not separately priced by Part B

I **S0342** Lifestyle modification program for management of coronary artery disease, including all supportive services; fourth quarter / stage
BETOS: Z2   Undefined codes
Service not separately priced by Part B

I **S0353** Treatment planning and care coordination management for cancer, initial treatment
BETOS: Z2   Undefined codes
Service not separately priced by Part B

I **S0354** Treatment planning and care coordination management for cancer, established patient with a change of regimen
BETOS: Z2   Undefined codes
Service not separately priced by Part B

I **S0390** Routine foot care; removal and/or trimming of corns, calluses and/or nails and preventive maintenance in specific medical conditions (e.g., diabetes), per visit
BETOS: Z2   Undefined codes
Service not separately priced by Part B

I **S0395** Impression casting of a foot performed by a practitioner other than the manufacturer of the orthotic
BETOS: Z2   Undefined codes
Service not separately priced by Part B

I **S0400** Global fee for extracorporeal shock wave lithotripsy treatment of kidney stone(s)
BETOS: Z2   Undefined codes
Service not separately priced by Part B

VISION SUPPLIES (S0500-S0596)

I **S0500** Disposable contact lens, per lens
BETOS: Z2   Undefined codes
Service not separately priced by Part B

I **S0504** Single vision prescription lens (safety, athletic, or sunglass), per lens
BETOS: Z2   Undefined codes
Service not separately priced by Part B

I **S0506** Bifocal vision prescription lens (safety, athletic, or sunglass), per lens
BETOS: Z2   Undefined codes
Service not separately priced by Part B

I **S0508** Trifocal vision prescription lens (safety, athletic, or sunglass), per lens
BETOS: Z2   Undefined codes
Service not separately priced by Part B

I **S0510** Non-prescription lens (safety, athletic, or sunglass), per lens
BETOS: Z2   Undefined codes
Service not separately priced by Part B

● New code   ▲ Revised code   **C** Carrier judgment   **D** Special coverage instructions apply
I Not payable by Medicare   **M** Non-covered by Medicare   **S** Non-covered by Medicare statute   *AHA Coding Clinic®*

S0512 Daily wear specialty contact lens, per lens
BETOS: Z2 Undefined codes
Service not separately priced by Part B

S0514 Color contact lens, per lens
BETOS: Z2 Undefined codes
Service not separately priced by Part B

S0515 Scleral lens, liquid bandage device, per lens
BETOS: Z2 Undefined codes
Service not separately priced by Part B

S0516 Safety eyeglass frames
BETOS: Z2 Undefined codes
Service not separately priced by Part B

S0518 Sunglasses frames
BETOS: Z2 Undefined codes
Service not separately priced by Part B

S0580 Polycarbonate lens (list this code in addition to the basic code for the lens)
BETOS: Z2 Undefined codes
Service not separately priced by Part B

S0581 Nonstandard lens (list this code in addition to the basic code for the lens)
BETOS: Z2 Undefined codes
Service not separately priced by Part B

S0590 Integral lens service, miscellaneous services reported separately
BETOS: Z2 Undefined codes
Service not separately priced by Part B

S0592 Comprehensive contact lens evaluation
BETOS: Z2 Undefined codes
Service not separately priced by Part B

S0595 Dispensing new spectacle lenses for patient supplied frame
BETOS: Z2 Undefined codes
Service not separately priced by Part B

S0596 Phakic intraocular lens for correction of refractive error
BETOS: Z2 Undefined codes
Service not separately priced by Part B

SCREENINGS AND EXAMINATIONS (S0601-S0622)

S0601 Screening proctoscopy
BETOS: Z2 Undefined codes
Service not separately priced by Part B

S0610 Annual gynecological examination, new patient ♀
BETOS: Z2 Undefined codes
Service not separately priced by Part B

S0612 Annual gynecological examination, established patient ♀
BETOS: Z2 Undefined codes
Service not separately priced by Part B

S0613 Annual gynecological examination; clinical breast examination without pelvic evaluation ♀
BETOS: Z2 Undefined codes
Service not separately priced by Part B

S0618 Audiometry for hearing aid evaluation to determine the level and degree of hearing loss
BETOS: Z2 Undefined codes
Service not separately priced by Part B

S0620 Routine ophthalmological examination including refraction; new patient
BETOS: Z2 Undefined codes
Service not separately priced by Part B

S0621 Routine ophthalmological examination including refraction; established patient
BETOS: Z2 Undefined codes
Service not separately priced by Part B

S0622 Physical exam for college, new or established patient (list separately in addition to appropriate evaluation and management code)
BETOS: Z2 Undefined codes
Service not separately priced by Part B

MISCELLANEOUS PROVIDER SERVICES AND SUPPLIES (S0630-S3722), SEE ALSO MISCELLANEOUS PROVIDER SERVICES (S0199-S0400)

S0630 Removal of sutures; by a physician other than the physician who originally closed the wound
BETOS: Z2 Undefined codes
Service not separately priced by Part B

S0800 Laser in situ keratomileusis (LASIK)
BETOS: Z2 Undefined codes
Service not separately priced by Part B

S0810 Photorefractive keratectomy (PRK)
BETOS: Z2 Undefined codes
Service not separately priced by Part B

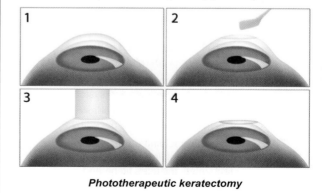

Phototherapeutic keratectomy

S0812 Phototherapeutic keratectomy (PTK)
BETOS: Z2 Undefined codes
Service not separately priced by Part B

S1001 Deluxe item, patient aware (list in addition to code for basic item)
BETOS: Z2   Undefined codes
Service not separately priced by Part B

S1002 Customized item (list in addition to code for basic item)
BETOS: Z2   Undefined codes
Service not separately priced by Part B

S1015 IV tubing extension set
BETOS: Z2   Undefined codes
Service not separately priced by Part B

S1016 Non-PVC (polyvinyl chloride) intravenous administration set, for use with drugs that are not stable in PVC e.g. paclitaxel
BETOS: Z2   Undefined codes
Service not separately priced by Part B

S1030 Continuous noninvasive glucose monitoring device, purchase (for physician interpretation of data, use CPT® code)
BETOS: Z2   Undefined codes
Service not separately priced by Part B

S1031 Continuous noninvasive glucose monitoring device, rental, including sensor, sensor replacement, and download to monitor (for physician interpretation of data, use CPT® code)
BETOS: Z2   Undefined codes
Service not separately priced by Part B

S1034 Artificial pancreas device system (e.g., low glucose suspend (LGS) feature) including continuous glucose monitor, blood glucose device, insulin pump and computer algorithm that communicates with all of the devices
BETOS: Z2   Undefined codes
Service not separately priced by Part B

S1035 Sensor; invasive (e.g., subcutaneous), disposable, for use with artificial pancreas device system
BETOS: Z2   Undefined codes
Service not separately priced by Part B

S1036 Transmitter; external, for use with artificial pancreas device system
BETOS: Z2   Undefined codes
Service not separately priced by Part B

S1037 Receiver (monitor); external, for use with artificial pancreas device system
BETOS: Z2   Undefined codes
Service not separately priced by Part B

S1040 Cranial remolding orthosis, pediatric, rigid, with soft interface material, custom fabricated, includes fitting and adjustment(s) Ⓐ
BETOS: Z2   Undefined codes
Service not separately priced by Part B

S2053 Transplantation of small intestine and liver allografts

BETOS: Z2   Undefined codes
Service not separately priced by Part B

S2054 Transplantation of multivisceral organs
BETOS: Z2   Undefined codes
Service not separately priced by Part B

S2055 Harvesting of donor multivisceral organs, with preparation and maintenance of allografts; from cadaver donor
BETOS: Z2   Undefined codes
Service not separately priced by Part B

S2060 Lobar lung transplantation
BETOS: Z2   Undefined codes
Service not separately priced by Part B

S2061 Donor lobectomy (lung) for transplantation, living donor
BETOS: Z2   Undefined codes
Service not separately priced by Part B

S2065 Simultaneous pancreas kidney transplantation
BETOS: Z2   Undefined codes
Service not separately priced by Part B

S2066 Breast reconstruction with gluteal artery perforator (GAP) flap, including harvesting of the flap, microvascular transfer, closure of donor site and shaping the flap into a breast, unilateral
BETOS: Z2   Undefined codes
Service not separately priced by Part B

S2067 Breast reconstruction of a single breast with "stacked" deep inferior epigastric perforator (DIEP) flap(s) and/or gluteal artery perforator (GAP) flap(s), including harvesting of the flap(s), microvascular transfer, closure of donor site(s) and shaping the flap into a breast, unilateral
BETOS: Z2   Undefined codes
Service not separately priced by Part B

S2068 Breast reconstruction with deep inferior epigastric perforator (DIEP) flap or superficial inferior epigastric artery (SIEA) flap, including harvesting of the flap, microvascular transfer, closure of donor site and shaping the flap into a breast, unilateral
BETOS: Z2   Undefined codes
Service not separately priced by Part B

S2070 Cystourethroscopy, with ureteroscopy and/or pyeloscopy; with endoscopic laser treatment of ureteral calculi (includes ureteral catheterization)
BETOS: Z2   Undefined codes
Service not separately priced by Part B

S2079 Laparoscopic esophagomyotomy (Heller type)
BETOS: Z2   Undefined codes
Service not separately priced by Part B

● New code   ▲ Revised code   **C** Carrier judgment   **D** Special coverage instructions apply
I Not payable by Medicare   **M** Non-covered by Medicare   **S** Non-covered by Medicare statute   AHA Coding Clinic®

S2080 Laser-assisted uvulopalatoplasty (LAUP)
BETOS: Z2 Undefined codes
Service not separately priced by Part B

S2083 Adjustment of gastric band diameter via subcutaneous port by injection or aspiration of saline
BETOS: Z2 Undefined codes
Service not separately priced by Part B

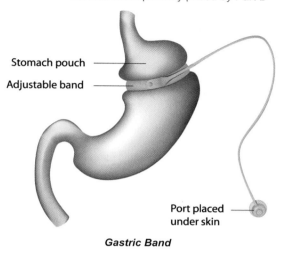

Stomach pouch

Adjustable band

Port placed under skin

Gastric Band

S2095 Transcatheter occlusion or embolization for tumor destruction, percutaneous, any method, using yttrium-90 microspheres
BETOS: Z2 Undefined codes
Service not separately priced by Part B

S2102 Islet cell tissue transplant from pancreas; allogeneic
BETOS: Z2 Undefined codes
Service not separately priced by Part B

S2103 Adrenal tissue transplant to brain
BETOS: Z2 Undefined codes
Service not separately priced by Part B

S2107 Adoptive immunotherapy i.e. development of specific anti-tumor reactivity (e.g., tumor-infiltrating lymphocyte therapy) per course of treatment
BETOS: Z2 Undefined codes
Service not separately priced by Part B

S2112 Arthroscopy, knee, surgical for harvesting of cartilage (chondrocyte cells)
BETOS: Z2 Undefined codes
Service not separately priced by Part B

S2115 Osteotomy, periacetabular, with internal fixation
BETOS: Z2 Undefined codes
Service not separately priced by Part B

S2117 Arthroereisis, subtalar
BETOS: Z2 Undefined codes
Service not separately priced by Part B

S2118 Metal-on-metal total hip resurfacing, including acetabular and femoral components
BETOS: Z2 Undefined codes
Service not separately priced by Part B

S2120 Low density lipoprotein (LDL) apheresis using heparin-induced extracorporeal LDL precipitation
BETOS: Z2 Undefined codes
Service not separately priced by Part B

S2140 Cord blood harvesting for transplantation, allogeneic ♀ Ⓐ
BETOS: Z2 Undefined codes
Service not separately priced by Part B

S2142 Cord blood-derived stem-cell transplantation, allogeneic ♀ Ⓐ
BETOS: Z2 Undefined codes
Service not separately priced by Part B

S2150 Bone marrow or blood-derived stem cells (peripheral or umbilical), allogeneic or autologous, harvesting, transplantation, and related complications; including: pheresis and cell preparation/storage; marrow ablative therapy; drugs, supplies, hospitalization with outpatient follow-up; medical/surgical, diagnostic, emergency, and rehabilitative services; and the number of days of pre-and post-transplant care in the global definition
BETOS: Z2 Undefined codes
Service not separately priced by Part B

S2152 Solid organ(s), complete or segmental, single organ or combination of organs; deceased or living donor(s), procurement, transplantation, and related complications; including: drugs; supplies; hospitalization with outpatient follow-up; medical/surgical, diagnostic, emergency, and rehabilitative services, and the number of days of pre- and post-transplant care in the global definition
BETOS: Z2 Undefined codes
Service not separately priced by Part B

S2202 Echosclerotherapy
BETOS: Z2 Undefined codes
Service not separately priced by Part B

S2205 Minimally invasive direct coronary artery bypass surgery involving mini-thoracotomy or mini-sternotomy surgery, performed under direct vision; using arterial graft(s), single coronary arterial graft [MIPS]
BETOS: Z2 Undefined codes
Service not separately priced by Part B

S2206 Minimally invasive direct coronary artery bypass surgery involving mini-thoracotomy or mini-sternotomy surgery, performed under direct vision; using arterial graft(s), two coronary arterial grafts [MIPS]
BETOS: Z2 Undefined codes
Service not separately priced by Part B

S2207 Minimally invasive direct coronary artery bypass surgery involving mini-thoracotomy or mini-sternotomy surgery, performed under direct vision; using venous graft only, single coronary venous graft **MIPS**
BETOS: Z2   Undefined codes
Service not separately priced by Part B

S2208 Minimally invasive direct coronary artery bypass surgery involving mini-thoracotomy or mini-sternotomy surgery, performed under direct vision; using single arterial and venous graft(s), single venous graft **MIPS**
BETOS: Z2   Undefined codes
Service not separately priced by Part B

S2209 Minimally invasive direct coronary artery bypass surgery involving mini-thoracotomy or mini-sternotomy surgery, performed under direct vision; using two arterial grafts and single venous graft **MIPS**
BETOS: Z2   Undefined codes
Service not separately priced by Part B

S2225 Myringotomy, laser-assisted
BETOS: Z2   Undefined codes
Service not separately priced by Part B

S2230 Implantation of magnetic component of semi-implantable hearing device on ossicles in middle ear
BETOS: Z2   Undefined codes
Service not separately priced by Part B

S2235 Implantation of auditory brain stem implant
BETOS: Z2   Undefined codes
Service not separately priced by Part B

S2260 Induced abortion, 17 to 24 weeks ♀ Ⓐ
BETOS: Z2   Undefined codes
Service not separately priced by Part B

S2265 Induced abortion, 25 to 28 weeks ♀ Ⓐ
BETOS: Z2   Undefined codes
Service not separately priced by Part B

S2266 Induced abortion, 29 to 31 weeks ♀ Ⓐ
BETOS: Z2   Undefined codes
Service not separately priced by Part B

S2267 Induced abortion, 32 weeks or greater ♀ Ⓐ
BETOS: Z2   Undefined codes
Service not separately priced by Part B

S2300 Arthroscopy, shoulder, surgical; with thermally-induced capsulorrhaphy
BETOS: Z2   Undefined codes
Service not separately priced by Part B

S2325 Hip core decompression
BETOS: Z2   Undefined codes
Service not separately priced by Part B
Coding Clinic: 2017, Q3

S2340 Chemodenervation of abductor muscle(s) of vocal cord
BETOS: Z2   Undefined codes
Service not separately priced by Part B

S2341 Chemodenervation of adductor muscle(s) of vocal cord
BETOS: Z2   Undefined codes
Service not separately priced by Part B

S2342 Nasal endoscopy for post-operative debridement following functional endoscopic sinus surgery, nasal and/or sinus cavity(s), unilateral or bilateral
BETOS: Z2   Undefined codes
Service not separately priced by Part B

S2348 Decompression procedure, percutaneous, of nucleus pulposus of intervertebral disc, using radiofrequency energy, single or multiple levels, lumbar
BETOS: Z2   Undefined codes
Service not separately priced by Part B

S2350 Diskectomy, anterior, with decompression of spinal cord and/or nerve root(s), including osteophytectomy; lumbar, single interspace
BETOS: Z2   Undefined codes
Service not separately priced by Part B

S2351 Diskectomy, anterior, with decompression of spinal cord and/or nerve root(s), including osteophytectomy; lumbar, each additional interspace (list separately in addition to code for primary procedure)
BETOS: Z2   Undefined codes
Service not separately priced by Part B

S2400 Repair, congenital diaphragmatic hernia in the fetus using temporary tracheal occlusion, procedure performed in utero ♀ Ⓐ
BETOS: Z2   Undefined codes
Service not separately priced by Part B

S2401 Repair, urinary tract obstruction in the fetus, procedure performed in utero ♀ Ⓐ
BETOS: Z2   Undefined codes
Service not separately priced by Part B

S2402 Repair, congenital cystic adenomatoid malformation in the fetus, procedure performed in utero ♀ Ⓐ
BETOS: Z2   Undefined codes
Service not separately priced by Part B

S2403 Repair, extralobar pulmonary sequestration in the fetus, procedure performed in utero ♀ Ⓐ
BETOS: Z2   Undefined codes
Service not separately priced by Part B

S2404 Repair, myelomeningocele in the fetus, procedure performed in utero ♀ Ⓐ
BETOS: Z2   Undefined codes
Service not separately priced by Part B

S2405 Repair of sacrococcygeal teratoma in the fetus, procedure performed in utero ♀ Ⓐ
BETOS: Z2   Undefined codes
Service not separately priced by Part B

● New code   ▲ Revised code   🄲 Carrier judgment   🄳 Special coverage instructions apply
🄸 Not payable by Medicare   🄼 Non-covered by Medicare   🅂 Non-covered by Medicare statute   AHA Coding Clinic®

CPT® is a registered trademark of the American Medical Association. All rights reserved.

S2409 Repair, congenital malformation of fetus, procedure performed in utero, not otherwise classified ♀ Ⓐ
BETOS: Z2 Undefined codes
Service not separately priced by Part B

S2411 Fetoscopic laser therapy for treatment of twin-to-twin transfusion syndrome
BETOS: Z2 Undefined codes
Service not separately priced by Part B

S2900 Surgical techniques requiring use of robotic surgical system (list separately in addition to code for primary procedure)
BETOS: Z2 Undefined codes
Service not separately priced by Part B
Coding Clinic: 2010, Q1

S3000 Diabetic indicator; retinal eye exam, dilated, bilateral
BETOS: Z2 Undefined codes
Service not separately priced by Part B

S3005 Performance measurement, evaluation of patient self assessment, depression
BETOS: Z2 Undefined codes
Service not separately priced by Part B

S3600 STAT laboratory request (situations other than S3601)
BETOS: Z2 Undefined codes
Service not separately priced by Part B

S3601 Emergency STAT laboratory charge for patient who is homebound or residing in a nursing facility
BETOS: Z2 Undefined codes
Service not separately priced by Part B

S3620 Newborn metabolic screening panel, includes test kit, postage and the laboratory tests specified by the state for inclusion in this panel (e.g., galactose; hemoglobin, electrophoresis; hydroxyprogesterone, 17-D; phenylalanine (PKU); and thyroxine, total)
BETOS: Z2 Undefined codes
Service not separately priced by Part B

S3630 Eosinophil count, blood, direct
BETOS: Z2 Undefined codes
Service not separately priced by Part B

S3645 HIV-1 antibody testing of oral mucosal transudate
BETOS: Z2 Undefined codes
Service not separately priced by Part B

S3650 Saliva test, hormone level; during menopause ♀ Ⓐ
BETOS: Z2 Undefined codes
Service not separately priced by Part B

S3652 Saliva test, hormone level; to assess preterm labor risk ♀ Ⓐ
BETOS: Z2 Undefined codes
Service not separately priced by Part B

S3655 Antisperm antibodies test (Immunobead®) ♂
BETOS: Z2 Undefined codes
Service not separately priced by Part B

S3708 Gastrointestinal fat absorption study
BETOS: Z2 Undefined codes
Service not separately priced by Part B

S3722 Dose optimization by area under the curve (AUC) analysis, for infusional 5-fluorouracil
BETOS: Z2 Undefined codes
Service not separately priced by Part B

GENETIC TESTING (S3800-S3870)

S3800 Genetic testing for amyotrophic lateral sclerosis (ALS)
BETOS: Z2 Undefined codes
Service not separately priced by Part B

S3840 DNA analysis for germline mutations of the RET proto-oncogene for susceptibility to multiple endocrine neoplasia type 2
BETOS: Z2 Undefined codes
Service not separately priced by Part B

S3841 Genetic testing for retinoblastoma
BETOS: Z2 Undefined codes
Service not separately priced by Part B

S3842 Genetic testing for Von Hippel-Lindau disease
BETOS: Z2 Undefined codes
Service not separately priced by Part B

S3844 DNA analysis of the Connexin 26 gene (GJB2) for susceptibility to congenital, profound deafness
BETOS: Z2 Undefined codes
Service not separately priced by Part B

S3845 Genetic testing for alpha-thalassemia
BETOS: Z2 Undefined codes
Service not separately priced by Part B

S3846 Genetic testing for hemoglobin E beta-thalassemia
BETOS: Z2 Undefined codes
Service not separately priced by Part B

S3849 Genetic testing for Niemann-Pick disease
BETOS: Z2 Undefined codes
Service not separately priced by Part B

S3850 Genetic testing for sickle cell anemia
BETOS: Z2 Undefined codes
Service not separately priced by Part B

S3852 DNA analysis for APOE epsilon 4 allele for susceptibility to Alzheimer's disease
BETOS: Z2 Undefined codes
Service not separately priced by Part B

S3853 Genetic testing for myotonic muscular dystrophy
BETOS: Z2 Undefined codes
Service not separately priced by Part B

♂ Male only   ♀ Female only   Ⓐ Age   A2 - Z3 = ASC Payment indicator   A - Y = APC Status indicator
ASC = ASC Approved Procedure   **DME** Paid under the DME fee schedule   **MIPS** MIPS code

S3854 Gene expression profiling panel for use in the management of breast cancer treatment
BETOS: Z2   Undefined codes
Service not separately priced by Part B
Coding Clinic: 2016, Q2

S3861 Genetic testing, sodium channel, voltage-gated, type V, alpha subunit (SCN5A) and variants for suspected brugada syndrome
BETOS: Z2   Undefined codes
Service not separately priced by Part B

S3865 Comprehensive gene sequence analysis for hypertrophic cardiomyopathy
BETOS: Z2   Undefined codes
Service not separately priced by Part B

S3866 Genetic analysis for a specific gene mutation for hypertrophic cardiomyopathy (HCM) in an individual with a known HCM mutation in the family
BETOS: Z2   Undefined codes
Service not separately priced by Part B

S3870 Comparative genomic hybridization (CGH) microarray testing for developmental delay, autism spectrum disorder and/or intellectual disability
BETOS: Z2   Undefined codes
Service not separately priced by Part B

MISCELLANEOUS TESTS (S3900-S3904)

S3900 Surface electromyography (EMG)
BETOS: Z2   Undefined codes
Service not separately priced by Part B

S3902 Ballistocardiogram
BETOS: Z2   Undefined codes
Service not separately priced by Part B

S3904 Masters two step
BETOS: Z2   Undefined codes
Service not separately priced by Part B

ASSORTED OBSTETRICAL AND FERTILITY SERVICES (S4005-S4989)

S4005 Interim labor facility global (labor occurring but not resulting in delivery) ♀
BETOS: Z2   Undefined codes
Service not separately priced by Part B

S4011 In vitro fertilization; including but not limited to identification and incubation of mature oocytes, fertilization with sperm, incubation of embryo(s), and subsequent visualization for determination of development ♀ A
BETOS: Z2   Undefined codes
Service not separately priced by Part B

S4013 Complete cycle, gamete intrafallopian transfer (GIFT), case rate ♀ A
BETOS: Z2   Undefined codes
Service not separately priced by Part B

S4014 Complete cycle, zygote intrafallopian transfer (ZIFT), case rate ♀ A
BETOS: Z2   Undefined codes
Service not separately priced by Part B

S4015 Complete in vitro fertilization cycle, not otherwise specified, case rate ♀ A
BETOS: Z2   Undefined codes
Service not separately priced by Part B

S4016 Frozen in vitro fertilization cycle, case rate ♀ A
BETOS: Z2   Undefined codes
Service not separately priced by Part B

S4017 Incomplete cycle, treatment cancelled prior to stimulation, case rate ♀
BETOS: Z2   Undefined codes
Service not separately priced by Part B

S4018 Frozen embryo transfer procedure cancelled before transfer, case rate ♀ A
BETOS: Z2   Undefined codes
Service not separately priced by Part B

S4020 In vitro fertilization procedure cancelled before aspiration, case rate ♀
BETOS: Z2   Undefined codes
Service not separately priced by Part B

S4021 In vitro fertilization procedure cancelled after aspiration, case rate ♀
BETOS: Z2   Undefined codes
Service not separately priced by Part B

S4022 Assisted oocyte fertilization, case rate ♀ A
BETOS: Z2   Undefined codes
Service not separately priced by Part B

S4023 Donor egg cycle, incomplete, case rate ♀ A
BETOS: Z2   Undefined codes
Service not separately priced by Part B

S4025 Donor services for in vitro fertilization (sperm or embryo), case rate ♀
BETOS: Z2   Undefined codes
Service not separately priced by Part B

S4026 Procurement of donor sperm from sperm bank ♂
BETOS: Z2   Undefined codes
Service not separately priced by Part B

S4027 Storage of previously frozen embryos ♀ A
BETOS: Z2   Undefined codes
Service not separately priced by Part B

S4028 Microsurgical epididymal sperm aspiration (MESA) ♂
BETOS: Z2   Undefined codes
Service not separately priced by Part B

S4030 Sperm procurement and cryopreservation services; initial visit ♂
BETOS: Z2   Undefined codes
Service not separately priced by Part B

● New code   ▲ Revised code   C Carrier judgment   D Special coverage instructions apply
I Not payable by Medicare   M Non-covered by Medicare   S Non-covered by Medicare statute   AHA Coding Clinic®

S4031 Sperm procurement and cryopreservation services; subsequent visit ♂
BETOS: Z2 Undefined codes
Service not separately priced by Part B

S4035 Stimulated intrauterine insemination (IUI), case rate ♀ Ⓐ
BETOS: Z2 Undefined codes
Service not separately priced by Part B

S4037 Cryopreserved embryo transfer, case rate ♀ Ⓐ
BETOS: Z2 Undefined codes
Service not separately priced by Part B

S4040 Monitoring and storage of cryopreserved embryos, per 30 days ♀ Ⓐ
BETOS: Z2 Undefined codes
Service not separately priced by Part B

S4042 Management of ovulation induction (interpretation of diagnostic tests and studies, non-face-to-face medical management of the patient), per cycle ♀ Ⓐ
BETOS: Z2 Undefined codes
Service not separately priced by Part B

S4981 Insertion of levonorgestrel-releasing intrauterine system ♀ Ⓐ
BETOS: Z2 Undefined codes
Service not separately priced by Part B

S4989 Contraceptive intrauterine device (e.g., Progestacert IUD), including implants and supplies ♀ Ⓐ
BETOS: Z2 Undefined codes
Service not separately priced by Part B

Intrauterine device

MISCELLANEOUS MEDICATIONS AND THERAPEUTIC SUBSTANCES (S4990-S5014)

S4990 Nicotine patches, legend
BETOS: Z2 Undefined codes
Service not separately priced by Part B

S4991 Nicotine patches, non-legend
BETOS: Z2 Undefined codes
Service not separately priced by Part B

S4993 Contraceptive pills for birth control ♀ Ⓐ
BETOS: Z2 Undefined codes
Service not separately priced by Part B

S4995 Smoking cessation gum
BETOS: Z2 Undefined codes
Service not separately priced by Part B

S5000 Prescription drug, generic
BETOS: Z2 Undefined codes
Service not separately priced by Part B

S5001 Prescription drug, brand name
BETOS: Z2 Undefined codes
Service not separately priced by Part B

S5010 5% dextrose and 0.45% normal saline, 1000 ml
BETOS: Z2 Undefined codes
Service not separately priced by Part B

S5012 5% dextrose with potassium chloride, 1000 ml
BETOS: Z2 Undefined codes
Service not separately priced by Part B

S5013 5% dextrose/0.45% normal saline with potassium chloride and magnesium sulfate, 1000 ml
BETOS: Z2 Undefined codes
Service not separately priced by Part B

S5014 5% dextrose/0.45% normal saline with potassium chloride and magnesium sulfate, 1500 ml
BETOS: Z2 Undefined codes
Service not separately priced by Part B

VARIOUS HOME CARE SERVICES (S5035-S5199)

S5035 Home infusion therapy, routine service of infusion device (e.g., pump maintenance)
BETOS: Z2 Undefined codes
Service not separately priced by Part B

S5036 Home infusion therapy, repair of infusion device (e.g., pump repair)
BETOS: Z2 Undefined codes
Service not separately priced by Part B

S5100 Day care services, adult; per 15 minutes Ⓐ
BETOS: Z2 Undefined codes
Service not separately priced by Part B

S5101 Day care services, adult; per half day Ⓐ
BETOS: Z2 Undefined codes
Service not separately priced by Part B

S5102 Day care services, adult; per diem Ⓐ
BETOS: Z2 Undefined codes
Service not separately priced by Part B

S5105 Day care services, center-based; services not included in program fee, per diem
BETOS: Z2 Undefined codes
Service not separately priced by Part B

♂ Male only ♀ Female only Ⓐ Age A2 - Z3 = ASC Payment indicator A - Y = APC Status indicator
ASC = ASC Approved Procedure **DME** Paid under the DME fee schedule **MIPS** MIPS code

S5108 Home care training to home care client, per 15 minutes
BETOS: Z2 Undefined codes
Service not separately priced by Part B

S5109 Home care training to home care client, per session
BETOS: Z2 Undefined codes
Service not separately priced by Part B

S5110 Home care training, family; per 15 minutes
BETOS: Z2 Undefined codes
Service not separately priced by Part B

S5111 Home care training, family; per session
BETOS: Z2 Undefined codes
Service not separately priced by Part B

S5115 Home care training, non-family; per 15 minutes
BETOS: Z2 Undefined codes
Service not separately priced by Part B

S5116 Home care training, non-family; per session
BETOS: Z2 Undefined codes
Service not separately priced by Part B

S5120 Chore services; per 15 minutes
BETOS: Z2 Undefined codes
Service not separately priced by Part B

S5121 Chore services; per diem
BETOS: Z2 Undefined codes
Service not separately priced by Part B

S5125 Attendant care services; per 15 minutes
BETOS: Z2 Undefined codes
Service not separately priced by Part B

S5126 Attendant care services; per diem
BETOS: Z2 Undefined codes
Service not separately priced by Part B

S5130 Homemaker service, NOS; per 15 minutes
BETOS: Z2 Undefined codes
Service not separately priced by Part B

S5131 Homemaker service, NOS; per diem
BETOS: Z2 Undefined codes
Service not separately priced by Part B

S5135 Companion care, adult (e.g., IADL/ADL); per 15 minutes Ⓐ
BETOS: Z2 Undefined codes
Service not separately priced by Part B

S5136 Companion care, adult (e.g., IADL/ADL); per diem Ⓐ
BETOS: Z2 Undefined codes
Service not separately priced by Part B

S5140 Foster care, adult; per diem Ⓐ
BETOS: Z2 Undefined codes
Service not separately priced by Part B

S5141 Foster care, adult; per month Ⓐ
BETOS: Z2 Undefined codes
Service not separately priced by Part B

S5145 Foster care, therapeutic, child; per diem Ⓐ
BETOS: Z2 Undefined codes
Service not separately priced by Part B

S5146 Foster care, therapeutic, child; per month Ⓐ
BETOS: Z2 Undefined codes
Service not separately priced by Part B

S5150 Unskilled respite care, not hospice; per 15 minutes
BETOS: Z2 Undefined codes
Service not separately priced by Part B

S5151 Unskilled respite care, not hospice; per diem
BETOS: Z2 Undefined codes
Service not separately priced by Part B

S5160 Emergency response system; installation and testing
BETOS: Z2 Undefined codes
Service not separately priced by Part B

S5161 Emergency response system; service fee, per month (excludes installation and testing)
BETOS: Z2 Undefined codes
Service not separately priced by Part B

S5162 Emergency response system; purchase only
BETOS: Z2 Undefined codes
Service not separately priced by Part B

S5165 Home modifications; per service
BETOS: Z2 Undefined codes
Service not separately priced by Part B

S5170 Home delivered meals, including preparation; per meal
BETOS: Z2 Undefined codes
Service not separately priced by Part B

S5175 Laundry service, external, professional; per order
BETOS: Z2 Undefined codes
Service not separately priced by Part B

S5180 Home health respiratory therapy, initial evaluation
BETOS: Z2 Undefined codes
Service not separately priced by Part B

S5181 Home health respiratory therapy, NOS, per diem
BETOS: Z2 Undefined codes
Service not separately priced by Part B

S5185 Medication reminder service, non-face-to-face; per month
BETOS: Z2 Undefined codes
Service not separately priced by Part B

S5190 Wellness assessment, performed by non-physician
BETOS: Z2 Undefined codes
Service not separately priced by Part B

S5199 Personal care item, NOS, each
BETOS: Z2 Undefined codes
Service not separately priced by Part B

● New code   ▲ Revised code   🄲 Carrier judgment   🄳 Special coverage instructions apply
🄸 Not payable by Medicare   🄼 Non-covered by Medicare   🅂 Non-covered by Medicare statute   AHA Coding Clinic®

HOME INFUSION THERAPY (S5497-S5523), SEE ALSO
HOME INFUSION THERAPY (S9325-S9379); HOME THERAPY
SERVICES (S9490-S9810)

S5497 Home infusion therapy, catheter care /
maintenance, not otherwise classified;
includes administrative services, professional
pharmacy services, care coordination,
and all necessary supplies and equipment
(drugs and nursing visits coded separately),
per diem
BETOS: Z2   Undefined codes
Service not separately priced by Part B

S5498 Home infusion therapy, catheter care /
maintenance, simple (single lumen), includes
administrative services, professional
pharmacy services, care coordination and
all necessary supplies and equipment,
(drugs and nursing visits coded separately),
per diem
BETOS: Z2   Undefined codes
Service not separately priced by Part B

S5501 Home infusion therapy, catheter care /
maintenance, complex (more than one
lumen), includes administrative services,
professional pharmacy services, care
coordination, and all necessary supplies and
equipment (drugs and nursing visits coded
separately), per diem
BETOS: Z2   Undefined codes
Service not separately priced by Part B

S5502 Home infusion therapy, catheter care /
maintenance, implanted access device,
includes administrative services, professional
pharmacy services, care coordination and all
necessary supplies and equipment, (drugs
and nursing visits coded separately), per
diem (use this code for interim maintenance
of vascular access not currently in use)
BETOS: Z2   Undefined codes
Service not separately priced by Part B

S5517 Home infusion therapy, all supplies
necessary for restoration of catheter patency
or declotting
BETOS: Z2   Undefined codes
Service not separately priced by Part B

S5518 Home infusion therapy, all supplies
necessary for catheter repair
BETOS: Z2   Undefined codes
Service not separately priced by Part B

S5520 Home infusion therapy, all supplies (including
catheter) necessary for a peripherally
inserted central venous catheter (PICC) line
insertion
BETOS: Z2   Undefined codes
Service not separately priced by Part B

S5521 Home infusion therapy, all supplies (including
catheter) necessary for a midline catheter
insertion
BETOS: Z2   Undefined codes
Service not separately priced by Part B

S5522 Home infusion therapy, insertion of
peripherally inserted central venous catheter
(PICC), nursing services only (no supplies or
catheter included)
BETOS: Z2   Undefined codes
Service not separately priced by Part B

S5523 Home infusion therapy, insertion of midline
venous catheter, nursing services only
(no supplies or catheter included)
BETOS: Z2   Undefined codes
Service not separately priced by Part B

INSULIN AND DELIVERY DEVICES (S5550-S5571)

S5550 Insulin, rapid onset, 5 units
BETOS: Z2   Undefined codes
Service not separately priced by Part B

S5551 Insulin, most rapid onset (Lispro or Aspart);
5 units
BETOS: Z2   Undefined codes
Service not separately priced by Part B

S5552 Insulin, intermediate acting (NPH or LENTE);
5 units
BETOS: Z2   Undefined codes
Service not separately priced by Part B

S5553 Insulin, long acting; 5 units
BETOS: Z2   Undefined codes
Service not separately priced by Part B

S5560 Insulin delivery device, reusable pen;
1.5 ml size
BETOS: Z2   Undefined codes
Service not separately priced by Part B

S5561 Insulin delivery device, reusable pen;
3 ml size
BETOS: Z2   Undefined codes
Service not separately priced by Part B

S5565 Insulin cartridge for use in insulin delivery
device other than pump; 150 units
BETOS: Z2   Undefined codes
Service not separately priced by Part B

S5566 Insulin cartridge for use in insulin delivery
device other than pump; 300 units
BETOS: Z2   Undefined codes
Service not separately priced by Part B

S5570 Insulin delivery device, disposable pen
(including insulin); 1.5 ml size
BETOS: Z2   Undefined codes
Service not separately priced by Part B

♂ Male only   ♀ Female only   **Ⓐ** Age   A2 - Z3 = ASC Payment indicator   A - Y = APC Status indicator
ASC = ASC Approved Procedure   **DME** Paid under the DME fee schedule   **MIPS** MIPS code

S5571 Insulin delivery device, disposable pen (including insulin); 3 ml size
BETOS: Z2   Undefined codes
Service not separately priced by Part B

IMAGING STUDIES (S8030-S8092), SEE ALSO CONTRAST AGENTS/DIAGNOSTIC IMAGING (Q9950-Q9992)

S8030 Scleral application of tantalum ring(s) for localization of lesions for proton beam therapy
BETOS: Z2   Undefined codes
Service not separately priced by Part B

S8035 Magnetic source imaging
BETOS: Z2   Undefined codes
Service not separately priced by Part B

S8037 Magnetic resonance cholangiopancreatography (MRCP)
BETOS: Z2   Undefined codes
Service not separately priced by Part B

S8040 Topographic brain mapping
BETOS: Z2   Undefined codes
Service not separately priced by Part B

S8042 Magnetic resonance imaging (MRI), low-field
BETOS: Z2   Undefined codes
Service not separately priced by Part B

S8055 Ultrasound guidance for multifetal pregnancy reduction(s), technical component (only to be used when the physician doing the reduction procedure does not perform the ultrasound, guidance is included in the CPT® code for multifetal pregnancy reduction - 59866) ♀ Ⓐ
BETOS: Z2   Undefined codes
Service not separately priced by Part B

S8080 Scintimammography (radioimmunoscintigraphy of the breast), unilateral, including supply of radiopharmaceutical
BETOS: Z2   Undefined codes
Service not separately priced by Part B

S8085 Fluorine-18 fluorodeoxyglucose (F-18 FDG) imaging using dual-head coincidence detection system (non-dedicated PET scan)
BETOS: Z2   Undefined codes
Service not separately priced by Part B

S8092 Electron beam computed tomography (also known as ultrafast CT, cine CT)
BETOS: Z2   Undefined codes
Service not separately priced by Part B

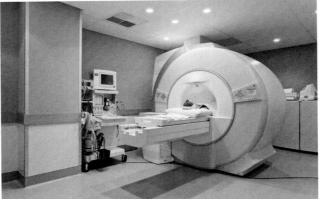

CT Scanner

ASSISTED BREATHING SUPPLIES (S8096-S8210), SEE ALSO BREATHING AIDS (A7000-A7048); INTERMITTENT POSITIVE PRESSURE BREATHING DEVICES (E0500); OTHER BREATHING AIDS (E0605, E0606)

S8096 Portable peak flow meter
BETOS: Z2   Undefined codes
Service not separately priced by Part B

S8097 Asthma kit (including but not limited to portable peak expiratory flow meter, instructional video, brochure, and/or spacer)
BETOS: Z2   Undefined codes
Service not separately priced by Part B

S8100 Holding chamber or spacer for use with an inhaler or nebulizer; without mask
BETOS: Z2   Undefined codes
Service not separately priced by Part B

S8101 Holding chamber or spacer for use with an inhaler or nebulizer; with mask
BETOS: Z2   Undefined codes
Service not separately priced by Part B

S8110 Peak expiratory flow rate (physician services)
BETOS: Z2   Undefined codes
Service not separately priced by Part B

S8120 Oxygen contents, gaseous, 1 unit equals 1 cubic foot
BETOS: Z2   Undefined codes
Service not separately priced by Part B

S8121 Oxygen contents, liquid, 1 unit equals 1 pound
BETOS: Z2   Undefined codes
Service not separately priced by Part B

S8130 Interferential current stimulator, 2 channel
BETOS: Z2   Undefined codes
Service not separately priced by Part B

S8131 Interferential current stimulator, 4 channel
BETOS: Z2   Undefined codes
Service not separately priced by Part B

● New code   ▲ Revised code   Ⓒ Carrier judgment   Ⓓ Special coverage instructions apply
Ⓘ Not payable by Medicare   Ⓜ Non-covered by Medicare   Ⓢ Non-covered by Medicare statute   AHA Coding Clinic®

     CPT® is a registered trademark of the American Medical Association. All rights reserved.

I **S8185** Flutter device
    BETOS: Z2   Undefined codes
    Service not separately priced by Part B

I **S8186** Swivel adapter
    BETOS: Z2   Undefined codes
    Service not separately priced by Part B

I **S8189** Tracheostomy supply, not otherwise classified
    BETOS: Z2   Undefined codes
    Service not separately priced by Part B

I **S8210** Mucus trap
    BETOS: Z2   Undefined codes
    Service not separately priced by Part B

MISCELLANEOUS SUPPLIES AND SERVICES (S8265-S9152), SEE ALSO MISCELLANEOUS SUPPLIES AND SERVICES (S9381-S9485)

I **S8265** Haberman feeder for cleft lip/palate
    BETOS: Z2   Undefined codes
    Service not separately priced by Part B

I **S8270** Enuresis alarm, using auditory buzzer and/or vibration device
    BETOS: Z2   Undefined codes
    Service not separately priced by Part B

I **S8301** Infection control supplies, not otherwise specified
    BETOS: Z2   Undefined codes
    Service not separately priced by Part B

I **S8415** Supplies for home delivery of infant
    BETOS: Z2   Undefined codes
    Service not separately priced by Part B

I **S8420** Gradient pressure aid (sleeve and glove combination), custom made
    BETOS: Z2   Undefined codes
    Service not separately priced by Part B

I **S8421** Gradient pressure aid (sleeve and glove combination), ready made
    BETOS: Z2   Undefined codes
    Service not separately priced by Part B

I **S8422** Gradient pressure aid (sleeve), custom made, medium weight
    BETOS: Z2   Undefined codes
    Service not separately priced by Part B

I **S8423** Gradient pressure aid (sleeve), custom made, heavy weight
    BETOS: Z2   Undefined codes
    Service not separately priced by Part B

I **S8424** Gradient pressure aid (sleeve), ready made
    BETOS: Z2   Undefined codes
    Service not separately priced by Part B

I **S8425** Gradient pressure aid (glove), custom made, medium weight
    BETOS: Z2   Undefined codes
    Service not separately priced by Part B

I **S8426** Gradient pressure aid (glove), custom made, heavy weight
    BETOS: Z2   Undefined codes
    Service not separately priced by Part B

I **S8427** Gradient pressure aid (glove), ready made
    BETOS: Z2   Undefined codes
    Service not separately priced by Part B

I **S8428** Gradient pressure aid (gauntlet), ready made
    BETOS: Z2   Undefined codes
    Service not separately priced by Part B

I **S8429** Gradient pressure exterior wrap
    BETOS: Z2   Undefined codes
    Service not separately priced by Part B

I **S8430** Padding for compression bandage, roll
    BETOS: Z2   Undefined codes
    Service not separately priced by Part B

I **S8431** Compression bandage, roll
    BETOS: Z2   Undefined codes
    Service not separately priced by Part B

I **S8450** Splint, prefabricated, digit (specify digit by use of modifier)
    BETOS: Z2   Undefined codes
    Service not separately priced by Part B

I **S8451** Splint, prefabricated, wrist or ankle
    BETOS: Z2   Undefined codes
    Service not separately priced by Part B

I **S8452** Splint, prefabricated, elbow
    BETOS: Z2   Undefined codes
    Service not separately priced by Part B

I **S8460** Camisole, post-mastectomy   ♀
    BETOS: Z2   Undefined codes
    Service not separately priced by Part B

I **S8490** Insulin syringes (100 syringes, any size)
    BETOS: Z2   Undefined codes
    Service not separately priced by Part B

I **S8930** Electrical stimulation of auricular acupuncture points; each 15 minutes of personal one-on-one contact with the patient
    BETOS: Z2   Undefined codes
    Service not separately priced by Part B

I **S8940** Equestrian/hippotherapy, per session
    BETOS: Z2   Undefined codes
    Service not separately priced by Part B

I **S8948** Application of a modality (requiring constant provider attendance) to one or more areas; low-level laser; each 15 minutes
    BETOS: Z2   Undefined codes
    Service not separately priced by Part B

I **S8950** Complex lymphedema therapy, each 15 minutes
    BETOS: Z2   Undefined codes
    Service not separately priced by Part B

♂ Male only   ♀ Female only   **A** Age   A2 - Z3 = ASC Payment indicator   A - Y = APC Status indicator
ASC = ASC Approved Procedure   **DME** Paid under the DME fee schedule   **MIPS** MIPS code

S8990 Physical or manipulative therapy performed for maintenance rather than restoration
BETOS: Z2   Undefined codes
Service not separately priced by Part B

S8999 Resuscitation bag (for use by patient on artificial respiration during power failure or other catastrophic event)
BETOS: Z2   Undefined codes
Service not separately priced by Part B

S9001 Home uterine monitor with or without associated nursing services ♀
BETOS: Z2   Undefined codes
Service not separately priced by Part B

S9007 Ultrafiltration monitor
BETOS: Z2   Undefined codes
Service not separately priced by Part B

S9024 Paranasal sinus ultrasound
BETOS: Z2   Undefined codes
Service not separately priced by Part B

S9025 Omnicardiogram/cardiointegram
BETOS: Z2   Undefined codes
Service not separately priced by Part B

S9034 Extracorporeal shockwave lithotripsy for gall stones (if performed with ERCP, use 43265)
BETOS: Z2   Undefined codes
Service not separately priced by Part B

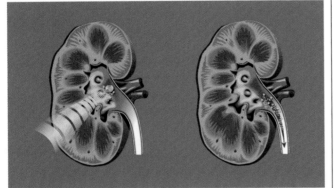

Extracorporeal shock wave lithotripsy

S9055 Procuren or other growth factor preparation to promote wound healing
BETOS: Z2   Undefined codes
Service not separately priced by Part B

S9056 Coma stimulation per diem
BETOS: Z2   Undefined codes
Service not separately priced by Part B

S9061 Home administration of aerosolized drug therapy (e.g., pentamidine); administrative services, professional pharmacy services, care coordination, all necessary supplies and equipment (drugs and nursing visits coded separately), per diem
BETOS: Z2   Undefined codes
Service not separately priced by Part B

S9083 Global fee urgent care centers
BETOS: Z2   Undefined codes
Service not separately priced by Part B

S9088 Services provided in an urgent care center (list in addition to code for service)
BETOS: Z2   Undefined codes
Service not separately priced by Part B

S9090 Vertebral axial decompression, per session
BETOS: Z2   Undefined codes
Service not separately priced by Part B

S9097 Home visit for wound care
BETOS: Z2   Undefined codes
Service not separately priced by Part B

S9098 Home visit, phototherapy services (e.g., Bili-lite), including equipment rental, nursing services, blood draw, supplies, and other services, per diem
BETOS: Z2   Undefined codes
Service not separately priced by Part B

S9110 Telemonitoring of patient in their home, including all necessary equipment; computer system, connections, and software; maintenance; patient education and support; per month
BETOS: Z2   Undefined codes
Service not separately priced by Part B

S9117 Back school, per visit
BETOS: Z2   Undefined codes
Service not separately priced by Part B

S9122 Home health aide or certified nurse assistant, providing care in the home; per hour
BETOS: Z2   Undefined codes
Service not separately priced by Part B

S9123 Nursing care, in the home; by registered nurse, per hour (use for general nursing care only, not to be used when CPT® codes 99500-99602 can be used)
BETOS: Z2   Undefined codes
Service not separately priced by Part B

S9124 Nursing care, in the home; by licensed practical nurse, per hour
BETOS: Z2   Undefined codes
Service not separately priced by Part B

S9125 Respite care, in the home, per diem
BETOS: Z2   Undefined codes
Service not separately priced by Part B

S9126 Hospice care, in the home, per diem
BETOS: Z2   Undefined codes
Service not separately priced by Part B

S9127 Social work visit, in the home, per diem
BETOS: Z2   Undefined codes
Service not separately priced by Part B

S9128 Speech therapy, in the home, per diem
BETOS: Z2   Undefined codes
Service not separately priced by Part B

S9129 Occupational therapy, in the home, per diem
BETOS: Z2   Undefined codes
Service not separately priced by Part B

S9131 Physical therapy; in the home, per diem
BETOS: Z2   Undefined codes
Service not separately priced by Part B

S9140 Diabetic management program, follow-up visit to non-MD provider
BETOS: Z2   Undefined codes
Service not separately priced by Part B

S9141 Diabetic management program, follow-up visit to MD provider
BETOS: Z2   Undefined codes
Service not separately priced by Part B

S9145 Insulin pump initiation, instruction in initial use of pump (pump not included)
BETOS: Z2   Undefined codes
Service not separately priced by Part B

S9150 Evaluation by ocularist
BETOS: Z2   Undefined codes
Service not separately priced by Part B

S9152 Speech therapy, re-evaluation
BETOS: Z2   Undefined codes
Service not separately priced by Part B

HOME MANAGEMENT OF PREGNANCY (S9208-S9214)

S9208 Home management of preterm labor, including administrative services, professional pharmacy services, care coordination, and all necessary supplies or equipment (drugs and nursing visits coded separately), per diem (do not use this code with any home infusion per diem code)
BETOS: Z2   Undefined codes
Service not separately priced by Part B

S9209 Home management of preterm premature rupture of membranes (PPROM), including administrative services, professional pharmacy services, care coordination, and all necessary supplies or equipment (drugs and nursing visits coded separately), per diem (do not use this code with any home infusion per diem code)
BETOS: Z2   Undefined codes
Service not separately priced by Part B

S9211 Home management of gestational hypertension, includes administrative services, professional pharmacy services, care coordination and all necessary supplies and equipment (drugs and nursing visits coded separately); per diem (do not use this code with any home infusion per diem code)   ♀ Ⓐ
BETOS: Z2   Undefined codes
Service not separately priced by Part B

S9212 Home management of postpartum hypertension, includes administrative services, professional pharmacy services, care coordination, and all necessary supplies and equipment (drugs and nursing visits coded separately), per diem (do not use this code with any home infusion per diem code)   ♀ Ⓐ
BETOS: Z2   Undefined codes
Service not separately priced by Part B

S9213 Home management of preeclampsia, includes administrative services, professional pharmacy services, care coordination, and all necessary supplies and equipment (drugs and nursing services coded separately); per diem (do not use this code with any home infusion per diem code)   ♀ Ⓐ
BETOS: Z2   Undefined codes
Service not separately priced by Part B

S9214 Home management of gestational diabetes, includes administrative services, professional pharmacy services, care coordination, and all necessary supplies and equipment (drugs and nursing visits coded separately); per diem (do not use this code with any home infusion per diem code)   ♀ Ⓐ
BETOS: Z2   Undefined codes
Service not separately priced by Part B

HOME INFUSION THERAPY (S9325-S9379), SEE ALSO HOME INFUSION THERAPY (S5497-S5523); HOME THERAPY SERVICES (S9490-S9810)

S9325 Home infusion therapy, pain management infusion; administrative services, professional pharmacy services, care coordination, and all necessary supplies and equipment, (drugs and nursing visits coded separately), per diem (do not use this code with S9326, S9327 or S9328)
BETOS: Z2   Undefined codes
Service not separately priced by Part B

S9326 Home infusion therapy, continuous (twenty-four hours or more) pain management infusion; administrative services, professional pharmacy services, care coordination and all necessary supplies and equipment (drugs and nursing visits coded separately), per diem
BETOS: Z2   Undefined codes
Service not separately priced by Part B

S9327 Home infusion therapy, intermittent (less than twenty-four hours) pain management infusion; administrative services, professional pharmacy services, care coordination, and all necessary supplies and equipment (drugs and nursing visits coded separately), per diem
BETOS: Z2   Undefined codes
Service not separately priced by Part B

S9328 Home infusion therapy, implanted pump pain management infusion; administrative services, professional pharmacy services, care coordination, and all necessary supplies and equipment (drugs and nursing visits coded separately), per diem
BETOS: Z2   Undefined codes
Service not separately priced by Part B

S9329 Home infusion therapy, chemotherapy infusion; administrative services, professional pharmacy services, care coordination, and all necessary supplies and equipment (drugs and nursing visits coded separately), per diem (do not use this code with S9330 or S9331)
BETOS: Z2   Undefined codes
Service not separately priced by Part B

S9330 Home infusion therapy, continuous (twenty-four hours or more) chemotherapy infusion; administrative services, professional pharmacy services, care coordination, and all necessary supplies and equipment (drugs and nursing visits coded separately), per diem
BETOS: Z2   Undefined codes
Service not separately priced by Part B

S9331 Home infusion therapy, intermittent (less than twenty-four hours) chemotherapy infusion; administrative services, professional pharmacy services, care coordination, and all necessary supplies and equipment (drugs and nursing visits coded separately), per diem
BETOS: Z2   Undefined codes
Service not separately priced by Part B

S9335 Home therapy, hemodialysis; administrative services, professional pharmacy services, care coordination, and all necessary supplies and equipment (drugs and nursing services coded separately), per diem
BETOS: Z2   Undefined codes
Service not separately priced by Part B

S9336 Home infusion therapy, continuous anticoagulant infusion therapy (e.g., Heparin), administrative services, professional pharmacy services, care coordination and all necessary supplies and equipment (drugs and nursing visits coded separately), per diem
BETOS: Z2   Undefined codes
Service not separately priced by Part B

S9338 Home infusion therapy, immunotherapy, administrative services, professional pharmacy services, care coordination, and all necessary supplies and equipment (drugs and nursing visits coded separately), per diem
BETOS: Z2   Undefined codes
Service not separately priced by Part B

S9339 Home therapy; peritoneal dialysis, administrative services, professional pharmacy services, care coordination and all necessary supplies and equipment (drugs and nursing visits coded separately), per diem
BETOS: Z2   Undefined codes
Service not separately priced by Part B

S9340 Home therapy; enteral nutrition; administrative services, professional pharmacy services, care coordination, and all necessary supplies and equipment (enteral formula and nursing visits coded separately), per diem
BETOS: Z2   Undefined codes
Service not separately priced by Part B

S9341 Home therapy; enteral nutrition via gravity; administrative services, professional pharmacy services, care coordination, and all necessary supplies and equipment (enteral formula and nursing visits coded separately), per diem
BETOS: Z2   Undefined codes
Service not separately priced by Part B

S9342 Home therapy; enteral nutrition via pump; administrative services, professional pharmacy services, care coordination, and all necessary supplies and equipment (enteral formula and nursing visits coded separately), per diem
BETOS: Z2   Undefined codes
Service not separately priced by Part B

S9343 Home therapy; enteral nutrition via bolus; administrative services, professional pharmacy services, care coordination, and all necessary supplies and equipment (enteral formula and nursing visits coded separately), per diem
BETOS: Z2   Undefined codes
Service not separately priced by Part B

S9345 Home infusion therapy, anti-hemophilic agent infusion therapy (e.g., Factor VIII); administrative services, professional pharmacy services, care coordination, and all necessary supplies and equipment (drugs and nursing visits coded separately), per diem
BETOS: Z2   Undefined codes
Service not separately priced by Part B

S9346 Home infusion therapy, alpha-1-proteinase inhibitor (e.g., Prolastin); administrative services, professional pharmacy services, care coordination, and all necessary supplies and equipment (drugs and nursing visits coded separately), per diem
BETOS: Z2   Undefined codes
Service not separately priced by Part B

● New code   ▲ Revised code   **C** Carrier judgment   **D** Special coverage instructions apply
I Not payable by Medicare   **M** Non-covered by Medicare   **S** Non-covered by Medicare statute   AHA Coding Clinic®

🔳 **S9347** Home infusion therapy, uninterrupted, long-term, controlled rate intravenous or subcutaneous infusion therapy (e.g., epoprostenol); administrative services, professional pharmacy services, care coordination, and all necessary supplies and equipment (drugs and nursing visits coded separately), per diem
BETOS: Z2   Undefined codes
Service not separately priced by Part B

🔳 **S9348** Home infusion therapy, sympathomimetic/inotropic agent infusion therapy (e.g., Dobutamine); administrative services, professional pharmacy services, care coordination, all necessary supplies and equipment (drugs and nursing visits coded separately), per diem
BETOS: Z2   Undefined codes
Service not separately priced by Part B

🔳 **S9349** Home infusion therapy, tocolytic infusion therapy; administrative services, professional pharmacy services, care coordination, and all necessary supplies and equipment (drugs and nursing visits coded separately), per diem
BETOS: Z2   Undefined codes
Service not separately priced by Part B

🔳 **S9351** Home infusion therapy, continuous or intermittent anti-emetic infusion therapy; administrative services, professional pharmacy services, care coordination, and all necessary supplies and equipment (drugs and visits coded separately), per diem
BETOS: Z2   Undefined codes
Service not separately priced by Part B

🔳 **S9353** Home infusion therapy, continuous insulin infusion therapy; administrative services, professional pharmacy services, care coordination, and all necessary supplies and equipment (drugs and nursing visits coded separately), per diem
BETOS: Z2   Undefined codes
Service not separately priced by Part B

🔳 **S9355** Home infusion therapy, chelation therapy; administrative services, professional pharmacy services, care coordination, and all necessary supplies and equipment (drugs and nursing visits coded separately), per diem
BETOS: Z2   Undefined codes
Service not separately priced by Part B

🔳 **S9357** Home infusion therapy, enzyme replacement intravenous therapy; (e.g., Imiglucerase); administrative services, professional pharmacy services, care coordination, and all necessary supplies and equipment (drugs and nursing visits coded separately), per diem
BETOS: Z2   Undefined codes
Service not separately priced by Part B

🔳 **S9359** Home infusion therapy, anti-tumor necrosis factor intravenous therapy; (e.g., Infliximab); administrative services, professional pharmacy services, care coordination, and all necessary supplies and equipment (drugs and nursing visits coded separately), per diem   MIPS
BETOS: Z2   Undefined codes
Service not separately priced by Part B

🔳 **S9361** Home infusion therapy, diuretic intravenous therapy; administrative services, professional pharmacy services, care coordination, and all necessary supplies and equipment (drugs and nursing visits coded separately), per diem
BETOS: Z2   Undefined codes
Service not separately priced by Part B

🔳 **S9363** Home infusion therapy, anti-spasmotic therapy; administrative services, professional pharmacy services, care coordination, and all necessary supplies and equipment (drugs and nursing visits coded separately), per diem
BETOS: Z2   Undefined codes
Service not separately priced by Part B

🔳 **S9364** Home infusion therapy, total parenteral nutrition (TPN); administrative services, professional pharmacy services, care coordination, and all necessary supplies and equipment including standard TPN formula (lipids, specialty amino acid formulas, drugs other than in standard formula and nursing visits coded separately), per diem (do not use with home infusion codes S9365-S9368 using daily volume scales)
BETOS: Z2   Undefined codes
Service not separately priced by Part B

🔳 **S9365** Home infusion therapy, total parenteral nutrition (TPN); one liter per day, administrative services, professional pharmacy services, care coordination, and all necessary supplies and equipment including standard TPN formula (lipids, specialty amino acid formulas, drugs other than in standard formula and nursing visits coded separately), per diem
BETOS: Z2   Undefined codes
Service not separately priced by Part B

🔳 **S9366** Home infusion therapy, total parenteral nutrition (TPN); more than one liter but no more than two liters per day, administrative services, professional pharmacy services, care coordination, and all necessary supplies and equipment including standard TPN formula (lipids, specialty amino acid formulas, drugs other than in standard formula and nursing visits coded separately), per diem
BETOS: Z2   Undefined codes
Service not separately priced by Part B

S9367 - S9433

TEMPORARY NATIONAL CODES (NON-MEDICARE) (S0012-S9999)

I **S9367** Home infusion therapy, total parenteral nutrition (TPN); more than two liters but no more than three liters per day, administrative services, professional pharmacy services, care coordination, and all necessary supplies and equipment including standard TPN formula (lipids, specialty amino acid formulas, drugs other than in standard formula and nursing visits coded separately), per diem
BETOS: Z2   Undefined codes
Service not separately priced by Part B

I **S9368** Home infusion therapy, total parenteral nutrition (TPN); more than three liters per day, administrative services, professional pharmacy services, care coordination, and all necessary supplies and equipment including standard TPN formula (lipids, specialty amino acid formulas, drugs other than in standard formula and nursing visits coded separately), per diem
BETOS: Z2   Undefined codes
Service not separately priced by Part B

I **S9370** Home therapy, intermittent anti-emetic injection therapy; administrative services, professional pharmacy services, care coordination, and all necessary supplies and equipment (drugs and nursing visits coded separately), per diem
BETOS: Z2   Undefined codes
Service not separately priced by Part B

I **S9372** Home therapy; intermittent anticoagulant injection therapy (e.g., Heparin); administrative services, professional pharmacy services, care coordination, and all necessary supplies and equipment (drugs and nursing visits coded separately), per diem (do not use this code for flushing of infusion devices with Heparin to maintain patency)
BETOS: Z2   Undefined codes
Service not separately priced by Part B

I **S9373** Home infusion therapy, hydration therapy; administrative services, professional pharmacy services, care coordination, and all necessary supplies and equipment (drugs and nursing visits coded separately), per diem (do not use with hydration therapy codes S9374-S9377 using daily volume scales)
BETOS: Z2   Undefined codes
Service not separately priced by Part B

I **S9374** Home infusion therapy, hydration therapy; one liter per day, administrative services, professional pharmacy services, care coordination, and all necessary supplies and equipment (drugs and nursing visits coded separately), per diem
BETOS: Z2   Undefined codes
Service not separately priced by Part B

I **S9375** Home infusion therapy, hydration therapy; more than one liter but no more than two liters per day, administrative services, professional pharmacy services, care coordination, and all necessary supplies and equipment (drugs and nursing visits coded separately), per diem
BETOS: Z2   Undefined codes
Service not separately priced by Part B

I **S9376** Home infusion therapy, hydration therapy; more than two liters but no more than three liters per day, administrative services, professional pharmacy services, care coordination, and all necessary supplies and equipment (drugs and nursing visits coded separately), per diem
BETOS: Z2   Undefined codes
Service not separately priced by Part B

I **S9377** Home infusion therapy, hydration therapy; more than three liters per day, administrative services, professional pharmacy services, care coordination, and all necessary supplies (drugs and nursing visits coded separately), per diem
BETOS: Z2   Undefined codes
Service not separately priced by Part B

I **S9379** Home infusion therapy, infusion therapy, not otherwise classified; administrative services, professional pharmacy services, care coordination, and all necessary supplies and equipment (drugs and nursing visits coded separately), per diem
BETOS: Z2   Undefined codes
Service not separately priced by Part B

MISCELLANEOUS SUPPLIES AND SERVICES (S9381-S9485), SEE ALSO MISCELLANEOUS SUPPLIES AND SERVICES (S8265-S9152)

I **S9381** Delivery or service to high risk areas requiring escort or extra protection, per visit
BETOS: Z2   Undefined codes
Service not separately priced by Part B

I **S9401** Anticoagulation clinic, inclusive of all services except laboratory tests, per session
BETOS: Z2   Undefined codes
Service not separately priced by Part B

I **S9430** Pharmacy compounding and dispensing services
BETOS: Z2   Undefined codes
Service not separately priced by Part B

I **S9433** Medical food nutritionally complete, administered orally, providing 100% of nutritional intake
BETOS: Z2   Undefined codes
Service not separately priced by Part B
Coding Clinic: 2008, Q4

● New code   ▲ Revised code   **C** Carrier judgment   **D** Special coverage instructions apply
I Not payable by Medicare   **M** Non-covered by Medicare   **S** Non-covered by Medicare statute   AHA Coding Clinic®

S9434 Modified solid food supplements for inborn errors of metabolism
BETOS: Z2   Undefined codes
Service not separately priced by Part B

S9435 Medical foods for inborn errors of metabolism
BETOS: Z2   Undefined codes
Service not separately priced by Part B

S9436 Childbirth preparation/lamaze classes, non-physician provider, per session   ♀ Ⓐ
BETOS: Z2   Undefined codes
Service not separately priced by Part B

S9437 Childbirth refresher classes, non-physician provider, per session   ♀ Ⓐ
BETOS: Z2   Undefined codes
Service not separately priced by Part B

S9438 Cesarean birth classes, non-physician provider, per session   ♀ Ⓐ
BETOS: Z2   Undefined codes
Service not separately priced by Part B

S9439 VBAC (vaginal birth after cesarean) classes, non-physician provider, per session   ♀ Ⓐ
BETOS: Z2   Undefined codes
Service not separately priced by Part B

S9441 Asthma education, non-physician provider, per session
BETOS: Z2   Undefined codes
Service not separately priced by Part B

S9442 Birthing classes, non-physician provider, per session   ♀ Ⓐ
BETOS: Z2   Undefined codes
Service not separately priced by Part B

S9443 Lactation classes, non-physician provider, per session   ♀ Ⓐ
BETOS: Z2   Undefined codes
Service not separately priced by Part B

S9444 Parenting classes, non-physician provider, per session
BETOS: Z2   Undefined codes
Service not separately priced by Part B

S9445 Patient education, not otherwise classified, non-physician provider, individual, per session
BETOS: Z2   Undefined codes
Service not separately priced by Part B

S9446 Patient education, not otherwise classified, non-physician provider, group, per session
BETOS: Z2   Undefined codes
Service not separately priced by Part B

S9447 Infant safety (including CPR) classes, non-physician provider, per session
BETOS: Z2   Undefined codes
Service not separately priced by Part B

S9449 Weight management classes, non-physician provider, per session
BETOS: Z2   Undefined codes
Service not separately priced by Part B

S9451 Exercise classes, non-physician provider, per session
BETOS: Z2   Undefined codes
Service not separately priced by Part B

S9452 Nutrition classes, non-physician provider, per session
BETOS: Z2   Undefined codes
Service not separately priced by Part B

S9453 Smoking cessation classes, non-physician provider, per session
BETOS: Z2   Undefined codes
Service not separately priced by Part B

S9454 Stress management classes, non-physician provider, per session
BETOS: Z2   Undefined codes
Service not separately priced by Part B

S9455 Diabetic management program, group session
BETOS: Z2   Undefined codes
Service not separately priced by Part B

S9460 Diabetic management program, nurse visit
BETOS: Z2   Undefined codes
Service not separately priced by Part B

S9465 Diabetic management program, dietitian visit
BETOS: Z2   Undefined codes
Service not separately priced by Part B

S9470 Nutritional counseling, dietitian visit
BETOS: Z2   Undefined codes
Service not separately priced by Part B

S9472 Cardiac rehabilitation program, non-physician provider, per diem
BETOS: Z2   Undefined codes
Service not separately priced by Part B

S9473 Pulmonary rehabilitation program, non-physician provider, per diem
BETOS: Z2   Undefined codes
Service not separately priced by Part B

S9474 Enterostomal therapy by a registered nurse certified in enterostomal therapy, per diem
BETOS: Z2   Undefined codes
Service not separately priced by Part B

S9475 Ambulatory setting substance abuse treatment or detoxification services, per diem
BETOS: Z2   Undefined codes
Service not separately priced by Part B

S9476 Vestibular rehabilitation program, non-physician provider, per diem
BETOS: Z2   Undefined codes
Service not separately priced by Part B

♂ Male only   ♀ Female only   Ⓐ Age   A2 - Z3 = ASC Payment indicator   A - Y = APC Status indicator
ASC = ASC Approved Procedure   **DME** Paid under the DME fee schedule   **MIPS** MIPS code

S9434 - S9476   TEMPORARY NATIONAL CODES (NON-MEDICARE) (S0012-S9999)

S9480 Intensive outpatient psychiatric services, per diem `MIPS`
BETOS: Z2   Undefined codes
Service not separately priced by Part B

S9482 Family stabilization services, per 15 minutes
BETOS: Z2   Undefined codes
Service not separately priced by Part B

S9484 Crisis intervention mental health services, per hour `MIPS`
BETOS: Z2   Undefined codes
Service not separately priced by Part B

S9485 Crisis intervention mental health services, per diem `MIPS`
BETOS: Z2   Undefined codes
Service not separately priced by Part B

HOME THERAPY SERVICES (S9490-S9810), SEE ALSO
HOME INFUSION THERAPY (S9325-S9379); HOME INFUSION
THERAPY (S5497-S5523)

S9490 Home infusion therapy, corticosteroid infusion; administrative services, professional pharmacy services, care coordination, and all necessary supplies and equipment (drugs and nursing visits coded separately), per diem
BETOS: Z2   Undefined codes
Service not separately priced by Part B

S9494 Home infusion therapy, antibiotic, antiviral, or antifungal therapy; administrative services, professional pharmacy services, care coordination, and all necessary supplies and equipment (drugs and nursing visits coded separately), per diem (do not use this code with home infusion codes for hourly dosing schedules S9497-S9504)
BETOS: Z2   Undefined codes
Service not separately priced by Part B

S9497 Home infusion therapy, antibiotic, antiviral, or antifungal therapy; once every 3 hours; administrative services, professional pharmacy services, care coordination, and all necessary supplies and equipment (drugs and nursing visits coded separately), per diem
BETOS: Z2   Undefined codes
Service not separately priced by Part B

S9500 Home infusion therapy, antibiotic, antiviral, or antifungal therapy; once every 24 hours; administrative services, professional pharmacy services, care coordination, and all necessary supplies and equipment (drugs and nursing visits coded separately), per diem
BETOS: Z2   Undefined codes
Service not separately priced by Part B

S9501 Home infusion therapy, antibiotic, antiviral, or antifungal therapy; once every 12 hours; administrative services, professional pharmacy services, care coordination, and all necessary supplies and equipment (drugs and nursing visits coded separately), per diem
BETOS: Z2   Undefined codes
Service not separately priced by Part B

S9502 Home infusion therapy, antibiotic, antiviral, or antifungal therapy; once every 8 hours, administrative services, professional pharmacy services, care coordination, and all necessary supplies and equipment (drugs and nursing visits coded separately), per diem
BETOS: Z2   Undefined codes
Service not separately priced by Part B

S9503 Home infusion therapy, antibiotic, antiviral, or antifungal; once every 6 hours; administrative services, professional pharmacy services, care coordination, and all necessary supplies and equipment (drugs and nursing visits coded separately), per diem
BETOS: Z2   Undefined codes
Service not separately priced by Part B

S9504 Home infusion therapy, antibiotic, antiviral, or antifungal; once every 4 hours; administrative services, professional pharmacy services, care coordination, and all necessary supplies and equipment (drugs and nursing visits coded separately), per diem
BETOS: Z2   Undefined codes
Service not separately priced by Part B

S9529 Routine venipuncture for collection of specimen(s), single home bound, nursing home, or skilled nursing facility patient
BETOS: Z2   Undefined codes
Service not separately priced by Part B

S9537 Home therapy; hematopoietic hormone injection therapy (e.g., erythropoietin, G-CSF, GM-CSF); administrative services, professional pharmacy services, care coordination, and all necessary supplies and equipment (drugs and nursing visits coded separately), per diem
BETOS: Z2   Undefined codes
Service not separately priced by Part B

S9538 Home transfusion of blood product(s); administrative services, professional pharmacy services, care coordination and all necessary supplies and equipment (blood products, drugs, and nursing visits coded separately), per diem
BETOS: Z2   Undefined codes
Service not separately priced by Part B

● New code   ▲ Revised code   **C** Carrier judgment   **D** Special coverage instructions apply
I Not payable by Medicare   **M** Non-covered by Medicare   **S** Non-covered by Medicare statute   AHA Coding Clinic®

I S9542 Home injectable therapy, not otherwise classified, including administrative services, professional pharmacy services, care coordination, and all necessary supplies and equipment (drugs and nursing visits coded separately), per diem
BETOS: Z2   Undefined codes
Service not separately priced by Part B

I S9558 Home injectable therapy; growth hormone, including administrative services, professional pharmacy services, care coordination, and all necessary supplies and equipment (drugs and nursing visits coded separately), per diem
BETOS: Z2   Undefined codes
Service not separately priced by Part B

I S9559 Home injectable therapy, interferon, including administrative services, professional pharmacy services, care coordination, and all necessary supplies and equipment (drugs and nursing visits coded separately), per diem
BETOS: Z2   Undefined codes
Service not separately priced by Part B

I S9560 Home injectable therapy; hormonal therapy (e.g., Leuprolide, Goserelin), including administrative services, professional pharmacy services, care coordination, and all necessary supplies and equipment (drugs and nursing visits coded separately), per diem
BETOS: Z2   Undefined codes
Service not separately priced by Part B

I S9562 Home injectable therapy, Palivizumab, including administrative services, professional pharmacy services, care coordination, and all necessary supplies and equipment (drugs and nursing visits coded separately), per diem
BETOS: Z2   Undefined codes
Service not separately priced by Part B

I S9590 Home therapy, irrigation therapy (e.g., sterile irrigation of an organ or anatomical cavity); including administrative services, professional pharmacy services, care coordination, and all necessary supplies and equipment (drugs and nursing visits coded separately), per diem
BETOS: Z2   Undefined codes
Service not separately priced by Part B

I S9810 Home therapy; professional pharmacy services for provision of infusion, specialty drug administration, and/or disease state management, not otherwise classified, per hour (do not use this code with any per diem code)
BETOS: Z2   Undefined codes
Service not separately priced by Part B

VARIOUS SERVICES, FEES, AND COSTS (S9900-S9999)

I S9900 Services by a Journal-listed Christian Science practitioner for the purpose of healing, per diem
BETOS: Z2   Undefined codes
Service not separately priced by Part B

I S9901 Services by a journal-listed Christian Science nurse, per hour
BETOS: Z2   Undefined codes
Service not separately priced by Part B

I S9960 Ambulance service, conventional air service, nonemergency transport, one-way (fixed wing)
BETOS: O1A   Ambulance
Service not separately priced by Part B

I S9961 Ambulance service, conventional air service, nonemergency transport, one-way (rotary wing)
BETOS: O1A   Ambulance
Service not separately priced by Part B

I S9970 Health club membership, annual
BETOS: Z2   Undefined codes
Service not separately priced by Part B

I S9975 Transplant related lodging, meals and transportation, per diem
BETOS: Z2   Undefined codes
Service not separately priced by Part B

I S9976 Lodging, per diem, not otherwise classified
BETOS: Z2   Undefined codes
Service not separately priced by Part B

I S9977 Meals, per diem, not otherwise specified
BETOS: Z2   Undefined codes
Service not separately priced by Part B

I S9981 Medical records copying fee, administrative
BETOS: Z2   Undefined codes
Service not separately priced by Part B

I S9982 Medical records copying fee, per page
BETOS: Z2   Undefined codes
Service not separately priced by Part B

I S9986 Not medically necessary service (patient is aware that service not medically necessary)
BETOS: Z2   Undefined codes
Service not separately priced by Part B

I S9988 Services provided as part of a Phase I clinical trial
BETOS: Z2   Undefined codes
Service not separately priced by Part B

I S9989 Services provided outside of the United States of America (list in addition to code(s) for service(s))
BETOS: Z2   Undefined codes
Service not separately priced by Part B

♂ Male only   ♀ Female only   Ⓐ Age   A2 - Z3 = ASC Payment indicator   A - Y = APC Status indicator
ASC = ASC Approved Procedure   **DME** Paid under the DME fee schedule   **MIPS** MIPS code

S9990 - S9999

▌ S9990 Services provided as part of a Phase II clinical trial

BETOS: Z2   Undefined codes
Service not separately priced by Part B

▌ S9991 Services provided as part of a Phase III clinical trial

BETOS: Z2   Undefined codes
Service not separately priced by Part B

▌ S9992 Transportation costs to and from trial location and local transportation costs (e.g., fares for taxicab or bus) for clinical trial participant and one caregiver/companion

BETOS: Z2   Undefined codes
Service not separately priced by Part B

▌ S9994 Lodging costs (e.g., hotel charges) for clinical trial participant and one caregiver/companion

BETOS: Z2   Undefined codes
Service not separately priced by Part B

▌ S9996 Meals for clinical trial participant and one caregiver/companion

BETOS: Z2   Undefined codes
Service not separately priced by Part B

▌ S9999 Sales tax

BETOS: Z2   Undefined codes
Service not separately priced by Part B
Coding Clinic: 2009, Q2

NATIONAL CODES ESTABLISHED FOR STATE MEDICAID AGENCIES (T1000-T5999)

NURSING SERVICES (T1000-T1005), SEE ALSO ADDITIONAL NURSING SERVICES (T1030-T1031)

T1000 Private duty / independent nursing service(s) - licensed, up to 15 minutes
BETOS: Z2   Undefined codes
Service not separately priced by Part B
Coding Clinic: 2009, Q2

T1001 Nursing assessment / evaluation
BETOS: Z2   Undefined codes
Service not separately priced by Part B

T1002 RN services, up to 15 minutes
BETOS: Z2   Undefined codes
Service not separately priced by Part B

T1003 LPN/LVN services, up to 15 minutes
BETOS: Z2   Undefined codes
Service not separately priced by Part B

T1004 Services of a qualified nursing aide, up to 15 minutes
BETOS: Z2   Undefined codes
Service not separately priced by Part B

T1005 Respite care services, up to 15 minutes
BETOS: Z2   Undefined codes
Service not separately priced by Part B

ALCOHOL AND SUBSTANCE ABUSE SERVICES (T1006-T1012)

T1006 Alcohol and/or substance abuse services, family/couple counseling
BETOS: Z2   Undefined codes
Service not separately priced by Part B

T1007 Alcohol and/or substance abuse services, treatment plan development and/or modification
BETOS: Z2   Undefined codes
Service not separately priced by Part B

T1009 Child sitting services for children of the individual receiving alcohol and/or substance abuse services   Ⓐ
BETOS: Z2   Undefined codes
Service not separately priced by Part B

T1010 Meals for individuals receiving alcohol and/or substance abuse services (when meals not included in the program)
BETOS: Z2   Undefined codes
Service not separately priced by Part B

T1012 Alcohol and/or substance abuse services, skills development
BETOS: Z2   Undefined codes
Service not separately priced by Part B

OTHER SERVICES (T1013-T1018)

T1013 Sign language or oral interpretive services, per 15 minutes
BETOS: Z2   Undefined codes
Service not separately priced by Part B

T1014 Telehealth transmission, per minute, professional services bill separately
BETOS: Z2   Undefined codes
Service not separately priced by Part B

T1015 Clinic visit/encounter, all-inclusive   MIPS
BETOS: Z2   Undefined codes
Service not separately priced by Part B
Coding Clinic: 2002, Q1

T1016 Case management, each 15 minutes
BETOS: Z2   Undefined codes
Service not separately priced by Part B

T1017 Targeted case management, each 15 minutes
BETOS: Z2   Undefined codes
Service not separately priced by Part B

T1018 School-based individualized education program (IEP) services, bundled
BETOS: Z2   Undefined codes
Service not separately priced by Part B

HOME HEALTH SERVICES (T1019-T1022)

T1019 Personal care services, per 15 minutes, not for an inpatient or resident of a hospital, nursing facility, ICF/MR or IMD, part of the individualized plan of treatment (code may not be used to identify services provided by home health aide or certified nurse assistant)
BETOS: Z2   Undefined codes
Service not separately priced by Part B

T1020 Personal care services, per diem, not for an inpatient or resident of a hospital, nursing facility, ICF/MR or IMD, part of the individualized plan of treatment (code may not be used to identify services provided by home health aide or certified nurse assistant)
BETOS: Z2   Undefined codes
Service not separately priced by Part B

T1021 Home health aide or certified nurse assistant, per visit
BETOS: Z2   Undefined codes
Service not separately priced by Part B

T1022 Contracted home health agency services, all services provided under contract, per day
BETOS: Z2   Undefined codes
Service not separately priced by Part B

♂ Male only   ♀ Female only   Ⓐ Age   A2 - Z3 = ASC Payment indicator   A - Y = APC Status indicator
ASC = ASC Approved Procedure   **DME** Paid under the DME fee schedule   **MIPS** MIPS code

SCREENINGS, ASSESSMENTS, AND TREATMENTS, INDIVIDUAL AND FAMILY (T1023-T1029)

I **T1023** Screening to determine the appropriateness of consideration of an individual for participation in a specified program, project or treatment protocol, per encounter
BETOS: Z2   Undefined codes
Service not separately priced by Part B

I **T1024** Evaluation and treatment by an integrated, specialty team contracted to provide coordinated care to multiple or severely handicapped children, per encounter   Ⓐ
BETOS: Z2   Undefined codes
Service not separately priced by Part B

I **T1025** Intensive, extended multidisciplinary services provided in a clinic setting to children with complex medical, physical, mental and psychosocial impairments, per diem   Ⓐ
BETOS: Z2   Undefined codes
Service not separately priced by Part B

I **T1026** Intensive, extended multidisciplinary services provided in a clinic setting to children with complex medical, physical, medical and psychosocial impairments, per hour   Ⓐ
BETOS: Z2   Undefined codes
Service not separately priced by Part B

I **T1027** Family training and counseling for child development, per 15 minutes   Ⓐ
BETOS: Z2   Undefined codes
Service not separately priced by Part B

I **T1028** Assessment of home, physical and family environment, to determine suitability to meet patient's medical needs
BETOS: Z2   Undefined codes
Service not separately priced by Part B

I **T1029** Comprehensive environmental lead investigation, not including laboratory analysis, per dwelling
BETOS: Z2   Undefined codes
Service not separately priced by Part B

ADDITIONAL NURSING SERVICES (T1030-T1031), SEE ALSO NURSING SERVICES (T1000-T1005)

I **T1030** Nursing care, in the home, by registered nurse, per diem
BETOS: Z2   Undefined codes
Service not separately priced by Part B

I **T1031** Nursing care, in the home, by licensed practical nurse, per diem
BETOS: Z2   Undefined codes
Service not separately priced by Part B

BEHAVIORAL HEALTH SERVICES (T1040-T1041)

I **T1040** Medicaid certified community behavioral health clinic services, per diem
BETOS: Z2   Undefined codes
Service not separately priced by Part B

I **T1041** Medicaid certified community behavioral health clinic services, per month
BETOS: Z2   Undefined codes
Service not separately priced by Part B

MISCELLANEOUS SERVICES AND SUPPLIES (T1502-T1999)

I **T1502** Administration of oral, intramuscular and/or subcutaneous medication by health care agency/professional, per visit
BETOS: Z2   Undefined codes
Service not separately priced by Part B

I **T1503** Administration of medication, other than oral and/or injectable, by a health care agency/professional, per visit
BETOS: Z2   Undefined codes
Service not separately priced by Part B

I **T1505** Electronic medication compliance management device, includes all components and accessories, not otherwise classified
BETOS: Z2   Undefined codes
Service not separately priced by Part B

I **T1999** Miscellaneous therapeutic items and supplies, retail purchases, not otherwise classified; identify product in "remarks"
BETOS: Z2   Undefined codes
Service not separately priced by Part B

TRANSPORTATION SERVICES (T2001-T2007)

I **T2001** Non-emergency transportation; patient attendant/escort
BETOS: Z2   Undefined codes
Service not separately priced by Part B

I **T2002** Non-emergency transportation; per diem
BETOS: Z2   Undefined codes
Service not separately priced by Part B

I **T2003** Non-emergency transportation; encounter/trip
BETOS: Z2   Undefined codes
Service not separately priced by Part B

I **T2004** Non-emergency transport; commercial carrier, multi-pass
BETOS: Z2   Undefined codes
Service not separately priced by Part B

I **T2005** Non-emergency transportation; stretcher van
BETOS: Z2   Undefined codes
Service not separately priced by Part B

● New code   ▲ Revised code   **C** Carrier judgment   **D** Special coverage instructions apply
I Not payable by Medicare   **M** Non-covered by Medicare   **S** Non-covered by Medicare statute   AHA Coding Clinic®

T2007 Transportation waiting time, air ambulance and non-emergency vehicle, one-half (1/2) hour increments
BETOS: Z2 Undefined codes
Service not separately priced by Part B

PREADMISSION SCREENING (T2010-T2011)

T2010 Preadmission screening and resident review (PASRR) level I identification screening, per screen
BETOS: Z2 Undefined codes
Service not separately priced by Part B

T2011 Preadmission screening and resident review (PASRR) level II evaluation, per evaluation
BETOS: Z2 Undefined codes
Service not separately priced by Part B

WAIVER SERVICES (T2012-T2041)

T2012 Habilitation, educational; waiver, per diem
BETOS: Z2 Undefined codes
Service not separately priced by Part B

T2013 Habilitation, educational, waiver; per hour
BETOS: Z2 Undefined codes
Service not separately priced by Part B

T2014 Habilitation, prevocational, waiver; per diem
BETOS: Z2 Undefined codes
Service not separately priced by Part B

T2015 Habilitation, prevocational, waiver; per hour
BETOS: Z2 Undefined codes
Service not separately priced by Part B

T2016 Habilitation, residential, waiver; per diem
BETOS: Z2 Undefined codes
Service not separately priced by Part B

T2017 Habilitation, residential, waiver; 15 minutes
BETOS: Z2 Undefined codes
Service not separately priced by Part B

T2018 Habilitation, supported employment, waiver; per diem
BETOS: Z2 Undefined codes
Service not separately priced by Part B

T2019 Habilitation, supported employment, waiver; per 15 minutes
BETOS: Z2 Undefined codes
Service not separately priced by Part B

T2020 Day habilitation, waiver; per diem
BETOS: Z2 Undefined codes
Service not separately priced by Part B

T2021 Day habilitation, waiver; per 15 minutes
BETOS: Z2 Undefined codes
Service not separately priced by Part B

T2022 Case management, per month
BETOS: Z2 Undefined codes
Service not separately priced by Part B

T2023 Targeted case management; per month
BETOS: Z2 Undefined codes
Service not separately priced by Part B

T2024 Service assessment/plan of care development, waiver
BETOS: Z2 Undefined codes
Service not separately priced by Part B

T2025 Waiver services; not otherwise specified (NOS)
BETOS: Z2 Undefined codes
Service not separately priced by Part B

T2026 Specialized childcare, waiver; per diem ⓐ
BETOS: Z2 Undefined codes
Service not separately priced by Part B

T2027 Specialized childcare, waiver; per 15 minutes ⓐ
BETOS: Z2 Undefined codes
Service not separately priced by Part B

T2028 Specialized supply, not otherwise specified, waiver
BETOS: Z2 Undefined codes
Service not separately priced by Part B

T2029 Specialized medical equipment, not otherwise specified, waiver
BETOS: Z2 Undefined codes
Service not separately priced by Part B

T2030 Assisted living, waiver; per month
BETOS: Z2 Undefined codes
Service not separately priced by Part B

T2031 Assisted living; waiver, per diem
BETOS: Z2 Undefined codes
Service not separately priced by Part B

T2032 Residential care, not otherwise specified (NOS), waiver; per month
BETOS: Z2 Undefined codes
Service not separately priced by Part B

T2033 Residential care, not otherwise specified (NOS), waiver; per diem
BETOS: Z2 Undefined codes
Service not separately priced by Part B

T2034 Crisis intervention, waiver; per diem
BETOS: Z2 Undefined codes
Service not separately priced by Part B

T2035 Utility services to support medical equipment and assistive technology/devices, waiver
BETOS: Z2 Undefined codes
Service not separately priced by Part B

T2036 Therapeutic camping, overnight, waiver; each session
BETOS: Z2 Undefined codes
Service not separately priced by Part B

♂ Male only   ♀ Female only   ⓐ Age   A2 - Z3 = ASC Payment indicator   A - Y = APC Status indicator
ASC = ASC Approved Procedure   **DME** Paid under the DME fee schedule   **MIPS** MIPS code

I T2037 Therapeutic camping, day, waiver; each session
BETOS: Z2   Undefined codes
Service not separately priced by Part B

I T2038 Community transition, waiver; per service
BETOS: Z2   Undefined codes
Service not separately priced by Part B

I T2039 Vehicle modifications, waiver; per service
BETOS: Z2   Undefined codes
Service not separately priced by Part B

I T2040 Financial management, self-directed, waiver; per 15 minutes
BETOS: Z2   Undefined codes
Service not separately priced by Part B

I T2041 Supports brokerage, self-directed, waiver; per 15 minutes
BETOS: Z2   Undefined codes
Service not separately priced by Part B

HOSPICE CARE (T2042-T2046)

I T2042 Hospice routine home care; per diem
BETOS: Z2   Undefined codes
Service not separately priced by Part B

I T2043 Hospice continuous home care; per hour
BETOS: Z2   Undefined codes
Service not separately priced by Part B

I T2044 Hospice inpatient respite care; per diem
BETOS: Z2   Undefined codes
Service not separately priced by Part B

I T2045 Hospice general inpatient care; per diem
BETOS: Z2   Undefined codes
Service not separately priced by Part B

I T2046 Hospice long term care, room and board only; per diem
BETOS: Z2   Undefined codes
Service not separately priced by Part B

PREVOCATIONAL HABILITATION WAIVER SERVICES (T2047)

● **I T2047** Habilitation, prevocational, waiver; per 15 minutes
BETOS: Z2   Undefined codes
Service not separately priced by Part B

LONG-TERM RESIDENTIAL CARE (T2048)

I T2048 Behavioral health; long-term care residential (non-acute care in a residential treatment program where stay is typically longer than 30 days), with room and board, per diem **MIPS**
BETOS: Z2   Undefined codes
Service not separately priced by Part B

NON-EMERGENCY TRANSPORTATION FEES (T2049)

I T2049 Non-emergency transportation; stretcher van, mileage; per mile
BETOS: Z2   Undefined codes
Service not separately priced by Part B

SERVICES RELATED TO BREAST MILK (T2101)

I T2101 Human breast milk processing, storage and distribution only   ♀ Ⓐ
BETOS: Z2   Undefined codes
Service not separately priced by Part B

INCONTINENCE SUPPLIES (T4521-T4545)

M T4521 Adult sized disposable incontinence product, brief/diaper, small, each   Ⓐ
BETOS: D1A   Medical/surgical supplies
Service not separately priced by Part B

M T4522 Adult sized disposable incontinence product, brief/diaper, medium, each   Ⓐ
BETOS: D1A   Medical/surgical supplies
Service not separately priced by Part B

M T4523 Adult sized disposable incontinence product, brief/diaper, large, each   Ⓐ
BETOS: D1A   Medical/surgical supplies
Service not separately priced by Part B

M T4524 Adult sized disposable incontinence product, brief/diaper, extra large, each   Ⓐ
BETOS: D1A   Medical/surgical supplies
Service not separately priced by Part B

M T4525 Adult sized disposable incontinence product, protective underwear/pull-on, small size, each   Ⓐ
BETOS: D1A   Medical/surgical supplies
Service not separately priced by Part B

M T4526 Adult sized disposable incontinence product, protective underwear/pull-on, medium size, each   Ⓐ
BETOS: D1A   Medical/surgical supplies
Service not separately priced by Part B

M T4527 Adult sized disposable incontinence product, protective underwear/pull-on, large size, each   Ⓐ
BETOS: D1A   Medical/surgical supplies
Service not separately priced by Part B

M T4528 Adult sized disposable incontinence product, protective underwear/pull-on, extra large size, each   Ⓐ
BETOS: D1A   Medical/surgical supplies
Service not separately priced by Part B

M T4529 Pediatric sized disposable incontinence product, brief/diaper, small/medium size, each   Ⓐ
BETOS: D1A   Medical/surgical supplies
Service not separately priced by Part B

● New code   ▲ Revised code   **C** Carrier judgment   **D** Special coverage instructions apply
I Not payable by Medicare   **M** Non-covered by Medicare   **S** Non-covered by Medicare statute   AHA Coding Clinic®

Ⓜ **T4530** Pediatric sized disposable incontinence product, brief/diaper, large size, each Ⓐ
BETOS: D1A Medical/surgical supplies
Service not separately priced by Part B

Ⓜ **T4531** Pediatric sized disposable incontinence product, protective underwear/pull-on, small/medium size, each Ⓐ
BETOS: D1A Medical/surgical supplies
Service not separately priced by Part B

Ⓜ **T4532** Pediatric sized disposable incontinence product, protective underwear/pull-on, large size, each Ⓐ
BETOS: D1A Medical/surgical supplies
Service not separately priced by Part B

Ⓜ **T4533** Youth-sized disposable incontinence product, brief/diaper, each
BETOS: D1A Medical/surgical supplies
Service not separately priced by Part B

Ⓜ **T4534** Youth-sized disposable incontinence product, protective underwear/pull-on, each
BETOS: D1A Medical/surgical supplies
Service not separately priced by Part B

Ⓜ **T4535** Disposable liner/shield/guard/pad/undergarment, for incontinence, each
BETOS: D1A Medical/surgical supplies
Service not separately priced by Part B

Ⓜ **T4536** Incontinence product, protective underwear/pull-on, reusable, any size, each
BETOS: D1A Medical/surgical supplies
Service not separately priced by Part B

Ⓜ **T4537** Incontinence product, protective underpad, reusable, bed size, each
BETOS: D1A Medical/surgical supplies
Service not separately priced by Part B

Ⓜ **T4538** Diaper service, reusable diaper, each diaper
BETOS: D1A Medical/surgical supplies
Service not separately priced by Part B

Ⓜ **T4539** Incontinence product, diaper/brief, reusable, any size, each
BETOS: D1A Medical/surgical supplies
Service not separately priced by Part B

Ⓜ **T4540** Incontinence product, protective underpad, reusable, chair size, each
BETOS: D1A Medical/surgical supplies
Service not separately priced by Part B

Ⅰ **T4541** Incontinence product, disposable underpad, large, each
BETOS: Z2 Undefined codes
Service not separately priced by Part B

Ⅰ **T4542** Incontinence product, disposable underpad, small size, each
BETOS: Z2 Undefined codes
Service not separately priced by Part B

Ⓜ **T4543** Adult sized disposable incontinence product, protective brief/diaper, above extra large, each Ⓐ
BETOS: D1A Medical/surgical supplies
Service not separately priced by Part B

Ⓜ **T4544** Adult sized disposable incontinence product, protective underwear/pull-on, above extra large, each Ⓐ
BETOS: D1A Medical/surgical supplies
Service not separately priced by Part B

Ⓜ **T4545** Incontinence product, disposable, penile wrap, each ♂
BETOS: D1A Medical/surgical supplies
Service not separately priced by Part B

OTHER AND UNSPECIFIED SUPPLIES (T5001-T5999)

Ⅰ **T5001** Positioning seat for persons with special orthopedic needs
BETOS: Z2 Undefined codes
Service not separately priced by Part B

Ⅰ **T5999** Supply, not otherwise specified
BETOS: Z2 Undefined codes
Service not separately priced by Part B

♂ Male only　　♀ Female only　　Ⓐ Age　　A2 - Z3 = ASC Payment indicator　　A - Y = APC Status indicator
ASC = ASC Approved Procedure　　**DME** Paid under the DME fee schedule　　**MIPS** MIPS code

NOTES

CORONAVIRUS DIAGNOSTIC PANEL
(U0001-U0005)

- **C** **U0001** CDC 2019 novel coronavirus (2019-nCoV) real-time RT-PCR diagnostic panel   A
  BETOS: T1H   Lab tests - other (non-Medicare fee schedule)
  Price established by carriers
  Coding Clinic: 2020, Q2

- **C** **U0002** 2019-nCoV Coronavirus, SARS-CoV-2/2019-nCoV (COVID-19), any technique, multiple types or subtypes (includes all targets), non-CDC   A
  BETOS: T1H   Lab tests - other (non-Medicare fee schedule)
  Price established by carriers
  Coding Clinic: 2020, Q2

- **C** **U0003** Infectious agent detection by nucleic acid (DNA or RNA); severe acute respiratory syndrome coronavirus 2 (SARS-CoV-2) (Coronavirus disease [COVID-19]), amplified probe technique, making use of high throughput technologies as described by CMS-2020-01-R   A
  BETOS: T1H   Lab tests - other (non-Medicare fee schedule)
  Price established by carriers
  Coding Clinic: 2020, Q2

- **C** **U0004** 2019-nCoV Coronavirus, SARS-CoV-2/2019-nCoV (COVID-19), any technique, multiple types or subtypes (includes all targets), non-CDC, making use of high throughput technologies as described by CMS-2020-01-R   A
  BETOS: T1H   Lab tests - other (non-Medicare fee schedule)
  Price established by carriers
  Coding Clinic: 2020, Q2

- **C** **U0005** Infectious agent detection by nucleic acid (DNA or RNA); severe acute respiratory syndrome coronavirus 2 (SARS-CoV-2) (coronavirus disease [COVID-19]), amplified probe technique, CDC or non-CDC, making use of high throughput technologies, completed within 2 calendar days from date of specimen collection (list separately in addition to either hcpcs code U0003 or U0004) as described by CMS-2020-01-r2   A
  BETOS: T1H   Lab tests - other (non-Medicare fee schedule)
  Price established by carriers

♂ Male only   ♀ Female only   **A** Age   A2 - Z3 = ASC Payment indicator   A - Y = APC Status indicator
ASC = ASC Approved Procedure   **DME** Paid under the DME fee schedule   **MIPS** MIPS code

NOTES

VISION SERVICES (V2020-V2799)

SPECTACLE FRAMES (V2020, V2025)

D **V2020** Frames, purchases `DME` A
BETOS: D1F   Prosthetic/Orthotic devices

M **V2025** Deluxe frame E1
BETOS: D1F   Prosthetic/Orthotic devices
Service not separately priced by Part B

LENSES, SINGLE VISION (V2100-V2199)

C **V2100** Sphere, single vision, plano to plus or minus 4.00, per lens `DME` A
BETOS: D1F   Prosthetic/Orthotic devices

C **V2101** Sphere, single vision, plus or minus 4.12 to plus or minus 7.00d, per lens `DME` A
BETOS: D1F   Prosthetic/Orthotic devices

C **V2102** Sphere, single vision, plus or minus 7.12 to plus or minus 20.00d, per lens `DME` A
BETOS: D1F   Prosthetic/Orthotic devices

C **V2103** Spherocylinder, single vision, plano to plus or minus 4.00d sphere, .12 to 2.00d cylinder, per lens `DME` A
BETOS: D1F   Prosthetic/Orthotic devices

C **V2104** Spherocylinder, single vision, plano to plus or minus 4.00d sphere, 2.12 to 4.00d cylinder, per lens `DME` A
BETOS: D1F   Prosthetic/Orthotic devices

C **V2105** Spherocylinder, single vision, plano to plus or minus 4.00d sphere, 4.25 to 6.00d cylinder, per lens `DME` A
BETOS: D1F   Prosthetic/Orthotic devices

C **V2106** Spherocylinder, single vision, plano to plus or minus 4.00d sphere, over 6.00d cylinder, per lens `DME` A
BETOS: D1F   Prosthetic/Orthotic devices

C **V2107** Spherocylinder, single vision, plus or minus 4.25 to plus or minus 7.00 sphere, .12 to 2.00d cylinder, per lens `DME` A
BETOS: D1F   Prosthetic/Orthotic devices

C **V2108** Spherocylinder, single vision, plus or minus 4.25d to plus or minus 7.00d sphere, 2.12 to 4.00d cylinder, per lens `DME` A
BETOS: D1F   Prosthetic/Orthotic devices

C **V2109** Spherocylinder, single vision, plus or minus 4.25 to plus or minus 7.00d sphere, 4.25 to 6.00d cylinder, per lens `DME` A
BETOS: D1F   Prosthetic/Orthotic devices

C **V2110** Spherocylinder, single vision, plus or minus 4.25 to 7.00d sphere, over 6.00d cylinder, per lens `DME` A
BETOS: D1F   Prosthetic/Orthotic devices

C **V2111** Spherocylinder, single vision, plus or minus 7.25 to plus or minus 12.00d sphere, .25 to 2.25d cylinder, per lens `DME` A
BETOS: D1F   Prosthetic/Orthotic devices

C **V2112** Spherocylinder, single vision, plus or minus 7.25 to plus or minus 12.00d sphere, 2.25d to 4.00d cylinder, per lens `DME` A
BETOS: D1F   Prosthetic/Orthotic devices

C **V2113** Spherocylinder, single vision, plus or minus 7.25 to plus or minus 12.00d sphere, 4.25 to 6.00d cylinder, per lens `DME` A
BETOS: D1F   Prosthetic/Orthotic devices

C **V2114** Spherocylinder, single vision, sphere over plus or minus 12.00d, per lens `DME` A
BETOS: D1F   Prosthetic/Orthotic devices

C **V2115** Lenticular, (Myodisc), per lens, single vision `DME` A
BETOS: D1F   Prosthetic/Orthotic devices

C **V2118** Aniseikonic lens, single vision `DME` A
BETOS: D1F   Prosthetic/Orthotic devices

D **V2121** Lenticular lens, per lens, single `DME` A
BETOS: D1F   Prosthetic/Orthotic devices

C **V2199** Not otherwise classified, single vision lens A
BETOS: D1F   Prosthetic/Orthotic devices

LENSES, BIFOCALS (V2200-V2299)

C **V2200** Sphere, bifocal, plano to plus or minus 4.00d, per lens `DME` A
BETOS: D1F   Prosthetic/Orthotic devices

C **V2201** Sphere, bifocal, plus or minus 4.12 to plus or minus 7.00d, per lens `DME` A
BETOS: D1F   Prosthetic/Orthotic devices

C **V2202** Sphere, bifocal, plus or minus 7.12 to plus or minus 20.00d, per lens `DME` A
BETOS: D1F   Prosthetic/Orthotic devices

C **V2203** Spherocylinder, bifocal, plano to plus or minus 4.00d sphere, 0.12 to 2.00d cylinder, per lens `DME` A
BETOS: D1F   Prosthetic/Orthotic devices

C **V2204** Spherocylinder, bifocal, plano to plus or minus 4.00d sphere, 2.12 to 4.00d cylinder, per lens `DME` A
BETOS: D1F   Prosthetic/Orthotic devices

C **V2205** Spherocylinder, bifocal, plano to plus or minus 4.00d sphere, 4.25 to 6.00d cylinder, per lens `DME` A
BETOS: D1F   Prosthetic/Orthotic devices

C **V2206** Spherocylinder, bifocal, plano to plus or minus 4.00d sphere, over 6.00d cylinder, per lens `DME` A
BETOS: D1F   Prosthetic/Orthotic devices

♂ Male only   ♀ Female only   **A** Age   A2 - Z3 = ASC Payment indicator   A - Y = APC Status indicator
ASC = ASC Approved Procedure   `DME` Paid under the DME fee schedule   `MIPS` MIPS code

C **V2207** Spherocylinder, bifocal, plus or minus 4.25 to plus or minus 7.00d sphere, .12 to 2.00d cylinder, per lens DME A
BETOS: D1F Prosthetic/Orthotic devices

C **V2208** Spherocylinder, bifocal, plus or minus 4.25 to plus or minus 7.00d sphere, 2.12 to 4.00d cylinder, per lens DME A
BETOS: D1F Prosthetic/Orthotic devices

C **V2209** Spherocylinder, bifocal, plus or minus 4.25 to plus or minus 7.00d sphere, 4.25 to 6.00d cylinder, per lens DME A
BETOS: D1F Prosthetic/Orthotic devices

C **V2210** Spherocylinder, bifocal, plus or minus 4.25 to plus or minus 7.00d sphere, over 6.00d cylinder, per lens DME A
BETOS: D1F Prosthetic/Orthotic devices

C **V2211** Spherocylinder, bifocal, plus or minus 7.25 to plus or minus 12.00d sphere, .25 to 2.25d cylinder, per lens DME A
BETOS: D1F Prosthetic/Orthotic devices

C **V2212** Spherocylinder, bifocal, plus or minus 7.25 to plus or minus 12.00d sphere, 2.25 to 4.00d cylinder, per lens DME A
BETOS: D1F Prosthetic/Orthotic devices

C **V2213** Spherocylinder, bifocal, plus or minus 7.25 to plus or minus 12.00d sphere, 4.25 to 6.00d cylinder, per lens DME A
BETOS: D1F Prosthetic/Orthotic devices

C **V2214** Spherocylinder, bifocal, sphere over plus or minus 12.00d, per lens DME A
BETOS: D1F Prosthetic/Orthotic devices

C **V2215** Lenticular (Myodisc), per lens, bifocal DME A
BETOS: D1F Prosthetic/Orthotic devices

C **V2218** Aniseikonic, per lens, bifocal DME A
BETOS: D1F Prosthetic/Orthotic devices

C **V2219** Bifocal seg width over 28mm DME A
BETOS: D1F Prosthetic/Orthotic devices

C **V2220** Bifocal add over 3.25d DME A
BETOS: D1F Prosthetic/Orthotic devices

D **V2221** Lenticular lens, per lens, bifocal DME A
BETOS: D1F Prosthetic/Orthotic devices

C **V2299** Specialty bifocal (by report) A
BETOS: D1F Prosthetic/Orthotic devices

LENSES, TRIFOCAL (V2300-V2399)

C **V2300** Sphere, trifocal, plano to plus or minus 4.00d, per lens DME A
BETOS: D1F Prosthetic/Orthotic devices

C **V2301** Sphere, trifocal, plus or minus 4.12 to plus or minus 7.00d, per lens DME A
BETOS: D1F Prosthetic/Orthotic devices

C **V2302** Sphere, trifocal, plus or minus 7.12 to plus or minus 20.00, per lens DME A
BETOS: D1F Prosthetic/Orthotic devices

C **V2303** Spherocylinder, trifocal, plano to plus or minus 4.00d sphere, .12-2.00d cylinder, per lens DME A
BETOS: D1F Prosthetic/Orthotic devices

C **V2304** Spherocylinder, trifocal, plano to plus or minus 4.00d sphere, 2.25-4.00d cylinder, per lens DME A
BETOS: D1F Prosthetic/Orthotic devices

C **V2305** Spherocylinder, trifocal, plano to plus or minus 4.00d sphere, 4.25 to 6.00 cylinder, per lens DME A
BETOS: D1F Prosthetic/Orthotic devices

C **V2306** Spherocylinder, trifocal, plano to plus or minus 4.00d sphere, over 6.00d cylinder, per lens DME A
BETOS: D1F Prosthetic/Orthotic devices

C **V2307** Spherocylinder, trifocal, plus or minus 4.25 to plus or minus 7.00d sphere, .12 to 2.00d cylinder, per lens DME A
BETOS: D1F Prosthetic/Orthotic devices

C **V2308** Spherocylinder, trifocal, plus or minus 4.25 to plus or minus 7.00d sphere, 2.12 to 4.00d cylinder, per lens DME A
BETOS: D1F Prosthetic/Orthotic devices

C **V2309** Spherocylinder, trifocal, plus or minus 4.25 to plus or minus 7.00d sphere, 4.25 to 6.00d cylinder, per lens DME A
BETOS: D1F Prosthetic/Orthotic devices

C **V2310** Spherocylinder, trifocal, plus or minus 4.25 to plus or minus 7.00d sphere, over 6.00d cylinder, per lens DME A
BETOS: D1F Prosthetic/Orthotic devices

C **V2311** Spherocylinder, trifocal, plus or minus 7.25 to plus or minus 12.00d sphere, .25 to 2.25d cylinder, per lens DME A
BETOS: D1F Prosthetic/Orthotic devices

C **V2312** Spherocylinder, trifocal, plus or minus 7.25 to plus or minus 12.00d sphere, 2.25 to 4.00d cylinder, per lens DME A
BETOS: D1F Prosthetic/Orthotic devices

C **V2313** Spherocylinder, trifocal, plus or minus 7.25 to plus or minus 12.00d sphere, 4.25 to 6.00d cylinder, per lens DME A
BETOS: D1F Prosthetic/Orthotic devices

C **V2314** Spherocylinder, trifocal, sphere over plus or minus 12 .00d, per lens DME A
BETOS: D1F Prosthetic/Orthotic devices

C **V2315** Lenticular, (Myodisc), per lens, trifocal DME A
BETOS: D1F Prosthetic/Orthotic devices

C **V2318** Aniseikonic lens, trifocal DME A
BETOS: D1F Prosthetic/Orthotic devices

● New code ▲ Revised code **C** Carrier judgment **D** Special coverage instructions apply
I Not payable by Medicare **M** Non-covered by Medicare **S** Non-covered by Medicare statute AHA Coding Clinic®

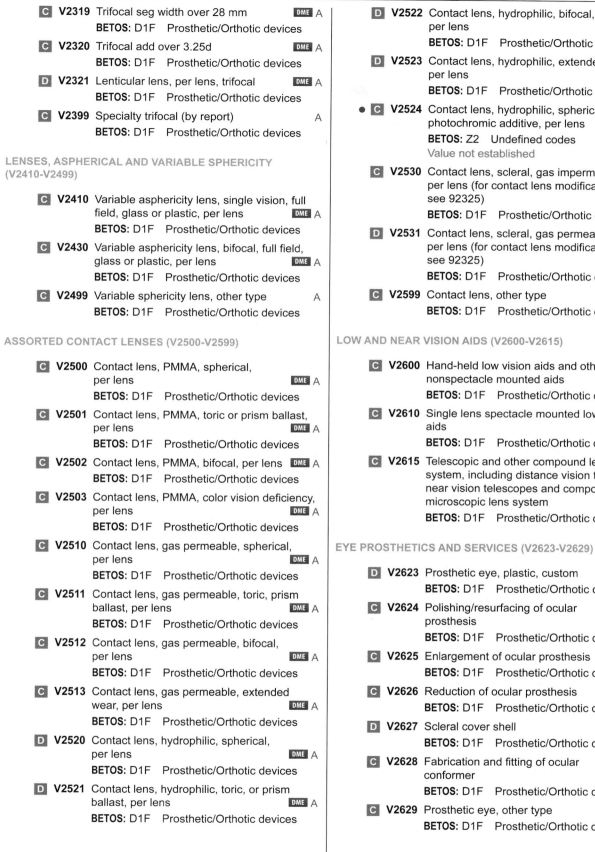

| | | |

C V2319 Trifocal seg width over 28 mm `DME` A
BETOS: D1F Prosthetic/Orthotic devices

C V2320 Trifocal add over 3.25d `DME` A
BETOS: D1F Prosthetic/Orthotic devices

D V2321 Lenticular lens, per lens, trifocal `DME` A
BETOS: D1F Prosthetic/Orthotic devices

C V2399 Specialty trifocal (by report) A
BETOS: D1F Prosthetic/Orthotic devices

LENSES, ASPHERICAL AND VARIABLE SPHERICITY (V2410-V2499)

C V2410 Variable asphericity lens, single vision, full field, glass or plastic, per lens `DME` A
BETOS: D1F Prosthetic/Orthotic devices

C V2430 Variable asphericity lens, bifocal, full field, glass or plastic, per lens `DME` A
BETOS: D1F Prosthetic/Orthotic devices

C V2499 Variable sphericity lens, other type A
BETOS: D1F Prosthetic/Orthotic devices

ASSORTED CONTACT LENSES (V2500-V2599)

C V2500 Contact lens, PMMA, spherical, per lens `DME` A
BETOS: D1F Prosthetic/Orthotic devices

C V2501 Contact lens, PMMA, toric or prism ballast, per lens `DME` A
BETOS: D1F Prosthetic/Orthotic devices

C V2502 Contact lens, PMMA, bifocal, per lens `DME` A
BETOS: D1F Prosthetic/Orthotic devices

C V2503 Contact lens, PMMA, color vision deficiency, per lens `DME` A
BETOS: D1F Prosthetic/Orthotic devices

C V2510 Contact lens, gas permeable, spherical, per lens `DME` A
BETOS: D1F Prosthetic/Orthotic devices

C V2511 Contact lens, gas permeable, toric, prism ballast, per lens `DME` A
BETOS: D1F Prosthetic/Orthotic devices

C V2512 Contact lens, gas permeable, bifocal, per lens `DME` A
BETOS: D1F Prosthetic/Orthotic devices

C V2513 Contact lens, gas permeable, extended wear, per lens `DME` A
BETOS: D1F Prosthetic/Orthotic devices

D V2520 Contact lens, hydrophilic, spherical, per lens `DME` A
BETOS: D1F Prosthetic/Orthotic devices

D V2521 Contact lens, hydrophilic, toric, or prism ballast, per lens `DME` A
BETOS: D1F Prosthetic/Orthotic devices

D V2522 Contact lens, hydrophilic, bifocal, per lens `DME` A
BETOS: D1F Prosthetic/Orthotic devices

D V2523 Contact lens, hydrophilic, extended wear, per lens `DME` A
BETOS: D1F Prosthetic/Orthotic devices

● **C V2524** Contact lens, hydrophilic, spherical, photochromic additive, per lens A
BETOS: Z2 Undefined codes
Value not established

C V2530 Contact lens, scleral, gas impermeable, per lens (for contact lens modification, see 92325) `DME` A
BETOS: D1F Prosthetic/Orthotic devices

D V2531 Contact lens, scleral, gas permeable, per lens (for contact lens modification, see 92325) `DME` A
BETOS: D1F Prosthetic/Orthotic devices

C V2599 Contact lens, other type A
BETOS: D1F Prosthetic/Orthotic devices

LOW AND NEAR VISION AIDS (V2600-V2615)

C V2600 Hand-held low vision aids and other nonspectacle mounted aids A
BETOS: D1F Prosthetic/Orthotic devices

C V2610 Single lens spectacle mounted low vision aids A
BETOS: D1F Prosthetic/Orthotic devices

C V2615 Telescopic and other compound lens system, including distance vision telescopic, near vision telescopes and compound microscopic lens system A
BETOS: D1F Prosthetic/Orthotic devices

EYE PROSTHETICS AND SERVICES (V2623-V2629)

D V2623 Prosthetic eye, plastic, custom `DME` A
BETOS: D1F Prosthetic/Orthotic devices

C V2624 Polishing/resurfacing of ocular prosthesis `DME` A
BETOS: D1F Prosthetic/Orthotic devices

C V2625 Enlargement of ocular prosthesis `DME` A
BETOS: D1F Prosthetic/Orthotic devices

C V2626 Reduction of ocular prosthesis `DME` A
BETOS: D1F Prosthetic/Orthotic devices

D V2627 Scleral cover shell `DME` A
BETOS: D1F Prosthetic/Orthotic devices

C V2628 Fabrication and fitting of ocular conformer `DME` A
BETOS: D1F Prosthetic/Orthotic devices

C V2629 Prosthetic eye, other type A
BETOS: D1F Prosthetic/Orthotic devices

♂ Male only   ♀ Female only   Ⓐ Age   A2 - Z3 = ASC Payment indicator   A - Y = APC Status indicator
ASC = ASC Approved Procedure   `DME` Paid under the DME fee schedule   `MIPS` MIPS code

LENSES, INTRAOCULAR (V2630-V2632)

D **V2630** Anterior chamber intraocular lens　　　N1 DME ASC N
BETOS: D1F　Prosthetic/Orthotic devices

D **V2631** Iris supported intraocular lens　N1 DME ASC N
BETOS: D1F　Prosthetic/Orthotic devices

D **V2632** Posterior chamber intraocular lens　　　N1 DME ASC N
BETOS: D1F　Prosthetic/Orthotic devices
Pub: 100-4, Chapter-32, 120.2

VISION SERVICES (V2700-V2799)

C **V2700** Balance lens, per lens　　　DME A
BETOS: D1F　Prosthetic/Orthotic devices

M **V2702** Deluxe lens feature　　　E1
BETOS: D1F　Prosthetic/Orthotic devices
Service not separately priced by Part B

C **V2710** Slab off prism, glass or plastic, per lens DME A
BETOS: D1F　Prosthetic/Orthotic devices

C **V2715** Prism, per lens　　　DME A
BETOS: D1F　Prosthetic/Orthotic devices

C **V2718** Press-on lens, Fresnell prism, per lens DME A
BETOS: D1F　Prosthetic/Orthotic devices

C **V2730** Special base curve, glass or plastic, per lens　　　DME A
BETOS: D1F　Prosthetic/Orthotic devices

D **V2744** Tint, photochromatic, per lens　DME A
BETOS: D1F　Prosthetic/Orthotic devices

D **V2745** Addition to lens; tint, any color, solid, gradient or equal, excludes photochromatic, any lens material, per lens DME A
BETOS: D1F　Prosthetic/Orthotic devices

D **V2750** Anti-reflective coating, per lens DME A
BETOS: D1F　Prosthetic/Orthotic devices

D **V2755** U-V lens, per lens　　　DME A
BETOS: D1F　Prosthetic/Orthotic devices

C **V2756** Eye glass case　　　E1
BETOS: Z2　Undefined codes
Service not separately priced by Part B

C **V2760** Scratch resistant coating, per lens DME E1
BETOS: D1F　Prosthetic/Orthotic devices

D **V2761** Mirror coating, any type, solid, gradient or equal, any lens material, per lens　　　B
BETOS: D1F　Prosthetic/Orthotic devices

D **V2762** Polarization, any lens material, per lens　　　DME E1
BETOS: D1F　Prosthetic/Orthotic devices

C **V2770** Occluder lens, per lens　　DME A
BETOS: D1F　Prosthetic/Orthotic devices

C **V2780** Oversize lens, per lens　　DME A
BETOS: D1F　Prosthetic/Orthotic devices

C **V2781** Progressive lens, per lens　　　B
BETOS: D1F　Prosthetic/Orthotic devices
Service not separately priced by Part B

D **V2782** Lens, index 1.54 to 1.65 plastic or 1.60 to 1.79 glass, excludes polycarbonate, per lens　　　DME A
BETOS: D1F　Prosthetic/Orthotic devices

D **V2783** Lens, index greater than or equal to 1.66 plastic or greater than or equal to 1.80 glass, excludes polycarbonate, per lens　　　DME A
BETOS: D1F　Prosthetic/Orthotic devices

D **V2784** Lens, polycarbonate or equal, any index, per lens　　　DME A
BETOS: D1F　Prosthetic/Orthotic devices

C **V2785** Processing, preserving and transporting corneal tissue　　　F4 ASC F
BETOS: D1F　Prosthetic/Orthotic devices
Pub: 100-4, Chapter-4, 200.1

D **V2786** Specialty occupational multifocal lens, per lens　　　DME E1
BETOS: D1F　Prosthetic/Orthotic devices

S **V2787** Astigmatism correcting function of intraocular lens　　　E1
BETOS: Z2　Undefined codes
Service not separately priced by Part B
Statute: 1862(a)(7)
Pub: 100-4, Chapter-14, 40.9; 100-4, Chapter-32, 120.1; 100-4, Chapter-32, 120.2

S **V2788** Presbyopia correcting function of intraocular lens　　　E1
BETOS: Z2　Undefined codes
Service not separately priced by Part B
Statute: 1862(a)(7)
Pub: 100-4, Chapter-14, 40.9; 100-4, Chapter-32, 120.1; 100-4, Chapter-32, 120.2

C **V2790** Amniotic membrane for surgical reconstruction, per procedure　N1 ASC N
BETOS: Z2　Undefined codes
Other carrier priced
Pub: 100-4, Chapter-4, 200.4

C **V2797** Vision supply, accessory and/or service component of another HCPCS vision code E1
BETOS: D1F　Prosthetic/Orthotic devices
Service not separately priced by Part B

C **V2799** Vision item or service, miscellaneous　　　A
BETOS: D1F　Prosthetic/Orthotic devices

● New code　　▲ Revised code　　**C** Carrier judgment　　**D** Special coverage instructions apply
I Not payable by Medicare　　**M** Non-covered by Medicare　　**S** Non-covered by Medicare statute　　AHA Coding Clinic®

HEARING SERVICES (V5008-V5364)

HEARING ASSESSMENTS AND EVALUATIONS (V5008-V5020)

M **V5008** Hearing screening   E1
BETOS: O1F   Hearing and speech services
Service not separately priced by Part B

S **V5010** Assessment for hearing aid   E1
BETOS: O1F   Hearing and speech services
Service not separately priced by Part B
Statute: 1862A7

S **V5011** Fitting/orientation/checking of hearing aid E1
BETOS: O1F   Hearing and speech services
Service not separately priced by Part B
Statute: 1862A7

S **V5014** Repair/modification of a hearing aid   E1
BETOS: O1F   Hearing and speech services
Service not separately priced by Part B
Statute: 1862A7

S **V5020** Conformity evaluation   E1
BETOS: O1F   Hearing and speech services
Service not separately priced by Part B
Statute: 1862A7

HEARING AID, MONAURAL (V5030-V5060)

S **V5030** Hearing aid, monaural, body worn, air conduction E1
BETOS: O1F   Hearing and speech services
Service not separately priced by Part B
Statute: 1862A7

S **V5040** Hearing aid, monaural, body worn, bone conduction E1
BETOS: O1F   Hearing and speech services
Service not separately priced by Part B
Statute: 1862A7

S **V5050** Hearing aid, monaural, in the ear   E1
BETOS: O1F   Hearing and speech services
Service not separately priced by Part B
Statute: 1862A7

S **V5060** Hearing aid, monaural, behind the ear E1
BETOS: O1F   Hearing and speech services
Service not separately priced by Part B
Statute: 1862A7

MISCELLANEOUS HEARING SERVICES AND SUPPLIES (V5070-V5110)

S **V5070** Glasses, air conduction   E1
BETOS: O1F   Hearing and speech services
Service not separately priced by Part B
Statute: 1862A7

S **V5080** Glasses, bone conduction   E1
BETOS: O1F   Hearing and speech services
Service not separately priced by Part B
Statute: 1862A7

S **V5090** Dispensing fee, unspecified hearing aid E1
BETOS: O1F   Hearing and speech services
Service not separately priced by Part B
Statute: 1862A7

S **V5095** Semi-implantable middle ear hearing prosthesis E1
BETOS: O1F   Hearing and speech services
Service not separately priced by Part B
Statute: 1862A7

S **V5100** Hearing aid, bilateral, body worn   E1
BETOS: O1F   Hearing and speech services
Service not separately priced by Part B
Statute: 1862A7

S **V5110** Dispensing fee, bilateral   E1
BETOS: O1F   Hearing and speech services
Service not separately priced by Part B
Statute: 1862A7

HEARING AIDS (V5120-V5267)

S **V5120** Binaural, body   E1
BETOS: O1F   Hearing and speech services
Service not separately priced by Part B
Statute: 1862A7

S **V5130** Binaural, in the ear   E1
BETOS: O1F   Hearing and speech services
Service not separately priced by Part B
Statute: 1862A7

S **V5140** Binaural, behind the ear   E1
BETOS: O1F   Hearing and speech services
Service not separately priced by Part B
Statute: 1862A7

S **V5150** Binaural, glasses   E1
BETOS: O1F   Hearing and speech services
Service not separately priced by Part B
Statute: 1862A7

S **V5160** Dispensing fee, binaural   E1
BETOS: O1F   Hearing and speech services
Service not separately priced by Part B
Statute: 1862A7

S **V5171** Hearing aid, contralateral routing device, monaural, in the ear (ITE) E1
BETOS: O1F   Hearing and speech services
Service not separately priced by Part B
Statute: 1862A7

S **V5172** Hearing aid, contralateral routing device, monaural, in the canal (ITC) E1
BETOS: O1F   Hearing and speech services
Service not separately priced by Part B
Statute: 1862A7

S **V5181** Hearing aid, contralateral routing device, monaural, behind the ear (BTE) E1
BETOS: O1F   Hearing and speech services
Service not separately priced by Part B
Statute: 1862A7

♂ Male only   ♀ Female only   **A** Age   A2 - Z3 = ASC Payment indicator   A - Y = APC Status indicator
ASC = ASC Approved Procedure   **DME** Paid under the DME fee schedule   **MIPS** MIPS code

[S] **V5190** Hearing aid, contralateral routing, monaural, glasses E1
BETOS: O1F Hearing and speech services
Service not separately priced by Part B
Statute: 1862A7

[S] **V5200** Dispensing fee, contralateral, monaural E1
BETOS: O1F Hearing and speech services
Service not separately priced by Part B
Statute: 1862A7

[S] **V5211** Hearing aid, contralateral routing system, binaural, ITE/ITE E1
BETOS: O1F Hearing and speech services
Service not separately priced by Part B
Statute: 1862A7

[S] **V5212** Hearing aid, contralateral routing system, binaural, ITE/ITC E1
BETOS: O1F Hearing and speech services
Service not separately priced by Part B
Statute: 1862A7

[S] **V5213** Hearing aid, contralateral routing system, binaural, ITE/BTE E1
BETOS: O1F Hearing and speech services
Service not separately priced by Part B
Statute: 1862A7

[S] **V5214** Hearing aid, contralateral routing system, binaural, ITC/ITC E1
BETOS: O1F Hearing and speech services
Service not separately priced by Part B
Statute: 1862A7

[S] **V5215** Hearing aid, contralateral routing system, binaural, ITC/BTE E1
BETOS: O1F Hearing and speech services
Service not separately priced by Part B
Statute: 1862A7

[S] **V5221** Hearing aid, contralateral routing system, binaural, BTE/BTE E1
BETOS: O1F Hearing and speech services
Service not separately priced by Part B
Statute: 1862A7

[S] **V5230** Hearing aid, contralateral routing system, binaural, glasses E1
BETOS: O1F Hearing and speech services
Service not separately priced by Part B
Statute: 1862A7

[S] **V5240** Dispensing fee, contralateral routing system, binaural E1
BETOS: O1F Hearing and speech services
Service not separately priced by Part B
Statute: 1862A7

[S] **V5241** Dispensing fee, monaural hearing aid, any type E1
BETOS: O1F Hearing and speech services
Service not separately priced by Part B
Statute: 1862A7
Coding Clinic: 2002, Q1

[S] **V5242** Hearing aid, analog, monaural, CIC (completely in the ear canal) E1
BETOS: O1F Hearing and speech services
Service not separately priced by Part B
Statute: 1862A7
Coding Clinic: 2002, Q1

[S] **V5243** Hearing aid, analog, monaural, ITC (in the canal) E1
BETOS: O1F Hearing and speech services
Service not separately priced by Part B
Statute: 1862A7
Coding Clinic: 2002, Q1

[S] **V5244** Hearing aid, digitally programmable analog, monaural, CIC E1
BETOS: O1F Hearing and speech services
Service not separately priced by Part B
Statute: 1862A7
Coding Clinic: 2002, Q1

[S] **V5245** Hearing aid, digitally programmable, analog, monaural, ITC E1
BETOS: O1F Hearing and speech services
Service not separately priced by Part B
Statute: 1862A7
Coding Clinic: 2002, Q1

[S] **V5246** Hearing aid, digitally programmable analog, monaural, ITE (in the ear) E1
BETOS: O1F Hearing and speech services
Service not separately priced by Part B
Statute: 1862A7
Coding Clinic: 2002, Q1

[S] **V5247** Hearing aid, digitally programmable analog, monaural, BTE (behind the ear) E1
BETOS: O1F Hearing and speech services
Service not separately priced by Part B
Statute: 1862A7
Coding Clinic: 2002, Q1

[S] **V5248** Hearing aid, analog, binaural, CIC E1
BETOS: O1F Hearing and speech services
Service not separately priced by Part B
Statute: 1862A7
Coding Clinic: 2002, Q1

[S] **V5249** Hearing aid, analog, binaural, ITC E1
BETOS: O1F Hearing and speech services
Service not separately priced by Part B
Statute: 1862A7
Coding Clinic: 2002, Q1

[S] **V5250** Hearing aid, digitally programmable analog, binaural, CIC E1
BETOS: O1F Hearing and speech services
Service not separately priced by Part B
Statute: 1862A7
Coding Clinic: 2002, Q1

● New code ▲ Revised code [C] Carrier judgment [D] Special coverage instructions apply
[I] Not payable by Medicare [M] Non-covered by Medicare [S] Non-covered by Medicare statute AHA Coding Clinic®

S **V5251** Hearing aid, digitally programmable analog, binaural, ITC   E1

    BETOS: O1F   Hearing and speech services
Service not separately priced by Part B
Statute: 1862A7
Coding Clinic: 2002, Q1

S **V5252** Hearing aid, digitally programmable, binaural, ITE   E1

    BETOS: O1F   Hearing and speech services
Service not separately priced by Part B
Statute: 1862A7
Coding Clinic: 2002, Q1

S **V5253** Hearing aid, digitally programmable, binaural, BTE   E1

    BETOS: O1F   Hearing and speech services
Service not separately priced by Part B
Statute: 1862A7
Coding Clinic: 2002, Q1

S **V5254** Hearing aid, digital, monaural, CIC   E1

    BETOS: O1F   Hearing and speech services
Service not separately priced by Part B
Statute: 1862A7
Coding Clinic: 2002, Q1

S **V5255** Hearing aid, digital, monaural, ITC   E1

    BETOS: O1F   Hearing and speech services
Service not separately priced by Part B
Statute: 1862A7
Coding Clinic: 2002, Q1

S **V5256** Hearing aid, digital, monaural, ITE   E1

    BETOS: O1F   Hearing and speech services
Service not separately priced by Part B
Statute: 1862A7
Coding Clinic: 2002, Q1

S **V5257** Hearing aid, digital, monaural, BTE   E1

    BETOS: O1F   Hearing and speech services
Service not separately priced by Part B
Statute: 1862A7
Coding Clinic: 2002, Q1

S **V5258** Hearing aid, digital, binaural, CIC   E1

    BETOS: O1F   Hearing and speech services
Service not separately priced by Part B
Statute: 1862A7
Coding Clinic: 2002, Q1

S **V5259** Hearing aid, digital, binaural, ITC   E1

    BETOS: O1F   Hearing and speech services
Service not separately priced by Part B
Statute: 1862A7
Coding Clinic: 2002, Q1

S **V5260** Hearing aid, digital, binaural, ITE   E1

    BETOS: O1F   Hearing and speech services
Service not separately priced by Part B
Statute: 1862A7
Coding Clinic: 2002, Q1

S **V5261** Hearing aid, digital, binaural, BTE   E1

    BETOS: O1F   Hearing and speech services
Service not separately priced by Part B
Statute: 1862A7
Coding Clinic: 2002, Q1

S **V5262** Hearing aid, disposable, any type, monaural   E1

    BETOS: O1F   Hearing and speech services
Service not separately priced by Part B
Statute: 1862A7
Coding Clinic: 2002, Q1

S **V5263** Hearing aid, disposable, any type, binaural   E1

    BETOS: O1F   Hearing and speech services
Service not separately priced by Part B
Statute: 1862A7
Coding Clinic: 2002, Q1

S **V5264** Ear mold/insert, not disposable, any type   E1

    BETOS: O1F   Hearing and speech services
Service not separately priced by Part B
Statute: 1862A7
Coding Clinic: 2002, Q1

S **V5265** Ear mold/insert, disposable, any type   E1

    BETOS: O1F   Hearing and speech services
Service not separately priced by Part B
Statute: 1862A7
Coding Clinic: 2002, Q1

S **V5266** Battery for use in hearing device   E1

    BETOS: O1F   Hearing and speech services
Service not separately priced by Part B
Statute: 1862A7
Coding Clinic: 2002, Q1

S **V5267** Hearing aid or assistive listening device/supplies/accessories, not otherwise specified   E1

    BETOS: O1F   Hearing and speech services
Service not separately priced by Part B
Statute: 1862A7
Coding Clinic: 2002, Q1

ASSISTIVE HEARING DEVICES (V5268-V5290)

S **V5268** Assistive listening device, telephone amplifier, any type   E1

    BETOS: O1F   Hearing and speech services
Service not separately priced by Part B
Statute: 1862A7
Coding Clinic: 2002, Q1

S **V5269** Assistive listening device, alerting, any type   E1

    BETOS: O1F   Hearing and speech services
Service not separately priced by Part B
Statute: 1862A7
Coding Clinic: 2002, Q1

♂ Male only   ♀ Female only   A Age   A2 - Z3 = ASC Payment indicator   A - Y = APC Status indicator
ASC = ASC Approved Procedure   **DME** Paid under the DME fee schedule   **MIPS** MIPS code

V5270 - V5362

HEARING SERVICES (V5008-V5364)

S **V5270** Assistive listening device, television amplifier, any type   E1
BETOS: O1F   Hearing and speech services
Service not separately priced by Part B
Statute: 1862A7
Coding Clinic: 2002, Q1

S **V5271** Assistive listening device, television caption decoder   E1
BETOS: O1F   Hearing and speech services
Service not separately priced by Part B
Statute: 1862A7
Coding Clinic: 2002, Q1

S **V5272** Assistive listening device, TDD   E1
BETOS: O1F   Hearing and speech services
Service not separately priced by Part B
Statute: 1862A7
Coding Clinic: 2002, Q1

S **V5273** Assistive listening device, for use with cochlear implant   E1
BETOS: O1F   Hearing and speech services
Service not separately priced by Part B
Statute: 1862A7
Coding Clinic: 2002, Q1

S **V5274** Assistive listening device, not otherwise specified   E1
BETOS: O1F   Hearing and speech services
Service not separately priced by Part B
Statute: 1862A7
Coding Clinic: 2002, Q1

S **V5275** Ear impression, each   E1
BETOS: O1F   Hearing and speech services
Service not separately priced by Part B
Statute: 1862A7
Coding Clinic: 2002, Q1

S **V5281** Assistive listening device, personal FM/DM system, monaural, (1 receiver, transmitter, microphone), any type   E1
BETOS: O1F   Hearing and speech services
Service not separately priced by Part B
Statute: 1862a7

S **V5282** Assistive listening device, personal FM/DM system, binaural, (2 receivers, transmitter, microphone), any type   E1
BETOS: O1F   Hearing and speech services
Service not separately priced by Part B
Statute: 1862a7

S **V5283** Assistive listening device, personal FM/DM neck, loop induction receiver   E1
BETOS: O1F   Hearing and speech services
Service not separately priced by Part B
Statute: 1862a7

S **V5284** Assistive listening device, personal FM/DM, ear level receiver   E1
BETOS: O1F   Hearing and speech services
Service not separately priced by Part B
Statute: 1862a7

S **V5285** Assistive listening device, personal FM/DM, direct audio input receiver   E1
BETOS: O1F   Hearing and speech services
Service not separately priced by Part B
Statute: 1862a7

S **V5286** Assistive listening device, personal blue tooth FM/DM receiver   E1
BETOS: O1F   Hearing and speech services
Service not separately priced by Part B
Statute: 1862a7

S **V5287** Assistive listening device, personal FM/DM receiver, not otherwise specified   E1
BETOS: O1F   Hearing and speech services
Service not separately priced by Part B
Statute: 1862a7

S **V5288** Assistive listening device, personal FM/DM transmitter assistive listening device   E1
BETOS: O1F   Hearing and speech services
Service not separately priced by Part B
Statute: 1862a7

S **V5289** Assistive listening device, personal FM/DM adapter/boot coupling device for receiver, any type   E1
BETOS: O1F   Hearing and speech services
Service not separately priced by Part B
Statute: 1862a7

S **V5290** Assistive listening device, transmitter microphone, any type   E1
BETOS: O1F   Hearing and speech services
Service not separately priced by Part B
Statute: 1862a7

OTHER AND MISCELLANEOUS HEARING SERVICES AND SUPPLIES (V5298, V5299)

S **V5298** Hearing aid, not otherwise classified   E1
BETOS: O1F   Hearing and speech services
Service not separately priced by Part B
Statute: 1862A7

D **V5299** Hearing service, miscellaneous   B
BETOS: O1F   Hearing and speech services
Price established by carriers

SPEECH-RELATED SCREENINGS AND COMMUNICATION DEVICE REPAIR (V5336-V5364)

S **V5336** Repair/modification of augmentative communicative system or device (excludes adaptive hearing aid)   E1
BETOS: O1F   Hearing and speech services
Service not separately priced by Part B
Statute: 1862A7

S **V5362** Speech screening   E1
BETOS: O1F   Hearing and speech services
Service not separately priced by Part B
Statute: 1862(a)(7)

● New code   ▲ Revised code   C Carrier judgment   D Special coverage instructions apply
I Not payable by Medicare   M Non-covered by Medicare   S Non-covered by Medicare statute   AHA Coding Clinic®

S **V5363** Language screening   E1
    BETOS: O1F   Hearing and speech services
    Service not separately priced by Part B
    Statute: 1862(a)(7)

S **V5364** Dysphagia screening   E1
    BETOS: O1F   Hearing and speech services
    Service not separately priced by Part B
    Statute: 1862(a)(7)

♂ Male only   ♀ Female only   **A** Age   A2 - Z3 = ASC Payment indicator   A - Y = APC Status indicator
ASC = ASC Approved Procedure   **DME** Paid under the DME fee schedule   **MIPS** MIPS code

NOTES

Appendix A
Table of Drugs and Biologicals

Generic and brand-name drugs found throughout the Table of Drugs and Biologicals are a representative sample of drugs and biologicals commonly associated with HCPCS Level II codes. Please check the CMS and FDA websites for the most up-to-date information on coverage, active brand names, and validity of drugs.

Caution: Never code directly from the Table of Drugs and Biologicals. Always cross-reference the code to the Tabular List before final code assignment. Questions regarding coding and billing guidance should be submitted to the insurer in whose jurisdiction a claim would be filed. For private sector health insurance systems, please contact the individual private insurance entity. For Medicaid systems, please contact the Medicaid Agency in the state in which the claim is being filed. For Medicare, contact the Medicare contractor.

Abbreviations used in the Table of Drugs and Biologicals

IA - Intra-arterial administration

IV - Intravenous administration

IM - Intramuscular administration

IT - Intrathecal

SC - Subcutaneous administration

INH - Administration by inhaled solution

VAR - Various routes of administration

OTH - Other routes of administration

ORAL - Administered orally

Intravenous administration includes all methods, such as gravity infusion, injections, and timed pushes into blood vessels, usually veins. IM refers to injections into muscles; IT to injections into the spinal column; and SC to injections into tissues (not muscle) under the skin. VAR denotes various routes of administration and is used for drugs that are commonly administered into joints, cavities, tissues, or topical applications, in addition to other parenteral administrations. OTH indicates other administration methods, such as intraocular injections, suppositories, or catheter injections.

Drug Name	Unit Per	Route	Code
ABATACEPT	10 mg	IV	J0129
ABCIXIMAB	10 mg	IV	J0130
ABELCET®	10 mg	IV	J0287
ABILIFY MAINTENA®	1 mg	IM	J0401
ABILIFY®	0.25 mg	IM	J0400
ABOBOTULINUM TOXIN A	5 IU	IM	J0586
ACCUNEB®	1 mg	INH	J7613
ACCUNEB® CONCENTRATED FORM	1 mg	INH	J7611
ACETADOTE®	100 mg	IV	J0132
ACETAMINOPHEN	10 mg	IV	J0131
ACETAZOLAMIDE SODIUM	up to 500 mg	IV, IM	J1120
ACETYLCYSTEINE	100 mg	IV	J0132
ACETYLCYSTEINE, UNIT DOSE, COMPOUNDED	1 gram	INH	J7604
ACETYLCYSTEINE, UNIT DOSE, NON-COMPOUNDED	1 gram	INH	J7608
ACLASTA®	1 mg	IV	J3489
ACOVA®	1 mg	IV	J0883
ACOVA®	1 mg	IV	J0884
ACTEMRA®	1 mg	IV	J3262
ACTHAR GEL, H.P.®	up to 40 IU	IV, IM, SC	J0800
ACTHREL®	1 mcg	IV, IM	J0795
ACTIMMUNE®	3 million IU	SC	J9216
ACTIVASE®	1 mg	IV	J2997
ACYCLOVIR	5 mg	IV	J0133
ADAGEN®	25 IU	IM	J2504
ADALIMUMAB	20 mg	SC	J0135
ADCETRIS®	1 mg	IV	J9042
ADENOCARD®	1 mg	IV	J0153
ADENOSINE	1 mg	IV	J0153
ADO-TRASTUZUMAB EMTANSINE	1 mg	IV	J9354
ADRENACLICK®	0.1 mg	SC, IM	J0171
ADRENALIN, EPINEPHRINE	0.1 mg	SC, IM	J0171

Drug Name	Unit Per	Route	Code
ADRENALIN®	0.1 mg	SC, IM	J0171
ADRIAMYCIN RDF®	10 mg	IV	J9000
ADRIAMYCIN®	10 mg	IV	J9000
ADVATE®	1 IU	IV	J7192
ADYNOVATE®	1 IU	IV	J7207
AFAMELANOTIDE IMPLANT	1 mg	OTH	J7352
AFLIBERCEPT	1 mg	OTH	J0178
AFSTYLA®	1 IU	IV	J7210
AGALSIDASE BETA	1 mg	IV	J0180
AGGRASTAT®	0.25 mg	IM, IV	J3246
AJOVY®	1 mg	SC	J3031
AKYNZEO®	300 mg and 0.5 mg	ORAL	J8655
ALA-TET®	up to 250 mg	IM, IV	J0120
ALATROFLOXACIN MESYLATE	100 mg	IV	J0200
ALBUTEROL AND IPRATROPIUM BROMIDE, NON-COMPOUNDED	up to 2.5 mg/ up to 0.5 mg	INH	J7620
ALBUTEROL, CONCENTRATED FORM, COMPOUNDED	1 mg	INH	J7610
ALBUTEROL, CONCENTRATED FORM, NON-COMPOUNDED	1 mg	INH	J7611
ALBUTEROL, UNIT DOSE, COMPOUNDED	1 mg	INH	J7609
ALBUTEROL, UNIT DOSE, NON-COMPOUNDED	1 mg	INH	J7613
ALDESLEUKIN	single use vial	IV	J9015
ALDURAZYME®	0.1 mg	IV	J1931
ALEFACEPT	0.5 mg	IM, IV	J0215
ALEMTUZUMAB	1 mg	IV	J0202
ALFERON N®	250,000 IU	OTH	J9215
ALGLUCERASE	10 IU	IV	J0205
ALGLUCOSIDASE ALFA	10 mg	IV	J0220
ALIMTA®	10 mg	IV	J9305
ALIQOPA®	1 mg	IV	J9057
ALKERAN®	2 mg	ORAL	J8600

Drug Name	Unit Per	Route	Code
ALKERAN I.V.®	50 mg	IV	J9245
ALOXI®	25 mcg	IV	J2469
ALPHA 1-PROTEINASE INHIBITOR, HUMAN	10 mg	IV	J0256
ALPHANATE®	1 IU	IV	J7186
ALPROLIX®	1 IU	IV	J7201
ALPROSTADIL, INJECTION	1.25 mcg	OTH	J0270
ALPROSTADIL, URETHRAL SUPPOSITORY	each	OTH	J0275
ALTEPLASE RECOMBINANT	1 mg	IV	J2997
AMBISOME®	10 mg	IV	J0289
AMELUZ®	10 mg	OTH	J7345
AMIFOSTINE	500 mg	IV	J0207
AMIKACIN SULFATE	100 mg	IV	J0278
AMIKIN PEDIATRIC®	100 mg	IV	J0278
AMIKIN®	100 mg	IV	J0278
AMINOLEVULINIC ACID HCL, 10% GEL, TOPICAL	10 mg	OTH	J7345
AMINOLEVULINIC ACID HCL, TOPICAL, 20%	unit dose (354 mg)	OTH	J7308
AMINOPHYLLINE	up to 250 mg	IV	J0280
AMIODARONE HCL	30 mg	IV	J0282
AMITRIPTYLINE HCL	up to 20 mg	IM	J1320
AMOBARBITAL	up to 125 mg	IM, IV	J0300
AMPHADASE®	up to 150 IU	SC, IV	J3470
AMPHOCIN®	50 mg	IV	J0285
AMPHOTERICIN B	50 mg	IV	J0285
AMPHOTERICIN B CHOLESTERYL SULFATE COMPLEX	10 mg	IV	J0288
AMPHOTERICIN B LIPOSOME	10 mg	IV	J0289
AMPHOTERICIN B, LIPID COMPLEX	10 mg	IV	J0287
AMPICILLIN SODIUM	500 mg	IM, IV	J0290
AMPICILLIN SODIUM/SULBACTAM SODIUM	1.5 gm	IM, IV	J0295
AMYTAL®	up to 125 mg	IM, IV	J0300
ANASCORP®	up to 120 mg	IV	J0716
ANASPAZ®	up to 0.25 mg	SC, IM, IV	J1980
ANAVIP®	120 mg	IV	J0841
ANCEF®	500 mg	IV, IM	J0690
ANDEXXA®	10mg	IV	J7169
ANECTINE®	up to 20 mg	IV, IM	J0330
ANESTACAINE®	10 mg	IV	J2001
ANGIOMAX®	1 mg	IV	J0583
ANIDULAFUNGIN	1 mg	IV	J0348
ANISTREPLASE	30 IU	IV	J0350
ANTI D (RHO) IMMUNOGLOBULIN®	50 mcg	IM	J2788
ANTI D (RHO) IMMUNOGLOBULIN®	1 dose package, 300 mcg	IM	J2790

Drug Name	Unit Per	Route	Code
ANTIEMETIC DRUG, NOT OTHERWISE SPECIFIED	-	ORAL	J8597
ANTIEMETIC DRUG, RECTAL/ SUPPOSITORY, NOT OTHERWISE SPECIFIED	-	OTH	J8498
ANTIFLEX®	up to 60 mg	IV, IM	J2360
ANTIHEMOPHILIC FACTOR VIII/ VON WILLEBRAND FACTOR COMPLEX (HUMAN)	1 IU	IV	J7186
ANTI-INHIBITOR COAGULANT COMPLEX	1 IU	IV	J7198
ANTI-NEOPLASTIC DRUGS, NOT OTHERWISE CLASSIFIED	-	-	J9999
ANTITHROMBIN III (HUMAN)	1 IU	IV	J7197
ANTITHROMBIN RECOMBINANT	50 IU	IV	J7196
ANTIVENIN POLYVALENT®	120 mg	IV	J0841
ANTIZOL®	15 mg	IV	J1451
APOKYN®	1 mg	SC	J0364
APOMORPHINE HYDROCHLORIDE	1 mg	SC	J0364
APREPITANT	1 mg	IV	J0185
APREPITANT	5 mg	ORAL	J8501
APRESOLINE®	up to 20 mg	IV, IM	J0360
APROTININ	10,000 kiu	INJ	J0365
ARALAST NP®	10 mg	IV	J0256
ARALAST®	10 mg	IV	J0256
ARANESP® (FOR ESRD)	1 mcg	IV, SC	J0882
ARANESP® (NON-ESRD)	1 mcg	IV, SC	J0881
ARBUTAMINE HCL	1 mg	IV	J0395
ARCALYST®	1 mg	SC	J2793
AREDIA®	30 mg	IV	J2430
ARFORMOTEROL	15 mcg	INH	J7605
ARGATROBAN (FOR ESRD)	1 mg	IV	J0884
ARGATROBAN (NON-ESRD USE)	1 mg	IV	J0883
ARIDOL®	5 mg	INH	J7665
ARIPIPRAZOLE	0.25 mg	IM	J0400
ARIPIPRAZOLE LAUROXIL	1 mg	IM	J1944
ARIPIPRAZOLE LAUROXIL (ARISTADA INITIO®)	1 mg	IM	J1943
ARIPIPRAZOLE, EXTENDED RELEASE	1 mg	IM	J0401
ARISTADA INITIO®	1 mg	IM	J1943
ARISTADA®	1 mg	IM	J1944
ARIXTRA®	0.5 mg	SC	J1652
ARRANON®	50 mg	IV	J9261
ARSENIC TRIOXIDE	1 mg	IV	J9017
ARZERRA®	10 mg	IV	J9302
ASPARAGINASE	1,000 IU	IV, IM	J9019
ASPARAGINASE, NOS	10,000 IU	IM, IV	J9020
ASPARLAS®	10 units	IV	J9118
ASTAGRAF XL®	0.1 mg	ORAL	J7508

Drug Name	Unit Per	Route	Code
ATEZOLIZUMAB	10 mg	IV	J9022
ATGAM®	250 mg	IV	J7504
ATIVAN®	2 mg	IM, IV	J2060
ATROPEN®	0.01 mg	IV	J0461
ATROPINE SULFATE	0.01 mg	IV	J0461
ATROPINE, CONCENTRATED FORM, COMPOUNDED	1 mg	INH	J7635
ATROPINE, UNIT DOSE FORM, COMPOUNDED	1 mg	INH	J7636
ATROVENT HFA®	1 mg	INH	J7644
ATRYN®	50 IU	IV	J7196
AUROTHIOGLUCOSE	up to 50 mg	IM	J2910
AUTOLOGOUS CULTURED CHONDROCYTES, IMPLANT	each	OTH	J7330
AUTOPLEX T®	1 IU	IV	J7198
AUVI-Q®	0.1 mg	SC, IM	J0171
AVASTIN®	0.25 mg	IV	C9257
AVASTIN®	10 mg	IV	J9035
AVEED®	1 mg	IM	J3145
AVELOX IV®	100 mg	IV	J2280
AVELOX®	100 mg	IV	J2280
AVELUMAB	10 mg	IV	J9023
AVONEX®	30 mcg	IM	J1826
AVYCAZ®	0.5 g/0.125 g	IV	J0714
AZACITIDINE	1 mg	SC, IV	J9025
AZASAN®	50 mg	ORAL	J7500
AZATHIOPRINE, ORAL	50 mg	ORAL	J7500
AZATHIOPRINE, PARENTERAL	100 mg	IV	J7501
AZITHROMYCIN	500 mg	IV	J0456
BACLOFEN	10 mg	IT	J0475
BACLOFEN FOR INTRATHECAL TRIAL	50 mcg	IT	J0476
BACTOCILL®	up to 250 mg	IM, IV	J2700
BAL IN OIL®	100 mg	IM	J0470
BANFLEX®	up to 60 mg	IV, IM	J2360
BASILIXIMAB	20 mg	IV	J0480
BAVENCIO®	10 mg	IV	J9023
BAXDELA®	1 mg	IV	C9462
BAYRHO D FULL DOSE®	1 dose package, 300 mcg	IM	J2790
BAYRHO D MINI-DOSE®	50 mcg	IM	J2788
BAYTET®	up to 250 IU	IM	J1670
BCG LIVE INTRAVESICAL INSTILLATION	1 mg	OTH	J9030
BEBULIN VH®	1 IU	IV	J7194
BEBULIN®	1 IU	IV	J7194
BECLOMETHASONE, UNIT DOSE FORM, COMPOUNDED	1 mg	INH	J7622
BELATACEPT	1 mg	IV	J0485

Drug Name	Unit Per	Route	Code
BELEODAQ®	10 mg	IV	J9032
BELIMUMAB	10 mg	IV	J0490
BELINOSTAT	10 mg	IV	J9032
BELRAPZO®	1 mg	IV	J9036
BENDAMUSTINE HCL, BENDEKA®	1 mg	IV	J9034
BENDAMUSTINE HCL, TREANDA®	1 mg	IV	J9033
BENDAMUSTINE HYDROCHLORIDE (BELRAPZO®)	1 mg	IV	J9036
BENDEKA®	1 mg	IV	J9034
BENEFIX®	1 IU	IV	J7195
BENLYSTA®	10 mg	IV	J0490
BENRALIZUMAB	1 mg	SC	J0517
BENTYL®	up to 20 mg	IM	J0500
BENZACOT®	up to 200 mg	IM	J3250
BENZTROPINE MESYLATE	1 mg	IM, IV	J0515
BEOVU®	1 mg	OTH	J0179
BERINERT®	10 IU	IV	J0597
BESPONSA®	0.1 mg	IV	J9229
BETAMETHASONE ACETATE AND BETAMETHASONE SODIUM PHOSPHATE	3 mg/3 mg	IM	J0702
BETAMETHASONE, UNIT DOSE FORM, COMPOUNDED	1 mg	INH	J7624
BETASERON®	0.25 mg	SC	J1830
BETHANECHOL CHLORIDE, MYOTONACHOL OR URECHOLINE	up to 5 mg	SC	J0520
BETHKIS®	300 mg	INH	J7682
BEVACIZUMAB	0.25 mg	IV	C9257
BEVACIZUMAB	10 mg	IV	J9035
BEZLOTOXUMAB	10 mg	IV	J0565
BICILLIN C-R®	100,000 IU	IM	J0558
BICILLIN L-A®	100,000 IU	IM	J0561
BICNU®	100 mg	IV	J9050
BIMATOPROST, INTRACAMERAL IMPLANT	1 mcg	OTH	J7351
BIPERIDEN LACTATE	5 mg	IV	J0190
BITOLTEROL MESYLATE, CONCENTRATED FORM, COMPOUNDED	1 mg	INH	J7628
BITOLTEROL MESYLATE, UNIT DOSE FORM, COMPOUNDED	1 mg	INH	J7629
BIVALIRUDIN	1 mg	IV	J0583
BIVIGAM®	500 mg	IV	J1556
BLEOMYCIN SULFATE	15 IU	IM, IV, SC	J9040
BLINATUMOMAB	1 mcg	IV	J9039
BLINCYTO®	1 mcg	IV	J9039
BLOXIVERZ®	up to 0.5 mg	IM, IV, SC	J2710
BONIVA®	1 mg	IV	J1740
BORTEZOMIB (VELCADE®)	0.1 mg	IV	J9041
BORTEZOMIB, NOS	0.1 mg	IV	J9044

Drug Name	Unit Per	Route	Code
BOTOX COSMETIC®	1 IU	IM	J0585
BOTOX®	1 IU	IM	J0585
BRAVELLE®	75 IU	SC	J3355
BRENTUXIMAB VEDOTIN	1 mg	IV	J9042
BREXANOLONE	1mg	IV	J1632
BRINEURA®	1 mg	IV	J0567
BROLUCIZUMAB-DBLL	1 mg	OTH	J0179
BROMPHENIRAMINE MALEATE	10 mg	IM, SC, IV	J0945
BROVANA®	15 mcg	INH	J7605
BUDESONIDE INHALATION SOLUTION, COMPOUNDED	0.5 mg	INH	J7627
BUDESONIDE INHALATION SOLUTION, COMPOUNDED	0.25 mg	INH	J7634
BUDESONIDE INHALATION SOLUTION, NON-COMPOUNDED	0.5 mg	INH	J7626
BUDESONIDE INHALATION SOLUTION, NON-COMPOUNDED	0.25 mg	INH	J7633
BUNAVAIL®	<=3 mg	ORAL	J0572
BUNAVAIL®	>3 mg but <=6 mg	ORAL	J0573
BUNAVAIL®	>6 mg but <=10 mg	ORAL	J0574
BUNAVAIL®	>10 mg	ORAL	J0575
BUPIVACAINE LIPOSOME	1 mg	IV	C9290
BUPRENEX®	0.1 mg	IM	J0592
BUPRENORPHINE	1 mg	ORAL	J0571
BUPRENORPHINE HYDROCHLORIDE	0.1 mg	IM	J0592
BUPRENORPHINE IMPLANT	74.2 mg	OTH	J0570
BUPRENORPHINE/NALOXONE	<=3 mg	ORAL	J0572
BUPRENORPHINE/NALOXONE	>3 mg but <=6 mg	ORAL	J0573
BUPRENORPHINE/NALOXONE	>6 mg but <=10 mg	ORAL	J0574
BUPRENORPHINE/NALOXONE	>10 mg	ORAL	J0575
BUROSUMAB-TWZA	1 mg	SC	J0584
BUSULFAN	1 mg	IV	J0594
BUSULFAN	2 mg	ORAL	J8510
BUSULFEX®	1 mg	IV	J0594
BUTORPHANOL TARTRATE	1 mg	IM	J0595
C-1 ESTERACE INHIBITOR, HUMAN, (BERINERT®)	10 IU	IV	J0597
C-1 ESTERACE INHIBITOR, HUMAN, (CINRYZE®)	10 IU	IV	J0598
C-1 ESTERACE INHIBITOR, HUMAN, (HAEGARDA®)	10 IU	IV	J0599
C-1 ESTERACE INHIBITOR, RECOMBINANT, (RUCONEST®)	10 IU	IV	J0596
CABAZITAXEL	1 mg	IV	J9043
CABERGOLINE	0.25 mg	ORAL	J8515
CABLIVI®	1 mg	IV	C9047

Drug Name	Unit Per	Route	Code
CAFFEINE CITRATE	5 mg	IV	J0706
CALASPARGASE-PEGOL-MKNL	10 units	IV	J9118
CALCITONIN-SALMON	up to 400 IU	SC, IM	J0630
CALCITRIOL	0.1 mcg	IM	J0636
CALCIUM DISODIUM VERSENATE®	up to 1000 mg	IV, SC, IM	J0600
CALCIUM GLUCONATE	10 ml	IV	J0610
CALCIUM GLYCEROPHOSPHATE AND CALCIUM LACTATE	10 ml	IM, SC	J0620
CALDOLOR®	100 mg	IV	J1741
CAMPATH®	1 mg	IV	J0202
CAMPTOSAR®	20 mg	IV	J9206
CANAKINUMAB	1 mg	SC	J0638
CANCIDAS®	5 mg	IV	J0637
CANGRELOR	1 mg	IV	C9460
CAPECITABINE	150 mg	ORAL	J8520
CAPECITABINE	500 mg	ORAL	J8521
CAPLACIZUMAB-YHDP	1 mg	IV	C9047
CAPSAICIN 8% PATCH	per sq cm	OTH	J7336
CARBACOT®	up to 10 ml	IV, IM	J2800
CARBIDOPA/LEVODOPA, ENTERAL SUSPENSION	100 ml	OTH	J7340
CARBOCAINE®	10 ml	VAR	J0670
CARBOPLATIN	50 mg	IV	J9045
CARBOPLATIN NOVAPLUS®	50 mg	IV	J9045
CARFILZOMIB	1 mg	IV	J9047
CARMUSTINE	100 mg	IV	J9050
CARNITOR®	1 gm	IV	J1955
CARTICEL®	each	OTH	J7330
CASPOFUNGIN ACETATE	5 mg	IV	J0637
CAVERJECT IMPULSE®	1.25 mcg	OTH	J0270
CAVERJECT®	1.25 mcg	OTH	J0270
CEFAZOLIN SODIUM	500 mg	IV, IM	J0690
CEFEPIME HYDROCHLORIDE	500 mg	IV	J0692
CEFIDEROCOL	5 mg	INJ	J0693
CEFOTAXIME SODIUM	1 g	IV, IM	J0698
CEFOXITIN SODIUM	1 g	IV, IM	J0694
CEFTAROLINE FOSAMIL	10 mg	IV	J0712
CEFTAZIDIME	500 mg	IV, IM	J0713
CEFTAZIDIME AND AVIBACTAM	0.5 g/0.125 g	IV	J0714
CEFTIZOXIME SODIUM	500 mg	IV, IM	J0715
CEFTOLOZANE AND TAZOBACTAM	50 mg/25 mg	IV	J0695
CEFTRIAXONE SODIUM	250 mg	IV, IM	J0696
CEFUROXIME SODIUM, STERILE	750 mg	IV, IM	J0697
CELLCEPT®	250 mg	ORAL	J7517
CEMIPLIMAB-RWLC	1 mg	IV	J9119
CENTRUROIDES IMMUNE F(AB)2	up to 120 mg	IV	J0716
CEPHALOTHIN SODIUM	up to 1 g	IM, IV	J1890
CEPHAPIRIN SODIUM	up to 1 g	IV, IM	J0710

Drug Name	Unit Per	Route	Code
CEPROTIN®	10 IU	IV	J2724
CEREZYME®	10 IU	IV	J1786
CERLIPONASE ALFA	1 mg	IV	J0567
CERTOLIZUMAB PEGOL	1 mg	SC	J0717
CERUBIDINE®	10 mg	IV	J9150
CESAMET®	1 mg	ORAL	J8650
CETIRIZINE HYDROCHLORIDE	0.5 mg	IV	J1201
CETRAXAL®	6 mg	OTH	J7342
CETUXIMAB	10 mg	IV	J9055
CHEMOTHERAPEUTIC, NOT OTHERWISE SPECIFIED	-	ORAL	J8999
CHLORAMPHENICOL SODIUM SUCCINATE	up to 1 g	IV	J0720
CHLORDIAZEPOXIDE	up to 100 mg	IM, IV	J1990
CHLOROMYCETIN SODIUM SUCCINATE®	up to 1 g	IV	J0720
CHLOROPROCAINE HCL	30 ml	VAR	J2400
CHLOROQUINE HCL	up to 250 mg	IM	J0390
CHLOROTHIAZIDE SODIUM	500 mg	IV	J1205
CHLORPROMAZINE HCL	up to 50 mg	IM, IV	J3230
CHORIONIC GONADOTROPIN	1,000 USP units	IM	J0725
CIDOFOVIR	375 mg	IV	J0740
CILASTATIN SODIUM, IMIPENEM	250 mg	IV, IM	J0743
CIMZIA®	1 mg	SC	J0717
CINACALCET, ORAL, (FOR ESRD ON DIALYSIS)	1 mg	ORAL	J0604
CINQAIR®	1 mg	IV	J2786
CINRYZE®	10 IU	IV	J0598
CINVANTI®	1 mg	IV	J0185
CIPRO I.V.®	200 mg	IV	J0744
CIPROFLOXACIN	200 mg	IV	J0744
CIPROFLOXACIN, OTIC SUSPENSION	6 mg	OTH	J7342
CISPLATIN, POWDER OR SOLUTION	10 mg	IV	J9060
CLADRIBINE	1 mg	IV	J9065
CLADRIBINE NOVAPLUS®	1 mg	IV	J9065
CLAFORAN®	1 g	IV, IM	J0698
CLEVIDIPINE BUTYRATE	1 mg	IV	C9248
CLEVIPREX®	1 mg	IV	C9248
CLEXANE FORTE®	10 mg	SC	J1650
CLEXANE®	10 mg	SC	J1650
CLOFARABINE	1 mg	IV	J9027
CLOLAR®	1 mg	IV	J9027
CLONIDINE HYDROCHLORIDE	1 mg	OTH	J0735
COAGADEX®	1 IU	IV	J7175
COAGULATION FACTOR XA (RECOMBINANT), INACTIVATED-ZHZO (ANDEXXA®)	10 mg	IV	J7169

Drug Name	Unit Per	Route	Code
COCAINE HYDROCHLORIDE NASAL SOLUTION	1 mg	OTH	C9046
CODEINE PHOSPHATE	30 mg	IV, IM, SC	J0745
COGENTIN®	1 mg	IM, IV	J0515
COLISTIMETHATE SODIUM	up to 150 mg	IV, IM	J0770
COLLAGENASE CLOSTRIDIUM HISTOLYTICUM	0.01 mg	OTH	J0775
COLY-MYCIN M®	up to 150 mg	IV, IM	J0770
COMBIVENT RESPIMAT®	0.5 mg	INH	J7620
COMPOUNDED DRUG, NOT OTHERWISE CLASSIFIED	-	VAR	J7999
CONIVAPTAN HYDROCHLORIDE	1 mg	IV	C9488
CONTRACEPTIVE SUPPLY, HORMONE CONTAINING PATCH	each	OTH	J7304
CONTRACEPTIVE SUPPLY, HORMONE CONTAINING VAGINAL RING	each	OTH	J7303
COPANLISIB	1 mg	IV	J9057
COPAXONE®	20 mg	SC	J1595
COPPER CONTRACEPTIVE, INTRAUTERINE	each	OTH	J7300
CORTICORELIN OVINE TRIFLUTATE	1 mcg	IV, IM	J0795
CORTICOTROPIN	up to 40 IU	IV, IM, SC	J0800
CORTROSYN®	0.25 mg	IV	J0834
CORVERT®	1 mg	IV	J1742
COSMEGEN®	0.5 mg	IV	J9120
COSYNTROPIN	0.25 mg	IV	J0834
CRESEMBA®	1 mg	IV	J1833
CRIZANLIZUMAB-TMCA	5 mg	IV	J0791
CROFAB®	up to 1 gram	IV	J0840
CROFAB®	120 mg	IV	J0841
CROMOLYN SODIUM, COMPOUNDED	10 mg	INH	J7632
CROMOLYN SODIUM, NON-COMPOUNDED	10 mg	INH	J7631
CROTALIDAE IMMUNE F(AB')2 (EQUINE)	120 mg	IV	J0841
CROTALIDAE POLYVALENT IMMUNE FAB (OVINE)	up to 1 gram	IV	J0840
CRYOSERV®	50%, 50 ml	OTH	J1212
CRYSVITA®	1 mg	SC	J0584
CUBICIN®	1 mg	IV	J0878
CUVITRU®	100 mg	IV	J1555
CYANOCOBALAMIN, VITAMIN B-12	up to 1,000 mcg	IM, SC	J3420
CYCLOPHOSPHAMIDE	25 mg	ORAL	J8530
CYCLOPHOSPHAMIDE	100 mg	IV	J9070
CYCLOSPORINE, ORAL	100 mg	ORAL	J7502
CYCLOSPORINE, ORAL	25 mg	ORAL	J7515
CYCLOSPORINE, PARENTERAL	250 mg	OTH	J7516

Drug Name	Unit Per	Route	Code
CYRAMZA®	5 mg	IV	J9308
CYTARABINE	100 mg	SC, IV	J9100
CYTARABINE LIPOSOME	10 mg	IT	J9098
CYTOGAM®	vial	IV	J0850
CYTOMEGALOVIRUS IMMUNE GLOBULIN INTRAVENOUS (HUMAN)	vial	IV	J0850
CYTOVENE®	500 mg	IV	J1570
D5W	1000 cc	IV	J7070
DACARBAZINE	100 mg	IV	J9130
DACLIZUMAB	25 mg	IV	J7513
DACOGEN®	1 mg	IV	J0894
DACTINOMYCIN	0.5 mg	IV	J9120
DALBAVANCIN	5 mg	IV	J0875
DALTEPARIN SODIUM	2500 IU	SC	J1645
DALVANCE®	5 mg	IV	J0875
DAPTOMYCIN	1 mg	IV	J0878
DARATUMUMAB	10 mg	IV	J9145
DARATUMUMAB AND HYALURONIDASE-FIHJ	10 mg	INJ	J9144
DARBEPOETIN ALFA (FOR ESRD)	1 mcg	IV, SC	J0882
DARBEPOETIN ALFA (NON-ESRD)	1 mcg	IV, SC	J0881
DARZALEX®	10 mg	IV	J9145
DAUNORUBICIN	10 mg	IV	J9150
DAUNORUBICIN CITRATE, LIPOSOMAL FORMULATION	10 mg	IV	J9151
DDAVP®	1 mcg	IV, SC	J2597
DECITABINE	1 mg	IV	J0894
DEFEROXAMINE MESYLATE	500 mg	IM, SC, IV	J0895
DEGARELIX	1 mg	SC	J9155
DEKPAK 13 DAY TAPERPAK®	0.25 mg	ORAL	J8540
DELAFLOXACIN	1 mg	IV	C9462
DELATESTRYL®	1 mg	IM	J3121
DELESTROGEN®	up to 10 mg	IM	J1380
DEMADEX®	10 mg/ml	IV	J3265
DEMEROL®	100 mg	IM, IV, SC	J2175
DENILEUKIN DIFTITOX	300 mcg	IV	J9160
DENOSUMAB	1 mg	SC	J0897
DEOXYCHOLIC ACID	1 mg	IV	J0591
DEPO ESTRADIOL®	up to 5 mg	IM	J1000
DEPO-ESTRADIOL CYPIONATE	up to 5 mg	IM	J1000
DEPO-MEDROL®	20 mg	IM	J1020
DEPO-MEDROL®	40 mg	IM	J1030
DEPO-MEDROL®	80 mg	IM	J1040
DEPO-PROVERA®	1 mg	IM	J1050
DEPO-TESTOSTERONE®	1 mg	IM	J1071
DESFERAL®	500 mg	IM, SC, IV	J0895
DESMOPRESSIN ACETATE	1 mcg	IV, SC	J2597

Drug Name	Unit Per	Route	Code
DEXAMETHASONE	0.25 mg	ORAL	J8540
DEXAMETHASONE 9 PERCENT, INTRAOCULAR	1mcg	OTH	J1095
DEXAMETHASONE ACETATE	1 mg	IM	J1094
DEXAMETHASONE INTENSOL®	0.25 mg	ORAL	J8540
DEXAMETHASONE SODIUM PHOSPHATE	1 mg	IM, IV, OTH	J1100
DEXAMETHASONE, CONCENTRATED FORM. COMPOUNDED	1 mg	INH	J7637
DEXAMETHASONE, INTRAVITREAL IMPLANT	0.1 mg	OTH	J7312
DEXAMETHASONE, LACRIMAL OPHTHALMIC INSERT	0.1 mg	OTH	J1096
DEXAMETHASONE, UNIT DOSE FORM, COMPOUNDED	1 mg	INH	J7638
DEXFERRUM®	50 mg	IV	J1750
DEXPAK®	0.25 mg	ORAL	J8540
DEXRAZOXANE HYDROCHLORIDE	250 mg	IV	J1190
DEXTRAN 40	500 ml	IV	J7100
DEXTRAN 75	500 ml	IV	J7110
DEXTROSE 5% IN LACTATED RINGERS	up to 1000 cc	IV	J7121
DEXTROSE 5% NORMAL SALINE SOLUTION	500 ml = 1 unit	IV	J7042
DEXTROSE/WATER (5%)	500 ml = 1 unit	IV	J7060
DEXYCU®	1mcg	OTH	J1095
D-GAM ANTI D®	1 dose package, 300 mcg	IM	J2790
D-GAM ANTI-D®	50 mcg	IM	J2788
DIAMOX®	up to 500 mg	IV, IM	J1120
DIAQUA-2®	up to 20 mg	IM, IV	J1940
DIAZEPAM	up to 5 mg	IM, IV	J3360
DIAZOXIDE	up to 300 mg	IV	J1730
DICLOFENAC SODIUM	0.5 mg	IV	J1130
DICYCLOMINE HCL	up to 20 mg	IM	J0500
DIETHYLSTILBESTROL DIPHOSPHATE	250 mg	IV	J9165
DIFLUCAN®	200 mg	IV	J1450
DIGIFAB®	vial	IV, IM	J1162
DIGOXIN	up to 0.5 mg	IV, IM	J1160
DIGOXIN IMMUNE FAB (OVINE)	vial	IV, IM	J1162
DIHYDROERGOTAMINE MESYLATE	1 mg	IV, IM	J1110
DILANTIN®	50 mg	IV, IM	J1165
DILAUDID®	up to 4 mg	SC, IM, IV	J1170
DIMENHYDRINATE	up to 50 mg	IM, IV	J1240
DIMERCAPROL	100 mg	IM	J0470
DIMETHYL SULFOXIDE (DMSO), 50%	50 ml	OTH	J1212
DIPHENHYDRAMINE	up to 50 mg	IV, IM	J1200

Drug Name	Unit Per	Route	Code
DIPRIVAN®	10 mg	IV	J2704
DIPYRIDAMOLE	10 mg	IV	J1245
DIURIL SODIUM®	500 mg	IV	J1205
DMSO, DIMETHYL SULFOXIDE, 50%	50 ml	OTH	J1212
DOBUTAMINE HCL	250 mg	IV	J1250
DOBUTREX®	250 mg	IV	J1250
DOCATAXEL	1 mg	IV	J9171
DOLASETRON MESYLATE	10 mg	IV	J1260
DOLOPHINE®	up to 10 mg	IM, SC	J1230
DOPAMINE HCL	40 mg	IV	J1265
DORIPENEM	10 mg	IV	J1267
DORNASE ALPHA, UNIT DOSE FORM, NON-COMPOUNDED	1 mg	INH	J7639
DOSTINEX®	0.25 mg	ORAL	J8515
DOXERCALCIFEROL	1 mcg	IV	J1270
DOXORUBICIN HCL	10 mg	IV	J9000
DRAMAMINE®	up to 50 mg	IM, IV	J1240
DRAMOJECT®	up to 50 mg	IM, IV	J1240
DROPERIDOL	up to 5 mg	IM, IV	J1790
DROPERIDOL AND FENTANYL CITRATE	up to 2 ml ampule	IM, IV	J1810
DUOPA®	100 ml	OTH	J7340
DURACLON®	1 mg	OTH	J0735
DURAMORPH®	up to 10 mg	IM, IV, SC	J2270
DUROLANE®	1 mg	IA	J7318
DURVALUMAB	10 mg	IV	J9173
DYMENATE®	up to 50 mg	IM, IV	J1240
DYNACIN®	1 mg	IV	J2265
DYPHYLLINE	up to 500 mg	IM	J1180
DYSPORT®	5 IU	IM	J0586
ECALLANTIDE	1 mg	SC	J1290
ECULIZUMAB	10 mg	IV	J1300
EDARAVONE	1 mg	IV	J1301
EDETATE CALCIUM DISODIUM	up to 1000 mg	IV, SC, IM	J0600
EDETATE DISODIUM	150 mg	IV	J3520
EDEX®	1.25 mcg	OTH	J0270
ELAPRASE®	1 mg	IV	J1743
ELELYSO®	10 IU	IV	J3060
ELIGARD®	1 mg	SC	J9218
ELITEK®	0.5 mg	IV	J2783
ELLENCE®	2 mg	IV	J9178
ELLIOTTS' B SOLUTION	1 ml	IT	J9175
ELOCTATE WITH FC FUSION PROTEIN®	1 IU	IV	J7192
ELOSULFASE ALFA	1 mg	IV	J1322
ELOTUZUMAB	1 mg	IV	J9176
ELOXATIN®	0.5 mg	IV	J9263
ELSPAR®	1,000 IU	IM, IV	J9019

Drug Name	Unit Per	Route	Code
ELZONRIS®	10 mcg	IV	J9269
EMAPALUMAB-LZSG	1 mg	IV	J9210
EMEND®	5 mg	ORAL	J8501
EMICIZUMAB-KXWH	0.5 mg	SC	J7170
EMPLICITI®	1 mg	IV	J9176
ENBREL®	25 mg	SC	J1438
ENDRATE®	150 mg	IV	J3520
ENFORTUMAB VEDOTIN-EJFV	0.25 mg	IV	J9177
ENFUVIRTIDE	1 mg	SC	J1324
ENOXAPARIN SODIUM	10 mg	SC	J1650
ENTYVIO®	1 mg	IV	J3380
ENVARSUS XR®	0.25mg	ORAL	J7503
EPINEPHRINE	0.1 mg	SC, IM	J0171
EPIPEN 2-PAK®	0.1 mg	SC, IM	J0171
EPIPEN JR 2-PAK®	0.1 mg	SC, IM	J0171
EPIRUBICIN HYDROCHLORIDE	2 mg	IV	J9178
EPOETIN ALFA (NON-ESRD)	1000 IU	IV, SC	J0885
EPOETIN BETA (FOR ESRD)	1 mcg	IV	J0887
EPOETIN BETA (NON-ESRD USE)	1 mcg	IV	J0888
EPOGEN®	1000 IU	IV, SC	J0885
EPOPROSTENOL	0.5 mg	IV	J1325
EPSOM SALT®	500 mg	IV, IM	J3475
EPTIFIBATIDE	5 mg	IM, IV	J1327
EPTINEZUMAB-JJMR	1 mg	IV	J3032
ERAVACYCLINE	1 mg	IV	J0122
ERAXIS®	1 mg	IV	J0348
ERBITUX®	10 mg	IV	J9055
ERGONOVINE MALEATE	up to 0.2 mg	IM, IV	J1330
ERIBULIN MESYLATE	0.1 mg	IV	J9179
ERTAPENEM SODIUM	500 mg	IM, IV	J1335
ERWINAZE®	1,000 IU	IV, IM	J9019
ERWINAZE®	10,000 IU	IM, IV	J9020
ERYTHROCIN LACTOBIONATE®	500 mg	IV	J1364
ERYTHROMYCIN LACTOBIONATE	500 mg	IV	J1364
ESTRADIOL VALERATE	up to 10 mg	IM	J1380
ESTROGEN, CONJUGATED	25 mg	IV, IM	J1410
ESTRONE	1 mg	IM	J1435
ETANERCEPT	25 mg	SC	J1438
ETELCALCETIDE	0.1 mg	IV	J0606
ETEPLIRSEN	10 mg	IV	J1428
ETHAMOLIN®	100 mg	IV	J1430
ETHANOLAMINE OLEATE	100 mg	IV	J1430
ETHYOL®	500 mg	IV	J0207
ETIDRONATE DISODIUM	300 mg	IV	J1436
ETONOGESTREL IMPLANT	each	OTH	J7307
ETOPOSIDE	10 mg	IV	J9181
ETOPOSIDE	50 mg	ORAL	J8560
EUFLEXXA®	dose	OTH	J7323

Drug Name	Unit Per	Route	Code
EVENITY®	1 mg	SC	J3111
EVEROLIMUS, ORAL	0.25 mg	ORAL	J7527
EVOMELA®	1 mg	IV	J9246
EVZIO®	1 mg	IM, IV, SC	J2310
EXONDYS 51®	10 mg	IV	J1428
EXPAREL®	1 mg	IV	C9290
EXTAVIA®	0.25 mg	SC	J1830
EYLEA®	1 mg	OTH	J0178
FABRAZYME®	1 mg	IV	J0180
FACTOR IX (ANTIHEMOPHILIC FACTOR, PURIFIED, NON-RECOMBINANT)	1 IU	IV	J7193
FACTOR IX (ANTIHEMOPHILIC FACTOR, RECOMBINANT), NOT OTHERWISE SPECIFIED	1 IU	IV	J7195
FACTOR IX (ANTIHEMOPHILIC FACTOR, RECOMBINANT), RIXUBIS®	1 IU	IV	J7200
FACTOR IX, (ANTIHEMOPHILIC FACTOR, RECOMBINANT), GLYCOPEGYLATED, REBINYN®	1 IU	IV	J7203
FACTOR IX, ALBUMIN FUSION PROTEIN, (RECOMBINANT), IDELVION®	1 IU	IV	J7202
FACTOR IX, COMPLEX	1 IU	IV	J7194
FACTOR IX, FC FUSION PROTEIN, (RECOMBINANT), ALPROLIX®	1 IU	IV	J7201
FACTOR VIIA (ANTIHEMOPHILIC FACTOR, RECOMBINANT), NOVOSEVEN RT®	1 mcg	IV	J7189
FACTOR VIIA (ANTIHEMOPHILIC FACTOR, RECOMBINANT) - JNCW (SEVENFACT®)	1 mcg	IV	J7212
FACTOR VIII (ANTIHEMOPHILIC FACTOR, (PORCINE))	1 IU	IV	J7191
FACTOR VIII (ANTIHEMOPHILIC FACTOR, HUMAN)	1 IU	IV	J7190
FACTOR VIII, (ANTIHEMOPHILIC FACTOR, RECOMBINANT), AFSTYLA®	1 IU	IV	J7210
FACTOR VIII, (ANTIHEMOPHILIC FACTOR RECOMBINANT), (ESPEROCT®), GLYCOPEGYLATED-EXEI	per IU	IV	J7204
FACTOR VIII, (ANTIHEMOPHILIC FACTOR, RECOMBINANT), KOVALTRY®	1 IU	IV	J7211
FACTOR VIII (ANTI-HEMOPHILIC FACTOR, RECOMBINANT), NOT OTHERWISE SPECIFIED	1 IU	IV	J7192
FACTOR VIII, (ANTI-HEMOPHILIC FACTOR, RECOMBINANT), NOVOEIGHT®	1 IU	IV	J7182
FACTOR VIII, (ANTIHEMOPHILIC FACTOR, RECOMBINANT), NUWIQ®	1 IU	IV	J7209
FACTOR VIII (ANTI-HEMOPHILIC FACTOR, RECOMBINANT), OBIZUR®	1 IU	IV	J7188

Drug Name	Unit Per	Route	Code
FACTOR VIII, (ANTIHEMOPHILIC FACTOR, RECOMBINANT), PEGYLATED	1 IU	IV	J7207
FACTOR VIII, (ANTIHEMOPHILIC FACTOR, RECOMBINANT), PEGYLATED-AUCL, (JIVI®)	1 IU	IV	J7208
FACTOR VIII, (ANTIHEMOPHILIC FACTOR, RECOMBINANT), XYNTHA®	1 IU	IV	J7185
FACTOR VIII FC FUSION (RECOMBINANT)	1 IU	IV	J7205
FACTOR X, (HUMAN)	1 IU	IV	J7175
FACTOR XIII A-SUBUNIT (RECOMBINANT)	1 IU	IV	J7181
FACTOR XIII, ANTIHEMOPHILIC FACTOR (HUMAN)	1 IU	IV	J7180
FAM-TRASTUZUMAB DERUXTECAN-NXKI	1 mg	IV	J9358
FASENRA®	1 mg	SC	J0517
FASLODEX®	25 mg	IM	J9395
FEIBA NF®	1 IU	IV	J7198
FEIBA VH IMMUNO®	1 IU	IV	J7198
FENTANYL CITRATE	0.1 mg	IM, IV	J3010
FERRIC CARBOXYMALTOSE	1 mg	IV	J1439
FERRIC DERISOMALTOSE	10 mg	IV	J1437
FERRIC PYROPHOSPHATE CITRATE POWDER	0.1 mg of iron	OTH	J1444
FERRIC PYROPHOSPHATE CITRATE SOLUTION	0.1 mg of iron	IV	J1443
FERRLECIT®	12.5 mg	IV	J2916
FIBRINOGEN CONCENTRATE (HUMAN), FIBRYGA®	1 mg	IV	J7177
FIBRINOGEN CONCENTRATE (HUMAN), NOS	1 mg	IV	J7178
FIBRYGA®	1 mg	IV	J7177
FILGRASTIM (G-CSF), EXCLUDES BIOSIMILARS	1 mcg	SC, IV	J1442
FIRAZYR®	1 mg	SC	J1744
FIRMAGON®	1 mg	SC	J9155
FIRST PROGESTERONE MC10®	50 mg	IM	J2675
FLEBOGAMMA DIF®	500 mg	IV	J1572
FLEBOGAMMA®	500 mg	IV	J1572
FLEXOJECT®	up to 60 mg	IV, IM	J2360
FLEXON®	up to 60 mg	IV, IM	J2360
FLOLAN®	0.5 mg	IV	J1325
FLOXURIDINE	500 mg	IA	J9200
FLUCONAZOLE	200 mg	IV	J1450
FLUDARABINE PHOSPHATE	50 mg	IV	J9185
FLUNISOLIDE, UNIT DOSE FORM, COMPOUNDED	1 mg	INH	J7641
FLUOCINOLONE ACETONIDE, (YUTIQ®)	0.01 mg	OTH	J7314
FLUOCINOLONE ACETONIDE, INTRAVITREAL IMPLANT (ILUVIEN®)	0.01 mg	OTH	J7313

Drug Name	Unit Per	Route	Code
FLUOCINOLONE ACETONIDE, INTRAVITREAL IMPLANT (RETISERT®)	0.01 mg	OTH	J7311
FLUOROURACIL	500 mg	IV	J9190
FLUPHENAZINE DECANOATE	up to 25 mg	IM	J2680
FOLOTYN®	1 mg	IV	J9307
FOMEPIZOLE	15 mg	IV	J1451
FOMIVIRSEN SODIUM, INTRAOCULAR	1.65 mg	OTH	J1452
FONDAPARINUX SODIUM	0.5 mg	SC	J1652
FORADIL AEROLIZER®	20 mcg	INH	J7606
FORMOTEROL FUMARATE, UNIT DOSE, NON-COMPOUNDED	20 mcg	INH	J7606
FORMOTEROL, UNIT DOSE FORM, COMPOUNDED	12 mcg	INH	J7640
FORTAZ®	500 mg	IV, IM	J0713
FORTEO®	10 mcg	SC	J3110
FOSAPREPITANT	1 mg	IV	J1453
FOSCARNET SODIUM	1,000 mg	IV	J1455
FOSCAVIR®	1,000 mg	IV	J1455
FOSNETUPITANT AND PALONOSETRON	235 mg and 0.25 mg	IV	J1454
FRAGMIN®	2500 IU	SC	J1645
FREMANEZUMAB-VFRM	1 mg	SC	J3031
FUDR®	500 mg	IA	J9200
FULVESTRANT	25 mg	IM	J9395
FUROSEMIDE	up to 20 mg	IM, IV	J1940
FUZEON®	1 mg	SC	J1324
GABLOFEN®	50 mcg	IT	J0476
GABLOFEN®	10 mg	IT	J0475
GALLIUM NITRATE	1 mg	IV	J1457
GALSULFASE	1 mg	IV	J1458
GAMIFANT®	1 mg	IV	J9210
GAMMA GLOBULIN	1 cc	IM	J1460
GAMMA GLOBULIN	over 10 cc	IM	J1560
GAMMAGARD LIQUID®	500 mg	IV	J1569
GAMMAKED®	500 mg	IV	J1561
GAMMAPLEX®	500 mg	IV	J1557
GAMULIN RH®	50 mcg	IM	J2788
GAMULIN RH®	1 dose package, 300 mcg	IM	J2790
GAMUNEX-C®	500 mg	IV	J1561
GANCICLOVIR SODIUM	500 mg	IV	J1570
GANCICLOVIR, IMPLANT	4.5 mg	OTH	J7310
GARAMYCIN®	up to 80 mg	IM, IV	J1580
GASTROCROM®	10 mg	INH	J7631
GAZYVA®	10 mg	INJ	J9301
GEFITINIB	250 mg	ORAL	J8565
GEL-ONE®	dose	OTH	J7326

Drug Name	Unit Per	Route	Code
GEL-SYN®	0.1 mg	OTH	J7328
GEMCITABINE HYDROCHLORIDE (INFUGEM®)	100 mg	IV	J9198
GEMCITABINE HYDROCHLORIDE, NOS	200 mg	IV	J9201
GEMTUZUMAB OZOGAMICIN	0.1 mg	IV	J9203
GENGRAF®	100 mg	ORAL	J7502
GENGRAF®	25 mg	ORAL	J7515
GENOTROPIN®	1 mg	SC	J2941
GENTAMICIN (GARAMYCIN®)	up to 80 mg	IM, IV	J1580
GENVISC 850®	1 mg	OTH	J7320
GEODON®	10 mg	IM	J3486
GIVOSIRAN	0.5 mg	IV	J0223
GLASSIA®	10 mg	IV	J0257
GLATIRAMER ACETATE	20 mg	SC	J1595
GLUCAGEN HYPOKIT®	1 mg	SC, IM, IV	J1610
GLUCAGEN®	1 mg	SC, IM, IV	J1610
GLUCAGON EMERGENCY KIT FOR LOW BLOOD SUGAR®	1 mg	SC, IM, IV	J1610
GLUCAGON HYDROCHLORIDE	1 mg	SC, IM, IV	J1610
GLUCARPIDASE	10 units	IV	C9293
GLYCOPYRROLATE, CONCENTRATED FORM, COMPOUNDED	1 mg	INH	J7642
GLYCOPYRROLATE, UNIT DOSE FORM, COMPOUNDED	1 mg	INH	J7643
GOLD SODIUM THIOMALATE	up to 50 mg	IM	J1600
GOLIMUMAB	1 mg	IV	J1602
GOLODIRSEN	10 mg	IV	J1429
GONADORELIN HYDROCHLORIDE	100 mcg	SC, IV	J1620
GOPRELTO®	1 mg	OTH	C9046
GOSERELIN ACETATE IMPLANT	3.6 mg	OTH	J9202
GRANISETRON HYDROCHLORIDE	100 mcg	IV	J1626
GRANISETRON, EXTENDED RELEASE	0.1 mg	IV	J1627
GRANIX®	1 mcg	SC, IV	J1447
GUSELKUMAB	1 mg	SC	J1628
HAEGARDA®	10 IU	IV	J0599
HALAVEN®	0.1 mg	IV	J9179
HALDOL DECANOATE®	50 mg	IM	J1631
HALDOL®	up to 5 mg	IM, IV	J1630
HALOPERIDOL	up to 5 mg	IM, IV	J1630
HALOPERIDOL DECANOATE	50 mg	IM	J1631
HECTOROL®	1 mcg	IV	J1270
HELIXATE FS®	1 IU	IV	J7192
HEMIN	1 mg	IV	J1640
HEMLIBRA®	0.5 mg	SC	J7170
HEMOFIL-M®	1 IU	IV	J7190

Drug Name	Unit Per	Route	Code
HEMOPHILIA CLOTTING FACTOR, NOT OTHERWISE CLASSIFIED	1 IU	IV	J7199
HEPAGAM B®	0.5 ml	IM	J1571
HEPAGAM B®	0.5 ml	IV	J1573
HEPARIN SODIUM	1,000 IU	IV, SC	J1644
HEPARIN SODIUM (HEPARIN LOCK FLUSH)	10 IU	IV	J1642
HERCEPTIN HYLECTA®	10 mg	SC	J9356
HERCEPTIN®	10 mg	IV	J9355
HISTAJECT®	10 mg	IM, SC, IV	J0945
HISTRELIN ACETATE	10 mcg	OTH	J1675
HISTRELIN IMPLANT	50 mg	OTH	J9225
HISTRELIN IMPLANT	50 mg	OTH	J9226
HIZENTRA®	100 mg	SC	J1559
HUMATE-P®	1 IU	IV	J7187
HUMATROPE®	1 mg	SC	J2941
HUMIRA®	20 mg	SC	J0135
HYALGAN®	dose	OTH	J7321
HYALURONAN OR DERIVATIVE, DUROLANE®	1 mg	IA	J7318
HYALURONAN OR DERIVATIVE, EUFLEXXA®	dose	OTH	J7323
HYALURONAN OR DERIVATIVE, GEL-ONE®	dose	OTH	J7326
HYALURONAN OR DERIVATIVE, GENVISC 850®	1 mg	OTH	J7320
HYALURONAN OR DERIVATIVE, HYALGAN®	dose	OTH	J7321
HYALURONAN OR DERIVATIVE, HYMOVIS®	1 mg	OTH	J7322
HYALURONAN OR DERIVATIVE, MONOVISC®	dose	IV	J7327
HYALURONAN OR DERIVATIVE, ORTHOVISC®	dose	OTH	J7324
HYALURONAN OR DERIVATIVE, SUPARTZ®	dose	OTH	J7321
HYALURONAN OR DERIVATIVE, SYNOJOYNT®	1 mg	OTH	J7331
HYALURONAN OR DERIVATIVE, SYNVISC®	1 mg	OTH	J7325
HYALURONAN OR DERIVATIVE, SYNVISC-ONE®	1 mg	OTH	J7325
HYALURONAN OR DERIVATIVE, TRILURON®	1 mg	OTH	J7332
HYALURONAN OR DERIVATIVE, TRIVISC®	1 mg	VAR	J7329
HYALURONAN OR DERIVATIVE, VISCO-3®	dose	OTH	J7333
HYALURONAN OR DERIVITIVE, GEL-SYN®	0.1 mg	OTH	J7328
HYALURONIDASE	up to 150 IU	SC, IV	J3470
HYALURONIDASE, OVINE, PRESERVATIVE FREE	up to 999 IU	VAR	J3471

Drug Name	Unit Per	Route	Code
HYALURONIDASE, OVINE, PRESERVATIVE FREE	1000 IU	VAR	J3472
HYALURONIDASE, RECOMBINANT	1 usp	SC	J3473
HYCAMTIN®	0.25 mg	ORAL	J8705
HYCAMTIN®	0.1 mg	IV	J9351
HYDRALAZINE HCL	up to 20 mg	IV, IM	J0360
HYDROCORTISONE ACETATE	up to 25 mg	IV, IM, SC	J1700
HYDROCORTISONE SODIUM PHOSPHATE	up to 50 mg	IV, IM, SC	J1710
HYDROCORTISONE SODIUM SUCCINATE	up to 100 mg	IV, IM, SC	J1720
HYDROMORPHONE	up to 4 mg	SC, IM, IV	J1170
HYDROXYPROGESTERONE CAPROATE, MAKENA®	10 mg	IV	J1726
HYDROXYPROGESTERONE CAPROATE, NOT OTHERWISE SPECIFIED	10 mg	IV	J1729
HYDROXYZINE HCL	up to 25 mg	IM	J3410
HYLENEX®	up to 150 IU	SC	J3470
HYLENEX®	1 usp	SC	J3473
HYMOVIS®	1 mg	OTH	J7322
HYOSCYAMINE SULFATE	up to 0.25 mg	SC, IM, IV	J1980
HYPERRHO S/D FULL DOSE®	1 dose package, 300 mcg	IM	J2790
HYPERRHO SD MINI DOSE®	50 mcg	IM	J2788
HYPERTET S/D®	up to 250 IU	IM	J1670
HYPERTONIC SALINE SOLUTION	1 ml	IV	J7131
HYQVIA®	100 mg	IV	J1575
IBALIZUMAB-UIYK	10 mg	IV	J1746
IBANDRONATE SODIUM	1 mg	IV	J1740
IBUPROFEN	100 mg	IV	J1741
IBUTILIDE FUMARATE	1 mg	IV	J1742
ICATIBANT	1 mg	SC	J1744
IDAMYCIN PFS®	5 mg	IV	J9211
IDARUBICIN HCL	5 mg	IV	J9211
IDELVION®	1 IU	IV	J7202
IDURSULFASE	1 mg	IV	J1743
IFEX®	1 g	IV	J9208
IFOSFAMIDE	1 g	IV	J9208
ILARIS®	1 mg	SC	J0638
ILUMYA®	1 mg	SC	J3245
ILUVIEN®	0.01 mg	OTH	J7313
IMFINZI®	10 mg	IV	J9173
IMIGLUCERASE	10 IU	IV	J1786
IMIPENEM 4 MG, CILASTATIN 4 MG, AND RELEBACTAM 2 MG	See Descriptor	IV	J0742
IMITREX STATDOSE®	6 mg	SC	J3030
IMLYGIC®	1 million PFU	OTH	J9325

Drug Name	Unit Per	Route	Code
IMMUNE GLOBULIN, BIVIGAM®	500 mg	IV	J1556
IMMUNE GLOBULIN, CUVITRU®	100 mg	IV	J1555
IMMUNE GLOBULIN, FLEBOGAMMA®/FLEBOGAMMA DIF®	500 mg	IV	J1572
IMMUNE GLOBULIN, GAMMAGARD LIQUID®	500 mg	IV	J1569
IMMUNE GLOBULIN, GAMMAPLEX®	500 mg	IV	J1557
IMMUNE GLOBULIN, GAMUNEX-C®/GAMMAKED®	500 mg	IV	J1561
IMMUNE GLOBULIN, HEPATITIS B, HEPAGAM B®	0.5 ml	IM	J1571
IMMUNE GLOBULIN, HEPATITIS B, HEPAGAM B®	0.5 ml	IV	J1573
IMMUNE GLOBULIN, HIZENTRA®	100 mg	SC	J1559
IMMUNE GLOBULIN, LYOPHILIZED	500 mg	IV	J1566
IMMUNE GLOBULIN, NON-LYOPHILIZED	500 mg	IV	J1599
IMMUNE GLOBULIN, OCTAGAM®	500 mg	IV	J1568
IMMUNE GLOBULIN, PRIVIGEN®	500 mg	IV	J1459
IMMUNE GLOBULIN, RHOPHYLAC®	100 IU	IM	J2791
IMMUNE GLOBULIN, VIVAGLOBIN®	100 mg	IV	J1562
IMMUNE GLOBULIN, XEMBIFY®	100 mg	IV	J1558
IMMUNE GLOBULIN/ HYALURONIDASE (HYQVIA®)	100 mg	IV	J1575
IMMUNOSUPPRESSIVE DRUG, NOT OTHERWISE CLASSIFIED	-	-	J7599
IMURAN®	50 mg	ORAL	J7500
INAPSINE®	up to 5 mg	IM, IV	J1790
INCOBOTULINUM TOXIN A	1 IU	IM	J0588
INCRELEX®	1 mg	SC	J2170
INDERAL®	up to 1 mg	IV	J1800
INEBILIZUMAB-CDON	1 mg	INJ	J1823
INFED®	50 mg	IV	J1750
INFLIXIMAB, EXCLUDES BIOSIMILAR	10 mg	IM, IV	J1745
INFUGEM®	100 mg	IV	J9198
INJECTAFER®	1 mg	IV	J1439
INOTUZUMAB OZOGAMICIN	0.1 mg	IV	J9229
INSULIN	5 IU	SC	J1815
INSULIN (ADMINISTERED THROUGH DME)	50 IU	SC	J1817
INTEGRILIN®	5 mg	IM, IV	J1327
INTERFERON ALFA-2A, RECOMBINANT	3 million IU	SC, IM	J9213
INTERFERON ALFA-2B, RECOMBINANT	1 million IU	VAR	J9214
INTERFERON ALFA-N3 (HUMAN LEUKOCYTE DERIVED)	250,000 IU	OTH	J9215
INTERFERON ALPHACON-1, RECOMBINANT	1 mcg	SC	J9212

Drug Name	Unit Per	Route	Code
INTERFERON BETA-1A	30 mcg	IM	J1826
INTERFERON BETA-1B	0.25 mg	SC	J1830
INTERFERON GAMMA-1B	3 million IU	SC	J9216
INTRON A ®	1 million IU	VAR	J9214
INTROPIN®	40 mg	IV	J1265
INVANZ®	500 mg	IM, IV	J1335
INVEGA SUSTENNA®	1 mg	IM	J2426
IPILIMUMAB	1 mg	IV	J9228
IPRATROPIUM BROMIDE, UNIT DOSE FORM, COMPOUNDED	1 mg	INH	J7645
IPRATROPIUM BROMIDE, UNIT DOSE FORM, NON-COMPOUNDED	1 mg	INH	J7644
IRESSA®	250 mg	ORAL	J8565
IRINOTECAN	20 mg	IV	J9206
IRINOTECAN LIPOSOME	1 mg	IV	J9205
IRON DEXTRAN	50 mg	IV	J1750
IRON SUCROSE	1 mg	IV	J1756
ISATUXIMAB-IRFC	10 mg	IV	J9227
ISAVUCONAZONIUM	1 mg	IV	J1833
ISOETHARINE HCL, CONCENTRATED FORM, COMPOUNDED	1 mg	INH	J7647
ISOETHARINE HCL, CONCENTRATED FORM, NON-COMPOUNDED	1 mg	INH	J7648
ISOETHARINE HCL, UNIT DOSE FORM, COMPOUNDED	1 mg	INH	J7650
ISOETHARINE HCL, UNIT DOSE FORM, NON-COMPOUNDED	1 mg	INH	J7649
ISOPROTERENOL HCL, CONCENTRATED FORM, COMPOUNDED	1 mg	INH	J7657
ISOPROTERENOL HCL, CONCENTRATED FORM, NON-COMPOUNDED	1 mg	INH	J7658
ISOPROTERENOL HCL, UNIT DOSE FORM, COMPOUNDED	1 mg	INH	J7660
ISOPROTERENOL HCL, UNIT DOSE FORM, NON-COMPOUNDED	1 mg	INH	J7659
ISTODAX®	1 mg	IV	J9315
ITRACONAZOLE	50 mg	IV	J1835
IXABEPILONE	1 mg	IV	J9207
IXEMPRA®	1 mg	IV	J9207
JETREA®	0.125 mg	IV	J7316
JEVTANA®	1 mg	IV	J9043
JIVI®	1 IU	IV	J7208
KADCYLA®	1 mg	IV	J9354
KALBITOR®	1 mg	SC	J1290
KANAMYCIN SULFATE	up to 75 mg	IM, IV	J1850
KANAMYCIN SULFATE	up to 500 mg	IM, IV	J1840
KANUMA®	1 mg	IV	J2840
KEFZOL®	500 mg	IV, IM	J0690

Drug Name	Unit Per	Route	Code
KENGREAL®	1 mg	IV	C9460
KEPIVANCE®	50 mcg	IV	J2425
KEPPRA®	10 mg	IV	J1953
KETOROLAC TROMETHAMINE	15 mg	IM, IV	J1885
KEYTRUDA®	1 mg	IV	J9271
KHAPZORY®	0.5 mg	IV	J0642
KINEVAC®	5 mcg	IV	J2805
KOATE-DVI®	1 IU	IV	J7190
KOGENATE FS®	1 IU	IV	J7192
KOVALTRY®	1 IU	IV	J7211
KRYSTEXXA®	1 mg	IV	J2507
KYLEENA®	19.5 mg	OTH	J7296
KYPROLIS®	1 mg	IV	J9047
LACOSAMIDE	1mg	IV	C9254
LACTATED RINGERS	up to 1,000 cc	IV	J7120
LACTATED RINGERS WITH DEXTROSE 5%	up to 1000 cc	IV	J7121
LAETRILE, AMYGDALIN, VITAMIN B-17	dose	VAR	J3570
LANADELUMAB-FLYO	1 mg	SC	J0593
LANOXIN®	up to 0.5 mg	IV, IM	J1160
LANREOTIDE	1 mg	SC	J1930
LARONIDASE	0.1 mg	IV	J1931
LARTRUVO™	10 mg	IV	J9285
LEFAMULIN	1mg	IV	J6091
LEMTRADA®	1 mg	IV	J0202
LEPIRUDIN	50 mg	IV	J1945
LEUCOVORIN CALCIUM	50 mg	IM, IV	J0640
LEUKINE®	50 mcg	IV	J2820
LEUPROLIDE ACETATE	1 mg	IM	J9218
LEUPROLIDE ACETATE, (FOR DEPOT SUSPENSION)	3.75 mg	IM	J1950
LEUPROLIDE ACETATE, (FOR DEPOT SUSPENSION)	7.5 mg	IM	J9217
LEUPROLIDE ACETATE, IMPLANT	65 mg	OTH	J9219
LEVALBUTEROL, CONCENTRATED FORM, COMPOUNDED	0.5 mg	INH	J7607
LEVALBUTEROL, CONCENTRATED FORM, NON-COMPOUNDED	0.5 mg	INH	J7612
LEVALBUTEROL, UNIT DOSE, COMPOUNDED	0.5 mg	INH	J7615
LEVALBUTEROL, UNIT DOSE, NON-COMPOUNDED	0.5 mg	INH	J7614
LEVAQUIN®	250 mg	IV	J1956
LEVETIRACETAM	10 mg	IV	J1953
LEVOCARNITINE	1 gm	IV	J1955
LEVOFLOXACIN	250 mg	IV	J1956
LEVOLEUCOVORIN (KHAPZORY®)	0.5 mg	IV	J0642
LEVOLEUCOVORIN, NOT OTHERWISE SPECIFIED	0.5 mg	IV	J0641
LEVONORGESTREL IMPLANT	each	OTH	J7306

Drug Name	Unit Per	Route	Code
LEVONORGESTREL-RELEASING INTRAUTERINE CONTRACEPTIVE SYSTEM, KYLEENA®	19.5 mg	OTH	J7296
LEVONORGESTREL-RELEASING INTRAUTERINE CONTRACEPTIVE SYSTEM, LILETTA®	52 mg	OTH	J7297
LEVONORGESTREL-RELEASING INTRAUTERINE CONTRACEPTIVE SYSTEM, MIRENA®	52 mg	OTH	J7298
LEVONORGESTREL-RELEASING INTRAUTERINE CONTRACEPTIVE SYSTEM, SKYLA®	13.5 mg	OTH	J7301
LEVORPHANOL TARTRATE	up to 2 mg	SC, IV	J1960
LEVULAN KERASTICK®	unit dose (354 mg)	OTH	J7308
LEXISCAN®	0.1 mg	IV	J2785
LIBERIM D®	50 mcg	IM	J2788
LIBERIM D®	1 dose package, 300 mcg	IM	J2790
LIBTAYO®	1 mg	IV	J9119
LIDOCAINE HCL	10 mg	IV	J2001
LIDOCAINE/TETRACAINE	per patch	OTH	C9285
LILETTA®	52 mg	OTH	J7297
LINCOCIN®	up to 300 mg	IV	J2010
LINCOMYCIN	up to 300 mg	IV	J2010
LINEZOLID	200 mg	IV	J2020
LIORESAL INTRATHECAL®	10 mg	IT	J0475
LIPOSOMAL, DAUNORUBICIN AND CYTARABINE	1 mg/2.27 mg	IV	J9153
LORAZEPAM	2 mg	IM, IV	J2060
LOVENOX HP®	10 mg	SC	J1650
LOVENOX®	10 mg	SC	J1650
LOXAPINE	1 mg	OTH	J2062
LUCENTIS®	0.1 mg	OTH	J2778
LUMINAL®	up to 120 mg	IM, IV	J2560
LUMIZYME®	10 mg	IV	J0221
LUMOXITI®	0.01 mg	IV	J9313
LUPRON DEPOT®	3.75 mg	IM	J1950
LUPRON DEPOT®	7.5 mg	IM	J9217
LUPRON®	1 mg	IM	J9218
LURBINECTEDIN	0.1 mg	INJ	J9223
LUSPATERCEPT-AAMT	0.25 mg	IV	J0896
LUXTURNA®	1 billion vector genomes	OTH	J3398
LYMPHOCYTE IMMUNE GLOBULIN, ANTI-THYMOCYTE GLOBULIN, EQUINE	250 mg	IV	J7504
LYMPHOCYTE IMMUNE GLOBULIN, ANTI-THYMOCYTE GLOBULIN, RABBIT	25 mg	OTH	J7511
MACUGEN®	0.3 mg	OTH	J2503
MAGNESIUM SULFATE	500 mg	IV, IM	J3475

Drug Name	Unit Per	Route	Code
MAKENA®	10 mg	IV	J1726
MANNITOL	25% in 50 ml	IV	J2150
MANNITOL	5 mg	INH	J7665
MARQIBO®	1 mg	IV	J9371
MAXIPIME®	500 mg	IV	J0692
MECASERMIN	1 mg	SC	J2170
MECHLORETHAMINE HCL (NITROGEN MUSTARD), HN2	10 mg	IV	J9230
MEDROL DOSEPAK®	4 mg	ORAL	J7509
MEDROL®	4 mg	ORAL	J7509
MEDROXYPROGESTERONE ACETATE	1 mg	IM	J1050
MEFOXIN®	1 g	IV, IM	J0694
MELOXICAM	1 mg	IV	J1738
MELPHALAN	2 mg	ORAL	J8600
MELPHALAN (EVOMELA®)	1 mg	IV	J9246
MELPHALAN HCL	50 mg	IV	J9245
MEPERIDINE AND PROMETHAZINE HCL	up to 50 mg	IM, IV	J2180
MEPERIDINE HYDROCHLORIDE	100 mg	IM, IV, SC	J2175
MEPIVACAINE HCL	10 ml	VAR	J0670
MEPOLIZUMAB	1 mg	IV	J2182
MEPSEVII®	1 mg	IV	J3397
MEROPENEM	100 mg	IV	J2185
MEROPENEM AND VABORBACTAM	10mg/10mg	IV	J2186
MERREM®	100 mg	IV	J2185
MESNA	200 mg	IV	J9209
MESNEX®	200 mg	IV, ORAL	J9209
METAPROTERENOL SULFATE, CONCENTRATED FORM, COMPOUNDED	10 mg	INH	J7667
METAPROTERENOL SULFATE, CONCENTRATED FORM, NON-COMPOUNDED	10 mg	INH	J7668
METAPROTERENOL SULFATE, UNIT DOSE FORM, COMPOUNDED	10 mg	INH	J7670
METAPROTERENOL SULFATE, UNIT DOSE FORM, NON-COMPOUNDED	10 mg	INH	J7669
METARAMINOL BITARTRATE	10 mg	IV, IM, SC	J0380
METHACHOLINE CHLORIDE	1 mg	INH	J7674
METHADONE HCL	up to 10 mg	IM, SC	J1230
METHERGINE®	0.2 mg	IV, IM	J2210
METHOCARBAMOL	up to 10 ml	IV, IM	J2800
METHOTREXATE	2.5 mg	ORAL	J8610
METHOTREXATE SODIUM	5 mg	IV, IM, IT, IA, SC	J9250
METHOTREXATE SODIUM	50 mg	IV, IM, IT, IA, SC	J9260
METHYL AMINOLEVULINATE, TOPICAL, 16.8%	1 gram	OTH	J7309

Drug Name	Unit Per	Route	Code
METHYLDOPATE HCL	up to 250 mg	IV	J0210
METHYLERGONOVINE MALEATE	UP TO 0.2 mg	IV, IM	J2210
METHYLNALTREXONE	0.1 mg	SC	J2212
METHYLPREDNISOLONE ACETATE	20 mg	IM	J1020
METHYLPREDNISOLONE ACETATE	40 mg	IM	J1030
METHYLPREDNISOLONE ACETATE	80 mg	IM	J1040
METHYLPREDNISOLONE SODIUM SUCCINATE	up to 40 mg	IM, IV	J2920
METHYLPREDNISOLONE SODIUM SUCCINATE	up to 125 mg	IM, IV	J2930
METHYLPREDNISOLONE, ORAL	4 mg	ORAL	J7509
METOCLOPRAMIDE HCL	up to 10 mg	IV	J2765
MIACALCIN®	up to 400 IU	SC, IM	J0630
MICAFUNGIN SODIUM	1 mg	IV	J2248
MICRHOGAM ULTRA FILTERED PLUS®	50 mcg	IM	J2788
MICRHOGAM ULTRA FILTERED PLUS®	1 dose package, 300 mcg	IM	J2790
MICRHOGAM®	50 mcg	IM	J2788
MICRHOGAM®	1 dose package, 300 mcg	IM	J2790
MIDAZOLAM HCL	1 mg	IM, IV	J2250
MILLIPRED DP®	5 mg	ORAL	J7510
MILLIPRED®	up to 1 ml	IM	J2650
MILLIPRED®	5 mg	ORAL	J7510
MILRINONE LACTATE	5 mg	IV	J2260
MINOCYCLINE HYDROCHLORIDE	1 mg	IV	J2265
MIO-REL®	up to 60 mg	IV, IM	J2360
MIRCERA® (FOR ESRD)	1 mcg	IV	J0887
MIRCERA® (NON-ESRD USE)	1 mcg	IV	J0888
MIRENA	52 mg	OTH	J7298
MITOMYCIN	5 mg	IV	J9280
MITOMYCIN, OPTHALMIC	0.2 mg	OTH	J7315
MITOMYCIN PYELOCALYCEAL INSTILLATION	1 mg	OTH	J9281
MITOSOL®	0.2 mg	OTH	J7315
MITOXANTRONE HCL	5 mg	IV	J9293
MOGAMULIZUMAB-KPKC	1 mg	IV	J9204
MOMETASONE FUROATE SINUS IMPLANT	10 mcg	OTH	J7401
MONOCLATE-P®	1 IU	IV	J7190
MONONINE®	1 IU	IV	J7193
MONOVISC®	dose	OTH	J7327
MORPHINE SULFATE	up to 10 mg	IM, IV, SC	J2270
MORPHINE SULFATE	10 mg	OTH	J2274
MOXETUMOMAB PASUDOTOX-TDFK	0.01 mg	IV	J9313

Drug Name	Unit Per	Route	Code
MOXIFLOXACIN	100 mg	IV	J2280
MOZOBIL®	1 mg	SC	J2562
MUROMONAB-CD3, PARENTERAL	5 mg	OTH	J7505
MUSE® URETHRAL SUPPOSITORY	each	OTH	J0275
MUTAMYCIN®	5 mg	IV	J9280
MYCAMINE®	1 mg	IV	J2248
MYCOPHENOLATE MOFETIL	250 mg	ORAL	J7517
MYCOPHENOLIC ACID, ORAL	180 mg	ORAL	J7518
MYFORTIC®	180 mg	ORAL	J7518
MYLERAN®	2 mg	ORAL	J8510
MYOBLOC®	100 IU	IM	J0587
MYOZYME®	10 mg	IV	J0220
NABILONE	1 mg	ORAL	J8650
NAGLAZYME®	1 mg	IV	J1458
NALBUPHINE HCL	10 mg	IM, IV, SC	J2300
NALOXONE HCL	1 mg	IM, IV, SC	J2310
NALTREXONE (DEPOT FORM)	1 mg	IM	J2315
NANDROLONE DECANOATE	up to 50 mg	IM	J2320
NAROPIN POLYAMP®	1 mg	OTH	J2795
NAROPIN SDV®	1 mg	OTH	J2795
NAROPIN®	1 mg	OTH	J2795
NASAL VACCINE INHALATION	dose	INH	J3530
NATALIZUMAB	1 mg	IV	J2323
NATRECOR®	0.1 mg	IV	J2325
NAVELBINE®	10 mg	IV	J9390
NEBUPENT®	300 mg	INH	J2545
NECITUMUMAB	1 mg	IV	J9295
NELARABINE	50 mg	IV	J9261
NEMBUTAL SODIUM®	50 mg	IM, IV	J2515
NEORAL®	25 mg	ORAL	J7515
NEORAL®	100 mg	ORAL	J7502
NEOSTIGMINE METHYLSULFATE	up to 0.5 mg	IM, IV, SC	J2710
NESIRITIDE	0.1 mg	IV	J2325
NETUPITANT AND PALONOSETRON	300 mg/0.5 mg	ORAL	J8655
NEULASTA®	6 mg	SC	J2505
NEUPOGEN®	1 mcg	SC, IV	J1442
NEXPLANON®	each	OTH	J7307
NIPENT®	10 mg	IV	J9268
NIVOLUMAB	1 mg	IV	J9299
NONCHEMOTHERAPEUTIC, NOT OTHERWISE SPECIFIED	-	ORAL	J8499
NORDITROPIN FLEXPRO PEN®	1 mg	SC	J2941
NOT OTHERWISE CLASSIFIED DRUGS	-	INH	J7699
NOT OTHERWISE CLASSIFIED DRUGS, ADMINISTERED THROUGH DME	-	OTH	J7799
NOT OTHERWISE CLASSIFIED DRUGS, CHEMOTHERAPEUTIC	-	ORAL	J8999

Drug Name	Unit Per	Route	Code
NOT OTHERWISE CLASSIFIED DRUGS, IMMUNOSUPPRESSIVE	-	-	J7599
NOT OTHERWISE CLASSIFIED DRUGS, NONCHEMOTHERAPEUTIC	-	ORAL	J8499
NOVAREL®	1,000 IU	IM	J0725
NOVOEIGHT®	1 IU	IV	J7182
NOVOSEVEN RT®	1 mcg	IV	J7189
NPLATE®	10 mcg	SC	J2796
NUCALA®	1 mg	IV	J2182
NULECIT®	12.5 mg	IV	J2916
NULOJIX®	1 mg	IV	J0485
NUSINERSEN	0.1 mg	IV	J2326
NUTROPIN AQ NUSPIN 10®	1 mg	SC	J2941
NUTROPIN AQ NUSPIN 5®	1 mg	SC	J2941
NUVARING®	each	OTH	J7303
NUWIQ®	1 IU	IV	J7209
NUZYRA®	1 mg	IV	J0121
OBINUTUZUMAB	10 mg	INJ	J9301
OBIZUR®	1 IU	IV	J7188
OCRELIZUMAB	1 mg	IV	J2350
OCREVUS®	1 mg	IV	J2350
OCRIPLASMIN	0.125 mg	IV	J7316
OCTAGAM®	500 mg	IV	J1568
OCTREOTIDE, DEPOT FORM	1 mg	IM	J2353
OCTREOTIDE, NON-DEPOT FORM	25 mcg	IV, SC	J2354
OFATUMUMAB	10 mg	IV	J9302
OFIRMEV®	10 mg	IV	J0131
OLANZAPINE	1 mg	IM	J2358
OLARATUMAB	10 mg	IV	J9285
OMACETAXINE MEPESUCCINATE	0.01 mg	IV	J9262
OMADACYCLINE	1 mg	IV	J0121
OMALIZUMAB	5 mg	SC	J2357
OMNITROPE®	1 mg	SC	J2941
ONABOTULINUM TOXIN A	1 IU	IM	J0585
ONASEMNOGENE ABEPARVOVEC-XIOI	up to 5x10^{15} vector genomes	IV	J3399
ONCASPAR®	single dose vial	IM, IV	J9266
ONDANSETRON HCl	1 mg	IV	J2405
ONIVYDE®	1 mg	IV	J9205
ONPATTRO®	0.1 mg	IV	J0222
ONTAK®	300 mcg	IV	J9160
OPANA®	up to 1 mg	IV, SC, IM	J2410
OPDIVO®	1 mg	IV	J9299
OPRELVEKIN	5 mg	SC	J2355
ORAPRED ODT®	5 mg	ORAL	J7510
ORAVERSE®	up to 5 mg	IM, IV	J2760
ORBACTIV®	10 mg	IV	J2407

Drug Name	Unit Per	Route	Code
ORENCIA®	10 mg	IV	J0129
ORENITRAM®	1 mg	IV, SC, INH	J3285
ORFRO®	up to 60 mg	IV, IM	J2360
ORITAVANCIN	10 mg	IV	J2407
ORPHENADRINE CITRATE	up to 60 mg	IV, IM	J2360
ORPHENATE®	up to 60 mg	IV, IM	J2360
ORTHOCLONE OKT3®	5 mg	OTH	J7505
ORTHOVISC®	dose	OTH	J7324
OSMITROL®	25% in 50 ml	IV	J2150
OTIPRIO®	6 mg	OTH	J7342
OXACILLIN SODIUM	up to 250 mg	IM, IV	J2700
OXALIPLATIN	0.5 mg	IV	J9263
OXYMORPHONE HCL	up to 1 mg	IV, SC, IM	J2410
OXYTETRACYCLINE HCL	up to 50 mg	IM	J2460
OXYTOCIN	up to 10 IU	IV, IM	J2590
OZURDEX®	0.1 mg	OTH	J7312
PACERONE®	30 mg	IV	J0282
PACLITAXEL	1 mg	IV	J9267
PACLITAXEL PROTEIN-BOUND PARTICLES	1 mg	IV	J9264
PALIFERMIN	50 mcg	IV	J2425
PALIPERIDONE PALMITATE, EXTENDED RELEASE	1 mg	IM	J2426
PALONOSETRON HCL	25 mcg	IV	J2469
PAMIDRONATE DISODIUM	30 mg	IV	J2430
PANHEMATIN®	1 mg	IV	J1640
PANITUMUMAB	10 mg	IV	J9303
PANMYCIN®	up to 250 mg	IM, IV	J0120
PANTOPRAZOLE SODIUM	per vial	IV	C9113
PAPAVERINE HCL	up to 60 mg	IV, IM	J2440
PARAGARD®	each	OTH	J7300
PARICALCITOL	1 mcg	IV, IM	J2501
PARSABIV®	0.1 mg	IV	J0606
PARTOBULIN SDF®	50 mcg	IM	J2788
PARTOBULIN SDF®	1 dose package, 300 mcg	IM	J2790
PASIREOTIDE LONG ACTING	1 mg	IV	J2502
PATISIRAN	0.1 mg	IV	J0222
PEDIAPRED®	5 mg	ORAL	J7510
PEGADEMASE BOVINE	25 IU	IM	J2504
PEGAPTANIB SODIUM	0.3 mg	OTH	J2503
PEGASPARGASE	single dose vial	IM, IV	J9266
PEGFILGRASTIM	6 mg	SC	J2505
PEGINESATIDE (FOR ESRD)	0.1 mg	IV, SC	J0890
PEGLOTICASE	1 mg	IV	J2507
PEMBROLIZUMAB	1 mg	IV	J9271
PEMETREXED	10 mg	IV	J9305

Drug Name	Unit Per	Route	Code
PEMETREXED (PEMFEXY®)	10 mg	IV	J9304
PEMFEXY®	10 mg	IV	J9304
PENICILLIN G BENZATHINE	100,000 IU	IM	J0561
PENICILLIN G BENZATHINE AND PENICILLIN G PROCAINE	100,000 IU	IM	J0558
PENICILLIN G POTASSIUM	up to 600,000 IU	IM, IV	J2540
PENICILLIN G PROCAINE, AQUEOUS	up to 600,000 IU	IM, IV	J2510
PENTAMIDINE ISETHIONATE, INHALATION SOLUTION, NON-COMPOUNDED	300 mg	INH	J2545
PENTAMIDINE, COMPOUNDED	300 mg	OTH	J7676
PENTASTARCH, 10% SOLUTION	100 ml	IV	J2513
PENTAZOCINE HCL	30 mg	IM, SC, IV	J3070
PENTOBARBITAL SODIUM	50 mg	IM, IV	J2515
PENTOSTATIN	10 mg	IV	J9268
PERAMIVIR	1 mg	IV	J2547
PERFOROMIST®	20 mcg	INH	J7606
PERJETA®	1 mg	IV	J9306
PERPHENAZINE	up to 5 mg	IM, IV	J3310
PERSANTINE IV®	10 mg	IV	J1245
PERSERIS®	0.5 mg	IM, SC	J2798
PERTUZUMAB	1 mg	IV	J9306
PERTUZUMAB, TRASTUZUMAB, AND HYALURONIDASE-ZZXF	10 mg	INJ	J9316
PFIZERPEN®	up to 600,000 IU	IM, IV	J2540
PHARMORUBICIN PFS®	2 mg	IV	J9178
PHARMORUBICIN RDF®	2 mg	IV	J9178
PHENERGAN®	up to 50 mg	IM, IV	J2550
PHENOBARBITAL SODIUM	up to 120 mg	IM, IV	J2560
PHENTOLAMINE MESYLATE	up to 5 mg	IM, IV	J2760
PHENYLEPHRINE AND KETOROLAC	1 ml	OTH	J1097
PHENYLEPHRINE HCL	up to 1 ml	SC, IM, IV	J2370
PHENYTOIN SODIUM	50 mg	IV, IM	J1165
PHOTOFRIN®	75 mg	IV	J9600
PHOTREXA VISCOUS®	up to 3mL	OTH	J2787
PHYTONADIONE, VITAMIN K	1 mg	IM, SC, IV	J3430
PIPERACILLIN/TAZOBACTAM SODIUM	1.125 g	IV	J2543
PITOCIN®	up to 10 IU	IV, IM	J2590
PLAZOMICIN	5 mg	IV	J0291
PLERIXAFOR	1 mg	SC	J2562
PLICAMYCIN	2,500 mcg	IV	J9270
POLATUZUMAB VEDOTIN-PIIQ	1 mg	IV	J9309
POLIVY®	1 mg	IV	J9309

Drug Name	Unit Per	Route	Code
POLOCAINE MPF®	10 ml	VAR	J0670
POLOCAINE®	10 ml	VAR	J0670
PORFIMER SODIUM	75 mg	IV	J9600
PORTRAZZA®	1 mg	IV	J9295
POTASSIUM CHLORIDE	2 mEq	IV	J3480
POTELIGEO®	1 mg	IV	J9204
PRALATREXATE	1 mg	IV	J9307
PRALIDOXIME CHLORIDE	up to 1 g	IV, IM, SC	J2730
PREDNISOLONE ACETATE	up to 1 ml	IM	J2650
PREDNISOLONE, ORAL	5 mg	ORAL	J7510
PREDNISONE, IMMEDIATE OR DELAYED RELEASE, ORAL	1 mg	ORAL	J7512
PREGNYL®	1,000 IU	IM	J0725
PRELONE®	5 mg	ORAL	J7510
PREMARIN®	25 mg	IV, IM	J1410
PRIALT®	1 mcg	OTH	J2278
PRIMAXIN IV®	250 mg	IV, IM	J0743
PRIVIGEN®	500 mg	IV	J1459
PROAIR HFA®	1 mg	INH	J7611
PROAIR HFA®	1 mg	INH	J7613
PROBUPHINE®	74.2 mg	OTH	J0570
PROCAINAMIDE HCL	up to 1 g	IM, IV	J2690
PROCHLORPERAZINE	up to 10 mg	IV, IM	J0780
PROCRIT®	1000 IU	IV, SC	J0885
PROFILNINE SD®	1 IU	IV	J7194
PROGESTERONE	50 mg	IM	J2675
PROGRAF®	1 mg	ORAL	J7507
PROGRAF®	5 mg	IV	J7525
PROLASTIN®	10 mg	IV	J0256
PROLASTIN-C®	10 mg	IV	J0256
PROLEUKIN®	single use vial	IV	J9015
PROLIXIN DECANOATE®	up to 25 mg	IM	J2680
PROMAZINE HCL	up to 25 mg	IM	J2950
PROMETHAZINE HCL	up to 50 mg	IM, IV	J2550
PROP-A-TANE®	10 mg	IM, SC, IV	J0945
PROPOFOL	10 mg	IV	J2704
PROPRANOLOL	up to 1 mg	IV	J1800
PROSTIN VR PEDIATRIC®	1.25 mcg	IV	J0270
PROTAMINE SULFATE	10 mg	IV	J2720
PROTEIN C CONCENTRATE	10 IU	IV	J2724
PROTIRELIN	250 mcg	IV	J2725
PROTOPAM CHLORIDE®	up to 1 g	IV, IM, SC	J2730
PROVOCHOLINE®	1 mg	INH	J7674
PULMOZYME®	1 mg	INH	J7639
PYRIDOXINE HCL	100 mg	IM, IV	J3415
QUELICIN®	up to 20 mg	IV, IM	J0330
QUINUPRISTIN/DALFOPRISTIN	500 mg (150/350)	IV	J2770

Drug Name	Unit Per	Route	Code
RADICAVA®	1 mg	IV	J1301
RAMUCIRUMAB	5 mg	IV	J9308
RANIBIZUMAB	0.1 mg	OTH	J2778
RANITIDINE HCL	25 mg	IV, IM	J2780
RAPAMUNE®	1 mg	ORAL	J7520
RAPIVAB®	1 mg	IV	J2547
RASBURICASE	0.5 mg	IV	J2783
RAVULIZUMAB-CWVZ	10 mg	IV	J1303
RAYOS®	1 mg	ORAL	J7512
REBIF®	30 mcg	IM	J1826
REBINYN®	1 IU	IV	J7203
RECLAST®	1 mg	IV	J3489
RECOMBINATE®	1 IU	IV	J7192
REGADENOSON	0.1 mg	IV	J2785
REGITINE®	up to 5 mg	IM, IV	J2760
REGLAN®	up to 10 mg	IV	J2765
RELISTOR®	0.1 mg	SC	J2212
REMICADE®	10 mg	IM, IV	J1745
REOPRO®	10 mg	IV	J0130
RESECTISOL®	25% in 50 ml	IV	J2150
RESLIZUMAB	1 mg	IV	J2786
RETAVASE®	18.1 mg	IV	J2993
RETEPLASE	18.1 mg	IV	J2993
RETISERT®	0.01 mg	OTH	J7311
RETROVIR®	10 mg	IV	J3485
REVEFENACIN, INHALATION SOLUTION	1 mcg	OTH	J7677
RHEUMATREX DOSE PACK®	2.5 mg	ORAL	J8610
RHO(D) IMMUNE GLOBULIN, HUMAN, FULL DOSE	1 dose package, 300 mcg	IM	J2790
RHO(D) IMMUNE GLOBULIN, HUMAN, MINI DOSE	50 mcg	IM	J2788
RHO(D) IMMUNE GLOBULIN, HUMAN, SOLVENT DETERGENT	100 IU	IM, IV	J2792
RHO(D) IMMUNE GLOBULIN, HUMAN, RHOPHYLAC®	100 IU	IM, IV	J2791
RHOGAM ULTRA FILTERED PLUS®	50 mcg	IM	J2788
RHOGAM ULTRA FILTERED PLUS®	1 dose package, 300 mcg	IM	J2790
RHOGAM®	50 mcg	IM	J2788
RHOGAM®	1 dose package, 300 mcg	IM	J2790
RHOPHYLAC®	50 mcg	IM	J2788
RHOPHYLAC®	1 dose package, 300 mcg	IM	J2790
RHOPHYLAC®	100 IU	IM, IV	J2791
RIASTAP®	1mg	IV	J7178

Drug Name	Unit Per	Route	Code
RIBOFLAVIN 5'-PHOSPHATE, OPHTHALMIC SOLUTION	up to 3mL	OTH	J2787
RILONACEPT	1 mg	SC	J2793
RIMABOTULINUM TOXIN B	100 IU	IM	J0587
RIMSO-50®	50%, 50 ml	OTH	J1212
RINGERS LACTATE INFUSION	up to 1,000 cc	IV	J7120
RISPERDAL CONSTA®	0.5 mg	IM	J2794
RISPERIDONE (PERSERIS®)	0.5 mg	IM, SC	J2798
RISPERIDONE (RISPERDAL CONSTA®)	0.5 mg	IM	J2794
RITUXAN HYCELA®	10 mg	SC	J9311
RITUXAN®	10 mg	IV	J9312
RITUXIMAB	10 mg	IV	J9312
RITUXIMAB AND HYALURONIDASE	10 mg	SC	J9311
RIXUBIS®	1 IU	IV	J7195
RIXUBIS®	1 IU	IV	J7200
ROBAXIN®	up to 10 ml	IV, IM	J2800
ROCALTROL®	0.1 mcg	IM	J0636
ROLAPITANT	0.5 mg	IV	J2797
ROLAPITANT, ORAL	1 mg	ORAL	J8670
ROMIDEPSIN	1 mg	IV	J9315
ROMIPLOSTIM	10 mcg	SC	J2796
ROMOSOZUMAB-AQQG	1 mg	SC	J3111
ROPIVACAINE HYDROCHLORIDE	1 mg	OTH	J2795
RUCONEST®	10 IU	IV	J0596
RUM-K®	2 mEq	IV	J3480
SACITUZUMAB GOVITECAN-HZIY	2.5 mg	INJ	J9317
SAIZEN®	1 mg	SC	J2941
SALINE SOLUTION, HYPERTONIC	1 ml	IV	J7131
SALINE SOLUTION, NORMAL	infusion, 250 cc	IV	J7050
SALINE SOLUTION, NORMAL	infusion, 1,000 cc	IV	J7030
SALINE SOLUTION, NORMAL DEXTROSE 5%	500 ml = 1 unit	IV	J7042
SALINE SOLUTION, STERILE	500 ml = 1 unit	IV, OTH	J7040
SANDIMMUNE®	100 mg	ORAL	J7502
SANDIMMUNE®	25 mg	ORAL	J7515
SANDIMMUNE®	250 mg	OTH	J7516
SANDOSTATIN LAR DEPOT®	1 mg	IM	J2353
SANDOSTATIN®	25 mcg	IV, SC	J2354
SARGRAMOSTIM (GM-CSF)	50 mcg	IV	J2820
SCANDONEST L®	10 ml	VAR	J0670
SEBELIPASE ALFA	1 mg	IV	J2840
SECREFLO®	1mcg	IV	J2850
SECRETIN, SYNTHETIC, HUMAN	1 mcg	IV	J2850
SENSIPAR®	1 mg	ORAL	J0604
SEROSTIM®	1 mg	SC	J2941
SIGNIFOR LAR®	1 mg	IV	J2502
SILTUXIMAB	10 mg	IV	J2860

Drug Name	Unit Per	Route	Code
SIMPONI ARIA®	1 mg	IV	J1602
SIMPONI®	1 mg	IV	J1602
SIMULECT®	20 mg	IV	J0480
SINCALIDE	5 mcg	IV	J2805
SIROLIMUS	1 mg	ORAL	J7520
SIVEXTRO®	1 mg	IV	J3090
SKELEX®	up to 10 ml	IV, IM	J2800
SKYLA®	13.5 mg	OTH	J7301
SODIUM FERRIC GLUCONATE COMPLEX IN SUCROSE	12.5 mg	IV	J2916
SOLFOTON®	up to 120 mg	IM, IV	J2560
SOLIRIS®	10 mg	IV	J1300
SOLU-CORTEF®	up to 100 mg	IV, IM, SC	J1720
SOLU-MEDROL®	up to 40 mg	IM, IV	J2920
SOLU-MEDROL®	up to 125 mg	IM, IV	J2930
SOMATREM	1 mg	SC	J2940
SOMATROPIN	1 mg	SC	J2941
SOMATULINE DEPOT®	1 mg	SC	J1930
SOTALOL HYDROCHLORIDE	1 mg	IV	C9482
SPECTINOMYCIN HCL	up to 2 g	IM	J3320
SPORANOX®	50 mg	IV	J1835
STELARA®	1 mg	SC	J3357
STELARA®	1 mg	IV	J3358
STREPTOKINASE	250,000 IU	IV	J2995
STREPTOMYCIN	up to 1 g	IM	J3000
STREPTOZOCIN	1 gm	IV	J9320
SUBLIMAZE®	0.1 mg	IM, IV	J3010
SUCCINYLCHOLINE CHLORIDE	up to 20 mg	IV, IM	J0330
SUMATRIPTAN SUCCINATE	6 mg	SC	J3030
SUMYCIN®	up to 250 mg	IM, IV	J0120
SUPARTZ®	dose	OTH	J7321
SUPPRELIN LA®	10 mcg	OTH	J1675
SUPPRELIN LA®	50 mg	OTH	J9226
SYLVANT®	10 mg	IV	J2860
SYNERCID®	500 mg	IV	J2770
SYNRIBO®	0.01 mg	IV	J9262
SYNVISC®	1 mg	OTH	J7325
SYNVISC-ONE®	1 mg	OTH	J7325
TACROLIMUS, ORAL, EXTENDED RELEASE, ASTAGRAF XL®	0.1 mg	ORAL	J7508
TACROLIMUS, ORAL, EXTENDED RELEASE, ENVARSUS XR®	0.25 mg	ORAL	J7503
TACROLIMUS, ORAL, IMMEDIATE RELEASE	1 mg	ORAL	J7507
TACROLIMUS, PARENTERAL	5 mg	IV	J7525
TAGRAXOFUSP-ERZS	10 mcg	IV	J9269
TAKHZYRO®	1 mg	SC	J0593
TALADINE®	25 mg	IV, IM	J2780
TALIGLUCERACE ALFA	10 IU	IV	J3060

Drug Name	Unit Per	Route	Code
TALIMOGENE LAHERPAREPVEC	1 million PFU	OTH	J9325
TAXOL®	1 mg	IV	J9264
TAXOL®	1 mg	IV	J9267
TAXOTERE®	1 mg	IV	J9171
TAZICEF®	500 mg	IV, IM	J0713
TBO-FILGRASTIM	1 mcg	SC, IV	J1447
TECENTRIQ™	10 mg	IV	J9022
TEDIZOLID PHOSPHATE	1 mg	IV	J3090
TEFLARO®	10 mg	IV	J0712
TELAVANCIN	10 mg	IV	J3095
TEMODAR®	5 mg	ORAL	J8700
TEMODAR®	1 mg	IV	J9328
TEMOZOLOMIDE	5 mg	ORAL	J8700
TEMOZOLOMIDE	1 mg	IV	J9328
TEMSIROLIMUS	1 mg	IV	J9330
TENECTEPLASE	1 mg	IV	J3101
TEPADINA®	15 mg	IV	J9340
TEPROTUMUMAB-TRBW	10 mg	IV	J3241
TERBUTALINE SULFATE	up to 1 mg	SC, IV	J3105
TERBUTALINE SULFATE, CONCENTRATED FORM, COMPOUNDED	1 mg	INH	J7680
TERBUTALINE SULFATE, UNIT DOSE FORM, COMPOUNDED	1 mg	INH	J7681
TERIPARATIDE	10 mcg	SC	J3110
TESTOSTERONE CYPIONATE	1 mg	IM	J1071
TESTOSTERONE ENANTHATE	1 mg	IM	J3121
TESTOSTERONE UNDECANOATE	1 mg	IM	J3145
TETANUS IMMUNE GLOBULIN, HUMAN	up to 250 IU	IM	J1670
TETRACYCLINE	up to 250 mg	IM, IV	J0120
THEOPHYLLINE	40 mg	IV	J2810
THIAMINE HCL	100 mg	IM, IV	J3411
THIETHYLPERAZINE MALEATE	up to 10 mg	IM, IV	J3280
THIOTEPA	15 mg	IV	J9340
THROMBATE III®	1 IU	IV	J7197
THYMOGLOBULIN®	25 mg	OTH	J7511
THYROGEN®	0.9 mg	IM, SC	J3240
THYROTROPIN ALFA	0.9 mg	IM, SC	J3240
TIGECYCLINE	1 mg	IV	J3243
TILDRAKIZUMAB	1 mg	SC	J3245
TINZAPARIN SODIUM	1000 IU	SC	J1655
TIROFIBAN HCL	0.25 mg	IM, IV	J3246
TNKASE®	1 mg	IV	J3101
TOBI PODHALER®	300 mg	INH	J7682
TOBI®	300 mg	INH	J7682
TOBRAMYCIN SULFATE	up to 80 mg	IM, IV	J3260
TOBRAMYCIN, UNIT DOSE, COMPOUNDED	300 mg	INH	J7685

Drug Name	Unit Per	Route	Code
TOBRAMYCIN, UNIT DOSE, NON-COMPOUNDED	300 mg	INH	J7682
TOCILIZUMAB	1 mg	IV	J3262
TOPOTECAN	0.25 mg	ORAL	J8705
TOPOTECAN	0.1 mg	IV	J9351
TORADOL®	15 mg	IM, IV	J1885
TORISEL®	1 mg	IV	J9330
TORSEMIDE	10 mg/ml	IV	J3265
TOTECT®	250 mg	IV	J1190
TRABECTEDIN	0.1 mg	IV	J9352
TRASTUZUMAB AND HYALURONIDASE-OYSK	10 mg	SC	J9356
TRASTUZUMAB, EXCLUDES BIOSIMILAR	10 mg	IV	J9355
TREANDA®	1 mg	IV	J9033
TRELSTAR DEPOT®	3.75 mg	IM	J3315
TRELSTAR LA®	3.75 mg	IM	J3315
TREMFYA®	1 mg	SC	J1628
TREPROSTINIL	1 mg	IV, SC, INH	J3285
TREPROSTNIL, UNIT DOSE, COMPOUND	1.74 mg	INH	J7686
TRETTEN®	1 IU	IV	J7181
TREXALL®	2.5 mg	ORAL	J8610
TRIAMCINOLONE ACETONIDE	1 mg	VAR	J3300
TRIAMCINOLONE ACETONIDE XR	1 mg	IV	J3304
TRIAMCINOLONE ACETONIDE, NOT OTHERWISE SPECIFIED	10 mg	VAR	J3301
TRIAMCINOLONE DIACETATE	5 mg	IM	J3302
TRIAMCINOLONE HEXACETONIDE	5 mg	VAR	J3303
TRIAMCINOLONE, CONCENTRATED FORM, COMPOUNDED	1 mg	INH	J7683
TRIAMCINOLONE, UNIT DOSE, COMPOUNDED	1 mg	INH	J7684
TRIFLUPROMAZINE HCL	up to 20 mg	IM, IV	J3400
TRILAFON®	up to 5 mg	IM, IV	J3310
TRIMETHOBENZAMIDE HCL	up to 200 mg	IM	J3250
TRIMETREXATE GLUCURONATE	25 mg	IV	J3305
TRIPTODUR®	3.75 mg	IM	J3316
TRIPTORELIN PAMOATE	3.75 mg	IM	J3315
TRIPTORELIN, EXTENDED-RELEASE	3.75 mg	IM	J3316
TRISENOX®	1 mg	IV	J9017
TRIVISC®	1 mg	VAR	J7329
TROGARZO®	10 mg	IV	J1746
TYGACIL®	1 mg	IV	J3243
TYSABRI®	1 mg	IV	J2323
TYVASO REFILL KIT®	1.74 mg	INH	J7686
TYVASO STARTER KIT®	1.74 mg	INH	J7686
TYVASO®	1.74 mg	INH	J7686

Drug Name	Unit Per	Route	Code
ULTOMIRIS®	10 mg	IV	J1303
UNASYN®	1.5 gm	IM, IV	J0295
UNCLASSIFIED BIOLOGICS	dose	VAR	J3590
UNCLASSIFIED DRUG OR BIOLOGICAL USED FOR ESRD ON DIALYSIS	dose	IV	J3591
UNCLASSIFIED DRUGS	-	-	J3490
UNCLASSIFIED DRUGS OR BIOLOGICALS	-	-	C9399
UNSPECIFIED DRUG ADMINISTERED THROUGH A METERED DOSE INHALER	dose	INH	J3535
UNSPECIFIED VACCINE, NASAL INHALATION	dose	INH	J3530
UREA	up to 40 g	IV	J3350
URECHOLINE®	up to 5 mg	SC	J0520
UROFOLLITROPIN	75 IU	SC	J3355
UROKINASE	5,000 IU vial	IV	J3364
UROKINASE	250,000 IU vial	IV	J3365
USTEKINUMAB	1 mg	SC	J3357
USTEKINUMAB	1 mg	IV	J3358
VABOMERE®	10mg/10mg	IV	J2186
VACCINE, NASAL INHALATION	dose	INH	J3530
VALIUM®	up to 5 mg	IM, IV	J3360
VALRUBICIN, INTRAVESICAL	200 mg	OTH	J9357
VALSTAR®	200 mg	OTH	J9357
VANCOMYCIN HCL	500 mg	IV, IM	J3370
VANTAS®	50 mg	OTH	J9225
VAPRISOL®	1 mg	IV	C9488
VARUBI®	1 mg	ORAL	J8670
VECTIBIX®	10 mg	IV	J9303
VEDOLIZUMAB	1 mg	IV	J3380
VELAGLUCERASE ALFA	100 IU	IV	J3385
VELCADE®	0.1 mg	IV, SC	J9041
VELCADE®	0.1 mg	IV	J9044
VELETRI®	0.5 mg	IV	J1325
VENOFER®	1 mg	IV	J1756
VENTOLIN HFA®	1 mg	INH	J7611
VENTOLIN HFA®	1 mg	INH	J7613
VERSED®	1 mg	IM, IV	J2250
VERTEPORFIN	0.1 mg	IV	J3396
VESTRONIDASE ALFA-VJBK	1 mg	IV	J3397
VFEND®	10 mg	IV	J3465
VIADUR®	65 mg	OTH	J9219
VIBATIV®	10 mg	IV	J3095
VIDAZA®	1 mg	SC, IV	J9025
VIMIZIM®	1 mg	IV	J1322
VINBLASTINE SULFATE	1 mg	IV	J9360
VINCRISTINE SULFATE	1 mg	IV	J9370
VINCRISTINE SULFATE LIPOSOME	1 mg	IV	J9371

Drug Name	Unit Per	Route	Code
VINORELBINE TARTRATE	10 mg	IV	J9390
VISCO-3®	dose	OTH	J7333
VISTACOT®	up to 25 mg	IM	J3410
VISUDYNE®	0.1 mg	IV	J3396
VITAMIN B1	100 mg	IM, IV	J3411
VITAMIN B-12, CYANOCOBALAMIN	up to 1,000 mcg	IM, SC	J3420
VITAMIN B-17	dose	VAR	J3570
VITAMIN K, PHYTONADIONE	1 mg	IM, SC, IV	J3430
VITELLE NESTREX®	100 mg	IM, IV	J3415
VITRASE®	up to 150 IU	SC, IV	J3470
VITRASE®	up to 999 IU	VAR	J3471
VITRASE®	1000 IU	VAR	J3472
VIVAGLOBIN®	100 mg	IV	J1562
VON WILLEBRAND FACTOR (RECOMBINANT), VONVENDI®	1 IU	IV	J7179
VON WILLEBRAND FACTOR COMPLEX (HUMAN), WILATE®	1 IU	IV	J7183
VON WILLEBRAND FACTOR COMPLEX, HUMATE-P®	1 IU	IV	J7187
VONVENDI®	1 IU	IV	J7179
VORAXAZE®	10 units	IV	C9293
VORETIGENE NEPARVOVEC-RZYL	1 billion vector genomes	OTH	J3398
VORICONAZOLE	10 mg	IV	J3465
VPRIV®	100 IU	IV	J3385
VYXEOS®	1 mg/2.27 mg	IV	J9153
WILATE®	1 IU	IV	J7183
WINRHO SDF®	50 mcg	IM	J2788
WINRHO SDF®	1 dose package, 300 mcg	IM	J2790
XELODA®	150 mg	ORAL	J8520
XELODA®	500 mg	ORAL	J8521
XEMBIFY®	100 mg	1 IV	J1558
XEOMIN®	1 IU	IM	J0588
XERVA®	1 mg	IV	J0122
XGEVA®	1 mg	SC	J0897
XIAFLEX®	0.01 mg	OTH	J0775
XOLAIR®	5 mg	SC	J2357
XOPENEX CONCENTRATE®	0.5 mg	INH	J7612
XOPENEX CONCENTRATE®	0.5 mg	INH	J7614
XOPENEX HFA®	0.5 mg	INH	J7612
XOPENEX HFA®	0.5 mg	INH	J7614
XOPENEX®	0.5 mg	INH	J7612
XOPENEX®	0.5 mg	INH	J7614
XULANE®	each	OTH	J7304
XYLOCAINE HCL®	10 mg	IV	J2001
XYNTHA®	1 IU	IV	J7185
YERVOY®	1 mg	IV	J9228

Drug Name	Unit Per	Route	Code
YONDELIS®	0.1 mg	IV	J9352
YUPELRI®	1 mcg	OTH	J7677
YUTIQ®	0.01 mg	OTH	J7314
ZALTRAP®	1 mg	IV	J9400
ZANOSAR®	1 gm	IV	J9320
ZEMAIRA®	10 mg	IV	J0256
ZEMDRI®	5 mg	IV	J0291
ZEMPLAR®	1 mcg	IV, IM	J2501
ZERBAXA®	50 mg/25 mg	IV	J0695
ZICONOTIDE	1 mcg	OTH	J2278
ZIDOVUDINE	10 mg	IV	J3485
ZINACEF®	750 mg	IV, IM	J0697
ZINECARD®	250 mg	IV	J1190
ZINPLAVA®	10 mg	IV	J0565
ZIPRASIDONE MESYLATE	10 mg	IM	J3486
ZITHROMAX IV®	500 mg	IV	J0456

Drug Name	Unit Per	Route	Code
ZIV-AFLIBERCEPT	1 mg	IV	J9400
ZOFRAN®	1 mg	IV	J2405
ZOLADEX®	3.6 mg	OTH	J9202
ZOLEDRONIC ACID	1 mg	IV	J3489
ZOMETA®	1 mg	IV	J3489
ZORBTIVE®	1 mg	SC	J2941
ZORTRESS®	0.25 mg	ORAL	J7527
ZOSYN®	1.125 g	IV	J2543
ZOVIRAX®	5 mg	IV	J0133
ZUBSOLV®	<=3 mg	ORAL	J0572
ZUBSOLV®	>3 mg but <=6 mg	ORAL	J0573
ZUBSOLV®	>6 mg but <=10 mg	ORAL	J0574
ZUBSOLV®	>10 mg	ORAL	J0575
ZYPREXA®	1 mg	IM	J2358
ZYVOX®	200 mg	IV	J2020

Appendix B
HCPCS Level II Modifiers, Lay Descriptions, and Tips

Mod	Modifier Description, Definition, Explanation, and Tips
A1	**Dressing for one wound** **Definition:** Append modifier A1 to identify a surgical dressing that a provider or a surgical supplier uses for dressing of a single wound. **Explanation:** This modifier indicates that a particular surgical supply that the provider uses is a dressing on a wound. It also indicates the number of wounds on which the provider is using the dressing, or the number of wounds for which a durable medical equipment supplier is providing a supply. Use A1 with the appropriate HCPCS code when the provider uses a surgical supply for dressing of one wound. The modifier number corresponds to the number of wounds a surgical dressing is applied to, meaning A1 is for one wound, A2 is for two wounds, A3 for three wounds and so on. The modifier a provider uses corresponds to the number of wounds on which the provider is using the dressing, not the total number of wounds that the provider treats. **Tips:** It is important to use modifier A1 to A9 appropriately with Healthcare Common Procedure Coding System, or HCPCS codes according to the number of surgical or debrided wounds for which the supplier is providing the surgical dressing. Incorrect use may lead to denial or underpayment.
A2	**Dressing for two wounds** **Definition:** Append modifier A2 to identify a surgical dressing that a provider or a surgical supplier uses for dressing of two wounds. **Explanation:** This modifier indicates that a particular surgical supply that the provider uses is a dressing on a wound. It also indicates the number of wounds on which the provider is using the dressing, or the number of wounds for which a durable medical equipment supplier is providing a supply. Use A2 with the appropriate HCPCS code when the provider uses a surgical supply for dressing of two wounds. The modifier number corresponds to the number of wounds a surgical dressing is applied to, meaning A1 is for one wound, A2 is for two wounds, A3 for three wounds and so on. The modifier a provider uses corresponds to the number of wounds on which the provider is using the dressing, not the total number of wounds that the provider treats. **Tips:** It is important to use modifier A1 to A9 appropriately with HCPCS codes according to the number of surgical or debrided wounds for which the supplier is providing the dressing. Incorrect use may lead to denial or underpayment.
A3	**Dressing for three wounds** **Definition:** Append modifier A3 to identify a surgical dressing that a provider or a surgical supplier uses for dressing of three wounds. **Explanation:** This modifier indicates that a particular surgical supply that the provider uses is a dressing on a wound. It also indicates the number of wounds on which the provider is using the dressing, or the number of wounds for which a durable medical equipment supplier is providing a supply. Use A3 with the appropriate HCPCS code when the provider uses a surgical supply for dressing of three wounds. The modifier number corresponds to the number of wounds a surgical dressing is applied to, meaning A1 is for one wound, A2 is for two wounds, A3 for three wounds and so on. The modifier a provider uses corresponds to the number of wounds on which the provider is using the dressing, not the total number of wounds that the provider treats. **Tips:** It is important to use modifier A1 to A9 appropriately with HCPCS codes according to the number of surgical or debrided wounds for which the supplier is providing the dressing. Incorrect use may lead to denial or underpayment.
A4	**Dressing for four wounds** **Definition:** Append modifier A4 to identify a surgical dressing that a provider or a surgical supplier uses for dressing of four wounds. **Explanation:** This modifier indicates that a particular surgical supply that the provider uses is a dressing on a wound. It also indicates the number of wounds on which the provider is using the dressing, or the number of wounds for which a durable medical equipment supplier is providing a supply. Use A4 with the appropriate HCPCS code when the provider uses a surgical supply for dressing of four wounds. The modifier number corresponds to the number of wounds a surgical dressing is applied to, meaning A1 is for one wound, A2 is for two wounds, A3 for three wounds and so on. The modifier a provider uses corresponds to the number of wounds on which the provider is using the dressing, not the total number of wounds that the provider treats. **Tips:** It is important to use modifier A1 to A9 appropriately with HCPCS codes according to the number of surgical or debrided wounds for which the supplier is providing the dressing. Incorrect use may lead to denial or underpayment.

Mod	Modifier Description, Definition, Explanation, and Tips
A5	**Dressing for five wounds**
	Definition: Append modifier A5 to identify a surgical dressing that a provider or a surgical supplier uses for dressing of five wounds.
	Explanation: This modifier indicates that a particular surgical supply that the provider uses is a dressing on a wound. It also indicates the number of wounds on which the provider is using the dressing, or the number of wounds for which a durable medical equipment supplier is providing a supply. Use A5 with the appropriate HCPCS code when the provider uses a surgical supply for dressing of five wounds.
	The modifier number corresponds to the number of wounds a surgical dressing is applied to, meaning A1 is for one wound, A2 is for two wounds, A3 for three wounds and so on. The modifier a provider uses corresponds to the number of wounds on which the provider is using the dressing, not the total number of wounds that the provider treats.
	Tips: It is important to use modifier A1 to A9 appropriately with HCPCS codes according to the number of surgical or debrided wounds for which the supplier is providing the dressing. Incorrect use may lead to denial or underpayment.
A6	**Dressing for six wounds**
	Definition: Append modifier A6 to identify a surgical dressing that a provider or a surgical supplier uses for dressing of six wounds.
	Explanation: This modifier indicates that a particular surgical supply that the provider uses is a dressing on a wound. It also indicates the number of wounds on which the provider is using the dressing, or the number of wounds for which a durable medical equipment supplier is providing a supply. Use A6 with the appropriate HCPCS code when the provider uses a surgical supply for dressing of six wounds.
	The modifier number corresponds to the number of wounds a surgical dressing is applied to, meaning A1 is for one wound, A2 is for two wounds, A3 for three wounds and so on. The modifier a provider uses corresponds to the number of wounds on which the provider is using the dressing, not the total number of wounds that the provider treats.
	Tips: It is important to use modifier A1 to A9 appropriately with HCPCS codes according to the number of surgical or debrided wounds for which the supplier is providing the dressing. Incorrect use may lead to denial or underpayment.
A7	**Dressing for seven wounds**
	Definition: Append modifier A7 to identify a surgical dressing that a provider or a surgical supplier uses for dressing of seven wounds.
	Explanation: This modifier indicates that a particular surgical supply that the provider uses is a dressing on a wound. It also indicates the number of wounds on which the provider is using the dressing, or the number of wounds for which a durable medical equipment supplier is providing a supply. Use A7 with the appropriate HCPCS code when the provider uses a surgical supply for dressing of seven wounds.
	The modifier number corresponds to the number of wounds a surgical dressing is applied to, meaning A1 is for one wound, A2 is for two wounds, A3 for three wounds and so on. The modifier a provider uses corresponds to the number of wounds on which the provider is using the dressing, not the total number of wounds that the provider treats.
	Tips: It is important to use modifier A1 to A9 appropriately with HCPCS codes according to the number of surgical or debrided wounds for which the supplier is providing the dressing. Incorrect use may lead to denial or underpayment.
A8	**Dressing for eight wounds**
	Definition: Append modifier A8 to identify a surgical dressing that a provider or a surgical supplier uses for dressing of eight wounds.
	Explanation: This modifier indicates that a particular surgical supply that the provider uses is a dressing on a wound. It also indicates the number of wounds on which the provider is using the dressing, or the number of wounds for which a durable medical equipment supplier is providing a supply. Use A8 with the appropriate HCPCS code when the provider uses a surgical supply for dressing of eight wounds.
	The modifier number corresponds to the number of wounds a surgical dressing is applied to, meaning A1 is for one wound, A2 is for two wounds, A3 for three wounds and so on. The modifier a provider uses corresponds to the number of wounds on which the provider is using the dressing, not the total number of wounds that the provider treats.
	Tips: It is important to use modifier A1 to A9 appropriately with HCPCS codes according to the number of surgical or debrided wounds for which the supplier is providing the dressing. Incorrect use may lead to denial or underpayment.

Mod	Modifier Description, Definition, Explanation, and Tips
A9	**Dressing for nine or more wounds** **Definition:** Append modifier A9 to identify a surgical dressing that a provider or a surgical supplier uses for dressing of nine or more wounds. **Explanation:** This modifier indicates that a particular surgical supply that the provider uses is a dressing on a wound. It also indicates the number of wounds on which the provider is using the dressing, or the number of wounds for which a durable medical equipment supplier is providing a supply. Use A9 with the appropriate HCPCS code when the provider uses a surgical supply for dressing of nine or more wounds. The modifier number corresponds to the number of wounds a surgical dressing is applied to, meaning A1 is for one wound, A2 is for two wounds, A3 for three wounds and so on. The modifier a provider uses corresponds to the number of wounds on which the provider is using the dressing, not the total number of wounds that the provider treats. **Tips:** It is important to use modifier A1 to A9 appropriately with HCPCS codes according to the number of surgical or debrided wounds for which the supplier is providing the dressing. Incorrect use may lead to denial or underpayment.
AA	**Anesthesia services performed personally by anesthesiologist** **Definition:** Append this modifier to anesthesia service codes when the provider personally performs the entire anesthesia service. **Explanation:** This modifier documents the service of the provider who personally provides the anesthesia during the entire surgical procedure. This modifier is also applicable when the provider is continuously supervising a student anesthetist during the procedure or when the procedure involves the provider with one resident. To report modifier AA, the provider continuously monitors a single case. The provider must remain physically present in the operating room during the entire procedure when billing the personally performed modifier AA. **Tips:** If the provider does not continuously monitor the single case, use another appropriate modifier such as AD, Medical supervision by a physician: more than four concurrent anesthesia procedures.
AD	**Medical supervision by a physician: more than four concurrent anesthesia procedures** **Definition:** Append this modifier to anesthesia service codes when the provider concurrently supervises anesthesia for more than four procedures. **Explanation:** This modifier documents the service when the provider oversees more than four concurrent anesthesia procedures or when he performs other services while directing concurrent procedures. Concurrent anesthesia procedures are those that occur at the same time or overlap even if only by a minute. The provider may also participate in induction of the anesthesia. **Tips:** If the provider continuously monitors a single case, personally performing the entire anesthesia service, use modifier AA, Anesthesia services performed personally by anesthesiologist.
AE	**Registered dietician** **Definition:** Append this modifier to indicate the services of a nutrition professional. **Explanation:** This modifier indicates the services of a nutrition professional or a registered dietician on claims with medical nutrition therapy codes such as 97802 to 97804, and G0270 to G0271. This code may also be applicable to Diabetes outpatient self management training services, or DSMT, reportable under G0108 individual, per 30 minutes and G0109, group session, 2 or more, per 30 minutes. **Tips:** Use this modifier to represent the professional services of a nutrition professional or a registered dietician in a critical access hospital, or CAH. An all inclusive rate payment methodology applies in the case of a CAH.
AF	**Specialty physician** **Definition:** Append this modifier to indicate the services of a specialty physician in a physician scarcity area. **Explanation:** Modifier AF is a Medicare use only modifier that represents the services of a specialty physician in a physician scarcity area, or a geographic area with a shortage of primary care doctors or specialists available to the Medicare population in that area. Use of this modifier provides for a quarterly bonus payment along with claim payment. Behavioral Medicine, Oncology, Endocrinology, Neurology, Neurosurgery, and Orthopedics, are some examples of specialty physicians. **Tips:** Use this modifier to represent professional services of a specialty physician in a physician scarcity area in a critical access hospital.
AG	**Primary physician** **Definition:** Append this modifier to indicate the services of a primary care physician in a physician scarcity area. **Explanation:** Modifier AG is a Medicare use only modifier that represents the services of a primary care physician in a physician scarcity area, or a geographic area with a shortage of primary care doctors or specialists available to the Medicare population in that area. Use of this modifier provides for a quarterly bonus payment along with claim payment. A primary care physician is typically defined as a general practitioner, family practice practitioner, general internist, pediatrician, obstetrician, or gynecologist. **Tips:** Use this modifier to represent professional services of a primary physician in a physician scarcity area in a critical access hospital.

Mod	Modifier Description, Definition, Explanation, and Tips
AH	**Clinical psychologist**
	Definition: Append this modifier to indicate the services of a clinical psychologist.
	Explanation: This modifier indicates the services the provider is reporting are for a qualified clinical psychologist for the psychiatric therapeutic procedures that he performs for a patient in a facility. The modifier indicates that a clinical psychologist, who qualifies as per Medicare guidelines to provide these services, is performing the service the facility is reporting under the CPT® code for the procedure.
	Tips: When the facility uses this modifier with any CPT® code, it lets the payer know that a qualified clinical psychologist handled the services and reimbursement can be made as per Medicare payment guidelines. If you fail to append the right modifier to the CPT® code, it may lead to incorrect payments and fraudulent claims.
AI	**Principal physician of record**
	Definition: Append this modifier to the initial hospital and nursing home visit codes to show that the provider is responsible for the overall care of the patient.
	Explanation: This modifier indicates the service by the admitting or attending provider who oversees the patient's care, as distinct from other providers who may furnish specialty care. The principal provider of record shall append modifier AI to the initial visit code. The primary purpose of this modifier is to identify the principal provider of record on the initial hospital and nursing home visit codes.
	Tips: Remember that modifier AI is for inpatient use only, not for outpatient evaluation and management, or E/M, codes.
	Modifier AI is informational only and does not impact the payment.
AJ	**Clinical social worker**
	Definition: Append this modifier to indicate the services of a clinical social worker.
	Explanation: This modifier indicates the services of a qualified clinical social worker for therapeutic procedures that he performs in the facility. The modifier indicates that a clinical social worker, who qualifies as per Medicare guidelines to provide these services, is performing the service the facility is reporting under the CPT® code for the procedure.
	Tips: When the facility uses this modifier with any CPT® code, it lets the payer know that a qualified clinical social worker handled the services and reimbursement can be made as per CMS payment guidelines. If you fail to append the right modifier to the CPT® code, it may lead to incorrect payments and fraudulent claims.
AK	**Non participating physician**
	Definition: Append this modifier to indicate the services of a non participating physician.
	Explanation: This modifier indicates the services of a non participating provider who chooses not to participate in the Medicare fee schedule reimbursement, meaning he does not accept the Medicare approved amount as full payment for covered service. Medicare does not reimburse non participating physicians directly. Instead Medicare reimburses the patient for the allowable costs. The provider has to arrange for payment directly from the patient.
	Tips: Use this modifier to represent the services of a non participating physician in a critical access hospital.
AM	**Physician, team member service**
	Definition: Append this modifier to indicate the services of a member of a provider's team, usually a physician assistant who is part of the provider's team.
	Explanation: Append modifier AM if a physician assistant or other team member of the provider's team renders service. Usually, the supervising provider bills these services and the provider uses this modifier to indicate that his team member performs the service.
	Tips: This modifier is informational only and should not impact reimbursement. It just identifies that during the procedure the provider is not rendering the actual service but he is supervising the service.
AO	**Alternate payment method declined by provider of service**
	Definition: Append this modifier to each line of service on a claim if the provider prefers to decline participation in an alternate payment method by the payer.
	Explanation: Modifier AO indicates that the provider declines an alternate payment methodology and wants to continue with the original method of reimbursement. Use this modifier if you do not prefer to participate in bundled payment program for example for a care improvement initiative under the Affordable care act and you would continue to receive the reimbursement according to regular fee for service payment rules.
	Tips: If the provider does not report the AO modifier on each line of service on the claim then the provider receives the claim back as unprocessable with instruction to rebill the services on separate claims.

Mod	Modifier Description, Definition, Explanation, and Tips
AP	**Determination of refractive state was not performed in the course of diagnostic ophthalmological examination**
	Definition: Append this modifier to eye examination codes to indicate that reimbursement of the code does not include a fee for determination of a refractive state, or the process that the provider performs to determine the patient's refractive error and need for glasses or contact lenses.
	Explanation: This is an informational modifier that indicates that determination of a refractive state was not part of the work effort that the provider puts in diagnostic ophthalmological examination and the overall value of the eye examination codes such as 92004, 92014, 92002, 92012, do not include the value of refraction.
	Tips: Modifier AP became unnecessary when the values for the eye exam codes no longer included payment for refraction. If an ophthalmologist performed an eye exam without refraction, he would append modifier AP to show that the fee did not include refraction. CPT® gave refraction its own code, 92015, Determination of refractive state, which Medicare will not reimburse for, and excluded that work from the value of the eye exam codes. Since Medicare does not consider refraction an intrinsic part of any code, modifier AP is no longer necessary.
AQ	**Physician providing a service in an unlisted health professional shortage area (HPSA)**
	Definition: Append this modifier to represent the services that the provider renders in zip code areas that do not fall within a listed health professional shortage area, or HPSA.
	Explanation: Modifier AQ represents the provider's service in a health professional shortage area that is not listed in Medicare's annual file for automated HPSA bonus payment. CMS posts a file annually of ZIP codes, within which the HPSA bonus payment is made automatically. An unlisted health professional shortage area includes zip code areas that fall partially within a full county HPSA but is not considered to be in that county based on the United States Postal Service dominance decision; is a zip code area that falls partially within a non full county HPSA; is a zip code area that was not included in the automated file of HPSA areas based on the date the file was run, and zip code areas that do not fall entirely in a designated full county HPSA.
	Tips: Do not use this modifier if the provider does not render the service in the health professional shortage area.
	Do not use this modifier with codes that represent only a technical component.
AR	**Physician provider services in a physician scarcity area**
	Definition: Append this modifier to represent the services of a physician provider in a physician scarcity area.
	Explanation: Modifier AR represents the services that a provider performs in a physician scarcity area, or an area which has a shortage of health professionals. It was a previously effective code until June of 2008 and was used by the provider to obtain a physician scarcity area bonus payment.
	Tips: Use this modifier only for dates of service January 1, 2005, through June 30, 2008.
AS	**Physician assistant, nurse practitioner, or clinical nurse specialist services for assistant at surgery**
	Definition: Append this modifier to represent the services of a healthcare professional acting as an assistant during a surgery.
	Explanation: Healthcare professionals like a physician assistant, nurse practitioner, or clinical nurse specialist who acts as an assistant during a surgery reports the identical procedure as the primary surgeon with a modifier AS. These professionals report these services under a surgeons' provider number. The main surgeon should clearly specify in the medical record the medical necessity for utilizing the service of an assistant.
AT	**Acute treatment (this modifier should be used when reporting service 98940, 98941, 98942)**
	Definition: Append this modifier with specific chiropractic manipulative treatment, or CMT, spinal codes when the provider performs treatment of the acute or chronic spinal subluxation.
	Explanation: The provider uses modifier AT with chiropractic manipulative treatment codes such as 98940 to 98942 to indicate the acute or active nature of treatment. The patient's medical record should also support the active nature of chiropractic treatment in that the record should reflect the anticipated result of the chiropractic manipulation is either an improvement in, or a complete arrest of the progression, of the patient's condition.
	Tips: This modifier is not applicable when the medical records suggest that the provider is performing a maintenance chiropractic service to maintain or further prevent deterioration of a chronic condition.
AU	**Item furnished in conjunction with a urological, ostomy, or tracheostomy supply**
	Definition: Append this modifier with Healthcare Common Procedure Coding System, or HCPCS codes that identify the supply associated with urological, ostomy, or tracheostomy procedures.
	Explanation: Use this modifier with Healthcare Common Procedure Coding System, or HCPCS codes that a provider reports for supplies associated with a urological procedure, or those for the male and female urinary tract system and the male reproductive organs; an ostomy, or a surgically created opening in a patient's body for the discharge of body wastes; or for a tracheostomy, an opening made in the patient's neck into the trachea, or windpipe to create an airway or to remove secretions from the patient's lungs.
	Tips: Use modifier AU with HCPCS codes such as A4217; Sterile water or saline, 500 ml, A4450; Surgical trays, A4452; Tape, waterproof, per 18 square inches, and A5120; Skin barrier, wipes or swabs, each.

Mod	Modifier Description, Definition, Explanation, and Tips
AV	**Item furnished in conjunction with a prosthetic device, prosthetic or orthotic** **Definition:** Append this modifier with Healthcare Common Procedure Coding System, or HCPCS codes that identify the supply associated with a prosthetic device, prosthetic, or orthotic. **Explanation:** Use this modifier with Healthcare Common Procedure Coding System, or HCPCS codes that a provider reports for supplies associated with a prosthetic device, prosthetic or orthotic, meaning an artificial or manmade replacement for a body part or a supportive device. **Tips:** Use modifier AV with HCPCS codes such as: A4450; Tape, non-waterproof, per 18 square inches, A4452; Tape, waterproof, per 18 square inches and A5120; Skin barrier, wipes or swabs, each. Providers can refer to the Medicare Durable Medical Equipment, Prosthetics or Orthotics and Supplies Fee Schedule on the Centers for Medicare and Medicaid Services, or CMS, website to determine which procedures are reportable with modifier AV. Allowable procedure codes for modifier AV appear on the file with modifier AV such as A4450 AV.
AW	**Item furnished in conjunction with a surgical dressing** **Definition:** Append this modifier with Healthcare Common Procedure Coding System, or HCPCS codes that identify the supply associated with a surgical dressing. **Explanation:** Use this modifier with Healthcare Common Procedure Coding System, or HCPCS codes that a provider reports for supplies associated with a surgical dressing, meaning a sterile bandage or compress applied to a wound to encourage healing and to prevent infection.
AX	**Item furnished in conjunction with dialysis services** **Definition:** Append this modifier to Healthcare Common Procedure Coding System, or HCPCS codes that identify a supply associated with a dialysis services. **Explanation:** Use this modifier for Healthcare Common Procedure Coding System, or HCPCS codes that a provider reports for items he furnishes that are dialysis supplies or equipment, but are not specifically identified as dialysis supplies or equipment in the code descriptor. Use modifier AX with dialysis supplies such as those codes in the ranges A4215 to A4217, A4244 to A4248, A4450, A4452, A4651 to A4670, A4927, A4928, A4930, A4931, A6216, A6250, A6260, and A6402. Use modifier AX also with dialysis equipment codes such as E0210, E1632, E1637, and E1639. **Tips:** A provider can report this code for items furnished in conjunction with home dialysis services too.
AY	**Item or service furnished to an ESRD patient that is not for the treatment of ESRD** **Definition:** Append this modifier to Healthcare Common Procedure Coding System, or HCPCS codes that represent an item or service she furnishes to an End Stage Renal Disease, or ESRD, patient that is not for the treatment of the ESRD. **Explanation:** This modifier was developed for only Medicare purposes. Under the bundled payment system, a single payment is made for renal dialysis services and other items and services for example, supplies and equipment the provider uses to administer dialysis, and the drugs, biologicals, laboratory tests, and support services related to home dialysis. However, if any End Stage Renal Disease, or ESRD facility provides any items or services to a beneficiary, which do not relate to the treatment of the patient's ESRD condition, then the ESRD facility submits those services using the AY modifier to allow for separate payment outside of ESRD bundled payment system. **Tips:** Use this modifier only when the documents clearly support that the service the provider performs for a reason unrelated to ESRD treatment.
AZ	**Physician providing a service in a dental health professional shortage area for the purpose of an electronic health record incentive payment** **Definition:** Append this modifier to represent the services that a provider renders in zip codes areas that fall within a designated dental health professional shortage area, or HPSA to obtain the electronic health record, or EHR, incentive payment. **Explanation:** Modifier AZ represents the services that a provider performs in a dental physician scarcity area, or a geographic area with a shortage of dental health professionals available to the Medicare population in that area. Append this modifier to report services the provider renders in a dental HPSA when the Zip code does not fully fall within that dental HPSA. Use of this modifier provides for an electronic health record incentive payment, made to eligible providers that adopt, implement, upgrade, or demonstrate meaningful use of certified EHR technology. **Tips:** This modifier does not impact the payment or calculation of the fee for service geographic quarterly HPSA, or health professional shortage area bonus.

Mod	Modifier Description, Definition, Explanation, and Tips
BA	**Item furnished in conjunction with parenteral enteral nutrition (PEN) services** **Definition:** Append modifier BA to represent an item or service a provider furnishes in conjunction with parenteral enteral nutrition, or PEN, services. **Explanation:** A provider reports the BA modifier for items that a provider furnishes for use with parenteral enteral nutrition services. For example, when the provider uses an intravenous, or IV pole in conjunction with parenteral nutrition, and reports E0776, IV pole, the provider appends the BA modifier. **Tips:** Use the BA modifier with E0776 exclusively.
BL	**Special acquisition of blood and blood products** **Definition:** Append this modifier to Healthcare Common Procedure Code System, or HCPCS codes that the provider reports for the actual blood or blood product. **Explanation:** Use this modifier with appropriate blood product Healthcare Common Procedure Code System, or HCPCS codes that a provider uses in an outpatient hospital setting for example when he purchases the products from a community blood bank or when he assess a charge for the blood or blood product that the provider collects in his own blood bank. **Tips:** The provider reports charges for the blood or blood product itself with the date of service, the number of units, and the appropriate blood product HCPCS code and modifier BL. He also reports the processing and storage services on a separate line the same line item date of service, the same number of units, and the same appropriate blood product HCPCS code and modifier BL. This modifier is applicable for blood products payment under the hospital outpatient prospective payment system. There is no requirement for use of this modifier by critical access hospitals, or CAHs.
BO	**Orally administered nutrition, not by feeding tube** **Definition:** Append this modifier to enteral nutrition Healthcare Common Procedure Code System, or HCPCS codes when the provider administers enteral nutrition products by mouth. **Explanation:** A provider appends this modifier with Healthcare Common Procedure Code System, or HCPCS codes that he reports for enteral nutrition therapy. He administers the enteral nutrition products to the patient orally, or by mouth, and not through a feeding tube. This modifier is applicable for enteral nutrients, reportable using HCPCS codes B4149 to B4162. **Tips:** This modifier is applicable for certain Home Health and Hospice services as well.
BP	**The beneficiary has been informed of the purchase and rental options and has elected to purchase the item** **Definition:** Append modifier BP to a code for durable medical equipment where the provider informs the beneficiary of the purchase and rental options and the beneficiary elects to purchase the item. **Explanation:** Modifier BP indicates that the patient chooses to purchase a durable medical equipment, or DME, item after the provider fully informs the recipient at the time the patient receives the item of the purchase and rental options for the item. A provider appends this modifier for durable medical equipment, or DME, items such as parenteral and enteral, or PEN pumps and electric wheelchairs, reportable with HCPCS K0835 thru K0891. **Tips:** Medicare discontinued the use of the following modifiers on claims for most capped rental items outside of those identified above: BP, The beneficiary has been informed of the purchase and rental options and has elected to purchase the item, modifier BR, and modifier BU, The beneficiary has been informed of the purchase and rental options and after 30 days has not informed the supplier of his/her decision. This change was due to the implementation of Section 5101 of the Deficit Reduction Act of 2005.
BR	**The beneficiary has been informed of the purchase and rental options and has elected to rent the item** **Definition:** Append modifier BR to a code for durable medical equipment, or DME, items where the provider informs the beneficiary of the differences between purchasing and renting of the DME item and the beneficiary chooses to rent the item. **Explanation:** Modifier BR identifies a code as an item where the beneficiary chooses to rent the item after the provider fully informs the recipient at the time the patient receives the item of the purchase and rental options available. A provider appends this modifier for durable medical equipment, or DME, items such as parenteral and enteral, or PEN pumps and electric wheelchairs, reportable with HCPCS K0835 through K0891. **Tips:** Medicare discontinued the use of the following modifiers on claims for most capped rental items outside of those identified above: BP, The beneficiary has been informed of the purchase and rental options and has elected to purchase the item, modifier BR, and modifier BU, The beneficiary has been informed of the purchase and rental options and after 30 days has not informed the supplier of his/her decision. This change was due to the implementation of Section 5101 of the Deficit Reduction Act of 2005.

Mod	Modifier Description, Definition, Explanation, and Tips
BU	**The beneficiary has been informed of the purchase and rental options and after 30 days has not informed the supplier of his/her decision** **Definition:** Append modifier BU to a code for durable medical equipment, or DME, items where the provider informs the beneficiary of the differences between purchasing and renting the item and after 30 days the beneficiary has not informed the supplier of his decision. **Explanation:** Modifier BU identifies a code for a durable medical equipment, or DME, item that a provider fully informs the recipient at the time the patient receives the item of the purchase and rental options available but the beneficiary does not inform the supplier of his decision to rent or purchase the item for 30 days or more. A provider appends this modifier for certain durable medical equipment, or DME, items such as parenteral and enteral, or PEN, pumps and electric wheelchairs regardless of the date of the first rental period, reportable with HCPCS K0835 thru K0891, and on all capped rental items where the first rental period began prior to January 1, 2006. **Tips:** Medicare discontinued the use of the following modifiers on claims for most capped rental items outside of those identified above: BP, The beneficiary has been informed of the purchase and rental options and has elected to purchase the item, modifier BR, and modifier BU, The beneficiary has been informed of the purchase and rental options and after 30 days has not informed the supplier of his/her decision. This change was due to the implementation of Section 5101 of the Deficit Reduction Act of 2005.
CA	**Procedure payable only in the inpatient setting when performed emergently on an outpatient who expires prior to admission** **Definition:** Append modifier CA when the patient is an outpatient, in an inpatient setting, and the patient passes away without being admitted as an inpatient. **Explanation:** In order to receive payment for the CA modifier with a Healthcare Common Procedure Coding System, or HCPCS code, the patient should be an emergency patient and must be an outpatient, the setting should be an inpatient setting only, and the patient passes away without being admitted as an inpatient. For outpatients who receive inpatient only procedures on an emergency basis and who expire before inpatient admittance to the hospital, the provider receives a specific outpatient Ambulatory Payment Classification, or APC payment as reimbursement for all the services on that day. The assignment of a modifier CA on an inpatient only procedure line identifies the service as such and assigns the specific payment, and turns on a packaging flag for all other line items on that claim with that date of service. Payment is only permissible for one procedure with a modifier of CA. **Tips:** Do not use modifier CA on more than one procedure on a claim. If a provider submits multiple inpatient only procedures with the modifier CA, the payer returns the claim back to the provider. If a provider applies a modifier CA on an inpatient only procedure code for a patient who did not expire, and the patient discharge status code is not 20, Expired, then the provider will also get the claim back.
CB	**Service ordered by a renal dialysis facility (RDF) physician as part of the ESRD beneficiary's dialysis benefit, is not part of the composite rate, and is separately reimbursable** **Definition:** A provider appends modifier CB to identify services ordered by a renal dialysis facility, or RDF, provider as part of the dialysis benefit of an end stage renal disease, or ESRD patient. This is not a part of the composite rate payment, and is separately reimbursable. **Explanation:** A provider appends modifier CB to services related to an ESRD patient's dialysis treatment and ordered by the dialysis facility physician. The test is not a part of the dialysis facility's composite rate payment, and is separately reimbursable. These services may include chest X-rays and other X-rays presumptively considered to be dialysis related and, therefore, appropriate for submission with the CB modifier; along with lab tests such as certain panel tests, urinalysis, and specific electrocardiogram, or ECG, tests and some vascular studies. **Tips:** Modifier CB affects consolidated billing rules for skilled nursing facilities for inpatients. Append modifier CB, only after determining that the patient has ESRD entitlement, he is undergoing the test for dialysis treatment for ESRD, the test is an order of the dialysis facility, the test is not a part of the composite rate, and is separately reimbursable. The patient should be in a Medicare Part A stay, Bill 21X or 22X.
CC	**Procedure code change (use 'CC' when the procedure code submitted was changed either for administrative reasons or because an incorrect code was filed)** **Definition:** A provider appends modifier CC to report a procedure code change, when the procedure code submitted changes either for administrative reasons, or due to filing of an incorrect code. **Explanation:** A provider appends modifier CC to a service when the procedure code submitted changes either for administrative reasons or due to incorrect code usage. Commonly, a contractor uses this modifier to identify when the procedure code submitted was changed by them. **Tips:** Providers should not use modifier CC. It is an internal modifier that identifies when the Medicare contractor changes the procedure code that the provider submitted.

Mod	Modifier Description, Definition, Explanation, and Tips
CD	**AMCC test has been ordered by an ESRD facility or MCP physician that is part of the composite rate and is not separately billable** **Definition:** Append modifier CD when the End Stage Renal Disease, or ESRD provider or any provider performs an automated multi channel laboratory test, or AMCC test on an ESRD patient who is undergoing maintenance dialysis. **Explanation:** Use this modifier when an End Stage Renal Disease, or ESRD provider or any provider performs an automated multi channel laboratory test, or AMCC, test on an ESRD patient who is undergoing maintenance dialysis. This modifier indicates that the test is a part of the composite rate and is not separately reimbursable. When a provider reports an individual laboratory code such as 82330, Calcium; ionized, as Monthly Capitation Payment, or MCP requires, rather than reporting the disease panel code, such as 82310, Calcium; total, he appends modifier CD, when the test is part of the composite rate or he appends CE, AMCC test has been ordered by an ESRD facility or MCP provider that is a composite rate test but is beyond the normal frequency covered under the rate and is separately reimbursable based on medical necessity. **Tips:** Providers billing AMCC ESRD related tests to Medicare must report CD, CE, or CF modifiers for each test. Beginning with dates of service on or after April 1, 2015, ESRD claims will no longer require ESRD facilities to submit theses three modifiers: CD, CE, AMCC test has been ordered by an ESRD facility or MCP physician that is a composite rate test but is beyond the normal frequency covered under the rate and is separately reimbursable based on medical necessity; or modifier CF, AMCC test has been ordered by an ESRD facility or MCP physician that is not part of the composite rate and is separately billable.
CE	**AMCC test has been ordered by an ESRD facility or MCP physician that is a composite rate test but is beyond the normal frequency covered under the rate and is separately reimbursable based on medical necessity** **Definition:** Append modifier CE when the End Stage Renal Disease, ESRD facility or another facility performs an automated multi channel laboratory, or AMCC test on an ESRD patient who is undergoing maintenance dialysis. This modifier indicates that the test is beyond the normal frequency limit the composite reimbursement covers so it is separately payable. **Explanation:** Use this modifier when either the ESRD facility or another facility performs an automated multi channel laboratory, or AMCC test on an ESRD patient who is undergoing maintenance dialysis. This modifier indicates that the test is reasonable and medically necessary, a part of the composite rate, but is beyond the frequency limits and is separately reimbursable. When a provider reports an individual laboratory code such as 82330. Calcium; ionized, as the Monthly Capitation Payment, or MCP requires, rather than reporting the disease panel code, such as 82310, Calcium; total, he appends modifier CD, AMCC test has been ordered by an ESRD facility or MCP physician that is part of the composite rate and is not separately billable, or he appends modifier CE when the code is separately reimbursable. **Tips:** Providers billing AMCC ESRD related tests to Medicare must report CD, CE, or CF modifiers for each test. Beginning with dates of service on or after April 1, 2015, ESRD claims will no longer require ESRD facilities to submit theses three modifiers: CD, AMCC test has been ordered by an ESRD facility or MCP physician that is part of the composite rate and is not separately billable; or modifier CE; or CF, AMCC test has been ordered by an ESRD facility or MCP physician that is not part of the composite rate and is separately billable.
CF	**AMCC test has been ordered by an ESRD facility or MCP physician that is not part of the composite rate and is separately billable** **Definition:** Append modifier CF when the End Stage Renal Disease, ESRD facility or an outside facility performs an automated multi channel laboratory, or AMCC, test on an ESRD patient undergoing maintenance dialysis. This modifier indicates that the test is not included in the composite rate and is separately reimbursable. **Explanation:** When submitting claims to Medicare for ESRD related automated multi channel chemistry tests, or AMCC tests, use modifier CF to identify which tests are not inclusive within the ESRD facility composite rate payment. Append modifier CF to identify tests that the provider orders that are not a part of the composite rate. These tests are separately reimbursable. Use modifier CF if the provider orders tests for chronic dialysis for ESRD such as an AMCC test that is not part of the composite rate and is separately billable and has been ordered by an ESRD facility or Monthly Capitation Payment, or MCP physician. You may submit this modifier with any of the AMCC codes. **Tips:** Providers billing AMCC ESRD related tests to Medicare must report CD, CE, or CF modifiers for each test. Beginning with dates of service on or after April 1, 2015, ESRD claims will no longer require ESRD facilities to submit these three modifiers: CD, AMCC test has been ordered by an ESRD facility or MCP physician that is part of the composite rate and is not separately billable; or CE, AMCC test has been ordered by an ESRD facility or MCP physician that is a composite rate test but is beyond the normal frequency covered under the rate and is separately reimbursable based on medical necessity; or modifier CF.

Mod	Modifier Description, Definition, Explanation, and Tips
CG	**Policy criteria applied** **Definition:** Append modifier CG to a code to identify a policy criteria applied. **Explanation:** For services reportable as an L3923 orthosis that has a rigid plastic or metal component, you must add the CG modifier. If you bill a claim for L3923 without a CG modifier, it will be denied. Similarly, if a spinal garment for example L0450, L0454, L0621, L0625, or L0628 is made primarily of a nonelastic material, such as canvas, cotton, or nylon, or has a rigid posterior panel, you must add the CG modifier or the service will be rejected or denied for incorrect coding. **Tips:** This modifier is informational only and you may submit it with all procedure codes.
CH	**0 percent impaired, limited or restricted** **Definition:** Append modifier CH to a code for a patient with a zero percent impairment, with limited or restricted movement. **Explanation:** Modifier CH identifies the extent of a patient's impairment. The severity of impairment to assign this modifier is zero percent impaired, with limited or restricted movement. CH is a severity modifier that a provider uses on specific therapy claims. Report only one functional limitation for each related therapy plan of care, or POC. In situations where a provider completes reporting on the first reportable functional limitation and the need for treatment continues, he reports a second functional limitation using another set of G codes. Functional reporting is necessary, at the beginning of a therapy episode of care, or on the date of service, or DOS, for the initial therapy service; at least once every ten treatment days; on the same DOS that a provider reports an evaluative or re evaluative on a claim; at the time of patient discharge from a therapy episode of care; and on the same DOS the reporting of a particular functional limitation ends, when further therapy is necessary. **Tips:** Use this modifier to report the severity or complexity for the functional measure for each non payable therapy G code. The severity modifiers reflect the patient's percentage of functional impairment as determined by the therapist, physician, or nonphysician practitioner who provides the therapy services. The appropriate severity modifiers report a patient's current status, the anticipated goal status, and the discharge status.
CI	**At least 1 percent but less than 20 percent impaired, limited or restricted** **Definition:** Append modifier CI to a code for a patient with an impairment of one to 20 percent, with limited or restricted movement. **Explanation:** Modifier CI identifies the extent of impairment in a patient. The severity of impairment may range from one percent to 20 percent, with limited or restricted movement. CI is a severity modifier that a provider uses on specific therapy claims. Report only one functional limitation for each related therapy plan of care, or POC. In situations where a provider completes reporting on the first reportable functional limitation and the need for treatment continues, he reports a second functional limitation using another set of G codes. Functional reporting is necessary, at the beginning of a therapy episode of care, or on the DOS for the initial therapy service; at least once every ten treatment days; on the same DOS that a provider reports an evaluative or re evaluative on a claim; at the time of patient discharge from a therapy episode of care; and on the same DOS the reporting of a particular functional limitation ends, when further therapy is necessary. **Tips:** Use this modifier to report the severity or complexity for the functional measure for each non payable therapy G code. The severity modifiers reflect the patient's percentage of functional impairment as determined by the therapist, physician, or nonphysician practitioner who provides the therapy services. The appropriate severity modifiers report a patient's current status, the anticipated goal status, and the discharge status.

Mod	Modifier Description, Definition, Explanation, and Tips
CJ	**At least 20 percent but less than 40 percent impaired, limited or restricted** **Definition:** Append modifier CJ to a code for a patient with an impairment of 20 to 40 percent, with limited or restricted movement. **Explanation:** Modifier CJ identifies the extent of impairment in a patient. The severity of impairment may range from 20 percent to 40 percent, with limited or restricted movement. CJ is a severity modifier that a provider uses on specific therapy claims. Report only one functional limitation for each related therapy plan of care, or POC. In situations where a provider completes reporting on the first reportable functional limitation and the need for treatment continues, he reports a second functional limitation using another set of G codes. Functional reporting is necessary, at the beginning of a therapy episode of care, or on the date of service, or DOS, for the initial therapy service; at least once every ten treatment days; on the same DOS that a provider reports an evaluative or re evaluative on a claim; at the time of patient discharge from a therapy episode of care; and on the same DOS the reporting of a particular functional limitation ends, when further therapy is necessary. **Tips:** Use this modifier to report the severity or complexity for the functional measure for each non payable therapy G code. The severity modifiers reflect the patient's percentage of functional impairment as determined by the therapist, physician, or nonphysician practitioner who provides the therapy services. The appropriate severity modifiers report a patient's current status, the anticipated goal status, and the discharge status.
CK	**At least 40 percent but less than 60 percent impaired, limited or restricted** **Definition:** Append modifier CK to a code for a patient with an impairment of 40 to 60 percent, with limited or restricted movement. **Explanation:** Modifier CK identifies the extent of impairment in a patient. The severity of impairment may range from 40 percent to 60 percent, with limited or restricted movement. CK is a severity modifier that a provider uses on specific therapy claims. Report only one functional limitation for each related therapy plan of care, or POC. In situations where a provider completes reporting on the first reportable functional limitation and the need for treatment continues, he reports a second functional limitation using another set of G codes. Functional reporting is necessary, at the beginning of a therapy episode of care, or on the date of service, or DOS, for the initial therapy service; at least once every ten treatment days; on the same DOS that a provider reports an evaluative or re evaluative on a claim; at the time of patient discharge from a therapy episode of care; and on the same DOS the reporting of a particular functional limitation ends, when further therapy is necessary. **Tips:** Use this modifier to report the severity or complexity for the functional measure for each non payable therapy G code. The severity modifiers reflect the patient's percentage of functional impairment as determined by the therapist, physician, or nonphysician practitioner who provides the therapy services. The appropriate severity modifiers report a patient's current status, the anticipated goal status, and the discharge status.
CL	**At least 60 percent but less than 80 percent impaired, limited or restricted** **Definition:** Append modifier CL to a code for a patient with an impairment of 60 to 80 percent, with limited or restricted movement. **Explanation:** Modifier CL identifies the extent of impairment in a patient. The severity of impairment may range from 60 percent to 80 percent, with limited or restricted movement. CL is a severity modifier that a provider uses on specific therapy claims. Report only one functional limitation for each related therapy plan of care, or POC. In situations where a provider completes reporting on the first reportable functional limitation and the need for treatment continues, he reports a second functional limitation using another set of G codes. Functional reporting is necessary, at the beginning of a therapy episode of care, or on the date of service, or DOS, for the initial therapy service; at least once every ten treatment days; on the same DOS that a provider reports an evaluative or re evaluative on a claim; at the time of patient discharge from a therapy episode of care; and on the same DOS the reporting of a particular functional limitation ends, when further therapy is necessary. **Tips:** Use this modifier to report the severity or complexity for the functional measure for each non payable therapy G code. The severity modifiers reflect the patient's percentage of functional impairment as determined by the therapist, physician, or nonphysician practitioner who provides the therapy services. The appropriate severity modifiers report a patient's current status, the anticipated goal status, and the discharge status.

Mod	Modifier Description, Definition, Explanation, and Tips
CM	**At least 80 percent but less than 100 percent impaired, limited or restricted** **Definition:** Append modifier CM to a code for a patient with an impairment of 80 to 100 percent, with limited or restricted movement. **Explanation:** Modifier CM identifies the extent of impairment in a patient. The severity of impairment may range from 80 percent to 100 percent, with limited or restricted movement. CM is a severity modifier that a provider uses on specific therapy claims. Report only one functional limitation for each related therapy plan of care, or POC. In situations where a provider completes reporting on the first reportable functional limitation and the need for treatment continues, he reports a second functional limitation using another set of G codes. Functional reporting is necessary, at the beginning of a therapy episode of care, or on the date of service, or DOS for the initial therapy service; at least once every ten treatment days; on the same DOS that a provider reports an evaluative or re evaluative on a claim; at the time of patient discharge from a therapy episode of care; and on the same DOS the reporting of a particular functional limitation ends, when further therapy is necessary. **Tips:** Use this modifier to report the severity or complexity for the functional measure for each non payable therapy G code. The severity modifiers reflect the patient's percentage of functional impairment as determined by the therapist, physician, or nonphysician practitioner who provides the therapy services. The appropriate severity modifiers report a patient's current status, the anticipated goal status, and the discharge status.
CN	**100 percent impaired, limited or restricted** **Definition:** Append modifier CN to a code for a patient with an impairment of 100 percent, with limited or restricted movement. **Explanation:** Modifier CN identifies the extent of impairment in a patient. The severity of impairment is 100 percent, with limited or restricted movement. CN is a severity modifier that a provider uses on specific therapy claims. Report only one functional limitation for each related therapy plan of care, or POC. In situations where a provider completes reporting on the first reportable functional limitation and the need for treatment continues, he reports a second functional limitation using another set of G codes. Functional reporting is necessary, at the beginning of a therapy episode of care, or on the date of service, or DOS, for the initial therapy service; at least once every ten treatment days; on the same DOS that a provider reports an evaluative or re evaluative on a claim; at the time of patient discharge from a therapy episode of care; and on the same DOS the reporting of a particular functional limitation ends, when further therapy is necessary. **Tips:** Use this modifier to report the severity or complexity for the functional measure for each non payable therapy G code. The severity modifiers reflect the patient's percentage of functional impairment as determined by the therapist, physician, or nonphysician practitioner who provides the therapy services. The appropriate severity modifiers report a patient's current status, the anticipated goal status, and the discharge status.
CO	**Outpatient occupational therapy services furnished in whole or in part by an occupational therapy assistant** **Definition:** Append modifier CO to codes for outpatient occupational therapy (OPT) when an OPT assistant performs all or a portion of the service. **Explanation:** Modifier CO denotes that some or all of a patient's outpatient occupational therapy (OPT) was performed by an OPT assistant. The OPT assistant performs the therapy in an outpatient setting, and the diagnosis code must be consistent with a condition that requires occupational therapy. OPT helps injured, ill, or disabled patients develop, recover, and improve skills needed for activities of daily living (ADLs),such as eating, bathing, dressing, toileting, and walking, and work-related activities, such as lifting, bending, sorting, and other skills depending on the type of work the patient performs. **Tips:** Append modifier CO only with codes on the list of applicable therapy services for occupational therapy and that are part of the plan of care for that patient.
CQ	**Outpatient physical therapy services furnished in whole or in part by a physical therapist assistant** **Definition:** Append modifier CQ to codes for outpatient physical therapy (PT) when an PT assistant performs all or a portion of the service. **Explanation:** Modifier CQ denotes that some or all of a patient's outpatient physical therapy (PT) was performed by a PT assistant. The PT assistant performs the therapy in an outpatient setting, and the diagnosis code must be consistent with a condition that requires occupational therapy. Physical therapy uses therapeutic exercises and equipment to help patients with physical dysfunction regain or improve their physical abilities. **Tips:** Append modifier CQ only with codes on the list of applicable therapy services for physical therapy and that are part of the plan of care for that patient.

Mod	Modifier Description, Definition, Explanation, and Tips
CR	**Catastrophe/disaster related** **Definition:** Append modifier CR to a code for services related to an emergency or disaster related condition. **Explanation:** Modifier CR identifies the services given to victims in the case of an emergency or disaster related condition such as a hurricane. In the event of a disaster or emergency, the Centers for Medicare and Medicaid Services, or CMS, issues specific guidance for use of this modifier. CMS provides information such as the geographic area the code is applicable to, and the beginning and end dates that apply to the use of the modifier and its related bill condition code, DR, Disaster related, which a provider also reports to identify the services are or may be impacted by specific policies related to a national or regional disaster. **Tips:** Use this modifier to code for catastrophe, disaster or emergency claims. You may use CR modifier for institutional or non institutional billing. One may use this modifier in case of an emergency disaster related condition and there is a condition levied on the payment of Medicare.
CS	**Cost-sharing waived for specified covid-19 testing-related services that result in and order for or administration of a covid-19 test and/or used for cost-sharing waived preventive services furnished via telehealth in rural health clinics and federally qualified health centers during the covid-19 public health emergency** **Definition:** Append modifier CS to indicate cost-sharing is waived for specified COVID-19 testing-related services. Rural health clinics and federally qualified health centers also use modifier CS to distinguish telehealth services that have cost-sharing waived during the COVID-19 public health emergency. **Explanation:** Modifier CS is appropriate with codes for specified COVID-19 test-related services, including applicable telehealth services, if those services meet certain requirements for waiving cost-sharing. Examples of requirements include codes for evaluation and management (E/M) services that result in an order for, or administration of, a COVID-19 lab test during the public health emergency. **Tips:** Payer rules may vary for use of this modifier. Medicare states cost-sharing does not apply for COVID-19 testing-related services, which are medical visits that are furnished between March 18, 2020, and the end of the COVID-19 public health emergency (PHE); result in an order for or administration of a COVID-19 test; are related to furnishing or administering such a test or to the evaluation of an individual for purposes of determining the need for such a test; and are in any of the following E/M categories: office and other outpatient services; hospital observation services; emergency department services; nursing facility services; domiciliary, rest home, or custodial care services; home services; and online digital evaluation and management services. Medicare provides lists of codes that modifier CS may apply to. For Medicare, cost-sharing does not apply to the specified medical visit services for which payment is made to hospital outpatient departments paid under the Outpatient Prospective Payment System (OPPS), physicians and other professionals under the Physician Fee Schedule, Critical Access Hospitals (CAHs), RHCs, and FQHCs. RHCs and FQHCs append CS to G2025 (Distant site telehealth services Rural Health Clinics or Federally Qualified Health Centers (RHC/FQHC)) when the code represents one of the services where coinsurance is waived. Providers who use modifier CS should not charge patients co-insurance and/or deductible amounts for those services.
CT	**Computed tomography services furnished using equipment that does not meet each of the attributes of the National Electrical Manufacturers Association (NEMA) XR-29-2013 standard** **Definition:** Append modifier CT when a provider renders computed tomography (CT) with equipment that doesn't meet the National Electrical Manufacturers' Association standard. **Explanation:** The National Electrical Manufacturers' Association (NEMA) represents U.S. electrical equipment and medical imaging manufacturers. These manufacturers produce products that generate and transmit electricity and can be used for medical, commercial, and industrial purposes. Modifier CT appended to a code indicates that CT equipment was used for the patient's services, but that equipment does not comply with NEMA standards.
DA	**Oral health assessment by a licensed health professional other than a dentist** Summary: Append modifier DA to a code for an oral health assessment that a licensed health professional, other than a dentist, performs. **Explanation:** Modifier DA identifies an oral health assessment for a patient with dental or oral health problems. A licensed health professional other than a dentist performs this assessment. An oral health assessment determines the level of a patient's oral hygiene such as healthy or unhealthy oral cleanliness, condition of the lips, tongue, saliva, gums and tissue, and caries risk, meaning the patient's risk of tooth decay. **Tips:** This modifier is informational only and may be submitted with any appropriate HCPCS code.

Mod	Modifier Description, Definition, Explanation, and Tips
E1	**Upper left, eyelid** **Definition:** Append modifier E1 when the provider performs a procedure on the left upper eyelid of a patient. **Explanation:** Modifier E1 illustrates a procedure that the provider performs on a patient's left upper eyelid. A provider uses modifier E1 to identify the left upper eyelid, instead of using modifier LT, Left side, which identifies a procedure the provider performs on the left side of the body. HCPCS level II modifiers apply to codes for procedures that the provider performs on paired organs, like eyelids, fingers, or toes. These modifiers help to prevent denials when the provider submits duplicate codes to report separate procedures on different sites or different sides of the body. **Tips:** If more than one modifier needs to be applied, you may need to repeat the HCPCS code on another line with the appropriate Level II modifier. When modifier E1 applies to the service, use it before selecting modifiers LT, RT, or 59, Distinct procedural service.
E2	**Lower left, eyelid** **Definition:** Append modifier E2 when the provider performs a procedure on the left lower eyelid of a patient. **Explanation:** Modifier E2 illustrates a procedure that the provider performs on the patient's left lower eyelid. A provider uses modifier E2 to identify the left lower eyelid, instead of using modifier LT, Left side, which identifies a procedure the provider performs on the left side of the body. HCPCS level II modifiers apply to codes for procedures that the provider performs on paired organs, like eyelids, fingers, or toes. These modifiers help to prevent denials when the provider submits duplicate codes to report separate procedures on different sites or different sides of the body. **Tips:** If more than one modifier needs to be applied, you may need to repeat the HCPCS code on another line with the appropriate Level II modifier.
E3	**Upper right, eyelid** **Definition:** Append modifier E3 when the provider performs a procedure on the right upper eyelid of a patient. **Explanation:** Modifier E3 illustrates a procedure that the provider performs on the patient's right upper eyelid. A provider uses modifier E3 to identify the right upper eyelid, instead of using modifier RT, Right side, which identifies a procedure the provider performs on the right side of the body. HCPCS level II modifiers apply to codes for procedures that the provider performs on paired organs, like eyelids, fingers, or toes. These modifiers help to prevent denials when the provider submits duplicate codes to report separate procedures on different sites or different sides of the body. **Tips:** If more than one modifier needs to be applied, repeat the HCPCS code on another line with the appropriate Level II modifier.
E4	**Lower right, eyelid** **Definition:** Append modifier E4 when the provider performs a procedure on the right lower eyelid of a patient. **Explanation:** Modifier E4 illustrates a procedure that the provider performs on the patient's right lower eyelid. A provider uses modifier E4 to identify the right lower eyelid, instead of using modifier RT, Right side, which identifies a procedure the provider performs on the right side of the body. HCPCS level II modifiers apply to codes for procedures that the provider performs on paired organs, like eyelids, fingers, or toes. These modifiers help to prevent denials when the provider submits duplicate codes to report separate procedures on different sites or different sides of the body. **Tips:** If more than one modifier needs to be applied, you may need to repeat the HCPCS code on another line with the appropriate Level II modifier.
EA	**Erythropoietic stimulating agent (ESA) administered to treat anemia due to anti-cancer chemotherapy** **Definition:** Append modifier EA when the provider administers an agent that stimulates red blood cell production. The provider administers an erythropoietic stimulating agent, or ESA to treat anemia, a condition of a lower than normal hemoglobin, or red blood cell count in the blood of a patient taking anti cancer chemical compounds or drugs. **Explanation:** Modifier EA depicts administration of erythropoietic stimulating agent, or ESA, to a patient who has taken or is taking anti cancer drugs. The provider administers ESA to enhance the stimulation of red blood cells to treat anemia or low hemoglobin. The medical record should justify the diagnosis that corresponds to the administration of ESA as well as the nature or extent of the anemia. **Tips:** If the provider administers ESA to treat anemia due to anticancer radiotherapy, append modifier EB, Erythropoietic stimulating agent or ESA administered to treat anemia due to anti cancer radiotherapy. If the provider administers ESA to treat anemia, not due to anti cancer radiotherapy or chemotherapy, append modifier EC, Erythropoietic stimulating agent or ESA, administered to treat anemia not due to anti cancer radiotherapy or anti cancer chemotherapy.

Mod	Modifier Description, Definition, Explanation, and Tips
EB	**Erythropoietic stimulating agent (ESA) administered to treat anemia due to anti-cancer radiotherapy** **Definition:** Append modifier EB when the provider administers an agent that stimulates red blood cell production. The provider administers an erythropoietic stimulating agent, or ESA to treat anemia, a condition of a lower than normal hemoglobin, or red blood cells count in the blood of a patient taking anti cancer radiotherapy. **Explanation:** Modifier EB identifies administration of erythropoietic stimulating agent, or ESA, to a patient who has received or is receiving anti cancer radiotherapy. The provider administers ESA to enhance the stimulation of red blood cells to treat anemia or low hemoglobin. The medical record should justify the diagnosis that corresponds to the administration of ESA as well as the nature or extent of the anemia. **Tips:** If the provider administers ESA to treat anemia due to anticancer chemotherapy, append modifier EA, Erythropoietic stimulating agent or ESA administered to treat anemia due to anti cancer chemotherapy. If the provider administers ESA to treat anemia, not due to anti cancer radiotherapy or chemotherapy, append modifier EC, Erythropoietic stimulating agent or ESA administered to treat anemia not due to anti cancer radiotherapy or anti cancer chemotherapy.
EC	**Erythropoietic stimulating agent (ESA) administered to treat anemia not due to anti-cancer radiotherapy or anti-cancer chemotherapy** **Definition:** Append modifier EC when the provider administers an agent that stimulates red blood cell production. The provider administers an erythropoietic stimulating agent, or ESA to treat anemia, a condition of a lower than normal red blood cell count or hemoglobin in the blood of a patient. The anemia is not because of taking anti cancer chemotherapy or radiotherapy. **Explanation:** Modifier EC identifies administration of erythropoietic stimulating agent, or ESA, to a patient to enhance the stimulation of red blood cells to treat anemia or low hemoglobin. The medical record should justify the diagnosis that corresponds to the administration of ESA as well as the nature or extent of the anemia. Append this modifier when anemia does not develop due to anti cancer chemotherapy or radiotherapy. **Tips:** If the provider administers ESA to treat anemia due to anticancer chemotherapy, append modifier EA, Erythropoietic stimulating agent or ESA administered to treat anemia due to anti cancer chemotherapy. If the provider administers ESA to treat anemia due to anticancer radiotherapy, append modifier EB, Erythropoietic stimulating agent or ESA administered to treat anemia due to anti cancer radiotherapy.
ED	**Hematocrit level has exceeded 39% (or hemoglobin level has exceeded 13.0 G/dl) for 3 or more consecutive billing cycles immediately prior to and including the current cycle** **Definition:** Append modifier ED to a code for hemodialysis patients when the provider measures the hematocrit level and it exceeds 39 percent or the hemoglobin level exceeds 13.0 g/dl, or grams per deciliter, for three or more consecutive billings immediately prior to and including the current service. **Explanation:** Modifier ED illustrates the measurement of a patient's hematocrit level which exceeds 39 percent or a hemoglobin level, which is greater than 13.0 g/dl, or grams per deciliter, in a patient undergoing hemodialysis for end stage renal disease, or ESRD. When the kidneys fail to perform their function, dialysis becomes important to remove waste products from the blood. The provider tests the patient's hemoglobin level in hemodialysis patients. He tests for three or more consecutive billing cycles immediately prior to and including the current cycle and appends this modifier when applicable. **Tips:** Requests for payments or claims for ESAs for ESRD patients receiving dialysis in renal dialysis facilities must report modifiers ED or EE, Hematocrit level has not exceeded 39% or hemoglobin level has not exceeded 13.0 g per dl for three or more consecutive billing cycles immediately prior to and including the current cycle. Providers may continue to report modifier GS, Dosage of erythropoietin stimulating agent has been reduced and maintained in response to hematocrit or hemoglobin level, when the provider reports that the hematocrit or hemoglobin levels exceed the monitoring threshold and a dose reduction has occurred. When the GS modifier is on a claim also reporting modifier EE, the claim will be paid in full. The GS modifier, however, has no effect on the 50 percent dosage reduction, on claims reporting modifier ED.

Mod	Modifier Description, Definition, Explanation, and Tips
EE	**Hematocrit level has not exceeded 39% (or hemoglobin level has not exceeded 13.0 G/dl) for 3 or more consecutive billing cycles immediately prior to and including the current cycle** **Definition:** Append modifier EE to a code for hemodialysis patients when the provider measures the hematocrit level which does not exceed 39 percent or the hemoglobin level does not exceed 13.0g/dl, or grams per deciliter, for three or more consecutive billings immediately prior to and including the current service. **Explanation:** Modifier EE illustrates the measurement of the hematocrit level which does not exceed 39 percent or a hemoglobin level, which is not greater than 13.0 g per dl, or grams per deciliter, in a patient undergoing hemodialysis for end stage renal disease, or ESRD. When the kidneys fail to perform their function, dialysis becomes important to remove waste products from the blood. The provider tests the patient's hemoglobin level in hemodialysis patients. He tests for three or more consecutive billing cycles immediately prior to and including the current cycle and appends this modifier when applicable. **Tips:** Requests for payments or claims for ESAs for ESRD patients must report modifiers ED, Hematocrit level has exceeded 39% or hemoglobin level has exceeded 13.0 g per dl for three or more consecutive billing cycles immediately prior to and including the current cycle, or append modifier EE. Providers may continue to report the modifier GS, Dosage of erythropoietin stimulating agent has been reduced and maintained in response to hematocrit or hemoglobin level, when the hematocrit or hemoglobin levels that the provider reports exceed the monitoring threshold and a dose reduction has occurred. When the GS modifier is on a claim also reporting modifier EE, the claim will be paid in full. The GS modifier, however, has no effect on the 50 percent dosage reduction, on claims reporting modifier ED.
EJ	**Subsequent claims for a defined course of therapy, e.g., EPO, sodium hyaluronate, infliximab** **Definition:** Append modifier EJ to a code for subsequent claims for a defined course of EPO, sodium hyaluronate, or infliximab therapy for a patient. **Explanation:** Modifier EJ illustrates the coding of subsequent claims for a defined course of therapy for a patient. The therapy may include EPO, or erythropoietin therapy, a growth factor that stimulates the production of red blood cells; sodium hyaluronate, a substance similar to a joints own natural protection that acts like a lubricant and or cushion when injected directly into a joint such as the knee; or infliximab, a manmade antibody given intravenously to treat various chronic inflammatory diseases. This modifier allows the easy identification of a subsequent claim, which does not require as much information as an initial claim and prevents unnecessary claim inquiries, letters, and questionnaires. One can submit subsequent claims electronically. **Tips:** Modifier EJ is an informational code for Medicare use. Because of this fact, submit this modifier in the last modifier position, after any other modifiers. The biller may also submit this modifier with many HCPCS J codes for injections.
EM	**Emergency reserve supply (for ESRD benefit only)** **Definition:** Append modifier EM to a code for an emergency reserve supply of an erythropoiesis stimulating agent, or ESA, for hemodialysis patients with end stage renal disease, or ESRD. **Explanation:** Modifier EM illustrates the measurement of the emergency reserve supply for an ESA, or erythropoiesis stimulating agent in a patient undergoing hemodialysis for end stage renal disease, or ESRD. When the kidneys fail to perform their function, dialysis becomes important to remove waste products from the blood. The provider tests the patient's blood to ensure that the dialysis is removing the waste products effectively. Use this code for ESRD patients beginning to self administer an ESA, or erythropoiesis stimulating agents, at home for the treatment of anemia due to the disease and who receive an extra month supply of the drug, this one month reserve supply is reportable on the claim line with modifier EM. **Tips:** Providers most commonly append this modifier to 90999, Unlisted dialysis procedure, inpatient or outpatient. It is not necessary to use the modifier on every claim line, but facilities should be sure to include the modifier on at least one revenue code claim line for Medicare. The modifier can affect the processing of the payment of the code.
EP	**Service provided as part of Medicaid early periodic screening diagnosis and treatment (EPSDT) program** **Definition:** Append modifier EP to a code for a service that the provider gives as part of the Medicaid early periodic screening diagnosis and treatment, or EPSDT program. **Explanation:** Modifier EP illustrates billing of the service that the provider delivers as part of the Medicaid early periodic screening diagnosis and treatment, or EPSDT, program. This includes preventive health checkups and treatments to children from birth to young adults. A few of the types of early preventative health screening and treatments include immunization, administration and health screenings for hearing and vision problems. Modifier EP can be appended to several of the immunization administration codes, and preventive medicine, periodic and interperiodic assessments. **Tips:** Only providers delivering EPSDT medical services should use the EP modifier code for billing purposes. The claim form must contain the procedure code to represent the type of medical service that the provider gives along with the EP modifier to show this was an early preventative service office visit.

Mod	Modifier Description, Definition, Explanation, and Tips
ER	**Items and services furnished by a provider-based, off-campus emergency department** **Definition:** Append modifier ER to codes for outpatient hospital services and items, such as drugs or bandages, furnished in an off-campus provider-based emergency department (ED). **Explanation:** Modifier ER denotes that an item or outpatient hospital service was provided by an off-campus provider-based emergency department. Off campus means a location physically separate from the immediate area of the hospital facility and or in a building located more than 250 yards away from the main hospital buildings. **Tips:** Critical access hospitals are not required to append this modifier. Modifier ER is used for informational purposes at its institution in 2019 and does not impact payment, but like other modifiers previously introduced for tracking outpatient services provided in other off-campus provider-based departments (PBDs), it may at some point affect payment. Individual providers should not append modifier ER and instead should use the appropriate place of service code to indicate outpatient services furnished in an on-campus, remote, or satellite location of a hospital or in an off-campus, provider-based hospital setting.
ET	**Emergency services** **Definition:** Append modifier ET to a code for the emergency services, including hospital emergency services, for multiple service dates, where the ER encounter spans more than one service date. **Explanation:** Modifier ET illustrates billing for the hospital emergency room, or ER, services when the provider delivers emergency services to a patient in that setting. This includes emergency department services for multiple service dates. ER services that a patient receives in a hospital are excluded from SNF Consolidated Billing, or SNF CB, for beneficiaries that are in a skilled Part A SNF stay. This code flags the service to bypass SNF Consolidated Billing, or CB, claim edits for the ER related service line items identified by the modifier ET. This code is not applicable for the services a patient receives in the Part A skilled nursing facility, or SNF. Append modifier ET with codes such as 99070, 99218, 99281 to 99285, and 99291 and 99292. **Tips:** Append modifier ET every time the patient visits the hospital emergency room, or ER. The services given in a hospital emergency room excludes the skilled nursing facility care. The service extends to multiple dates of service. Append this modifier to a code for an emergency dental procedures as well.
EX	**Expatriate beneficiary** **Definition:** This modifier designates a non-U.S. citizen working in his home country. **Explanation:** The Centers for Medicare and Medicaid Services (CMS) identify expatriates as insureds who are non-U.S. citizens working in their home country.
EY	**No physician or other licensed healthcare provider order for this item or service** **Definition:** Append modifier EY to items or services without an order or prescription from the treating provider. This informational modifier notifies insurer that the provider is requesting a denial for secondary billing. For Medicare this is under the Coordination of Benefit, or COB guidelines. A provider appends this code when they issue durable medical equipment, prosthetic and orthotic supplies, or DMEPOS, without an order. **Explanation:** For Coordination of Benefit, or COB, purposes, the suppliers use the modifier EY, No licensed healthcare provider order for this item or service, on each line item on the claim and report their own name and National Provider Identifier, or NPI, as the ordering or referring provider. This is done to obtain a Medicare denial, under COB guidelines, which is where two or more insurances work together to pay for a service when a patient has more than one health insurance plan. Failure to include the EY modifier with all codes results in the return of the claim as unprocessable. If a provider has an order for some, but not all, of the items or services the provider furnishes to the Medicare beneficiary, the provider submits a separate claim for the items the provider dispenses to the patient without the treating physician's order. **Tips:** Medicare coverage requires an order by the provider, with the exception of some preventive screenings, or else the service is denied.
F1	**Left hand, second digit** **Definition:** Append modifier F1 when the provider performs a procedure on the second digit, or finger, of the left hand. **Explanation:** Modifier F1 identifies a procedure that the provider performs on the second, or index, finger of the left hand. This modifier is appropriate for surgical and diagnostic services but is not appropriate for Evaluation and Management, or E/M services. HCPCS level II modifiers apply to codes for procedures that the provider performs on paired organs, like eyelids, fingers, or toes. These modifiers help to prevent denials when the provider submits duplicate codes to report separate procedures on different sites or different sides of the body. **Tips:** For Medicare purposes, all line items with identical modifiers are subject to policies for proper coding except line items with the modifiers F1 to F9, which are not subject to the edit. However, they are subject to additional edits based on the specific use of the modifier as defined in other instructions from the Centers for Medicare and Medicaid Services, or CMS.

Mod	Modifier Description, Definition, Explanation, and Tips
F2	**Left hand, third digit**
	Definition: Append modifier F2 when the provider performs a procedure on the third digit, or finger of the left hand.
	Explanation: Modifier F2 illustrates a procedure that the provider performs on the third digit of the left hand. This modifier is appropriate for surgical and diagnostic services but is not appropriate for Evaluation and Management, or E/M services.
	HCPCS level II modifiers apply to codes for procedures that the provider performs on paired organs, like eyelids, fingers, or toes. These modifiers help to prevent denials when the provider submits duplicate codes to report separate procedures on different sites or different sides of the body.
	Tips: For Medicare purposes, all line items with identical modifiers are subject to policies for proper coding except line items with the modifiers F1 to F9, which are not subject to the edit. However, they are subject to additional edits based on the specific use of the modifier as defined in other instructions from the Centers for Medicare and Medicaid Services, or CMS.
F3	**Left hand, fourth digit**
	Definition: Append modifier F3 when the provider performs a procedure on the fourth digit, or finger, of the left hand.
	Explanation: Modifier F3 illustrates a procedure that the provider performs on the fourth finger of the left hand. This modifier is appropriate for surgical and diagnostic services but not appropriate for Evaluation and Management, or E/M services.
	HCPCS level II modifiers apply to codes for procedures that the provider performs on paired organs, like eyelids, fingers, or toes. These modifiers help to prevent denials when the provider submits duplicate codes to report separate procedures on different sites or different sides of the body.
	Tips: For Medicare purposes, all line items with identical modifiers are subject to policies for proper coding except line items with the modifiers F1 to F9, which are not subject to the edit. However, they are subject to additional edits based on the specific use of the modifier as defined in other instructions from the Centers for Medicare and Medicaid Services, or CMS.
F4	**Left hand, fifth digit**
	Definition: Append modifier F4 when the provider performs a procedure on the fifth digit, or finger of the left hand.
	Explanation: Modifier F4 illustrates a procedure that the provider performs on the fifth finger of the left hand. This modifier is applicable usually to surgical and diagnostic services but not appropriate for Evaluation and Management, or EM, services.
	HCPCS level II modifiers apply to codes for procedures that the provider performs on paired organs, like eyelids, fingers, or toes. These modifiers help to prevent denials when the provider submits duplicate codes to report separate procedures on different sites or different sides of the body.
	Tips: For Medicare purposes, all line items with identical modifiers are subject to policies for proper coding except line items with the modifiers F1 to F9, which are not subject to the edit. However, they are subject to additional edits based on the specific use of the modifier as defined in other instructions from the Centers for Medicare and Medicaid Services, or CMS.
F5	**Right hand, thumb**
	Definition: Append modifier F5 when the provider performs a procedure on the thumb of the right hand.
	Explanation: Modifier F5 illustrates a procedure that the provider performs on the thumb of the right hand. This modifier is appropriate for surgical and diagnostic services but not appropriate for Evaluation and management, or E/M, services.
	HCPCS level II modifiers apply to codes for procedures that the provider performs on paired organs, like eyelids, fingers, or toes. These modifiers help to prevent denials when the provider submits duplicate codes to report separate procedures on different sites or different sides of the body.
	Tips: For Medicare purposes, all line items with identical modifiers are subject to policies for proper coding except line items with the modifiers F1 to F9, which are not subject to the edit. However, they are subject to additional edits based on the specific use of the modifier as defined in other instructions from the Centers for Medicare and Medicaid Services, or CMS.

Mod	Modifier Description, Definition, Explanation, and Tips
F6	**Right hand, second digit** **Definition:** Append modifier F6 when the provider performs a procedure on the second digit, or finger, of the right hand. **Explanation:** Modifier F6 illustrates a procedure that the provider performs on the second finger of the right hand. This modifier is appropriate for surgical and diagnostic services but not appropriate for Evaluation and Management, or E/M services. HCPCS level II modifiers apply to codes for procedures that the provider performs on paired organs, like eyelids, fingers, or toes. These modifiers help to prevent denials when the provider submits duplicate codes to report separate procedures on different sites or different sides of the body. **Tips:** For Medicare purposes, all line items with identical modifiers are subject to policies for proper coding except line items with the modifiers F1 to F9, which are not subject to the edit. However, they are subject to additional edits based on the specific use of the modifier as defined in other instructions from the Centers for Medicare and Medicaid Services, or CMS.
F7	**Right hand, third digit** **Definition:** Append modifier F7 when the provider performs a procedure on the third digit, or finger, of the right hand. **Explanation:** Modifier F7 illustrates a procedure that the provider performs on the third finger of the right hand. This modifier is appropriate for surgical and diagnostic services but not appropriate for Evaluation and Management, or E/M services. HCPCS level II modifiers apply to codes for procedures that the provider performs on paired organs, like eyelids, fingers, or toes. These modifiers help to prevent denials when the provider submits duplicate codes to report separate procedures on different sites or different sides of the body. **Tips:** For Medicare purposes, all line items with identical modifiers are subject to policies for proper coding except line items with the modifiers F1 to F9, which are not subject to the edit. However, they are subject to additional edits based on the specific use of the modifier as defined in other instructions from the Centers for Medicare and Medicaid Services, or CMS.
F8	**Right hand, fourth digit** **Definition:** Append modifier F8 when the provider performs a procedure on the fourth digit, or finger, of the right hand. **Explanation:** Modifier F8 illustrates a procedure that the provider performs on the fourth digit of the right hand. This modifier is appropriate for surgical and diagnostic services but not appropriate for Evaluation and Management, or E/M services. HCPCS level II modifiers apply to codes for procedures that the provider performs on paired organs, like eyelids, fingers, or toes. These modifiers help to prevent denials when the provider submits duplicate codes to report separate procedures on different sites or different sides of the body. **Tips:** For Medicare purposes, all line items with identical modifiers are subject to policies for proper coding except line items with the modifiers F1 to F9, which are not subject to the edit. However, they are subject to additional edits based on the specific use of the modifier as defined in other instructions from the Centers for Medicare and Medicaid Services, or CMS.
F9	**Right hand, fifth digit** **Definition:** Append modifier F9 when the provider performs a procedure on the fifth digit, or finger, of the right hand. **Explanation:** Modifier F9 illustrates a procedure that the provider performs on the fifth digit of the right hand. This modifier is appropriate for surgical and diagnostic services but not appropriate for Evaluation and Management, or E/M services. HCPCS level II modifiers apply to codes for procedures that the provider performs on paired organs, like eyelids, fingers, or toes. These modifiers help to prevent denials when the provider submits duplicate codes to report separate procedures on different sites or different sides of the body. **Tips:** For Medicare purposes, all line items with identical modifiers are subject to policies for proper coding except line items with the modifiers F1 to F9, which are not subject to the edit. However, they are subject to additional edits based on the specific use of the modifier as defined in other instructions from the Centers for Medicare and Medicaid Services, or CMS.

Mod	Modifier Description, Definition, Explanation, and Tips
FA	**Left hand, thumb**
	Definition: Append modifier FA when the provider performs a procedure on the thumb of the left hand.
	Explanation: Modifier FA illustrates a procedure that the provider performs on the thumb of the left hand. This modifier is appropriate for surgical and diagnostic services but not appropriate for Evaluation and Management, or E/M, services.
	HCPCS level II modifiers apply to codes for procedures that the provider performs on paired organs, like eyelids, fingers, or toes. These modifiers help to prevent denials when the provider submits duplicate HCPCS codes to report separate procedures on different sites or different sides of the body.
	Tips: For Medicare purposes, all line items with identical modifiers are subject to policies for proper coding except line items with the modifiers F1 to F9, which are not subject to the edit. However, they are subject to additional edits based on the specific use of the modifier as defined in other instructions from the Centers for Medicare and Medicaid Services, or CMS.
FB	**Item provided without cost to provider, supplier or practitioner, or full credit received for replaced device (examples, but not limited to, covered under warranty, replaced due to defect, free samples)**
	Definition: Append modifier FB with the facility charge for a surgery when a provider furnishes a device at no cost or when there is a full credit for a replacement device. This modifier triggers a reduced Ambulatory Payment Classification, or APC, payment when a provider reports the code on claims subject to the outpatient prospective payment system, or OPPS.
	Explanation: Modifier FB identifies the replacement of an implanted item or device with a device for which the provider incurs no cost or when the provider replaces an implanted device with a device for which they receive a full credit in the amount of the cost of the replaced device. Modifier FB may extend to nuclear medicine procedures when the provider obtains the associated diagnostic radiopharmaceutical at no cost. Append this modifier only when the supplier or provider makes the item available without cost or the facility receives an entire credit for the cost of the item.
	Always append modifier FB to the surgical procedure code, and not the item code. If the provider reports the modifier with the device code instead of the procedure code, the entire claim will be returned.
	Tips: Report modifier FC when the facility does not receive full credit for the cost of the item but receives a partial credit for the replaced device.
FC	**Partial credit received for replaced device**
	Definition: Append modifier FC when a facility furnishes a device and does not incur the full cost of the device such as when the provider receives a manufacturer credit of 50 percent or more of the cost of the device.
	Explanation: Modifier FC identifies that the provider receives a partial credit of 50 percent or more of the cost of a device for a replaced device. A provider appends this modifier for a new replacement device where the provider receives a discount of at least half or more of the cost of an item such as those under warranty, recall, or field action. Always append modifier FB to the surgical procedure code, and not the item code.
	At the time of device replacement, the provider may not know the amount of credit the manufacturer will provide for the device, or whether he will provide any discount at all. The facility has the option of either submitting the claim immediately without the FC modifier, or submitting a claim adjustment with the FC modifier at a later date once the credit determination is made. Or the facility may hold the claim until it is sure of the status of the credit.
	Tips: Medicare reduces their payment by 50 percent of the estimated cost of the device included in the procedure payment in cases in which the facility reports that it receives a credit of 50 percent or more of the cost of the new replacement device by appending the FC modifier to the device implantation procedure HCPCS code.
FP	**Service provided as part of family planning program**
	Definition: Append modifier FP to a code when reporting an annual family planning examination.
	Explanation: Modifier FP identifies that the services the provider furnishes is part of a family planning program. As a rule, providers append modifier FP only when reporting for the annual family planning examination. The provider reports the FP modifier with the code he reports for the family planning service.
	Tips: A provider omits modifier FP when reporting for all other family planning services, such as evaluation and management services, laboratory services, and anesthesia services.
FX	**X-ray taken using film**
	Definition: Append modifier FX to a radiology code to indicate that an X-ray is film.
	Explanation: Modifier FX indicates that the provider took an X-ray using film, as opposed to digital radiography, which uses digital X-ray sensors to produce an X-ray image.
	Tips: Append modifier FY to a radiology code to indicate that a CT scan was performed using cassette-based (film) imaging.
	For any radiology service, be sure to determine if you need to append other modifiers to the radiology code, such as modifiers LT (left), RT (right), 50 (bilateral), 26 (professional component), or TC (technical component). The circumstances of each encounter will dictate appropriate modifier usage, along with each payer's requirements. Be sure to check specific payer guidelines for acceptable modifiers.

                CPT® is a registered trademark of the American Medical Association. All rights reserved.

Mod	Modifier Description, Definition, Explanation, and Tips
FY	**X-ray taken using computed radiography technology/cassette-based imaging** **Definition:** Append modifier FY to a radiology code to indicate that a digital image was created using cassette-based imaging, such as a phosphor imaging plate (IP), rather than conventional film. **Explanation:** Providers are required to append modifier FY to a radiology code when the imaging involves cassette-based imaging. Medicare payments for cassette-based imaging are reduced by 7% until 2023 and 10% thereafter. The imaging plate is reusable and requires no chemicals or darkroom. Cassette-based imaging involves using an imaging plate that has a phosphorus layer which, when exposed to X-ray or gamma radiation, captures and stores the image. The plate is placed in a scanner, and the image is released when a laser beam is focused on the plate. The image data is converted into electrical signals which are digitized and displaced on a monitor for the radiologist to read (interpret) the image. The digitized image can be saved like any digital file, and the plate is erased to be reused. **Tips:** Append modifier FY to a radiology code to indicate that imaging was performed using a phosphor imaging plate or cassette-based imaging. For any radiology service, be sure to determine if you need to append other modifiers to the radiology code, such as modifiers LT (left), RT (right), 50 (bilateral), 26 (professional component), or TC (technical component). The circumstances of each encounter will dictate appropriate modifier usage, along with each payer's requirements. Be sure to check specific payer guidelines for acceptable modifiers.
G0	**Telehealth services for diagnosis, evaluation, or treatment, of symptoms of an acute stroke** **Definition:** Append modifier G0 (G-zero) to codes for diagnosis, evaluation, or treatment of an acute stroke via an audio or video telecommunications system. **Explanation:** Modifier G0 (G-zero) denotes that a provider diagnosed, evaluated, or treated a patient for an acute stroke remotely using an audio and/or video telecommunication system. **Tips:** CMS removed restrictions on geographic locations and types of sites where acute stroke telehealth services can be furnished, so telehealth services for acute stroke may be provided to patients in both rural and urban areas. In addition, mobile stroke units may qualify as originating sites for purposes of diagnosis, evaluation, or treatment of symptoms of an acute stroke. Whether an ambulance equipped with an audio and/or video telecommunication system qualifies as a mobile stroke unit is uncertain. Check with CMS and payers if uncertain that a code qualifies for this modifier.
G1	**Most recent URR reading of less than 60** **Definition:** Append modifier G1 to a code for a hemodialysis patient when the provider measures the urea reduction ratio, or URR, and the reading is less than 60. **Explanation:** Modifier G1 illustrates the measurement of the urea reduction ratio, or URR, in a patient undergoing hemodialysis for end stage renal disease, or ESRD. When the kidneys fail to perform their function, dialysis becomes important to remove waste products from the blood. The provider tests the patient's blood to ensure that the dialysis is removing the waste products effectively. The provider takes two blood samples, one at the beginning of treatment and the second at the end of dialysis, and compares them. Any reduction in urea due to dialysis is known as the urea reduction ratio, or URR. Use G1 to report a reading of less than 60. Providers most commonly append this modifier to 90999, Unlisted dialysis procedure, inpatient or outpatient. It is not necessary to use the modifier on every code, but facilities should be sure to include the modifier on at least one claim line for Medicare. The modifier can affect the processing of the payment of the code. **Tips:** Select the proper modifier from G1 to G5 based on the reading. When using modifier G1, you should remember that the provider measures the ratio of urea reduction in a patient undergoing hemodialysis, and the reading is less than 60. Watch situations where G1 to G5 are not applicable because of the number of dialysis sessions. For example, when modifier G6, ESRD patient for whom less than six dialysis sessions have been provided in a month, applies for Medicare claims instead of the G1 to G5 modifiers due to the number of patient dialysis sessions. Medicare requires all hemodialysis claims to show the most recent urea reduction ratio for a patient undergoing dialysis. The dialysis facility should monitor the URR monthly in patients who are admitted in the facility. Monitoring of URR in home patients should take place at least quarterly.

Mod	Modifier Description, Definition, Explanation, and Tips
G2	**Most recent URR reading of 60 to 64.9** **Definition:** Append modifier G2 to a code for hemodialysis patients when the provider measures the urea reduction ratio and the reading is 60 to 64.9. **Explanation:** Modifier G2 illustrates the measurement of urea reduction ratio, or URR, in a patient undergoing hemodialysis for end stage renal disease, called ESRD. When the kidneys fail to perform their function, dialysis becomes important to remove waste products from the blood. The provider tests the patient's blood to ensure that the dialysis is removing the waste products effectively. The provider takes two blood samples, one at the beginning and the second at the end of dialysis, and compares them. Any reduction in urea due to dialysis is known as urea reduction ratio, URR. Use G2 for a reading of 60 to 64.9. **Tips:** Select the proper modifier from G1 to G5 based on the reading. When using modifier G2, you should remember that the provider measures the ratio of urea reduction in a patient undergoing hemodialysis, and the reading ranges from 60 to 64.9. Watch for when G6, ESRD patient for whom less than six dialysis sessions have been provided in a month, applies for Medicare claims instead of G1 to G5 based on the number of dialysis sessions. Medicare requires all hemodialysis claims to show the most recent urea reduction ratio for a patient undergoing dialysis. The dialysis facility should monitor the URR monthly in patients who are admitted in the facility. Monitoring of URR in home patients should take place at least quarterly. Providers most commonly append this modifier to 90999, Unlisted dialysis procedure, inpatient or outpatient. It is not necessary to use the modifier on every claim line, but facilities should be sure to include the modifier on at least one revenue code claim line for Medicare. The modifier can affect the processing of the payment of the code.
G3	**Most recent URR reading of 65 to 69.9** **Definition:** Append modifier G3 to a code for hemodialysis patients when the provider measures the urea reduction ratio and the reading is 65 to 69.9. **Explanation:** Modifier G3 illustrates the measurement of urea reduction ratio, or URR, in a patient undergoing hemodialysis for end stage renal disease, called ESRD. When the kidneys fail to perform their function, dialysis becomes important to remove waste products from the blood. The provider tests the patient's blood to ensure that the dialysis is removing the waste products effectively. The provider takes two blood samples, one at the beginning and the second at the end of dialysis, and compares them. Any reduction in urea due to dialysis is known as urea reduction ratio, URR. Use G3 for a reading of 65 to 69.9. **Tips:** Select the proper modifier from G1 to G5 based on the reading. When using modifier G3, you should remember that the provider measures the ratio of urea reduction in a patient undergoing hemodialysis, and the reading ranges from 65 to 65.9. Watch for when G6, ESRD patient for whom less than six dialysis sessions have been provided in a month, applies for Medicare claims instead of G1 to G5 based on the number of dialysis sessions. Medicare requires all hemodialysis claims to show the most recent urea reduction ratio for a patient undergoing dialysis. The dialysis facility should monitor the URR monthly in patients who are admitted in the facility. Monitoring of URR in home patients should take place at least quarterly. Providers most commonly append this modifier to 90999, Unlisted dialysis procedure, inpatient or outpatient. It is not necessary to use the modifier on every claim line, but facilities should be sure to include the modifier on at least one revenue code claim line for Medicare. The modifier can affect the processing of the payment of the code.
G4	**Most recent URR reading of 70 to 74.9** **Definition:** Append modifier G4 to a code for hemodialysis patients when the provider measures the urea reduction ratio and the reading is 70 to 74.9. **Explanation:** Modifier G4 illustrates the measurement of urea reduction ratio, or URR, in a patient undergoing hemodialysis for end stage renal disease, called ESRD. When the kidneys fail to perform their function, dialysis becomes important to remove waste products from the blood. The provider tests the patient's blood to ensure that the dialysis is removing the waste products effectively. The provider takes two blood samples, one at the beginning and the second at the end of dialysis, and compares them. Any reduction in urea due to dialysis is known as urea reduction ratio, URR. Use G4 for a reading of 70 to 74.9. **Tips:** Select the proper modifier from G1 to G5 based on the reading. When using modifier G4, you should remember that the provider measures the ratio of urea reduction in a patient undergoing hemodialysis, and the reading ranges from 70 to 74.9. Watch for when G6, ESRD patient for whom less than six dialysis sessions have been provided in a month, applies for Medicare claims instead of G1 to G5 based on the number of dialysis sessions. Medicare requires all hemodialysis claims to show the most recent urea reduction ratio for a patient undergoing dialysis. The dialysis facility should monitor the URR monthly in patients who are admitted in the facility. Monitoring of URR in home patients should take place at least quarterly. Providers most commonly append this modifier to 90999, Unlisted dialysis procedure, inpatient or outpatient. It is not necessary to use the modifier on every claim line, but facilities should be sure to include the modifier on at least one revenue code claim line for Medicare. The modifier can affect the processing of the payment of the code.

Mod	Modifier Description, Definition, Explanation, and Tips
G5	**Most recent URR reading of 75 or greater** **Definition:** Append modifier G5 to a code for hemodialysis patients when the provider measures the urea reduction ratio and the reading is greater than 75. **Explanation:** Modifier G5 illustrates the measurement of urea reduction ratio, or URR, in a patient undergoing hemodialysis for end stage renal disease, called ESRD. When the kidneys fail to perform their function, dialysis becomes important to remove waste products from the blood. The provider tests the patient's blood to ensure that the dialysis is removing the waste products effectively. The provider takes two blood samples, one at the beginning and the second at the end of dialysis, and compares them. Any reduction in urea due to dialysis is known as urea reduction ratio, URR. Use G5 for a reading greater than 75. **Tips:** Select the proper modifier from G1 to G5 based on the reading. When using modifier G5, you should remember that the provider measures the ratio of urea reduction in a patient undergoing hemodialysis, and the reading is greater than 75. Watch for when G6, ESRD patient for whom less than six dialysis sessions have been provided in a month, applies for Medicare claims instead of G1 to G5 based on the number of dialysis sessions. Medicare requires all hemodialysis claims to show the most recent urea reduction ratio for a patient undergoing dialysis. The dialysis facility should monitor the URR monthly in patients who are admitted in the facility. Monitoring of URR in home patients should take place at least quarterly. Providers most commonly append this modifier to 90999, Unlisted dialysis procedure, inpatient or outpatient. It is not necessary to use the modifier on every claim line, but facilities should be sure to include the modifier on at least one revenue code claim line for Medicare. The modifier can affect the processing of the payment of the code.
G6	**ESRD patient for whom less than six dialysis sessions have been provided in a month** **Definition:** Append modifier G6 to a code to show that the patient has had fewer than six sessions of dialysis in a month. Use this modifier for patients with end stage renal disease, or ESRD. **Explanation:** Modifier G6 represents that a patient has undergone fewer than six sessions of dialysis in a month for ESRD. When the kidneys fail to perform their function, dialysis becomes important to remove waste products from the blood. **Tips:** If the provider confirms the patient had dialysis on fewer than six days in a month, modifier G6 applies. Watch for when G6 applies for Medicare claims instead of G1 to G5 for urea reduction ratio based on the number of dialysis sessions. Medicare requires a modifier from G1 to G6 for all hemodialysis claims as part of data collection on the most recent urea reduction ratio for a patient undergoing dialysis. The dialysis facility should monitor the URR monthly in patients who are admitted in the facility. Monitoring of URR in home patients should take place at least quarterly. Providers most commonly append this modifier to 90999, Unlisted dialysis procedure, inpatient or outpatient. It is not necessary to use the modifier on every claim line, but facilities should be sure to include the modifier on at least one revenue code claim line for Medicare. The modifier can affect the processing of the payment of the code.
G7	**Pregnancy resulted from rape or incest or pregnancy certified by physician as life threatening** **Definition:** Append modifier G7 to an abortion code in cases of pregnancy that result from rape or incest, or when the provider confirms the pregnancy is dangerous for the patient's life. **Explanation:** Modifier G7 represents pregnancy due to rape or incest, or pregnancy that may pose a threat to the woman's life for reasons such as illness or injury. Medicare covers abortions when the patient's life is in danger, and the medical documentation should justify that the pregnancy was a danger to the patient's life. Medicare also covers abortions in cases of rape or incest. **Tips:** Check payer requirements for the codes to which modifier G7 applies. Typical codes include induced abortion codes 59840 to 59857 and 59866, Multifetal pregnancy reduction. If the provider bills these codes without modifier G7, Medicare will not reimburse the claims. Medicare will not reimburse abortions unless the pregnancy is the result of rape or incest, or the pregnancy is life threatening due to patient illness or condition, which may be the result of the pregnancy.

Mod	Modifier Description, Definition, Explanation, and Tips
G8	**Monitored anesthesia care (MAC) for deep complex, complicated, or markedly invasive surgical procedure** **Definition:** Append modifier G8 when the provider performs monitored anesthesia care, called MAC, for a procedure that is deep complex, complicated, or distinctly invasive. **Explanation:** Modifier G8 depicts monitored anesthesia care, or MAC, for a patient undergoing an invasive and complex surgical procedure. The provider administers MAC during a diagnostic or therapeutic procedure. He regularly monitors the physiologic functions during the administration of MAC. The medical record should justify the diagnosis that corresponds to the administration of monitored anesthesia as well as the complex or particularly invasive nature of the surgical procedure. **Tips:** Payers may define the codes the provider may use this modifier with certain anesthesia codes. Examples may include only certain anesthesia codes, 00300, 00400, and 00920. Check payer policies for specific codes. Providers generally report G8 secondary to modifiers AA, Anesthesia services performed personally by anesthesiologist, and QX, CRNA service: with medical direction by a physician. You should not use modifier QS, Monitored anesthesia care service, along with G8 because the latter indicates that the provider has given MAC.
G9	**Monitored anesthesia care for patient who has history of severe cardio-pulmonary condition** **Definition:** Append modifier G9 when the provider performs monitored anesthesia care, called MAC, for a patient with a severe condition relating to the heart and lungs. **Explanation:** Modifier G9 depicts monitored anesthesia care, or MAC, for a patient who has a history of a severe cardiopulmonary condition. The provider administers MAC during a diagnostic or therapeutic procedure. He regularly monitors the physiologic functions during the administration of MAC. The medical record should justify the diagnosis that corresponds to the administration of monitored anesthesia as well as the nature of the cardiopulmonary condition. **Tips:** You should report this modifier with anesthesia codes when appropriate for the patient. Providers generally report G9 secondary to modifiers AA, Anesthesia service performed personally by anesthesiologist, and QX, CRNA service: with medical direction by a physician. You should not use modifier QS, Monitored anesthesia care service, along with G9 because the latter indicates that the provider has given MAC.
GA	**Waiver of liability statement issued as required by payer policy, individual case** **Definition:** Append modifier GA to a code when a payer requires the provider to present an advance beneficiary notice, or ABN, before the patient receives an item or service the provider expects Medicare not to cover. **Explanation:** The provider appends modifier GA to a code to indicate the patient's receipt of an advance beneficiary notice, or ABN, also known as a waiver of liability, for items or services for which the provider believes Medicare will not consider reasonable and necessary and thus deny payment. Medicare denial may involve services subject to a local coverage determination, or LCD, a denial based on the policies of a particular intermediary or carrier. The intent of the ABN is to inform the patient that Medicare certainly or most probably will not pay for an item or service and will assign financial responsibility to the patient for the charges. **Tips:** You can append modifier GA with a code even when the patient refuses to sign an ABN. Medicare prohibits the routine use of an ABN except for certain services that have a frequency limit on coverage.
GB	**Claim being resubmitted for payment because it is no longer covered under a global payment demonstration** **Definition:** Append modifier GB to a code when the provider resubmits a claim for payment because a global payment demonstration, a type of bundling program, does not cover the service anymore. **Explanation:** Modifier GB identifies services for which a provider submits a claim under a global payment demonstration and later determines the patient or the service did not qualify for inclusion, so he resubmits the claim under the traditional fee for service program. Global payment demonstration projects reimburse a package price for a group of services based on the expected costs for an episode of care, as a combined quality improvement and cost reduction measure. The original claim may have been a no pay claim, one that identifies services or items for informational purposes without expectation of reimbursement. **Tips:** If another modifier defines the services more distinctly, use GB as the secondary modifier. Modifier GB is an informational modifier, and the provider may submit it with any HCPCS or CPT® code.

Mod	Modifier Description, Definition, Explanation, and Tips
GC	**This service has been performed in part by a resident under the direction of a teaching physician**
	Definition: Append modifier GC to a code when a resident performs any portion of a service under the guidance of a teaching provider.
	Explanation: Modifier GC denotes that a resident, a medical graduate working in a teaching facility and under the supervision of a teaching provider, performs a billable service. The teaching provider must be present during the major part of the service and be readily available for other parts of the service. The medical record must include notes from both the resident and the teaching provider, with the teaching provider's notes commenting on the resident's documentation, attesting to the resident's findings, correcting or elaborating as necessary, also known as an attestation. Both the resident and the teaching provider must sign and date the documentation.
	Tips: Modifier GC is an informational modifier, and the provider may submit it with any CPT® or HCPCS code.
	A cosignature alone does not satisfy CMS guidelines for documenting the presence and extent of involvement of the teaching provider.
	You can report a service with modifier GC when the teaching provider assists the resident during an entire procedure and reexamines the patient after the procedure, as well.
	Medicare does not consider a lab pathologist as a teaching provider.
GE	**This service has been performed by a resident without the presence of a teaching physician under the primary care exception**
	Definition: Append modifier GE to a code when a resident sees a patient in an outpatient, or primary care, setting in the absence of a teaching provider.
	Explanation: Modifier GE denotes that the resident renders the services under Medicare's primary care exception rule, which reduces the restrictions on the physical presence requirement for teaching providers. Under certain conditions, Medicare will pay for the three lowest levels of Evaluation and Management, or E/M, services for outpatients seen by a resident without the presence of a teaching provider. The medical record has to demonstrate that the resident observes and appropriately documents the patient's present illness and physical examination and follows a plan of care. The resident must sign the medical documentation. Although the resident provides the E/M service in the absence of the teaching provider, the teaching provider reviews the patient's records and discusses the case with the resident.
	Tips: For new patients, append modifier GE to New Patient Office or Other Outpatient Services codes 99202, and 99203. For existing patients, append this modifier to Established Patient Office or Other Outpatient Services codes 99211, 99212 and 99213.
	Medicare does not reimburse the service if the provider bills modifier GE with CPT® codes other than those given above.
	Medicare does not reimburse modifier GE if the provider bills it with HCPCS codes G0438, Annual wellness visit, including personal preventive plan service, first visit, or G0439, Annual wellness visit, including personal preventive plan service, subsequent visit.
GF	**Non-physician (e.g., nurse practitioner (NP), certified registered nurse anesthetist (CRNA), certified registered nurse (CRN), clinical nurse specialist (CNS), physician assistant (PA)) services in a critical access hospital**
	Definition: Append modifier GF to a code when a nonphysician provider performs a service in a critical access hospital.
	Explanation: Modifier GF denotes that a nonphysician provider, such as a nurse practitioner, certified registered nurse anesthetist, certified registered nurse, clinical nurse practitioner, or a physician assistant, renders a service in critical access hospital, a facility Medicare certifies under different conditions of participation in the Medicare program than an acute care facility. The nonphysician provider delivers the service in the absence of a physician provider. The medical record must show adequate documentation of the patient's present illness and physical examination and follow a plan of care. The nonphysician provider must sign the medical documentation.
	Tips: Modifier GF is an informational modifier, and the provider may submit it with any CPT® or HCPCS codes.
	Medicare reimburses 85 percent of the actual service charges to a nonphysician provider.
	The guidelines for reporting the services of a certified registered nurse anesthetist, or CRNA, may change, so check with your payer for specific information.

Mod	Modifier Description, Definition, Explanation, and Tips
GG	**Performance and payment of a screening mammogram and diagnostic mammogram on the same patient, same day** **Definition:** Append modifier GG to a code when the provider performs two distinct mammograms, both screening and diagnostic, on a patient on the same date of service. **Explanation:** Modifier GG denotes that the provider performs screening mammography, an X-ray of the breast done for early detection of breast cancer, and during that exam detects an abnormality for which he performs diagnostic mammography on the same date of service to confirm the presence of cancer or any other defect. The provider does not require a separate order from the treating provider to perform the diagnostic mammography. **Tips:** If the provider converts a screening mammography to a diagnostic mammography but does not perform separate mammography exams, append to the relevant code modifier GH, Diagnostic mammogram converted from screening mammogram on same day. Medicare reimburses both screening and diagnostic mammography services as the modifier is for the purpose of discovering any abnormality in the breast. Medicare denies reimbursement for an add on code if the provider bills it without an appropriate mammography code. Both mammography codes with the appropriate add on code should appear on the same claim. Also, Medicare does not reimburse the service if the provider performs the second mammography only as a quality check or because of a system failure. If the screening services are self referred, the provider should give his own national provider identifier, or NPI, and not the referring provider's NPI for the service to be reimbursable. If the provider takes additional views on the same date of service because of the presence of an implant, payers may consider it as diagnostic views done on the same date. Payers may restrict the codes the provider may use with this modifier to certain mammography codes. Check payer policies for specific codes.
GH	**Diagnostic mammogram converted from screening mammogram on same day** **Definition:** Append modifier GH to a code when the provider performs a single mammogram that begins as a screening mammogram but converts it to a diagnostic mammogram. **Explanation:** Modifier GH denotes that the provider converts a screening mammography, an X-ray of the breast done for early detection of breast cancer, to a diagnostic mammography in a patient on the same date of service as a single exam This may occur if the patient presents for a screening mammogram due to an abnormality, and the provider changes the study from screening to diagnostic. The provider does not take any additional views during the exam. **Tips:** Append modifier GH to a single diagnostic mammography code. Medicare will pay for the diagnostic mammography only and not the screening mammography. If separate mammograms are performed on the same date of service, both screening and diagnostic, due to the discovery of an abnormality on a screening mammogram that requires further delineation, for example, report both exams and append modifier GG to the add on mammography code. Payers may restrict the use of this modifier to certain mammography codes. Check payer policies for specific codes.
GJ	**"Opt-out" physician or practitioner emergency or urgent service** **Definition:** Append modifier GJ to a code when a provider who has elected not to participate in the Medicare program renders services to a patient who presents with an emergency situation. **Explanation:** Modifier GJ denotes a service by a provider rendering emergency treatment to a Medicare patient and has no personal contract with the patient. The provider must submit the claim to Medicare on the patient's behalf and may not bill the patient more than Medicare's limiting charge. Medicare reimburses the patient directly for an unassigned claim. To submit an assigned claim, a provider can complete a CMS855 enrollment without impact on his opt out status for other services. The medical documentation must justify the emergency or urgent nature of the services to the patient. **Tips:** If the opt out provider asks the patient to return for a followup visit, he must ask the patient to sign a personal contract for these services in order to charge the patient for services Medicare will not pay. However, if the patient requires followup of the emergency care, Medicare would continue to pay until the time the patient no longer requires such care.

Mod	Modifier Description, Definition, Explanation, and Tips
GK	**Reasonable and necessary item/service associated with a GA or GZ modifier** **Definition:** Append modifier GK to a code, in addition to modifier GA or GZ, for upgrades to durable medical equipment, or DME, items or services that the provider deems medically necessary but exceed medical necessity under Medicare's coverage requirements. **Explanation:** The provider appends modifier GK to a code for an item or service associated with modifier GA, Carrier judgment Waiver of liability statement issued as required by payer policy, individual case, or GZ, Item or service expected to be denied as not reasonable and necessary, such as an upgrade to DME. If the provider expects to bill the patient for the difference in the cost, he presents an advance beneficiary notice, or ABN, to the patient and submits the claim with both modifiers. Medicare automatically denies the claim line with modifier GA on the basis of medical necessity but processes the claim line with modifier GK to allow the provider to bill the usual and customary fee for the upgraded items he supplies. Use modifier GZ in association with GK when an ABN is neither obtained nor required. **Tips:** If the provider doesn't intend to charge the patient for the difference in the cost of an upgrade, append modifier GL, Medically unnecessary upgrade provided instead of nonupgraded item, no charge, no advance beneficiary notice, or ABN. Do not use modifier GK for institutional claims that include the use of equipment and supplies, lab and radiology services, and other included items or services. You should append HCPCS modifiers in order on the claim, with GA or GZ before the use of GK. Always give a detailed description of the DME along with the manufacturer and the model number in the claim. Individual payers may specify use of modifier KX, Requirements specified in the medical policy have been met, along with modifier GK. Check with the payer to be sure. Medicare will reject a claim with modifier GK when modifier GA or GZ does not accompany it.
GL	**Medically unnecessary upgrade provided instead of non-upgraded item, no charge, no advance beneficiary notice (ABN)** **Definition:** Append modifier GL to a code for an upgrade to durable medical equipment, or DME, items that the provider deems medically necessary but exceed medical necessity under Medicare's coverage requirements. The provider does not charge the patient for the difference in cost and does not present an advance beneficiary notice, or ABN. **Explanation:** Modifier GL denotes that the provider upgrades a DME item but does not plan to charge the patient for the difference in the cost. The provider essentially bills Medicare for the cost of a nonupgraded item instead of the item he actually provides. The provider adds modifier GL to the HCPCS code that represents the nonupgraded item. **Tips:** Modifier GL does not require submission of an ABN. Individual payers may specify use of modifier KX, Requirements specified in the medical policy have been met, along with modifier GK. Check with the payer to be sure.
GM	**Multiple patients on one ambulance trip** **Definition:** Append modifier GM to a code for the transport of a patient by an ambulance that transports additional patients during the same trip. **Explanation:** Modifier GM denotes the situation in which an ambulance transports multiple patients during a single trip. The medical documentation must include the total number of patients and the particulars of each. The provider should submit the number of miles traveled by each patient along with the origin and destination modifier in the primary position and append modifier GM as the secondary modifier. **Tips:** You should append modifier GM only with ambulance transport claims. Append modifier GM even when only one of the transported patients is a Medicare beneficiary.
GN	**Services delivered under an outpatient speech language pathology plan of care** **Definition:** Append modifier GN to a code when the provider renders services that are part of a speech and language pathology plan of care for an outpatient. **Explanation:** Modifier GN denotes services that are part of an outpatient speech and language pathology plan of care. The provider carries out the service in an outpatient setting. The medical documentation must include a diagnosis code that indicates the patient is suffering from a speech disorder. **Tips:** Append modifier GN only with codes on the list of applicable therapy services for speech and language pathology and that are part of the plan of care for that patient. Medicare pays for services with modifier GN only when the patient receives these services as an outpatient.

Mod	Modifier Description, Definition, Explanation, and Tips
GO	**Services delivered under an outpatient occupational therapy plan of care** **Definition:** Append modifier GO to a code when the provider renders services that are part of an occupational therapy plan of care for an outpatient. **Explanation:** Modifier GO denotes services that are part of an outpatient occupational therapy plan of care. The provider carries out the service in an outpatient setting. The medical documentation must include a diagnosis code that is consistent with a condition that requires occupational therapy. **Tips:** Append modifier GO only with codes on the list of applicable therapy services for occupational therapy and that are part of the plan of care for that patient. Medicare pays for services with modifier GO only when the patient receives these services as an outpatient.
GP	**Services delivered under an outpatient physical therapy plan of care** **Definition:** Append modifier GP to a code when the provider renders services that are part of a physical therapy plan of care for an outpatient. **Explanation:** Modifier GP denotes services that are part of an outpatient physical therapy plan of care. The provider carries out the service in an outpatient setting. The medical documentation must include a diagnosis code that is consistent with a condition that requires physical therapy. **Tips:** Append modifier GP only with codes on the list of applicable therapy services for physical therapy and that are part of the plan of care for that patient. Medicare pays for services with modifier GP only when the patient receives these services as an outpatient.
GQ	**Via asynchronous telecommunications system** **Definition:** Append modifier GQ for services rendered to a patient via an asynchronous telecommunications system, one that does not involve live two way communication. **Explanation:** Modifier GQ denotes healthcare services provided via an asynchronous communication method. Asynchronous communication does not take place in real time. An example of delivery of a service via asynchronous communication includes a provider at a distant location, even in another state, who receives X-ray images transmitted across a secure network and then transmits the report of his reading of the images for later review by the patient's primary care provider. An exchange of email between a patient and a provider also constitute asynchronous telecommunication services. **Tips:** See payer guidelines for specific codes that require or are eligible for the GQ modifier.
GR	**This service was performed in whole or in part by a resident in a department of veterans affairs medical Centers or clinic, supervised in accordance with VA policy** **Definition:** Append modifier GR to codes for services rendered to a patient by a resident provider in a Veterans Administration, or VA, facility. **Explanation:** Modifier GR denotes services rendered in a VA facility by a resident provider, a medical graduate working under the supervision of an attending provider. The VA facility appends modifier GR to the appropriate HCPCS code for the service and submits the claim under the name of the attending provider. **Tips:** Modifier GR on VA claims has the same consequences as modifier GC, This service has been performed in part by a resident under the direction of a teaching physician, and modifier GE, This service has been performed by a resident without the presence of a teaching physician under the primary care exception. VA claims do not use modifier GC, This service has been performed in part by a resident under the direction of a teaching physician, or modifier GE, This service has been performed by a resident without the presence of a teaching physician under the primary care exception modifiers.
GS	**Dosage of erythropoietin stimulating agent has been reduced and maintained in response to hematocrit or hemoglobin level** **Definition:** Append modifier GS to a code when the provider reduces and maintains the dosage of erythropoietin, a hormone that stimulates the production of red blood cells, in response to an elevation in the level of hematocrit or hemoglobin in a patient with anemia of chronic kidney disease. **Explanation:** Modifier QS denotes a reduction in the dose of erythropoietin, or EPO, in response to an elevation in hematocrit, which measures the volume of red blood cells, or hemoglobin, which measures the amount of hemoglobin, a protein in red blood cells, for the treatment of anemia of chronic kidney disease. Medicare closely monitors the administration of erythropoietin stimulating agents, or ESAs, which at higher levels than necessary are ineffective and lead to complications, such as blood clots. **Tips:** Payers may designate only specific codes the provider may use with this modifier, such as injection codes J0881, J0882, J0885, and Q4081. Check payer policies for specific codes. Reimbursement depends upon the dosage reported, but Medicare automatically reduces reimbursement by 25 percent if the provider submits the claim without modifier GS.

Mod	Modifier Description, Definition, Explanation, and Tips
GT	**Via interactive audio and video telecommunication systems** **Definition:** Append modifier GT for telehealth, the use of an interactive audio and video communication system between a distant provider and the patient to execute a plan of care. **Explanation:** Modifier GT denotes a telehealth system, real time audiovisual conferencing between a patient and provider, in which a provider at a distant site provides healthcare services for a patient at a different location, including an examination. The patient must be an active participant in a telehealth visit, but it is not necessary for the provider to personally perform all portions of a telehealth service, as his clinical staff may provide some services. **Tips:** Providers most commonly append this modifier to HCPCS code Q3014, Telehealth originating site facility fee. It is not necessary to use the modifier on every claim line, but facilities should be sure to include the modifier on at least one revenue code claim line for Medicare. The modifier can affect the processing of the payment of the code. Medicare reimburses modifier GT to only providers who have a license to provide telehealth services under the laws of their state. Payers may designate only specific codes the provider may use with this modifier, such as office visit codes 99202 through 99215, neurobehavioral status exam code 96116, and individual medical nutrition therapy codes G0270, 97802, and 97803. Check payer policies for specific codes.
GU	**Waiver of liability statement issued as required by payer policy, routine notice** **Definition:** Append modifier GU to a code when a payer requires the provider to present an advance beneficiary notice, or ABN, as a routine notice before the patient receives an item or service the provider expects Medicare not to cover. **Explanation:** Modifier GU indicates the patient's receipt of an advance beneficiary notice, or ABN, also known as a waiver of liability, as a routine notice for items or services that the provider believes Medicare will not consider reasonable and necessary and thus deny payment. The intent of the ABN is to inform the patient that Medicare certainly or most probably will not pay for an item or service and will assign financial responsibility to the patient for the charges. Medicare generally prohibits routine notices except for items and services that are experimental, subject to frequency limitations for coverage, or always denied for medical necessity. Durable medical equipment and supplies without a supplier number also fall under this exception. **Tips:** For an ABN issued for a specific item or service, rather than as a routine notice, report modifier GA, Waiver of liability statement issued as required by payer policy, individual case.
GV	**Attending physician not employed or paid under arrangement by the patient's hospice provider** **Definition:** A provider appends modifier GV to report that the patient's attending physician, is not an employee, or is not volunteering at the hospice provider of the patient. The attending physician may be a doctor specialized in a particular field, or a nurse practitioner. **Explanation:** A provider appends modifier GV when a provider performs a service related to the problem for which a patient was admitted into hospice. This provider is not a part of the hospice provider or their employee and provides services independently of the hospice. **Tips:** A patient, who opts for hospice coverage, waives his Medicare Part B payment for any treatment of terminal illness during the hospice period. However, there is an exception for the provider who attends the patient, referred to as attending physician in the modifier descriptor, who is not an employee of the hospice and is in no way attached to the hospice. The attending provider may also include a nurse practitioner, besides specific specialty providers.
GW	**Service not related to the hospice patient's terminal condition** **Definition:** A provider appends modifier GW to identify a service that the provider renders to a patient that is not related to the patient's terminal condition. **Explanation:** A provider appends modifier GW when the provider delivers a service, not related to the problem for which the patient was admitted into the hospice. This provider is not a part of the hospice or an employee of the hospice and provides the services independently. **Tips:** For Medicare payment, report modifier GW, if the patient's condition for hospice care is not related to the service.
GX	**Notice of liability issued, voluntary under payer policy** **Definition:** Append modifier GX to report issuance of a voluntary, or optional, advance beneficiary notice, or ABN, for any service not covered. **Explanation:** Modifier GX indicates the patient's receipt of a notice of liability, usually in the form of an advance beneficiary notice, or ABN, that is not required by payer policy, to let the patient know of his financial responsibility for items or services that Medicare never covers. The provider can bill the patient for items and services not subject to Medicare coverage whether or not the provider issues an ABN. **Tips:** Medicare reimburses modifier GX only if it is used secondary to modifier TS, Followup service, or modifier GY, Item or service statutorily excluded, does not meet the definition of any Medicare benefit, or for nonMedicare insurers, is not a contract benefit. If the patient has a secondary insurance that pays for the service, Medicare denies the reimbursement so that the provider can then submit the claim to the second payer. Medicare denies the reimbursement of modifier GX if the service is not covered by medical necessity.

Mod	Modifier Description, Definition, Explanation, and Tips
GY	**Item or service statutorily excluded, does not meet the definition of any Medicare benefit or, for Non-Medicare insurers, is not a contract benefit** **Definition:** Append modifier GY to report services and supplies excluded by Medicare regulations or which are not a contract benefit for other payers. **Explanation:** Modifier GY denotes items or services not covered by Medicare under any circumstance, and the provider expects a denial. Medicare does not require the provider to present an advance beneficiary notice, or ABN, to bill the patient for these items or services. Some examples of items and services statutorily excluded by Medicare include acupuncture, cosmetic surgery, hearing aids, and most types of dental care. **Tips:** Modifier GY indicates that a particular service is not covered by Medicare. There is no need to submit an ABN to use modifier GY. You should not use modifier GY with add on codes.
GZ	**Item or service expected to be denied as not reasonable and necessary** **Definition:** Append modifier GZ when the provider expects a Medicare denial for an item or service as not a medical necessity but does not provide the patient with an advance beneficiary notice, or ABN. **Explanation:** Modifier GZ denotes an item or service for which the provider expects Medicare to deny reimbursement as not meeting the requirements of Medicare for medical necessity but for which the provider does not present the patient with an ABN. The provider may not bill the patient for the denied charges but can request a review. **Tips:** This is an informational modifier. Medicare processes claims with modifier GZ just like other claims. If the provider appends both modifier GZ and modifier GA, Waiver of liability statement issued as required by payer policy, individual case, on the same claim line, it is invalid and the claim is not reimbursable.
H9	**Court-ordered** **Definition:** Append modifier H9 to a code to indicate that a particular service was ordered by the court. **Explanation:** Modifier H9 denotes any service a patient undergoes by court order, such as a psychiatric evaluation, substance abuse treatment, foster care services, and others. **Tips:** For court ordered medical testimony, append modifier H9 to 99075, Medical testimony.
HA	**Child/adolescent program** **Definition:** Append modifier HA to designate the delivery of services through a program specifically designed for children and or adolescents. **Explanation:** Modifier HA denotes services a provider renders to a child or adolescent as part of a program designed specifically for children and or adolescents. Medicare does not cover this modifier, but Medicaid programs typically require modifier HA to indicate services provided to a child or adolescent. Specific use of the HA modifier may vary depending upon the program. **Tips:** See payer guidelines for specific codes that require or are eligible for the HA modifier.
HB	**Adult program, non-geriatric** **Definition:** Append modifier HB to designate the delivery of services to adult individuals, not including the elderly, as part of a care program for adults. **Explanation:** Modifier HB denotes services rendered to an adult participant a medical or psychiatric care program designed for adults. These include programs funded by Medicaid and other agencies. Use of the HB modifier may vary depending upon the program. **Tips:** See payer guidelines for specific codes that require or are eligible for the HB modifier.
HC	**Adult program, geriatric** **Definition:** Append modifier HC to designate services given to adult participants in a care program specifically designed for the elderly. **Explanation:** Modifier HC denotes services rendered to adults in a geriatric medical or psychiatric care program. These include programs funded by Medicaid and other agencies. Use of the HC modifier may vary depending upon the program. **Tips:** See payer guidelines for specific codes that require or are eligible for the HC modifier.

Mod	Modifier Description, Definition, Explanation, and Tips
HD	**Pregnant/parenting women's program** **Definition:** A provider appends modifier HD to services designed for pregnant women or women with dependent children. **Explanation:** A provider appends this modifier to identify the services that he provides as a part of a program for women who are pregnant or women who have children. The services may include treatment for postpartum depression screening, or antepartum visits as well as alcohol and or drug detoxification, and behavioral health. **Tips:** Modifier HD is not payable by Medicare.
HE	**Mental health program** **Definition:** Append modifier HE when the provider provides a particular service through a program specifically designed for the provision of mental health services. **Explanation:** Modifier HE denotes a service provided to a participant in a mental health services program, including those administered by state and local agencies. Use of the HE modifier may vary depending upon the program. **Tips:** See payer guidelines for specific codes that require or are eligible for the HE modifier.
HF	**Substance abuse program** **Definition:** Append modifier HF when the provider performs services for a participant in a substance abuse program. **Explanation:** Modifier HF denotes services provided to a participant in a substance abuse program. Specific use of the HF modifier varies depending upon the program and its sponsoring agency and payer. **Tips:** See payer guidelines for specific codes that require or are eligible for the HF modifier.
HG	**Opioid addiction treatment program** **Definition:** Append modifier HG when the provider performs services for a participant in an opioid addiction treatment program. **Explanation:** Modifier HG denotes services provided to a participant in an opioid addiction treatment program, including long term residential programs, outpatient programs, and methadone clinics. Specific use of the HG modifier varies depending upon the program and its sponsoring agency and payer. **Tips:** See payer guidelines for specific codes that require or are eligible for the HG modifier.
HH	**Integrated mental health/substance abuse program** **Definition:** Append modifier HH when the provider performs services for a participant in a combined mental health and substance abuse program. **Explanation:** Modifier HH denotes services provided to a participant in an integrated mental health and substance abuse program, including long term residential programs, outpatient programs, and others. Specific use of the HH modifier varies depending upon the program and its sponsoring agency and payer. **Tips:** See payer guidelines for specific codes that require or are eligible for the HH modifier.
HI	**Integrated mental health and intellectual disability/developmental disabilities program** **Definition:** Append modifier HI when the provider performs services for a participant in a program specifically for individuals with intellectual and or developmental disabilities. **Explanation:** Modifier HI denotes services provided to a participant in an intellectual disability and or developmental disabilities program. Specific use of the HI modifier varies depending upon the program and its sponsoring agency and payer. **Tips:** See payer guidelines for specific codes that require or are eligible for the HI modifier.
HJ	**Employee assistance program** **Definition:** Append modifier HJ when the provider performs services for a participant in an employee assistance program. **Explanation:** Modifier HJ denotes services provided to a participant in an employee assistance program, or EAP. Specific use of the HJ modifier varies depending upon the EAP and its sponsoring agency and payer, which may be a state Medicaid program. **Tips:** See payer guidelines for specific codes that require or are eligible for the HJ modifier.

Mod	Modifier Description, Definition, Explanation, and Tips
HK	**Specialized mental health programs for high-risk populations** **Definition:** Append modifier HK when the provider performs services for a participant in a mental health program designed for groups of people who are at greater risk for mental illness. **Explanation:** Modifier HK denotes services provided to individuals who participate in a specialized mental health program for high risk populations, such as the elderly, low income families, substance abusers, and people with a history of mental illness. Specific use of the HK modifier varies depending upon the program and its sponsoring agency and payer. **Tips:** See payer guidelines for specific codes that require the HK modifier.
HL	**Intern** **Definition:** Append modifier HL to the code when an intern performs a behavioral health service. **Explanation:** Append this modifier to a behavioral health service code to show that the provider is an intern. The condition of the patient may require an intern to render the service. **Tips:** HCPCS modifiers HL through HP identify the level of education of a provider who performs psychological or psychiatric services. These codes are not covered by Medicare, but some carriers may base payment for services on the provider's education level.
HM	**Less than bachelor degree level** **Definition:** Append modifier HM to the code when a provider with less than a bachelor's degree level of education performs a behavioral health service. **Explanation:** Append this modifier to a behavioral health service code to show that the provider holds less than a bachelor's degree level of education. The condition of the patient may require a provider with less than a bachelor's degree level of education to render the service. **Tips:** HCPCS modifiers HL through HP identify the level of education of a provider who performs psychological or psychiatric services. These codes are not covered by Medicare, but some carriers may base payment for services on the provider's education level.
HN	**Bachelor's degree level** **Definition:** Append modifier HN to the code when a provider who holds a bachelor's degree performs a behavioral health service. **Explanation:** Append this modifier to a behavioral health service code to show that the provider holds a bachelor's degree. The condition of the patient may require a provider with a bachelor's degree level of education to render the service. **Tips:** HCPCS modifiers HL through HP identify the level of education of a provider who performs psychological or psychiatric services. These codes are not covered by Medicare, but some carriers may base payment for services on the provider's education level.
HO	**Master's degree level** **Definition:** Append modifier HO to the bill for any behavioral health service by a provider with a master's degree. **Explanation:** Append this modifier to a behavioral health service code to show that the provider holds a master's degree. The condition of the patient may require the provider of master's degree level to render the service. **Tips:** HCPCS modifiers HL through HP identify the level of education of the provider who performs psychological or psychiatric services. These codes are not covered by Medicare, but some carriers do base payment for services on the provider's education level. If the provider is an intern, use modifier HL, Intern. If the provider holds less than a bachelor's degree, append modifier HM, Less than bachelor degree level. If the provider holds a bachelor's degree, append modifier HN, Bachelors degree level. If the provider is of a doctoral level, use modifier HP, Doctoral level. You should append modifier HO with the code H2011, Crisis intervention service, per 15 minutes. This code includes crisis intervention in an emergency setting for patients and the families of patients who exhibit extreme mental duress with disturbed thoughts, mood, or behavior.

Mod	Modifier Description, Definition, Explanation, and Tips
HP	**Doctoral level**
	Definition: Append modifier HP to a bill for any behavioral health service that a provider with a doctoral degree, e.g., PhD, provides to the patient.
	Explanation: Append this modifier to a behavioral health service code to show that the provider holds a doctoral level degree, i.e., PhD.
	The medical documentation should justify the treatment by a provider who holds a doctoral degree. The condition of the patient may require the provider of doctoral level to render the service.
	The doctoral level provider offers services to improve the mental health of the patient.
	Tips: HCPCS modifiers HL through HP identify the level of education of the provider who performs psychological or psychiatric services. These codes are not covered by Medicare, but some carriers do base payment for services on the provider's education level. When using the modifier HP, you should remember that the provider, who renders the service for behavioral health, must be of doctoral level.
	If the provider is an intern, use modifier HL, Intern.
	If the provider holds less than a bachelor's degree, append modifier HM, Less than bachelor degree level.
	If the provider holds a bachelor's degree, append modifier HN, Bachelors degree level.
	If the provider is of a masters degree level, use modifier HO, Masters degree level.
HQ	**Group setting**
	Definition: Append modifier HQ to a service when the provider renders service for behavioral care to patients in a group setting.
	Explanation: Append this modifier to a behavioral health service code to show that the provider rendered the behavioral health services in a group setting.
	The medical documentation should justify the treatment of the patients in a group setting by a provider who is not a physician. The patient's condition may necessitate the service for behavioral healthcare.
	The provider offers this service to improve the mental and behavioral health of the patient in a group setting.
	Tips: You should append modifier HQ with codes that include services such as comprehensive community support, psychosocial rehabilitation, family training, developmental therapy, or group supported living.
HR	**Family/couple with client present**
	Definition: Append modifier HR to a service in which the provider renders therapy to the family or couples in the presence of a client.
	Explanation: Append this modifier to a behavioral health service code to show that the provider offers therapy to a family or couple in the presence of a client.
	The medical documentation must justify the mental health therapy for the family or couple with the client present. The client refers to the patient who requires the therapy. The provider offers mental health therapy to the patient in the presence of his family.
	The provider renders this service to improve the mental and behavioral health of the patient.
	Tips: If the patient is not present at the therapy session, use the modifier HS, Family or couple without client present.
	You should append modifier HR to the services that include services such as mental health therapy, psychiatry, activity therapy, or other health services.
HS	**Family/couple without client present**
	Definition: Append modifier HR to a service in which the provider renders therapy to the family or couple in the absence of a client.
	Explanation: Append this modifier to a behavioral health service code to show that the provider met with the family or partner of a client without the client present.
	The medical documentation must justify the mental health therapy of the families or couple in the absence of a client. The client refers to the patient who needs the therapy.
	The provider renders this service to improve the mental and behavioral health of the patient.
	Tips: If the patient is present for the therapy session, use the modifier HR, Family or couple with client present.
	You should append modifier HS to the services that include services such as mental health therapy, psychiatry, activity therapy, or other health services.

Mod	Modifier Description, Definition, Explanation, and Tips
HT	**Multi-disciplinary team**
	Definition: Append modifier HT to a service when a multidisciplinary team renders service for behavioral care to the patient.
	Explanation: Append this modifier to a behavioral health service code to show that a team of providers with different areas of expertise treated the patient.
	The medical documentation should justify the treatment of the patients by a multidisciplinary team of providers, who are not physicians. The patient's condition may necessitate the service for behavioral healthcare. The multidisciplinary team refers to the group of individuals from different fields and come together for assessment and consultations of patients.
	The providers offer this service to improve the mental and behavioral health of the patient in a multidisciplinary team.
	Tips: You should append modifier HT with codes that include services such as comprehensive community support, psychosocial rehabilitation, family training, developmental therapy, or group supported living.
HU	**Funded by child welfare agency**
	Definition: Append modifier HU to the service when the provider receives funds from a child welfare agency for therapy provided to a patient.
	Explanation: Append this modifier to a behavioral health service code to show that the provider receives funds from a child welfare agency for therapy that he provides patients.
	The medical documentation must validate that the child welfare agency funds the treatment service for the patient. It is the agency that arranges the financing for the therapy that the patient undergoes.
	The provider utilizes the resources from a child welfare agency and offers mental and behavioral healthcare to the patient.
	Tips: HCPCS modifiers HU through HZ identify government and other agency funding for mental health services. When using the modifier HU, you should remember that the child welfare agency funds the service.
	If the state addictions agency funds the service code, use modifier HV, Funded state addictions agency.
	If the provider receives funds from state mental health agency, use modifier HW, Funded by state mental health agency.
	If the county or local agency finances the service code, append modifier HX, Funded by county or local agency.
	If the juvenile justice agency offers money for the service code, append modifier HY, Funded by juvenile justice agency.
	If the criminal justice agency funds the service code, use modifier HZ, Funded by criminal justice agency.
HV	**Funded state addictions agency**
	Definition: Append modifier HV to the service when the provider receives funds from a state addictions agency, to offer therapy to the patients.
	Explanation: Append this modifier to a behavioral health service code to show that the provider receives funds from a state addictions agency for therapy that he offers patients.
	The medical documentation must validate that the state addictions agency funds the treatment service for the patient. It is the agency that arranges the financing for the therapy that the patient undergoes.
	The provider utilizes the resources from a state addictions agency and offers mental and behavioral healthcare to the patient.
	Tips: HCPCS modifiers HU through HZ identify government and other agency funding for mental health services. When using the modifier HV, you should remember that the state addictions agency funds the service.
	If the child welfare agency funds the service code, use modifier HU, Funded by child welfare agency.
	If the provider receives funds from state mental health agency, use modifier HW, Funded by state mental health agency.
	If the county or local agency finances the service code, append modifier HX, Funded by county or local agency.
	If the juvenile justice agency offers money for the service code, append modifier HY, Funded by juvenile justice agency.
	If the criminal justice agency funds the service code, use modifier HZ, Funded by criminal justice agency.

Mod	Modifier Description, Definition, Explanation, and Tips
HW	**Funded by state mental health agency** **Definition:** Append modifier HW to the service when the provider receives funds from a state mental health agency to provide therapy for a patient. **Explanation:** Append this modifier to a behavioral health service code to show that the provider receives funds from a state mental health agency for therapy that he provides patients. The medical documentation must validate that the state mental health agency funds the treatment service for the patient. It is the agency that arranges the financing for the therapy that the patient undergoes. The provider utilizes the resources from state mental health agency and offers mental and behavioral healthcare to the patient. **Tips:** HCPCS modifiers HU through HZ identify government and other agency funding for mental health services. When using the modifier HW, you should remember that the state mental health agency funds the service. If the child welfare agency funds the service code, use modifier HU, Funded by child welfare agency. If the state addictions agency funds the service code, use modifier HV, Funded state addictions agency. If the county or local agency finances the service code, append modifier HX, Funded by county or local agency. If the juvenile justice agency offers money for the service code, append modifier HY, Funded by juvenile justice agency. If the criminal justice agency funds the service code, use modifier HZ, Funded by criminal justice agency.
HX	**Funded by county/local agency** **Definition:** Append modifier HX to the service when the provider receives funds from a county or local agency to provide therapy to a patient. **Explanation:** Append this modifier to a behavioral health service code to show that the provider receives funds from a county or local agency for therapy that he provides patients. The medical documentation must validate that the county or local agency funds the treatment service for the patient. It is the agency that arranges the financing for the therapy that the patient undergoes. The provider utilizes the resources from county or local agency and offers mental and behavioral healthcare to the patient. **Tips:** HCPCS modifiers HU through HZ identify government and other agency funding for mental health services. When using the modifier HX, you should remember that the county or local agency funds the service. If the child welfare agency funds the service code, use modifier HU, Funded by child welfare agency. If the state addictions agency funds the service code, use modifier HV, Funded state addictions agency. If the provider receives funds from state mental health agency, use modifier HW, Funded by state mental health agency. If the juvenile justice agency offers money for the service code, append modifier HY, Funded by juvenile justice agency. If the criminal justice agency funds the service code, use modifier HZ, Funded by criminal justice agency.
HY	**Funded by juvenile justice agency** **Definition:** Append modifier HY to the service when the provider receives funds from a juvenile justice agency to provide therapy to a patient. **Explanation:** Append this modifier to a behavioral health service code to show that the provider receives funds from a juvenile justice agency for therapy that he provides patients. The medical documentation must validate that the juvenile justice agency funds the treatment service for the patient. It is the agency that arranges the financing for the therapy that the patient undergoes. The provider utilizes the resources from juvenile justice agency and offers mental and behavioral healthcare to the patient. **Tips:** HCPCS modifiers HU through HZ identify government and other agency funding for mental health services. When using the modifier HY, you should remember that the juvenile justice agency funds the service. If the child welfare agency funds the service code, use modifier HU, Funded by child welfare agency. If the state addictions agency funds the service code, use modifier HV, Funded state addictions agency. If the provider receives funds from state mental health agency, use modifier HW, Funded by state mental health agency. If the county or local agency finances the service code, append modifier HX, Funded by county or local agency. If the criminal justice agency funds the service code, use modifier HZ, Funded by criminal justice agency.

Mod	Modifier Description, Definition, Explanation, and Tips
HZ	**Funded by criminal justice agency**
	Definition: Append modifier HZ to the service when the provider receives funds from the criminal justice agency to provide therapy to a patient.
	Explanation: Append this modifier to a behavioral health service code to show that the provider receives funds from a criminal justice agency for therapy that he provides patients.
	The medical documentation must validate that the criminal justice agency funds the treatment service for the patient. It is the agency that arranges the financing for the therapy that the patient undergoes.
	The provider utilizes the resources from criminal justice agency and offers mental and behavioral healthcare to the patient.
	Tips: HCPCS modifiers HU through HZ identify government and other agency funding for mental health services. When using the modifier HZ, you should remember that the criminal justice agency funds the service.
	If the child welfare agency funds the service code, use modifier HU, Funded by child welfare agency.
	If the state addictions agency funds the service code, use modifier HV, Funded state addictions agency.
	If the provider receives funds from state mental health agency, use modifier HW, Funded by state mental health agency.
	If the county or local agency finances the service code, append modifier HX, Funded by county or local agency.
	If the juvenile justice agency offers money for the service code, append modifier HY, Funded by juvenile justice agency.
J1	**Competitive acquisition program no-pay submission for a prescription number**
	Definition: Providers enrolled in the Competitive Acquisition Program, or CAP, for drugs and biologicals append modifier J1 to the code for a drug, along with number of prescriptions.
	Explanation: The medical documentation should justify the number of prescriptions of a drug that the provider administers to the patient. Modifier J1 indicates that the drug is a no pay item and the provider obtains it through CAP. This reflects that the patient does not pay for the drug.
	Competitive Acquisition Program refers to a program in which the provider buys and bills for certain drugs and biologicals obtained from approved CAP vendors and administer them to the beneficiary patient.
	Although this modifier is still active, the CAP program was suspended at the end of 2008.
	Tips: When using modifier J1, the provider who prescribes the drug must be enrolled in the Competitive Acquisition Program.
	You can combine the modifier J1 with modifier J2, Competitive Acquisition Program, restocking of emergency drugs after emergency administration, on the same line.
	The CAP is an alternative to the average sales price, or ASP, methodology for acquiring certain Part B drugs administered in physicians' offices. Participating CAP providers must obtain all CAP drugs from an Approved CAP Vendor. Drugs that are not available through the CAP can be purchased through the ASP methodology. The CAP program was suspended on December 31, 2008.
J2	**Competitive acquisition program, restocking of emergency drugs after emergency administration**
	Definition: Providers enrolled in the Competitive Acquisition Program, or CAP, for drugs and biologicals append modifier J2 when the provider restocks drugs administered in an emergency situation.
	Explanation: The medical documentation should justify that the patient had an immediate requirement for the drug, which the provider administers to the patient. Modifier J2 indicates that the provider needs to restock the emergency drugs for when the vendor cannot deliver the drug on time or when an urgent need for the drug occurs.
	Competitive Acquisition Program refers to a program in which the provider buys and bills for certain drugs and biologicals obtained from approved CAP vendors and administer them to the beneficiary patient.
	Although this modifier is still active, the CAP program was suspended at the end of 2008.
	Tips: When using modifier J2, the provider who prescribes the drug must be enrolled in the competitive acquisition program.
	You can combine the modifier J2 with modifier J1, Competitive acquisition program no pay submission for a prescription number, on the same line.
	The CAP is an alternative to the average sales price, or ASP, methodology for acquiring certain Part B drugs administered in physicians' offices. Participating CAP providers must obtain all CAP drugs from an Approved CAP Vendor. Drugs that are not available through the CAP can be purchased through the ASP methodology. The CAP program was suspended on December 31, 2008.

Mod	Modifier Description, Definition, Explanation, and Tips
J3	**Competitive acquisition program (CAP), drug not available through CAP as written, reimbursed under average sales price methodology** **Definition:** Append modifier J3 when the provider is enrolled in the Competitive Acquisition Program, or CAP, for drugs and biologicals, but the drug is not available from a CAP vendor; reimbursement will be made using the average sales price, or ASP, methodology. **Explanation:** The medical documentation should justify that the drug is not available from the approved CAP vendor, and the CAP enrolled provider orders and purchases the drug or biological from a source other than the approved CAP vendor. Competitive Acquisition Program refers to a program in which the provider buys and bills for certain drugs and biologicals obtained from approved CAP vendors and administer them to the beneficiary patient. Although this modifier is still active, the CAP program was suspended at the end of 2008. **Tips:** When using modifier J3, the provider who prescribes the drug must be enrolled in the Competitive Acquisition Program. You cannot combine modifier J3 with modifier J1, Competitive Acquisition Program no pay submission for a prescription number, or modifier J2, Competitive Acquisition Program, restocking of emergency drugs after emergency administration, on the same line. If the provider orders the drug from an alternate method, i.e., other than the approved CAP vendor, and the patient is a primary Medicare beneficiary, use modifier M2, Medicare secondary payer, MSP. The CAP is an alternative to the average sales price, or ASP, methodology for acquiring certain Part B drugs administered in physicians' offices. Participating CAP physicians must obtain all CAP drugs from an Approved CAP Vendor. Drugs that are not available through the CAP can be purchased through the ASP methodology. The CAP program was suspended on December 31, 2008.
J4	**DMEPOS item subject to DMEPOS competitive bidding program that is furnished by a hospital upon discharge** **Definition:** Append modifier J4 when the provider supplies durable medical equipment, prosthetics, orthotics, and supplies, or DMEPOS, to a Medicare patient upon discharge from the hospital. Report this modifier only if the patient's permanent residence is in a competitive bidding area, or CBA. **Explanation:** Modifier J4 indicates that a Medicare patient received DMEPOS, such as a walker or related accessories, upon discharge from the hospital. Patients may use the equipment in their homes, since part A payment for inpatient hospital services includes the payment for these items. The competitive bidding program covers the changes for certain durable medical equipment, prosthetics, orthotics, and supplies for payment by Medicare to the suppliers. It converts outdated prices to lower and more accurate prices. **Tips:** When using modifier J4, the provider who offers the DMEPOS to the patient on discharge from the hospital cannot be a contract supplier. Providers most commonly append this modifier to HCPCS codes that refer to the use of durable medical equipment. Use the modifier J4 if the patient, who receives the DMEPOS, permanently resides in a competitive bidding area, even if the provider who supplies the equipment is outside the competitive bidding area.
J5	**Off-the-shelf orthotic subject to dmepos competitive bidding program that is furnished as part of a physical therapist or occupational therapist professional service** **Definition:** Append modifier J5 when the provider supplies an off-the-shelf orthotic subject to the Medicare Durable Medical Equipment, Prosthetics, Orthotics, and Supplies (DMEPOS) Competitive Bidding Program. Report this modifier when the orthotic is furnished as part of a physical therapist or occupational therapist professional service. **Explanation:** Modifier J5 indicates that a Medicare patient received an off-the-shelf orthotic as a part of a physical therapist or occupational therapist professional service. Off-the-shelf orthotics are prefabricated supplies that require minimal self-adjustment to fit the patient and ensure that the treatment goals are met. Examples are certain leg, arm, back, and neck braces. The orthotic must be subject to the DMEPOS Competitive Bidding Program for the modifier to apply. Under the program, certain items are subject to competitive bidding, and Medicare awards contracts to suppliers who offer the best price and meet quality and financial standards. **Tips:** Medicare identifies the specific off-the-shelf (OTS) orthotic codes included in a competitive bidding program.

Mod	Modifier Description, Definition, Explanation, and Tips
JA	**Administered intravenously**
	Definition: CMS encourages providers to append modifier JA to all intravenous injection codes, but especially when the provider administers erythropoiesis stimulating agents, or ESAs, intravenously to patients with end stage renal disease, or ESRD. Modifier JA is informational and does not affect payment.
	Explanation: Use modifier JA to report the administration of drugs covered by HCPCS intravenous injection codes. CMS encourages providers who intravenously administer erythropoiesis stimulating agents to patients with end stage renal disease to append this modifier for tracking purposes.
	Any claim for erythropoiesis stimulating agents or ESA administration, ESRD facilities must include the hemoglobin and or hematocrit values, the route of administration using the JA or JB modifier code, and the Kt/V, calculated using a specified formula, to indicate the adequacy of dialysis.
	When the kidneys fail to function, the patient undergoes dialysis to remove waste products from the blood. The provider collects a blood sample to measure the level of hemoglobin and hematocrit before the dialysis treatment. If the patient is found to be anemic, the provider administers intravenous or subcutaneous ESAs.
	ESAs stimulate red blood cell production in patients with anemia that results from conditions such as chronic kidney failure, chemotherapy, and other treatments. It includes agents like epoetin alfa and darbepoetin alfa.
	Tips: If the provider uses subcutaneous route to administer the ESAs, append modifier JB, Administered subcutaneously, with the code.
	Failure to include the JA or JB modifier for ESA route of administration when reporting Q4081, Injection, epoetin alfa, 100 units, for ESRD on dialysis, or J0882, Injection, darbepoetin alfa, 1 mcg, for ESRD on dialysis, on a 72X type of bill will result in that bill being returned to the provider.
JB	**Administered subcutaneously**
	Definition: CMS encourages providers to append modifier JB to all subcutaneous injection codes, but especially when the provider administers erythropoiesis stimulating agents, or ESAs, intravenously to patients with end stage renal disease, or ESRD. Modifier JB is informational and does not affect payment.
	Explanation: Use modifier JB to report the administration of drugs covered by HCPCS subcutaneous injection codes. CMS encourages providers who subcutaneously administer erythropoiesis stimulating agents to patients with end stage renal disease to append this modifier for tracking purposes.
	Any claim for erythropoiesis stimulating agents or ESA administration, ESRD facilities must include the hemoglobin and or hematocrit values, the route of administration using the JA or JB modifier code, and the Kt/V, calculated using a specified formula, to indicate the adequacy of dialysis.
	When the kidneys fail to function, the patient undergoes dialysis to remove waste products from the blood. The provider collects a blood sample to measure the level of hemoglobin and hematocrit before the dialysis treatment. If the patient is found to be anemic, the provider administers intravenous or subcutaneous ESAs.
	ESAs stimulate red blood cell production in patients with anemia that results from conditions such as chronic kidney failure, chemotherapy, and other treatments. It includes agents like epoetin alfa and darbepoetin alfa.
	Tips: If the provider uses intravenous route to administer the ESAs, append modifier JA, Administered intravenously, with the code.
	Failure to include the JA or JB modifier for ESA route of administration when reporting Q4081, Injection, epoetin alfa, 100 units, for ESRD on dialysis, or J0882, Injection, darbepoetin alfa, 1 microgram, for ESRD on dialysis, on a 72X type of bill will result in that bill being returned to the provider.
JC	**Skin substitute used as a graft**
	Definition: Append modifier JC to codes when the provider uses a skin substitute as a graft to replace debrided tissue in a wound.
	Explanation: Modifier JC indicates that the provider replaced debrided tissue in a wound with a skin substitute. The medical documentation should justify the use of a skin substitute as a graft to replace the debrided tissue in a wound. The provider implants or inserts the skin substitute into the wound to aid healing, and replace the devitalized or nonviable tissue.
	Tips: Providers most commonly append this modifier to HCPCS codes for skin substitutes when used to treat wounds, infections, or ulcers. The substitute typically replaces the dermal and epidermal layers of the skin.
	If the provider uses the skin substitute as a covering, and not as a graft, append modifier JD, Skin substitute not used as a graft.
	Submit HCPCS modifier JC or HCPCS modifier JD with HCPCS codes Q4100, Skin substitute, not otherwise specified as well as Q4101 through Q4121 and Q4136 to Q4137, codes that specify brands or types of skin substitutes.

Mod	Modifier Description, Definition, Explanation, and Tips
JD	**Skin substitute not used as a graft** **Definition:** Append modifier JD when the provider uses a skin substitute to cover wound due to inadequate skin available for coverage. **Explanation:** Modifier JD indicates that the provider used a skin substitute because of inadequate skin available to cover the wound. The medical documentation should justify the use of skin substitute to cover the wound. The provider uses the skin substitute as a dressing to cover the wound, to help protect it from contamination, and to replace defective tissue. The provider repairs or replaces the defective tissue with an artificial skin substitute, which aids in the healing process. **Tips:** When using the modifier JD, the skin substitute fits over the wound site. Providers most commonly append this modifier to HCPCS codes for skin substitutes when used to treat wounds, infections, or ulcers. The substitute typically replaces the dermal and epidermal layers of the skin. If the provider uses the skin substitute as a graft, and not as a covering, append modifier JC, Skin substitute used as a graft. Submit HCPCS modifier JC or HCPCS modifier JD with HCPCS codes Q4100, Skin substitute, not otherwise specified as well as Q4101 through Q4121 and Q4136 to Q4137, codes that specify brands or types of skin substitutes.
JE	**Administered via dialysate** **Definition:** Append modifier JE when the provider administers drugs and biologicals mixed in the dialysate solution, through any route of dialysate administration, to patients with end stage renal disease, or ESRD. **Explanation:** Modifier JE indicates that the provider administered drugs or biologicals to a patient with end stage renal disease, or ESRD, via the dialysate. The provider compounds the dialysate with injectable drugs and biologicals to administer to the patient. When the kidneys fail to function properly, patients undergo dialysis to remove waste products from the blood. The process of dialysis uses a fluid, called dialysate, which contains soluble substances and helps to remove toxic products from the blood. **Tips:** If the provider administers drugs or biologicals to a patient without ESRD, append modifier AY, Item or service furnished to an ESRD patient that is not for the treatment of ESRD.
JG	**Drug or biological acquired with 340b drug pricing program discount** **Definition:** Append modifier JG to a code for a drug or biological (a drug derived from a living organism using biotechnology) administered in a hospital outpatient department and purchased under a discount pricing program known as 340B. **Explanation:** Modifier JG indicates that a provider dispensed a drug that was purchased through the 340B Drug Pricing Program. The 340B Drug Pricing Program refers to a program under which certain drugs and biologicals, except for vaccines, administered in a hospital outpatient department can be purchased by certain hospitals and other healthcare providers from drug manufacturers at discounted prices. Biological refers to a drug derived from human, animal, or microorganism components using biotechnology; examples include cells, genes, tissues, recombinant proteins, vaccines, allergens, and blood and blood components. **Tips:** The price of drugs covered by the Drug Pricing Program is calculated based on a formula contained in section 340B(a)(2) of the Public Health Service Act. Participating providers in this program who may purchase drugs at these significantly lower prices are registered with DHHS/HRSA's Office of Pharmacy Affairs (www.hrsa.gov/opa).
JW	**Drug amount discarded/not administered to any patient** **Definition:** Append modifier JW when billing for a drug or biological for which the provider discards the remainder of a single dose vial after administering a portion of the drug to the patient. **Explanation:** Append this modifier to the drugs and biologicals codes to show that the provider administers the necessary or prescribed amount of a drug supplied in a single dose vial and discards the remaining amount of the drug. The medical documentation must include the amount of the drug that the provider discards, along with the reason for the same. **Tips:** Some drugs are billed by dose, so if the dose administered is less than the amount of a drug supplied in a single use vial, append modifier JW to bill the amount of the drug discarded. You must bill the amount of drug used and the amount discarded separately. Other drugs are billed by units, as specified in the code's official descriptor. For these drugs, if the administered dose is less than the amount specified in the OD, the provider bills for the unit specified in the OD. Do not append the JW modifier in this case because the provider is paid by the unit specified in the OD and not the amount actually administered.

Mod	Modifier Description, Definition, Explanation, and Tips
K0	**Lower extremity prosthesis functional level 0 - does not have the ability or potential to ambulate or transfer safely with or without assistance and a prosthesis does not enhance their quality of life or mobility** **Definition:** Append modifier K0 to cover the use of lower limb prosthetic device that does not contribute to the patient's ability to move safely with or without any support, nor does the prosthetic device enhance the patient's quality of life or mobility. **Explanation:** Append this modifier to a claim for a lower limb prosthesis to indicate a functional state of zero for the patient for whom the provider supplies the prosthesis. The medical documentation must illustrate that the functional level of the patient, even with the lower limb prosthesis, is zero, i.e., the patient cannot move about independently, or even with assistance, and the prosthesis device does not improve the quality of life of the patient. CMS requires that documentation for a claim for lower limb prosthesis should accurately reflect the beneficiary's medical conditions that necessitate the use of the specific lower limb prosthesis as well as medical conditions that would impact the beneficiary's ability to effectively utilize the device in achieving a defined functional state. **Tips:** HCPCS modifiers K0 through K4 apply to the supply of lower limb prostheses and identify the functional level that a patient motivated to ambulate reaches or maintains within a reasonable time period. Modifier K1 indicates that the patient has the ability or potential to use prosthesis for transfers or ambulation on level surfaces at fixed cadence, typical of the limited and unlimited household ambulator. Modifier K2 indicates that the patient has the ability or potential for ambulation with the ability to traverse low level environmental barriers such as curbs, stairs or uneven surfaces, typical of the limited community ambulator. Modifier K3 indicates that the patient has the ability or potential for ambulation with variable cadence. Typical of the community ambulator who has the ability to traverse most environmental barriers and may have vocational, therapeutic, or exercise activity that demands prosthetic utilization beyond simple locomotion. Modifier K4 indicates that the patient has the ability or potential for prosthetic ambulation that exceeds basic ambulation skills, exhibiting high impact, stress, or energy levels, typical of the prosthetic demands of the child, active adult, or athlete.
K1	**Lower extremity prosthesis functional level 1 - has the ability or potential to use a prosthesis for transfers or ambulation on level surfaces at fixed cadence, typical of the limited and unlimited household ambulator** **Definition:** Append modifier K1 to cover the use of lower limb prosthetic device that contributes to the patient's ability to move safely on level surface at a fixed pace, typical of a patient who goes about his normal activities within his home. **Explanation:** Append this modifier to a claim for lower limb prosthesis to indicate a functional state of one for the patient for whom the provider supplies the prosthesis. The medical documentation must illustrate that the functional level of the patient with the lower limb prosthesis is one, i.e., the patient is able to move about independently on level surfaces at a fixed rhythm with the help of the prosthetic device. CMS requires that documentation for a claim for lower limb prosthesis should accurately reflect the beneficiary's medical conditions that necessitate the use of the specific lower limb prosthesis as well as medical conditions that would impact the beneficiary's ability to effectively utilize the device in achieving a defined functional state. **Tips:** HCPCS modifiers K0 through K4 apply to the supply of lower limb prosthesis and identify the functional level that a patient motivated to ambulate reaches or maintains within a reasonable time period. Modifier K0 indicates that the patient has a functional level of zero, i.e., the patient cannot move about independently, or even with assistance, and the prosthetic device does not improve the quality of life of the patient. Modifier K2 indicates that the patient has the ability or potential for ambulation with the ability to traverse low level environmental barriers such as curbs, stairs or uneven surfaces, typical of the limited community ambulator. Modifier K3 indicates that the patient has the ability or potential for ambulation with variable cadence. Typical of the community ambulator who has the ability to traverse most environmental barriers and may have vocational, therapeutic, or exercise activity that demands prosthetic utilization beyond simple locomotion. Modifier K4 indicates that the patient has the ability or potential for prosthetic ambulation that exceeds basic ambulation skills, exhibiting high impact, stress, or energy levels, typical of the prosthetic demands of the child, active adult, or athlete.

Mod	Modifier Description, Definition, Explanation, and Tips
K2	**Lower extremity prosthesis functional level 2 - has the ability or potential for ambulation with the ability to traverse low level environmental barriers such as curbs, stairs or uneven surfaces, typical of the limited community ambulator** **Definition:** Append modifier K2 to a code for a lower limb prosthetic device that contributes to the patient's ability to move safely over low level barriers, such as stairs or other uneven surfaces. **Explanation:** Append this modifier to a claim for lower limb prosthesis to indicate a functional state of two for a patient for whom the provider supplies lower limb prosthesis. The medical documentation must illustrate that the functional level of the patient with the lower limb prosthesis is two, i.e., the patient can move about independently over low level surfaces, such as stairs, and even control his motion, with the help of the prosthetic device. CMS requires that support of a claim for lower limb prosthesis should accurately reflect the beneficiary's medical conditions that necessitate the use of the specifically ordered lower limb prosthesis as well as beneficiary's medical conditions that would impact the beneficiary's ability to effectively utilize the specifically ordered lower limb prosthesis in achieving a defined functional state. **Tips:** HCPCS modifiers K0 through K4 apply to the supply of lower limb prosthesis and identify the functional level that a patient motivated to ambulate reaches or maintains within a reasonable time period. Modifier K0 indicates that the patient does not have the ability or potential to ambulate or transfer safely with or without assistance and prosthesis does not enhance their quality of life or mobility. Modifier K1 indicates that the patient has the ability or potential to use prosthesis for transfers or ambulation on level surfaces at fixed cadence, typical of the limited and unlimited household ambulator. Modifier K3 indicates that the patient has the ability or potential for ambulation with variable cadence. Typical of the community ambulator who has the ability to traverse most environmental barriers and may have vocational, therapeutic, or exercise activity that demands prosthetic utilization beyond simple locomotion. Modifier K4 indicates that the patient has the ability or potential for prosthetic ambulation that exceeds basic ambulation skills, exhibiting high impact, stress, or energy levels, typical of the prosthetic demands of the child, active adult, or athlete.
K3	**Lower extremity prosthesis functional level 3 - has the ability or potential for ambulation with variable cadence, typical of the community ambulator who has the ability to transverse most environmental barriers and may have vocational, therapeutic, or exercise activity that demands prosthetic utilization beyond simple locomotion** **Definition:** Append modifier K3 to the code for a lower limb prosthetic device that contributes to the patient's ability to move safely over most barriers with a variable pace and to perform certain activities that are beyond the use of the device. **Explanation:** Append this modifier to a claim for lower limb prosthesis to identify a functional state of three for a patient for whom the provider supplies lower limb prosthesis. The medical documentation must illustrate that the functional level of the patient with the lower limb prosthesis is three, i.e., the patient can move about independently over most barriers with variable rhythm. The patient employs the prosthetic device to perform activities, such as exercise, vocational activities, and therapeutic activities, as well as ambulation. CMS requires that documentation for a claim for lower limb prosthesis should accurately reflect the beneficiary's medical conditions that necessitate the use of the specific lower limb prosthesis as well as medical conditions that would impact the beneficiary's ability to effectively utilize the device in achieving a defined functional state. **Tips:** HCPCS modifiers K0 through K4 apply to the supply of lower limb prosthesis and identify the functional level that a patient motivated to ambulate reaches or maintains within a reasonable time period. Modifier K0 indicates that the patient does not have the ability or potential to ambulate or transfer safely with or without assistance and prosthesis does not enhance their quality of life or mobility. Modifier K1 indicates that the patient has the ability or potential to use prosthesis for transfers or ambulation on level surfaces at fixed cadence, typical of the limited and unlimited household ambulator. Modifier K2 indicates that the patient has the ability or potential for ambulation with the ability to traverse low level environmental barriers such as curbs, stairs or uneven surfaces, typical of the limited community ambulator. Modifier K4 indicates that the patient has the ability or potential for prosthetic ambulation that exceeds basic ambulation skills, exhibiting high impact, stress, or energy levels, typical of the prosthetic demands of the child, active adult, or athlete.

Mod	Modifier Description, Definition, Explanation, and Tips
K4	**Lower extremity prosthesis functional level 4 - has the ability or potential for prosthetic ambulation that exceeds the basic ambulation skills, exhibiting high impact, stress, or energy levels, typical of the prosthetic demands of the child, active adult, or athlete**
	Definition: Append modifier K4 to the code for a lower limb prosthetic device that contributes to the patient's ability to move about safely and engage in high energy activities typical of the prosthetic demands of a child, active adult, or athlete.
	Explanation: Append this modifier to a claim for lower limb prosthesis to identify a functional state of four for a patient for whom the provider supplies the lower limb prosthesis. The medical documentation must illustrate that the functional level of the lower limb prosthesis is four, i.e., the patient can move about independently and engage in high energy activities, such as those of a healthy child, active adult, or athlete.
	CMS requires that documentation for a claim for lower limb prosthesis should accurately reflect the beneficiary's medical conditions that necessitate the use of the specific lower limb prosthesis as well as medical conditions that would impact the beneficiary's ability to effectively utilize the device in achieving a defined functional state.
	Tips: HCPCS modifiers K0 through K4 apply to the supply of lower limb prosthesis and identify the functional level that a patient motivated to ambulate reaches or maintains within a reasonable time period.
	Modifier K0 indicates that the patient does not have the ability or potential to ambulate or transfer safely with or without assistance and prosthesis does not enhance their quality of life or mobility.
	Modifier K1 indicates that the patient has the ability or potential to use prosthesis for transfers or ambulation on level surfaces at fixed cadence, typical of the limited and unlimited household ambulator.
	Modifier K2 indicates that the patient has the ability or potential for ambulation with the ability to traverse low level environmental barriers such as curbs, stairs or uneven surfaces, typical of the limited community ambulator.
	Modifier K3 indicates that the patient has the ability or potential for ambulation with variable cadence. Typical of the community ambulator who has the ability to traverse most environmental barriers and may have vocational, therapeutic, or exercise activity that demands prosthetic utilization beyond simple locomotion.
KA	**Add on option/accessory for wheelchair**
	Definition: Append this modifier to wheelchair codes for the supply of accessories and options.
	Explanation: Append modifier KA to show that the provider supplies accessories and options for a wheelchair to a patient. Numerous HCPCS codes exist for wheelchair options and accessories, for purchase or rental.
	Tips: Append this modifier to HCPCS codes E0955, Wheelchair accessory, headrest, cushioned, any type, including fixed mounting hardware, each; E0985 through E2378 for wheelchair accessories, with the exception of codes for power wheelchair interfaces for which you would append modifier KC. You may also append modifier KA to K0015, Detachable nonadjustable height armrest and K0070, Rear wheel assembly, complete, with pneumatic tire, spokes or molded, each.
KB	**Beneficiary requested upgrade for ABN, more than 4 modifiers identified on claim**
	Definition: Append modifier KB to a claim for durable medical equipment, prosthetics, orthotics, and supplies, or DMEPOS, when an advanced beneficiary notice, or ABN, applies when there are more than four modifiers on a claim line.
	Explanation: Append this modifier to a claim for DMEPOS items that require an advance beneficiary notice or ABN, for line items that need more than four modifiers on the claim.
	An Advance Beneficiary Notice refers to a standardized notice that the provider or supplier issues to a Medicare beneficiary before providing certain outpatient or hospice, home health agencies, and religious nonmedical healthcare institutions items or services. An ABN must be issued when the provider believes Medicare may not pay for an item or service that Medicare usually covers and that Medicare may not consider medically reasonable and necessary for the patient in this particular instance. Additional guidelines apply to hospices, home health agencies, and durable medical equipment suppliers.
	The patient must have original Medicare rather than Medicare Advantage plans. The KB modifier only applies to claims for DMEPOS where the supplier obtained an ABN. If providers or suppliers do not issue a valid ABN to the beneficiary when Medicare requires it, they cannot bill the beneficiary for the service and may be financially liable if Medicare doesn't pay.
	Tips: When reporting the modifier KB, you should remember that an ABN applies when more than four modifiers are present on the claim line.
	In cases when the supplier does not issue an ABN, and the provider reports more than four modifiers, append modifier 99, Multiple modifiers.

Mod	Modifier Description, Definition, Explanation, and Tips
KC	**Replacement of special power wheelchair interface** **Definition:** Append modifier KC to a claim for the replacement of the interface for a power mobility device, i.e., the wheelchair, in a multiple competitive bidding product category. **Explanation:** Append this modifier when the interface is used with a competitively bid complex rehabilitative power mobility device base code. Interface refers to the way the patient causes a power wheelchair to move, such as a hand or chin control interface, sip and puff tube, or compact remote joystick. As a patient's physical condition deteriorates, he may require a change in the control interface. CMS added the KC modifier to cover the full cost of a special power wheelchair interface replacement when a change in the patient's medical condition makes the existing interface difficult or impossible for the patient to use or in cases where the existing interface is irreparably damaged or has exceeded its reasonable useful lifetime, when the interface is supplied through competitive bidding complex categories. **Tips:** When using the modifier KC, you should remember that the code identifies only competitive bidding complex categories. If the code covers both competitive and noncompetitive bidding categories, append modifier KE, Bid under round one of the DMEPOS competitive bidding program for use with noncompetitive bid base equipment. Append modifier KC to HCPCS codes for various types of power wheelchair interfaces when the accessory supplied with a competitively bid complex rehabilitative PMD base code. These include E2321 to E2330, Power wheelchair accessories, etc.; E2312, Power wheelchair accessory, hand or chin control interface, mini proportional remote joystick, proportional, including fixed mounting hardware; E2351, Power wheelchair accessory, electronic interface to operate speech generating device using power wheelchair control interface; E2373, Power wheelchair accessory, hand or chin control interface, compact remote joystick, proportional, including fixed mounting hardware; E2374, Power wheelchair accessory, hand or chin control interface, standard remote joystick, not including controller, proportional, including all related electronics and fixed mounting hardware, replacement only; and K0835 thru K0864, Power wheelchair, groups two and three.
KD	**Drug or biological infused through DME** **Definition:** Append modifier KD to a code for a drug or biological, which the provider infuses through a durable medical equipment, or DME, such as an implanted infusion pump. **Explanation:** Append this modifier for drugs and biologicals to show that the provider instills the drug through an implanted infusion pump categorized as a DME. Providers surgically implant infusion pumps in patients who need long term medication. The pump can deliver the drug in a measured dose at a continuous rate or intermittently. Medicare covers the intravenous, intraarterial, subcutaneous, intrathecal, or epidural administration of certain drugs via an infusion pump, such as those used for heart failure and pulmonary arterial hypertension, immunoglobulin for primary immune deficiency, insulin for diabetes, antifungals, antivirals, and narcotics to treat severe pain unrelieved by other methods, and chemotherapy, with modifier KD. Append this modifier to drug and biological codes administered via the above routes through an infusion pump. The medical documentation must illustrate that a medically necessary drug is administered via an implanted DME, i.e., an infusion pump.
KE	**Bid under round one of the DMEPOS competitive bidding program for use with non-competitive bid base equipment** **Definition:** Append modifier KE to codes for competitively bid wheelchair accessory claims when the accessory will be used with a noncompetitive bid wheelchair. **Explanation:** Append this modifier to codes for accessory items to be used with a noncompetitive bid base item. The modifier indicates an accessory code that can be billed with either competitive or noncompetitive base items when the accessory is to be used with a noncompetitive bid item. The competitive bidding program sets payment amounts for certain durable medical equipment, prosthetics, orthotics, and supplies, or DMEPOS to reduce beneficiary copays and save Medicare money while ensuring beneficiary access to quality items and services. **Tips:** The KE modifier is a pricing modifier that suppliers must use to identify when the same accessory HCPCS code can be furnished in multiple competitive and noncompetitive bidding product categories. For competitively bid accessories used with competitively bid base equipment supplied to beneficiaries living in competitive bid areas, the supplier should submit modifier KG, DMEPOS item subject to DMEPOS competitive bidding program number one, or KK, DMEPOS item subject to DMEPOS competitive bidding program number two, as appropriate.

Mod	Modifier Description, Definition, Explanation, and Tips
KF	**Item designated by FDA as class III device** **Definition:** Append modifier KF to a code for a device that the Food and Drug Administration, or FDA, has designated as a class III device. **Explanation:** Append this modifier for durable medical equipment designated as a class III device by the FDA. This pricing modifier identifies class III devices on the durable medical equipment, prosthetics, orthotics, and supplies, or DMEPOS, fee schedule. Append modifier KF with claims for investigational FDA designated class III devices, such as intraspinal catheter with infusion pump, electrodes of an external defibrillator, stair climbing power wheelchairs, and other devices. Class III devices are investigational devices still in clinical trials. The FDA designates as Class III those devices which cannot be classified into class I, i.e., those subject only to general controls, such as good manufacturing practice regulations, or class II, i.e., those which require additional performance review or postmarket surveillance to assure safety and effectiveness, because insufficient information exists to determine safety and effectiveness. These devices require FDA premarket approval to be released in the market. The FDA designates class III devices as category A for which initial questions of safety and effectiveness have not been resolved and the FDA is unsure whether the device type is safe and effective or category B which the FDA believes to be class I or II type devices for which underlying questions of safety and effectiveness have been resolved or safety and effectiveness have been demonstrated because other manufacturers have obtained FDA approval for that device type. Medicare does not pay for category A devices. The provider participating in the clinical trial must furnish all necessary information concerning the device, the clinical trial, and participating Medicare beneficiaries that the contractor deems necessary for a coverage determination and claims processing. Medicare contractors make the coverage determinations on all FDA approved category B devices by applying Medicare's longstanding criteria and procedures for making coverage decisions. Coverage decisions should be made for FDA approved investigational device exemptions, or IDEs, as they currently are made for FDA approved devices.
KG	**DMEPOS item subject to DMEPOS competitive bidding program number 1** **Definition:** Append modifier KG to a code for a claim for durable medical equipment, prosthetics, orthotics, and supplies, or DMEPOS, which the supplier provides in a multiple competitive bidding product category for a standard product category. **Explanation:** Append this modifier when the supplier delivers the same DMEPOS item in multiple competitive bidding product categories for a standard product category. The competitive bidding program sets payment amounts for certain durable medical equipment, prosthetics, orthotics, and supplies, or DMEPOS to reduce beneficiary copays and save Medicare money while ensuring beneficiary access to quality items and services. **Tips:** Failure to report this modifier may result in claim denial, Medicare overpayments, and other penalties that may lead to termination of the contract. The KG and KK modifiers are used in the round one rebid of the competitive bidding program as pricing modifiers and the KU and KW modifiers are reserved for future program use. The modifier KY indicates a claim for a beneficiary who resides in a competitive bidding area and purchases accessories and supplies for use with durable medical equipment. The competitive bidding program includes nine DMEPOS product categories; the number in the descriptor is the round number and indicates an expansion of the program to designated geographical boundaries. These modifiers are described as follows: KG: DMEPOS item subject to DMEPOS competitive bidding program number one. KK: DMEPOS item subject to DMEPOS competitive bidding program number two. KU: DMEPOS item subject to DMEPOS competitive bidding program number three. KW: DMEPOS item subject to DMEPOS competitive bidding program number four. KY: DMEPOS item subject to DMEPOS competitive bidding program number five.
KH	**DMEPOS item, initial claim, purchase or first month rental** **Definition:** Append modifier KH to the code for a claim for the first rental month or purchase option of durable medical equipment, prosthetics, orthotics, and supplies, or DMEPOS. The beneficiary may decide to purchase the item at any time during the rental period. **Explanation:** Append this modifier to DMEPOS claims for the first month of a capped rental period. Capped rental involves the payment of rent for 13 consecutive months to the supplier of the item, while the beneficiary uses the equipment. It covers all the costs including reasonable repairs, maintenance, replacement, or other costs. **Tips:** You should append the modifier KH with modifier RR, Rental; use the RR modifier when DME is to be rented. The KH modifier may also be used in conjunction with HCPCS modifier NU, New equipment, and UE, Used durable medical equipment. These modifiers do not need to be submitted on claims for oxygen and oxygen equipment.

Mod	Modifier Description, Definition, Explanation, and Tips
KI	**DMEPOS item, second or third month rental** **Definition:** Append modifier KI to identify the second or third rental month or purchase option for durable medical equipment, prosthetics, orthotics, and supplies, or DMEPOS. The beneficiary may decide to purchase the item at any time of the rental period. **Explanation:** Append this modifier to DMEPOS claims for the second or third month of the capped rental period. Capped rental involves the payment of rent for 13 consecutive months to the supplier of the item, while the beneficiary uses the equipment. It covers all the costs including reasonable repairs, maintenance, replacement, or other costs. **Tips:** Use the modifier KI for the second or third month's rent of the DMEPOS items. You should append the modifier KI with modifier RR, Rental; use the RR modifier when DME is to be rented. These modifiers do not need to be submitted on claims for oxygen and oxygen equipment. For the first month rental period, use modifier KH, DMEPOS item, initial claim, purchase or first month rental. If the rental period continues past the third month, append modifier KJ, DMEPOS item, parenteral enteral nutrition, pen, pump or capped rental, months four to 15.
KJ	**DMEPOS item, parenteral enteral nutrition (PEN) pump or capped rental, months four to fifteen** **Definition:** Append modifier KJ to identify the fourth to 15th rental month purchase option for durable medical equipment, prosthetics, orthotics, and supplies, or DMEPOS; parenteral enteral nutrition pump rental, or capped rental. The beneficiary may purchase the item at any time of the rental period. **Explanation:** Append this modifier to DMEPOS, parenteral enteral nutrition pump, or capped rental claims for the fourth to 15th month of the capped rental period. Capped rental involves the payment of rent for 13 consecutive months to the supplier of the item, while the beneficiary uses the DMEPOS equipment and up to 15 months for parenteral enteral nutrition pump or other capped rental items. It covers all the costs including reasonable repairs, maintenance, replacement, or other costs. **Tips:** Use modifier KJ for each month of rental past the third month and up to the 13th month for DMEPOS items and up to the 15th month for a parenteral enteral nutrition pump You should append the modifier KJ with modifier RR, Rental; use the RR modifier when DME is to be rented. These modifiers do not need to be submitted on claims for oxygen and oxygen equipment. For the first month rental period, use modifier KH, DMEPOS item, initial claim, purchase or first month rental, and for the second and third rental months, append modifier KI, DMEPOS item, second or third month rental.
KK	**DMEPOS item subject to DMEPOS competitive bidding program number 2** **Definition:** Append modifier KK to code for durable medical equipment, prosthetics, orthotics, and supplies, or DMEPOS, which the supplier provides in a multiple competitive bidding product category for a complex product category. **Explanation:** Append this modifier when the supplier delivers the same DMEPOS item in multiple competitive bidding product categories for a complex product category. The competitive bidding program sets payment amounts for certain durable medical equipment, prosthetics, orthotics, and supplies, or DMEPOS to reduce beneficiary copays and save Medicare money while ensuring beneficiary access to quality items and services. **Tips:** Modifier KK is a pricing modifier for DMEPOS item claims that the supplier provides the beneficiary. Failure to report this modifier may result in claim denial, Medicare overpayments, and other penalties that may lead to termination of the contract. The KG and KK modifiers are used in the round one rebid of the competitive bidding program as pricing modifiers and the KU and KW modifiers are reserved for future program use. The modifier KY indicates a claim for a beneficiary who resides in a competitive bidding area and purchases accessories and supplies for use with durable medical equipment. The competitive bidding program includes nine DMEPOS product categories; the number in the descriptor is the round number and indicates an expansion of the program to designated geographical boundaries. These modifiers are described as follows: KG: DMEPOS item subject to DMEPOS competitive bidding program number one. KK: DMEPOS item subject to DMEPOS competitive bidding program number two. KU: DMEPOS item subject to DMEPOS competitive bidding program number three. KW: DMEPOS item subject to DMEPOS competitive bidding program number four. KY: DMEPOS item subject to DMEPOS competitive bidding program number five.

Mod	Modifier Description, Definition, Explanation, and Tips
KL	**DMEPOS item delivered via mail** **Definition:** Append modifier KL to the claim for a mail order supply of durable medical equipments, prosthetics, orthotics, and supplies, or DMEPOS. **Explanation:** Append this modifier to indicate that the DMEPOS supplies were delivered to the beneficiary's residence through the mail and not from a local supplier storefront. Currently, this modifier applies to claims for only diabetic supply codes that a beneficiary receives through mail order. **Tips:** Failure to report this modifier may result in claim denial, Medicare overpayments, and other penalties that may lead to termination of the contract.
KM	**Replacement of facial prosthesis including new impression/moulage** **Definition:** Append modifier KM to the claim for the fabrication of any replacement of a prosthesis for any part of the face; this includes a new impression or mold, i.e., a moulage, of the face to be treated with the prosthesis. **Explanation:** Append this modifier to the claim for the replacement of a facial prosthesis; this includes the mold or impression if the provider needs one to fabricate the prosthesis, so do not bill the mold separately. **Tips:** If the provider uses a previously created mold to fabricate the replacement facial prosthesis, append modifier KN, Replacement of facial prosthesis using previous master model. Modifiers KM and KN must be appended to claims for replacement of facial prostheses provided by a nonphysician reported with codes L8040 through L8047. These codes include prosthetic procedures over various regions of the face like nasal prosthesis, midfacial prosthesis, orbital prosthesis, and others.
KN	**Replacement of facial prosthesis using previous master model** **Definition:** Append modifier KN to the claim for the fabrication of any replacement prosthesis for any part of the face that the provider fabricated using a previously created mold. **Explanation:** Append this modifier to the claim for a replacement facial prosthesis when the provider uses a previously created mold to fabricate the prosthesis. **Tips:** If the provider uses a new impression or mold of the face to replace a facial prosthesis, append modifier KM, Replacement of facial prosthesis including new impression or moulage. Modifiers KM and KN must be appended to claims for replacement of facial prostheses provided by a nonphysician reported with codes L8040 through L8047. These codes include prosthetic procedures over various regions of the face like nasal prosthesis, midfacial prosthesis, orbital prosthesis, and others.
KO	**Single drug unit dose formulation** **Definition:** Append modifier KO to the code for a single drug supplied in a unit dose container, which the provider administers to a patient. **Explanation:** Append this modifier to a drug code to show that the provider administers a single drug that was supplied as a unit dose to the patient. **Tips:** Do not append this modifier to drug codes that are not supplied in a unit dose vial or container. Drugs supplied in unit dose form consist of inhalation drugs administered via a device classified as durable medical equipment, or DME. However, do not append modifier KO to J2545, Pentamidine isethionate, inhalation solution, FDA approved final product, noncompounded, administered through DME, unit dose form, per 300 mg or Q4074, Iloprost, inhalation solution, FDA approved final product, noncompounded, administered through DME, unit dose form, up to 20 mcg. Do not append the modifier to codes for the concentrated form of a drug. If the provider dispenses the first drug of the multiple drug in unit dose, append modifier KP, First drug of a multiple drug unit dose formulation. If the provider dispenses second or subsequent dose of a multiple drug in unit dose, append modifier KQ, Second or subsequent drug of a multiple drug unit dose formulation. If you do not append modifier KO, KP, or KQ to a code for a unit dose of a drug, Medicare will deny the claim.

Mod	Modifier Description, Definition, Explanation, and Tips
KP	**First drug of a multiple drug unit dose formulation** **Definition:** Append modifier KP to the drug code for the first drug that the provider includes in a multiple drug formulation compounded from drugs supplied in a unit dose form or for the first dose of a single drug supplied in a unit dose form when the total dose is greater than the amount supplied in a single vial or container. **Explanation:** Append this modifier to a code for the first drug that that the provider uses to compound a multiple drug unit dose formulation composed of more than one drug dispensed in a unit dose form. Also, append this modifier to the code for the first dose of a drug when the provider administers a single drug in a dose greater than the amount supplied in the unit dose form. **Tips:** Do not append this modifier to drug codes that are not supplied in a unit dose vial or container. Do not append the modifier to drug codes for a concentrated form of the drug. For the first dose, when the provider compounds a multiple drug formulation from two or more drugs dispensed in single drug unit form or when the provider administers a larger dose of a drug than that supplied in single unit dose form, append modifier KQ, Second or subsequent drug of a multiple drug unit dose formulation. If more than two drugs are compounded from drugs dispensed in unit dose form, no modifier is appended to the codes for the additional drugs. If the provider dispenses a unit dose of a single drug, append modifier KO, Single drug unit dose formulation. Use the modifier JW to identify unused drugs or biologicals from single use vials or single use packages that are appropriately discarded in order to receive payment for the amount of discarded drug or biological. If you do not append modifier KO, KP, or KQ to a code for a unit dose of a drug, Medicare will deny the claim.
KQ	**Second or subsequent drug of a multiple drug unit dose formulation** **Definition:** Append modifier KQ to the drug code for the second drug that the provider includes in a multiple drug formulation compounded from drugs supplied in a unit dose form or for the second dose of a single drug supplied in a unit dose form when the total dose is greater than the amount supplied in a single vial or container. **Explanation:** Append this modifier to a code for the second drug that that the provider uses to compound a multiple drug unit dose formulation composed of more than one drug dispensed in a unit dose form. Also, append this modifier to the code for the second dose of a drug when the provider administers a single drug in a dose greater than the amount supplied in the unit dose form. **Tips:** Do not append this modifier to drug codes that are not supplied in a unit dose vial or container. Do not append the modifier to drug codes for a concentrated form of the drug. For the first dose, when the provider compounds a multiple drug formulation from two or more drugs dispensed in single drug unit form or when the provider administers a larger dose of a drug than that supplied in single unit dose form, append modifier KP, First drug of a multiple drug unit dose formulation. If more than two drugs are compounded from drugs dispensed in unit dose form, no modifier is appended to the codes for the additional drugs. If the provider dispenses a unit dose of a single drug, append modifier KO, Single drug unit dose formulation. Use the modifier JW to identify unused drugs or biologicals from single use vials or single use packages that are appropriately discarded in order to receive payment for the amount of discarded drug or biological. If you do not append modifier KO, KP, or KQ to a code for a unit dose of a drug, Medicare will deny the claim.
KR	**Rental item, billing for partial month** **Definition:** Append modifier KR to the code for a claim for a partial month rental for durable medical equipment, prosthetics, orthotics, and supplies, or DMEPOS. **Explanation:** Append this modifier to DMEPOS claims for a partial month of the capped rental period. The supplier submits the code for a month's rental of the DMEPOS and appends this modifier when the rental period was less than the month claimed. Capped rental involves the payment of rent for 13 consecutive months to the supplier of the item, while the beneficiary uses the equipment. It covers all the costs including reasonable repairs, maintenance, replacement, or other costs. **Tips:** You should append the modifier KR with modifier RR, Rental; use the RR modifier when DME is to be rented. For the first month rental period, use modifier KH, DMEPOS item, initial claim, purchase or first month rental. If the rental period continues to a second or third rental month, append modifier KI, DMEPOS item, second or third month rental. If the rental period continues for a fourth to 15th month, append modifier KJ, DMEPOS item, parenteral enteral nutrition, pen, pump or capped rental, months four to 15.

Mod	Modifier Description, Definition, Explanation, and Tips
KS	**Glucose monitor supply for diabetic beneficiary not treated with insulin** **Definition:** Append modifier KS when the provider supplies a glucose monitor to a patient who is not being treated with insulin injections. **Explanation:** The provider appends modifier KS when he dispenses all diabetic supplies to a patient per his order. The documentation must include the diagnosis of diabetes in order for the supplies to be covered. Append modifier KS on every claim for a glucose monitor and related supplies for patients not receiving insulin injections. **Tips:** The provider must have a record for the supplies that exceed the utilization guideline. New documentation should be presented at least every six months if the patient regularly uses the supplies.
KT	**Beneficiary resides in a competitive bidding area and travels outside that competitive bidding area and receives a competitive bid item** **Definition:** Append modifier KT when a beneficiary residing in a competitive bidding area, or CBA, receives a competitive bid item while traveling outside that competitive bidding area. **Explanation:** The supplier appends modifier KT for competitive bidding items, such as durable medical equipment, prosthetics, orthotics, and similar supplies, or DMEPOS, which he supplies to beneficiaries traveling outside the CBA in which they reside. Append the KT modifier to claims for nonmail order durable medical equipment, prosthetics, orthotics, and supplies when supplying these items to beneficiaries who require these items when traveling outside their resident CBA. If a CBA resident obtains a CBA item in a nonCBA area while traveling, the noncontract supplier must append modifier KT to the claim. Similarly, if a CBA resident obtains a CBA item from a contract supplier in a different CBA, the contract CBA supplier must append modifier KT to the claim. **Tips:** Important questions that need to be answered when a beneficiary needs a competitively bid item while traveling include the following: Is the beneficiary's permanent residence inside or outside a CBA? To verify a beneficiary's permanent CBA address, enter the beneficiary's permanent residence ZIP code into the CBA finder tool on the home page of the competitive bidding implementation contractor, or CBIC. Is the item being obtained inside or outside a CBA? If the beneficiary whose permanent address is inside a CBA travels to another CBA and the required item is a competitively bid item, the beneficiary must obtain the item from a CBA contractor who must append modifier KT to the claim. If the beneficiary needs a noncompetitive bid item, any Medicare enrolled supplier can provide the item. If the beneficiary whose permanent address is inside a CBA travels to nonCBA and needs a competitive bid item, the beneficiary may obtain the item from any Medicare enrolled supplier, and the supplier must affix the KT modifier to the claim. If the beneficiary's permanent residence is not in a CBA and the beneficiary travels to a CBA and requires a competitive bid item, the beneficiary must obtain the item from a contract supplier for the area where he or she is visiting. If the beneficiary needs a nonbid item, he or she may obtain the item from any Medicare enrolled supplier. In both cases, the supplier will be paid the fee schedule amount for the area where the patient permanently resides. If the beneficiary's permanent residence is not in a CBA and the beneficiary travels to an area that is not in a CBA and requires a competitive bid item, the beneficiary may obtain the item from any Medicare enrolled supplier. The supplier will be paid the fee schedule amount for the state where the beneficiary permanently resides. Claims submitted without the KT modifier by skilled nursing facilities, or SNFs, and other nursing facilities that are not located in a CBA and are not contract suppliers will be denied for residents who receive enteral nutrition items while in the facility if their permanent home address is in a CBA. Mail order CBA diabetic supplies claims with the KT modifier will be denied for traveling beneficiaries unless the supplies are shipped to the beneficiary's permanent CBA home address.

Mod	Modifier Description, Definition, Explanation, and Tips
KU	**DMEPOS item subject to DMEPOS competitive bidding program number 3** **Definition:** Append this modifier to indicate a durable medical equipment item depending upon the DMEPOS competitive bidding program number three, i.e., reserved for future program use. **Explanation:** Append modifier KU when the supplier supplies the same durable medical equipment, prosthetics, orthotics, and similar supplies, or DMEPOS, in multiple competitive bidding product categories or when the same code can be used to describe both competitively and noncompetitively bid items. The KU modifier is reserved for future use. **Tips:** The KG, KK, KU and KW modifiers are pricing modifiers that identify when the same supply or accessory HCPCS code is furnished in multiple competitive bidding product categories or when the same code can be used to describe both competitively and noncompetitively bid items. The KG and KK modifiers are used in the Round I Rebid of the competitive bidding program as pricing modifiers and the KU and KW modifiers are reserved for future program use. The competitive bid modifiers KG, KK, KU, and KW are only used on claims for beneficiaries that live in a Competitive Bidding Area, or CBA. Competitive Bidding Program pricing modifiers KE, KG, KK, KU, KW, or KY, NU, RR or UE modifier should be placed in the first position following the HCPCS code and the KE modifier should be placed in the second position.
KV	**DMEPOS item subject to DMEPOS competitive bidding program that is furnished as part of a professional service** **Definition:** Append modifier KV, when professional providers, who are not contract suppliers, supply walkers and related accessories to beneficiaries in a competitive bidding area or CBA. **Explanation:** The noncontract professional provider appends modifier KV when he or she supplies walkers and other accessories to beneficiaries in a competitive bidding area or CBA. Contract suppliers should not append modifier KV. **Tips:** Walkers that are appropriately supplied in accordance with this exception will be paid at the single payment amount. The provider, as a noncontract supplier, should append modifier KV in combination with the following HCPCS codes: A4636, Replacement, handgrip, cane, crutch, or walker, each; A4637, Replacement, tip, cane, crutch, walker, each; and E0130 to E0159 for walkers and replacement parts. On the claim billed to the Durable Medical Equipment Medicare Administrative Contractor or DME MAC, the walker line item must have the same date of service as the professional service office visit billed to the Part A or Part B MAC. The provider and treating practitioners should submit the office visit claim and the walker claim on the same day to ensure timely and accurate claims processing.
KW	**DMEPOS item subject to DMEPOS competitive bidding program number 4** **Definition:** Append this modifier to indicate a durable medical equipment item depending upon the DMEPOS competitive bidding program number four, i.e., reserved for future program use. **Explanation:** Append modifier KW when the supplier supplies the same DMEPOS item in multiple competitive bidding product categories. This modifier is reserved for future use. **Tips:** The KG, KK, KU and KW modifiers are pricing modifiers that identify when the same supply or accessory HCPCS code is furnished in multiple competitive bidding product categories or when the same code can be used to describe both competitively and noncompetitively bid items. The KG and KK modifiers are used in the Round I Rebid of the competitive bidding program as pricing modifiers and the KU and KW modifiers are reserved for future program use. The competitive bid modifiers, KG, KK, KU, and KW, are only used on claims for beneficiaries that live in a Competitive Bidding Area, or CBA. Competitive Bidding Program pricing modifiers KE, KG, KK, KU, KW, or KY, the NU, RR or UE modifier should be placed in the first position following the HCPCS code and the KE modifier should be placed in the second position.

Mod	Modifier Description, Definition, Explanation, and Tips
KX	**Requirements specified in the medical policy have been met** **Definition:** The provider should append modifier KX when exceptions are in effect and the beneficiary qualifies for a therapy cap exception. **Explanation:** Append modifier KX on claims for physical therapy, occupational therapy or speech language pathology services when therapy exceeds the caps listed in the medical policy. When you append modifier KX, it means that the provider attests that the requirements in the medical policy that relate to therapy cap exceptions have been met. In addition, it means the medical record documents that the additional therapy was medically necessary. The beneficiary may qualify for use of the cap exceptions at any time during the episode when documented medically necessary services exceed caps. All covered and medically necessary services qualify for exceptions to caps. All requests for exception require that the KX modifier be added to the claim. By appending the KX modifier, the provider attests that the services billed are reasonable and necessary services, that they require the skills of a therapist, that the medical record justifies the services, and that they qualify for an exception using the automatic process exception. **Tips:** The following CPT® codes for evaluation procedures may qualify for requests for exception with the addition of modifier KX: 97161-97172. If a physical therapy, occupational therapy, or speech language pathology service would be payable before the cap is reached and can be justified as still medically necessary after the cap is reached, that service should be covered. Contact your contractor for interpretation if you are not sure that a service qualifies for exception. It is very important to recognize that most conditions would not ordinarily result in services exceeding the cap. Use the KX modifier only when therapy that exceeds the cap can be justified and documented. Routine use of the KX modifier for all patients with these conditions will likely show up on data analysis as aberrant and invite inquiry. Ensure that the medical record includes sufficient detail to support the use of the modifier. Documentation does not have to be provided unless requested, however. In addition to its other existing uses, the KX modifier should also be used to identify services that are gender specific, i.e., services that are considered female or male only, which includes transgender patients or patients with ambiguous genitalia; that the physician or practitioner is performing a service on a patient for whom gender specific editing may apply; and that the service should be allowed to continue with normal processing. Payment will be made if the coverage and reporting criteria have been met for the service. Justification for exceptions to therapy caps include medical diagnoses and complications that might directly and significantly influence the amount of treatment required. Other variables, such as the availability of a caregiver at home, that affect appropriate treatment may also justify an exception. Published research, clinical guidelines from professional sources, and or clinical or common sense should support the request for an exception to therapy caps. The patient's lack of access to outpatient hospital therapy services alone, when outpatient hospital therapy services are excluded from the limitation, does not constitute justification for exceptions to therapy caps. Residents of skilled nursing facilities prevented by consolidated billing from accessing hospital services, debilitated patients for whom transportation to the hospital is a physical hardship, or lack of therapy services at hospitals in the beneficiary's county may or may not qualify as justification for continued services above the caps. The patient's condition and complexities might justify extended services, but their location does not.

Mod	Modifier Description, Definition, Explanation, and Tips
KY	**DMEPOS item subject to DMEPOS competitive bidding program number 5** **Definition:** Append modifier KY to codes for a claim for competitive bid, or CB, wheelchair accessories in the durable medical equipment, prosthetics, orthotics, and supplies, or DMEPOS, competitive bidding program number five. **Explanation:** Append this modifier when the supplier delivers the same DMEPOS item in multiple competitive bidding product categories for complex product category. The KY modifier should only be appended to competitive bid, or CB, wheelchair accessories. The competitive bidding program sets payment amounts for certain durable medical equipment, prosthetics, orthotics, and supplies, or DMEPOS to reduce beneficiary copays and save Medicare money while ensuring beneficiary access to quality items and services. **Tips:** Failure to report this modifier may result in claim denial, Medicare overpayments, and other penalties that may lead to termination of the contract. The KG and KK modifiers are used in the round one rebid of the competitive bidding program as pricing modifiers and the KU and KW modifiers are reserved for future program use. The modifier KY indicates a claim for a beneficiary who resides in a competitive bidding area and purchases accessories and supplies for use with durable medical equipment. The competitive bidding program includes nine DMEPOS product categories; the number in the descriptor is the round number and indicates an expansion of the program to designated geographical boundaries. These modifiers are described as follows: KG: DMEPOS item subject to DMEPOS competitive bidding program number one. KK: DMEPOS item subject to DMEPOS competitive bidding program number two. KU: DMEPOS item subject to DMEPOS competitive bidding program number three. KW: DMEPOS item subject to DMEPOS competitive bidding program number four. KY: DMEPOS item subject to DMEPOS competitive bidding program number five.
KZ	**New coverage not implemented by managed care** **Definition:** Append modifier KZ when the provider implants a defibrillator in a patient for a new indication not previously included in managed care or Medicare Advantage plan guidelines for implantation of a defibrillator. **Explanation:** Append modifier KZ to the claim when the provider implants a cardioverter defibrillator, or ICD, based on an indication or condition not previously included in managed care guidelines. Append modifier KZ to codes for ICDs placed on Medicare Managed Care claims for the new coverage guidelines. However, make sure you report implants performed under the older guidelines without this modifier. Medicare does not require an advanced beneficiary notice or ABN to reimburse the services given by the provider. **Tips:** CPT® codes to which HCPCS modifier KZ may be appended include 33240 through 33241; 33243 and 33244; 33249 and 33979.
LC	**Left circumflex coronary artery** **Definition:** Append modifier LC to a code for procedures on the left circumflex coronary artery. **Explanation:** Append this modifier to codes when the provider performs a procedure on the left circumflex coronary artery. The left circumflex coronary artery supplies blood to the left atrium and left ventricle of the heart, i.e., the upper and the lower chambers of the heart respectively. **Tips:** The various types of procedures on the left circumflex coronary artery include angioplasty, atherectomy, stent placement, or grafting. If the provider performs a procedure on the right coronary artery, append modifier RC, right coronary artery. If the provider performs a procedure on the left anterior descending artery, use modifier LD, Left anterior descending coronary artery. If the provider targets the left main coronary artery, use modifier LM, Left main coronary artery. If the provider performs a procedure on ramus intermedius coronary artery, use modifier RI, Ramus intermedius coronary artery.

Mod	Modifier Description, Definition, Explanation, and Tips
LD	**Left anterior descending coronary artery** **Definition:** Append modifier LD to a code for procedures on the left anterior descending coronary artery. **Explanation:** Append this modifier to codes when the provider performs a procedure on the left anterior descending coronary artery, also known as the anterior interventricular artery. The left anterior descending coronary artery supplies blood to the left ventricle, the left lower chamber of the heart that pumps blood out of the heart to the rest of the body. **Tips:** The various types of procedures on the left anterior descending coronary artery include angioplasty, atherectomy, stent placement, or grafting. If the provider performs a procedure on the right coronary artery, append modifier RC, right coronary artery. If the provider performs a procedure on the left circumflex coronary artery, append modifier LC, left circumflex coronary artery. If the provider targets the left main coronary artery, use modifier LM, Left main coronary artery. If the provider performs a procedure on ramus intermedius coronary artery, use modifier RI, Ramus intermedius coronary artery.
LL	**Lease/rental (use the 'll' modifier when DME equipment rental is to be applied against the purchase price)** **Definition:** A provider appends modifier LL to durable medical equipment, or DME, rental items that he applies the rental payments against the purchase price. DME is medical equipment that helps a patient to manage his activities of daily living, or ADL, in an easier way or that provides therapeutic benefits to a patient. **Explanation:** A provider appends modifier LL to codes for DME rental that he applies the rental payments against the purchase price for the item. DME helps the patient to manage his activities of daily living in an easier way. A few examples of DME's are crutches, wheelchairs, commodes, canes, walkers, hospital beds, patient safety equipment, and fracture and traction apparatus. **Tips:** A provider uses modifier RR, Rented item, if the DME item is being rented by the patient, modifier NU, New purchased item, if the DME item is purchased new by the patient, and modifier NR, New when rented, when the DME, which was new at the time of rental is subsequently purchased.
LM	**Left main coronary artery** **Definition:** Append modifier LM to a code for procedures on the left main coronary artery. **Explanation:** Append this modifier to codes when the provider performs a procedure on the left main coronary artery. The left main coronary artery supplies blood to a large portion of the heart and the arteries branching off the heart. **Tips:** The various types of procedures on the left main coronary artery include angioplasty, atherectomy, stent placement, or grafting. If the provider performs a procedure on the right coronary artery, append modifier RC, right coronary artery. If the provider performs a procedure on the left circumflex coronary artery, append modifier LC, left circumflex coronary artery. If the provider performs a procedure on the left anterior descending artery, use modifier LD, Left anterior descending coronary artery. If the provider performs a procedure on ramus intermedius coronary artery, use modifier RI, Ramus intermedius coronary artery.
LR	**Laboratory round trip** **Definition:** Append modifier LR to a code for travel costs involved with obtaining a diagnostic laboratory service from either a nursing home patient or homebound patient. **Explanation:** Modifier LR identifies a code for a diagnostic or a laboratory procedure that requires round trip travel to acquire the specimen. The provider identifies the round trip travel by use of the LR modifier. Independent clinical laboratories may append this modifier to a HCPCS code such as P9604, Travel allowance one way in connection with a medically necessary laboratory specimen collection drawn from home bound or nursing home bound patient; prorated trip charge. **Tips:** Not using modifier LR should have no effect on payment.
LS	**FDA-monitored intraocular lens implant** **Definition:** Append modifier LS to a code for a patient undergoing surgery and fitted with an intraocular lens implant, or IOL. **Explanation:** Modifier LS illustrates a code for a patient undergoing surgery and fitting with an intraocular lens implant, or IOL. The provider surgically places an intraocular lens in the eye of a patient with eye disorders such as cataracts or myopia. A cataract is an eye condition in which the lens of the eye becomes opaque gradually, leading to blurred vision. Myopia causes the patient to lose focus of distant objects, and he is only able to see nearby objects clearly. Modifier LS provides additional information to the payer when billing eye procedures that the provider places an IOL that is being monitored by the Food and Drug Administration, or FDA. **Tips:** Append this modifier on provider claims for eye surgery in patients with IOL implants.

Mod	Modifier Description, Definition, Explanation, and Tips
LT	**Left side (used to identify procedures performed on the left side of the body)** **Definition:** Append modifier LT to specify the procedure that the provider performs is on the left side of the body. **Explanation:** Modifier LT illustrates that a provider performs a procedure on the left side of a patient's body. LT represents the left anatomical side of the body, when the body contains the same anatomical part on both the right and left side of the body. The provider applies LT in the case of procedures he performs on the left side of a paired organ such as the kidneys, lungs, legs, or ears. A provider does not append this modifier when a procedure code specifies bilateral, or modifier 50, Bilateral Procedure, as they are not compatible or if the code specifies a particular side of the body. **Tips:** Modifier LT does not affect the allowed amount on a claim; however, lack of the modifier can lead to denials. Some private payers do not recognize the LT and RT, Right side modifiers. For these procedures, a provider may use a single code with modifier 50, Bilateral Procedure, to denote a bilateral procedure. When using more than one modifier, place a pricing modifier, or a modifier that affects reimbursement, in the first modifier position. Then place the informational modifier in the second modifier position. For example if a provider uses a procedure code with modifier 22, Increased Procedural Services and modifier LT, then place modifier 22 first and modifier LT second.
M2	**Medicare secondary payer (MSP)** **Definition:** Append modifier M2 to specify that Medicare is the secondary payer for a drug procured outside of the Competitive Acquisition Program, or CAP, for drugs and biological. **Explanation:** The M2 modifier is only for the submission of claims by providers, enrolled in the Competitive Acquisition Program, or CAP, for drugs and biological, an alternative reimbursement methodology to the Average Sales Price, or ASP payment method. The provider appends this modifier when he incorrectly identifies the patient's main insurer and procures a CAP drug for a Medicare patient from a source other than the CAP vendor. The CAP provider later determines that Medicare is primary and that the drug should have been ordered through the approved CAP vendor. The provider appends the M2 modifier to the drug, which allows the local carrier's claims processing system to make a payment under ASP. The participating CAP provider maintains documentation in the beneficiary's medical record to provide further information if necessary as to why they made the initial determination that Medicare is secondary to another payer. The local carrier may request this documentation for review purposes. **Tips:** Modifier M2 is no longer effective for services after December 31, 2008.
MA	**Ordering professional is not required to consult a clinical decision support mechanism due to service being rendered to a patient with a suspected or confirmed emergency medical condition** **Definition:** Append modifier MA to a code for services when the provider did not consult a clinical decision support mechanism because the patient had a suspected or confirmed emergency medical condition. **Explanation:** Modifier MA indicates that a provider did not access or receive support from a qualified clinical decision support mechanism for a service he provided due to the patient having or suspected to have an emergency medical condition. Qualified clinical decision support mechanisms (CDSM) factor into appropriate use criteria (AUC) and quality measures required by certain Medicare/CMS participation programs. Ordinarily, registered qualified clinical decision support mechanism providers must meet certain requirements, but this is an exception to the rule. The AUC program establishes criteria for ordering of advanced diagnostic imaging services, such as CTs, PET scans, MRI, and nuclear imaging studies, for a Medicare beneficiary. The ordering professional must consult a qualified CDSM, which is an electronic portal through which appropriate use criteria (AUC) are accessed. The CDSM determines whether the advanced imaging order adheres to AUC. If the AUC consulted was not applicable (e.g., no AUC is available to address the patient's clinical condition), the ordering professional must consult with another professional at the time of the order for imaging services. The program is set to be fully implemented 1 January 2021, when claims that do meet AUC criteria will not be paid. The program impacts anyone who orders or furnishes advances diagnostic imaging services and whose claims are paid under the physician fee schedule (PFS), hospital outpatient prospective payment system (OPPS) or ambulatory surgical center (ASS) payment system. In the meantime, an Education and Operations Testing Period begins 1 January 2020. Before that date, participation is voluntary. **Tips:** For other instances when the ordering professional is not required to consult a clinical decision support mechanism, see modifiers MB through MD.

Mod	Modifier Description, Definition, Explanation, and Tips
MB	**Ordering professional is not required to consult a clinical decision support mechanism due to the significant hardship exception of insufficient internet access** **Definition:** Append modifier MB to a code for services when the provider did not consult a clinical decision support mechanism because he had insufficient Internet access. **Explanation:** Modifier MB indicates that a provider did not access or receive support from a qualified clinical decision support mechanism for a service he provided due to not having sufficient access to the Internet. Qualified clinical decision support mechanisms (CDSM) factor into appropriate use criteria (AUC) and quality measures required by certain Medicare/CMS participation programs. Ordinarily, registered qualified clinical decision support mechanism providers must meet certain requirements, but this is an exception to the rule. The AUC program establishes criteria for ordering of advanced diagnostic imaging services, such as CTs, PET scans, MRI, and nuclear imaging studies, for a Medicare beneficiary. The ordering professional must consult a qualified CDSM, which is an electronic portal through which appropriate use criteria (AUC) are accessed. The CDSM determines whether the advanced imaging order adheres to AUC. If the AUC consulted was not applicable (e.g., no AUC is available to address the patient's clinical condition), the ordering professional must consult with another professional at the time of the order for imaging services. The program is set to be fully implemented 1 January 2021, when claims that do meet AUC criteria will not be paid. The program impacts anyone who orders or furnishes advances diagnostic imaging services and whose claims are paid under the physician fee schedule (PFS), hospital outpatient prospective payment system (OPPS) or ambulatory surgical center (ASS) payment system. In the meantime, an Education and Operations Testing Period begins 1 January 2020. Before that date, participation is voluntary. **Tips:** For other instances when the ordering professional is not required to consult a clinical decision support mechanism, see modifiers MA through MD.
MC	**Ordering professional is not required to consult a clinical decision support mechanism due to the significant hardship exception of electronic health record or clinical decision support mechanism vendor issues** **Definition:** Append modifier MC to a code for services when the provider did not consult a clinical decision support mechanism (CDSM) because of HER or CDSM issues. **Explanation:** Modifier MC indicates that a provider did not access or receive support from a qualified clinical decision support mechanism for a service he provided due to issues with the electronic health record (EHR) or clinical decision support mechanism (CDSM) vendor issues. Qualified clinical decision support mechanisms (CDSM) factor into appropriate use criteria (AUC) and quality measures required by certain Medicare/CMS participation programs. Ordinarily, registered qualified clinical decision support mechanism providers must meet certain requirements, but this is an exception to the rule. The AUC program establishes criteria for ordering of advanced diagnostic imaging services, such as CTs, PET scans, MRI, and nuclear imaging studies, for a Medicare beneficiary. The ordering professional must consult a qualified CDSM, which is an electronic portal through which appropriate use criteria (AUC) are accessed. The CDSM determines whether the advanced imaging order adheres to AUC. If the AUC consulted was not applicable (e.g., no AUC is available to address the patient's clinical condition), the ordering professional must consult with another professional at the time of the order for imaging services. The program is set to be fully implemented 1 January 2021, when claims that do meet AUC criteria will not be paid. The program impacts anyone who orders or furnishes advances diagnostic imaging services and whose claims are paid under the physician fee schedule (PFS), hospital outpatient prospective payment system (OPPS) or ambulatory surgical center (ASS) payment system. In the meantime, an Education and Operations Testing Period begins 1 January 2020. Before that date, participation is voluntary. **Tips:** For other instances when the ordering professional is not required to consult a clinical decision support mechanism, see modifiers MA through MD.

Mod	Modifier Description, Definition, Explanation, and Tips
MD	**Ordering professional is not required to consult a clinical decision support mechanism due to the significant hardship exception of extreme and uncontrollable circumstances** **Definition:** Append modifier MD to a code for services when the provider did not consult a clinical decision support mechanism because of uncontrollable circumstances or because doing so would represent a significant hardship. **Explanation:** Modifier MD indicates that a provider did not access or receive support from a qualified clinical decision support mechanism (CDSM) for a service he provided due to circumstances beyond his control or because accessing or receiving support from a CDSM would represent a significant hardship. Qualified clinical decision support mechanisms (CDSM) factor into appropriate use criteria (AUC) and quality measures required by certain Medicare/CMS participation programs. Ordinarily, registered qualified clinical decision support mechanism providers must meet certain requirements, but this is an exception to the rule. The AUC program establishes criteria for ordering of advanced diagnostic imaging services, such as CTs, PET scans, MRI, and nuclear imaging studies, for a Medicare beneficiary. The ordering professional must consult a qualified CDSM, which is an electronic portal through which appropriate use criteria (AUC) are accessed. The CDSM determines whether the advanced imaging order adheres to AUC. If the AUC consulted was not applicable (e.g., no AUC is available to address the patient's clinical condition), the ordering professional must consult with another professional at the time of the order for imaging services. The program is set to be fully implemented 1 January 2021, when claims that do meet AUC criteria will not be paid. The program impacts anyone who orders or furnishes advances diagnostic imaging services and whose claims are paid under the physician fee schedule (PFS), hospital outpatient prospective payment system (OPPS) or ambulatory surgical center (ASS) payment system. In the meantime, an Education and Operations Testing Period begins 1 January 2020. Before that date, participation is voluntary. **Tips:** For other instances when the ordering professional is not required to consult a clinical decision support mechanism, see modifiers MA through MC.
ME	**The order for this service adheres to appropriate use criteria in the clinical decision support mechanism consulted by the ordering professional** **Definition:** Append modifier ME to a code for services that meet appropriate use criteria according to the clinical decision support mechanism consulted. **Explanation:** Modifier ME indicates that the ordering professional consulted a qualified clinical decision support mechanism (CDSM) prior to ordering advanced diagnostic imaging services and that said services meet the appropriate use criteria (AUC). Qualified clinical decision support mechanisms (CDSMs) factor into appropriate use criteria (AUC) and quality measures required by certain Medicare/CMS participation programs. Ordinarily, registered qualified clinical decision support mechanism providers must meet certain requirements. The AUC program establishes criteria for ordering of advanced diagnostic imaging services, such as CTs, PET scans, MRI, and nuclear imaging studies, for a Medicare beneficiary. The ordering professional must consult a qualified CDSM, which is an electronic portal through which appropriate use criteria (AUC) are accessed. The CDSM determines whether the advanced imaging order adheres to AUC. If the AUC consulted was not applicable (e.g., no AUC is available to address the patient's clinical condition), the ordering professional must consult with another professional at the time of the order for imaging services. The program is set to be fully implemented 1 January 2021, when claims that do meet AUC criteria will not be paid. The program impacts anyone who orders or furnishes advances diagnostic imaging services and whose claims are paid under the physician fee schedule (PFS), hospital outpatient prospective payment system (OPPS) or ambulatory surgical center (ASS) payment system. In the meantime, an Education and Operations Testing Period begins 1 January 2020. Before that date, participation is voluntary. **Tips:** When the advanced diagnostic imaging service requested by an ordering professional does not meet AUC, append modifier MF.

Mod	Modifier Description, Definition, Explanation, and Tips
MF	**The order for this service does not adhere to the appropriate use criteria in the clinical decision support mechanism consulted by the ordering professional** **Definition:** Append modifier MF to a code for services that DO NOT meet appropriate use criteria according to the clinical decision support mechanism consulted. **Explanation:** Modifier MF indicates that the ordering professional consulted a qualified clinical decision support mechanism (CDSM) prior to ordering advanced diagnostic imaging services but said services DO NOT meet the appropriate use criteria (AUC). Qualified clinical decision support mechanisms (CDSMs) factor into appropriate use criteria (AUC) and quality measures required by certain Medicare/CMS participation programs. Ordinarily, registered qualified clinical decision support mechanism providers must meet certain requirements. The AUC program establishes criteria for ordering of advanced diagnostic imaging services, such as CTs, PET scans, MRI, and nuclear imaging studies, for a Medicare beneficiary. The ordering professional must consult a qualified CDSM, which is an electronic portal through which appropriate use criteria (AUC) are accessed. The CDSM determines whether the advanced imaging order adheres to AUC. If the AUC consulted was not applicable (e.g., no AUC is available to address the patient's clinical condition), the ordering professional must consult with another professional at the time of the order for imaging services. The program is set to be fully implemented 1 January 2021, when claims that do meet AUC criteria will not be paid. The program impacts anyone who orders or furnishes advances diagnostic imaging services and whose claims are paid under the physician fee schedule (PFS), hospital outpatient prospective payment system (OPPS) or ambulatory surgical center (ASS) payment system. In the meantime, an Education and Operations Testing Period begins 1 January 2020. Before that date, participation is voluntary. **Tips:** When an ordering professional consults a CDSM and the advanced diagnostic imaging services DO meet AUC, append modifier ME.
MG	**The order for this service does not have applicable appropriate use criteria in the qualified clinical decision support mechanism consulted by the ordering professional** **Definition:** Append modifier MG to a code for services when the ordering professional consults the clinical decision support mechanism (CDSM), but the CDSM does not have applicable appropriate use criteria. **Explanation:** Modifier MG indicates that the ordering professional consulted a qualified clinical decision support mechanism (CDSM) prior to ordering advanced diagnostic imaging services but the CDSM did have appropriate use criteria (AUC) that applied to the situation. Qualified clinical decision support mechanisms (CDSMs) factor into appropriate use criteria (AUC) and quality measures required by certain Medicare/CMS participation programs. Ordinarily, registered qualified clinical decision support mechanism providers must meet certain requirements. The AUC program establishes criteria for ordering of advanced diagnostic imaging services, such as CTs, PET scans, MRI, and nuclear imaging studies, for a Medicare beneficiary. The ordering professional must consult a qualified CDSM, which is an electronic portal through which appropriate use criteria (AUC) are accessed. The CDSM determines whether the advanced imaging order adheres to AUC. If the AUC consulted was not applicable (e.g., no AUC is available to address the patient's clinical condition), the ordering professional must consult with another professional at the time of the order for imaging services. The program is set to be fully implemented 1 January 2021, when claims that do meet AUC criteria will not be paid. The program impacts anyone who orders or furnishes advances diagnostic imaging services and whose claims are paid under the physician fee schedule (PFS), hospital outpatient prospective payment system (OPPS) or ambulatory surgical center (ASS) payment system. In the meantime, an Education and Operations Testing Period begins 1 January 2020. Before that date, participation is voluntary.

Mod	Modifier Description, Definition, Explanation, and Tips
MH	**Unknown if ordering professional consulted a clinical decision support mechanism for this service, related information was not provided to the furnishing professional or provider** **Definition:** Append modifier MH to a code for services when it is not known whether the ordering professional consulted the clinical decision support mechanism (CDSM) or whether related information was not provided to the professional or provider who furnishes the services. **Explanation:** Modifier MH applies to advanced diagnostic imaging services for which it is unknown if the ordering professional consulted a qualified clinical decision support mechanism (CDSM) prior to ordering the services or if the furnishing provider was not provided the related information. Qualified clinical decision support mechanisms (CDSMs) factor into appropriate use criteria (AUC) and quality measures required by certain Medicare/CMS participation programs. Ordinarily, registered qualified clinical decision support mechanism providers must meet certain requirements. The AUC program establishes criteria for ordering of advanced diagnostic imaging services, such as CTs, PET scans, MRI, and nuclear imaging studies, for a Medicare beneficiary. The ordering professional must consult a qualified CDSM, which is an electronic portal through which appropriate use criteria (AUC) are accessed. The CDSM determines whether the advanced imaging order adheres to AUC. If the AUC consulted was not applicable (e.g., no AUC is available to address the patient's clinical condition), the ordering professional must consult with another professional at the time of the order for imaging services. The program is set to be fully implemented 1 January 2021, when claims that do meet AUC criteria will not be paid. The program impacts anyone who orders or furnishes advances diagnostic imaging services and whose claims are paid under the physician fee schedule (PFS), hospital outpatient prospective payment system (OPPS) or ambulatory surgical center (ASS) payment system. In the meantime, an Education and Operations Testing Period begins 1 January 2020. Before that date, participation is voluntary.
MS	**Six month maintenance and servicing fee for reasonable and necessary parts and labor which are not covered under any manufacturer or supplier warranty** **Definition:** Append modifier MS to a code to identify the service is for a six month periodic, in home visit by the provider for inspection and servicing of equipment. The service the provider performs includes the general maintenance and servicing to the item as well as costs not covered by a manufacturer or supplier warranty for reasonable and necessary parts to service the equipment. **Explanation:** Modifier MS illustrates a code for the routine maintenance and performance checks a provider performs every six months on DME, or durable medical equipment such as oxygen equipment. This maintenance and servicing typically includes the labor time spent and any reasonable and necessary parts he uses to keep the equipment in good working order, and which are not covered under any manufacturer or supplier warranty. The provider appends this modifier to Healthcare Common Procedure Coding System, or HCPCS, codes such as oxygen concentrator codes E1390 to E1392, and K0738, Portable gaseous oxygen system, rental; home compressor used to fill portable oxygen cylinders; includes portable containers, regulator, flowmeter, humidifier, cannula or mask, and tubing. **Tips:** Medicare no longer pays for maintenance and servicing of capped rental items every six months with the exception of oxygen equipment. For other capped rental items, Medicare typically covers reasonable and necessary repairs and servicing once the beneficiary owns the capped rental item.
NB	**Nebulizer system, any type, FDA-cleared for use with specific drug** **Definition:** Append modifier NB to a code for any type of nebulizer system that is cleared by the Food and Drug Administration, or FDA, for use with specific drugs. **Explanation:** Modifier NB illustrates the use of a nebulizer system of any type. The nebulizer system that the provider appends the modifier to is a system cleared by the Food and Drug Administration, or FDA, for use with specific drugs. This modifier may be applicable to Healthcare Common Procedure Coding System, or HCPCS, codes E0550 through E0585, which identify different types of nebulizer systems. **Tips:** Append this modifier for Medicare services that the facility submits to a durable medical equipment, or DME Medicare Administrative Contractor, a DME MAC.
NR	**New when rented (use the 'NR' modifier when DME which was new at the time of rental is subsequently purchased)** **Definition:** A provider appends modifier NR to identify durable medical equipment, or DME, that was new at the time of rental, and a patient subsequently purchases it. DME is medical equipment that helps a patient to manage his activities of daily living in an easier way or that provides therapeutic benefits to a patient. **Explanation:** A provider appends modifier NR to a code to indicate that a DME item that the patient purchases was new DME when the patient first received the item at the time of rental. DME helps the patient to manage his activities of daily living in an easier way. A few examples of DME's are crutches, wheelchairs, commodes, canes, walkers, hospital beds, patient safety equipment, and fracture and traction apparatus. **Tips:** A provider uses the modifier RR, Rented item, if the item is being rented by the patient and modifier NU, New purchased item, if the item is purchased new by the patient.

Mod	Modifier Description, Definition, Explanation, and Tips
NU	**New equipment** **Definition:** Append modifier NU to a code for new durable medical equipment item. **Explanation:** Modifier NU identifies that the beneficiary has received new or fresh durable medical equipment, or DME, that is equipment which has never been used before. The DME codes the provider may most often append this modifier to, are items that are inexpensive or routinely purchased items, capped rental items, items requiring frequent and substantial servicing, or oxygen equipment. The codes that may apply include HCPCS E codes and K codes items including complex rehabilitative power wheelchairs, K0835 through K0891. **Tips:** Append this modifier to identify new durable medical equipment, or DME, items.
P1	**A normal healthy patient** **Definition:** The provider administers anesthesia to a normal healthy individual. **Explanation:** The anesthesia provider appends this modifier to an anesthesia code to show that the provider administers anesthesia to a normal healthy individual during any procedure. A normal healthy individual includes patients with no physiologic or psychiatric disorder and patients with a good level of exercise tolerance. It does not include very young and very old individuals. The medical record should justify the diagnosis that corresponds to the individual being normal and healthy. **Tips:** The anesthesia modifiers P1 to P6 identify the health condition of the patient in whom the provider is going to administer the anesthesia. The identification of the health condition helps the payer to determine the complexity of the anesthesia case. Many payers will reimburse more for anesthesia identified with modifiers P2 to P5 because the patient's case is likely more complex. Payers will not reimburse more for modifier P1 because the patient is normal and healthy or for P6 because the patient is brain dead. The provider uses this modifier only with anesthesia codes that range from 00100 to 01999. Coders will not append this modifier; only the anesthesia provider will append it.
P2	**A patient with mild systemic disease** **Definition:** The provider administers anesthesia to an individual with mild systemic disease. Patients with mild systemic disease have a well controlled disease of one body system. **Explanation:** The anesthesia provider appends this modifier to an anesthesia code to show that the provider administers anesthesia to an individual with mild systemic disease during any procedure. Patients with mild systemic disease have a well controlled disease of one body system, for example, controlled hypertension, controlled diabetes mellitus, mild obesity, or a smoking history with no symptoms of chronic obstructive pulmonary disease. Mild systemic disease does not affect the activities of daily living. The medical record should justify the diagnosis that corresponds to mild systemic disease. **Tips:** The anesthesia modifiers P1 to P6 identify the health condition of the patient in whom the provider is going to administer the anesthesia. The identification of the health condition helps the payer to determine the complexity of the anesthesia case. Many payers will reimburse more for anesthesia identified with modifiers P2 to P5 because the patient's case is likely more complex. Payers will not reimburse more for modifier P1 because the patient is normal and healthy or for P6 because the patient is brain dead. The provider uses this modifier only with anesthesia codes that range from 00100 to 01999. Coders will not append this modifier; only the anesthesia provider will append it.

Mod	Modifier Description, Definition, Explanation, and Tips
P3	**A patient with severe systemic disease** **Definition:** The provider administers anesthesia to an individual with severe systemic disease. Patients with severe systemic disease have some limitation in activities and well controlled disease of more than one body system or one major body system. **Explanation:** The anesthesia provider appends this modifier to an anesthesia code to show that the provider administers anesthesia to an individual with severe systemic disease. Patients with severe systemic disease have some limitation in activities and well controlled disease of more than one body system or one major body system. For example, the category includes patients with stable angina, controlled congestive heart failure, poorly controlled hypertension, type 1 diabetes that has affected the vascular system, and moderate obesity. In severe systemic disease, there is no immediate danger of death. The medical record should justify the diagnosis that corresponds to severe systemic disease. **Tips:** The anesthesia modifiers P1 to P6 identify the health condition of the patient in whom the provider is going to administer the anesthesia. The identification of the health condition helps the payer to determine the complexity of the anesthesia case. Many payers will reimburse more for anesthesia identified with modifiers P2 to P5 because the patient's case is likely more complex. Payers will not reimburse more for modifier P1 because the patient is normal and healthy or for P6 because the patient is brain dead. The provider uses this modifier only with anesthesia codes that range from 00100 to 01999. Coders will not append this modifier; only the anesthesia provider will append it.
P4	**A patient with severe systemic disease that is a constant threat to life** **Definition:** The provider administers anesthesia in an individual with severe systemic disease that is a constant threat to the life of the patient. **Explanation:** The anesthesia provider appends this modifier to an anesthesia code to show that the provider administers anesthesia to an individual with severe systemic disease that is a constant threat to life. Patients with severe systemic disease have a poorly controlled disease of more than one body system or one major body system. For example, the category includes patients with unstable angina, chronic renal failure, or symptomatic congestive heart failure. There is a possible risk and danger of death. The medical record should justify the diagnosis that corresponds to severe systemic disease that has a possible risk of death. **Tips:** The anesthesia modifiers P1 to P6 identify the health condition of the patient in whom the provider is going to administer the anesthesia. The identification of the health condition helps the payer to determine the complexity of the anesthesia case. Many payers will reimburse more for anesthesia identified with modifiers P2 to P5 because the patient's case is likely more complex. Payers will not reimburse more for modifier P1 because the patient is normal and healthy or for P6 because the patient is brain dead. The provider uses this modifier only with anesthesia codes that range from 00100 to 01999. Coders will not append this modifier; only the anesthesia provider will append it.
P5	**A moribund patient who is not expected to survive without the operation** **Definition:** The provider administers anesthesia to a terminally ill individual who will not survive without the operative procedure. **Explanation:** The provider administers anesthesia in a critically ill patient who will not survive without the operation. The medical record should justify the diagnosis that corresponds to a critically ill or injured patient who requires a life saving surgery. **Tips:** The anesthesia modifiers P1 to P6 identify the health condition of the patient in whom the provider is going to administer the anesthesia. The identification of the health condition helps the payer to determine the complexity of the anesthesia case. Many payers will reimburse more for anesthesia identified with modifiers P2 to P5 because the patient's case is likely more complex. Payers will not reimburse more for modifier P1 because the patient is normal and healthy or for P6 because the patient is brain dead. The provider uses this modifier only with anesthesia codes that range from 00100 to 01999. Coders will not append this modifier; only the anesthesia provider will append it.

Mod	Modifier Description, Definition, Explanation, and Tips
P6	**A declared brain-dead patient whose organs are being removed for donor purposes** **Definition:** The provider administers anesthesia in a brain dead individual undergoing organ removal for donor purposes. **Explanation:** The anesthesia provider appends this modifier to an anesthesia code to show that the provider administers anesthesia to a brain dead individual undergoing organ removal for donor purposes. Brain death is the complete and irreversible cessation of brain function as determined by two doctors not associated with the transplant team. The medical record should justify the diagnosis that corresponds to a brain dead individual for organ donor purposes. **Tips:** The anesthesia modifiers P1 to P6 identify the health condition of the patient in whom the provider is going to administer the anesthesia. The identification of the health condition helps the payer to determine the complexity of the anesthesia case. Many payers will reimburse more for anesthesia identified with modifiers P2 to P5 because the patient's case is likely more complex. Payers will not reimburse more for modifier P1 because the patient is normal and healthy or for P6 because the patient is brain dead. The provider uses this modifier only with anesthesia codes that range from 00100 to 01999. Coders will not append this modifier; only the anesthesia provider will append it.
PA	**Surgical or other invasive procedure on wrong body part** **Definition:** Append this modifier to indicate an adverse event when the provider performs a surgical or other invasive procedure on the wrong body part. **Explanation:** The provider appends modifier PA to surgical codes when he performs a surgical or other invasive procedure on the wrong body part due to an error. He appends this modifier so that the insurer including Medicare knows not to provide reimbursement. Not adhering to the Centers for Medicare and Medicaid Services, or CMS, guidelines of appending this modifier in situations where a provider performs a surgical or other invasive procedure on a body part that is not consistent with the correct documentation on the patient consent form may result in payment by the insurer and recoupment of the payment later on. Typically, the insurer considers all services the provider delivers in the operating room when an error occurs as related and considers them non covered as well. All other providers in the operating room when the error occurs, who bill individually for their services, are also not eligible for payment. Finally, all related services the patient receives during the same hospitalization in which the error occurs are usually not covered. **Tips:** Modifier PA notifies the insurer of the situation and ensures that the provider will not receive payment for the procedure done in error. Medicare also will not cover services related to the error. Using this modifier may increase malpractice risk. Use this modifier only with surgical codes.
PB	**Surgical or other invasive procedure on wrong patient** **Definition:** Append the PB modifier to indicate an adverse event when the provider performs a surgical or other invasive procedure on the wrong patient. **Explanation:** The provider appends modifier PB to codes when he performs a surgical or other invasive procedure on the wrong patient. He appends this modifier so that the insurer including Medicare knows not to provide reimbursement. Not adhering to the Centers for Medicare and Medicaid Services, or CMS, guidelines of appending this modifier in situations where a provider performs a surgical or other invasive procedure on the wrong patient may result in payment by the insurer and recoupment of the payment later on. Typically, the insurer considers all services the provider delivers in the operating room when an error occurs as related and considers them non covered as well. All other providers in the operating room when the error occurs, who bill individually for their services, are also not eligible for payment. Finally, all related services the patient receives during the same hospitalization in which the error occurs are usually not covered. **Tips:** Modifier PB notifies the insurer of the situation and ensures that the provider will not receive payment for the procedure done in error. Medicare also will not cover services related to the error. Using this modifier may increase malpractice risk.

Mod	Modifier Description, Definition, Explanation, and Tips
PC	**Wrong surgery or other invasive procedure on patient** **Definition:** Append the PC modifier to indicate an adverse event when the provider performs the wrong surgery or other invasive procedure on a patient. **Explanation:** The provider appends modifier PC to codes when he performs the wrong surgery or other invasive procedure on a patient. He appends this modifier so that the insurer including Medicare knows not to provide reimbursement. Not adhering to the Centers for Medicare and Medicaid Services, or CMS, guidelines of appending this modifier in situations where a provider performs wrong surgery or other invasive procedure on patient may result in wrong payment by insurer and recoupment of the payment later on. Typically, the insurer considers all services the provider delivers in the operating room when an error occurs as related and considers them non covered as well. All other providers in the operating room when the error occurs, who bill individually for their services, are also not eligible for payment. Finally, all related services the patient receives during the same hospitalization in which the error occurs are usually not covered. **Tips:** Modifier PC will ensure that you will not receive reimbursement for the procedure done in error and Medicare also will not cover services related to the error. Using this modifier may increase malpractice risk.
PD	**Diagnostic or related non diagnostic item or service provided in a wholly owned or operated entity to a patient who is admitted as an inpatient within 3 days** **Definition:** Modifier PD is a payment modifier that a provider uses with diagnostic or related non diagnostic items or services that a provider delivers in a wholly owned or operated entity to a patient who becomes an inpatient within three days. **Explanation:** Append this modifier with Healthcare Common Procedure Code System, or HCPCS codes that the provider and supplier use to report preadmission diagnostic and non diagnostic services that relate to the admission. Use this modifier to identify that the entity providing the service is wholly owned or operated by the hospital and the patient who receives the services becomes an inpatient within three days. An entity is wholly owned by the hospital if the hospital is the sole owner of the entity. And, an entity is wholly operated by a hospital if the hospital has exclusive responsibility for conducting and overseeing the entity's routine operations, regardless of whether the hospital also has policymaking authority over the entity. **Tips:** If the entity is not wholly owned or operated by a hospital, do not append modifier PD. Medicare will pay for the professional component of codes with a technical professional split that a provider delivers within three calendar days. When practices append PD to a code that doesn't have both professional and technical components, Medicare will pay for the service based on the facility rate.
PI	**Positron emission tomography (PET) or PET/computed tomography (CT) to inform the initial treatment strategy of tumors that are biopsy proven or strongly suspected of being cancerous based on other diagnostic testing** **Definition:** Append modifier PI to a code for positron emission tomography, PET or PET computed tomography, CT imaging studies that a provider performs to help plan the initial treatment strategy in patients with tumors, suspected to be cancerous by other diagnostic testing or proven to be cancerous through a biopsy. The provider uses the study to determine the location or extent of the tumor. **Explanation:** Modifier PI illustrates the use of imaging studies such as positron emission tomography, PET, or PET computed tomography, CT, in patients known or strongly suspected of having a cancerous tumor, an abnormal growth of tissue that rapidly multiples and spreads throughout the body destroying normal cells. Computed tomography is when the provider rotates an X-ray tube and detectors around a patient, which produces a tomogram, a computer generated cross sectional image, which providers use to diagnose, manage, and treat the disease. These studies enable the provider to plan an initial treatment strategy for patients with tumors that are proven on biopsy or suspected of being cancerous by other diagnostic tests. **Tips:** Append modifier PI when services are related to F 18 fluoro D glucose or FDG PET imaging study. Append modifier PI for procedure codes, such as 78608, Brain imaging, positron emission tomography or PET; metabolic evaluation, and the PET range of codes 78811 through 78816.
PL	**Progressive addition lenses** **Definition:** Append modifier PL to a code for a patient undergoing eye procedures for progressive additional lenses. **Explanation:** Modifier PL illustrates an eye procedure in a patient for the fitting of progressive additional lenses. **Tips:** HCPCS Level II codes represent implantable materials used in the treatment of eye and ear disorders. These codes also report the supplies of visual aids such as contact lenses and glasses.

Mod	Modifier Description, Definition, Explanation, and Tips
PM	**Post mortem** **Definition:** Append modifier PM to a code to identify post mortem visits to a patient. **Explanation:** Modifier PM identifies visits that occur after the death of a patient and on the same day as the patient's death, from visits occurring before death. Providers append the PM modifier for post mortem visits, on the date of death, regardless of the patient's level of care or site of service. The date of death is the date of death reported on the death certificate. Hospice providers are to report hospice visits that occur before death separately from those which occur after death. **Tips:** Do not report post mortem visits occurring on a date subsequent to the date of death, due to system limitations with reporting services after the date of the death. Report modifier PM when billing post mortem visits provided on the date of death beginning with services on or after April 1, 2014.
PN	**Non-excepted service provided at an off-campus, outpatient, provider-based department of a hospital** **Definition:** Modifier PN represents the technical component of non-excepted items and services. **Explanation:** With this modifier, hospitals are paid under the MPFS for non-excepted items and services, which are billed on the institutional claim and must be billed with a new claim line modifier PN to indicate that an item or service is a non-excepted item or service. The payment rate for these services will generally be 50 percent of the OPPS rate with some exceptions. Packaging, and certain other OPPS policies, will continue to apply to such services. Check the CMS website for specific reimbursement information related to services with modifier PN appended, as certain non-excepted services may be paid under MPFS. Do not append modifier PN to excepted items and services – Certain off-campus provider-based departments (PBDs) are permitted to continue to bill Medicare for excepted items and services under the OPPS. Excepted items and services are: All items and services furnished in a dedicated emergency department. Items and services that were furnished and billed by an off-campus PBD prior to November 2, 2015. Items and services furnished in a hospital department within 250 yards of a remote location of the hospital.
PO	**Excepted service provided at an off-campus, outpatient, provider-based department of a hospital** **Definition:** Append the PO modifier to indicate a service, procedure, or surgery that takes place at a provider based hospital outpatient department, off campus. **Explanation:** A hospital facility appends modifier PO to a code for each service, procedure, or surgery that takes place at an off campus location in a provider based outpatient department. Off campus means a location physically separate from the immediate area of the hospital facility and or in a building located more than 250 yards away from the main hospital buildings. This is an informational modifier for data collection purposes. **Tips:** Individual providers should not append modifier PO and instead should use the appropriate place of service code to indicate outpatient services furnished in an on campus, remote, or satellite location of a hospital or in an off campus, provider based hospital setting.
PS	**Positron emission tomography (PET) or PET/computed tomography (CT) to inform the subsequent treatment strategy of cancerous tumors when the beneficiary's treating physician determines that the pet study is needed to inform subsequent anti-tumor strategy** **Definition:** A provider appends modifier PS to a positron emission tomography, or PET, or computed tomography, or CT scan to determine a subsequent treatment strategy of cancerous tumors when the provider determines he needs the PET study to determine a subsequent antitumor strategy for the patient. **Explanation:** Modifier PS illustrates the use of imaging studies such as positron emission tomography, PET, or computed tomography, CT, in patients having a cancerous tumor, or an abnormal growth of tissue that rapidly multiplies and spreads throughout the body destroying normal cells. A positron emission tomography, or PET scan is a nuclear medicine imaging technique, which produces a three dimensional image of functional processes in the body; the system detects pairs of gamma rays emitted indirectly by a positron emitting radionuclide, or tracer, which is introduced into the body on a biologically active molecule, or glucose. A computed tomography, or CT scan is when the provider rotates an X-ray tube and detectors around a patient, which produces a tomogram, a computer generated cross sectional image, which providers use to diagnose, manage, and treat the disease. These studies enable the provider to determine a subsequent treatment strategy for patients with cancerous tumors. **Tips:** Append modifier PS to all procedure codes that the provider bills with a cancer diagnosis codes such as, 78608, Brain imaging, positron emission tomography or PET; metabolic evaluation, and code range 78811 to 78816. While submitting claim for the professional component only, append modifier 26 first, and then append modifier PS. While submitting claim for the technical component only, append modifier TC first, and then append modifier PS.

Mod	Modifier Description, Definition, Explanation, and Tips
PT	**Colorectal cancer screening test; converted to diagnostic test or other procedure** **Definition:** Append this modifier when a colorectal cancer screening test converts to a diagnostic or therapeutic procedure. **Explanation:** Append modifier PT when the provider performs screening colonoscopy, flexible sigmoidoscopy, or barium enema and finds and or removes a lesion or performs a biopsy during the same encounter. **Tips:** Modifier PT waives the deductible for services furnished in connection with or in relation to a colorectal cancer screening test furnished on the same date and in the same encounter as a colonoscopy, flexible sigmoidoscopy, or barium enema that were initiated as colorectal cancer screening services and that became diagnostic or therapeutic. Codes associated with this modifier fall in the range of 10021-69990, Surgery.
Q0	**Investigational clinical service provided in a clinical research study that is in an approved clinical research study** **Definition:** Append modifier Q0 for a service which the provider performs for an approved investigative clinical research study. **Explanation:** Approved investigational clinical services consist of services that the provider investigates as an objective within the study. Not all investigational clinical services are approved. Investigational clinical services may include services that are approved, unapproved, or otherwise covered or not covered under Medicare. **Tips:** Append modifiers Q0 and Q1 on outpatient provider claims for services provided in Medicare qualified clinical trials studies. These include trials that fall under the 2007 Medicare Clinical Trial Policy, trials that a specific National Coverage Determination or NCD, and investigational device exemption or IDE trials requires.
Q1	**Routine clinical service provided in a clinical research study that is in an approved clinical research study** **Definition:** Append modifier Q1 for a routine clinical service that the provider performs for a patient enrolled in an approved clinical research study. **Explanation:** The CMS defines routine clinical services as those items and services that Medicare typically covers for beneficiaries outside of the clinical research study that the provider uses for direct patient management within the study and that do not meet the definition of investigational clinical services. Routine clinical services may include items or services required solely for the provision of the investigational clinical services, e.g., administration of a chemotherapeutic agent; clinically appropriate monitoring, whether or not required by the investigational clinical service, e.g., blood tests to measure tumor markers; and items or services required for the prevention, diagnosis, or treatment of research related adverse events, e.g., blood levels of various parameters to measure kidney function. **Tips:** Append modifiers Q0 and Q1 on outpatient provider claims for services provided in Medicare qualified clinical trials studies. These include trials that fall under the 2007 Medicare Clinical Trial Policy, trials that a specific National Coverage Determination or NCD, and investigational device exemption or IDE trials requires.
Q2	**Demonstration procedure/service** **Definition:** Append modifier Q2 to services billed in conjunction with a demonstration procedure or service. **Explanation:** CMS conducts and sponsors demonstration projects to test and measure the effect of potential program changes. The demonstrations study the likely impact of new methods of service delivery, coverage of new types of service, and new payment approaches on beneficiaries, providers, health plans, states, and the Medicare Trust Funds. Append modifier Q2 when the services involve demonstration of a procedure/service to allow accurate identification and documentation of payment for Medicare beneficiaries enrolled in the demonstration.
Q3	**Live kidney donor surgery and related services** **Definition:** Append modifier Q3 when the provider performs services related to care for a live kidney donor. **Explanation:** The provider appends modifier Q3 for care for a live kidney donor to receive 100 percent reimbursement of the allowed charge. Live kidney donor services include those services which the provider performs during the preoperative, intraoperative, and postoperative periods. The provider bills these services to the carrier under the name and health insurance claim number of the kidney recipient. **Tips:** Medicare part B reimburses for services reported with modifier Q3 if the provider bills the transplant surgery codes 50320, Donor nephrectomy including cold preservation; open, from living donor or 50547, Laparoscopy, surgical; donor nephrectomy including cold preservation, from living donor.

Mod	Modifier Description, Definition, Explanation, and Tips
Q4	**Service for ordering/referring physician qualifies as a service exemption** **Definition:** Append this modifier when a provider orders a service from or refers a Medicare beneficiary to another service provider with whom the original provider has a financial relationship if the service provided qualifies as a service related exemption. **Explanation:** Service related exemptions permit a provider to refer a Medicare beneficiary to a service entity with whom the referring provider has a financial relationship. Append modifier Q4 to the code for the service when an exemption applies. This modifier is for informational purposes only and does not affect the reimbursement. **Tips:** Unless an exception applies, if a physician or a member of a physician's immediate family has a financial relationship with a healthcare entity, the physician may not make referrals to that entity for the furnishing of designated health services, or DHS under the Medicare program. The following services are DHS: clinical laboratory services; physical therapy services; occupational therapy services; radiology services, including magnetic resonance imaging, computerized axial tomography scans, and ultrasound services; radiation therapy services and supplies; durable medical equipment and supplies; parenteral and enteral nutrients, equipment, and supplies; prosthetics, orthotics, and prosthetic devices and supplies; home health services; outpatient prescription drugs; and inpatient and outpatient hospital services. Individual payers may have policies that specify which nonphysicians you may use this modifier for. Check the payer's individual policy to be sure.
Q5	**Service furnished under a reciprocal billing arrangement by a substitute physician or by a substitute physical therapist furnishing outpatient physical therapy services in a health professional shortage area, a medically underserved area, or a rural area** **Definition:** Append modifier Q5 when a substitute provider (physician or physical therapist) evaluates a patient under a reciprocal billing arrangement in a rural area or an area with a shortage of healthcare professionals or medical services. **Explanation:** Modifier Q5 denotes when another provider examines or treats a patient due to absence of the regular provider and based on a prior agreement to cover for one another, when the care takes place in a rural or underserved area. The alternate provider should sign any reports documenting the care he provided. **Tips:** The patient's regular physician may submit the claim, and, if assignment is accepted, receive the Part B payment, for covered visit services, including emergency visits and related services, which the regular physician arranges to be provided by a substitute physician on an occasional reciprocal basis under the following conditions: The regular physician must not be available to provide the visit services; and The Medicare patient needs to arrange or seek to receive the visit services from the regular physician; and This modifier is to be used by providers who render services to patients in a rural area, an area where there is a shortage of healthcare professionals, or an otherwise underserved area. The substitute physician may not provide the visit services to Medicare patients over a continuous period of longer than 60 days subject with an exception for the provider being on active military duty; and The regular physician must identify the services as substitute physician services by entering HCPCS code Q5 modifier, service furnished by a substitute physician under a reciprocal billing arrangement, after the procedure code. The regular physician must keep on file a record of each service provided by the substitute physician, associated with the substitute physician's UPIN or NPI when required, and make this record available to the carrier upon request. If the only substitution services a physician performs in connection with an operation are postoperative services furnished during the period covered by the global fee, these services need not be identified on the claim as substitution services. A physician may have reciprocal arrangements with more than one physician. The arrangements need not be in writing. The regular physician is not entitled to bill and receive direct payment for substitute provider services furnished after the expiration of 60 days of the period. The substitute physician must bill for these services in his or her own name. The regular physician may, however, bill and receive payment for the services that the substitute physician provides on his or her behalf during the 60 day the period. The provider should append modifier Q5 with the supporting documentation providing the reason for the service.

Mod	Modifier Description, Definition, Explanation, and Tips
Q6	**Service furnished under a fee-for-time compensation arrangement by a substitute physician or by a substitute physical therapist furnishing outpatient physical therapy services in a health professional shortage area, a medically underserved area, or a rural area** **Definition:** Append this modifier when a locum tenens, or substitute, provider (physician or physical therapist) performs the services under a fee-for-time compensation agreement, in a rural area or an area with a shortage of healthcare professionals or medical services. **Explanation:** Append modifier Q6 when a locum tenens, or substitute, provider performs healthcare services in the absence of the original provider. Criteria for this modifier include that the regular physician is unavailable to provide the visit services; the Medicare beneficiary has arranged or seeks to receive the visit services from the regular physician; the regular physician pays the locum tenens for his or her services on a per diem or similar fee for time basis; the substitute physician does not provide the visit services to Medicare patients over a continuous period of longer than 60 days subject to some exceptions; the provider renders services to patients in a rural area, an area where there is a shortage of healthcare professionals, or an otherwise underserved area.; and the regular physician identifies the services as substitute physician services meeting the requirements of this section by entering HCPCS code modifier Q6. **Tips:** The locum tenens provider provides a service when the original provider is not present to provide due to any illness, pregnancy, vacation or continuation of medical education. If a provider leaves a medical group and the group hires a locum tenens physician, the medical group must keep on file a record of each service which the substitute provider assumes and also takes a note of the substitute provider's PIN or NPI. Also, the provider identification number PIN or NPI of the provider who has left the medical group is written on the claim to indicate who the locum tenens provider is substituting for. This modifier is to be used by providers who render services to patients in a rural area, an area where there is a shortage of healthcare professionals, or an otherwise underserved area. This modifier has no effect on payment.
Q7	**One class A finding** **Definition:** Append this modifier for foot care that involves at least one class A findings. The provider uses class findings to determine the level of foot care. Medicare does not cover routine foot care unless the patient is suffering from systemic conditions which lead to decreased sensation over the area of foot and leg or when the foot care is essential. **Explanation:** Append modifier Q7 when the provider identifies one class A finding. The provider uses class findings to determine the level of foot care. Class A findings include nontraumatic amputation of foot or integral skeletal portion thereof. Medicare covers the service when the provider renders foot care and identifies one class A finding. Medicare does not cover routine foot care unless the patient is suffering from systemic conditions which lead to decreased sensation over the area of foot and leg or when the foot care is essential. Services ordinarily considered routine might also be covered if they are performed as a necessary and integral part of otherwise covered services, such as diagnosis and treatment of diabetic ulcers, wounds, and infections or if the patient has peripheral neuropathy, i.e., decreased sensation in the extremities that might result in injury if the patient tries to take care of his or her nails. Routine foot care involves excision of corns or calluses, maintenance of cleanliness of foot in bedridden patient, and trimming or debridement of nails. **Tips:** Append modifier Q9, One class B and two class C findings, when the provider identifies one class B and two class C findings. Append modifier Q8, Two class B findings, when the provider identifies two class B findings. Modifiers Q7, Q8, and Q9 should usually be used with HCPCS code G0127, Trimming of dystrophic nails, any number, or CPT® codes 11055 to 11057, Paring or cutting of benign hyperkeratotic lesion, e.g., corn or callus, depending on number of lesions; 11719, Trimming of nondystrophic nails, any number; and when appropriate, 11720, Debridement of nails by any methods; 1 to 5; or 11721, Debridement of nails by any methods; 6 or more.

Mod	Modifier Description, Definition, Explanation, and Tips
Q8	**Two class B findings** **Definition:** Append this modifier for foot care required because of two class B findings. The provider uses class findings to determine the level of foot care. Medicare does not cover routine foot care unless the patient has systemic conditions which lead to decreased sensation over the area of foot and leg or when the foot care is essential. **Explanation:** Append modifier Q8 when the provider identifies two class B findings. The provider uses class findings to determine the level of foot care. Class B findings include absent posterior tibial pulse, absent dorsalis pedis pulse, advanced trophic changes which include any three of the following conditions, such as increased or decreased hair growth; nail thickening; or changes in color, texture, or reddening of the skin. Medicare does not cover routine foot care unless the patient has systemic conditions which lead to decreased sensation over the area of foot and leg or when the foot care is essential. Services ordinarily considered routine might also be covered if they are performed as a necessary and integral part of otherwise covered services, such as diagnosis and treatment of diabetic ulcers, wounds, and infections or if the patient has peripheral neuropathy, i.e., decreased sensation in the extremities that might result in injury if the patient tries to take care of his or her nails. Routine foot care involves excision of corns or calluses, maintenance of cleanliness of foot in bedridden patient, and trimming or debridement of nails. **Tips:** Append modifier Q9, One class B and two class C findings, when the provider identifies one class B and two class C findings. Append modifier Q7, One class A finding, when the provider identifies one class A finding. Modifiers Q7, Q8, and Q9 should usually be used with HCPCS code G0127, Trimming of dystrophic nails, any number, or CPT® codes 11055 to 11057, Paring or cutting of benign hyperkeratotic lesion, e.g., corn or callus, depending on number of lesions; 11719, Trimming of nondystrophic nails, any number; and when appropriate, 11720, Debridement of nails by any methods; 1 to 5; or 11721, Debridement of nails by any methods; 6 or more.
Q9	**One class B and two class C findings** **Definition:** Append this modifier for routine foot care services for one class B finding and two class C findings. The provider uses class findings to determine the level of foot care. Medicare does not cover routine foot care unless the patient has systemic conditions which lead to decreased sensation over the area of foot and leg or when the foot care is essential. **Explanation:** Append modifier Q9 when the provider identifies one class B and two class C findings. The provider uses class findings to determine the level of foot care. Class B findings include absent posterior tibial pulse, absent dorsalis pedis pulse, advanced trophic changes which include any three of the following conditions, such as increased or decreased hair growth; nail thickening; or changes in color, texture, or reddening of the skin. Class C findings include claudication, burning, coldness of the feet, edema, tingling or abnormal spontaneous sensations in the feet. Medicare does not cover routine foot care unless the patient has systemic conditions which lead to decreased sensation over the area of foot and leg or when the foot care is essential. Services ordinarily considered routine might also be covered if they are performed as a necessary and integral part of otherwise covered services, such as diagnosis and treatment of diabetic ulcers, wounds, and infections or if the patient has peripheral neuropathy, i.e., decreased sensation in the extremities that might result in injury if the patient tries to take care of his or her nails. Routine foot care involves excision of corns or calluses, maintenance of cleanliness of foot in bedridden patient, and trimming or debridement of nails. **Tips:** Append modifier Q8, Two class B findings, when the provider identifies two class B findings. Append modifier Q7, One class A finding, when the provider identifies one class A finding. Modifiers Q7, Q8, and Q9 should usually be used with HCPCS code G0127, Trimming of dystrophic nails, any number, or CPT® codes 11055 to 11057, Paring or cutting of benign hyperkeratotic lesion, e.g., corn or callus, depending on number of lesions; 11719, Trimming of nondystrophic nails, any number; and when appropriate, 11720, Debridement of nails by any methods; 1 to 5; or 11721, Debridement of nails by any methods; 6 or more.
QA	**Prescribed amounts of stationary oxygen for daytime use while at rest and nighttime use differ and the average of the two amounts is less than 1 liter per minute (LPM)** **Definition:** Add modifier QA to a code when a patient at rest requires different amounts of stationary oxygen during the daytime and nighttime but the average of the two amounts is less than 1 L per minute (LPM). **Explanation:** Use this modifier when the provider prescribes two different amounts of stationary oxygen for daytime and nighttime use for a patient at rest but the averaged amounts equal less than 1 L per minute. The prescribed oxygen amount depends upon the severity of disease. In severe conditions like chronic obstructive pulmonary disease (COPD) or chronic respiratory failure (CRF) the lungs fail to provide sufficient oxygen to the body tissues. Sufficient oxygen is essential for all normal physiological functions. **Tips:** See QB, QE, QF, QG, QH and QR for other oxygen-related modifiers.

Mod	Modifier Description, Definition, Explanation, and Tips
QB	**Prescribed amounts of stationary oxygen for daytime use while at rest and nighttime use differ and the average of the two amounts exceeds 4 liters per minute (LPM) and portable oxygen is prescribed** **Definition:** Append modifier QB when a provider prescribes different amounts of stationary oxygen for daytime and nighttime use for a patient at rest and the average of the two amounts is greater than 4 L per minute (LPM), when the patient also has portable oxygen prescribed. **Explanation:** Use this modifier when a patient at rest receives different amounts of provider-prescribed stationary oxygen for daytime and nighttime use and the two amounts average out to greater than 4 L per minute, and the patient also has portable oxygen. The prescribed oxygen amount depends upon the severity of disease. In severe conditions like chronic obstructive pulmonary disease (COPD) or chronic respiratory failure (CRF) the lungs fail to provide sufficient oxygen to the body tissues. Sufficient oxygen is essential for all normal physiological functions. **Tips:** Proper use of QB is important because Medicare increases monthly payment for oxygen when the patient has a prescription for portable oxygen in addition to stationary oxygen. See QA, QE, QF, QG, QH and QR for other oxygen-related modifiers.
QC	**Single channel monitoring** **Definition:** Append this modifier for single channel monitoring. Report this modifier for informational purposes only; it does not affect payment. **Explanation:** Append modifier QC when the provider performs single channel monitoring. Report this modifier for informational purposes only; it does not affect payment. Providers routinely monitor patients in the ICU using single-channel electrocardiogram, or ECG, monitoring. **Tips:** Individual payers may have policies that specify which nonphysicians you may use this modifier for. Check the payer's individual policy to be sure.
QD	**Recording and storage in solid state memory by a digital recorder** **Definition:** Append this modifier for recording and storage by a digital recorder in solid state memory. Report this modifier for informational purposes only; it does not affect payment. **Explanation:** Append modifier QD when the provider records and stores the voice data by a digital recorder in a solid state memory. Report this modifier for informational purposes only; it does not affect payment. **Tips:** Individual payers may have policies that specify which nonphysicians you may use this modifier for. Check the payer's individual policy to be sure.
QE	**Prescribed amount of stationary oxygen while at rest is less than 1 liter per minute (LPM)** **Definition:** Append this modifier when a provider prescribes oxygen at less than 1 L per minute (LPM) to a patient. This modifier may be appended only to HCPCS codes for stationary oxygen systems. **Explanation:** Append modifier QE when the supplier prescribes oxygen at less than 1 LPM using a stationary oxygen system for a patient. You should not append this modifier with codes for portable systems or oxygen contents. **Tips:** Append modifier QE with stationary gaseous E0424, Stationary compressed gaseous oxygen system, rental; includes container, contents, regulator, flow meter, humidifier, nebulizer, cannula or mask, and tubing or liquid E0439, Stationary liquid oxygen system, rental; includes container, contents, regulator, flowmeter, humidifier, nebulizer, cannula or mask, & tubing systems or with an oxygen concentrator E1390, Oxygen concentrator, single delivery port, capable of delivering 85 percent or greater oxygen concentration at the prescribed flow rate and E1391, Oxygen concentrator, dual delivery port, capable of delivering 85 percent or greater oxygen concentration at the prescribed flow rate, each. Fee schedule payments for stationary oxygen system rentals are all inclusive and represent a monthly allowance per beneficiary. Accordingly, a supplier must bill on a monthly basis for stationary oxygen equipment and contents furnished during a rental month. The monthly payment of stationary oxygen decreases by 50 percent if the home health agency supplies stationary oxygen. The suppliers bill this service by appending modifier QE. See QA, QB, QF, QG, QH and QR for other oxygen-related modifiers.

Mod	Modifier Description, Definition, Explanation, and Tips
QF	**Prescribed amount of stationary oxygen while at rest exceeds 4 liters per minute (LPM) and portable oxygen is prescribed** **Definition:** Append modifier QF to a code for a patient who is oxygen dependent at rest and receiving more than 4 L of oxygen per minute via a stationary oxygen supply, and who has a provider-prescribed portable oxygen device. **Explanation:** Modifier QF illustrates the quantity of oxygen prescribed, more than 4 L per minute (LPM) to the lungs via a stationary oxygen supply for a patient at rest, as well as prescription of a portable oxygen device. The prescribed oxygen amount depends upon the severity of disease. In severe conditions like chronic obstructive pulmonary disease (COPD) or chronic respiratory failure (CRF) the lungs fail to provide sufficient oxygen to the body tissues. Sufficient oxygen is essential for all normal physiological functions. **Tips:** When the oxygen supply is greater than 4 LPM without use of portable oxygen, use modifier QG (Prescribed Amount Of Stationary Oxygen While At Rest Is Greater Than 4 Liters Per Minute [LPM]). Proper use of QF is important because Medicare increases monthly payment for oxygen when the patient has a prescription for portable oxygen in addition to stationary oxygen. See QA, QB, QE, QG, QH and QR for other oxygen-related modifiers.
QG	**Prescribed amount of stationary oxygen while at rest is greater than 4 liters per minute (LPM)** **Definition:** Append modifier QG to a code for a patient who is oxygen dependent at rest, and the provider prescribes oxygen via stationary supply at more than 4 L per minute. **Explanation:** Modifier QG illustrates the quantity of oxygen prescribed via a stationary supply at more than 4 L per minute (LPM) for a patient at rest. The prescribed oxygen amount depends upon the severity of disease. In severe conditions like chronic obstructive pulmonary disease (COPD) or chronic respiratory failure (CRF), the lungs fail to provide sufficient oxygen to the body tissues. Sufficient oxygen is essential for all normal physiological functions. **Tips:** When the oxygen supply is greater than 4 LPM using a stationary supply, and the patient also has use of a portable oxygen supply, use modifier QG. Proper use of QG is important because Medicare increases monthly payment for oxygen when the patient has a prescription for portable oxygen in addition to stationary oxygen at greater than 4 LPM. See QA, QB, QE, QF, QH and QR for other oxygen-related modifiers.
QH	**Oxygen conserving device is being used with an oxygen delivery system** **Definition:** Append modifier QH to indicate the patient uses a device that controls oxygen flow from an oxygen cylinder based on the rate of inhalation or by delivering pulses of oxygen at fixed volumes per breath. **Explanation:** Modifier QH represents use of an oxygen conserving device with an oxygen delivery system. Patients who are unable to breathe properly due to severe lung disease need supplemental oxygen. The oxygen conserving device, OCD, on a tank or portable oxygen concentrator makes the oxygen supply last longer. It makes oxygen therapy more efficient, more portable. and more cost effective. **Tips:** Medicare requires home health agencies and other suppliers to use modifier QH to indicate the use of an oxygen conserving device. See QE to QH for the range of oxygen related modifiers.
QJ	**Services/items provided to a prisoner or patient in state or local custody, however the state or local government, as applicable, meets the requirements in 42 CFR 411.4 (b)** **Definition:** Append modifier QJ to a code when the provider supplies the service or item to a patient in jail or custody, subject to the regulations at 42 CFR 411.4 (b). The regulations state Medicare may provide payment if the patient in custody has to repay the cost of the service or item provided to him. **Explanation:** Append modifier QJ only if a medical service or item goes to a prisoner or patient in custody whose state or local law requires him to pay for his own medical care, meeting the conditions of 42 CFR411.4b. Typically the state or local government is responsible for covering the costs of patients in custody, but those regulations say that Medicare may pay for services provided to a person in custody if the situation meets two conditions. The first condition is that state or local law requires the person to repay the cost of medical service she received while in custody. The second condition is that the state or local government bills individuals who received medical care, whether under Medicare or not, and then the government follows the same debt collection practices it uses for other debts. **Tips:** You cannot use modifier QJ with service codes when the patient is not in jail or custody. It is incorrect to use modifier QJ if the patient is in jail but state or local government pays the medical bills. If Medicare denies a modifier QJ claim, you may appeal either by showing that the claim meets the conditions of 42 CFR 411.4b or by showing that the patient was not in custody under authority of penal statute.

Mod	Modifier Description, Definition, Explanation, and Tips
QK	**Medical direction of two, three, or four concurrent anesthesia procedures involving qualified individuals** **Definition:** Append modifier QK to the anesthesia code when an anesthesiologist supervises and participates in two to four procedures that overlap each other. **Explanation:** Use modifier QK when the provider performs medical direction for two, three, or four concurrent procedures that involve qualified individuals. The qualified individuals may be Certified Registered Nurse Anesthetists, called CRNAs, Anesthesiologist Assistants, called AAs, interns, residents, or a combination of these individuals. For example, suppose the first procedure begins at 9 a.m. and finishes at 9:30 a.m., the second procedure begins at 9:15 a.m. and finishes at 10 a.m., and the third procedure begins at 9:10 a.m. and finishes at 10:10 a.m. This means when the provider begins the second and third procedure, he is directing more than one procedure at a time. In such a case, the provider appends modifier QK to bill for this service. **Tips:** If a payer receives two anesthesia service claims for the same patient, same date of service, with no medical direction or supervision modifiers, the payer will allow the first claim processed and will deny the second claim, and you will have to appeal with the proper modifiers appended, such as QK, QX, CRNA service: with medical direction by a physician, or QY, Medical direction of one certified registered nurse anesthetist by an anesthesiologist. If you are submitting multiple modifiers, submit modifier QK first.
QL	**Patient pronounced dead after ambulance called** **Definition:** Append modifier QL to an ambulance code when an ambulance arrives and the patient has died on scene. **Explanation:** Modifier QL applies to those ambulance services in which the ambulance reaches the site where the patient is, such as the accident site or home, and a qualified provider declares the patient legally dead before transport in the ambulance. **Tips:** If a provider declares a patient is dead after ambulance dispatch but before ambulance transport, use modifier QL to ensure proper payment. Medicare payment will reflect the basic life support base rate but not mileage or the adjustment for rural services. For payers other than Medicare, check their specific policies.
QM	**Ambulance service provided under arrangement by a provider of services** **Definition:** Append QM modifier to ambulance codes for ambulance services provided under arrangement between the provider and an ambulance company. **Explanation:** When the provider has an arrangement with an ambulance company for ambulance services, then provider appends modifier QM with such ambulance services. **Tips:** If the requesting provider and ambulance service provider are one and the same, append modifier QN, Ambulance service furnished directly by a provider of services. All HCPCS ambulance codes must have a QM or QN modifier.
QN	**Ambulance service furnished directly by a provider of services** **Definition:** Append modifier QN to codes for ambulance services supplied directly by the provider. **Explanation:** Use modifier QN to identify ambulance services the provider supplies directly rather than under financial arrangement with outside ambulance service providers. **Tips:** When the provider has an arrangement with an ambulance company for ambulance services, then provider appends modifier QM, Ambulance service provided under arrangement by a provider of services. When ambulance services are provided by another service provider, it may affect reimbursement for these services from outside vendor. All HCPCS ambulance codes must have a QN or QM modifier.
QP	**Documentation is on file showing that the laboratory test(s) was ordered individually or ordered as a CPT®-recognized panel other than automated profile codes 80002-80019, G0058, G0059, and G0060.** **Definition:** Append modifier QP to laboratory service codes when the clinician orders the test as a single test, whether as an individual test or as a panel. **Explanation:** Laboratory providers append modifier QP to those single laboratory CPT® codes for individual tests or panel tests. For example, if the lab performs many tests like total serum cholesterol, triglycerides, and high density lipid profile, the lab may report them with the single laboratory code 80061, Lipid panel, with modifier QP. When you append this modifier, you're letting the payer know that you have documentation available that the clinician ordered an individual test or a panel represented by a single CPT® code. **Tips:** Modifier QP is an informational modifier that does not affect payment. Note: Codes 80002-80019, G0058, G0059, and G0060 are deleted CPT® and HCPCS codes, but are still included in this official descriptor from CMS.

Mod	Modifier Description, Definition, Explanation, and Tips
QQ	**Ordering professional consulted a qualified clinical decision support mechanism for this service and the related data was provided to the furnishing professional** **Definition:** Append modifier QQ to a code for services for which the provider consulted and received qualified decision support in determining appropriate use criteria (AUC) before ordering an advanced imaging procedure. **Explanation:** Modifier QQ indicates that a provider accessed and received support from a qualified clinical decision support mechanism for a service he provided. Qualified clinical decision support mechanisms factor into appropriate use criteria (AUC) and quality measures required by certain Medicare/CMS participation programs. Qualified clinical decision support mechanism providers must meet certain requirements and be registered by CMS. **Tips:** A list of qualified clinical decision support mechanisms can be found at https://www.cms.gov/Medicare/Quality-Initiatives-Patient-Assessment-Instruments/Appropriate-Use-Criteria-Program/CDSM.html. Beginning in January 2019, physicians must use AUC when ordering advanced imaging procedures such as CT, MRI, and PET for certain specific conditions. Providers can earn points for quality by employing AUC earlier than this deadline.
QR	**Prescribed amounts of stationary oxygen for daytime use while at rest and nighttime use differ and the average of the two amounts is greater than 4 liters per minute (LPM)** **Definition:** Add modifier QR to a code when a patient at rest requires different amounts of stationary oxygen during the daytime and nighttime and the average of the two amounts is greater than 4 L per minute (LPM). **Explanation:** Use this modifier when the provider prescribes two different amounts of stationary oxygen for daytime and nighttime use for a patient at rest and the two amounts average greater than 4 L per minute. The prescribed oxygen amount depends upon the severity of disease. In severe conditions like chronic obstructive pulmonary disease (COPD) or chronic respiratory failure (CRF) the lungs fail to provide sufficient oxygen to the body tissues. Sufficient oxygen is essential for all normal physiological functions. **Tips:** When the daytime and nighttime oxygen supply averages greater than 4 LPM and the patient also has a prescribed portable oxygen supply, use modifier QB. See QA, QB, QE, QF, QG, and QH for other oxygen-related modifiers.
QS	**Monitored anesthesia care service** **Definition:** Append modifier QS to an anesthesia code when the anesthesia provider's services meet the definition of monitored anesthesia care, or MAC. MAC refers a combination of a local anesthetic with sedation generally administered by a provider who is qualified to provide general anesthesia. **Explanation:** Modifier QS indicates that the anesthesia provider, who may be an anesthesiologist or other qualified individual such as a Certified Registered Nurse Anesthetist, CRNA, or Anesthesiologist Assistant, AA, performs monitored anesthesia care. MAC involves monitoring the patient's vital signs while in the operating room, examination prior to anesthesia, the prescription for anesthesia care, and postoperative care. **Tips:** This modifier does not impact reimbursement; it is informational only. Use this modifier in addition to P modifiers for anesthesia codes. If anesthesia provider provides monitored anesthesia care for deep complex, complicated, or markedly invasive surgical procedure, use modifier G8. If anesthesia provider provides monitored anesthesia care for a patient who has history of severe cardiopulmonary condition, use modifier G9. Some payers may pay more for this modifier as long as reasons for providing MAC are medically necessary and documented in the record.
QT	**Recording and storage on tape by an analog tape recorder** **Definition:** Append modifier QT to any CPT® or HCPCS code when a recording is made on analog tape while performing any procedure. **Explanation:** Append this modifier when the provider records any procedure or part of a procedure on analog tape. This modifier does not impact reimbursement, it is purely informational only. **Tips:** You can use this modifier at the last modifier position after all other important modifiers.
QW	**CLIA waived test** **Definition:** Append modifier QW to a laboratory test which has been waived from Clinical Laboratory Improvement Amendments requirements. It is compulsory to have CLIA number for such Centers. **Explanation:** Append this modifier to codes for individual laboratory tests that have been waived by the FDA from CLIA requirements. All medical laboratories, including physician office laboratories, must have CLIA certification in order to receive payments from Medicare and Medicaid. The FDA waives some individual tests from CLIA requirements, and CMS publishes a list of these CLIA waived tests quarterly. Lists of waived tests may be obtained from the CMS CLIA web page and clicking on Categorization of Tests in the menu and downloading Tests Granted Waived Status Under CLIA. Providers may use this list to determine if a particular test product can be appropriately performed by a laboratory with a CLIA waiver and is eligible to be billed using the QW modifier.

Mod	Modifier Description, Definition, Explanation, and Tips
QX	**CRNA service: with medical direction by a physician**
	Definition: Append modifier QX to codes for anesthesia services when a Certified Registered Nurse Anesthetist, CRNA, provides anesthesia under the supervision of a physician provider other than an anesthesiologist.
	Explanation: When a CRNA performs an anesthesia service under supervision of a provider who is not an anesthesiologist, append modifier QX.
	Tips: If a CRNA performs anesthesia services without supervision, use modifier QZ, CRNA service; without medical direction by a physician.
	IF a CRNA performs anesthesia services under the supervision of an anesthesiologist, use modifier QY: Medical direction of one certified registered nurse anesthetist or CRNA by an anesthesiologist.
	This modifier can only be appended to anesthesia codes; if appended to any other code, CMS will deny the claim.
QY	**Medical direction of one certified registered nurse anesthetist (CRNA) by an anesthesiologist**
	Definition: Append modifier QY to codes for anesthesia services when one Certified Registered Nurse Anesthetist, CRNA, provides anesthesia under the supervision of an anesthesiologist provider.
	Explanation: When one CRNA performs anesthesia services under supervision of anesthesiologist provider, append modifier QY.
	Tips: If a CRNA performs anesthesia services with supervision of a physician provider other than an anesthesiologist, use modifier QX, CRNA service; with medical direction by a physician.
	If a CRNA performs anesthesia services without the supervision of a provider, use modifier QZ: CRNA service; without medical direction by a physician.
	This modifier can only be appended to anesthesia codes; if appended to any other code, CMS will deny the claim.
QZ	**CRNA service: without medical direction by a physician**
	Definition: Append modifier QZ to codes for anesthesia services when a Certified Registered Nurse Anesthetist, CRNA, provides anesthesia without supervision.
	Explanation: When a CRNA performs anesthesia services independently without supervision of any provider, append modifier QZ.
	Tips: If a CRNA performs anesthesia services with supervision of a physician provider other than an anesthesiologist, use modifier QX, CRNA service: with medical direction by a physician.
	If a CRNA performs anesthesia service with supervision of an anesthesiologist, use modifier QY, Medical direction of one certified registered nurse anesthetist, CRNA, by an anesthesiologist.
	If a CRNA performs anesthesia services without the supervision of a provider, use modifier QZ: CRNA service; without medical direction by a physician.
	This modifier can only be appended to anesthesia codes; if appended to any other code, CMS will deny the claim.
RA	**Replacement of a DME, orthotic or prosthetic item**
	Definition: Append the modifier RA when the provider replaces the durable medical equipment, prosthetics, or orthotics, and supplies, or DMEPOS, when the beneficiary loses the item or damages it in such a way that it can't be repaired.
	Explanation: Append this modifier to the claim for the replacement of DMEPOS when the supplier furnishes the beneficiary with a new item, identical to the original item, to replace a lost, stolen, or irreparably damaged item. Irreparable damage refers to the wear and tear of the equipment due to an accident, disaster, day to day use, or other event. The medical documentation must include the details related to the replacement of the item.
	Append the RA modifier on all DMEPOS claims where an item replaces the same item which has been lost, stolen, or irreparably damaged prior to the equipment's reasonable useful lifetime and also for billing replacement claims when the DMEPOS item has met its reasonable useful lifetime. CMS encourages suppliers to enter the abbreviation RUL which indicates reasonable useful lifetime and the date the beneficiary received the original equipment that is being replaced when billing for an item that has met its reasonable useful lifetime use.
	Tips: If the supplier replaces only a part of the item to repair it, use modifier RB, Replacement of a part of a DME, orthotic or prosthetic item furnished as part of a repair.

Mod	Modifier Description, Definition, Explanation, and Tips
RB	**Replacement of a part of a DME, orthotic or prosthetic item furnished as part of a repair** **Definition:** Append the modifier RB when the provider replaces a part of the durable medical equipment, prosthetics, orthotics, and supplies, or DMEPOS, to repair the item. **Explanation:** Append this modifier to the claim for the replacement of a part of the DMEPOS, so as to repair the damage. The supplier furnishes the beneficiary with a new replacement part for a damaged or worn out part of the item. The medical documentation must include the details related to the replacement of the part of the item, including the amount of time the repair takes, the HCPCS code for the base equipment, that the patient owns the equipment, and the date the patient acquired the equipment. This modifier applies only to items that the beneficiary owns. If the beneficiary rents the DMEPOS item, the rental amount includes the cost of repair and maintenance. **Tips:** If the provider replaces the item completely, use modifier RA, Replacement of a DME, orthotic or prosthetic item.
RC	**Right coronary artery** **Definition:** Append modifier RC to a code for procedures on the right coronary artery. **Explanation:** Append this modifier to codes when the provider performs a procedure on the right coronary artery. The right coronary artery supplies blood to the right atrium and ventricle of the heart, i.e., the upper and the lower chamber of the heart respectively. **Tips:** The various types of procedures on the right coronary artery include angioplasty, atherectomy, stent placement, or grafting. If the provider performs a procedure on the left circumflex, append modifier LC, Left circumflex coronary artery. If the provider performs a procedure on the left anterior descending artery, use modifier LD, Left anterior descending coronary artery. If the provider targets the main coronary artery, use modifier LM, Left main coronary artery. If the provider performs a procedure on ramus intermedius coronary artery, use modifier RI, Ramus intermedius coronary artery.
RD	**Drug provided to beneficiary, but not administered "incident-to"** **Definition:** Append modifier RD to a claim for a drug that the provider supplies to the beneficiary and the beneficiary may administer the drug on his own. **Explanation:** Report this modifier when the provider supplies a drug to the beneficiary which he may administer on his own. The phrase incident to refers to when the provider administers or supplies a drug as part of his services, such as those necessary to accomplish a primary procedure.
RE	**Furnished in full compliance with FDA-mandated risk evaluation and mitigation strategy (REMS)** **Definition:** Append modifier RE to report extended release or long acting opioid drugs that the provider supplies in compliance with the Food and Drug Administration, or FDA, risk evaluation and mitigation strategy, or REMS. **Explanation:** Append this modifier to the code for an extended release, ER, or long acting, LA, opioid drug, which the provider supplies in compliance with the FDA's risk evaluation and mitigation strategy. ER, LA opioids are highly potent FDA approved drugs, such as morphine sulfate, fentanyl, oxycodone, and hydrocodone, used to treat moderate to severe persistent pain for serious and chronic conditions. The misuse and abuse of these drugs have resulted in a serious public health crisis of addiction, overdose, and death. The REMS is part of a multiagency federal effort to address the growing problem of prescription drug abuse and misuse. The REMS introduces new safety measures to reduce risks and improve safe use of ER, LA opioids while continuing to provide access to these medications for patients in pain.
RI	**Ramus intermedius coronary artery** **Definition:** Append modifier RI to the codes for a procedure on the ramus intermedius coronary artery. **Explanation:** Append this modifier to the code when the provider performs a procedure on the ramus intermedius coronary artery. The ramus intermedius coronary artery branches off the left coronary artery, one of the major arteries that supplies blood to the left atrium and ventricle of the heart, i.e., the upper and the lower chambers of the heart respectively. **Tips:** The various types of procedures on the coronary artery include angioplasty, atherectomy, stent placement, or grafting. If the provider performs a procedure on the left circumflex, append modifier LC, Left circumflex coronary artery. If the provider performs a procedure on the left anterior descending artery, use modifier LD, Left anterior descending coronary artery. If the provider targets the main coronary artery, use modifier LM, Left main coronary artery. If the provider performs a procedure on right coronary artery, use modifier RC, Right coronary artery.

Mod	Modifier Description, Definition, Explanation, and Tips
RR	**Rental (use the 'RR' modifier when DME is to be rented)** **Definition:** A provider appends modifier RR to identify the use of rented durable medical equipment, or DME, items. **Explanation:** Append modifier RR for rented DME's. Durable medical equipments is medical equipment that helps a patient to manage his activities of daily living in an easier way or that provides therapeutic benefits to a patient. The equipment this modifier is typically applicable to may be inexpensive or other routinely purchased DME, frequent or substantial servicing, certain customized items, or oxygen equipment. A few examples of DME's are crutches, wheelchairs, commodes, canes, walkers, hospital beds, patient safety equipment, and fracture and traction apparatus. **Tips:** Append modifier RR for certain services that the provider submits to durable medical equipment Medicare Administrative Contractors.
RT	**Right side (used to identify procedures performed on the right side of the body)** **Definition:** Append this modifier to the code for a procedure that a provider performs on the patient's right side. **Explanation:** Use this modifier to identify a procedure on the right side of the body. This modifier usually applies to procedures on paired organs, such as eyes, nostrils, ears, ovaries, lungs, and kidneys. **Tips:** If the provider performs the procedure on the left side of the body, append modifier LT, Left side, to identify procedures performed on the left side of the body. If the provider carries out a procedure on both sides, i.e., on each organ of an organ pair, append modifier 50, Bilateral procedure. If the provider performs the service on an organ which is not paired, such as the right side of the back, do not append modifier RT, since there is only one back.
SA	**Nurse practitioner rendering service in collaboration with a physician** **Definition:** Append modifier SA when a nurse practitioner assists the provider in a procedure, other than a surgery. **Explanation:** Use this modifier to show that a nurse practitioner assists the provider in performing a procedure. This modifier should not be used with a surgery code. Nurse practitioner may refer to a certified registered nurse or an assistant. Nurse practitioners are graduates of a nursing program. **Tips:** Use this modifier when the provider bills a service on behalf of the nurse practitioner, who assists the provider during nonsurgical services. If a nurse midwife assists the provider, append modifier SB, Nurse midwife.
SB	**Nurse midwife** **Definition:** Append modifier SB when a nurse midwife performs a service, other than a surgery. **Explanation:** Use this modifier to show that a nurse midwife assists the provider in performing a nonsurgical procedure. This modifier should not be appended to a surgery code. Nurse midwives are certified graduates of a nursing program, who specialize in midwifery i.e., those who provide patient care during pregnancy and childbirth. **Tips:** Use this modifier when the provider bills a service on behalf of the nurse midwife, who assists the provider during nonsurgical services. If a nurse practitioner assists the provider, append modifier SA, Nurse practitioner rendering service in collaboration with a physician.
SC	**Medically necessary service or supply** **Definition:** Append modifier SC to codes for services or supplies deemed medically necessary under Medicare's coverage requirements. **Explanation:** The provider appends this modifier for the supply of medically necessary services. Medically necessary services and supplies are those that help to diagnose and treat a medical condition and meet the standard care of medical practice.

Mod	Modifier Description, Definition, Explanation, and Tips
SD	**Services provided by registered nurse with specialized, highly technical home infusion training** **Definition:** Append modifier SD to infusion codes when a registered nurse or RN provides infusion services to a patient with a chronic illness who continues to need intravenous infusions at home after discharge from a hospital or rehabilitation Centers. **Explanation:** Append this modifier to infusion codes when a patient, who has a chronic illness and requires intravenous therapy for long term care, receives the service from a trained infusion nurse. Services include administering intravenous therapies, monitoring the patient's condition at home, and training the patient or caregiver how to properly clean and adjust intravenous tubes. Registered nurses are graduates of a nursing program who have passed a national licensing exam. Infusion nurses obtain specialized training and credentials to administer intravenous medications. **Tips:** Do not use modifier SD with infusion codes when the infusion is administered in a hospital setting.
SE	**State and/or federally-funded programs/services** **Definition:** Append modifier SE to codes for services that are paid by state or federal government. **Explanation:** Use modifier SE for those CPT® and HCPCS codes where the state or federal government pays the bills for the services or programs.
SF	**Second opinion ordered by a professional review organization (PRO) per section 9401, p.l. 99-272 (100% reimbursement - no Medicare deductible or coinsurance)** **Definition:** Append modifier SF to such CPT® codes where a quality improvement organization or QIO, also known as peer review organization or PRO, asks a provider to give a second opinion to confirm the decision of another provider. Codes with the SF modifier are reimbursed at 100% with no Medicare deductible or coinsurance if approved. **Explanation:** Append this code when a QIO or PRO asks a provider to give a second opinion for a decision or diagnosis made by another provider. When this modifier is applied, the patient does not pay a deducible or have to use coinsurance, and Medicare pays the provider 100% per section 9401, p.l. 99-272. **Tips:** You can use modifier SF only with certain eye surgery codes.
SG	**Ambulatory surgical Centers (ASC) facility service** **Definition:** Modifier SG appended to CPT® codes identified services provided by an ambulatory surgical Centers, which means facility fee only. Effective for services on or after January 1, 2008, the SG modifier is no longer applicable for Medicare services. ASC providers should discontinue applying the SG modifier on ASC facility claims. **Explanation:** Effective for services on or after January 1, 2008, the SG modifier is no longer applicable for Medicare services. ASC providers should discontinue applying the SG modifier on ASC facility claims.
SH	**Second concurrently administered infusion therapy** **Definition:** Append modifier SH to infusion codes for the second drug when a provider administers more than one drug at the same time by intravenous infusion. Use this code for intravenous infusion therapy codes administered in the patient's home. **Explanation:** When the provider administers two drugs at the same time by intravenous infusion in the patient's home, append this code. This modifier applies only to home infusion therapy. **Tips:** If provider administers three or more drugs by infusion therapy at the same time, use modifier SJ, Third or more concurrently administered infusion therapy.
SJ	**Third or more concurrently administered infusion therapy** **Definition:** Append modifier SJ to home infusion codes for each additional drug after the second when the provider administers multiple drugs at the same time by intravenous infusion. Use this code for intravenous infusion therapy codes administered in the patient's home. **Explanation:** When the provider administers three or more drugs at the same time by intravenous drug infusion in the patient's home, append modifier SH. This modifier applies only to home infusion therapy. **Tips:** If provider administers two drugs at the same time by intravenous infusion, use modifier SH, Second concurrently administered infusion therapy.
SK	**Member of high risk population (use only with codes for immunization)** **Definition:** Append modifier SK to immunization codes that are identified for those people who are at high risk for getting a disease, e.g., underlying medical conditions, weakened immune systems, work related, or other special circumstances that increase risk of illness. **Explanation:** When the provider provides immunization to people that he identifies as high risk, he appends modifier SK to such codes. High risk includes those with underlying medical conditions, weakened immune systems, work related, or other special circumstances that increase risk of illness. Identification of high risk individuals is determined by clinical expertise. Decisions regarding whether an individual is part of a high risk population and should receive a specific preventive item or service identified for those at high risk should be made by the attending provider. **Tips:** Do not use modifier SK for immunization codes that are given to patients who are not at high risk.

Mod	Modifier Description, Definition, Explanation, and Tips
SL	**State supplied vaccine** **Definition:** Append modifier SL to vaccine codes that a state supplies and a provider administers at no cost to eligible individuals. **Explanation:** Each state provides some vaccines free of cost. Use modifier SL with immunization procedure codes to identify those immunization materials obtained from the state Department of Health to identify that the vaccine itself was obtained at no cost to the provider or patient. **Tips:** You may use this modifier with CPT® codes in the range of 90460 to 90474, Immunization administration for vaccines and toxoids that accurately reflects the administration of the vaccines. Do not append modifier SL to the administration procedure codes. Both the procedure code for the vaccine itself and the code for administration must be submitted, and all vaccines administered on a single date of service must be reported on the same claim.
SM	**Second surgical opinion** **Definition:** Append modifier SM to evaluation and management codes for claims by a consulting provider, when another provider has requested a second opinion. **Explanation:** Use this modifier when you submit an evaluation and management code for a second opinion. The provider performing the second opinion submits the code with the modifier. **Tips:** This modifier may be used with CPT® and HCPCS level II codes. Patient initiated second opinions that relate to the medical need for surgery or for major nonsurgical diagnostic and therapeutic procedures, e.g., invasive diagnostic techniques such as cardiac catheterization and gastroscopy, are covered under Medicare. In the event that the recommendation of the first and second physician differs regarding the need for surgery, or other major procedure, a third opinion is also covered. Second and third opinions are covered even though the surgery or other procedure, if performed, is determined not covered. Payment may be made for the history and examination of the patient and for other covered diagnostic services required to properly evaluate the patient's need for a procedure and to render a professional opinion. In some cases, the results of tests done by the first physician may be available to the second physician.
SN	**Third surgical opinion** **Definition:** Use this modifier when you submit an evaluation and management code for a third opinion. The provider performing the third opinion submits the code with the modifier. **Explanation:** Use this modifier when you submit an evaluation and management code for a third opinion. The provider performing the third opinion submits the code with the modifier. A third opinion might be requested when the original provider and the consultant come to different conclusions. **Tips:** Patient initiated second opinions that relate to the medical need for surgery or for major nonsurgical diagnostic and therapeutic procedures, e.g., invasive diagnostic techniques such as cardiac catheterization and gastroscopy, are covered under Medicare. In the event that the recommendation of the first and second physician differs regarding the need for surgery, or other major procedure, a third opinion is also covered. Second and third opinions are covered even though the surgery or other procedure, if performed, is determined not covered. Payment may be made for the history and examination of the patient and for other covered diagnostic services required to properly evaluate the patient's need for a procedure and to render a professional opinion. In some cases, the results of tests done by the first physician may be available to the second physician.
SQ	**Item ordered by home health** **Definition:** Append this modifier to indicate that the item the provider orders is for home health service in a patient's home. **Explanation:** Append modifier SQ for an item ordered for a patient receiving home health services such as home infusion therapy, catheter care or maintenance, and respiratory therapy equipment and services. A provider may need to use the SQ modifier for medical and dressing supplies, or durable medical equipment, DME to indicate that the item is for home health use. For coverage of an item, medical documentation for the item and a dated order is generally necessary, with some items requiring preauthorization. **Tips:** This modifier is not covered by Medicare. However, some other payers may allow the claim to process under their home care benefit without a copayment when the provider appends this modifier. For rented durable medical equipment, or DME, use modifier RR, Rented equipment.

Mod	Modifier Description, Definition, Explanation, and Tips
SS	**Home infusion services provided in the infusion suite of the IV therapy provider** **Definition:** Append modifier SS when the therapy provider introduces a requisite drug at a specific dosage and at a specific rate into the patient's blood vessels at the infusion therapy providers outpatient infusion suite, a medical office that provides outpatient infusion services. **Explanation:** Append modifier SS when the provider prepares the infusion equipment or provides administration and supplies using the provider's own infusion suite. For example, a typical infusion may involve the provider using an intravenous line connected to a small mechanical pump to administer the drug at the prescribed rate for the prescribed length of time. The time recorded is for the duration of the patient service in the suite. Providers append the modifier to applicable HCPCS codes, which may include: S5522, PICC line insertion, supplies catheter excluded; S5520, PICC line kit; S5523, Midline insertion, supplies catheter excluded and S5521, Midline kit. **Tips:** This modifier is not covered by Medicare. However, some other payers may allow the claim to process under the home care benefit without a copayment. If a nurse does the infusion, use modifier SD, Services provided by registered nurse with specialized, highly technical home infusion training.
ST	**Related to trauma or injury** **Definition:** Append modifier ST to services the provider performs in the case of trauma or injury. **Explanation:** Append modifier ST to report procedures or services which the provider performs on a patient who has undergone a trauma or injury. **Tips:** This modifier is not covered by Medicare but other payers may allow the addition of the ST modifier to codes associated with a trauma patient's care, as long as the care is related to the trauma. The ST modifier may permit a supplemental payment for designated trauma Centers and enhanced rates to providers for trauma cases that meet specific criteria. If a trauma response team associated with hospital provides intensive level of examination and care that a Medicare patient requires, use code G0390, Trauma services associated with critical care services. Medicare policies provide coverage for critical care services of less than 30 minutes provided to the beneficiaries.
SU	**Procedure performed in physician's office (to denote use of facility and equipment)** **Definition:** A provider appends modifier SU to indicate where the provider performs the service in order to show that the provider uses his own facility and equipment while performing a procedure on the patient. **Explanation:** A provider appends modifier SU as an informational modifier to show the location of the service relative to the costs associated with the procedure that the provider performs for the patient. This may include the costs of running an office such as rent, equipment, supplies, and nonphysician staff costs, which may be referred to as the practice expense. **Tips:** Modifier SU is not payable by Medicare.
SV	**Pharmaceuticals delivered to patient's home but not utilized** **Definition:** A provider appends modifier SV to the pharmaceuticals or drugs that a patient receives in the home but the patient never uses them. **Explanation:** A provider appends modifier SV as an informational modifier to indicate drugs that a patient receives in his home setting but never uses them. There are various reasons for the patient not using the drugs, such as a change in the patient's condition, the patient dies, or the patient is admitted to a hospital or skilled nursing facility, or other facility. **Tips:** Modifier SV is not payable by Medicare.
SW	**Services provided by a certified diabetic educator** **Definition:** Append modifier SW to identify services that a certified diabetic educator provides to a diabetic patient. **Explanation:** Append modifier SW to denote services that a certified diabetic educator provides to a diabetic patient about lifestyle modification and self management. He may give training to the patient on how to monitor blood glucose levels, educate the patient about diet and exercise, and provide awareness about insulin treatment plans. The educator provides these services according to the instruction of the provider, who is managing the patient's diabetes condition. Certification from the provider, who is managing the patient's condition, is necessary regarding the patient's needs and implementation for the coverage of the service. **Tips:** Medicare provides coverage for diabetes self management education and training, which is provided by a certified provider in accordance with Medicare policies. Reimbursement is based on carrier judgment.

Mod	Modifier Description, Definition, Explanation, and Tips
SY	**Persons who are in close contact with member of high-risk population (use only with codes for immunization)**
	Definition: Append this modifier to codes for immunizations a patient receives who either cares for or works closely with patient who are highly prone to infection or a disease.
	Explanation: Append this informational modifier with codes for immunization of persons in close contact with patients who come under the category of high risk population, meaning patients who may have a preexisting risk factor, pathology, or decreased immunity and are more likely to be affected with an infection or disease.
	Append this modifier with codes for immunizations such as G0008, Administration of influenza virus vaccine, or CPT® 90371, Hepatitis B immune globulin (HBIg), human, for intramuscular use. This code includes the provider counseling the patient or family.
	Tips: Medicare does not pay for this modifier.
	For immunizations of a member of a high risk population, use modifier SK, Member of high risk population, use only with codes for immunization.
T1	**Left foot, second digit**
	Definition: Append modifier T1 to identify that the provider performs the procedure on the second digit, or toe, of the left foot.
	Explanation: This modifier identifies services that the provider performs on the second digit, or toe, of a patient's left foot. Use this modifier for services such as amputation, arthrodesis, or fusion of joints of the toe, a repair, revision or reconstruction procedure, removal of foreign body from within the toe and nail bed procedures.
	HCPCS level II modifiers apply to codes for procedures that the provider performs on paired organs, like eyelids, fingers, or toes. These modifiers help to prevent denials when the provider submits duplicate codes to report separate procedures on different sites or different sides of the body.
	Tips: The reimbursement for this code depends on carrier judgment.
	For nail debridement, there is no need to add toe modifiers since up to five nails are included in the nail debridement code 11720, Debridement of nails by any method; one to five. You could include the T modifiers to be more specific to the carrier.
	For avulsion of ingrown toe nails, use the CPT® code 11730, Avulsion of nail plate, partial or complete, simple; single. Append the appropriate toe modifier depending on which toe nail the provider treats. If the provider treats two or more nails, report each with appropriate T modifier separately.
	For biopsy of a nail unit use CPT® code 11755, Biopsy of nail unit, and append appropriate T modifier. For example, for biopsy of the fourth digit, or the toe, on the left foot report 11755 T3.
	A patient presents with five ingrown toenails. The provider completes simple avulsion on both sides of left foot, great toe and right foot, great toe, and one side of left foot, second digit. Report 11730 TA, left foot, great toe; 11732 T5 59, Avulsion of nail plate, partial or complete, simple; each additional nail plate, right foot, great toe; 11732 T1 59, left foot, second digit. 11732 is used for each additional nail plate after the first 11730.
	Use amputation codes 28810, Amputation, metatarsal, with toe, single for amputation of the metatarsal ray along with the attached toe; or code 28825, Amputation, toe; interphalangeal joint, when the provider removes a toe from its interphalangeal joint. Append the T modifier according to the toe the provider removes.

Mod	Modifier Description, Definition, Explanation, and Tips
T2	**Left foot, third digit**

Definition: Append modifier T2 to identify that the provider performs a procedure on the third digit, or toe, of the left foot.

Explanation: This modifier identifies services that a provider performs on the third digit, or toe, of a patient's left foot. Use this modifier for services such as amputation, arthrodesis or fusion of joints of the toe, a repair, revision or reconstruction procedure, removal of foreign body from within the toe and nail bed procedures.

HCPCS level II modifiers apply to codes for procedures that the provider performs on paired organs, like eyelids, fingers, or toes. These modifiers help to prevent denials when the provider submits duplicate codes to report separate procedures on different sites or different sides of the body.

Tips: The reimbursement for this code depends on carrier judgment.

For nail debridement, there is no need to add toe modifiers since up to five nails are included in the nail debridement code 11720, Debridement of nails by any method; one to five. You could include the T modifiers to be more specific to the carrier.

For avulsion of ingrown toe nails, use the CPT® code 11730, Avulsion of nail plate, partial or complete, simple; single. Append the appropriate toe modifier depending on which toe nail the provider treats. If the provider treats two or more nails, report each with appropriate T modifier separately.

For biopsy of a nail unit use CPT® code 11755, Biopsy of nail unit, and append appropriate T modifier. For example, for biopsy of the fourth digit, or the toe, on the left foot report 11755 T3.

A patient presents with five ingrown toenails. The provider completes simple avulsion on both sides of left foot, great toe and right foot, great toe, and one side of left foot, second digit. Report 11730 TA, left foot, great toe; 11732 T5 59, Avulsion of nail plate, partial or complete, simple; each additional nail plate, right foot, great toe; 11732 T1 59, left foot, second digit. 11732 is used for each additional nail plate after the first 11730.

Use amputation codes 28810, Amputation, metatarsal, with toe, single for amputation of the metatarsal ray along with the attached toe; or code 28825, Amputation, toe; interphalangeal joint, when the provider removes a toe from its interphalangeal joint. Append the T modifier according to the toe the provider removes.

T3	**Left foot, fourth digit**

Definition: Append modifier T3 to identify that the provider performs a procedure on the fourth digit, or toe, of the left foot.

Explanation: This modifier identifies services that the provider performs on the fourth digit, or toe, of a patient's left foot. Use this modifier for services such as amputation, arthrodesis or fusion of joints of the toe, a repair, revision or reconstruction procedure, removal of foreign body from within the toe and nail bed procedures.

HCPCS level II modifiers apply to codes for procedures that the provider performs on paired organs, like eyelids, fingers, or toes. These modifiers help to prevent denials when the provider submits duplicate codes to report separate procedures on different sites or different sides of the body.

Tips: The reimbursement for this code depends on carrier judgment.

For nail debridement, there is no need to add toe modifiers since up to five nails are included in the nail debridement code 11720, Debridement of nails by any method; one to five. You could include the T modifiers to be more specific to the carrier.

For avulsion of ingrown toe nails, use the CPT® code 11730, Avulsion of nail plate, partial or complete, simple; single. Append the appropriate toe modifier depending on which toe nail the provider treats. If the provider treats two or more nails, report each with appropriate T modifier separately.

For biopsy of a nail unit use CPT® code 11755, Biopsy of nail unit, and append appropriate T modifier. For example, for biopsy of the fourth digit, or the toe, on the left foot report 11755 T3.

A patient presents with five ingrown toenails. The provider completes simple avulsion on both sides of left foot, great toe and right foot, great toe, and one side of left foot, second digit. Report 11730 TA, left foot, great toe; 11732 T5 59, Avulsion of nail plate, partial or complete, simple; each additional nail plate, right foot, great toe; 11732 T1 59, left foot, second digit. 11732 is used for each additional nail plate after the first 11730.

Use amputation codes 28810, Amputation, metatarsal, with toe, single for amputation of the metatarsal ray along with the attached toe; or code 28825, Amputation, toe; interphalangeal joint, when the provider removes a toe from its interphalangeal joint. Append the T modifier according to the toe the provider removes.

Mod	Modifier Description, Definition, Explanation, and Tips
T4	**Left foot, fifth digit** **Definition:** Append modifier T4 to identify that the provider performs a procedure on the fifth digit, or toe, of the left foot. **Explanation:** This modifier identifies services that a provider performs on the fifth digit, or toe, of a patient's left foot. Use this modifier for services such as amputation, arthrodesis or fusion of joints of the toe, a repair, revision or reconstruction procedure, removal of foreign body from within the toe and nail bed procedures. HCPCS level II modifiers apply to codes for procedures that the provider performs on paired organs, like eyelids, fingers, or toes. These modifiers help to prevent denials when the provider submits duplicate codes to report separate procedures on different sites or different sides of the body. **Tips:** The reimbursement for this code depends on carrier judgment. For nail debridement, there is no need to add toe modifiers since up to five nails are included in the nail debridement code 11720, Debridement of nails by any method; one to five. You could include the T modifiers to be more specific to the carrier. For avulsion of ingrown toe nails, use the CPT® code 11730, Avulsion of nail plate, partial or complete, simple; single. Append the appropriate toe modifier depending on which toe nail the provider treats. If the provider treats two or more nails, report each with appropriate T modifier separately. For biopsy of a nail unit use CPT® code 11755, Biopsy of nail unit, and append appropriate T modifier. For example, for biopsy of the fourth digit, or the toe, on the left foot report 11755 T3. A patient presents with five ingrown toenails. The provider completes simple avulsion on both sides of left foot, great toe and right foot, great toe, and one side of left foot, second digit. Report 11730 TA, left foot, great toe; 11732 T5 59, Avulsion of nail plate, partial or complete, simple; each additional nail plate, right foot, great toe; 11732 T1 59, left foot, second digit. 11732 is used for each additional nail plate after the first 11730. Use amputation codes 28810, Amputation, metatarsal, with toe, single for amputation of the metatarsal ray along with the attached toe; or code 28825, Amputation, toe; interphalangeal joint, when the provider removes a toe from its interphalangeal joint. Append the T modifier according to the toe the provider removes.
T5	**Right foot, great toe** **Definition:** Append modifier T5 to identify that the provider performs a procedure on the great toe of the right foot. **Explanation:** This modifier identifies services that a provider performs on the great toe of a patient's right foot. Use this modifier for services such as amputation, arthrodesis or fusion of joints of the toe, a repair, revision or reconstruction procedure, removal of foreign body from within the toe and nail bed procedures. HCPCS level II modifiers apply to codes for procedures that the provider performs on paired organs, like eyelids, fingers, or toes. These modifiers help to prevent denials when the provider submits duplicate codes to report separate procedures on different sites or different sides of the body. **Tips:** The reimbursement for this code depends on carrier judgment. For nail debridement, there is no need to add toe modifiers since up to five nails are included in the nail debridement code 11720, Debridement of nails by any method; one to five. You could include the T modifiers to be more specific to the carrier. For avulsion of ingrown toe nails, use the CPT® code 11730, Avulsion of nail plate, partial or complete, simple; single. Append the appropriate toe modifier depending on which toe nail the provider treats. If the provider treats two or more nails, report each with appropriate T modifier separately. For biopsy of a nail unit use CPT® code 11755, Biopsy of nail unit, and append appropriate T modifier. For example, for biopsy of the fourth digit, or the toe, on the left foot report 11755 T3. A patient presents with five ingrown toenails. The provider completes simple avulsion on both sides of left foot, great toe and right foot, great toe, and one side of left foot, second digit. Report 11730 TA, left foot, great toe; 11732 T5 59, Avulsion of nail plate, partial or complete, simple; each additional nail plate, right foot, great toe; 11732 T1 59, left foot, second digit. 11732 is used for each additional nail plate after the first 11730. Use amputation codes 28810, Amputation, metatarsal, with toe, single for amputation of the metatarsal ray along with the attached toe; or code 28825, Amputation, toe; interphalangeal joint, when the provider removes a toe from its interphalangeal joint. Append the T modifier according to the toe the provider removes.

Mod	Modifier Description, Definition, Explanation, and Tips
T6	**Right foot, second digit** **Definition:** Append modifier T6 to identify that the provider performs a procedure on the second digit, or toe, of the right foot. **Explanation:** This modifier identifies services that a provider performs on the second digit, or toe, of a patient's right foot. Use this modifier for services such as amputation, arthrodesis or fusion of joints of the toe, a repair, revision or reconstruction procedure, removal of foreign body from within the toe and nail bed procedures. HCPCS level II modifiers apply to codes for procedures that the provider performs on paired organs, like eyelids, fingers, or toes. These modifiers help to prevent denials when the provider submits duplicate codes to report separate procedures on different sites or different sides of the body. **Tips:** The reimbursement for this code depends on carrier judgment. For nail debridement, there is no need to add toe modifiers since up to five nails are included in the nail debridement code 11720, Debridement of nails by any method; one to five. You could include the T modifiers to be more specific to the carrier. For avulsion of ingrown toe nails, use the CPT® code 11730, Avulsion of nail plate, partial or complete, simple; single. Append the appropriate toe modifier depending on which toe nail the provider treats. If the provider treats two or more nails, report each with appropriate T modifier separately. For biopsy of a nail unit use CPT® code 11755, Biopsy of nail unit, and append appropriate T modifier. For example, for biopsy of the fourth digit, or the toe, on the left foot report 11755 T3. A patient presents with five ingrown toenails. The provider completes simple avulsion on both sides of left foot, great toe and right foot, great toe, and one side of left foot, second digit. Report 11730 TA, left foot, great toe; 11732 T5 59, Avulsion of nail plate, partial or complete, simple; each additional nail plate, right foot, great toe; 11732 T1 59, left foot, second digit. 11732 is used for each additional nail plate after the first 11730. Use amputation codes 28810, Amputation, metatarsal, with toe, single for amputation of the metatarsal ray along with the attached toe; or code 28825, Amputation, toe; interphalangeal joint, when the provider removes a toe from its interphalangeal joint. Append the T modifier according to the toe the provider removes.
T7	**Right foot, third digit** **Definition:** Append modifier T7 to identify that the provider performs a procedure on the third digit, or toe, of the right foot. **Explanation:** This modifier identifies that the provider performs the procedure on the third digit, or toe, of a patient's right foot. Use this modifier for services such as amputation, arthrodesis or fusion of joints of the toe, a repair, revision or reconstruction procedure, removal of foreign body from within the toe and nail bed procedures. HCPCS level II modifiers apply to codes for procedures that the provider performs on paired organs, like eyelids, fingers, or toes. These modifiers help to prevent denials when the provider submits duplicate codes to report separate procedures on different sites or different sides of the body. **Tips:** The reimbursement for this code depends on carrier judgment. For nail debridement, there is no need to add toe modifiers since up to five nails are included in the nail debridement code 11720, Debridement of nails by any method; one to five. You could include the T modifiers to be more specific to the carrier. For avulsion of ingrown toe nails, use the CPT® code 11730, Avulsion of nail plate, partial or complete, simple; single. Append the appropriate toe modifier depending on which toe nail the provider treats. If the provider treats two or more nails, report each with appropriate T modifier separately. For biopsy of a nail unit use CPT® code 11755, Biopsy of nail unit, and append appropriate T modifier. For example, for biopsy of the fourth digit, or the toe, on the left foot report 11755 T3. A patient presents with five ingrown toe nails. The provider completes simple avulsion on both sides of left foot, great toe and right foot, great toe, and one side of left foot, second digit. Report 11730 TA, left foot, great toe; 11732 T5 59, Avulsion of nail plate, partial or complete, simple; each additional nail plate, right foot, great toe; 11732 T1 59, left foot, second digit. 11732 is used for each additional nail plate after the first 11730. Use amputation codes 28810, Amputation, metatarsal, with toe, single for amputation of the metatarsal ray along with the attached toe; or code 28825, Amputation, toe; interphalangeal joint, when the provider removes a toe from its interphalangeal joint. Append the T modifier according to the toe the provider removes.

Mod	Modifier Description, Definition, Explanation, and Tips
T8	**Right foot, fourth digit** **Definition:** Append modifier T8 to identify that the provider performs a procedure on the fourth digit, or toe, of the right foot. **Explanation:** This modifier identifies services that the provider performs on the fourth digit, or toe, of a patient's right foot. Use this modifier for services such as amputation, arthrodesis or fusion of joints of the toe, a repair, revision or reconstruction procedure, removal of foreign body from within the toe and nail bed procedures. HCPCS level II modifiers apply to codes for procedures that the provider performs on paired organs, like eyelids, fingers, or toes. These modifiers help to prevent denials when the provider submits duplicate codes to report separate procedures on different sites or different sides of the body. **Tips:** The reimbursement for this code depends on carrier judgment. For nail debridement, there is no need to add toe modifiers since up to five nails are included in the nail debridement code 11720, Debridement of nails by any method; one to five. You could include the T modifiers to be more specific to the carrier. For avulsion of ingrown toe nails, use the CPT® code 11730, Avulsion of nail plate, partial or complete, simple; single. Append the appropriate toe modifier depending on which toe nail the provider treats. If the provider treats two or more nails, report each with appropriate T modifier separately. For biopsy of a nail unit use CPT® code 11755, Biopsy of nail unit, and append appropriate T modifier. For example, for biopsy of the fourth digit, or the toe, on the left foot report 11755 T3. A patient presents with five ingrown toenails. The provider completes simple avulsion on both sides of left foot, great toe and right foot, great toe, and one side of left foot, second digit. Report 11730 TA, left foot, great toe; 11732 T5 59, Avulsion of nail plate, partial or complete, simple; each additional nail plate, right foot, great toe; 11732 T1 59, left foot, second digit. 11732 is used for each additional nail plate after the first 11730. Use amputation codes 28810, Amputation, metatarsal, with toe, single for amputation of the metatarsal ray along with the attached toe; or code 28825, Amputation, toe; interphalangeal joint, when the provider removes a toe from its interphalangeal joint. Append the T modifier according to the toe the provider removes.
T9	**Right foot, fifth digit** **Definition:** Append modifier T9 to identify that the provider performs a procedure on the fifth digit, or toe, of the right foot. **Explanation:** This modifier identifies services that the provider performs on the fifth digit, or toe, of a patient's right foot. Use this modifier for services such as amputation, arthrodesis or fusion of joints of the toe, a repair, revision or reconstruction procedure, removal of foreign body from within the toe and nail bed procedures. HCPCS level II modifiers apply to codes for procedures that the provider performs on paired organs, like eyelids, fingers, or toes. These modifiers help to prevent denials when the provider submits duplicate codes to report separate procedures on different sites or different sides of the body. **Tips:** The reimbursement for this code depends on carrier judgment. For nail debridement, there is no need to add toe modifiers since up to five nails are included in the nail debridement code 11720, Debridement of nails by any method; one to five. You could include the T modifiers to be more specific to the carrier. For avulsion of ingrown toe nails, use the CPT® code 11730, Avulsion of nail plate, partial or complete, simple; single. Append the appropriate toe modifier depending on which toe nail the provider treats. If the provider treats two or more nails, report each with appropriate T modifier separately. For biopsy of a nail unit use CPT® code 11755, Biopsy of nail unit, and append appropriate T modifier. For example, for biopsy of the fourth digit, or the toe, on the left foot report 11755 T3. A patient presents with five ingrown toenails. The provider completes simple avulsion on both sides of left foot, great toe and right foot, great toe, and one side of left foot, second digit. Report 11730 TA, left foot, great toe; 11732 T5 59, Avulsion of nail plate, partial or complete, simple; each additional nail plate, right foot, great toe; 11732 T1 59, left foot, second digit. 11732 is used for each additional nail plate after the first 11730. Use amputation codes 28810, Amputation, metatarsal, with toe, single for amputation of the metatarsal ray along with the attached toe; or code 28825, Amputation, toe; interphalangeal joint, when the provider removes a toe from its interphalangeal joint. Append the T modifier according to the toe the provider removes.

Mod	Modifier Description, Definition, Explanation, and Tips
TA	**Left foot, great toe** **Definition:** Append modifier TA to identify that the provider performs a procedure on the great toe of the left foot. **Explanation:** This modifier identifies services that the provider performs on the great toe of a patient's left foot. Use this modifier for services such as amputation, arthrodesis or fusion of joints of the toe, a repair, revision or reconstruction procedure, removal of foreign body from within the toe and nail bed procedures. HCPCS level II modifiers apply to codes for procedures that the provider performs on paired organs, like eyelids, fingers, or toes. These modifiers help to prevent denials when the provider submits duplicate codes to report separate procedures on different sites or different sides of the body. **Tips:** The reimbursement for this code depends on carrier judgment. For Mitchell osteotomy in the left first metatarsal use 28296, Correction, hallux valgus or bunion, with or without sesamoidectomy; with metatarsal osteotomy, e.g., Mitchell, Chevron, or concentric type procedures and append modifier TA. Use code 28750 Arthrodesis, great toe; metatarsophalangeal joint for Arthrodesis or fusion of the joint connecting the great toe to the foot. For arthrodesis of the left foot with great toe therefore use 28750 TA. Use code 28755 Arthrodesis, great toe; interphalangeal joint for Arthrodesis or fusion of the joint connecting the small bones within the great toe to the foot. For arthrodesis of the small joints within the left great toe therefore use 28755 TA. For nail debridement, do not add toe modifiers since up to five nails are included in the nail debridement code 11720, Debridement of nails by any method; one to five. You could include the T modifiers to be more specific to the carrier. For avulsion of ingrown toe nails, use the CPT® code 11730, Avulsion of nail plate, partial or complete, simple; single. Append the appropriate toe modifier depending on which toe nail the provider treats. If the provider treats two or more nails, report each with appropriate T modifier separately. For biopsy of a nail unit use CPT® code 11755, Biopsy of nail unit, and append appropriate T modifier. For example for biopsy of left great toe, report 11755 TA. A patient presents with five ingrown toenails. The provider completes simple avulsion on both sides of left foot, great toe and right foot, great toe, and one side of left foot, second digit. Report 11730 TA, left foot, great toe; 11732 T5 59, Avulsion of nail plate, partial or complete, simple; each additional nail plate, right foot, great toe; 11732 T1 59, left foot, second digit. 11732 is used for each additional nail plate after the first 11730. Use amputation codes 28810, Amputation, metatarsal, with toe, single for amputation of the metatarsal ray along with the attached toe; or code 28825, Amputation, toe; interphalangeal joint, when the provider removes a toe from its interphalangeal joint. Append the T modifier according to the toe the provider removes.
TB	**Drug or biological acquired with 340b drug pricing program discount, reported for informational purposes** **Definition:** Append modifier TB for informational purposes to a code for a drug or biological (a drug derived from a living organism using biotechnology) purchased at a discount as determined by the 340b Drug Pricing Program. **Explanation:** Modifier TB indicates that a drug was purchased at a discount as determined under the 340B Drug Pricing Program. This modifier is for informational purposes, meaning that although the drug was purchased at a discount, other conditions stipulated by the 340B Drug Pricing Program may not apply. Biological refers to a drug derived from human, animal, or microorganism components using biotechnology; examples include cells, genes, tissues, recombinant proteins, vaccines, allergens, and blood and blood components. **Tips:** The price of drugs covered by the Drug Pricing Program is calculated based on a formula contained in section 340B(a)(2) of the Public Health Service Act. Participating providers in this program who may purchase drugs at these significantly lower prices are registered with DHHS/HRSA's Office of Pharmacy Affairs (www.hrsa.gov/opa).
TC	**Technical component; under certain circumstances, a charge may be made for the technical component alone; under those circumstances the technical component charge is identified by adding modifier 'TC' to the usual procedure number; technical component charges are institutional charges and not billed separately by physicians; however, portable X-ray suppliers only bill for technical component and should utilize modifier TC; the charge data from portable X-ray suppliers will then be used to build customary and prevailing profiles** **Definition:** A provider appends modifier TC to bill for the technical component of a test only. **Explanation:** Append modifier TC to report the technical component of a procedure that has both a technical and professional component, the payment for which consists of the practice and the malpractice expenses. The provider commonly appends this modifier to procedures such as injection administration, laboratory, radiology, surgery, and radiation therapy. **Tips:** Append modifier TC if the procedure reads as 1, in the PC or TC indicator on the Medicare physician fee schedule database, or MPFSDB. As modifier TC is a payment modifier, report this modifier as the first modifier.

Mod	Modifier Description, Definition, Explanation, and Tips
TD	**RN** **Definition:** A provider appends this license level modifier TD when a registered nurse, or RN, provides services to a patient. A license level modifier such as TD represents the treating provider's license level that some payers base reimbursement upon. **Explanation:** A provider may use this modifier to show that a registered nurse helps the provider perform a service. This modifier should not be used with a surgery code. The modifier may also be applicable for behavioral health use, or for home health billing. The nurses may only provide services and bill for codes that fall within the scope of practice allowed by their professional training and state licensure. Check state specific requirements and payer's guidelines for all applicable uses for this code. **Tips:** If a nurse midwife assists the provider, append modifier SB, Nurse midwife. If a nurse practitioner assists the provider with a service, append modifier SA, Nurse practitioner rendering service in collaboration with a physician.
TE	**LPN/LVN** **Definition:** Append this license level modifier TE when a licensed practical nurse, LPN, or a licensed vocational nurse, LVN, provides services to a patient. A license level modifier represents the treating provider's license level that some payers base reimbursement upon. **Explanation:** A provider may use this modifier to show that a licensed practical nurse or a licensed vocational nurse helps the provider perform a service. This modifier stands for a licensed practical nurse, or LPN, in most of the United States. In other areas such as California and Texas, they are also known as a licensed vocational nurse, or LVN. An LPN or LVN takes care of patients who are ill, disabled, or injured. They work under the direction of a supervising physician. This modifier should not be used with a surgery code. The modifier may also be applicable for behavioral health use, or for home health billing. The nurses may only provide services and bill for codes that fall within the scope of practice allowed by their professional training and state licensure. Check state specific requirements and payer's guidelines for all applicable uses for this code. **Tips:** Medicare does not pay for this modifier. If a nurse midwife assists the provider, append modifier SB, Nurse midwife. If a nurse practitioner assists the provider with a service, append modifier SA, Nurse practitioner rendering service in collaboration with a physician. If a registered nurse assists the provider, append the modifier TD, RN.
TF	**Intermediate level of care** **Definition:** A provider may append this tier level modifier of TF when the patient receives services at an intermediate level of care. **Explanation:** This modifier indicates that the patient receives an intermediate level of care. A provider determines a patient's level of care by the type and amount of assistance or care the patient requires. An intermediate level is physician supervised service of a patient that typically does not need continuous care or daily therapeutic treatment. Some payers also require this modifier for physical, and or occupational therapy services, home management activities assistance, and even when reporting some tiered office level services. Medicare may even require this modifier at times such as on provider claims for demonstration services to indicate a level of complexity. **Tips:** Medicare does not pay for this modifier. If the patient receives a complex or high level of care, append modifier TG, Complex high level of care.
TG	**Complex/high tech level of care** **Definition:** A provider appends modifier TG when a patient receives a complex or high level of care. **Explanation:** This modifier indicates that the patient receives a complex or high level of care. A provider determines a patient's level of care by the type and amount of assistance or care the patient requires. The patient with a complex or high level of care may have multiple conditions simultaneously, or a critical condition that necessitates a highly skilled and complex level of care, which one or more multispecialty providers may render in a well equipped facility. This may be combined with behavioral health problems, limited functional capabilities, and other patient needs. A provider uses this code to indicate a more intense level of service and a higher complexity of treatment. **Tips:** Medicare does not pay for this modifier. If the patient receives an intermediate level of care, append modifier TF, Intermediate level of care.

Mod	Modifier Description, Definition, Explanation, and Tips
TH	**Obstetrical treatment/services, prenatal or postpartum** **Definition:** A provider appends modifier TH when a female patient receives medical care for problems related to her pregnancy and following the birth of the child. **Explanation:** This modifier indicates that a female patient receives medical care for problems related to her pregnancy and following the birth of the child. The provider may render requisite treatment for the various aspects of pregnancy, including monitoring the health of the mother and providing medical support for the recovery of the mother following a cesarean or normal delivery. **Tips:** Medicare does not pay for this modifier.
TJ	**Program group, child and/or adolescent** **Definition:** Append modifier TJ when a group of children or adolescents receive a treatment or therapy program together as a group. **Explanation:** This modifier indicates that the provider renders a service or provides therapy to a group of children or adolescent patients together at the same session. Some states may use to flag service for children's screening exams or mental health services, too. **Tips:** Medicare does not pay for this modifier.
TK	**Extra patient or passenger, non-ambulance** **Definition:** A provider appends modifier TK for a nonambulance vehicle transport of a patient with the patient's caregiver or parent, or an extra patient or passenger. **Explanation:** Use this modifier when a non ambulance vehicle such as a wheel chair van, mini bus or mobility van carries a patient and their caregiver or parent, or an extra patient or passenger. A multiple carry trip for example typically consists of two or more patients who a provider transports on the same trip. **Tips:** Medicare does not pay for this modifier.
TL	**Early intervention/individualized family service plan (IFSP)** **Definition:** A provider appends modifier TL when the provider charts out an early intervention or an individualized service plan for a patient. **Explanation:** Use modifier TL if the provider suggests an early intervention plan for a patient with a condition such as developmental delay, one of a group of disorders a patient can develop in childhood, affecting behavioral growth and development skills. The provider may also offer a customized plan that he charts out according to the specific needs of the patient and family. This type of service is often known as an individualized family service plan, or IFSP. **Tips:** The T modifiers are the HCPCS modifiers for procedures, supplies and durable medical equipment codes. Medicare does not pay for this modifier.
TM	**Individualized education program (IEP)** **Definition:** A provider appends modifier TM when the provider charts out an individualized service plan, or IEP for a patient. **Explanation:** Use modifier TM if the provider suggests a customized patient education plan that he charts out according to the specific needs of the patient and family. A comprehensive IEP treatment plan developed for a specific child may include behavior health, physical therapy, occupational therapy, speech therapy, and audiology services along with screening and assessment services and even IEP specialized transportation. **Tips:** The T modifiers are the HCPCS modifiers for procedures, supplies, and durable medical equipment codes. Medicare does not pay for this modifier.
TN	**Rural/outside providers' customary service area** **Definition:** A provider appends this modifier to services he provides in a rural area or an area outside his normal service area. **Explanation:** A provider appends modifier TN as an informational modifier to identify services he provides in a rural area or area outside his normal service area such as outside the county in which the provider is located. This modifier may also identify such services as nonambulance transportation services, home health or hospice services, respite care services, and nursing care, or therapy services a provider renders outside their regular service area. **Tips:** This modifier may be applicable with certain transportation codes.

Mod	Modifier Description, Definition, Explanation, and Tips
TP	**Medical transport, unloaded vehicle** **Definition:** A provider appends modifier TP to indicate mileage when a patient is not present in the vehicle. **Explanation:** Use this informational modifier to indicate unloaded mileage when submitting claims for nonemergency transport services such as a wheelchair van, mini bus, or mobility van. Transportation providers are normally paid for loaded mileage, or the time a patient is actually in the vehicle. An unloaded vehicle usually refers to when a patient is not present in the vehicle. Any unloaded mileage is usually inclusive in the base rate for these services. **Tips:** The T modifiers are the HCPCS modifiers for procedures, supplies, and durable medical equipment codes. Medicare does not pay for this modifier. Some payers may also require use of modifier TP with procedure codes A0021 to A0999, which identify all transportation services, including ambulance.
TQ	**Basic life support transport by a volunteer ambulance provider** **Definition:** A provider appends modifier TQ when a volunteer ambulance provider performs a basic life support transport. **Explanation:** Use this modifier when a volunteer ambulance provider performs a basic life support level of service patient transport to the requisite destination. Basic life support services, or BLS services, require the ambulance provider meet certain guidelines, which may include at least two attendants in the ambulance, one of which must be a certified emergency medical technician, or EMT, legally approved to operate all lifesaving and life-sustaining equipment. **Tips:** The T modifiers are the HCPCS modifiers for procedures, supplies, and durable medical equipment codes. Medicare does not pay for this modifier. Some payers may also require use of modifier TP with procedure codes A0021 to A0999, which identify all transportation services, including ambulance.
TR	**School-based individualized education program (IEP) services provided outside the public school district responsible for the student** **Definition:** A provider appends modifier TR when the provider performs school based customized education program services. He provides these services outside the public school district responsible for the student. **Explanation:** Use HCPCS modifier TR when the provider renders a personalized school based education program for a student. He provides this individualized education service, or IEP, outside the public school district responsible for the student. A comprehensive IEP treatment plan developed for a specific child may include behavior health, physical therapy, occupational therapy, speech therapy, and audiology services, along with screening and assessment services, and even IEP specialized transportation. **Tips:** The T modifiers are the HCPCS modifiers for procedures, supplies, and durable medical equipment codes. Medicare does not pay for this modifier.
TS	**Follow-up service** **Definition:** A provider appends modifier TS for a follow up service for a patient after a first or initial service or procedure. **Explanation:** Use this HCPCS modifier when the provider renders follow up service subsequent to the initial service or procedure. In the follow up service, the provider monitors the recovery or prognosis of the patient's condition. He may also advise additional measures to manage new symptoms that may emerge since the patient's last visit. **Tips:** The T modifiers are the HCPCS modifiers for procedures, supplies, and durable medical equipment codes. Medicare individuals with a diagnosis of prediabetes and certain risk factors may receive up to two screening tests per year and one screening test every six months. A provider reports these screening services with the appropriate Glucose code from the range 82947 to 82951 and modifier TS to indicate the service is a follow up service.
TT	**Individualized service provided to more than one patient in same setting** **Definition:** A provider appends modifier TT when the provider offers an individualized service to more than one patient in the same setting. **Explanation:** Use the HCPCS modifier TT when the provider renders personalized service to each of two or more patients in the same setting. This modifier may identify services provided to two patients who reside in the same residence. The provider generally delivers the service simultaneously. The services can range from nursing services, to multiple passenger transports, to behavior therapy services. **Tips:** The T modifiers are the HCPCS modifiers for procedures, supplies, and durable medical equipment codes. Medicare does not pay for this modifier.

Mod	Modifier Description, Definition, Explanation, and Tips
TU	**Special payment rate, overtime** **Definition:** A provider appends modifier TU for a special payment rate when the provider performs overtime work, or time worked before or after normally scheduled hours. **Explanation:** Use HCPCS modifier TU to denote the special payment rate that applies when the provider performs services overtime. For example some payers may reimburse for after hours care provided outside the normal business hours, including weekends or holidays and before 8 am and after 5 pm; Monday through Friday. In these situations the payer may require the provider to report the services with the TU modifier in order to receive the special rate. **Tips:** The T modifiers are the HCPCS modifiers for procedures, supplies, and durable medical equipment codes. Medicare does not pay for this modifier.
TV	**Special payment rates, holidays/weekends** **Definition:** A provider appends modifier TV to all services that a patient receives on holidays or weekends, to advise the payer that special payment rates may apply. **Explanation:** Append modifier TV for additional reimbursement for delivery of service at times other than regularly scheduled office hours. This may include, such situations as off hours care, or extended care on a weekend or holiday, when the office is normally closed. **Tips:** Modifier TV is not payable by Medicare. A provider may use modifier TV for a patient who requires seven day per week home care service. Medicaid and other insurers may pay a higher rate for home care visits made on recognized holidays if they are preauthorized.
TW	**Back-up equipment** **Definition:** A provider appends modifier TW to report all types of back up durable medical equipment, or DME. Back up DME, is a secondary piece of equipment that is identical or similar to DME that is already in use. It meets the same medical need for a patient but is provided as a precaution for an emergency situation in case the primary piece of equipment fails. **Explanation:** A provider appends modifier TW for back up durable medical equipment. DME is medical equipment that helps a patient to manage his activities of daily living in an easier way or that provides therapeutic benefits to a patient. A few examples of back up DME's are wheelchairs, oxygen and other respiratory apparatus such as a backup ventilator, other patient monitoring devices, patient safety equipment, ambulatory infusion pumps, fracture and traction apparatus, and artificial kidney machines. **Tips:** Payers may require providers to append modifier TW to identify back up DME when requesting prior authorization for the item, as well as when submitting claims. Some payers may also request the TW modifier for Orthotic and Prosthetic Devices. Modifier TW is not payable by Medicare.
U1	**Medicaid level of care 1, as defined by each state** **Definition:** A provider appends modifier U1 to report the services related to a Medicaid level of care 1, as defined by each state. The level of care may relate to the amount of assistance a patient requires, or the complexity of care. A state may also use this code to have the provider identify a type of service or patient situation. See state specific requirements for use of this code. **Explanation:** A provider appends modifier U1 according to their states specific requirements. The code often defines a tiered service based upon complexity of care but a provider may need to apply the modifier to identify a type of service such as a healthcare home programs, comprehensive care, coordination and planning, and initial plan; or skilled nursing services A or B level of care. A provider may also use this code when he does not identify any behavioral health need during screening or evaluation of a patient. Identification of behavioral health need means that the provider, who is evaluating the patient, identifies a patient who is typically a child with a significant or potential behavioral health services need. **Tips:** The definition of modifier U1 may depend upon the procedure code the provider appends the modifier to. For example, in Minnesota the U1 modifier may define Care coordination, basic complexity level when a provider reports with Medical home program, comprehensive care coordination and planning codes S0280 or S0281, but it may mean substance abuse treatment for a special population or clients with children when the provider reports the modifier with H2035, Alcohol And/Or Other Drug Treatment Program, Per Hour. In compliance with Texas, or TX Medicaid, a provider appends modifier U1 to U3, with all delivery claims with codes, 59409, Vaginal delivery only, with or without episiotomy and or forceps, 59612, Vaginal delivery only, after previous cesarean delivery with or without episiotomy and or forceps, 59514, Cesarean delivery only, and 59620, Cesarean delivery only, following attempted vaginal delivery after previous cesarean delivery. Providers in Minnesota follow healthcare homes payment methodology to determine whether a patient's condition meets the requirement for a major chronic condition. At this time, the tier reflects the number of major chronic condition groups the patient has and a provider uses a modifier to reflect the projected intensity of care coordination services the patient will require. A provider uses modifier U1 for patients who have one to three major chronic condition groups, to indicate the patient is in Tier one.

Mod	Modifier Description, Definition, Explanation, and Tips
U2	**Medicaid level of care 2, as defined by each state** **Definition:** A provider appends modifier U2 to report the services related to a Medicaid level of care 2, as defined by each state. The level of care may relate to the amount of assistance a patient requires, or the complexity of care. A state may also use this code to have the provider identify a type of service or patient situation. See state specific requirements for use of this code. **Explanation:** A provider appends modifier U2 according to their states specific requirements. The code often defines a tiered service based upon complexity of care but a provider may need to apply the modifier to identify a type of service such as a healthcare home programs, comprehensive care, coordination and planning, and initial plan; or skilled nursing services A or B level of care. A provider may also use this code when he identifies any behavioral health need during screening or evaluation of a patient. Identification of behavioral health need means that the provider, who is evaluating the patient, identifies a patient who is typically a child with a significant or potential behavioral health services need. **Tips:** In compliance with Texas, or TX Medicaid, a provider appends modifier U1 to U3, with all delivery claims with codes, 59409, Vaginal delivery only, with or without episiotomy and or forceps, 59612, Vaginal delivery only, after previous cesarean delivery with or without episiotomy and or forceps, 59514, Cesarean delivery only, and 59620, Cesarean delivery only, following attempted vaginal delivery after previous cesarean delivery. Providers in Minnesota follow healthcare homes payment methodology to determine whether a patient's condition meets the requirement for a major chronic condition. At this time, the tier reflects the number of major chronic condition groups the patient has and a provider uses a modifier to reflect the projected intensity of care coordination services the patient will require. A provider uses modifier U2 for patients who have seven to nine major chronic condition groups, to indicate the patient is in Tier three.
U3	**Medicaid level of care 3, as defined by each state** **Definition:** A provider appends modifier U3 to report the services related to a Medicaid level of care 3, as defined by each state. The level of care may relate to the amount of assistance a patient requires, or the complexity of care. A state may also use this code to have the provider identify a type of service or patient situation. See state specific requirements for use of this code. **Explanation:** A provider appends modifier U3 according to their states specific requirements. The code often defines a tiered service based upon complexity of care but a provider may need to apply the modifier to identify a type of service or situation such as a healthcare home programs, comprehensive care, coordination and planning, and initial plan; or skilled nursing services A or B level of care. A provider may use this code for a mental health services encounter when he performs a behavioral health screening or evaluation of a patient. Identification of behavioral health need means that the provider, who is evaluating the patient, identifies a patient who is typically a child with a significant or potential behavioral health services need. **Tips:** Professional claims for Medicare demonstration services may include optional supplemental factor modifier U3. Supplemental complexity modifiers means that the provider will be eligible to receive a 15 percent or 30 percent increase in his healthcare homes care coordination payment for certain more complex patients. To indicate complexity, providers in Minnesota may use modifier U3, Primary language non English. This means that the English language skills are not sufficient to discuss and create complicated care plans, complex care choices, and options. This may apply to the patient or to a caregiver of a dependent patient. This also includes those patients or caregivers who are hearing impaired and require a sign language interpreter or use an augmentative communication device. Providers must consider whether the language barrier is significant enough to prevent a discussion with a patient's care team for care coordination services and report this modifier.

Mod	Modifier Description, Definition, Explanation, and Tips
U4	**Medicaid level of care 4, as defined by each state** **Definition:** A provider appends modifier U4 to report the services related to a Medicaid level of care 4, as defined by each state. The level of care may relate to the amount of assistance a patient requires, or the complexity of care. A state may also use this code to have the provider identify a type of service or patient situation. See state specific requirements for use of this code. **Explanation:** A provider appends modifier U4 according to their states specific requirements. A provider may use this code when he identifies any behavioral health need during screening or evaluation of a patient. Identification of behavioral health need means that the provider, who is evaluating the patient, identifies a patient who is a child with a significant or potential behavioral health services need. **Tips:** Professional claims for Medicare demonstration services may include optional supplemental factor modifier U4. Supplemental complexity modifiers mean that the provider will be eligible to receive a 15 percent or 30 percent increase in his healthcare homes care coordination payment for certain more complex patients. To indicate complexity, providers in Minnesota may use modifier U4 for severe and persistent mental illness. This means the patient has an active diagnosis of schizophrenia, bipolar disorder, major depression, or borderline personality disorder as per Minnesota statute. This may apply to the patient or to a caregiver of a dependent patient. If a patient has either one of the supplemental complexity modifiers, the allowable charge for the tier payment at this time increases by 15 percent. If both complexity modifiers are present, the allowable charge for the tier payment increases by 30 percent. Providers follow the guidelines provided by the Minnesota healthcare homes payment methodology to determine whether a patient's situation meets the level of warranting a supplemental complexity factor.
U5	**Medicaid level of care 5, as defined by each state** **Definition:** A provider appends modifier U5 to report the services related to a Medicaid level of care 5, as defined by each state. The level of care may relate to the amount of assistance a patient requires, or the complexity of care. A state may also use this code to have the provider identify a type of service or patient situation. See state specific requirements for use of this code. **Explanation:** A provider appends modifier U5 according to their states specific requirements. The code often defines a tiered service based upon complexity of care but a provider may need to apply the modifier to identify a type of service or situation such as a healthcare home programs, comprehensive care, coordination and planning, and initial plan, or an increased substance abuse treatment with medical services. A provider may use this code for a mental health services encounter when he performs a behavioral health screening or evaluation of a patient. Identification of behavioral health need means that the provider, who is evaluating the patient, identifies a patient who is typically a child with a significant or potential behavioral health services need. **Tips:** A provider uses U5 as a local modifier with codes for obstetrical and gynecological services in Illinois. The modifier flags the services as Direct Access services, or service available without a referral. For the Kansas Medical Assistance Program, or KMAP, a provider can append the U5 modifier to identify a Targeted Case Management service when appropriate, typically in the case of the frail and elderly who require a higher level of service. Modifier U5 is not payable by Medicare.
U6	**Medicaid level of care 6, as defined by each state** **Definition:** A provider appends modifier U6 to report the services related to a Medicaid level of care 6, as defined by each state. The level of care may relate to the amount of assistance a patient requires, or the complexity of care. A state may also use this code to have the provider identify a type of service or patient situation. See state specific requirements for use of this code. **Explanation:** A provider appends modifier U6 according to their states specific requirements. The code often defines a tiered service based upon complexity of care but a provider may need to apply the modifier to identify a type of service or situation such as a healthcare home programs, comprehensive care, coordination and planning, and initial plan; or for increased service such as an authorized podiatry encounter. A provider may use this code when he identifies any behavioral health need during screening or evaluation of a patient. Identification of behavioral health need means that the provider, who is evaluating the patient, identifies a patient who is a child with a significant or potential behavioral health services need. **Tips:** An Illinois provider may use U6 as a local modifier with codes for service provided within 60 days of hospital discharge such as a therapy visit within 60 days of hospital discharge. One use of the modifier for California Medicaid is to indicate EC pills, or emergency contraceptive pills. When filing Arkansas Medicaid family planning claims for provider services in an outpatient clinic, the modifier U6, identifies a basic family planning visit, Modifier U6 is not payable by Medicare.

Mod	Modifier Description, Definition, Explanation, and Tips
U7	**Medicaid level of care 7, as defined by each state** **Definition:** A provider appends modifier U7 to report the services related to a Medicaid level of care 7, as defined by each state. The level of care may relate to the amount of assistance a patient requires, or the complexity of care. A state may also use this code to have the provider identify a type of service or patient situation. See state specific requirements for use of this code. **Explanation:** A provider appends modifier U7 according to their states specific requirements. The code often defines a tiered service based upon complexity of care but a provider may need to apply the modifier to identify a type of service or situation such as a healthcare home programs, comprehensive care, coordination and planning, and initial plan; or an increased service such as an All-inclusive Clinic Visit. A provider may use this code for a mental health services encounter when he performs a behavioral health screening or evaluation of a patient. Identification of behavioral health need means that the provider, who is evaluating the patient, identifies a patient who is typically a child with a significant or potential behavioral health services need. **Tips:** Illinois uses U7 as a local modifier to flag the services for pregnancy resulting from incest. California Medicaid, applies the U7 modifier to denote services rendered by a Physician Assistant, PA. A provider appends the U7 modifier in Indiana for all waiver services. Modifier U7 is not payable by Medicare.
U8	**Medicaid level of care 8, as defined by each state** **Definition:** A provider appends modifier U8 to report the services related to a Medicaid level of care 8, as defined by each state. The level of care may relate to the amount of assistance a patient requires, or the complexity of care. A state may also use this code to have the provider identify a type of service or patient situation. See state specific requirements for use of this code. **Explanation:** A provider appends modifier U8 according to their states specific requirements. The code often defines a tiered service based upon complexity of care but a provider may need to apply the modifier to identify a type of service or situation such as a healthcare home programs, comprehensive care, coordination and planning, and initial plan; or an all inclusive service. A provider may use this code when he identifies any behavioral health need during screening or evaluation of a patient. Identification of behavioral health need means that the provider, who is evaluating the patient, identifies a patient who is a child with a significant or potential behavioral health services need. **Tips:** Illinois uses U8 as a local modifier with codes for pregnancy threatening the mother's life; where New York uses the modifier to flag a delivery prior to 39 weeks of gestation. Modifier U8 is not payable by Medicare.
U9	**Medicaid level of care 9, as defined by each state** **Definition:** A provider appends modifier U9 to report the services related to a Medicaid level of care 9, as defined by each state. The level of care may relate to the amount of assistance a patient requires, or the complexity of care. A state may also use this code to have the provider identify a type of service or patient situation. See state specific requirements for use of this code. **Explanation:** A provider appends modifier U9 according to their states specific requirements. The code often defines a tiered service based upon complexity of care but a provider may need to apply the modifier to identify a type of service or situation such as a healthcare home programs, comprehensive care, coordination and planning, and initial plan; or for such services as when he evaluates, diagnoses, and treats patients with vision problems, for example. **Tips:** Although Medicaid pays for routine vision care services, such as eyeglasses and routine eye care exams, Medicare generally does not. Therefore, Medicaid requires providers to apply the Medicaid standard fee schedule amounts when submitting claims for routine vision care services to recipients who are enrolled in both Medicaid and Medicare.

Mod	Modifier Description, Definition, Explanation, and Tips
UA	**Medicaid level of care 10, as defined by each state** **Definition:** A provider appends modifier UA to report the services related to a Medicaid level of care 10, as defined by each state. The level of care may relate to the amount of assistance a patient requires, or the complexity of care. A state may also use this code to have the provider identify a type of service or patient situation. See state specific requirements for use of this code. **Explanation:** A provider appends modifier UA according to their states specific requirements. The code often defines a tiered service based upon complexity of care but a provider may need to apply the modifier to identify a type of service or situation such to designate that the patient was admitted to the hospital or transferred to another hospital from the ED. **Tips:** Modifier UA is a Medicaid only modifier. Claims using this modifier submitted for members of plans other than Medicaid will be denied. Some providers use the UA modifier for surgical or nongeneral anesthesia related supplies and drugs, including surgical trays and plaster casting supplies, provided in conjunction with a surgical procedure code. However, when a provider reports this modifier with heroin detoxification code, H0014, Alcohol and/or drug services; ambulatory detoxification, the UA modifier indicates the outpatient heroin detoxification services per visit, days 1 – 7; something completely different.
UB	**Medicaid level of care 11, as defined by each state** **Definition:** A provider appends modifier UB to report the services related to a Medicaid level of care 11, as defined by each state. The level of care may relate to the amount of assistance a patient requires, or the complexity of care. A state may also use this code to have the provider identify a type of service or patient situation. See state specific requirements for use of this code. **Explanation:** A provider appends modifier UB according to their state specific requirements. The code often defines a tiered service based upon complexity of care but a provider may need to apply the modifier to identify a type of service or situation such as identifying that a transport is of a critically ill or injured patient over 24 months of age. The UB modifier can also indicate that the age of the patient is less than 21 or greater than 59, as for some Vision care services. **Tips:** Ohio for example uses the UB modifier to describe a Comprehensive ophthalmologic service for an individual younger than 21 or older than 59. In this situation the modifier is applicable only to CPT® procedure codes 92004, Ophthalmological services: medical examination and evaluation with initiation of diagnostic and treatment program; comprehensive, new patient, one or more visits, and 92014, Ophthalmological services: medical examination and evaluation, with initiation or continuation of diagnostic and treatment program; comprehensive, established patient, one or more visits. In California, a provider uses this code to identify surgical or general anesthesia related supplies and drugs, including surgical trays and plaster casting supplies, provided in conjunction with a surgical procedure code. However, when a provider reports this modifier with heroin detoxification code, H0014, Alcohol and/or drug services; ambulatory detoxification, the UB modifier indicates outpatient heroin detoxification services per visit, days 8 – 21. In Georgia, modifier UB indicates a delivery is a medically necessary delivery prior to 39 weeks of gestation. Wisconsin providers append the UB modifier to some Mental Health, Telemedical and Health and Behavior procedure codes to indicate an Advanced Practice Nurse provides the service.
UC	**Medicaid level of care 12, as defined by each state** **Definition:** A provider appends modifier UC to report the services related to the Medicaid level of care 12, as defined by each state. The level of care may relate to the amount of assistance a patient requires, or the complexity of care. A state may also use this code to have the provider identify a type of service or patient situation. See state specific requirements for use of this code. **Explanation:** A provider appends modifier UC according to their state specific requirements. The code often defines a tiered service based upon complexity of care but a provider may need to apply the modifier to identify a type of service or situation such as identifying a Clinical Nurse Specialist performs the service or to ensure payment goes to a Community Mental Health Services Program Provider, or CMHSP, and not to the rendering provider as this modifier indicates the CMHSP is billing Medicaid fee for service for a Community Based Services Waiver Program, or CWP beneficiary. **Tips:** Medicaid rules governing professional services within the Ohio Administrative Code, or OAC, indicate that one may report modifier UC along with 26 if the professional component for radiology procedure codes is provided by an advanced practice nurse, or APN, operating within the APN's scope of practice.

Mod	Modifier Description, Definition, Explanation, and Tips
UD	**Medicaid level of care 13, as defined by each state** **Definition:** A provider appends modifier UD to report the services related to a Medicaid level of care 13, as defined by each state. A state may also use this code to have the provider identify a type of service or patient situation. The level of care may relate to the amount of assistance a patient requires, or the complexity of care. See state specific requirements for use of this code. **Explanation:** A provider appends modifier UD according to their state specific requirements. The code often defines a tiered service based upon complexity of care but a provider may need to apply the modifier to identify a type of service or situation such as to denote services provided or drugs purchased under a particular program or when billing for an attending ED provider evaluation and management, or E and M service, to designate that the patient was discharged from the hospital and not admitted. **Tips:** Modifier UD is a Medicaid only modifier. Claims using this modifier submitted for members of plans other than Medicaid will be denied.
UE	**Used durable medical equipment** **Definition:** A provider appends modifier UE to identify an item as used durable medical equipment, or DME, that a patient purchases. DME is medical equipment that helps a patient to manage his activities of daily living in an easier way or that provides therapeutic benefits to a patient. **Explanation:** A provider appends modifier UE to codes for used DME. DME helps the patient to manage his activities of daily living in an easier way. The codes this modifier is typically applicable to are defined as Inexpensive or Routinely Purchased Items, or IRP Items, Capped Rental Items, Items Requiring Frequent and Substantial Servicing, or Oxygen Equipment. A few examples of DME's are crutches, wheelchairs, commodes, canes, walkers, hospital beds, patient safety equipment, and fracture and traction apparatus. **Tips:** Using modifier UE indicates that the provider is furnishing the patient with purchased used durable medical equipment. A provider uses modifier RR, Rented item, if the item is being rented by the patient and modifier NU, New purchased item, if the item is purchased new by the patient.
UF	**Services provided in the morning** **Definition:** A provider appends modifier UF to report that the services that the patient receives from the provider are occurring the morning. **Explanation:** Append modifier UF to identify that the provider sees the patient in the morning. This modifier typically defines services the patient receives between 6 a.m. to 11:59 a.m. and can include such services as provider professional services as well as home visits for mechanical ventilation care; nursing care, assessment or evaluation. **Tips:** Modifier UF is not payable by Medicare.
UG	**Services provided in the afternoon** **Definition:** A provider appends modifier UG to report that the services that the patient receives from the provider occur in the afternoon. **Explanation:** Append modifier UG to cover services that the patient receives by the provider in the afternoon. This modifier typically defines services the patient receives between 12 p.m. to 5:59 p.m. and can include such services as provider professional services as well as home visits for mechanical ventilation care; nursing care, assessment or evaluation. **Tips:** Modifier UG is not payable by Medicare.
UH	**Services provided in the evening** **Definition:** A provider appends modifier UH to report that the services that the patient receives from the provider occur in the evening. **Explanation:** Append modifier UH to identify that the provider sees the patient in the evening. This modifier typically defines services the patient receives between 6 p.m. to 11:59 p.m. and can include such services as provider professional services as well as home visits for mechanical ventilation care; nursing care, assessment or evaluation. **Tips:** Modifier UH is not payable by Medicare.
UJ	**Services provided at night** **Definition:** A provider appends modifier UJ to report that the services that the patient receives from the provider occur at night. **Explanation:** Append modifier UJ to cover services that the patient receives by the provider at night. This modifier typically defines services the patient receives between 12 a.m. to 5:59 a.m. and can include such services as provider professional services as well as home visits for mechanical ventilation care; nursing care, assessment or evaluation. **Tips:** Modifier UJ is not payable by Medicare.

Mod	Modifier Description, Definition, Explanation, and Tips
UK	**Services provided on behalf of the client to someone other than the client (collateral relationship)** **Definition:** A provider appends modifier UK to report services that the provider performs for someone other than the client, on behalf of the client. **Explanation:** Append modifier UK to cover the services that the provider renders to someone other than the client, on behalf of the client. A provider may need to report this modifier for mental health services such as, a family or couple visit without the client present; or when using H0046, Mental health services, not otherwise specified. This code may also be necessary if submitting newborn care services under the mother's ID information. **Tips:** Modifier UK is not payable by Medicare.
UN	**Two patients served** **Definition:** A provider appends modifier UN when two patients receive services at the same location such as portable X-ray services for two Medicare patients at the same location. The provider serves the patients during a single trip that the portable X-ray supplier makes to a particular location. **Explanation:** A provider reports this modifier when he provides services to patients at the same location. A provider may for example append the modifier with HCPCS code R0075, Transportation of portable X-ray equipment and personnel to home or nursing home, per trip to facility or location, more than one patient seen, when submitting Medicare portable X-rays. When you report this code combination, R0075 with modifier UN, the total Medicare payment for a single patient service covers both patients. **Tips:** If the provider serves only one patient in the example given, he reports a different HCPCS code R0070, Transportation of portable X-ray equipment and personnel to home or nursing home, per trip to facility or location, one patient seen, and no modifier, since the descriptor for this code states that the service is for one patient seen. Medicare allows a single transportation payment for each trip the portable X-ray supplier makes to a particular location.
UP	**Three patients served** **Definition:** A provider appends modifier UP when three patients receive services at the same location such as for portable X-ray services for three Medicare patients at the same location. The provider serves the patients during a single trip that the portable X-ray supplier makes to a particular location. **Explanation:** A provider reports this modifier when he provides services to three patients at the same location. A provider may for example append the modifier with HCPCS code R0075, Transportation of portable X-ray equipment and personnel to home or nursing home, per trip to facility or location, more than one patient seen, when submitting Medicare portable X-rays. **Tips:** If the provider serves only one patient, he reports a different HCPCS code R0070, Transportation of portable X-ray equipment and personnel to home or nursing home, per trip to facility or location, one patient seen, and no modifier, since the descriptor for this code states that the service is for one patient seen. Medicare allows a single transportation payment for each trip the portable X-ray supplier makes to a particular location.
UQ	**Four patients served** **Definition:** A provider appends modifier UQ when four patients receive services at the same location such as for portable X-ray services for four Medicare patients at the same location. The provider serves the patients during a single trip that the portable X-ray supplier makes to a particular location. **Explanation:** A provider reports this modifier when he provides services to four patients at the same location. A provider may for example append the modifier with HCPCS code R0075, Transportation of portable X-ray equipment and personnel to home or nursing home, per trip to facility or location, more than one patient seen, when submitting Medicare portable X-rays. **Tips:** If the provider serves only one patient, he reports a different HCPCS code R0070, Transportation of portable X-ray equipment and personnel to home or nursing home, per trip to facility or location, one patient seen, and no modifier, since the descriptor for this code states that the service is for one patient seen. Medicare allows a single transportation payment for each trip the portable X-ray supplier makes to a particular location.

Mod	Modifier Description, Definition, Explanation, and Tips
UR	**Five patients served**
	Definition: A provider appends modifier UR when five patients receive services at the same location such as for portable X-ray services for five Medicare patients at the same location. The provider serves the patients during a single trip that the portable X-ray supplier makes to a particular location.
	Explanation: A provider reports this modifier when he provides services to five patients at the same location. A provider may for example append the modifier with HCPCS code R0075, Transportation of portable X-ray equipment and personnel to home or nursing home, per trip to facility or location, more than one patient seen, when submitting Medicare portable X-rays.
	Tips: If the provider serves only one patient, he reports a different HCPCS code R0070, Transportation of portable X-ray equipment and personnel to home or nursing home, per trip to facility or location, one patient seen, and no modifier, since the descriptor for this code states that the service is for one patient seen.
	Medicare allows a single transportation payment for each trip the portable X-ray supplier makes to a particular location.
US	**Six or more patients served**
	Definition: A provider appends modifier US when six patients receive services at the same location such as for portable X-ray services for six Medicare patients at the same location. The provider serves the patients during a single trip that the portable X-ray supplier makes to a particular location.
	Explanation: A provider reports this modifier when he provides services to six patients at the same location. A provider may for example append the modifier with HCPCS code R0075, Transportation of portable X-ray equipment and personnel to home or nursing home, per trip to facility or location, more than one patient seen, when submitting Medicare portable X-rays.
	Tips: If the provider serves only one patient, he reports a different HCPCS code R0070, Transportation of portable X-ray equipment and personnel to home or nursing home, per trip to facility or location, one patient seen, and no modifier, since the descriptor for this code states that the service is for one patient seen.
	Medicare allows a single transportation payment for each trip the portable X-ray supplier makes to a particular location.
V1	**Demonstration modifier 1**
	Definition: Append modifier V1 to indicate that the service/procedure is part of a demonstration.
	Explanation: Modifier V1 was created with the series of V1, V2, and V3, all to indicate demonstration services/procedures. It is advisable to check Medicare's reimbursement guidelines for use of any of these modifiers.
	CMS conducts and sponsors demonstration projects to test and measure the effect of potential program changes. The demonstrations study the likely impact of new methods of service delivery, coverage of new types of service, and new payment approaches on beneficiaries, providers, health plans, states, and the Medicare Trust Funds. Append modifiers V1, V2, and V3 when the services involve demonstration of a procedure/service to allow accurate identification and documentation of payment for Medicare beneficiaries enrolled in the demonstration.
V2	**Demonstration modifier 2**
	Definition: Append modifier V2 to indicate that the service/procedure is part of a demonstration.
	Explanation: Modifier V2 was created with the series of V1, V2, and V3, all to indicate demonstration services/procedures. It is advisable to check Medicare's reimbursement guidelines for use of any of these modifiers.
	CMS conducts and sponsors demonstration projects to test and measure the effect of potential program changes. The demonstrations study the likely impact of new methods of service delivery, coverage of new types of service, and new payment approaches on beneficiaries, providers, health plans, states, and the Medicare Trust Funds. Append modifiers V1, V2, and V3 when the services involve demonstration of a procedure/service to allow accurate identification and documentation of payment for Medicare beneficiaries enrolled in the demonstration.
V3	**Demonstration modifier 3**
	Definition: Append modifier V3 to indicate that the service/procedure is part of a demonstration.
	Explanation: Modifier V3 was created with the series of V1, V2, and V3, all to indicate demonstration services/procedures. It is advisable to check Medicare's reimbursement guidelines for use of any of these modifiers.
	CMS conducts and sponsors demonstration projects to test and measure the effect of potential program changes. The demonstrations study the likely impact of new methods of service delivery, coverage of new types of service, and new payment approaches on beneficiaries, providers, health plans, states, and the Medicare Trust Funds. Append modifiers V1, V2, and V3 when the services involve demonstration of a procedure/service to allow accurate identification and documentation of payment for Medicare beneficiaries enrolled in the demonstration.

Mod	Modifier Description, Definition, Explanation, and Tips
V4	**Demonstration modifier 4** **Definition:** Append modifier V4 to indicate that the service/procedure is part of a demonstration. **Explanation:** CMS conducts and sponsors demonstration projects to test and measure the effect of potential program changes. The demonstrations study the likely impact of new methods of service delivery, coverage of new types of service, and new payment approaches on beneficiaries, providers, health plans, states, and the Medicare Trust Funds. Append the appropriate modifier when the services involve demonstration of a procedure/service to allow accurate identification and documentation for Medicare beneficiaries enrolled in the demonstration. **Tips:** This modifier is part of a series of similar modifiers that indicates demonstration services/procedures. It is advisable to check payer guidelines for use of any of these modifiers.
V5	**Vascular catheter (alone or with any other vascular access)** **Definition:** A provider appends modifier V5 to report a vascular catheter he uses to perform hemodialysis for a patient such as one with end stage renal disease, or ESRD. The provider may use the catheter alone or with another vascular access. **Explanation:** A provider appends this modifier to report the type of vascular access he uses for the delivery of hemodialysis to an ESRD patient. The provider uses the V5 modifier when he uses a vascular catheter for the ESRD patient's hemodialysis service and he uses this access with or without another vascular access to perform the service. ESRD defines the final stage of kidney failure where a patient is not able to live without dialysis or a transplant because of the complete or nearly complete irreversible loss of renal function. ESRD is also referred to as end stage kidney disease, end stage kidney failure, and end stage renal failure. Hemodialysis is a blood filtration procedure for a patient with this advanced, permanent kidney failure. During typical hemodialysis, a dialysis machine removes harmful wastes, salts, and fluid from the blood that would normally be eliminated in the urine. A provider uses a vascular catheter, or a flexible tube that he inserts into a blood vessel through which he can remove and return blood during hemodialysis, or perform other services such as pass instruments, draw blood, or instill fluids. **Tips:** ESRD claims for hemodialysis must indicate the type of vascular access the provider uses for the delivery of the hemodialysis at the last hemodialysis session of the month. Append modifier V5 when billing for hemodialysis revenue code 0821, Hemodialysis, composite or other rate. If the latest line item date of service billing for revenue code 0821 does not contain either modifier, V5, V6, Arteriovenous graft, or other vascular access not including a vascular catheter, or V7, Arteriovenous fistula only, in use with two needles, Medicare will return the claim to the provider 72x bill types, billing for hemodialysis.
V6	**Arteriovenous graft (or other vascular access not including a vascular catheter)** **Definition:** A provider appends modifier V6 to report an arteriovenous graft, or other vascular access he uses to perform hemodialysis for a patient such as one with end stage renal disease, or ESRD. The provider may use the graft alone or with another vascular access but he does not use a vascular catheter for this service. **Explanation:** A provider appends this modifier to report the type of vascular access he uses for the delivery of hemodialysis to a patient such as an ESRD patient. The provider uses the V6 modifier when he uses an arteriovenous graft, or other vascular access but not a vascular catheter to perform an ESRD patient's hemodialysis service. The provider uses an arteriovenous graft, for the hemodialysis service by surgically connecting a vein to an artery using a soft plastic tube, or an organic material from a person or animal. The provider then uses this access to remove and return blood during the hemodialysis service. ESRD defines the final stage of kidney failure where a patient is not able to live without dialysis or a transplant because of the complete or nearly complete irreversible loss of renal function. ESRD is also referred to as end stage kidney disease, end stage kidney failure, and end stage renal failure. Hemodialysis is a blood filtration procedure for a patient with this advanced, permanent kidney failure. During typical hemodialysis, a dialysis machine removes harmful wastes, salts, and fluid from the blood that would normally be eliminated in the urine. **Tips:** ESRD claims for hemodialysis with must indicate the type of vascular access the provider uses for the delivery of the hemodialysis at the last hemodialysis session of the month. If the latest line item date of service billing for revenue code 0821 does not contain either modifier, V5, V6, Arteriovenous graft, or other vascular access not including a vascular catheter, or V7, Arteriovenous fistula only, in use with two needles, Medicare will return the claim to the provider 72x bill types billing for hemodialysis.

Mod	Modifier Description, Definition, Explanation, and Tips
V7	**Arteriovenous fistula only (in use with two needles)**
	Definition: A provider appends modifier V7 to represent an arteriovenous fistula, in use with two needles to perform hemodialysis for a patient such as one with end stage renal disease, or ESRD. The provider does not use a vascular catheter, arteriovenous graft, or other vascular access when he reports this service.
	Explanation: A provider appends this modifier to report the type of vascular access he uses for the delivery of hemodialysis to a patient such as an ESRD patient. A provider appends modifier V7 to represent an arteriovenous fistula, in use with two needles. The provider then uses this access to remove and return blood during the hemodialysis service.
	ESRD defines the final stage of kidney failure where a patient is not able to live without dialysis or a transplant because of the complete or nearly complete irreversible loss of renal function. ESRD is also referred to as end stage kidney disease, end stage kidney failure, and end stage renal failure.
	Hemodialysis is a blood filtration procedure for a patient with this advanced, permanent kidney failure. During typical hemodialysis, a dialysis machine removes harmful wastes, salts, and fluid from the blood that would normally be eliminated in the urine. An arteriovenous fistula is a tract or abnormal passageway that is not supposed to be there that connects a coronary artery to the pulmonary venous circulation.
	Tips: Append modifier V7 when billing for hemodialysis revenue code 0821, Hemodialysis, Outpatient or Home, Hemodialysis Composite.
	If the latest line item date of service billing for revenue code 0821 does not contain either modifier, V5, Vascular catheter, alone or with any other vascular access, V6, Arteriovenous graft, or other vascular access not including a vascular catheter, or V7, Medicare will return the claim to the provider 72x bill types, billing for hemodialysis.
VM	**Medicare diabetes prevention program (MDPP) virtual make-up session**
	Definition: Append modifier VM to a code when a provider delivers an in-person virtual make-up session to a beneficiary who missed a group-based, classroom-style, core Medicare diabetes prevention program (MDPP) session.
	Explanation: Modifier VM indicates that the provider electronically delivered a make-up session as part of an established MDPP curriculum to a patient who missed a face-to-face group class.
	Tips: The MDPP is a six-month CDC-approved curriculum consisting of a minimum of 16 intensive "core" educational sessions delivered to a group of patients with prediabetes in a classroom-style setting aimed at preventing progression to type 2 diabetes mellitus. The curriculum provides training in long-term dietary change, increased physical activity, and behavior modification strategies for weight control. Less intensive follow-up monthly sessions help ensure that the participants maintain healthy behaviors. The primary goal of the expanded model is at least 5 percent average weight loss by participants.
VP	**Aphakic patient**
	Definition: A provider appends modifier VP to represent an aphakic patient, or a patient without a lens in the eye.
	Explanation: A provider appends modifier VP to represent an aphakic patient. An aphakic patient is one who has lost the lens of his eye, due to reasons such as surgical removal, an intervening ulcer, or an anomaly from birth. This may lead to problems related to the eye, such as, far sightedness and a loss of accommodation, or adjustment of the eye to view different objects. There may be complications which arise due to aphakia. These may include detachment of the retina and glaucoma.
	Tips: Modifier VP is informational only and you may report it with different types of service such as medical care, surgery, consultation, diagnostic radiology, anesthesia, assistant at surgery, other medical items or services, ambulatory surgical Centers, or facility usage for surgical services.
	If you report modifier VP with codes for any other types of service, the payer may return the claim as unprocessable. The provider may need to resubmit as a new claim without the modifier.
X1	**Continuous/broad services:** for reporting services by clinicians, who provide the principal care for a patient, with no planned endpoint of the relationship; services in this category represent comprehensive care, dealing with the entire scope of patient problems, either directly or in a care coordination role; reporting clinician service examples include, but are not limited to: primary care, and clinicians providing comprehensive care to patients in addition to specialty care
	Definition: Append modifier X1 to a code for continuing, broad or comprehensive care services, typically for a patient with multiple chronic conditions, with no anticipated endpoint, provided by primary care and specialty providers.
	Explanation: Modifier X1 defines a patient relationship category in which either a primary care physician or specialist, either directly or coordinating care by others, provide continuous broad or comprehensive care, potentially dealing with multiple chronic health issues, and the patient's health problems are such that no endpoint (cure or other endpoint) is anticipated.
	Tips: Patient relationship categories facilitate the attribution of patients and care episodes to clinicians who serve patients in different roles as part of the assessment of the cost of care.

Mod	Modifier Description, Definition, Explanation, and Tips
X2	**Continuous/focused services:** for reporting services by clinicians whose expertise is needed for the ongoing management of a chronic disease or a condition that needs to be managed and followed with no planned endpoint to the relationship; reporting clinician service examples include but are not limited to: a rheumatologist taking care of the patient's rheumatoid arthritis longitudinally but not providing general primary care services **Definition:** Append modifier X2 to a code for ongoing management of a chronic disease with no anticipated endpoint, typically provided by a specialist. **Explanation:** Modifier X2 defines a patient relationship category in which typically a specialist provides ongoing care and management for a specific chronic health issue, such as rheumatoid arthritis, heart disease, or diabetes, and no endpoint (cure or other endpoint) is anticipated. **Tips:** Patient relationship categories facilitate the attribution of patients and care episodes to clinicians who serve patients in different roles as part of the assessment of the cost of care.
X3	**Episodic/broad services:** for reporting services by clinicians who have broad responsibility for the comprehensive needs of the patient that is limited to a defined period and circumstance such as a hospitalization; reporting clinician service examples include but are not limited to the hospitalist's services rendered providing comprehensive and general care to a patient while admitted to the hospital **Definition:** Append modifier X3 to a code for services rendered by a provider with broad responsibility (i.e., oversight/management) for comprehensive and general care limited to a specific period or circumstance, such as a hospital admission. **Explanation:** Modifier X3 defines a patient relationship category in which a provider, such as a hospitalist, renders general and comprehensive care and management to a patient for a limited period of time, such as a hospitalization. **Tips:** Patient relationship categories facilitate the attribution of patients and care episodes to clinicians who serve patients in different roles as part of the assessment of the cost of care.
X4	**Episodic/focused services:** for reporting services by clinicians who provide focused care on particular types of treatment limited to a defined period and circumstance; the patient has a problem, acute or chronic, that will be treated with surgery, radiation, or some other type of generally time-limited intervention; reporting clinician service examples include but are not limited to, the orthopedic surgeon performing a knee replacement and seeing the patient through the postoperative period **Definition:** Append modifier X4 to a code for focused care services, such as surgical intervention or radiotherapy, for acute or chronic conditions rendered by a provider for a limited or defined period of time. **Explanation:** Modifier X4 defines a patient relationship category in which a provider, such as a surgeon or radiation oncologist, renders care and management or intervention to a patient for a specific chronic or acute condition over a defined or limited period of time. **Tips:** Patient relationship categories facilitate the attribution of patients and care episodes to clinicians who serve patients in different roles as part of the assessment of the cost of care.
X5	**Diagnostic services requested by another clinician:** for reporting services by a clinician who furnishes care to the patient only as requested by another clinician or subsequent and related services requested by another clinician; this modifier is reported for patient relationships that may not be adequately captured by the above alternative categories; reporting clinician service examples include but are not limited to, the radiologist's interpretation of an imaging study requested by another clinician **Definition:** Append modifier X5 to a code for primarily diagnostic services, such as interpreting an imaging study, rendered by a provider only as ordered by another clinician. **Explanation:** Modifier X5 indicates that a provider renders a service, primarily diagnostic, to a patient only at the request or order of another provider. The service could be something like interpretation of an imaging study, EKG, or laboratory test. The services may also be subsequent or related services as requested or ordered by another provider. **Tips:** This patient relationship category is reported for patient relationships that may not be adequately captured by modifiers X1-X4. Patient relationship categories facilitate the attribution of patients and care episodes to clinicians who serve patients in different roles as part of the assessment of the cost of care.

Mod	Modifier Description, Definition, Explanation, and Tips
XE	**Separate encounter, a service that is distinct because it occurred during a separate encounter** **Definition:** Append modifier XE to services that the provider performs for a patient at separate encounters on the same date of service. **Explanation:** A provider appends this modifier when the provider performs services on a patient at separate patient encounters that occur on the same date of service. Modifier XE defines a subset of the modifier 59, Distinct Procedural Service. CPT® instructions state that a provider should not use modifier 59 when a more descriptive modifier is available, such as modifier XE, for billing certain codes at high risk for incorrect billing. For example, a provider may identify a particular code pair as payable only with modifier XE but not modifier 59. Modifier XE is a more selective version of modifier 59 so it would be incorrect to include both modifiers on the same line. The combination of an alternative specific modifier with a general less specific modifier creates additional evaluation for both reporting and editing. Modifier XE is a valid modifier even before national edits are in place, so contractors are not prohibited from requiring the use of this selective modifier as an alternative to the general modifier 59 when necessary by local program integrity and compliance needs. **Tips:** Contractors recognize modifier XE as a separate modifier and the system allows a provider to report multiple lines with modifier 59 and the XE modifier. However, the system aggregates lines with the XE modifier along with lines containing modifier 59, whenever it collects the modifier 59 lines.
XP	**Separate practitioner, a service that is distinct because it was performed by a different practitioner** **Definition:** Append modifier XP to identify a service that a different provider performs on the patient. **Explanation:** A provider appends this modifier to identify a distinct service that a patient receives from a different provider who performs the service on the patient. Modifier XP defines a subset of the modifier 59, Distinct Procedural Service. CPT® instructions state that a provider should not use modifier 59 when a more descriptive modifier is available, such as modifier XP, for billing certain codes at high risk for incorrect billing. Modifier XP is a more selective version of modifier 59 so it would be incorrect to include both modifiers on the same line. The combination of an alternative specific modifier with a general less specific modifier creates additional evaluation for both reporting and editing. Modifier XP is a valid modifier even before national edits are in place, so contractors are not prohibited from requiring the use of these selective modifiers an alternative to the general modifier 59 when necessary by local program integrity and compliance needs. **Tips:** Contractors recognize modifier XP as a separate modifier and the system allows a provider to report multiple lines with modifier 59 and XP modifier. However, the system aggregates lines with the XP modifier along with lines containing modifier 59 whenever it collects modifier 59 lines.
XS	**Separate structure, a service that is distinct because it was performed on a separate organ/structure** **Definition:** Append modifier XS to a service that the provider performs for a patient on a separate organ or structure. **Explanation:** A provider appends this modifier to identify a distinct service when the provider performs services on a patient on different organs or structures. Modifier XS defines a subset of the modifier 59, Distinct Procedural Service. CPT® instructions state that a provider should not use modifier 59 when a more descriptive modifier is available, such as modifier XS, for billing certain codes at high risk for incorrect billing. Modifier XS is a more selective version of modifier 59 so it would be incorrect to include both modifiers on the same line. The combination of an alternative specific modifier with a general less specific modifier creates additional evaluation for both reporting and editing. Modifier XS is a valid modifier even before national edits are in place, so contractors are not prohibited from requiring the use of this selective modifier as an alternative to the general modifier 59 when necessary by local program integrity and compliance needs. **Tips:** Contractors recognize modifier XS as a separate modifier and the system allows a provider to report multiple lines with modifier 59 and XS modifier. However, the system aggregates lines with the XS modifier along with lines containing modifier 59 whenever it collects the modifier 59 lines.

Mod	Modifier Description, Definition, Explanation, and Tips
XU	**Unusual non-overlapping service, the use of a service that is distinct because it does not overlap usual components of the main service** **Definition:** Append modifier XU to a service that is distinct because it does not overlap with the usual components of the main service. **Explanation:** A provider appends this modifier to identify the service as a distinct service, as the service the provider performs does not overlap with the unusual components of the main, or primary, service he renders to a patient. Modifier XU defines a subset of the modifier 59, Distinct Procedural Service. CPT® instructions state that a provider should not use modifier 59 when a more descriptive modifier is available, such as modifier XU, for billing certain codes at high risk for incorrect billing. Modifier XU is a more selective version of modifier 59 so it would be incorrect to include both modifiers on the same line. The combination of an alternative specific modifier with a general less specific modifier creates additional evaluation for both reporting and editing. Modifier XU is a valid modifier even before national edits are in place, so contractors are not prohibited from requiring the use of this selective modifier as an alternative to the general modifier 59 when necessary by local program integrity and compliance needs. **Tips:** Contractors recognize modifier XU as a separate modifier and the system allows a provider to report multiple lines with modifier 59 and XU modifier. However, the system aggregates lines with the XU modifier along with lines containing modifier 59 whenever it collects modifier 59 lines.

Appendix C
List of Abbreviations

Abbreviation	Description
/	or
<	less than
<=	less than equal to
>	greater than
>=	greater than equal to
AAA	abdominal aortic aneurysm
AC	alternating current
ACE	Angiotensin converting enzyme
AFO	ankle-foot orthosis
AICC	anti-inhibitor coagulant complex
AK	above the knee
AKA	above knee amputation
ALS	advanced life support
AMP	ampule
ARB	Angiotensin receptor blocker
ART	arterial
ASC	ambulatory surgery center
ATT	attached
A-V	arteriovenous
AVF	arteriovenous fistula
BICROS	bilateral routing of signals
BK	below the knee
BKA	below knee amputation
BLS	basic life support
BMI	body mass index
BP	blood pressure
BTE	behind the ear (hearing aid)
CAD	coronary artery disease
CAPD	continuous ambulatory peritoneal dialysis
Carb	carbohydrate
CBC	complete blood count
cc	cubic centimeter
CCPD	continuous cycling peritoneal dialysis
CGH	comparative genomic hybridization
CHF	congestive heart failure
CIC	completely in the canal (hearing aid)
CIM	Coverage Issue Manual
CISD	critical incident stress debriefing
cm	centimeter
CMN	certificate of medical necessity
CMS	Centers for Medicare & Medicaid Services

Abbreviation	Description
CMV	Cytomegalovirus
Conc	concentrate(d)
Cont	continuous
CP	clinical psychologist
CPAP	continuous positive airway pressure
CPT®	Current Procedural Terminology
CRF	chronic renal failure
CRNA	certified registered nurse anesthetist
CROS	contralateral routing of signals
CSW	clinical social worker
CT	computed tomography
CTLSO	cervical-thoracic-lumbar-sacral orthosis
cu	cubic centimeter
DC	direct current
DI	diabetes insipidus
DLI	donor leukocyte infusion
DME	durable medical equipment
DME MAC	durable medical equipment Medicare administrative contractor
DMEPOS	durable medical equipment; prosthetic, orthotics, and other supplies
DMERC	durable medical equipment regional carrier
DR	diagnostic radiology
Dx	diagnosis
DXA	dual-energy X-ray absorptiometry
e.g.	for example
Ea	each
ECF	extended care facility
EEG	electroencephalogram
EKG	electrocardiogram
EMG	electromyography
EO	elbow orthosis
EP	electrophysiologic
EPO	epoetin alfa
EPSDT	early periodic screening, diagnosis and treatment
ESRD	end-stage renal disease
Ex	extended
EXPER	experimental
Ext	external
FDA	Food and Drug Administration

Abbreviation	Description
FDG-PET	positron emission with tomography with 18 fluorodeoxyglucose
Fem	female
FO	finger orthosis
FPD	fixed partial denture
Fr	french
ft	foot
G-CSF	filgrastim (granulocyte colony-stimulating factor)
gm or g	gram
H2O	water
HCL	hydrochloric acid
HCPCS	Healthcare Common Procedural Coding System
HCT	hematocrit
HCV	Hepatitis C virus
HDL-C	high density lipoprotein- cholesterol
HF	heart failure
HFO	hand-finger orthosis
HHA	home health agency
HI	high
HI-LO	high-low
HIT	home infusion therapy
HKAFO	hip-knee-ankle foot orthosis
HLA	human leukocyte antigen
HMES	heat and moisture exchange system
HNPCC	hereditary non-polyposis colorectal cancer
HO	hip orthosis
HPSA	health professional shortage area
HST	home sleep test
I-131	Iodine 131
IA	intra- arterial administration
lbs	pounds
ICF	intermediate care facility
ICU	intensive care unit
IM	intramuscular
in	inch
INF	infusion
INH	inhalation solution
INJ	injection
IOL	intraocular lens
ip	interphalangeal
IPD	intermittent peritoneal dialysis
IPPB	intermittent positive pressure breathing
IT	intrathecal administration
ITC	in the canal (hearing aid)

Abbreviation	Description
ITE	in the ear (hearing aid)
IU	international units
IV	intravenous
IVF	in vitro fertilization
IVP	Intrauterine pregnancy
KAFO	knee-ankle-foot orthosis
KO	knee orthosis
KOH	potassium hydroxide
L	left
LASIK	laser in situ keratomileusis
LAUP	laser assisted uvulopalatoplasty
LDL	low density lipoprotein
lbs	pounds
LDS	lipodystrophy syndrome
Lo	low
LOPS	loss of protective sensation
LPM	liters per minute
LPN/LVN	Licensed Practical Nurse/Licensed Vocational Nurse
LSO	lumbar-sacral orthosis
LTC	long term care facility
LVEF	left ventricular ejection fraction
MAC	Medicare administrative contractor
mcg	microgram
mCi	millicurie
MCM	Medicare Carriers Manual
MCP	metacarpophalangeal joint
mEq	milliequivalent
MESA	microsurgical epididymal sperm aspiration
mg	milligram
mgs	milligrams
MHT	megahertz
ml	milliliter
mm	millimeter
mmHg	millimeters of Mercury
mp	metacarpophalangeal
MRA	magnetic resonance angiography
MRI	magnetic resonance imaging
NA	sodium
NCI	National Cancer Institute
NEC	not elsewhere classified
NG	nasogastric
NH	nursing home
NMES	neuromuscular electrical stimulation
NOC	not otherwise classified
NOS	not otherwise specified

Abbreviation	Description
NSR	normal sinus rhythm
O2	oxygen
OBRA	Omnibus Budget Reconciliation Act
OMT	osteopathic manipulation therapy
OPPS	outpatient prospective payment system
ORAL	oral administration
OSA	obstructive sleep apnea
Ost	ostomy
OTH	other routes of administration
oz	ounce
PA	physician's assistant
PAR	parenteral
PCA	patient controlled analgesia
PCH	pouch
PEN	parenteral and enteral nutrition
PENS	percutaneous electrical nerve stimulation
PET	positron emission tomography
PHP	pre-paid health plan
PHP	physician hospital plan
PI	paramedic intercept
PICC	peripherally inserted central venous catheter
PKR	photorefractive keratotomy
PNB	peripheral nerve block
Pow	powder
PPPS	personalized prevention plan of service
PQRS	physician quality reporting system
PRK	photoreactive keratectomy
PRO	peer review organization
PSA	prostate specific antigen
PTB	patellar tendon bearing
PTK	phototherapeutic keratectomy
PVC	polyvinyl chloride
R	right
Repl	replace
RN	registered nurse
RP	retrograde pyelogram
Rx	prescription
SACH	solid ankle, cushion heel
SC	subcutaneous
SCT	specialty care transport
SEO	shoulder-elbow orthosis
SEWHO	shoulder-elbow-wrist-hand orthosis
SEXA	single energy X-ray absorptiometry
SGD	speech generating device
SM	samarium

Abbreviation	Description
SNCT	sensory nerve conduction test
SNF	skilled nursing facility
SO	sacroiliac orthosis
SO	shoulder orthosis
Sol	solution
SQ	square
SR	screen
ST	standard
SR	sustained release
Syr	syrup
TABS	tablets
Tc	Technetium
Tc 99m	Technetium isotope
TD	diphtheria toxoids vaccine
TDAP	diphtheria toxoids and acellular pertussis vaccine
TEE	transesophageal echocardiography
TENS	transcutaneous electrical nerve stimulator
THKAO	thoracic-hip-knee-ankle orthosis
TLSO	thoracic-lumbar-sacral-orthosis
TM	temporomandibular
TMJ	temporomandibular joint
TPN	total parenteral nutrition
U	unit
uCi	microcurie
VAR	various routes of administration
w	with
w/	with
w/o	without
WAK	wearable artificial kidney
wc	wheelchair
WHFO	wrist-hand-finger orthotic
wk	week
Xe	Xenon (isotope mass of xenon 133)

This page intentionally left blank

Appendix D
Place of Service/Type of Service

Place of Service

Code	Place of Service	Place of Service Description
1	Pharmacy	A facility or location where drugs and other medically related items and services are sold, dispensed, or otherwise provided directly to patients.
2	Telehealth	The location where health services and health related services are provided or received, through a telecommunication system.
3	School	A facility whose primary purpose is education.
4	Homeless Shelter	A facility or location whose primary purpose is to provide temporary housing to homeless individuals (e.g., emergency shelters, individual or family shelters).
5	Indian Health Service Free-standing Facility	A facility or location, owned and operated by the Indian Health Service, which provides diagnostic, therapeutic (surgical and non-surgical), and rehabilitation services to American Indians and Alaska Natives who do not require hospitalization.
6	Indian Health Service Provider-based Facility	A facility or location, owned and operated by the Indian Health Service, which provides diagnostic, therapeutic (surgical and non-surgical), and rehabilitation services rendered by, or under the supervision of, physicians to American Indians and Alaska Natives admitted as inpatients or outpatients.
7	Tribal 638 Free-standing Facility	A facility or location owned and operated by a federally recognized American Indian or Alaska Native tribe or tribal organization under a 638 agreement, which provides diagnostic, therapeutic (surgical and non-surgical), and rehabilitation services to tribal members who do not require hospitalization.
8	Tribal 638 Provider-based Facility	A facility or location owned and operated by a federally recognized American Indian or Alaska Native tribe or tribal organization under a 638 agreement, which provides diagnostic, therapeutic (surgical and non-surgical), and rehabilitation services to tribal members admitted as inpatients or outpatients.
9	Prison/Correctional Facility	A prison, jail, reformatory, work farm, detention center, or any other similar facility maintained by either Federal, State or local authorities for the purpose of confinement or rehabilitation of adult or juvenile criminal offenders.
11	Office	Location, other than a hospital, skilled nursing facility (SNF), military treatment facility, community health center, State or local public health clinic, or intermediate care facility (ICF), where the health professional routinely provides health examinations, diagnosis, and treatment of illness or injury on an ambulatory basis.
12	Home	Location, other than a hospital or other facility, where the patient receives care in a private residence.
13	Assisted Living Facility	Congregate residential facility with self-contained living units providing assessment of each resident's needs and on-site support 24 hours a day, 7 days a week, with the capacity to deliver or arrange for services including some health care and other services.
14	Group Home	A residence, with shared living areas, where clients receive supervision and other services such as social and/or behavioral services, custodial service, and minimal services (e.g., medication administration).
15	Mobile Unit	A facility/unit that moves from place-to-place equipped to provide preventive, screening, diagnostic, and/or treatment services.
16	Temporary Lodging	A short term accommodation such as a hotel, camp ground, hostel, cruise ship or resort where the patient receives care, and which is not identified by any other POS code.
17	Walk-in Retail Health Clinic	A walk-in health clinic, other than an office, urgent care facility, pharmacy or independent clinic and not described by any other Place of Service code, that is located within a retail operation and provides, on an ambulatory basis, preventive and primary care services.
18	Place of Employment-Worksite	A location, not described by any other POS code, owned or operated by a public or private entity where the patient is employed, and where a health professional provides on-going or episodic occupational medical, therapeutic or rehabilitative services to the individual.
19	Off Campus-Outpatient Hospital	A portion of an off-campus hospital provider based department which provides diagnostic, therapeutic (both surgical and nonsurgical), and rehabilitation services to sick or injured persons who do not require hospitalization or institutionalization.

Code	Place of Service	Place of Service Description
20	Urgent Care Facility	Location, distinct from a hospital emergency room, an office, or a clinic, whose purpose is to diagnose and treat illness or injury for unscheduled, ambulatory patients seeking immediate medical attention.
21	Inpatient Hospital	A facility, other than psychiatric, which primarily provides diagnostic, therapeutic (both surgical and nonsurgical), and rehabilitation services by, or under, the supervision of physicians to patients admitted for a variety of medical conditions.
22	On Campus-Outpatient Hospital	A portion of a hospital's main campus which provides diagnostic, therapeutic (both surgical and nonsurgical), and rehabilitation services to sick or injured persons who do not require hospitalization or institutionalization.
23	Emergency Room - Hospital	A portion of a hospital where emergency diagnosis and treatment of illness or injury is provided.
24	Ambulatory Surgical Center	A freestanding facility, other than a physician's office, where surgical and diagnostic services are provided on an ambulatory basis.
25	Birthing Center	A facility, other than a hospital's maternity facilities or a physician's office, which provides a setting for labor, delivery, and immediate post- partum care as well as immediate care of newborn infants.
26	Military Treatment Facility	A medical facility operated by one or more of the Uniformed Services. Military Treatment Facility (MTF) also refers to certain former U.S. Public Health Service (USPHS) facilities now designated as Uniformed Service Treatment Facilities (USTF).
31	Skilled Nursing Facility	A facility which primarily provides inpatient skilled nursing care and related services to patients who require medical, nursing, or rehabilitative services but does not provide the level of care or treatment available in a hospital.
32	Nursing Facility	A facility which primarily provides to residents skilled nursing care and related services for the rehabilitation of injured, disabled, or sick persons, or, on a regular basis, health-related care services above the level of custodial care to other than mentally retarded individuals.
33	Custodial Care Facility	A facility which provides room, board and other personal assistance services, generally on a long- term basis, and which does not include a medical component.
34	Hospice	A facility, other than a patient's home, in which palliative and supportive care for terminally ill patients and their families are provided.
41	Ambulance - Land	A land vehicle specifically designed, equipped and staffed for lifesaving and transporting the sick or injured.
42	Ambulance - Air or Water	An air or water vehicle specifically designed, equipped and staffed for lifesaving and transporting the sick or injured.
49	Independent Clinic	A location, not part of a hospital and not described by any other Place of Service code, that is organized and operated to provide preventive, diagnostic, therapeutic, rehabilitative, or palliative services to outpatients only.
50	Federally Qualified Health Center	A facility located in a medically underserved area that provides Medicare beneficiaries preventive primary medical care under the general direction of a physician.
51	Inpatient Psychiatric Facility	A facility that provides inpatient psychiatric services for the diagnosis and treatment of mental illness on a 24-hour basis, by or under the supervision of a physician.
52	Psychiatric Facility-Partial Hospitalization	A facility for the diagnosis and treatment of mental illness that provides a planned therapeutic program for patients who do not require full time hospitalization, but who need broader programs than are possible from outpatient visits to a hospital-based or hospital-affiliated facility.
53	Community Mental Health Center	A facility that provides the following services: outpatient services, including specialized outpatient services for children, the elderly, individuals who are chronically ill, and residents of the CMHC's mental health services area who have been discharged from inpatient treatment at a mental health facility; 24 hour a day emergency care services; day treatment, other partial hospitalization services, or psychosocial rehabilitation services; screening for patients being considered for admission to State mental health facilities to determine the appropriateness of such admission; and consultation and education services.
54	Intermediate Care Facility/Mentally Retarded	A facility which primarily provides health-related care and services above the level of custodial care to mentally retarded individuals but does not provide the level of care or treatment available in a hospital or SNF.
55	Residential Substance Abuse Treatment Facility	A facility which provides treatment for substance (alcohol and drug) abuse to live-in residents who do not require acute medical care. Services include individual and group therapy and counseling, family counseling, laboratory tests, drugs and supplies, psychological testing, and room and board.

Code	Place of Service	Place of Service Description
56	Psychiatric Residential Treatment Center	A facility or distinct part of a facility for psychiatric care which provides a total 24-hour therapeutically planned and professionally staffed group living and learning environment.
57	Non-residential Substance Abuse Treatment Facility	A location which provides treatment for substance (alcohol and drug) abuse on an ambulatory basis. Services include individual and group therapy and counseling, family counseling, laboratory tests, drugs and supplies, and psychological testing.
58	Non-residential Opioid Treatment Facility	A location that provides treatment for opioid use disorder on an ambulatory basis. Services include methadone and other forms of Medication Assisted Treatment (MAT).
60	Mass Immunization Center	A location where providers administer pneumococcal pneumonia and influenza virus vaccinations and submit these services as electronic media claims, paper claims, or using the roster billing method. This generally takes place in a mass immunization setting, such as, a public health center, pharmacy, or mall but may include a physician office setting.
61	Comprehensive Inpatient Rehabilitation Facility	A facility that provides comprehensive rehabilitation services under the supervision of a physician to inpatients with physical disabilities. Services include physical therapy, occupational therapy, speech pathology, social or psychological services, and orthotics and prosthetics services.
62	Comprehensive Outpatient Rehabilitation Facility	A facility that provides comprehensive rehabilitation services under the supervision of a physician to outpatients with physical disabilities. Services include physical therapy, occupational therapy, and speech pathology services.
65	End-Stage Renal Disease Treatment Facility	A facility other than a hospital, which provides dialysis treatment, maintenance, and/or training to patients or caregivers on an ambulatory or home-care basis.
71	Public Health Clinic	A facility maintained by either State or local health departments that provides ambulatory primary medical care under the general direction of a physician.
72	Rural Health Clinic	A certified facility which is located in a rural medically underserved area that provides ambulatory primary medical care under the general direction of a physician.
81	Independent Laboratory	A laboratory certified to perform diagnostic and/or clinical tests independent of an institution or a physician's office.
99	Other Place of Service	Other place of service not identified above.

Type of Service

Code	Type of Service Description
0	Whole Blood
1	Medical Care
2	Surgery
3	Consultation
4	Diagnostic Radiology
5	Diagnostic Laboratory
6	Therapeutic Radiology
7	Anesthesia
8	Assistant at Surgery
9	Other Medical Items or Services
A	Used DME
B	High Risk Screening Mammography
C	Low Risk Screening Mammography
D	Ambulance
E	Enteral/Parenteral Nutrients/Supplies
F	Ambulatory Surgical Center (Facility Usage for Surgical Services)

Code	Type of Service Description
G	Immunosuppressive Drugs
H	Hospice
J	Diabetic Shoes
K	Hearing Items and Services
L	ESRD Supplies
M	Monthly Capitation Payment for Dialysis
N	Kidney Donor
P	Lump Sum Purchase of DME, Prosthetics, Orthotics
Q	Vision Items or Services
R	Rental of DME
S	Surgical Dressings or Other Medical Supplies
T	Outpatient Mental Health Treatment Limitation
U	Occupational Therapy
V	Pneumococcal/Flu Vaccine
W	Physical Therapy

Appendix E
APC Status Indicators

This status indicator list reflects proposed OPPS payment status indicators for CY 2021 available when this book was sent to print.

Status Indicator	Definition
A	Services furnished to a hospital outpatient that are paid under a fee schedule or payment system other than OPPS*, for example: • Ambulance Services • Separately Payable Clinical Diagnostic Laboratory Services • Separately Payable Non-Implantable Prosthetics and Orthotics • Physical, Occupational, and Speech Therapy • Diagnostic Mammography • Screening Mammography
B	Codes that are not recognized by OPPS when submitted on an outpatient hospital Part B bill type (12x and 13x).
C	Inpatient Procedures
D	Discontinued Codes
E1	Items, Codes, and Services: • Not covered by any Medicare outpatient benefit category • Statutorily excluded by Medicare • Not reasonable and necessary
E2	Items, Codes, and Services: For which pricing information and claims data are not available
F	Corneal Tissue Acquisition; Certain CRNA Services and Hepatitis B Vaccines
G	Pass-Through Drugs and Biologicals
H	Pass-Through Device Categories
J1	Hospital Part B Services Paid Through a Comprehensive APC
J2	Hospital Part B Services That May Be Paid Through a Comprehensive APC
K	Nonpass-Through Drugs and Nonimplantable Biologicals, Including Therapeutic Radiopharmaceuticals
L	Influenza Vaccine; Pneumococcal Pneumonia Vaccine
M	Items and Services Not Billable to the MAC
N	Items and Services Packaged Into APC Rates
P	Partial Hospitalization
Q1	STV-Packaged Codes
Q2	T-Packaged Codes
Q3	Codes That May Be Paid Through a Composite APC
Q4	Conditionally Packaged Laboratory Tests
R	Blood and Blood Products
S	Procedure or Service, Not Discounted When Multiple
T	Procedure or Service, Multiple Procedure Reduction Applies
U	Brachytherapy Sources
V	Clinic or Emergency Department Visit
Y	Non-Implantable Durable Medical Equipment

* Note — Payments under a fee schedule or payment system other than OPPS may be contractor priced.

This page intentionally left blank

Appendix F
ASC Payment Indicators

Proposed ASC Payment Indicators for CY 2021 Proposed ASC Payment (Addendum DD1)
This payment indicator list reflects proposed OPPS/ASC payment indicators for CY 2021 available when
this book was sent to print. Be sure to check the CMS website at www.cms.gov for final changes.

Indicator	Payment Indicator Definition
A2	Surgical procedure on ASC list in CY 2007; payment based on OPPS relative payment weight.
B5	Alternative code may be available; no payment made
D5	Deleted/discontinued code; no payment made.
F4	Corneal tissue acquisition, hepatitis B vaccine; paid at reasonable cost.
G2	Non office-based surgical procedure added in CY 2008 or later; payment based on OPPS relative payment weight.
H2	Brachytherapy source paid separately when provided integral to a surgical procedure on ASC list; payment based on OPPS rate.
J7	OPPS pass-through device paid separately when provided integral to a surgical procedure on ASC list; payment contractor-priced.
J8	Device-intensive procedure; paid at adjusted rate.
K2	Drugs and biologicals paid separately when provided integral to a surgical procedure on ASC list; payment based on OPPS rate.
K5	Drugs and biologicals for which pricing information is not yet available.
K7	Unclassified drugs and biologicals; payment contractor-priced.
L1	Influenza vaccine; pneumococcal vaccine. Packaged item/service; no separate payment made.
L6	New Technology Intraocular Lens (NTIOL); special payment.
N1	Packaged service/item; no separate payment made.
P2	Office-based surgical procedure added to ASC list in CY 2008 or later with MPFS nonfacility PE RVUs; payment based on OPPS relative payment weight.
P3	Office-based surgical procedure added to ASC list in CY 2008 or later with MPFS nonfacility PE RVUs; payment based on MPFS nonfacility PE RVUs.
R2	Office-based surgical procedure added to ASC list in CY 2008 or later without MPFS nonfacility PE RVUs; payment based on OPPS relative payment weight.
Z2	Radiology or diagnostic service paid separately when provided integral to a surgical procedure on ASC list; payment based on OPPS relative payment weight.
Z3	Radiology or diagnostic service paid separately when provided integral to a surgical procedure on ASC list; payment based on MPFS nonfacility PE RVUs.

This page intentionally left blank

Appendix G
Column 1 and Column 2 Correct Coding Edits

Column 1	Column 2	Modifier	Column 1	Column 2	Modifier	Column 1	Column 2	Modifier
A9500	A9512	1	C5276	J0670	1	C9603	G0471	1
A9501	A9512	0	C5276	J2001	1	C9604	G0269	1
A9502	A9512	0	C5277	G0168	1	C9604	G0471	1
A9503	A9512	0	C5277	G0471	1	C9605	G0269	1
A9504	A9512	0	C5277	J0670	1	C9605	G0471	1
A9510	A9512	0	C5277	J2001	1	C9606	G0269	1
A9521	A9512	0	C5278	G0168	1	C9606	G0471	1
A9536	A9512	0	C5278	G0471	1	C9607	G0269	1
A9537	A9512	0	C5278	J0670	1	C9607	G0471	1
A9538	A9512	0	C5278	J2001	1	C9608	G0269	1
A9539	A9512	0	C8906	C8903	1	C9608	G0471	1
A9540	A9512	1	C8906	C8905	1	C9738	G0463	1
A9541	A9512	1	C8908	C8903	1	C9738	G0471	0
A9550	A9512	0	C8908	C8905	1	C9738	J2001	1
A9551	A9512	0	C8921	C8922	1	C9738	P9612	0
A9557	A9512	0	C8923	C8924	1	C9739	G0463	1
A9560	A9512	0	C8923	C8929	0	C9739	G0471	0
A9561	A9512	0	C8928	C8923	1	C9739	J2001	1
A9562	A9512	0	C8928	C8924	1	C9739	P9612	0
A9566	A9512	0	C8928	C8925	1	C9740	C9739	0
A9567	A9512	0	C8928	C8927	0	C9740	G0463	1
A9568	A9512	0	C8928	C8929	1	C9740	G0471	0
A9569	A9512	0	C8928	C8930	0	C9740	J2001	1
C5271	G0168	1	C8929	C8924	1	C9740	P9612	0
C5271	G0471	1	C8930	C8929	1	C9745	G0463	1
C5271	J0670	1	C8931	C8932	0	C9745	G0471	1
C5271	J2001	1	C8931	J1642	1	C9745	J0670	1
C5272	G0168	1	C8932	J1642	1	C9745	J2001	1
C5272	G0471	1	C8933	C8931	0	C9747	G0463	1
C5272	J0670	1	C8933	C8932	0	C9747	G0471	1
C5272	J2001	1	C8933	J1642	1	C9747	J0670	1
C5273	G0168	1	C8934	C8935	0	C9747	J2001	1
C5273	G0471	1	C8934	J1642	1	C9751	G0297	0
C5273	J0670	1	C8935	J1642	1	C9751	G0463	1
C5273	J2001	1	C8936	C8934	0	C9751	G0471	1
C5274	G0168	1	C8936	C8935	0	C9751	J0670	1
C5274	G0471	1	C8936	J1642	1	C9751	J2001	1
C5274	J0670	1	C8957	G0463	1	C9752	G0453	0
C5274	J2001	1	C9600	G0269	1	C9752	G0463	1
C5275	G0168	1	C9600	G0471	1	C9752	G0471	1
C5275	G0471	1	C9601	G0269	1	C9752	J0670	1
C5275	J0670	1	C9601	G0471	1	C9752	J2001	1
C5275	J2001	1	C9602	G0269	1	C9753	G0453	0
C5276	G0168	1	C9602	G0471	1	C9753	G0463	1
C5276	G0471	1	C9603	G0269	1	C9753	G0471	1

Column 1	Column 2	Modifier	Column 1	Column 2	Modifier	Column 1	Column 2	Modifier
C9753	J0670	1	G0105	G0408	1	G0120	G0509	1
C9753	J2001	1	G0105	G0425	1	G0121	G0105	0
E0781	E0782	1	G0105	G0426	1	G0121	G0380	1
G0101	G0181	1	G0105	G0427	1	G0121	G0381	1
G0101	G0182	1	G0105	G0463	1	G0121	G0382	1
G0101	G0380	1	G0105	G0471	1	G0121	G0383	1
G0101	G0381	1	G0105	G0508	1	G0121	G0384	1
G0101	G0382	1	G0105	G0509	1	G0121	G0406	1
G0101	G0383	1	G0106	G0105	0	G0121	G0407	1
G0101	G0384	1	G0106	G0121	0	G0121	G0408	1
G0101	G0406	1	G0106	G0181	1	G0121	G0425	1
G0101	G0407	1	G0106	G0182	1	G0121	G0426	1
G0101	G0408	1	G0106	G0380	1	G0121	G0427	1
G0101	G0425	1	G0106	G0381	1	G0121	G0463	1
G0101	G0426	1	G0106	G0382	1	G0121	G0471	1
G0101	G0427	1	G0106	G0383	1	G0121	G0508	1
G0101	G0463	1	G0106	G0384	1	G0121	G0509	1
G0101	G0508	1	G0106	G0406	1	G0123	P3000	0
G0101	G0509	1	G0106	G0407	1	G0124	G0141	0
G0104	G0105	0	G0106	G0408	1	G0124	G0147	0
G0104	G0106	1	G0106	G0425	1	G0124	G0148	0
G0104	G0120	1	G0106	G0426	1	G0124	P3000	0
G0104	G0121	0	G0106	G0427	1	G0124	P3001	0
G0104	G0181	1	G0106	G0463	1	G0127	G0380	1
G0104	G0182	1	G0106	G0508	1	G0127	G0381	1
G0104	G0380	1	G0106	G0509	1	G0127	G0382	1
G0104	G0381	1	G0108	G0270	0	G0127	G0383	1
G0104	G0382	1	G0108	G0271	0	G0127	G0384	1
G0104	G0383	1	G0109	G0270	0	G0127	G0406	1
G0104	G0384	1	G0109	G0271	0	G0127	G0407	1
G0104	G0406	1	G0117	G0118	0	G0127	G0408	1
G0104	G0407	1	G0120	G0105	0	G0127	G0425	1
G0104	G0408	1	G0120	G0106	0	G0127	G0426	1
G0104	G0425	1	G0120	G0121	0	G0127	G0427	1
G0104	G0426	1	G0120	G0181	1	G0127	G0463	1
G0104	G0427	1	G0120	G0182	1	G0127	G0471	1
G0104	G0463	1	G0120	G0380	1	G0127	G0508	1
G0104	G0471	1	G0120	G0381	1	G0127	G0509	1
G0104	G0508	1	G0120	G0382	1	G0141	G0123	0
G0104	G0509	1	G0120	G0383	1	G0141	G0143	0
G0105	G0181	1	G0120	G0384	1	G0141	G0144	0
G0105	G0182	1	G0120	G0406	1	G0141	P3000	0
G0105	G0380	1	G0120	G0407	1	G0145	G0147	0
G0105	G0381	1	G0120	G0408	1	G0145	G0148	0
G0105	G0382	1	G0120	G0425	1	G0148	G0147	0
G0105	G0383	1	G0120	G0426	1	G0151	G0281	1
G0105	G0384	1	G0120	G0427	1	G0151	G0283	1
G0105	G0406	1	G0120	G0463	1	G0151	G0329	1
G0105	G0407	1	G0120	G0508	1	G0157	G0281	1

Column 1	Column 2	Modifier
G0157	G0283	1
G0157	G0329	1
G0159	G0281	1
G0159	G0283	1
G0159	G0329	1
G0162	G0008	1
G0162	G0009	1
G0162	G0010	1
G0162	G0128	1
G0162	P9612	1
G0162	P9615	1
G0168	G0463	1
G0168	G0471	1
G0168	J0670	1
G0168	J2001	1
G0179	G0180	0
G0181	G0102	1
G0181	G0182	1
G0181	G0506	0
G0181	G0511	0
G0182	G0102	1
G0182	G0506	0
G0182	G0511	0
G0239	G0237	1
G0239	G0238	1
G0245	G0127	0
G0245	G0246	0
G0246	G0127	0
G0247	G0127	0
G0257	G0491	1
G0257	G0492	1
G0259	G0471	1
G0260	G0259	0
G0260	G0471	1
G0268	G0463	1
G0268	G0471	1
G0270	G0271	0
G0276	G0453	0
G0281	G0283	1
G0281	G0329	0
G0302	G0303	0
G0302	G0304	0
G0302	G0380	1
G0302	G0381	1
G0302	G0382	1
G0302	G0383	1
G0302	G0384	1
G0302	G0406	1
G0302	G0407	1

Column 1	Column 2	Modifier
G0302	G0408	1
G0302	G0425	1
G0302	G0426	1
G0302	G0427	1
G0302	G0463	1
G0302	G0508	1
G0302	G0509	1
G0303	G0304	0
G0303	G0380	1
G0303	G0381	1
G0303	G0382	1
G0303	G0383	1
G0303	G0384	1
G0303	G0406	1
G0303	G0407	1
G0303	G0408	1
G0303	G0425	1
G0303	G0426	1
G0303	G0427	1
G0303	G0463	1
G0303	G0508	1
G0303	G0509	1
G0304	G0380	1
G0304	G0381	1
G0304	G0382	1
G0304	G0383	1
G0304	G0384	1
G0304	G0406	1
G0304	G0407	1
G0304	G0408	1
G0304	G0425	1
G0304	G0426	1
G0304	G0427	1
G0304	G0463	1
G0304	G0508	1
G0304	G0509	1
G0305	G0380	1
G0305	G0381	1
G0305	G0382	1
G0305	G0383	1
G0305	G0384	1
G0305	G0406	1
G0305	G0407	1
G0305	G0408	1
G0305	G0425	1
G0305	G0426	1
G0305	G0427	1
G0305	G0463	1
G0305	G0508	1

Column 1	Column 2	Modifier
G0305	G0509	1
G0306	G0307	0
G0329	G0283	1
G0337	G0101	0
G0337	G0102	0
G0337	G0104	0
G0337	G0105	0
G0337	G0106	0
G0337	G0117	0
G0337	G0118	0
G0337	G0120	0
G0337	G0121	0
G0337	G0245	0
G0337	G0246	0
G0337	G0248	0
G0337	G0250	1
G0337	G0270	0
G0337	G0271	0
G0337	G0410	1
G0337	G0411	1
G0337	G0459	0
G0337	G0463	0
G0337	P3000	0
G0337	P3001	0
G0337	Q0091	0
G0339	G0340	1
G0339	G0459	0
G0339	G0463	0
G0339	G0471	0
G0339	G0500	0
G0339	G6002	0
G0339	G6003	1
G0339	G6004	1
G0339	G6005	1
G0339	G6006	1
G0339	G6007	1
G0339	G6008	1
G0339	G6009	1
G0339	G6010	1
G0339	G6011	1
G0339	G6012	1
G0339	G6013	1
G0339	G6014	1
G0340	G0459	0
G0340	G0463	0
G0340	G0471	0
G0340	G0500	0
G0340	G6002	0
G0340	G6003	1

Column 1	Column 2	Modifier
G0340	G6004	1
G0340	G6005	1
G0340	G6006	1
G0340	G6007	1
G0340	G6008	1
G0340	G6009	1
G0340	G6010	1
G0340	G6011	1
G0340	G6012	1
G0340	G6013	1
G0340	G6014	1
G0341	G0463	1
G0341	G0471	1
G0341	J0670	1
G0341	J1642	1
G0341	J1644	1
G0341	J2001	1
G0342	G0341	0
G0342	G0463	1
G0342	G0471	1
G0343	G0341	0
G0343	G0342	0
G0343	G0463	1
G0343	G0471	1
G0380	G0102	1
G0380	G0245	1
G0380	G0246	1
G0380	G0270	1
G0380	G0271	1
G0380	G0459	1
G0380	G0498	1
G0381	G0102	1
G0381	G0245	1
G0381	G0246	1
G0381	G0270	1
G0381	G0271	1
G0381	G0380	1
G0381	G0459	1
G0381	G0498	1
G0382	G0102	1
G0382	G0245	1
G0382	G0246	1
G0382	G0270	1
G0382	G0271	1
G0382	G0380	1
G0382	G0381	1
G0382	G0459	1
G0382	G0498	1
G0383	G0102	1

Column 1	Column 2	Modifier
G0383	G0245	1
G0383	G0246	1
G0383	G0270	1
G0383	G0271	1
G0383	G0380	1
G0383	G0381	1
G0383	G0382	1
G0383	G0459	1
G0383	G0498	1
G0384	G0102	1
G0384	G0245	1
G0384	G0246	1
G0384	G0270	1
G0384	G0271	1
G0384	G0380	1
G0384	G0381	1
G0384	G0382	1
G0384	G0383	1
G0384	G0459	1
G0384	G0498	1
G0396	G0442	0
G0396	G2011	0
G0397	G0396	0
G0397	G0442	0
G0397	G2011	0
G0398	G0399	0
G0398	G0400	0
G0399	G0400	0
G0402	G0250	1
G0402	G0270	0
G0402	G0271	0
G0402	G0380	1
G0402	G0381	1
G0402	G0382	1
G0402	G0383	1
G0402	G0384	1
G0402	G0438	0
G0402	G0439	0
G0402	G0444	0
G0402	G0459	1
G0402	G0463	1
G0403	G0404	0
G0403	G0405	0
G0406	G0102	0
G0406	G0245	0
G0406	G0246	0
G0406	G0250	0
G0406	G0270	0
G0406	G0271	0

Column 1	Column 2	Modifier
G0406	G0459	0
G0406	G0498	1
G0407	G0102	0
G0407	G0245	0
G0407	G0246	0
G0407	G0250	0
G0407	G0270	0
G0407	G0271	0
G0407	G0406	0
G0407	G0459	0
G0407	G0498	1
G0408	G0102	0
G0408	G0245	0
G0408	G0246	0
G0408	G0250	0
G0408	G0270	0
G0408	G0271	0
G0408	G0406	0
G0408	G0407	0
G0408	G0459	0
G0408	G0498	1
G0409	G0155	1
G0409	G0176	1
G0409	G0177	1
G0409	G0459	1
G0410	G0176	1
G0410	G0177	1
G0410	G0270	0
G0410	G0271	0
G0410	G0380	1
G0410	G0381	1
G0410	G0382	1
G0410	G0383	1
G0410	G0384	1
G0410	G0459	0
G0410	G0463	1
G0411	G0176	1
G0411	G0177	1
G0411	G0270	0
G0411	G0271	0
G0411	G0380	1
G0411	G0381	1
G0411	G0382	1
G0411	G0383	1
G0411	G0384	1
G0411	G0410	1
G0411	G0459	0
G0411	G0463	1
G0412	G0463	1

Column 1	Column 2	Modifier
G0412	G0471	1
G0413	G0463	1
G0413	G0471	1
G0414	G0463	1
G0414	G0471	1
G0415	G0413	1
G0415	G0463	1
G0415	G0471	1
G0420	G0421	1
G0422	G0423	1
G0422	G0471	1
G0423	G0471	1
G0424	G0237	0
G0424	G0238	0
G0424	G0239	0
G0424	G0406	1
G0424	G0407	1
G0424	G0408	1
G0424	G0422	1
G0424	G0423	1
G0424	G0471	1
G0425	G0102	0
G0425	G0245	0
G0425	G0246	0
G0425	G0250	1
G0425	G0270	0
G0425	G0271	0
G0425	G0406	0
G0425	G0407	0
G0425	G0408	0
G0425	G0424	1
G0425	G0459	0
G0425	G0498	1
G0426	G0102	0
G0426	G0245	0
G0426	G0246	0
G0426	G0250	1
G0426	G0270	0
G0426	G0271	0
G0426	G0406	0
G0426	G0407	0
G0426	G0408	0
G0426	G0424	1
G0426	G0425	0
G0426	G0459	0
G0426	G0498	1
G0426	G0508	0
G0426	G0509	0
G0427	G0102	0

Column 1	Column 2	Modifier
G0427	G0245	0
G0427	G0246	0
G0427	G0250	1
G0427	G0270	0
G0427	G0271	0
G0427	G0406	0
G0427	G0407	0
G0427	G0408	0
G0427	G0424	1
G0427	G0425	0
G0427	G0426	0
G0427	G0459	0
G0427	G0498	1
G0427	G0508	0
G0427	G0509	0
G0428	G0471	1
G0429	G0463	1
G0429	G0471	1
G0429	J2001	1
G0438	G0250	1
G0438	G0270	0
G0438	G0271	0
G0438	G0380	1
G0438	G0381	1
G0438	G0382	1
G0438	G0383	1
G0438	G0384	1
G0438	G0439	0
G0438	G0444	0
G0438	G0459	1
G0438	G0463	1
G0439	G0250	1
G0439	G0270	0
G0439	G0271	0
G0439	G0380	1
G0439	G0381	1
G0439	G0382	1
G0439	G0383	1
G0439	G0384	1
G0439	G0459	1
G0439	G0463	1
G0442	G0250	1
G0442	G0270	0
G0442	G0271	0
G0442	G0380	1
G0442	G0381	1
G0442	G0382	1
G0442	G0383	1
G0442	G0384	1

Column 1	Column 2	Modifier
G0442	G0459	1
G0443	G0250	1
G0443	G0270	0
G0443	G0271	0
G0443	G0380	1
G0443	G0381	1
G0443	G0382	1
G0443	G0383	1
G0443	G0384	1
G0443	G0396	0
G0443	G0397	0
G0443	G0459	1
G0443	G2011	0
G0444	G0250	1
G0444	G0270	0
G0444	G0271	0
G0444	G0380	1
G0444	G0381	1
G0444	G0382	1
G0444	G0383	1
G0444	G0384	1
G0445	G0250	1
G0445	G0270	0
G0445	G0271	0
G0445	G0380	1
G0445	G0381	1
G0445	G0382	1
G0445	G0383	1
G0445	G0384	1
G0445	G0444	0
G0447	G0473	1
G0448	G0471	1
G0455	G0463	1
G0458	G0471	0
G0458	G0500	0
G0458	P9612	0
G0459	G0250	1
G0459	G0270	0
G0459	G0271	0
G0459	G0444	1
G0459	G0445	1
G0459	G0446	1
G0459	G0447	1
G0459	G0473	1
G0460	P9020	1
G0463	G0102	0
G0463	G0117	0
G0463	G0118	0
G0463	G0245	0

Column 1	Column 2	Modifier
G0463	G0246	0
G0463	G0248	1
G0463	G0250	1
G0463	G0270	0
G0463	G0271	0
G0463	G0396	1
G0463	G0397	1
G0463	G0442	1
G0463	G0443	1
G0463	G0444	1
G0463	G0445	1
G0463	G0446	1
G0463	G0447	1
G0463	G0459	0
G0463	G0473	1
G0463	G2011	1
G0471	G0463	1
G0471	J0670	1
G0471	J2001	1
G0471	P9612	0
G0471	P9615	0
G0475	G0432	0
G0475	G0433	0
G0480	G0659	0
G0481	G0480	0
G0481	G0659	0
G0482	G0480	0
G0482	G0481	0
G0482	G0659	0
G0483	G0480	0
G0483	G0481	0
G0483	G0482	0
G0483	G0659	0
G0491	G0270	0
G0491	G0271	0
G0491	G0380	1
G0491	G0381	1
G0491	G0382	1
G0491	G0383	1
G0491	G0384	1
G0491	G0406	1
G0491	G0407	1
G0491	G0408	1
G0491	G0425	1
G0491	G0426	1
G0491	G0427	1
G0491	G0463	1
G0491	G0471	1
G0491	G0508	1

Column 1	Column 2	Modifier
G0491	G0509	1
G0492	G0270	0
G0492	G0271	0
G0492	G0380	1
G0492	G0381	1
G0492	G0382	1
G0492	G0383	1
G0492	G0384	1
G0492	G0406	1
G0492	G0407	1
G0492	G0408	1
G0492	G0425	1
G0492	G0426	1
G0492	G0427	1
G0492	G0463	1
G0492	G0471	1
G0492	G0508	1
G0492	G0509	1
G0498	G0463	1
G0498	J1644	1
G0500	G0380	1
G0500	G0381	1
G0500	G0382	1
G0500	G0383	1
G0500	G0384	1
G0500	G0406	1
G0500	G0407	1
G0500	G0408	1
G0500	G0425	1
G0500	G0426	1
G0500	G0427	1
G0500	G0463	1
G0508	G0102	0
G0508	G0245	0
G0508	G0246	0
G0508	G0250	1
G0508	G0270	0
G0508	G0271	0
G0508	G0406	0
G0508	G0407	0
G0508	G0408	0
G0508	G0424	1
G0508	G0459	0
G0508	G0509	0
G0509	G0102	0
G0509	G0245	0
G0509	G0246	0
G0509	G0250	1
G0509	G0270	0

Column 1	Column 2	Modifier
G0509	G0271	0
G0509	G0406	0
G0509	G0407	0
G0509	G0408	0
G0509	G0424	1
G0509	G0459	0
G0512	G0181	0
G0512	G0182	0
G0516	J0670	1
G0516	J2001	1
G0517	J0670	1
G0517	J2001	1
G0518	J0670	1
G0518	J2001	1
G2001	G0076	0
G2001	G0077	0
G2001	G0078	0
G2001	G0079	0
G2001	G0080	0
G2001	G0081	0
G2001	G0082	0
G2001	G0083	0
G2001	G0084	0
G2001	G0085	0
G2001	G0086	0
G2001	G0087	0
G2002	G0076	0
G2002	G0077	0
G2002	G0078	0
G2002	G0079	0
G2002	G0080	0
G2002	G0081	0
G2002	G0082	0
G2002	G0083	0
G2002	G0084	0
G2002	G0085	0
G2002	G0086	0
G2002	G0087	0
G2003	G0076	0
G2003	G0077	0
G2003	G0078	0
G2003	G0079	0
G2003	G0080	0
G2003	G0081	0
G2003	G0082	0
G2003	G0083	0
G2003	G0084	0
G2003	G0085	0
G2003	G0086	0

Column 1	Column 2	Modifier
G2003	G0087	0
G2004	G0076	0
G2004	G0077	0
G2004	G0078	0
G2004	G0079	0
G2004	G0080	0
G2004	G0081	0
G2004	G0082	0
G2004	G0083	0
G2004	G0084	0
G2004	G0085	0
G2004	G0086	0
G2004	G0087	0
G2005	G0076	0
G2005	G0077	0
G2005	G0078	0
G2005	G0079	0
G2005	G0080	0
G2005	G0081	0
G2005	G0082	0
G2005	G0083	0
G2005	G0084	0
G2005	G0085	0
G2005	G0086	0
G2005	G0087	0
G2006	G0076	0
G2006	G0077	0
G2006	G0078	0
G2006	G0079	0
G2006	G0080	0
G2006	G0081	0
G2006	G0082	0
G2006	G0083	0
G2006	G0084	0
G2006	G0085	0
G2006	G0086	0
G2006	G0087	0
G2007	G0076	0
G2007	G0077	0
G2007	G0078	0
G2007	G0079	0
G2007	G0080	0
G2007	G0081	0
G2007	G0082	0
G2007	G0083	0
G2007	G0084	0
G2007	G0085	0
G2007	G0086	0
G2007	G0087	0

Column 1	Column 2	Modifier
G2008	G0076	0
G2008	G0077	0
G2008	G0078	0
G2008	G0079	0
G2008	G0080	0
G2008	G0081	0
G2008	G0082	0
G2008	G0083	0
G2008	G0084	0
G2008	G0085	0
G2008	G0086	0
G2008	G0087	0
G2009	G0076	0
G2009	G0077	0
G2009	G0078	0
G2009	G0079	0
G2009	G0080	0
G2009	G0081	0
G2009	G0082	0
G2009	G0083	0
G2009	G0084	0
G2009	G0085	0
G2009	G0086	0
G2009	G0087	0
G2011	G0442	0
G2013	G0076	0
G2013	G0077	0
G2013	G0078	0
G2013	G0079	0
G2013	G0080	0
G2013	G0081	0
G2013	G0082	0
G2013	G0083	0
G2013	G0084	0
G2013	G0085	0
G2013	G0086	0
G2013	G0087	0
G2014	G0076	0
G2014	G0077	0
G2014	G0078	0
G2014	G0079	0
G2014	G0080	0
G2014	G0081	0
G2014	G0082	0
G2014	G0083	0
G2014	G0084	0
G2014	G0085	0
G2014	G0086	0
G2014	G0087	0

Column 1	Column 2	Modifier
G2015	G0076	0
G2015	G0077	0
G2015	G0078	0
G2015	G0079	0
G2015	G0080	0
G2015	G0081	0
G2015	G0082	0
G2015	G0083	0
G2015	G0084	0
G2015	G0085	0
G2015	G0086	0
G2015	G0087	0
G6001	G6017	1
G6002	G0459	0
G6002	G0463	1
G6002	G0471	0
G6002	G0500	0
G6002	G6001	0
G6002	G6017	1
G6003	G0459	0
G6003	G0463	1
G6003	G0471	0
G6003	G0500	0
G6004	G0459	0
G6004	G0463	1
G6004	G0471	0
G6004	G0500	0
G6004	G6003	1
G6005	G0459	0
G6005	G0463	1
G6005	G0471	0
G6005	G0500	0
G6005	G6003	1
G6005	G6004	1
G6006	G0459	0
G6006	G0463	1
G6006	G0471	0
G6006	G0500	0
G6006	G6003	1
G6006	G6004	1
G6006	G6005	1
G6007	G0459	0
G6007	G0463	1
G6007	G0471	0
G6007	G0500	0
G6007	G6003	1
G6007	G6004	1
G6007	G6005	1
G6007	G6006	1

Column 1	Column 2	Modifier
G6008	G0459	0
G6008	G0463	1
G6008	G0471	0
G6008	G0500	0
G6008	G6003	1
G6008	G6004	1
G6008	G6005	1
G6008	G6006	1
G6008	G6007	1
G6009	G0459	0
G6009	G0463	1
G6009	G0471	0
G6009	G0500	0
G6009	G6003	1
G6009	G6004	1
G6009	G6005	1
G6009	G6006	1
G6009	G6007	1
G6009	G6008	1
G6010	G0459	0
G6010	G0463	1
G6010	G0471	0
G6010	G0500	0
G6010	G6003	1
G6010	G6004	1
G6010	G6005	1
G6010	G6006	1
G6010	G6007	1
G6010	G6008	1
G6010	G6009	1
G6011	G0459	0
G6011	G0463	1
G6011	G0471	0
G6011	G0500	0
G6011	G6003	1
G6011	G6004	1
G6011	G6005	1
G6011	G6006	1
G6011	G6007	1
G6011	G6008	1
G6011	G6009	1
G6011	G6010	1
G6012	G0459	0
G6012	G0463	1
G6012	G0471	0
G6012	G0500	0
G6012	G6003	1
G6012	G6004	1
G6012	G6005	1

Column 1	Column 2	Modifier
G6012	G6006	1
G6012	G6007	1
G6012	G6008	1
G6012	G6009	1
G6012	G6010	1
G6012	G6011	1
G6013	G0459	0
G6013	G0463	1
G6013	G0471	0
G6013	G0500	0
G6013	G6003	1
G6013	G6004	1
G6013	G6005	1
G6013	G6006	1
G6013	G6007	1
G6013	G6008	1
G6013	G6009	1
G6013	G6010	1
G6013	G6011	1
G6013	G6012	1
G6014	G0459	0
G6014	G0463	1
G6014	G0471	0
G6014	G0500	0
G6014	G6003	1
G6014	G6004	1
G6014	G6005	1
G6014	G6006	1
G6014	G6007	1
G6014	G6008	1
G6014	G6009	1
G6014	G6010	1
G6014	G6011	1
G6014	G6012	1
G6014	G6013	1
G6015	G0339	0
G6015	G0340	0
G6015	G0459	0
G6015	G0463	1
G6015	G0471	0
G6015	G0500	0
G6015	G6003	0
G6015	G6004	0
G6015	G6005	0
G6015	G6006	0
G6015	G6007	0
G6015	G6008	0
G6015	G6009	0
G6015	G6010	0

Column 1	Column 2	Modifier
G6015	G6011	0
G6015	G6012	0
G6015	G6013	0
G6015	G6014	0
G6015	G6016	0
G6016	G0339	0
G6016	G0340	0
G6016	G0459	0
G6016	G0463	0
G6016	G0471	0
G6016	G6003	1
G6016	G6004	1
G6016	G6005	1
G6016	G6006	1
G6016	G6007	1
G6016	G6008	1
G6016	G6009	1
G6016	G6010	1
G6016	G6011	1
G6016	G6012	1
G6016	G6013	1
G6016	G6014	1
G6017	G0459	1
G6017	G0463	1
G6017	G0471	1
G6017	G0500	1
J1560	J1460	0
J2790	J2792	1
J7298	J7297	0
P3000	G0380	1
P3000	G0381	1
P3000	G0382	1
P3000	G0383	1
P3000	G0384	1
P3000	G0406	1
P3000	G0407	1
P3000	G0408	1
P3000	G0425	1
P3000	G0426	1
P3000	G0427	1
P3000	G0463	1
P3000	G0508	1
P3000	G0509	1
P3001	G0123	0
P3001	G0141	0
P3001	G0143	0
P3001	G0144	0
P3001	G0145	0
P3001	G0147	0

Column 1	Column 2	Modifier	Column 1	Column 2	Modifier	Column 1	Column 2	Modifier
P3001	G0148	0	P9036	P9011	1	P9040	P9073	1
P3001	G0380	1	P9036	P9016	1	P9603	P9604	1
P3001	G0381	1	P9036	P9019	1	P9612	P9615	0
P3001	G0382	1	P9036	P9020	1	Q0091	G0181	1
P3001	G0383	1	P9036	P9021	1	Q0091	G0182	1
P3001	G0384	1	P9036	P9022	1	Q0091	G0380	1
P3001	G0406	1	P9036	P9031	1	Q0091	G0381	1
P3001	G0407	1	P9036	P9034	1	Q0091	G0382	1
P3001	G0408	1	P9036	P9035	1	Q0091	G0383	1
P3001	G0425	1	P9036	P9039	1	Q0091	G0384	1
P3001	G0426	1	P9036	P9073	1	Q0091	G0406	1
P3001	G0427	1	P9037	P9010	1	Q0091	G0407	1
P3001	G0463	1	P9037	P9011	1	Q0091	G0408	1
P3001	G0508	1	P9037	P9016	1	Q0091	G0425	1
P3001	G0509	1	P9037	P9019	1	Q0091	G0426	1
P9011	P9010	1	P9037	P9020	1	Q0091	G0427	1
P9011	P9021	0	P9037	P9021	1	Q0091	G0463	1
P9011	P9022	0	P9037	P9022	1	Q0091	G0508	1
P9011	P9039	0	P9037	P9031	1	Q0091	G0509	1
P9022	P9010	1	P9037	P9034	1	Q1004	Q1005	1
P9022	P9016	1	P9037	P9035	1	Q2035	Q2034	0
P9022	P9021	1	P9037	P9039	1	Q2035	Q2036	0
P9022	P9039	1	P9037	P9073	1	Q2035	Q2037	0
P9032	P9010	1	P9038	P9010	1	Q2035	Q2038	0
P9032	P9011	1	P9038	P9011	1	Q2035	Q2039	0
P9032	P9016	1	P9038	P9016	1	Q2036	Q2034	0
P9032	P9019	1	P9038	P9019	1	Q2036	Q2037	0
P9032	P9020	1	P9038	P9020	1	Q2036	Q2038	0
P9032	P9021	1	P9038	P9021	1	Q2036	Q2039	0
P9032	P9022	1	P9038	P9022	1	Q2037	Q2034	0
P9032	P9031	1	P9038	P9031	1	Q2037	Q2038	0
P9032	P9034	1	P9038	P9034	1	Q2037	Q2039	0
P9032	P9035	1	P9038	P9035	1	Q2038	Q2034	0
P9032	P9039	1	P9038	P9039	1	Q2038	Q2039	0
P9032	P9073	1	P9038	P9073	1	Q2039	Q2034	0
P9033	P9010	1	P9039	P9010	1	Q2043	G0380	1
P9033	P9011	1	P9039	P9016	1	Q2043	G0381	1
P9033	P9016	1	P9039	P9021	1	Q2043	G0382	1
P9033	P9019	1	P9040	P9010	1	Q2043	G0383	1
P9033	P9020	1	P9040	P9011	1	Q2043	G0384	1
P9033	P9021	1	P9040	P9016	1	Q2043	G0463	1
P9033	P9022	1	P9040	P9019	1	Q2043	G0471	1
P9033	P9031	1	P9040	P9020	1	Q9951	Q9959	0
P9033	P9034	1	P9040	P9021	1	Q9951	Q9964	0
P9033	P9035	1	P9040	P9022	1	Q9958	Q9951	0
P9033	P9039	1	P9040	P9031	1	Q9958	Q9959	0
P9033	P9073	1	P9040	P9034	1	Q9958	Q9964	0
P9034	P9073	1	P9040	P9035	1	Q9958	Q9965	1
P9036	P9010	1	P9040	P9039	1	Q9958	Q9966	1

Column 1	Column 2	Modifier
Q9958	Q9967	1
Q9959	Q9964	0
Q9960	Q9951	0
Q9960	Q9958	1
Q9960	Q9959	0
Q9960	Q9964	0
Q9960	Q9965	1
Q9960	Q9966	1
Q9960	Q9967	1
Q9961	Q9951	0
Q9961	Q9958	1
Q9961	Q9959	0
Q9961	Q9960	1
Q9961	Q9964	0
Q9961	Q9965	1
Q9961	Q9966	1
Q9961	Q9967	1

Column 1	Column 2	Modifier
Q9962	Q9951	0
Q9962	Q9958	1
Q9962	Q9959	0
Q9962	Q9960	1
Q9962	Q9961	1
Q9962	Q9964	0
Q9962	Q9965	1
Q9962	Q9966	1
Q9962	Q9967	1
Q9963	Q9951	0
Q9963	Q9958	1
Q9963	Q9959	0
Q9963	Q9960	1
Q9963	Q9961	1
Q9963	Q9962	1
Q9963	Q9964	0
Q9963	Q9965	1

Column 1	Column 2	Modifier
Q9963	Q9966	1
Q9963	Q9967	1
Q9965	Q9951	0
Q9965	Q9959	0
Q9965	Q9964	0
Q9966	Q9951	0
Q9966	Q9959	0
Q9966	Q9964	0
Q9966	Q9965	1
Q9967	Q9951	0
Q9967	Q9959	0
Q9967	Q9964	0
Q9967	Q9965	1
Q9967	Q9966	1
R0075	R0070	1

Disclaimer: The information contained in this appendix was the most current information from the CMS website at the time of printing. For the most up-to-date information, visit www.cms.gov.

CHAPTER XII
SUPPLEMENTAL SERVICES

HCPCS LEVEL II CODES A0000 - V9999 FOR NATIONAL CORRECT CODING INITIATIVE POLICY MANUAL FOR MEDICARE SERVICES

Current Procedural Terminology (CPT®) codes, descriptions and other data only are copyright 2019 American Medical Association. All rights reserved.

CPT® is a registered trademark of the American Medical Association.

Applicable FARS\DFARS Restrictions Apply to Government Use.

Fee schedules, relative value units, conversion factors, prospective payment systems, and/or related components are not assigned by the AMA, are not part of CPT®, and the AMA is not recommending their use. The AMA does not directly or indirectly practice medicine or dispense medical services. The AMA assumes no liability for the data contained or not contained herein.

TABLE OF CONTENTS

Chapter XII 568

Supplemental Services.. 568

HCPCS Level II Codes A0000 - V9999 568

A. Introduction 568

B. Evaluation and Management (E&M) Services 568

C. NCCI Procedure-to-Procedure (PTP) Edit Specific Issues.. 568

D. Medically Unlikely Edits (MUEs) 571

E. General Policy Statements.. 573

Chapter XII

Supplemental Services

HCPCS Level II Codes A0000 - V9999

A. Introduction

The principles of correct coding discussed in Chapter I apply to HCPCS codes in the range A0000-V9999. Several general guidelines are repeated in this chapter. However, those general guidelines from Chapter I not discussed in this chapter are nonetheless applicable.

Physicians shall report the HCPCS/CPT® code that describes the procedure performed to the greatest specificity possible. A HCPCS/CPT® code shall be reported only if all services described by the code are performed. A physician shall not report multiple HCPCS/CPT® codes if a single HCPCS/CPT® code exists that describes the services. This type of unbundling is incorrect coding.

HCPCS/CPT® codes include all services usually performed as part of the procedure as a standard of medical/surgical practice. A physician shall not separately report these services simply because HCPCS/CPT® codes exist for them.

Specific issues unique to HCPCS Level II codes are clarified in this chapter.

The HCPCS Level II codes are alpha-numeric codes developed by the Centers for Medicare & Medicaid Services (CMS) as a complementary coding system to the *CPT® Manual*. These codes describe physician and non-physician services not included in the *CPT® Manual*, supplies, drugs, durable medical equipment, ambulance services, etc. The correct coding edits and policy statements that follow address those HCPCS Level II codes that are reported to MACs for Part B services.

B. Evaluation and Management (E&M) Services

Medicare Global Surgery Rules define the rules for reporting evaluation and management (E&M) services with procedures covered by these rules. This section summarizes some of the rules.

All procedures on the Medicare Physician Fee Schedule are assigned a global period of 000, 010, 090, XXX, YYY, ZZZ, or MMM.

The global concept does not apply to XXX procedures. The global period for YYY procedures is defined by the MAC. All procedures with a global period of ZZZ are related to another procedure, and the applicable global period for the ZZZ code is determined by the related procedure. Procedures with a global period of MMM are maternity procedures.

Since NCCI PTP edits are applied to same day services by the same provider to the same beneficiary, certain Global Surgery Rules are applicable to NCCI. An E&M service is separately reportable on the same date of service as a procedure with a global period of 000, 010, or 090 days under limited circumstances.

If a procedure has a global period of 090 days, it is defined as a major surgical procedure. If an E&M service is performed on the same date of service as a major surgical procedure for the purpose of deciding whether to perform this surgical procedure, the E&M service is separately reportable with modifier 57. Other preoperative E&M services on the same date of service as a major surgical procedure are included in the global payment for the procedure and are not separately reportable. NCCI does not contain edits based on this rule because MACs have separate edits.

If a procedure has a global period of 000 or 010 days, it is defined as a minor surgical procedure. In general, E&M services on the same date of service as the minor surgical procedure are included in the payment for the procedure. The decision to perform a minor surgical procedure is included in the payment for the minor surgical procedure and shall not be reported separately as an E&M service. However, a significant and separately identifiable E&M service unrelated to the decision to perform the minor surgical procedure is separately reportable with modifier 25. The E&M service and minor surgical procedure do not require different diagnoses. If a minor surgical procedure is performed on a new patient, the same rules for reporting E&M services apply. The fact that the patient is "new" to the provider is not sufficient alone to justify reporting an E&M service on the same date of service as a minor surgical procedure. NCCI contains many, but not all, possible edits based on these principles.

Example: If a physician determines that a new patient with head trauma requires sutures, confirms the allergy and immunization status, obtains informed consent, and performs the repair, an E&M service is not separately reportable. However, if the physician also performs a medically reasonable and necessary full neurological examination, an E&M service may be separately reportable.

For major and minor surgical procedures, postoperative E&M services related to recovery from the surgical procedure during the postoperative period are included in the global surgical package as are E&M services related to complications of the surgery. Postoperative visits unrelated to the diagnosis for which the surgical procedure was performed unless related to a complication of surgery may be reported separately on the same day as a surgical procedure with modifier 24 ("Unrelated Evaluation and Management Service by the Same Physician or Other Qualified Health Care Professional During a Postoperative Period").

Procedures with a global surgery indicator of "XXX" are not covered by these rules. Many of these "XXX" procedures are performed by physicians and have inherent pre-procedure, intra- procedure, and post-procedure work usually performed each time the procedure is completed. This work shall **not** be reported as a separate E&M code. Other "XXX" procedures are not usually performed by a physician and have no physician work relative value units associated with them. A physician shall **not** report a separate E&M code with these procedures for the supervision of others performing the procedure or for the interpretation of the procedure. With most "XXX" procedures, the physician may, however, perform a significant and separately identifiable E&M service on the same date of service which may be reported by appending modifier 25 to the E&M code. This E&M service may be related to the same diagnosis necessitating performance of the "XXX" procedure but cannot include any work inherent in the "XXX" procedure, supervision of others performing the "XXX" procedure, or time for interpreting the result of the "XXX" procedure. Appending modifier 25 to a significant, separately identifiable E&M service when performed on the same date of service as an "XXX" procedure is correct coding.

C. NCCI Procedure-to-Procedure (PTP) Edit Specific Issues

1. HCPCS code Q0091 (Screening Papanicolaou smear; obtaining, preparing and conveyance of cervical or vaginal smear to laboratory) describes the services necessary to procure and transport a pap smear specimen to the laboratory. If an E&M service is performed at the same patient encounter solely for the purpose of performing a

screening pap smear, the E&M service is not separately reportable. However, if a significant, separately identifiable E&M service is performed to evaluate other medical problems, both the screening pap smear and the E&M service may be reported separately. Modifier 25 should be appended to the E&M CPT® code indicating that a significant, separately identifiable E&M service was rendered.

2. HCPCS code G0101 (Cervical or vaginal cancer screening; pelvic and clinical breast examination may be reported with E&M services under certain circumstances. If a Medicare covered reasonable and medically necessary E&M service requires breast and/or pelvic examination, HCPCS code G0101 shall not be additionally reported. However, if the Medicare covered reasonable and medically necessary E&M service and the screening service, G0101, are unrelated to one another, both HCPCS code G0101 and the E&M service may be reported appending modifier 25 to the E&M service CPT® code. Use of modifier 25 indicates that the E&M service is significant and separately identifiable from the screening service, G0101.

3. HCPCS code G0102 (Prostate cancer screening; digital rectal examination) is not separately payable with an E&M code (CPT® codes 99201-99499). CMS published this policy in the "Federal Register", November 2, 1999, Page 59414 as follows:

> "As stated in the July 1999 proposed rule, a digital rectal exam (DRE) is a very quick and simple examination taking only a few seconds. We believe it is rarely the sole reason for a physician encounter and is usually part of an E/M encounter. In those instances when it is the only service furnished or it is furnished as part of an otherwise non- covered service, we will pay separately for code G0102. In those instances when it is furnished on the same day as a covered E/M service, we believe it is appropriate to bundle it into the payment for the covered E/M encounter."

4. Positron emission tomography (PET) imaging requires use of a radiopharmaceutical diagnostic imaging agent. HCPCS codes A9555 (Rubidium Rb-82...) and A9526 (Nitrogen N-13 Ammonia...) may only be reported with PET scan CPT® codes 78491 and 78492. HCPCS code A9552 (Fluorodeoxyglucose F-18, FDG,...) may only be reported with PET scan CPT® codes 78459, 78608, and 78811-78816.

5. HCPCS code A9512 (Technetium Tc-99m pertechnetate, diagnostic...) describes a radiopharmaceutical used for nuclear medicine studies. Technetium Tc-99m pertechnetate is also a component of other Technetium Tc-99m radiopharmaceuticals with separate AXXXX codes. Code A9512 shall not be reported with other AXXXX radiopharmaceuticals containing Technetium Tc-99m for a single nuclear medicine study. However, if two separate nuclear medicine studies are performed on the same date of service, one with the radiopharmaceutical described by HCPCS code A9512 and one with another AXXXX radiopharmaceutical labeled with Technetium Tc-99m, both codes may be reported using an NCCI- associated modifier. HCPCS codes A9500, A9540, and A9541 describe radiopharmaceuticals labeled with Technetium Tc-99m that may be used for separate nuclear medicine studies on the same date of service as a nuclear medicine study using the radiopharmaceutical described by HCPCS code A9512.

6. NCCI contains procedure-to-procedure (PTP) edits that bundle some radiopharmaceutical codes into nuclear medicine procedure codes. These code pairs represent radiopharmaceuticals that should not be reported with the nuclear medicine procedure since it is inappropriate to use that radiopharmaceutical for that procedure. In some situations where a patient has two nuclear medicine procedures performed on the same date of service, the radiopharmaceutical used for one procedure may be incompatible with the second nuclear medicine procedure. In this circumstance, it may be appropriate to report the radiopharmaceutical with modifiers 59 or X{EPSU}.

7. HCPCS code A4220 describes a refill kit for an implantable pump. It shall not be reported separately with CPT® codes 95990 (Refilling and maintenance of implantable pump..., spinal... or brain...) or 95991 (Refilling and maintenance of implantable pump,... spinal... or brain... requiring skill of physician or other qualified health care professional) since Medicare payment for these two CPT® codes includes the refill kit.

Similarly, HCPCS code A4220 shall not be reported separately with CPT® codes 62369 (Electronic analysis of programmable, implanted pump for intrathecal or epidural drug infusion (includes evaluation of reservoir status, alarm status, drug prescription status); with reprogramming and refill) or 62370 (Electronic analysis of programmable, implanted pump for intrathecal or epidural drug infusion (includes evaluation of reservoir status, alarm status, drug prescription status); with reprogramming and refill (requiring skill of a physician or other qualified health care professional)) since Medicare payment for these two CPT® codes includes the refill kit.

8. HCPCS code E0781 describes an ambulatory infusion pump used by a patient for infusions outside the physician office or clinic. It is a misuse of this code to report the infusion pump typically used in the physician office or clinic.

9. HCPCS codes G0422 and G0423 (Intensive cardiac rehabilitation;...per session) include the same services as the cardiac rehabilitation CPT® codes 93797 and 93798, but at a greater frequency. Intensive cardiac rehabilitation may be reported with as many as six hourly sessions on a single date of service. Cardiac rehabilitation services include medical nutrition services to reduce cardiac disease risk factors. Medical nutrition therapy (CPT® codes 97802-97804) shall not be reported separately for the same patient encounter. However, medical nutrition therapy services provided under the Medicare benefit for patients with diabetes or chronic renal failure performed at a separate patient encounter on the same date of service may be reported separately. The Medicare covered medical nutrition service cannot be provided at the same patient encounter as the cardiac rehabilitation service.

Physical or occupational therapy services performed at the same patient encounter as cardiac rehabilitation services are included in the cardiac rehabilitation benefit and are not separately reportable. (CMS Final Rule ("Federal Register", Vol. 74, No. 226, November 25, 2009, pages 61884-61885)). If physical therapy or occupational therapy services are performed at a separate, medically reasonable and necessary patient encounter on the same date of service as cardiac rehabilitation services, both types of services may be reported using an NCCI PTP-associated modifier.

10. Pulmonary rehabilitation (HCPCS code G0424) includes therapeutic services and all related monitoring services to improve respiratory function. It requires measurement of patient outcome which includes, but is not limited to, pulmonary function testing (e.g., pulmonary stress testing (CPT® code 94618), cardiopulmonary exercise testing (CPT® code 94621)). Pulmonary rehabilitation shall not be reported with HCPCS codes G0237 (Therapeutic procedures to increase strength or endurance of respiratory muscles... (includes monitoring)), G0238 (Therapeutic procedures to improve respiratory function... (includes monitoring)), or G0239 (Therapeutic procedures to improve respiratory function or increase strength... (includes monitoring)). The services are mutually exclusive. The procedures described by HCPCS codes G0237-G0239 include therapeutic procedures as well as all related monitoring services, the latter including, but not limited to, pulmonary function testing (e.g., pulmonary stress testing (CPT® code 94618), cardiopulmonary exercise testing (CPT® code 94621)).

Physical or occupational therapy services performed at the same patient encounter as pulmonary rehabilitation services are included in the pulmonary rehabilitation benefit and are not separately reportable. (CMS Final Rule ("Federal Register", Vol. 74, No. 226, November 25, 2009, Pages 61884-61885)). If physical therapy or occupational therapy services are performed at a separate, medically reasonable and necessary patient encounter on the same date of service as pulmonary rehabilitation services, both types of services may be reported using an NCCI PTP-associated modifier. Similarly, physical and occupational therapy services are not separately reportable with therapeutic pulmonary procedures for the same patient encounter.

Medical nutrition therapy services (CPT® codes 97802-97804) performed at the same patient encounter as a pulmonary rehabilitation or pulmonary therapeutic service are included in the pulmonary rehabilitation or pulmonary therapeutic service and are not separately reportable. The Medicare program provides a medical nutrition therapy benefit to beneficiaries for medical nutrition therapy related to diabetes mellitus or renal disease. If a physician provides a Medicare-covered medical nutrition service to a beneficiary with diabetes mellitus or renal disease on the same date of service as a pulmonary rehabilitation or pulmonary therapeutic service but at a separate patient encounter, the medical nutrition therapy service may be separately reportable with an NCCI-associated modifier. The Medicare-covered medical nutrition service cannot be provided at the same patient encounter as the pulmonary rehabilitation or pulmonary therapeutic service.

11. HCPCS code G0434 (Drug screen..., by CLIA waived test or moderate complexity test, per patient encounter) is used to report drug screening performed by a test that is CLIA waived or CLIA moderate complex. The code is reported with only one unit of service regardless of the number of drugs screened. HCPCS code G0431 (Drug screen... by high complexity test method..., per patient encounter) is used to report drug screening performed by a CLIA high complexity test method. This code is also reported with only one unit of service regardless of the number of drugs screened. If a provider performs drug screening, it is generally not necessary for that provider to send an additional specimen from the patient to another laboratory for drug screening for the same drugs.

For a single patient encounter, only G0431 or G0434 may be reported. The testing described by G0431 includes all CLIA high complexity drug screen testing as well as any less complex drug screen testing performed at the same patient encounter. HCPCS code G0431 describes a more extensive procedure than HCPCS code G0434. Physicians should not unbundle drug screen testing and report HCPCS codes G0431 and G0434 for the same patient encounter. (HCPCS codes G0431 and G0434 were deleted January 1, 2016.)

For Calendar Year 2016, presumptive drug testing should have been reported with HCPCS codes G0477-G0479. These codes differed based on the level of complexity of the testing methodology. Only one code from this code range should have been reported per date of service. These codes were deleted January 1, 2017.

Beginning January 1, 2017, presumptive drug testing may be reported with CPT® codes 80305-80307. These codes differ based on the level of complexity of the testing methodology. Only one code from this code range may be reported per date of service.

Beginning January 1, 2016, definitive drug testing may be reported with HCPCS codes G0480-G0483. These codes differ based on the number of drug classes including metabolites tested. On January 1, 2017, HCPCS code G0659 defining a different type of definitive drug testing was added. Only one code from this group of codes may be reported per date of service.

12. In accordance with code descriptor changes for HCPCS codes G0416 effective January 1, 2015, CMS requires that surgical pathology, including gross and microscopic examination, of any and all submitted prostate needle biopsy specimens from a single patient be reported with one unit of service of HCPCS code G0416 rather than CPT® code 88305.

Instructions for HCPCS codes G0416-G0419 in this Manual have undergone changes from year to year. For historical purposes, the prior instructions may be found at https://www.cms.gov/Medicare/Coding/NationalCorrectCodInitEd/NCCI-Manual-Archive.html

13. Blood products are described by HCPCS Level II P codes. If a P code describes an irradiated blood product, CPT® code 86945 (Irradiation of blood product, each unit) shall not be reported separately since the P code includes irradiation of the blood product. If a P code describes a CMV negative blood product, CPT® codes 86644 and/or 86645 (CMV antibody) shall not be reported separately for that blood product since the P code includes the CMV antibody testing. If a P code describes a deglycerolized blood product, CPT® codes 86930 (Frozen blood, each unit; freezing...), 86931 (Frozen blood, each unit; thawing), and/or 86932 (Frozen blood, each unit; freezing (includes preparation) and thawing) shall not be reported separately since the P code includes the freezing and thawing processes. If a P code describes a pooled blood product, CPT® code 86965 (Pooling of platelets or other blood products) shall not be reported separately since the P code includes the pooling of the blood products. If the P code describes a "frozen" plasma product, CPT® code 86927 (Fresh frozen plasma, thawing, each unit) shall not be reported separately since the P code includes the thawing process.

14. HCPCS codes G0396 and G0397 describe alcohol and/or substance (other than tobacco) abuse structured assessment and intervention services. These codes

shall not be reported separately with an E&M, psychiatric diagnostic, or psychotherapy service code for the same work/time. If the E&M, psychiatric diagnostic, or psychotherapy service would normally include assessment and/or intervention of alcohol or substance abuse based on the patient's clinical presentation, HCPCS G0396 or G0397 shall not be additionally reported. If a physician reports either of these G codes with an E&M, psychiatric diagnostic, or psychotherapy code using an NCCI PTP-associated modifier, the physician is certifying that the G code service is a distinct and separate service performed during a separate time period (not necessarily a separate patient encounter) than the E&M, psychiatric diagnostic, or psychotherapy service and is a service that is not included in the E&M, psychiatric diagnostic, or psychotherapy service based on the clinical reason for the E&M, psychiatric diagnostic, or psychotherapy service.

CPT® codes 99408 and 99409 describe services which are similar to those described by HCPCS codes G0396 and G0397, but are "screening" services which are not covered under the Medicare program. Where CPT® codes 99408 and 99409 are covered by State Medicaid programs, the policies explained in the previous paragraph for G0396/G0397 also apply to 99408/99409.

The same principles apply to separate reporting of E&M services with other screening, intervention, or counseling service HCPCS codes (e.g., G0442 (Annual alcohol misuse screening, 15 minutes), G0443 (Brief face-to-face behavioral counseling for alcohol misuse, 15 minutes), and G0444 (Annual depression screening, 15 minutes). If an E&M, psychiatric diagnostic, or psychotherapy service is related to a problem which would normally require evaluation and management duplicative of the HCPCS code, the HCPCS code is not separately reportable. For example, if a patient presents with symptoms suggestive of depression, the provider shall not report G0444 in addition to the E&M, psychiatric diagnostic, or psychotherapy service code. The time and work effort devoted to the HCPCS code screening, intervention, or counseling service must be distinct and separate from the time and work of the E&M, psychiatric diagnostic, or psychotherapy service. Both services may occur at the same patient encounter.

15. HCPCS code G0269 describes placement of an occlusive device into a venous or arterial access site after an open or percutaneous vascular procedure. Since this code is status "B" on the Medicare Physician Fee Schedule Database, payment for this service is included in the payment for the vascular procedure. Under the Outpatient Prospective Payment System (OPPS), HCPCS code G0269 has a payment status indicator of "N," indicating that payment is packaged into the payment for other services paid. Providers reporting services under Medicare's hospital OPPS should report all services in accordance with appropriate Medicare "Internet-Only Manual (IOM)" instructions.

16. HCPCS code V2790 (Amniotic membrane for surgical reconstruction, per procedure) shall not be reported separately with CPT® codes 65778 (Placement of amniotic membrane on the ocular surface; without sutures) or 65779 (Placement of amniotic membrane on the ocular surface; single layer, sutured) since Medicare payment for these two CPT® codes includes the amniotic membrane.

17. HCPCS code G0515 (Development of cognitive skills to improve...) was implemented January 1, 2018. It has the same code descriptor as CPT® code 97129, which was deleted effective January 1, 2018. All NCCI PTP and MUE issues that were relevant to CPT® code 97129 are also similarly relevant to HCPCS code G0515. (CPT® code 97532 was deleted on January 1, 2018)

D. Medically Unlikely Edits (MUEs)

1. MUEs are described in Chapter I, Section V.

2. Providers/suppliers should be cautious about reporting services on multiple lines of a claim using modifiers to bypass MUEs. MUE values are set so that such occurrences should be uncommon. If a provider/supplier does this frequently for any HCPCS/CPT® code, the provider/supplier may be coding units of service incorrectly. The provider/supplier should consider contacting their national healthcare organization or the national medical/surgical society whose members commonly perform the procedure to clarify the correct reporting of UOS. A national healthcare organization, provider/supplier, or other interested third party may request a reconsideration of the MUE value of a HCPCS/CPT® code by submitting a written request to: NCCIPTPMUE@cms.hhs. The written request should include a rationale for reconsideration, as well as a suggested remedy.

3. MUE values of HCPCS codes for discontinued drugs are zero.

4. The MUE value of HCPCS codes describing compounded inhalation drugs is zero, because compounded drugs are not FDA approved. The CMS "Internet-Only Manual", "Medicare Benefit Policy Manual", Chapter 15, Section 50.4.1 requires that claims processing contractors only pay for FDA approved drugs unless CMS issues other instructions.

5. HCPCS code J0171 (Injection, adrenalin, epinephrine, 0.1 mg) may be reported incorrectly. A one ml ampule of adrenalin/epinephrine contains 1.0 mg of adrenalin/epinephrine in a 1:1,000 solution. However, a 10 ml prefilled syringe with a 1:10,000 solution of adrenalin/epinephrine also contains only 1.0 mg of adrenalin/epinephrine. Thus a physician must recognize that ten UOS for HCPCS code J0171 correspond to a one ml ampule or 10 ml of a prefilled syringe (1:10,000 (0.1 mg/ml) solution).

6. There are two HCPCS codes describing injectable dexamethasone. HCPCS code J1094 (Injection, dexamethasone acetate, 1 mg) is no longer manufactured and has an MUE value of zero. HCPCS code J1100 (Injection, dexamethasone sodium phosphate, 1 mg) is currently available. When billing for dexamethasone, physicians should be careful to report the correct formulation with the correct HCPCS code.

7. Based on the code descriptor, HCPCS code J3471 (Injection, hyaluronidase, ovine, preservative free, per 1 USP unit (up to 999 units)) shall not be reported with more than 999 UOS. Per the CMS ASP (Average Sale Price) NDC (National Drug Code) HCPCS Crosswalk table, HCPCS code J3472 (Injection, hyaluronidase, ovine, preservative free, per 1000 USP units) should be reported for a product that is no longer available. Therefore, if a physician uses more than 999 USP units of the product described by J3471, the physician may report HCPCS code J3471 on more than one line of a claim appending modifier 59 or XU to additional claim lines and should report no more than 999 UOS on any one claim line.

8. The Medically Unlikely Edit (MUE) values for practitioner services for oral immunosuppressive, oral anti- cancer, and oral anti-emetic drugs are set at zero. Practitioners providing these medications to patients must bill the Durable Medical Equipment Medicare Administrative Contractors (DME MACs), rather than the Part A/Part B Medicare Administrative Contractors (A/B MACs), using the National Drug Codes(NDC). A/B MACs do not pay codes for these oral medications when submitted on practitioner claims. The MUE values for outpatient hospital services are based on the amount of drug that might be administered to a patient on a single date of service. Facilities may not report to the A/B MAC more than a one-day supply of any of these drugs for a single date of service. Outpatient hospital facilities may submit claims to DME MACs for a multiple-day supply of these drugs provided on a single date of service.

9. If a HCPCS drug code descriptor defines the unit of service as "per dose", only one unit of service may be reported per drug administration procedure even if more than the usual amount of drug is administered. For example, HCPCS code J7321 (Hyaluronan or derivative, Hyalgan, Supartz or VISCO-3, for intra-articular injection, per dose) describes a drug that may be injected into the knee joint. Only one unit of service may be reported for injection of the drug into each knee joint, even if the amount of injected drug exceeds the usual amount of drug injected.

10. The MUE values for HCPCS codes G0431 (Drug screen, qualitative; multiple drug classes by high complexity test method (e.g., immunoassay, enzyme assay), per patient encounter) and G0434 (Drug screen, other than chromatographic; any number of drug classes, by CLIA waived test or moderate complexity test, per patient encounter) are one since the unit of service for each code is defined as "per patient encounter" and the likelihood that a patient needs this type of testing at more than one encounter on a single date of service is very small. These codes include all drug screening at the patient encounter and should not be reported with multiple UOS at the same patient encounter. (HCPCS codes G0431 and G0434 were deleted January 1, 2016.)

For Calendar Year 2016, presumptive drug testing should have been reported with HCPCS codes G0477-G0479. These codes differed based on the level of complexity of the testing methodology. Only one code from this code range should have been reported per date of service. These codes were deleted January 1, 2017.

Beginning January 1, 2017, presumptive drug testing may be reported with CPT® codes 80305-80307. These codes differ based on the level of complexity of the testing methodology. Only one code from this code range may be reported per date of service.

Beginning January 1, 2016, definitive drug testing may be reported with HCPCS codes G0480-G0483. These codes are reported "per day" and shall not be reported with more than one unit of service per day. Definitive drug testing HCPCS code G0659 was implemented January 1, 2017. This code is reported "per day" and shall not be reported with more than one unit of service per day.

11. HCPCS codes Q9951 and Q9965-Q9967 describe low osmolar contrast material with different iodine concentrations. The appropriate code to report is based on the iodine concentration in the contrast material administered. The MUE value for HCPCS code Q9951 (Low osmolar contrast material, 400 or greater mg/ml iodine concentration, per ml) is zero. When this MUE value was established, no low osmolar contrast material products with iodine concentration of 400 mg iodine or greater per ml were identified. HCPCS code Q9951 is often incorrectly reported for low osmolar contrast material products with lower iodine concentrations. Similarly, HCPCS codes Q9958-Q9964 describe high osmolar contrast material with different iodine concentrations. The appropriate code to report is based on the iodine concentration in the contrast material administered.

12. HCPCS code K0462 (Temporary replacement for patient owned equipment being repaired, any type) may be reported with one unit of service for each item of patient-owned equipment that is being repaired. Component parts of a patient-owned piece of equipment being repaired shall not be reported separately. For example, if a patient-owned CPAP (continuous positive airway pressure) blower requires repair, the supplier may report one unit of service for K0462. The supplier shall not report an additional unit of service for an integral humidifier even if it also requires repair. Additionally, the supplier shall not report an additional UOS for a detachable humidifier unless it also requires repair at the same time.

13. Generally, only one unit of service for an item of durable medical equipment (DME) (e.g., oxygen concentrator, wheelchair base) may be paid on a single date of service. Medicare does not allow payment for backup or duplicate durable medical equipment. More than one unit of service may be paid on a single date of service for accessories and supplies related to DME when appropriate. Prosthetics and orthotics may also be paid with more than one unit of service on a single date of service when appropriate.

14. HCPCS code P9604 describes a flat rate, one way travel allowance for collection of medically necessary laboratory specimen(s) drawn from a home bound or nursing home bound patient. A round trip should be reported with modifier LR and one unit of service rather than two UOS. The reported UOS shall be prorated for multiple patients drawn at the same address and for stops at the homes of Medicare and non-Medicare patients, as described in the "Medicare Internet-Only Manual", Publication 100-04 ("Medicare Claims Processing Manual"), Chapter 16 (Laboratory Services), Section 60.2.

15. The CMS "Internet-only Manual" (Publication 100-04 "Medicare Claims Processing Manual", Chapter 12 (Physicians/Nonphysician Practitioners), Section 40.7.B. and Chapter 4 (Part B Hospital (Including Inpatient Hospital Part B and OPPS)), Section 20.6.2 requires that practitioners and outpatient hospitals report bilateral surgical procedures with modifier 50 and one unit of service on a single claim line unless the code descriptor defines the procedure as "bilateral". If the code descriptor defines the procedure as a "bilateral" procedure, it shall be reported with one unit of service without modifier 50. MUE values for surgical procedures that may be performed bilaterally are based on this reporting requirement. Since this reporting requirement does not apply to an ambulatory surgical center (ASC), an ASC should report a bilateral surgical procedure on two claim lines, each with one unit of service using modifiers LT and RT on different claim lines. This reporting requirement does not apply to non-surgical diagnostic procedures.

16. HCPCS codes G0406-G0408 describe follow-up inpatient consultation services via telehealth, and HCPCS codes G0425-G0427 describe emergency or initial inpatient telehealth consultation services via telehealth. These codes shall not be reported by a practitioner on the same date of service that the practitioner reports a face-to-face E&M code. These codes are used to report telehealth services that, if performed with the patient physically present, would be reported with corresponding CPT® codes.

Since follow-up inpatient consultation services with a patient present are reported using per diem CPT® codes 99231-99233, HCPCS codes G0406-G0408 may only be reported with a single unit of service per day.

Since initial inpatient consultation services with a patient present are reported using per diem CPT® codes 99231-99233, HCPCS codes G0425-G0427 may only be reported with a single unit of service per day when reporting inpatient telehealth consultation services. However, if HCPCS codes G0425-G0427 are used to report emergency department services, reporting rules are comparable to CPT® codes 99281-99285.

E. General Policy Statements

1. MUE and NCCI PTP edits are based on services provided by the same physician to the same beneficiary on the same date of service. Physicians shall not inconvenience beneficiaries nor increase risks to beneficiaries by performing services on different dates of service to avoid MUE or NCCI PTP edits.

2. In this Manual, many policies are described using the term "physician". Unless indicated differently the use of this term does not restrict the policies to physicians only but applies to all practitioners, hospitals, providers, or suppliers eligible to bill the relevant HCPCS/CPT® codes pursuant to applicable portions of the Social Security Act (SSA) of 1965, the Code of Federal Regulations (CFR), and Medicare rules. In some sections of this Manual, the term "physician" would not include some of these entities because specific rules do not apply to them. For example, Anesthesia Rules [e.g., CMS "Internet-Only Manual", Publication 100-04 ("Medicare Claims Processing Manual"), Chapter 12 (Physician/ Nonphysician Practitioners), Section 50(Payment for Anesthesiology Services)] and Global Surgery Rules [e.g., CMS "Internet-Only Manual", Publication 100-04 ("Medicare Claims Processing Manual"), Chapter 12 (Physician/Nonphysician Practitioners), Section 40 (Surgeons and Global Surgery)] do not apply to hospitals.

3. Providers reporting services under Medicare's hospital Outpatient Prospective Payment System (OPPS) shall report all services in accordance with appropriate Medicare "Internet-Only Manual (IOM)" instructions.

4. In 2010, the "CPT® Manual" modified the numbering of codes so that the sequence of codes as they appear in the "CPT® Manual" does not necessarily correspond to a sequential numbering of codes. In the "National Correct Coding Initiative Policy Manual for Medicare Services," use of a numerical range of codes reflects all codes that numerically fall within the range regardless of their sequential order in the "CPT® Manual."

5. With few exceptions, the payment for a surgical procedure includes payment for dressings, supplies, and local anesthesia. These items are not separately reportable under their own HCPCS/CPT® codes. Wound closures using adhesive strips or tape alone are not separately reportable. In the absence of an operative procedure, these types of wound closures are included in an E&M service. Under limited circumstances, wound closure using tissue adhesive may be reported separately. If a practitioner uses a tissue adhesive alone for a wound closure, it may be reported separately with HCPCS code G0168 (Wound closure utilizing tissue adhesive (s) only). If a practitioner uses tissue adhesive in addition to staples or sutures to close a wound, HCPCS code G0168 is not separately reportable but is included in the tissue repair. Under the OPPS, HCPCS code G0168 is not recognized and paid. Facilities may report wound closure using sutures, staples, or tissue adhesives, either singly or in combination with each other, with the appropriate CPT® code in the "Repair (Closure)" section of the "CPT® Manual."

6. With limited exceptions, Medicare Anesthesia Rules prevent separate payment for anesthesia for a medical or surgical procedure when provided by the physician performing the procedure. The physician shall not report CPT® codes 00100-01999, 62320-62327, or 64400-64530 for anesthesia for a procedure. Additionally, the physician shall not unbundle the anesthesia procedure and report component codes individually. For example, introduction of a needle or intracatheter into a vein (CPT® code 36000), venipuncture (CPT® code 36410), drug administration (CPT® codes 96360-96377) or cardiac assessment (e.g., CPT® codes 93000- 93010, 93040- 93042) shall not be reported when these procedures are related to the delivery of an anesthetic agent.

Medicare allows separate reporting for moderate conscious sedation services (CPT® codes 99151-99153) when provided by the same physician performing a medical or surgical procedure.

Under Medicare Global Surgery Rules, drug administration services (CPT® codes 96360-96377) are not separately reportable by the physician performing a procedure for drug administration services related to the procedure.

Under the OPPS, drug administration services related to operative procedures are included in the associated procedural HCPCS/CPT® codes. Examples of such drug administration services include, but are not limited to, anesthesia (local or other), hydration, and medications such as anxiolytics or antibiotics. Providers shall not report CPT® codes 96360-96377 for these services.

Medicare Global Surgery Rules prevent separate payment for postoperative pain management when provided by the physician performing an operative procedure. CPT® codes 36000, 36410, 62320-62327, 64400-64450, and 96360-96377 describe some services that may be used for postoperative pain management. The services described by these codes may be reported by the physician performing the operative procedure only if provided for purposes unrelated to the postoperative pain management, the operative procedure, or anesthesia for the procedure.

If a physician performing an operative procedure provides a drug administration service (CPT® codes 96360-96375) for a purpose unrelated to anesthesia, intra-operative care, or post-procedure pain management, the drug administration service (CPT® codes 96360-96375) may be reported with an NCCI PTP-associated modifier if performed in a non-facility site of service.

7. The Medicare global surgery package includes insertion of urinary catheters. CPT® codes 51701-51703 (Insertion of bladder catheters) shall not be reported with any procedure with a global period of 000, 010, or 090 days, nor with some procedures with a global period of MMM.

8. Closure/repair of a surgical incision is included in the global surgical package except as noted below. Wound repair CPT® codes 12001-13153 shall not be reported separately to describe closure of surgical incisions for procedures with global surgery indicators of 000, 010, 090, or MMM. Simple, intermediate, and complex wound repair codes may be reported with Mohs surgery (CPT® codes 17311-17315). Intermediate and complex repair codes may be reported with excision of benign lesions (CPT® codes 11401-11406, 11421-11426, 11441-11471) and excision of malignant lesions (CPT® codes 11600-11646). Wound repair codes (CPT® codes 12001-13153) not be reported with excisions of benign lesions with an excised diameter of 0.5 cm or less (CPT® codes 11400, 11420, 11440).

9. Control of bleeding during an operative procedure is an integral component of a surgical procedure, and is not separately reportable. Postoperative control of bleeding not requiring return to the operating room is included in the global surgical package, and is not separately reportable. However, control of bleeding requiring return to the operating room in the postoperative period is separately reportable using modifier 78.

10. A biopsy performed at the time of another more extensive procedure (e.g., excision, destruction, removal) is separately reportable under specific circumstances.

    If the biopsy is performed on a separate lesion, it is separately reportable. This situation may be reported with anatomic modifiers or modifier 59 or XS.

    The biopsy is not separately reportable if used for the purpose of assessing margins of resection or verifying resectability.

    If a biopsy is performed and submitted for pathologic evaluation that will be completed after the more extensive procedure is performed, the biopsy is not separately reportable with the more extensive procedure.

11. Most NCCI PTP edits for codes describing procedures that may be performed on bilateral organs or structures (e.g., arms, eyes, kidneys, lungs) allow use of NCCI PTP-associated modifiers (modifier indicator of "1") because the two codes of the code pair edit may be reported if the two procedures are performed on contralateral organs or structures. Most of these code pairs should not be reported with NCCI PTP-associated modifiers when the corresponding procedures are performed on the ipsilateral organ or structure unless there is a specific coding rationale to bypass the edit. The existence of the NCCI PTP edit indicates that the two codes generally should not be reported together unless the two corresponding procedures are performed at two separate patient encounters or two separate anatomic sites. However, if the corresponding procedures are performed at the same patient encounter and in contiguous structures, NCCI PTP-associated modifiers should generally not be used.

12. If fluoroscopy is performed during an endoscopic procedure, it is integral to the procedure. This principle applies to all endoscopic procedures including, but not limited to, laparoscopy, hysteroscopy, thoracoscopy, arthroscopy, esophagoscopy, colonoscopy, other GI endoscopy, laryngoscopy, bronchoscopy, and cystourethroscopy.

13. If the code descriptor for a HCPCS/CPT® code, "CPT® Manual" instruction for a code, or CMS instruction for a code indicates that the procedure includes radiologic guidance, a physician shall not separately report a HCPCS/CPT® code for radiologic guidance including, but not limited to, fluoroscopy, ultrasound, computed tomography, or magnetic resonance imaging codes. If the physician performs an additional procedure on the same date of service for which a radiologic guidance or imaging code may be separately reported, the radiologic guidance or imaging code appropriate for that additional procedure may be reported separately with an NCCI PTP-associated modifier if appropriate.

14. CPT® code 36591 describes "collection of blood specimen from a completely implantable venous access device." CPT® code 36592 describes "collection of blood specimen using an established central or peripheral venous catheter, not otherwise specified." These codes shall not be reported with any service other than a laboratory service. That is, these codes may be reported if the only non-laboratory service performed is the collection of a blood specimen by one of these methods.

15. CPT® code 96523 describes "irrigation of implanted venous access device for drug delivery system." This code may be reported only if no other service is reported for the patient encounter.

Appendix I Publication 100 References

Disclaimer: This appendix includes relevant sections of the CMS Medicare and Medicaid Publication 100 information but is not an all-inclusive document. CMS updates policies and procedures frequently. The information contained here was the most up-to-date information on the CMS website at the time of printing. For more recent updates, visit the CMS website.

100-1, Chapter-1, 10.1

Hospital Insurance (Part A) for Inpatient Hospital, Hospice, Home Health and Skilled Nursing Facility (SNF) Services - A Brief Description

Hospital insurance is designed to help patients defray the expenses incurred by hospitalization and related care. In addition to inpatient hospital benefits, hospital insurance covers post hospital extended care in SNFs and post hospital care furnished by a home health agency in the patient's home. Blood clotting factors, for hemophilia patients competent to use such factors to control bleeding without medical or other supervision, and items related to the administration of such factors, are also a Part A benefit for beneficiaries in a covered Part A stay. The purpose of these additional benefits is to provide continued treatment after hospitalization and to encourage the appropriate use of more economical alternatives to inpatient hospital care. Program payments for services rendered to beneficiaries by providers (i.e., hospitals, SNFs, and home health agencies) are generally made to the provider. In each benefit period, payment may be made for up to 90 inpatient hospital days, and 100 days of post hospital extended care services.

Hospices also provide Part A hospital insurance services such as short-term inpatient care. In order to be eligible to elect hospice care under Medicare, an individual must be entitled to Part A of Medicare and be certified as being terminally ill. An individual is considered to be terminally ill if the individual has a medical prognosis that his or her life expectancy is 6 months or less if the illness runs its normal course.

The Part A benefit categories of inpatient hospital services and SNF services are each subject to separate and mutually exclusive day limits, so that the use of benefit days under one of these benefits does not affect the number of benefit days that remain available under the other. Accordingly, the 90 days of inpatient hospital benefits (plus 60 nonrenewable lifetime reserve days — see Pub. 100-02, Medicare Benefit Policy Manual, chapter 5) that are available to a beneficiary in a hospital do not count against the 100 days of posthospital extended care benefits that are available in a SNF, and vice-versa.

100-1, Chapter-3, 20.5

Blood Deductibles (Part A and Part B)

Program payment may not be made for the first 3 pints of whole blood or equivalent units of packed red cells received under Part A and Part B combined in a calendar year. However, blood processing (e.g., administration, storage) is not subject to the deductible.

The blood deductibles are in addition to any other applicable deductible and coinsurance amounts for which the patient is responsible.

The deductible applies only to the first 3 pints of blood furnished in a calendar year, even if more than one provider furnished blood.

100-1, Chapter-3, 20.5.2

Part B Blood Deductible

Blood is furnished on an outpatient basis or is subject to the Part B blood deductible and is counted toward the combined limit. It should be noted that payment for blood may be made to the hospital under Part B only for blood furnished in an outpatient setting. Blood is not covered for inpatient Part B services.

100-1, Chapter-3, 20.5.3

Items Subject to Blood Deductibles

The blood deductibles apply only to whole blood and packed red cells. The term whole blood means human blood from which none of the liquid or cellular components have been removed. Where packed red cells are furnished, a unit of packed red cells is considered equivalent to a pint of whole blood. Other components of blood such as platelets, fibrinogen, plasma, gamma globulin, and serum albumin are not subject to the blood deductible. However, these components of blood are covered as biological.

Refer to Pub. 100-04, Medicare Claims Processing Manual, chapter 4, §231 regarding billing for blood and blood products under the Hospital Outpatient Prospective Payment System (OPPS).

100-1, Chapter-3, 30

Outpatient Mental Health Treatment Limitation

Regardless of the actual expenses a beneficiary incurs in connection with the treatment of mental, psychoneurotic, and personality disorders while the beneficiary is not an inpatient of a hospital at the time such expenses are incurred, the amount of those expenses that may be recognized for Part B deductible and payment purposes is limited to 62.5 percent of the Medicare approved amount for those services. The limitation is called the outpatient mental health treatment limitation (the limitation). The 62.5 percent limitation has been in place since the inception of the Medicare Part B program and it will remain effective at this percentage amount until January 1, 2010. However, effective January 1, 2010, through January 1, 2014, the limitation will be phased out as follows:

- January 1, 2010 –December 31, 2011, the limitation percentage is 68.75%.
  (Medicare pays 55% and the patient pays 45%).
- January 1, 2012 –December 31, 2012, the limitation percentage is 75%
  (Medicare pays 60% and the patient pays 40%).
- January 1, 2013 –December 31, 2013, the limitation percentage is 81.25%.
  (Medicare pays 65% and the patient pays 35%).
- January 1, 2014 –onward, the limitation percentage is 100% (Medicare pays 65% and the patient pays 35%).
- January 1, 2014 –onward, the limitation percentage is 100% (Medicare pays 80% and the patient pays 20%).

For additional details concerning the outpatient mental health treatment limitation, please see the Medicare Claims Processing Manual, Publication 100-04, chapter 9, section 60 and chapter 12, section 210.

100-1, Chapter-5, 90.2

Laboratory Defined

Laboratory means a facility for the biological, microbiological, serological, chemical, immuno-hematological, hematological, biophysical, cytological, pathological, or other examination of materials derived from the human body for the purpose of providing information for the diagnosis, prevention, or treatment of any disease or impairment of, or the assessment of the health of, human beings. These examinations also include procedures to determine, measure, or otherwise describe the presence or absence of various substances or organisms in the body. Facilities only collecting or preparing specimens (or both) or only serving as a mailing service and not performing testing are not considered laboratories.

100-2, Chapter-1, 10

Covered Inpatient Hospital Services Covered Under Part A

Patients covered under hospital insurance are entitled to have payment made on their behalf for inpatient hospital services. (Inpatient hospital services do not include extended care services provided by hospitals pursuant to swing bed approvals. See Pub. 100-02, Chapter 8, §10.3, "Hospital Providers of Extended Care Services."). However, both inpatient hospital and inpatient SNF benefits are provided under Part A - Hospital Insurance Benefits for the Aged and Disabled, of Title XVIII).

Additional information concerning the following topics can be found in the following chapters of this manual:

- Benefit Period is found in Chapter 3
- Counting Inpatient Days is found in Chapter 3
- Lifetime reserve days is found in Chapter 5
- Related payment information is housed in the Provider Reimbursement Manual

Blood must be furnished on a day which counts as a day of inpatient hospital services to be covered as a Part A service and to count toward the blood deductible. Thus, blood is not covered under Part A and does not count toward the Part A blood deductible when furnished to an inpatient after the inpatient has exhausted all benefit days in a benefit period, or where the individual has elected not to use lifetime reserve days. However, where the patient is discharged on their first day of entitlement or on the hospital's first day of participation, the hospital is permitted to submit a billing form with no accommodation charge, but with ancillary charges including blood.

The records for all Medicare hospital inpatient discharges are maintained in CMS for statistical analysis and use in determining future Prospective Payment System (PPS) Diagnosis Related Group (DRG) classifications and rates.

Non-PPS hospitals do not pay for noncovered services generally excluded from coverage in the Medicare Program. This may result in denial of a part of the billed charges or in denial of the entire admission, depending upon circumstance. In PPS hospitals, the following are also possible:

1. In appropriately admitted cases where a noncovered procedure was performed, denied services may result in payment of a different DRG (i.e., one which excludes payment for the noncovered procedure); or
2. In appropriately admitted cases that become cost outlier cases, denied services may lead to denial of some or all of an outlier payment.

The following examples illustrate this principle. If care is noncovered because a patient does not need to be hospitalized, the A/B MAC Part A denies the admission and makes no Part A (i.e., PPS) payment unless paid under limitation on liability. Under limitation on liability, Medicare payment may be made when the provider and the beneficiary were not aware the services were not necessary and could not reasonably be expected to know that the services were not necessary. For detailed instructions, see Pub. 100-04, Medicare Claims Processing Manual, Chapter 30,"Limitation on Liability" section 20. If a patient is appropriately hospitalized but receives (beyond routine services) only noncovered care, the admission is denied.

NOTE: The A/B MAC Part A does not deny an admission that includes covered care, even if noncovered care was also rendered. Under PPS, Medicare assumes that it is paying for only the covered care rendered whenever covered services needed to treat and/or diagnose the illness were in fact provided.

If a noncovered procedure is provided along with covered nonroutine care, a DRG change rather than an admission denial might occur. If noncovered procedures are elevating costs into the cost outlier category, outlier payment is denied in whole or in part.

When the hospital is included in PPS, most of the subsequent discussion regarding coverage of inpatient hospital services is relevant only in the context of determining the appropriateness of admissions, which DRG, if any, to pay, and the appropriateness of payment for any outlier cases.

If a patient receives items or services in excess of, or more expensive than, those for which payment can be made, payment is made only for the covered items or services or for only the appropriate prospective payment amount. This provision applies not only to inpatient services, but also to all hospital services under Parts A and B of the program. If the items or services were requested by the patient, the hospital may charge him or her the difference between the amount customarily charged for the services requested and the amount customarily charged for covered services.

An inpatient is a person who has been admitted to a hospital for bed occupancy for purposes of receiving inpatient hospital services (see §10.2 below). Generally, a patient is considered an inpatient if formally admitted as inpatient with the expectation that he or she will require hospital care that is expected to span at least two midnights and occupy a bed even though it later develops that the patient can be discharged or transferred to another hospital and not actually use a hospital bed overnight.

The physician or other practitioner responsible for a patient's care at the hospital is also responsible for deciding whether the patient should be admitted as an inpatient. Physicians should use the expectation of the patient to require hospital care that spans at least two midnights period as a benchmark, i.e., they should order admission for patients who are expected to require a hospital stay that crosses two midnights and the medical record supports that reasonable expectation. However, the decision to admit a patient is a complex medical judgment which can be made only after the physician has considered a number of factors, including the patient's medical history and current medical needs, the types of facilities available to inpatients and to outpatients, the hospital's by-laws and admissions policies, and the relative appropriateness of treatment in each setting. Factors to be considered when making the decision to admit include such things as:

- The severity of the signs and symptoms exhibited by the patient;

- The medical predictability of something adverse happening to the patient;

- The need for diagnostic studies that appropriately are outpatient services (i.e., their performance does not ordinarily require the patient to remain at the hospital for 24 hours or more) to assist in assessing whether the patient should be admitted; and

- The availability of diagnostic procedures at the time when and at the location where the patient presents.

Admissions of particular patients are not covered or noncovered solely on the basis of the length of time the patient actually spends in the hospital. In certain specific situations coverage of services on an inpatient or outpatient basis is determined by the following rules:

Minor Surgery or Other Treatment - When patients with known diagnoses enter a hospital for a specific minor surgical procedure or other treatment that is expected to keep them in the hospital for only a few hours (less than 24), they are considered outpatients for coverage purposes regardless of: the hour they came to the hospital, whether they used a bed, and whether they remained in the hospital past midnight.

Renal Dialysis - Renal dialysis treatments are usually covered only as outpatient services but may under certain circumstances be covered as inpatient services depending on the patient's condition. Patients staying at home, who are ambulatory, whose conditions are stable and who come to the hospital for routine chronic dialysis treatments, and not for a diagnostic workup or a change in therapy, are considered outpatients. On the other hand, patients undergoing short-term dialysis until their kidneys recover from an acute illness (acute dialysis), or persons with borderline renal failure who develop acute renal failure every time they have an illness and require dialysis (episodic dialysis) are usually inpatients. A patient may begin dialysis as an inpatient and then progress to an outpatient status.

Under original Medicare, the Quality Improvement Organization (QIO), for each hospital is responsible for deciding, during review of inpatient admissions on a case-by-case basis, whether the admission was medically necessary. Medicare law authorizes the QIO to make these judgments, and the judgments are binding for purposes of Medicare coverage. In making these judgments, however, QIOs consider only the medical evidence which was available to the physician at the time an admission decision had to be made. They do not take into account other information (e.g., test results) which became available only after admission, except in cases where considering the post-admission information would support a finding that an admission was medically necessary.

Refer to chapters 4 and 7 of Pub. 100-10, Quality Improvement Organization Manual with regard to initial determinations for these services. The QIO will review the swing bed services in these PPS hospitals as well.

NOTE: When patients requiring extended care services are admitted to beds in a hospital, they are considered inpatients of the hospital. In such cases, the services furnished in the hospital will not be considered extended care services, and payment may not be made under the program for such services unless the services are extended care services furnished pursuant to a swing bed agreement granted to the hospital by the Secretary of Health and Human Services.

100-2, Chapter-1, 10.1.4

Charges for Deluxe Private Room

Beneficiaries found to need a private room (either because they need isolation for medical reasons or because they need immediate admission when no other accommodations are available) may be assigned to any of the provider's private rooms. They do not have the right to insist on the private room of their choice, but their preferences should be given the same consideration as if they were paying all provider charges themselves. The program does not, under any circumstances, pay for personal comfort items. Thus, the program does not pay for deluxe accommodations and/or services. These would include a suite, or a room substantially more spacious than is required for treatment, or specially equipped or decorated, or serviced for the comfort and convenience of persons willing to pay a differential for such amenities. If the beneficiary (or representative) requests such deluxe accommodations, the provider should advise that there will be a charge, not covered by Medicare, of a specified amount per day (not exceeding the differential defined in the next sentence); and may charge the beneficiary that amount for each day he/she occupies the deluxe accommodations. The maximum amount the provider may charge the beneficiary for such accommodations is the differential between the most prevalent private room rate at the time of admission and the customary charge for the room occupied. Beneficiaries may not be charged this differential if they (or their representative) do not request the deluxe accommodations.

The beneficiary may not be charged such a differential in private room rates if that differential is based on factors other than personal comfort items. Such factors might include differences between older and newer wings, proximity to lounge, elevators or nursing stations, desirable view, etc. Such rooms are standard 1-bed units and not deluxe rooms for purposes of these instructions, even though the provider may call them deluxe and have a higher customary charge for them. No additional charge may be imposed upon the beneficiary who is assigned to a room that may be somewhat more desirable because of these factors.

100-2, Chapter-1, 40

Supplies, Appliances, and Equipment

Supplies, appliances, and equipment, which are ordinarily furnished by the hospital for the care and treatment of the beneficiary solely during the inpatient hospital stay, are covered inpatient hospital services.

Under certain circumstances, supplies, appliances, and equipment used during the beneficiary's inpatient stay are covered under Part A even though the supplies, appliances and equipment leave the hospital with the patient upon discharge. These are circumstances in which it would be unreasonable or impossible from a medical standpoint to limit the patient's use of the item to the periods during which the individual is an inpatient. Examples of items covered under this rule are:

- Items permanently installed in or attached to the patient's body while an inpatient, such as cardiac valves, cardiac pacemakers, and artificial limbs; and

- Items which are temporarily installed in or attached to the patient's body while an inpatient, and which are also necessary to permit or facilitate the patient's release from the hospital, such as tracheotomy or drainage tubes.

Hospital "admission packs" containing primarily toilet articles, such as soap, toothbrushes, toothpaste, and combs, are covered under Part A if routinely furnished by the hospital to all its inpatients. If not routinely furnished to all patients, the packs are not covered.

In that situation, the hospital may charge beneficiaries for the pack, but only if they request it with knowledge of what they are requesting and what the charge to them will be.

Supplies, appliances, and equipment furnished to an inpatient for use Only outside the hospital are not, in general, covered as inpatient hospital services. However, a temporary or disposable item, which is medically necessary to permit or facilitate the patient's departure from the hospital and is required until the patient can obtain a continuing supply, is covered as an inpatient hospital service.

Oxygen furnished to hospital inpatients is covered under Part A as an inpatient supply.

100-2, Chapter-1, 70

Inpatient Services in Connection With Dental Services

When a patient is hospitalized for a dental procedure and the dentist's service is covered under Part B, the inpatient hospital services furnished are covered under Part A. For example, both the professional services of the dentist and the inpatient hospital expenses are covered when the Dentist reduces a jaw fracture of an inpatient at a participating hospital. In addition, hospital inpatient services, which are necessary because of the patient's underlying medical condition and clinical status or the severity of a non covered dental procedure, are covered.

When the hospital services are covered, all ancillary services such as X-rays, administration of anaesthesia, use of the operating room, etc., are covered.

Regardless of whether the inpatient hospital services are covered, the medical services of physicians furnished in connection with non covered dental services are not covered. The services of an anaesthesiologist, radiologist, or pathologist whose services are performed in connection with the care, treatment, filling, removal, or replacement of teeth or structures directly supporting teeth are not covered.

100-2, Chapter-6, 10

Medical and Other Health Services Furnished to Inpatients of Participating Hospitals

Payment may be made under Part B for physician services and for the nonphysician medical and other health services as provided in this section when furnished by a participating hospital (either directly or under arrangements) to an inpatient of the hospital, but only if payment for these services cannot be made under Part A. This policy applies to all hospitals and critical access hospitals (CAHs) participating in Medicare, including those paid under a prospective payment system or alternative payment methodology such as State cost control systems, and to emergency hospital services furnished by nonparticipating hospitals. In this section, the term "hospital" includes all hospitals and CAHs, regardless of payment methodology, unless otherwise specified.

For services to be covered under Part A or Part B, a hospital must furnish nonphysician services to its inpatients directly or under arrangements (see chapter 16, §170 of this manual, "Inpatient Hospital or SNF Services Not Delivered Directly or Under Arrangement by the Provider"). A nonphysician service is one which does not meet the criteria defining physicians' services specifically provided for in regulation at 42 CFR 415.102. Services "incident to" physicians' services (except for the services of nurse anesthetists employed by anesthesiologists) are nonphysician services for purposes of this provision.

100-2, Chapter-6, 20.6

Outpatient Observation Services

A. Outpatient Observation Services Defined

Observation care is a well-defined set of specific, clinically appropriate services, which include ongoing short term treatment, assessment, and reassessment before a decision can be made regarding whether patients will require further treatment as hospital inpatients or if they are able to be discharged from the hospital. Observation services are commonly ordered for patients who present to the emergency department and who then require a significant period of treatment or monitoring in order to make a decision concerning their admission or discharge.

Observation services are covered only when provided by the order of a physician or another individual authorized by State licensure law and hospital staff bylaws to admit patients to the hospital or to order outpatient tests. In the majority of cases, the decision whether to discharge a patient from the hospital following resolution of the reason for the observation care or to admit the patient as an inpatient can be made in less than 48 hours, usually in less than 24 hours. In only rare and exceptional cases do reasonable and necessary outpatient observation services span more than 48 hours.

Hospitals may bill for patients who are directly referred to the hospital for outpatient observation services. A direct referral occurs when a physician in the community refers a patient to the hospital for outpatient observation, bypassing the clinic or emergency department (ED) visit. Effective for services furnished on or after January 1, 2003, hospitals may bill for patients directly referred for observation services.

See, Pub. 100-04, Medicare Claims Processing Manual, chapter 4, section 290, at http://www.cms.hhs.gov/manuals/downloads/clm104c04.pdf for billing and payment instructions for outpatient observation services.

Future updates will be issued in a Recurring Update Notification.

B. Coverage of Outpatient Observation Services

When a physician orders that a patient receive observation care, the patient's status is that of an outpatient. The purpose of observation is to determine the need for further treatment or for inpatient admission. Thus, a patient receiving observation services may improve and be released, or be admitted as an inpatient (see Pub. 100-02, Medicare Benefit Policy Manual, Chapter 1, Section 10 "Covered Inpatient Hospital Services Covered Under Part A" at https://www.cms.gov/Regulations-andGuidance/Guidance/Manuals/Downloads/bp102c01.pdf). For more information on correct reporting of observation services, see Pub. 100-04, Medicare Claims Processing Manual, chapter 4, section 290.2.2.)

All hospital observation services, regardless of the duration of the observation care, that are medically reasonable and necessary are covered by Medicare. Observation services are reported using HCPCS code G0378 (Hospital observation service, per hour). As of January 1, 2008, HCPCS code G0378 for hourly observation services is assigned status indicator N, signifying that its payment is always packaged. No separate payment is made for observation services reported with HCPCS code G0378. In most circumstances, observation services are supportive and ancillary to the other separately payable services provided to a patient. Beginning January 1, 2016, in certain circumstances when observation care is billed in conjunction with a clinic visit, Type A emergency department visit (Level 1 through 5), Type B emergency department visit (Level 1 through 5), critical care services, or direct referral for observation services as an integral part of a patient's extended encounter of care, comprehensive payment may be made for all services on the claim including, the entire extended care encounter when certain criteria are met. For information about billing and payment methodology for observation services in years prior to CY 2008, see Pub. 100-04, Medicare Claims Processing Manual, Chapter 4, §§290.3-290.4. For information about payment for extended assessment and management under composite APCs and comprehensive APCs, see §290.5.

Payment for all reasonable and necessary observation services is packaged into the payments for other separately payable services provided to the patient in the same encounter. Observation services packaged through assignment of status indicator N are covered OPPS services. Since the payment for these services is included in the APC payment for other separately payable services on the claim, hospitals must not bill Medicare beneficiaries directly for the packaged services.

C. Services Not Covered by Medicare and Notification to the Beneficiary

In making the determination whether an ABN can be used to shift liability to a beneficiary for the cost of non-covered items or services related to an encounter that includes observation care, the provider should follow a two-step process. First, the provider must decide whether the item or service meets either the definition of observation care or would be otherwise covered. If the item or service does not meet the definitional requirements of any Medicare-covered benefit under Part B, then the item or service is not covered by Medicare and an ABN is not required to shift the liability to the beneficiary. However, the provider may choose to provide voluntary notification for these items or services.

Second, if the item or service meets the definition of observation services or would be otherwise covered, then the provider must decide whether the item or service is "reasonable and necessary" for the beneficiary on the occasion in question, or if the item or service exceeds any frequency limitation for the particular benefit or falls outside of a timeframe for receipt of a particular benefit. In these cases, the ABN would be used to shift the liability to the beneficiary (see Pub. 100-04, Medicare Claims Processing Manual; Chapter 30, "Financial Liability Protections," Section 20, at https://www.cms.gov/Regulations-andGuidance/Guidance/Manuals/Downloads/clm104c30.pdf for information regarding Limitation On Liability (LOL) Under §1879 Where Medicare Claims Are Disallowed).

If an ABN is not issued to the beneficiary, the provider may be held liable for the cost of the item or service unless the provider/supplier is able to demonstrate that they did not know and could not have reasonably been expected to know that Medicare would not pay for the item or service.

100-2, Chapter-10, 10.2.2

Reasonableness of the Ambulance Trip

Under the FS payment is made according to the level of medically necessary services actually furnished. That is, payment is based on the level of service furnished (provided they were medically necessary), not simply on the vehicle used. Even if a local government requires an ALS response for all calls, payment under the FS is made only for the level of service furnished, and then only when the service is medically necessary.

100-2, Chapter-10,10.3.3

Separately Payable Ambulance Transport Under Part B versus Patient Transportation that is Covered Under a Packaged Institutional Service

Transportation of a beneficiary from his or her home, an accident scene, or any other point of origin is covered under Part B as an ambulance service only to the nearest hospital, critical access hospital (CAH), or skilled nursing facility (SNF) that is capable of furnishing the required level and type of care for the beneficiary's illness or injury and only if medical necessity and other program coverage criteria are met. An ambulance transport from a SNF to the nearest supplier of medically necessary services not available at the SNF where the beneficiary is a resident and not in a covered Part A stay, including the return trip, is covered under Part B provided that the ambulance transportation was medically reasonable and necessary and all other coverage requirements are met.

Medicare-covered ambulance services are paid either as separately billed services, in which case the entity furnishing the ambulance service bills Part B of the program, or as a packaged service, in which case the entity furnishing the ambulance service must seek payment from the provider who is responsible for the beneficiary's care. If either the origin or the destination of the ambulance transport is the beneficiary's home, then the ambulance transport is paid separately by Medicare Part B, and the entity that furnishes the ambulance transport may bill its A/B MAC (A) or (B) directly. If both the origin and destination of the ambulance transport are providers, e.g., a hospital, critical access hospital (CAH), skilled nursing facility (SNF), then responsibility for payment for the ambulance transport is determined in accordance with the following sequential criteria.

NOTE: These criteria must be applied in sequence as a flow chart and not independently of one another.

1. Provider Numbers:

   If the Medicare-assigned provider numbers of the two providers are different, then the ambulance service is separately billable to the program. If the provider number of both providers is the same, then consider criterion 2, "campus".

2. Campus:

   Following criterion 1, if the campuses of the two providers (sharing the same provider numbers) are the same, then the transport is not separately billable to the program. In this case the provider is responsible for payment. If the campuses of the two providers are different, then consider criterion 3, "patient status." "Campus" means the physical area immediately adjacent to the provider's main buildings, other areas and structures that are not strictly contiguous to the main buildings, but are located within 250 yards of the main buildings, and any of the other areas determined on an individual case basis by the CMS regional office to be part of the provider's campus.

3. Patient Status:

   Inpatient vs. Outpatient Following criteria 1 and 2, if the patient is an inpatient at both providers (i.e., inpatient status both at the origin and at the destination, providers sharing the same provider number but located on different campuses), then the transport is not separately billable. In this case the provider is responsible for payment. All other combinations (i.e., outpatient-to-inpatient, inpatient-to-outpatient, outpatient-to-outpatient) are separately billable to the program.

In the case where the point of origin is not a provider, Part A coverage is not available because, at the time the beneficiary is being transported, the beneficiary is not an inpatient of any provider paid under Part A of the program and ambulance services are excluded from the 3-day preadmission payment window.

The transfer, i.e., the discharge of a beneficiary from one provider with a subsequent admission to another provider, is also payable as a Part B ambulance transport, provided all program coverage criteria are met, because, at the time that the beneficiary is in transit, the beneficiary is not a patient of either provider and not subject to either the inpatient preadmission payment window or outpatient payment packaging requirements. This includes an outpatient transfer from a remote, off-campus emergency department (ER) to becoming an inpatient or outpatient at the main campus hospital, even if the ER is owned and operated by the hospital.

Once a beneficiary is admitted to a hospital, CAH, or SNF, it may be necessary to transport the beneficiary to another hospital or other site temporarily for specialized care while the beneficiary maintains inpatient status with the original provider. This movement of the patient is considered "patient transportation" and is covered as an inpatient hospital or CAH service and as a SNF service when the SNF is furnishing it as a covered SNF service and payment is made under Part A for that service. (If the beneficiary is a resident of a SNF and must be transported by ambulance to receive dialysis or certain other high-end outpatient hospital services, the ambulance

transport may be separately payable under Part B. Also, if the beneficiary is a SNF resident and not in a Part A covered stay and must be transported by ambulance to the nearest supplier of medically necessary services not available at the SNF, the ambulance transport, including the return trip, may be covered under Part B.) Because the service is covered and payable as a beneficiary transportation service under Part A, the service cannot be classified and paid for as an ambulance service under Part B. This includes intra-campus transfers between different departments of the same hospital, even where the departments are located in separate buildings. Such intra-campus transfers are not separately payable under the Part B ambulance benefit. Such costs are accounted for in the same manner as the costs of such a transfer within a single building.

100-2, Chapter-10, 20

Coverage Guidelines for Ambulance Service Claims

Payment may be made for expenses incurred by a patient for ambulance service provided conditions l, 2, and 3 in the left-hand column have been met. The right-hand column indicates the documentation needed to establish that the condition has been met.

Conditions	Review Action
1. Patient was transported by an approved supplier of ambulance services.	1. Ambulance suppliers are explained in greater detail in §10.1.3
2. The patient was suffering from an illness or injury, which contraindicated transportation by other means. (§10.2)	2. (a) The contractor presumes the requirement was met if the submitted documentation indicates that the patient: • Was transported in an emergency situation, e.g., as a result of an accident, injury or acute illness, or • Needed to be restrained to prevent injury to the beneficiary or others; or • Was unconscious or in shock; or • Required oxygen or other emergency treatment during transport to the nearest appropriate facility; or • Exhibits signs and symptoms that indicate the possibility of acute stroke; or • Had to remain immobile because of a fracture that had not been set or the possibility of a fracture; or • Was experiencing severe hemorrhage; or • Could be moved only by stretcher; or • Was bed-confined before and after the ambulance trip.
	b. In the absence of any of the conditions listed in (a) above additional documentation should be obtained to establish medical need where the evidence indicates the existence of the circumstances listed below: i. Patient's condition would not ordinarily require movement by stretcher, or ii. The individual was not admitted as a hospital inpatient (except in accident cases), or iii. The ambulance was used solely because other means of transportation were unavailable, or iv. The individual merely needed assistance in getting from his room or home to a vehicle. c. Where the information indicates a situation not listed in 2(a) or 2(b) above, refer the case to your supervisor.
3. The patient was transported from and to points listed below. a. From patient's residence (or other place where need arose) to hospital or skilled nursing facility.	3. Claims should show the ZIP Code of the point of pickup. a. i. Condition met if trip began within the institution's service area as shown in the carrier's locality guide. ii. Condition met where the trip began outside the institution's service area if the institution was the nearest one with appropriate facilities.

NOTE: A patient's residence is the place where he or she makes his/her home and dwells permanently, or for an extended period of time. A skilled nursing facility is one, which is listed in the Directory of Medical Facilities as a participating SNF or as an institution which meets §1861(j)(1) of the Act.

NOTE: A claim for ambulance service to a participating hospital or skilled nursing facility should not be denied on the grounds that there is a nearer nonparticipation institution having appropriate facilities.

b. Skilled nursing facility to a hospital or hospital to a skilled nursing facility.	b. i. Condition met if the ZIP Code of the pickup point is within the service area of the destination as shown in the carrier's locality guide. ii. Condition met where the ZIP Code of the pickup point is outside the service area of the destination if the destination institution was the nearest appropriate facility.
c. Hospital to hospital or skilled nursing facility to skilled nursing facility.	c. Condition met if the discharging institution was not an appropriate facility and the admitting institution was the nearest appropriate facility.
d. From a hospital or skilled nursing facility to patient's residence.	d. i. Condition met if patient's residence is within the institution's service area as shown in the carrier's locality guide. ii. Condition met where the patient's residence is outside the institution's service area if the institution was the nearest appropriate facility.
e. Round trip for hospital or participating skilled nursing facility inpatients to the nearest hospital or nonhospital treatment facility.	e. Condition met if the reasonable and necessary diagnostic or therapeutic service required by patient's condition is not available at the institution where the beneficiary is an inpatient.

NOTE: Ambulance service to a physician's office or a physician- directed clinic is not covered. See §10.3.8 above, where a stop is made at a physician's office en route to a hospital and §10.3.3 for additional exceptions.)

4. Ambulance services involving hospital admissions in Canada or Mexico are covered (Medicare Claims Processing Manual, Chapter 1, "General Billing Requirements," §10.1.3.) if the following conditions are met :	4. a. The foreign hospitalization has been determined to be covered; and b. The ambulance service meets the coverage requirements set forth in §§10-10.3. If the foreign hospitalization has been determined to be covered on the basis of emergency services (See the Medicare Claims Processing Manual, Chapter 1, "General Billing Requirements," §10.1.3), the necessity requirement (§10.2) and the destination requirement (§10.3) are considered met.
5. The carrier will make partial payment for otherwise covered ambulance service, which exceeded limits defined in item	5 & 6 (a) From the pickup point to the nearest appropriate facility, or 5 & 6 (b) From the nearest appropriate facility to the beneficiary's residence where he or she is being returned home from a distant institution.
6. The carrier will base the payment on the amount payable had the patient been transported:	

100-2, Chapter-10, 30.1.1

Ground Ambulance Services

Basic Life Support (BLS)

Definition: Basic life support (BLS) is transportation by ground ambulance vehicle and the provision of medically necessary supplies and services, including BLS ambulance services as defined by the State. The ambulance must be staffed by an individual who is qualified in accordance with State and local laws as an emergency medical technician-basic (EMT-Basic). These laws may vary from State to State or within a State. For example, only in some jurisdictions is an EMT-Basic permitted to operate limited equipment onboard the vehicle, assist more qualified personnel in performing assessments and interventions, and establish a peripheral intravenous (iv) line.

Basic Life Support (BLS) –Emergency

Definition: When medically necessary, the provision of BLS services, as specified above, in the context of an emergency response. An emergency response is one that, at the time the ambulance provider or supplier is called, it responds immediately. An immediate response is one in which the ambulance provider/supplier begins as quickly as possible to take the steps necessary to respond to the call.

Application: The determination to respond emergently with a BLS ambulance must be in accord with the local 911 or equivalent service dispatch protocol. If the call came in directly to the ambulance provider/supplier, then the provider's/supplier's dispatch protocol must meet, at a minimum, the standards of the dispatch protocol of the local 911 or equivalent service. In areas that do not have a local 911 or equivalent service, then the protocol must meet, at a minimum, the standards of a dispatch protocol in another similar jurisdiction within the State or, if there is no similar jurisdiction within the State, then the standards of any other dispatch protocol within the State. Where the dispatch was inconsistent with this standard of protocol, including where no protocol was used, the beneficiary's condition (for example, symptoms) at the scene determines the appropriate level of payment.

Advanced Life Support, Level 1 (ALS1)

Definition: Advanced life support, level 1 (ALS1) is the transportation by ground ambulance vehicle and the provision of medically necessary supplies and services including the provision of an ALS assessment or at least one ALS intervention.

Advanced Life Support Assessment

Definition: An advanced life support (ALS) assessment is an assessment performed by an ALS crew as part of an emergency response that was necessary because the patient's reported condition at the time of dispatch was such that only an ALS crew was qualified to perform the assessment. An ALS assessment does not necessarily result in a determination that the patient requires an ALS level of service.

Application: The determination to respond emergently with an ALS ambulance must be in accord with the local 911 or equivalent service dispatch protocol. If the call came in directly to the ambulance provider/supplier, then the provider's/supplier's dispatch protocol must meet, at a minimum, the standards of the dispatch protocol of the local 911 or equivalent service. In areas that do not have a local 911 or equivalent service, then the protocol must meet, at a minimum, the standards of a dispatch protocol in another similar jurisdiction within the State or, if there is no similar jurisdiction within the State, then the standards of any other dispatch protocol within the State. Where the dispatch was inconsistent with this standard of protocol, including where no protocol was used, the beneficiary's condition (for example, symptoms) at the scene determines the appropriate level of payment.

Advanced Life Support Intervention

Definition: An advanced life support (ALS) intervention is a procedure that is in accordance with State and local laws, required to be done by an emergency medical technician-intermediate (EMT-Intermediate) or EMT-Paramedic.

Application: An ALS intervention must be medically necessary to qualify as an intervention for payment for an ALS level of service. An ALS intervention applies only to ground transports.

Advanced Life Support, Level 1 (ALS1) –Emergency

Definition: When medically necessary, the provision of ALS1 services, as specified above, in the context of an emergency response. An emergency response is one that, at the time the ambulance provider or supplier is called, it responds immediately. An immediate response is one in which the ambulance provider/supplier begins as quickly as possible to take the steps necessary to respond to the call.

Application: The determination to respond emergently with an ALS ambulance must be in accord with the local 911 or equivalent service dispatch protocol. If the call came in directly to the ambulance provider/supplier, then the provider's/supplier's dispatch protocol must meet, at a minimum, the standards of the dispatch protocol of the local 911 or equivalent service. In areas that do not have a local 911 or equivalent service, then the protocol must meet, at a minimum, the standards of a dispatch protocol in another similar jurisdiction within the State or, if there is no similar jurisdiction within the State, then the standards of any other dispatch protocol within the State. Where the dispatch was inconsistent with this standard of protocol, including where no protocol was used, the beneficiary's condition (for example, symptoms) at the scene determines the appropriate level of payment.

Advanced Life Support, Level 2 (ALS2)

Definition: Advanced life support, level 2 (ALS2) is the transportation by ground ambulance vehicle and the provision of medically necessary supplies and services including (1) at least three separate administrations of one or more medications by intravenous push/bolus or by continuous infusion (excluding crystalloid fluids) or (2) ground ambulance transport, medically necessary supplies and services, and the provision of at least one of theALS2 procedures listed below:

  a. Manual defibrillation/cardioversion;

  b. Endo tracheal intubation;

  c. Central venous line;

  d. Cardiac pacing;

  e. Chest decompression;

  f. Surgical airway; or

  g. Intraosseous line.

Application: Crystalloid fluids include fluids such as 5 percent Dextrose in water, Saline and Lactated Ringer's. Medications that are administered by other means, for example: intramuscular/subcutaneous injection, oral, sublingually or nebulized, do not qualify to determine whether theALS2 level rate is payable. However, this is not an all-inclusive list. Likewise, a single dose of medication administered fractionally (i.e., one-third of a single dose quantity) on three separate occasions does not qualify for the ALS2 payment rate. The criterion of multiple administrations of the same drug requires a suitable quantity and amount of time between administrations that is in accordance with standard medical practice guidelines. The fractional administration of a single dose (for this purpose meaning a standard or protocol dose) on three separate occasions does not qualify for ALS2 payment.

In other words, the administration of 1/3of a qualifying dose 3 times does not equate to three qualifying doses for purposes of indicating ALS2 care. One-third of X given 3 times might = X (where X is a standard/protocol drug amount), but the same sequence does not equal 3 times X. Thus, if 3 administrations of the same drug are required to show that ALS2 care was given, each of those administrations must be in accord with local protocols. The run will not qualify on the basis of drug administration if that administration was not according to protocol.

An example of a single dose of medication administered fractionally on three separate occasions that would not qualify for the ALS2 payment rate would be the use of Intravenous (IV) Epinephrine in the treatment of pulse less Ventricular Tachycardia/Ventricular Fibrillation (VF/VT) in the adult patient. Administering this medication in increments of 0.25 mg, 0.25 mg, and 0.50 mg would not qualify for the ALS2 level of payment. This medication, according to the American Heart Association (AHA), Advanced Cardiac Life Support (ACLS) protocol, calls for Epinephrine to be administered in 1 mg increments every 3 to 5minutes. Therefore, in order to receive payment for an ALS2 level of service, based in part on the administration of Epinephrine, three separate administrations of Epinephrine in 1 mg increments must be administered for the treatment of pulse less VF/VT.

A second example that would not qualify for the ALS2 payment level is the use of Adenosine in increments of 2 mg, 2 mg, and 2 mg for a total of 6 mg in the treatment of an adult patient with Paroxysmal Supra ventricular Tachycardia (PSVT). According to ACLS guidelines, 6 mg of Adenosine should be given by rapid intravenous push (IVP) over 1 to 2 seconds. If the first dose does not result in the elimination of the supra ventricular tachycardia within 1 to 2 minutes, 12 mg of Adenosine should be administered IVP. If the supra ventricular tachycardia persists, a second 12 mg dose of Adenosine can be administered for a total of 30 mg of Adenosine. Three separate Administrations of the drug Adenosine in the dosage amounts outlined in the later case would qualify forALS2 payment.

Endotracheal intubation is one of the services that qualifies for the ALS2 level of payment; therefore, it is not necessary to consider medications administered by Endo tracheal intubation for the purpose of determining whether the ALS2 rate is payable. The monitoring and maintenance of an end tracheal tube that was previously inserted prior to transport also qualifies as an ALS2 procedure.

Advanced Life Support (ALS) Personnel

Definition: ALS personnel are individuals trained to the level of the emergency medical technician-intermediate (EMT-Intermediate) or paramedic.

Specialty Care Transport (SCT)

Definition: Specialty care transport (SCT) is the inter facility transportation of a critically injured or ill beneficiary by a ground ambulance vehicle, including the provision of medically necessary supplies and services, at a level of service beyond the scope of the EMT-Paramedic. SCT is necessary when a beneficiary's condition requires ongoing care that must be furnished by one or more health professionals in an appropriate specialty area, for example, emergency or critical care nursing, emergency medicine, respiratory care, cardiovascular care, or a paramedic with additional training.

Application: The EMT-Paramedic level of care is set by each State. SCT is necessary when a beneficiary's condition requires ongoing care that must be furnished by one or more health professionals in an appropriate specialty area. Care above that level that is medically necessary and that is furnished at a level of service above the EMT-Paramedic level of care is considered SCT. That is to say, if EMT-Paramedics -without specialty care certification or qualification -are permitted to furnish a given service in a State, then that service does not qualify for SCT. The phrase "EMT-Paramedic with additional training" recognizes that a State may permit a person who is not only certified as an EMT-Paramedic, but who also has successfully completed additional education as determined by the State in furnishing higher level medical services required by critically ill or critically injured patients, to furnish a level of service that otherwise would require a health professional in an appropriate specialty care area (for example, a nurse) to provide. "Additional training" means the specific additional training that a State requires a paramedic to complete in order to qualify to furnish specialty care to a critically ill or injured patient during an SCT.

Paramedic Intercept (PI)

Definition: Paramedic Intercept services are ALS services provided by an entity that does not provide the ambulance transport. This type of service is most often provided for an emergency ambulance transport in which a local volunteer ambulance that can provide only basic life support (BLS) level of service is dispatched to transport a patient. If the patient needs ALS services such as EKG monitoring, chest decompression, or I.V. therapy, another entity dispatches a paramedic to meet the BLS ambulance at the scene or once the ambulance is on the way to the hospital. The ALS paramedics then provide services to the patient.

This tiered approach to life saving is cost effective in many areas because most volunteer ambulances do not charge for their services and one paramedic service can cover many communities. Prior to March 1, 1999, Medicare payment could be made for these services, but only when the claim was submitted by the entity that actually furnished the ambulance transport. Payment could not be made directly to the intercept service provider. In those areas where State laws prohibit volunteer ambulances from billing Medicare and other health insurance, the intercept service could not receive payment for treating a Medicare beneficiary and was forced to bill the beneficiary for the entire service.

Paramedic intercept services furnished on or after March 1, 1999, may be payable separate from the ambulance transport, subject to the requirements specified below.

The intercept service(s) is:

- Furnished in a rural area;
- Furnished under a contract with one or more volunteer ambulance services; and,
- Medically necessary based on the condition of the beneficiary receiving the ambulance service.

- In addition, the volunteer ambulance service involved must:
- Meet the program's certification requirements for furnishing ambulance services;
- Furnish services only at the BLS level at the time of the intercept; and,
- Be prohibited by State law from billing anyone for any service. Finally, the entity furnishing the ALS paramedic intercept service must:
- Meet the program's certification requirements for furnishing ALS services, and,
- Bill all recipients who receive ALS paramedic intercept services from the entity, regardless of whether or not those recipients are Medicare beneficiaries.

For purposes of the paramedic intercept benefit, a rural area is an area that is designated as rural by a State law or regulation or any area outside of a Metropolitan Statistical Area or in New England, outside a New England County Metropolitan Area as defined by the Office of Management and Budget. The current list of these areas is periodically published in the Federal Register.

See the Medicare Claims Processing Manual, Chapter 15, "Ambulance," §20.1.4 for payment of paramedic intercept services.

Services in a Rural Area

Definition: Services in a rural area are services that are furnished (1) in an area outside a Metropolitan Statistical Area (MSA); or, (2) in New England, outside a New England County Metropolitan Area (NECMA); or, (3) an area identified as rural using the Goldsmith modification even though the area is within an MSA.

Emergency Response

Definition: Emergency response is a BLS or ALS1 level of service that has been provided in immediate response to a 911 call or the equivalent. An immediate response is one in which the ambulance provider/supplier begins as quickly as possible to take the steps necessary to respond to the call.

Application: The phrase "911 call or equivalent" is intended to establish the standard that the nature of the call at the time of dispatch is the determining factor. Regardless of the medium by which the call is made (e.g., a radio call could be appropriate) the call is of an emergent nature when, based on the information available to the dispatcher at the time of the call, it is reasonable for the dispatcher to issue an emergency dispatch in light of accepted, standard dispatch protocol. An emergency call need not come through 911 even in areas where a 911 call system exists. However, the determination to respond emergently must be in accord with the local 911 or equivalent service dispatch protocol. If the call came in directly to the ambulance provider/supplier, then the provider's/supplier's dispatch protocol and the dispatcher's actions must meet, at a minimum, the standards of the dispatch protocol of the local 911 or equivalent service. In areas that do not have a local 911 or equivalent service, then both the protocol and the dispatcher's actions must meet, at a minimum, the standards of the dispatch protocol in another similar jurisdiction within the State, or if there is no similar jurisdiction, then the standards of any other dispatch protocol within the State. Where the dispatch was inconsistent with this standard of protocol, including where no protocol was used, the beneficiary's condition (for example, symptoms) at the scene determines the appropriate level of payment.

EMT-Intermediate

Definition: EMT-Intermediate is an individual who is qualified, in accordance with State and local laws, as an EMT-Basic and who is also certified in accordance with State and local laws to perform essential advanced techniques and to administer a limited number of medications.

EMT-Paramedic

Definition: EMT-Paramedic possesses the qualifications of the EMT-Intermediate and, in accordance with State and local laws, has enhanced skills that include being able to administer additional interventions and medications.

Relative Value Units

Definition: Relative value units (RVUs) measure the value of ambulance services relative to the value of a base level ambulance service.

Application: The RVUs for the ambulance fee schedule are as follows:

> Service Level RVUs
> BLS 1.00
> BLS –Emergency 1.60
> ALS1 1.20
> ALS1 –Emergency 1.90
> ALS2 2.75
> SCT 3.25
> PI 1.75
> RVUs are not applicable to FW and RW services.

100-2, Chapter-12, 30.1

Rules for Payment of CORF Services

The payment basis for CORF services is 80 percent of the lesser of: (1) the actual charge for the service or (2) the physician fee schedule amount for the service when the physician fee schedule establishes a payment amount for such service. Payment for CORF services under the physician fee schedule is made for physical therapy, occupational therapy, speech-language pathology and respiratory therapy services, as well as the nursing and social and/or psychological services, which are a part of, or directly relate to, the rehabilitation plan of treatment.

Payment for covered durable medical equipment, orthotic and prosthetic (DMEPOS) devices and supplies provided by a CORF is based upon: the lesser of 80 percent of actual charges or the payment amount established under the DMEPOS fee schedule; or, the single payment amount established under the DMEPOS competitive bidding program, provided that payment for such an item is not included in the payment amount for other CORF services.

If there is no fee schedule amount for a covered CORF item or service, payment should be based on the lesser of 80 percent of the actual charge for the service provided or an amount determined by the local Medicare contractor.

The following conditions apply to CORF physical therapy, occupational therapy, and speech-language pathology services;

- Claims must contain the required functional reporting. (Reference: Sections 42 CFR 410.105.) Refer to Pub. 100-04, Medicare Claims Processing Manual, chapter 5, section 10.6.

NOTE: Functional reporting and documentation requirements are no longer applicable for claims for dates of service on and after January 1, 2019. For more information, refer to subsection F in section 30 above.

- The functional reporting on claims must be consistent with the functional limitations identified as part of the patient's therapy plan of care and expressed as part of the patient's therapy goals; effective for claims with dates of service on and after January, 1, 2013. (Reference: 42 CFR 410.105.) See Pub. 100-04, Medicare Claims Processing Manual, chapter 5, section 10.6.

NOTE: Functional reporting and documentation requirements are no longer applicable for claims for dates of service on and after January 1, 2019. For more information, refer to subsection F in section 30 above

- The National Provider Identifier (NPI) of the certifying physician identified for a CORF physical therapy, occupational therapy, and speech-language pathology plan of treatment must be included on the therapy claim. This requirement is effective for claims with dates of service on or after October 1, 2012. (See Pub. 100-04, Medicare Claims Processing Manual, chapter 5, section 10.3.)

Payment for CORF social and/or psychological services is made under the physician fee schedule only for HCPCS code G0409, as appropriate, and only when billed using revenue codes 0560, 0569, 0910, 0911, 0914 and 0919.

Payment for CORF respiratory therapy services is made under the physician fee schedule when provided by a respiratory therapist as defined at 42CFR485.70(j) and, only to the extent that these services support or are an adjunct to the rehabilitation plan of treatment, when billed using revenue codes 0410, 0412 and 0419. Separate payment is not made for diagnostic tests or for services related to physiologic monitoring services which are bundled into other respiratory therapy services appropriately performed by a respiratory therapist, such as HCPCS codes G0237, G0238 and G0239.

Payment for CORF nursing services is made under the physician fee schedule only when provided by a registered nurse as defined at 42CFR485.70(h) for nursing services only to the extent that these services support or are an adjunct to the rehabilitation plan of treatment. In addition, payment for CORF nursing services is made only when provided by a registered nurse. HCPCS code G0128 is used to bill for these services and only with revenue codes 0550 and 0559.

For specific payment requirements for CORF items and services see Pub. 100-04, Medicare Claims Processing Manual, Chapter 5, Part B Outpatient Rehabilitation and CORF/OPT Services.

100-2, Chapter-12, 40.5

Respiratory Therapy Services

A respiratory therapy plan of treatment is wholly established and signed by the referring physician before the respiratory therapist initiates the actual treatment.

A. Definition

Respiratory therapy services include only those services that can be appropriately provided to CORF patients by a qualified respiratory therapist, as defined at 42CFR485.70 (j), under a physician-established respiratory therapy plan of treatment. The facility physician must be present in the facility for a sufficient time to provide, in accordance with accepted principles of medical practice, medical direction, medical care services and consultation. Respiratory therapy services include the physiological monitoring necessary to furnish these services. Payment for these services is bundled into the payment for respiratory therapy services and is not payable separately. Diagnostic and other medical services provided in the CORF setting are not considered CORF services, and therefore may not be included in a respiratory therapy plan of treatment because these are covered under separate benefit categories.

The respiratory therapist assesses the patient to determine the appropriateness of pursed lip breathing activity and may check the patient's oxygen saturation level (via pulse oximetry). If appropriate, the respiratory therapist then provides the initial training in order to ensure that the patient can accurately perform the activity. The respiratory therapist may again check the patient's oxygen saturation level, or perform peak respiratory flow, or check other respiratory parameters. These types of services are considered "physiological monitoring" and are bundled into the payment for HCPCS codes G0237, G0238 and G0239. Physiological monitoring also includes the provision of a 6-minute walk test that is typically conducted before the start of the patient's respiratory therapy activities. The time to provide this walk "test" assessment is included as part of the HCPCS code G0238. When provided as part of a CORF respiratory therapy plan of treatment, payment for these monitoring activities is bundled into the payment for other services provided by the respiratory therapist, such as the three respiratory therapy specific G-codes.

B. Guidelines for Applying Coverage Criteria

There are some conditions for which respiratory therapy services may be indicated. However, respiratory therapy performed as part of a standard protocol without regard to the individual patient's actual condition, capacity for improving, and the need for such services as established, is not reasonable and medically necessary. All respiratory therapy services must meet the test of being "reasonable and medically necessary" pursuant to §1862(a)(1)(A) of the Act. Determinations of medical necessity are made based on local contractor decisions on a claim-by-claim basis.

The three HCPCS codes G0237, G0238, and G0239 are specific to services provided under the respiratory therapy plan of treatment and, as such, are not designated as subject to the therapy caps.

C. Patient Education Programs

Instructing a patient in the use of equipment, breathing exercises, etc. may be considered reasonable and necessary to the patient's respiratory therapy plan of treatment and can usually be given to a patient during the course of treatment by the respiratory therapist.

These educational instructions are bundled into the covered service and separate payment is not made.

100-2, Chapter-12, 40.8

Nursing Services

CORF nursing services may only be provided by an individual meeting the qualifications of a registered nurse, as defined at 42CFR485.70 (h). They must relate to, or be a part of, the rehabilitation plan of treatment.

CORF nursing services must be reasonable and medically necessary and are provided as an adjunct to the rehabilitation plan of treatment. For example, a registered nurse may perform or instruct a patient, as appropriate, in the proper procedure of "in and out" urethral catheterization,

tracheostomy tube suctioning, or the cleaning for ileostomy or colostomy bags.

Nursing services may not substitute for or supplant the services of physical therapists, occupational therapists, speech-language pathologists and respiratory therapists, but instead must support or further the services and goals provided in the rehabilitation plan of treatment.

CORF nursing services must be provided by a registered nurse and may only be coded as HCPCS code G0128 indicating that CORF "nursing services" were provided.

100-2, Chapter-12, 40.11

Vaccines

A CORF may provide pneumococcal pneumonia, influenza virus, and Hepatitis B vaccines to its patients. While not included as a service under the CORF benefit, Medicare will make payment to the CORF for certain vaccines and their administration provided to CORF patients (CY 2008 PFS Rule 72 FR 66293).

The following three vaccinations are covered in a CORF if a physician who is a doctor of medicine or osteopathy orders it for a CORF patient:

- Pneumococcal pneumonia vaccine and its administration;
- Hepatitis B vaccine and its administration furnished to a beneficiary who is at high or intermediate risk of contracting Hepatitis B; and
- Influenza virus vaccine and its administration

Payment for covered pneumococcal pneumonia, influenza virus, and Hepatitis B vaccines provided in the CORF setting is based on 95 percent of the average wholesale price. The CORF registered nurse provides administration of any of these vaccines using HCPCS codes G0008, G0009 or G0010 with payment based on CPT® code 90471.

100-2, Chapter-15, 50

Drugs and Biologicals

The Medicare program provides limited benefits for outpatient drugs. The program covers drugs that are furnished "incident to" a physician's service provided that the drugs are not usually self-administered by the patients who take them.

Generally, drugs and biologicals are covered only if all of the following requirements are met:

- They meet the definition of drugs or biologicals (see §50.1);
- They are of the type that are not usually self-administered. (see §50.2);
- They meet all the general requirements for coverage of items as incident to a physician's services (see §§50.1 and 50.3);
- They are reasonable and necessary for the diagnosis or treatment of the illness or injury for which they are administered according to accepted standards of medical practice (see §50.4);
- They are not excluded as non covered immunizations (see §50.4.4.2); and
- They have not been determined by the FDA to be less than effective. (See §§50.4.4)

Medicare Part B does generally not cover drugs that can be self-administered, such as those in pill form, or are used for self-injection. However, the statute provides for the coverage of some self-administered drugs. Examples of self-administered drugs that are covered include blood-clotting factors, drugs used in immunosuppressive therapy, erythropoietin for dialysis patients, osteoporosis drugs for certain homebound patients, and certain oral cancer drugs. (See §110.3for coverage of drugs, which are necessary to the effective use of Durable Medical Equipment (DME) or prosthetic devices.)

100-2, Chapter-15, 50.2

Determining Self-Administration of Drug or Biological

The Medicare program provides limited benefits for outpatient prescription drugs. The program covers drugs that are furnished "incident to" a physician's service provided that the drugs are not usually self-administered by the patients who take them. Section 112 of the Benefits, Improvements & Protection Act of 2000 (BIPA) amended sections 1861(s)(2)(A) and 1861(s)(2)(B) of the Act to redefine this exclusion. The prior statutory language referred to those drugs "which cannot be self-administered." Implementation of the BIPA provision requires interpretation of the phrase "not usually self-administered by the patient"

A. Policy

Fiscal intermediaries, carriers and Medicare Administrative Contractors (MACs) are instructed to follow the instructions below when applying the exclusion for drugs that are usually self-administered by the patient. Each individual contractor must make its own individual determination on each drug. Contractors must continue to apply the policy that not only the drug is medically reasonable and necessary for any individual claim, but also that the route of administration is medically reasonable and necessary. That is, if a drug is available in both oral and injectable forms, the injectable form of the drug must be medically reasonable and necessary as compared to using the oral form.

For certain injectable drugs, it will be apparent due to the nature of the condition(s) for which they are administered or the usual course of treatment for those conditions, they are, or are not, usually self-administered. For example, an injectable drug used to treat migraine headaches is usually self-administered. On the other hand, an injectable drug, administered at the same time as chemotherapy, used to treat anemia secondary to chemotherapy is not usually self-administered.

B. Administered

The term "administered" refers only to the physical process by which the drug enters the patient's body. It does not refer to whether the process is supervised by a medical professional (for example, to observe proper technique or side-effects of the drug). Injectable drugs, including intravenously administered drugs, are typically eligible for inclusion under the "incident to" benefit. With limited exceptions, other routes of administration including, but not limited to, oral drugs, suppositories, topical medications are considered to be usually self-administered by the patient.

C. Usually

For the purposes of applying this exclusion, the term "usually" means more than 50 percent of the time for all Medicare beneficiaries who use the drug. Therefore, if a drug is self-administered by more than 50 percent of Medicare beneficiaries, the drug is excluded from coverage and the contractor may not make any Medicare payment for it. In arriving at a single determination as to whether a drug is usually self-administered, contractors should make a separate determination for each indication for a drug as to whether that drug is usually self-administered.

After determining whether a drug is usually self-administered for each indication, contractors should determine the relative

contribution of each indication to total use of the drug (i.e., weighted average) in order to make an overall determination as to whether the drug is usually self-administered. For example, if a drug has three indications, is not self-administered for the first indication, but is self-administered for the second and third indications, and the first indication makes up 40 percent of total usage, the second indication makes up 30 percent of total usage, and the third indication makes up 30 percent of total usage, then the drug would be considered usually self-administered.

Reliable statistical information on the extent of self-administration by the patient may not always be available. Consequently, CMS offers the following guidance for each contractor's consideration in making this determination in the absence of such data:

1. Absent evidence to the contrary, presume that drugs delivered intravenously are not usually self- administered by the patient.

2. Absent evidence to the contrary, presume that drugs delivered by intramuscular injection are not usually self-administered by the patient. (Avonex, for example, is delivered by intramuscular injection, not usually self-administered by the patient.) The contractor may consider the depth and nature of the particular intramuscular injection in applying this presumption. In applying this presumption, contractors should examine the use of the particular drug and consider the following factors:

3. Absent evidence to the contrary, presume that drugs delivered by subcutaneous injection are self-administered by the patient. However, contractors should examine the use of the particular drug and consider the following factors:

   A. **Acute Condition -** Is the condition for which the drug is used an acute condition? If so, it is less likely that a patient would self-administer the drug. If the condition were longer term, it would be more likely that the patient would self-administer the drug.

   B. **Frequency of Administration** -How often is the injection given? For example, if the drug is administered once per month, it is less likely to be self-administered by the patient. However, if it is administered once or more per week, it is likely that the drug is self-administered by the patient.

In some instances, carriers may have provided payment for one or perhaps several doses of a drug that would otherwise not be paid for because the drug is usually self-administered. Carriers may have exercised this discretion for limited coverage, for example, during a brief time when the patient is being trained under the supervision of a physician in the proper technique for self-administration. Medicare will no longer pay for such doses. In addition, contractors may no longer pay for any drug when it is administered on an outpatient emergency basis, if the drug is excluded because it is usually self-administered by the patient.

D. Definition of Acute Condition

For the purposes of determining whether a drug is usually self-administered, an acute condition means a condition that begins over a short time period, is likely to be of short duration and/or the expected course of treatment is for a short, finite interval. A course of treatment consisting of scheduled injections lasting less than 2 weeks, regardless of frequency or route of administration, is considered acute. Evidence to support this may include Food and Drug Administration (FDA) approval language, package inserts, drug compendia, and other information.

E. By the Patient

The term "by the patient" means Medicare beneficiaries as a collective whole. The carrier includes only the patients themselves and not other individuals (that is, spouses, friends, or other care- givers are not considered the patient). The determination is based on whether the drug is self-administered by the patient a majority of the time that the drug is used on an outpatient basis by Medicare beneficiaries for medically necessary indications. The carrier ignores all instances when the drug is administered on an inpatient basis.

The carrier makes this determination on a drug-by-drug basis, not on a beneficiary-by-beneficiary basis. In evaluating whether beneficiaries as a collective whole self-administer, individual beneficiaries who do not have the capacity to self-administer any drug due to a condition other than the condition for which they are taking the drug in question are not considered. For example, an individual afflicted with paraplegia or advanced dementia would not have the capacity to self-administer any injectable drug, so such individuals would not be included in the population upon which the determination for self-administration by the patient was based. Note that some individuals afflicted with a less severe stage of an otherwise debilitating condition would be included in the population upon which the determination for "self-administered by the patient" was based; for example, an early onset of dementia.

F. Evidentiary Criteria

Contractors are only required to consider the following types of evidence: peer reviewed medical literature, standards of medical practice, evidence-based practice guidelines, FDA approved label, and package inserts. Contractors may also consider other evidence submitted by interested individuals or groups subject to their judgment.

Contractors should also use these evidentiary criteria when reviewing requests for making a determination as to whether a drug is usually self-administered, and requests for reconsideration of a pending or published determination.

Note that prior to August 1, 2002, one of the principal factors used to determine whether a drug was subject to the self-administered exclusion was whether the FDA label contained instructions for self-administration. However, CMS notes that under the new standard, the fact that the FDA label includes instructions for self-administration is not, by itself, a determining factor that a drug is subject to this exclusion.

G. Provider Notice of Noncovered Drugs

Contractors must describe on their Web site the process they will use to determine whether a drug is usually self-administered and thus does not meet the "incident to" benefit category. Contractors must publish a list of the injectable drugs that are subject to the self-administered exclusion on their Web site, including the data and rationale that led to the determination. Contractors will report the workload associated with developing new coverage statements in CAFM 21208.

Contractors must provide notice 45 days prior to the date that these drugs will not be covered. During the 45-day time period, contractors will maintain existing medical review and payment procedures. After the 45-day notice, contractors may deny payment for the drugs subject to the notice.

Contractors must not develop local coverage determinations (LCDs) for this purpose because further elaboration to describe drugs that do not meet the 'incident to' and the 'not usually self-administered' provisions of the statute are unnecessary. Current LCDs based solely on these provisions must be withdrawn. LCDs that address the self-administered

exclusion and other information may be reissued absent the self-administered drug exclusion material. Contractors will report this workload in CAFM 21206. However, contractors may continue to use and write LCDs to describe reasonable and necessary uses of drugs that are not usually self-administered.

H. Conferences Between Contractor

Contractors' Medical Directors may meet and discuss whether a drug is usually self-administered without reaching a formal consensus. Each contractor uses its discretion as to whether or not it will participate in such discussions. Each contractor must make its own individual determinations, except that fiscal intermediaries may, at their discretion, follow the determinations of the local carrier with respect to the self-administered exclusion.

I. Beneficiary Appeals

If a beneficiary's claim for a particular drug is denied because the drug is subject to the "Self-administered drug" exclusion, the beneficiary may appeal the denial. Because it is a "benefit category" denial and not a denial based on medical necessity, an Advance Beneficiary Notice (ABN) is not required. A "benefit category" denial (i.e., a denial based on the fact that there is no benefit category under which the drug may be covered) does not trigger the financial liability protection provisions of Limitation On Liability (under §1879 of the Act). Therefore, physicians or providers may charge the beneficiary for an excluded drug.

J. Provider and Physician Appeals

A physician accepting assignment may appeal a denial under the provisions found in Pub. 100-04, Medicare Claims Processing Manual, chapter 29.

K. Reasonable and Necessary

Contractors will make the determination of reasonable and necessary with respect to the medical appropriateness of a drug to treat the patient's condition. Contractors will continue to make the determination of whether the intravenous or injection form of a drug is appropriate as opposed to the oral form. Contractors will also continue to make the determination as to whether a physician's office visit was reasonable and necessary. However, contractors should not make a determination of whether it was reasonable and necessary for the patient to choose to have his or her drug administered in the physician's office or outpatient hospital setting. That is, while a physician's office visit may not be reasonable and necessary in a specific situation, in such a case an injection service would be payable.

L. Reporting Requirements

Each carrier, intermediary and Medicare Administrative Contractor (MAC) must report to CMS its complete list of injectable drugs that the contractor has determined are excluded when furnished incident to a physician's service on the basis that the drug is usually self-administered. The CMS expects that contractors will review injectable drugs on a rolling basis and update their list of excluded drugs as it is developed and no less frequently than annually. For example, contractors should not wait to publish this list until every drug has been reviewed. Contractors must enter their self-administered drug exclusion list to the Medicare Coverage Database (MCD). This database can be accessed at www.cms.hhs.gov/mcd. See Pub.100-08, Medicare Program Integrity Manual, Chapter 3, Section 3.3, "Policies and Guidelines Applied During Review", for instructions on submitting these lists to the MCD.

M. Drugs Treated as Hospital Outpatient Supplies

In certain circumstances, Medicare pays for drugs that may be considered usually self-administered by the patient when such drugs function as supplies. This is the case when the drugs provided are an integral component of a procedure or are directly related to it, i.e., when they facilitate the performance of or recovery from a particular procedure. Except for the applicable copayment, hospitals may not bill beneficiaries for these types of drugs because their costs, as supplies, are packaged into the payment for the procedure with which they are used. Listed below are examples of when drugs are treated as supplies and hospitals should bill Medicare for the drug as a supply and should not separately bill the beneficiary.

- Sedatives administered to a patient while he or she is in the preoperative area being prepared for a procedure.
- Mydriatic drops instilled into the eye to dilate the pupils, anti-inflammatory drops, antibiotic drops/ointments, and ocular hypotensives that are administered to a patient immediately before, during, or immediately following an ophthalmic procedure. This does not refer to the patient's eye drops that the patient uses pre-and postoperatively.
- Barium or low osmolar contrast media provided integral to a diagnostic imaging procedure.
- Topical solution used with photodynamic therapy furnished at the hospital to treat nonhyperkeratotic actinic keratosis lesions of the face or scalp.
- Antibiotic ointments such as bacitracin, placed on a wound or surgical incision at the completion of a procedure.

The following are examples of when a drug is not directly related or integral to a procedure, and does not facilitate the performance of or recovery from a procedure. Therefore the drug is not considered a packaged supply. In many of these cases the drug itself is the treatment instead of being integral or directly related to the procedure, or facilitating the performance of or recovery from a particular procedure.

- Drugs given to a patient for his or her continued use at home after leaving the hospital.
- Oral pain medication given to an outpatient who develops a headache while receiving chemotherapy administration treatment.
- Daily routine insulin or hypertension medication given preoperatively to a patient.
- A fentanyl patch or oral pain medication such as hydrocodone, given to an outpatient presenting with pain.
- A laxative suppository for constipation while the patient waits to receive an unrelated X-ray.

These two lists of examples may serve to guide hospitals in deciding which drugs are supplies packaged as a part of a procedure, and thus may be billed under Part B. Hospitals should follow CMS' guidance for billing drugs that are packaged and paid as supplies, reporting coded and uncoded drugs with their charges under the revenue code associated with the cost center under which the hospital accumulates the costs for the drugs.

100-2, Chapter-15, 50.4.2

Unlabeled Use of Drug

An unlabeled use of a drug is a use that is not included as an indication on the drugs label as approved by the FDA. FDA approved drugs used for indications other than what is indicated on the official label may be covered under Medicare if the carrier determines the use to be medically accepted, taking into consideration the major drug compendia, authoritative medical literature and/or accepted standards of medical practice. In the case of drugs used in an anti-cancer chemotherapeutic regimen, unlabeled uses are covered for a medically accepted indication as defined in §50.5.

These decisions are made by the contractor on a case-by-case basis.

100-2, Chapter-15, 50.4.4.2

Immunizations

Vaccinations or inoculations are excluded as immunizations unless they are directly related to the treatment of an injury or direct exposure to a disease or condition, such as anti-rabies treatment, tetanus antitoxin or booster vaccine, botulin antitoxin, antivenin sera, or immune globulin. In the absence of injury or direct exposure, preventive immunization (vaccination or inoculation) against such diseases as smallpox, polio, diphtheria, etc., is not covered. However, pneumococcal, Hepatitis B, and influenza virus vaccines are exceptions to this rule. (See items A, B, and C below.) In cases where a vaccination or inoculation is excluded from coverage, related charges are also not covered.

A. Pneumococcal Pneumonia Vaccinations

1. **Background and History of Coverage:**

   Section 1861(s)(10)(A) of the Social Security Act and regulations at 42 CFR 410.57 authorize Medicare coverage under Part B for pneumococcal vaccine and its administration.

   For services furnished on or after May 1, 1981 through September 18, 2014, the Medicare Part B program covered pneumococcal pneumonia vaccine and its administration when furnished in compliance with any applicable State law by any provider of services or any entity or individual with a supplier number. Coverage included an initial vaccine administered only to persons at high risk of serious pneumococcal disease (including all people 65 and older; immunocompetent adults at increased risk of pneumococcal disease or its complications because of chronic illness; and individuals with compromised immune systems), with revaccination administered only to persons at highest risk of serious pneumococcal infection and those likely to have a rapid decline in pneumococcal antibody levels, provided that at least 5 years had passed since the previous dose of pneumococcal vaccine.

   Those administering the vaccine did not require the patient to present an immunization record prior to administering the pneumococcal vaccine, nor were they compelled to review the patient's complete medical record if it was not available, relying on the patient's verbal history to determine prior vaccination status.

   Effective July 1, 2000, Medicare no longer required for coverage purposes that a doctor of medicine or osteopathy order the vaccine. Therefore, a beneficiary could receive the vaccine upon request without a physician's order and without physician supervision.

2. **Coverage Requirements:**

   Effective for claims with dates of service on and after September 19, 2014, an initial pneumococcal vaccine may be administered to all Medicare beneficiaries who have never received a pneumococcal vaccination under

Medicare Part B. A different, second pneumococcal vaccine may be administered 1 year after the first vaccine was administered (i.e., 11 full months have passed following the month in which the last pneumococcal vaccine was administered).

Those administering the vaccine should not require the patient to present an immunization record prior to administering the pneumococcal vaccine, nor should they feel compelled to review the patient's complete medical record if it is not available. Instead, provided that the patient is competent, it is acceptable to rely on the patient's verbal history to determine prior vaccination status.

Medicare does not require for coverage purposes that a doctor of medicine or osteopathy order the vaccine. Therefore, the beneficiary may receive the vaccine upon request without a physician's order and without physician supervision. B. Hepatitis B Vaccine Effective for services furnished on or after September 1, 1984, P.L. 98-369 provides coverage under Part B for Hepatitis B vaccine and its administration, furnished to a Medicare beneficiary who is at high or intermediate risk of contracting Hepatitis B. High-risk groups currently identified include (see exception below):

- ESRD patients;
- Hemophiliacs who receive Factor VIII or IX concentrates;
- Clients of institutions for the mentally retarded;
- Persons who live in the same household as a Hepatitis B Virus (HBV) carrier;
- Homosexual men;
- Illicit injectable drug abusers; and

Persons diagnosed with diabetes mellitus. Intermediate risk groups currently identified include:

- Staff in institutions for the mentally retarded; and
- Workers in health care professions who have frequent contact with blood or blood-derived body fluids during routine work.

EXCEPTION: Persons in both of the above-listed groups in paragraph B, would not be considered at high or intermediate risk of contracting Hepatitis B, however, if there were laboratory evidence positive for antibodies to Hepatitis B. (ESRD patients are routinely tested for Hepatitis B antibodies as part of their continuing monitoring and therapy.)

For Medicare program purposes, the vaccine may be administered upon the order of a doctor of medicine or osteopathy, by a doctor of medicine or osteopathy, or by home health agencies, skilled nursing facilities, ESRD facilities, hospital outpatient departments, and persons recognized under the incident to physicians' services provision of law.

A charge separate from the ESRD composite rate will be recognized and paid for administration of the vaccine to ESRD patients.

B. Hepatitis B Vaccine

Effective for services furnished on or after September 1, 1984, P.L. 98-369 provides coverage under Part B for Hepatitis B vaccine and its administration, furnished to a Medicare beneficiary who is at high or intermediate risk of contracting Hepatitis B. This coverage is effective for services furnished on or after September 1, 1984. High-risk groups currently identified include (see exception below):

- ESRD patients;
- Hemophiliacs who receive Factor VIII or IX concentrates;
- Clients of institutions for the mentally retarded;
- Persons who live in the same household as a Hepatitis B Virus (HBV) carrier;
- Homosexual men;
- Illicit injectable drug abusers; and
- Persons diagnosed with diabetes mellitus.

Intermediate risk groups currently identified include:

- Staff in institutions for the mentally retarded; and
- Workers in health care professions who have frequent contact with blood or blood-derived body fluids during routine work.

EXCEPTION: Persons in both of the above-listed groups in paragraph B, would not be considered at high or intermediate risk of contracting Hepatitis B, however, if there were laboratory evidence positive for antibodies to Hepatitis B. (ESRD patients are routinely tested for Hepatitis B antibodies as part of their continuing monitoring and therapy.)

For Medicare program purposes, the vaccine may be administered upon the order of a doctor of medicine or osteopathy, by a doctor of medicine or osteopathy, or by home health agencies, skilled nursing facilities, ESRD facilities, hospital outpatient departments, and persons recognized under the incident to physicians' services provision of law.

A charge separate from the ESRD composite rate will be recognized and paid for administration of the vaccine to ESRD patients.

C. Influenza Virus Vaccine

Effective for services furnished on or after May 1, 1993, the Medicare Part B program covers influenza virus vaccine and its administration when furnished in compliance with any applicable State law by any provider of services or any entity or individual with a supplier number. Typically, these vaccines are administered once a flu season. Medicare does not require, for coverage purposes, that a doctor of medicine or osteopathy order the vaccine. Therefore, the beneficiary may receive the vaccine upon request without a physician's order and without physician supervision.

100-2, Chapter-15, 100

Surgical Dressings, Splints, Casts, and Other Devices Used for Reductions of Fractures and Dislocations

Surgical dressings are limited to primary and secondary dressings required for the treatment of a wound caused by, or treated by, a surgical procedure that has been performed by a physician or other health care professional to the extent permissible under State law. In addition, surgical dressings required after debridement of a wound are also covered, irrespective of the type of debridement, as long as the debridement was reasonable and necessary and was performed by a health care professional acting within the scope of his/her legal authority when performing this function. Surgical dressings are covered for as long as they are medically necessary.

Primary dressings are therapeutic or protective coverings applied directly to wounds or lesions either on the skin or caused by an opening to the skin. Secondary dressing materials that serve a therapeutic or protective function and that are needed to secure a primary dressing are also covered. Items such as adhesive tape, roll gauze, bandages, and disposable compression material are examples of secondary dressings. Elastic stockings, support hose, foot coverings, leotards, knee supports, surgical leggings, gauntlets, and pressure garments for the arms and hands are examples of items that are not ordinarily covered as surgical dressings. Some items, such as transparent film, may be used as a primary or secondary dressing.

If a physician, certified nurse midwife, physician assistant, nurse practitioner, or clinical nurse specialist applies surgical dressings as part of a professional service that is billed to Medicare, the surgical dressings are considered incident to the professional services of the health care practitioner. (See §§60.1, 180, 190, 200, and 210.) When surgical dressings are not covered incident to the services of a health care practitioner and are obtained by the patient from a supplier (e.g., a drugstore, physician, or other health care practitioner that qualifies as a supplier) on an order from a physician or other health care professional authorized under State law or regulation to make such an order, the surgical dressings are covered separately under Part B.

Splints and casts, and other devices used for reductions of fractures and dislocations are covered under Part B of Medicare. This includes dental splints.

100-2, Chapter-15, 110

Durable Medical Equipment -General

Expenses incurred by a beneficiary for the rental or purchases of durable medical equipment (DME) are reimbursable if the following three requirements are met:

- The equipment meets the definition of DME (§110.1);
- The equipment is necessary and reasonable for the treatment of the patient's illness or injury or to improve the functioning of his or her malformed body member (§110.1); and
- The equipment is used in the patient's home.

The decision whether to rent or purchase an item of equipment generally resides with the beneficiary, but the decision on how to pay rests with CMS. For some DME, program payment policy calls for lump sum payments and in others for periodic payment. Where covered DME is furnished to a beneficiary by a supplier of services other than a provider of services, the DMERC makes the reimbursement. If a provider of services furnishes the equipment, the intermediary makes the reimbursement. The payment method is identified in the annual fee schedule update furnished by CMS.

The CMS issues quarterly updates to a fee schedule file that contains rates by HCPCS code and also identifies the classification of the HCPCS code within the following categories.

Category Code	Definition
IN	Inexpensive and Other Routinely Purchased Items
FS	Frequently Serviced Items
CR	Capped Rental Items
OX	Oxygen and Oxygen Equipment
OS	Ostomy, Tracheostomy & Urological Items
SD	Surgical Dressings
PO	Prosthetics & Orthotics
SU	Supplies
TE	Transcutaneous Electrical Nerve Stimulators

The DMERCs, carriers, and intermediaries, where appropriate, use the CMS files to determine payment rules. See the Medicare Claims Processing Manual, Chapter 20, "Durable

Medical Equipment, Surgical Dressings and Casts, Orthotics and Artificial Limbs, and Prosthetic Devices," for a detailed description of payment rules for each classification.

Payment may also be made for repairs, maintenance, and delivery of equipment and for expendable and nonreusable items essential to the effective use of the equipment subject to the conditions in §110.2.

See the Medicare Benefit Policy Manual, Chapter 11, "End Stage Renal Disease," for hemodialysis equipment and supplies.

100-2, Chapter-15, 110.1

Definition of Durable Medical Equipment

Durable medical equipment is equipment which:

- Can withstand repeated use;
- Is primarily and customarily used to serve a medical purpose;
- Generally is not useful to a person in the absence of an illness or injury; and
- Is appropriate for use in the home.

All requirements of the definition must be met before an item can be considered to be durable medical equipment.

The following describes the underlying policies for determining whether an item meets the definition of DME and may be covered.

A. Durability

An item is considered durable if it can withstand repeated use, i.e., the type of item that could normally be rented. Medical supplies of an expendable nature, such as incontinent pads, lamb's wool pads, catheters, ace bandages, elastic stockings, surgical facemasks, irrigating kits, sheets, and bags are not considered "durable" within the meaning of the definition. There are other items that, although durable in nature, may fall into other coverage categories such as supplies, braces, prosthetic devices, artificial arms, legs, and eyes.

B. Medical Equipment

Medical equipment is equipment primarily and customarily used for medical purposes and is not generally useful in the absence of illness or injury. In most instances, no development will be needed to determine whether a specific item of equipment is medical in nature. However, some cases will require development to determine whether the item constitutes medical equipment. This development would include the advice of local medical organizations (hospitals, medical schools, medical societies) and specialists in the field of physical medicine and rehabilitation. If the equipment is new on the market, it may be necessary, prior to seeking professional advice, to obtain information from the supplier or manufacturer explaining the design, purpose, effectiveness and method of using the equipment in the home as well as the results of any tests or clinical studies that have been conducted.

1. Equipment Presumptively Medical

Items such as hospital beds, wheelchairs, hemodialysis equipment, iron lungs, respirators, intermittent positive pressure breathing machines, medical regulators, oxygen tents, crutches, canes, trapeze bars, walkers, inhalators, nebulizers, commodes, suction machines, and traction equipment presumptively constitute medical equipment. (Although hemodialysis equipment is covered as a prosthetic device (§120), it also meets the definition of DME, and reimbursement for the rental or purchase of such equipment for use in the beneficiary's home will be made only under the provisions for payment applicable to DME. See the Medicare Benefit Policy Manual, Chapter 11, "End Stage Renal Disease" §30.1, for coverage of home use of hemodialysis.)

NOTE: There is a wide variety in types of respirators and suction machines. The DMERC's medical staff should determine whether the apparatus specified in the claim is appropriate for home use.

2. Equipment Presumptively Nonmedical

Equipment which is primarily and customarily used for a nonmedical purpose may not be considered "medical" equipment for which payment can be made under the medical insurance program. This is true even though the item has some remote medically related use. For example, in the case of a cardiac patient, an air conditioner might possibly be used to lower room temperature to reduce fluid loss in the patient and to restore an environment conducive to maintenance of the proper fluid balance. Nevertheless, because the primary and customary use of an air conditioner is a nonmedical one, the air conditioner cannot be deemed to be medical equipment for which payment can be made.

Other devices and equipment used for environmental control or to enhance the environmental setting in which the beneficiary is placed are not considered covered DME. These include, for example, room heaters, humidifiers, dehumidifiers, and electric air cleaners. Equipment which basically serves comfort or convenience functions or is primarily for the convenience of a person caring for the patient, such as elevators, stairway elevators, and posture chairs, do not constitute medical equipment. Similarly, physical fitness equipment (such as an exercycle), first-aid or precautionary-type equipment (such as preset portable oxygen units), self-help devices (such as safety grab bars), and training equipment (such as Braille training texts) are considered nonmedical in nature.

3. Special Exception Items

Specified items of equipment may be covered under certain conditions even though they do not meet the definition of DME because they are not primarily and customarily used to serve a medical purpose and/or are generally useful in the absence of illness or injury. These items would be covered when it is clearly established that they serve a therapeutic purpose in an individual case and would include:

a. Gel pads and pressure and water mattresses (which generally serve a preventive purpose) when prescribed for a patient who had bed sores or there is medical evidence indicating that they are highly susceptible to such ulceration; and

b. Heat lamps for a medical rather than a soothing or cosmetic purpose, e.g., where the need for heat therapy has been established.

In establishing medical necessity for the above items, the evidence must show that the item is included in the physician's course of treatment and a physician is supervising its use.

NOTE: The above items represent special exceptions and no extension of coverage to other items should be inferred

C. Necessary and Reasonable

Although an item may be classified as DME, it may not be covered in every instance. Coverage in a particular case is subject to the requirement that the equipment be necessary and reasonable for treatment of an illness or injury, or to improve the functioning of a malformed body member. These considerations will bar payment for equipment which cannot reasonably be expected to perform a therapeutic function in an

individual case or will permit only partial therapeutic function in an individual case or will permit only partial payment when the type of equipment furnished substantially exceeds that required for the treatment of the illness or injury involved.

See the Medicare Claims Processing Manual, Chapter 1, "General Billing Requirements;" §60, regarding the rules for providing advance beneficiary notices (ABNs) that advise beneficiaries, before items or services actually are furnished, when Medicare is likely to deny payment for them. ABNs allow beneficiaries to make an informed consumer decision about receiving items or services for which they may have to pay out-of-pocket and to be more active participants in their own health care treatment decisions.

1. Necessity for the Equipment

Equipment is necessary when it can be expected to make a meaningful contribution to the treatment of the patient's illness or injury or to the improvement of his or her malformed body member. In most cases the physician's prescription for the equipment and other medical information available to the DMERC will be sufficient to establish that the equipment serves this purpose.

2. Reasonableness of the Equipment

Even though an item of DME may serve a useful medical purpose, the DMERC or intermediary must also consider to what extent, if any, it would be reasonable for the Medicare program to pay for the item prescribed. The following considerations should enter into the determination of reasonableness:

1. Would the expense of the item to the program be clearly disproportionate to the therapeutic benefits which could ordinarily be derived from use of the equipment?

2. Is the item substantially more costly than a medically appropriate and realistically feasible alternative pattern of care?

3. Does the item serve essentially the same purpose as equipment already available to the beneficiary?

3. Payment Consistent With What is Necessary and Reasonable

Where a claim is filed for equipment containing features of an aesthetic nature or features of a medical nature which are not required by the patient's condition or where there exists a reasonably feasible and medically appropriate alternative pattern of care which is less costly than the equipment furnished, the amount payable is based on the rate for the equipment or alternative treatment which meets the patient's medical needs.

The acceptance of an assignment binds the supplier-assignee to accept the payment for the medically required equipment or service as the full charge and the supplier-assignee cannot charge the beneficiary the differential attributable to the equipment actually furnished.

4. Establishing the Period of Medical Necessity

Generally, the period of time an item of durable medical equipment will be considered to be medically necessary is based on the physician's estimate of the time that his or her patient will need the equipment. See the Medicare Program Integrity Manual, Chapters 5 and 6, for medical review guidelines.

D. Definition of a Beneficiary's Home

For purposes of rental and purchase of DME a beneficiary's home may be his/her own dwelling, an apartment, a relative's home, a home for the aged, or some other type of institution (such as an assisted living facility, or an intermediate care facility for the mentally retarded (ICF/MR)). However, an institution may not be considered a beneficiary's home if it:

- Meets at least the basic requirement in the definition of a hospital, i.e., it is primarily engaged in providing by or under the supervision of physicians, to inpatients, diagnostic and therapeutic services for medical diagnosis, treatment, and care of injured, disabled, and sick persons, or rehabilitation services for the rehabilitation of injured, disabled, or sick persons; or

- Meets at least the basic requirement in the definition of a skilled nursing facility, i.e., it is primarily engaged in providing to inpatients skilled nursing care and related services for patients who require medical or nursing care, or rehabilitation services for the rehabilitation of injured, disabled, or sick persons.

Thus, if an individual is a patient in an institution or distinct part of an institution which provides the services described in the bullets above, the individual is not entitled to have separate Part B payment made for rental or purchase of DME. This is because such an institution may not be considered the individual's home. The same concept applies even if the patient resides in a bed or portion of the institution not certified for Medicare.

If the patient is at home for part of a month and, for part of the same month is in an institution that cannot qualify as his or her home, or is outside the U.S., monthly payments may be made for the entire month. Similarly, if DME is returned to the provider before the end of a payment month because the beneficiary died in that month or because the equipment became unnecessary in that month, payment may be made for the entire month.

100-2, Chapter-15, 110.2

Repairs, Maintenance, Replacement, and Delivery

Under the circumstances specified below, payment may be made for repair, maintenance, and replacement of medically required DME, including equipment which had been in use before the user enrolled in Part B of the program. However, do not pay for repair, maintenance, or replacement of equipment in the frequent and substantial servicing or oxygen equipment payment categories. In addition, payments for repair and maintenance may not include payment for parts and labor covered under a manufacturer's or supplier's warranty.

A. Repairs

To repair means to fix or mend and to put the equipment back in good condition after damage or wear. Repairs to equipment which a beneficiary owns are covered when necessary to make the equipment serviceable. However, do not pay for repair of previously denied equipment or equipment in the frequent and substantial servicing or oxygen equipment payment categories. If the expense for repairs exceeds the estimated expense of purchasing or renting another item of equipment for the remaining period of medical need, no payment can be made for the amount of the excess. (See subsection C where claims for repairs suggest malicious damage or culpable neglect.)

Since renters of equipment recover from the rental charge the expenses they incur in maintaining in working order the equipment they rent out, separately itemized charges for repair of rented equipment are not covered. This includes items in the frequent and substantial servicing, oxygen equipment, capped rental, and inexpensive or routinely purchased payment categories which are being rented.

A new Certificate of Medical Necessity (CMN) and/or physician's order is not needed for repairs.

For replacement items, see Subsection C below.

B. Maintenance

Routine periodic servicing, such as testing, cleaning, regulating, and checking of the beneficiary's equipment, is not covered. The owner is expected to perform such routine maintenance rather than a retailer or some other person who charges the beneficiary. Normally, purchasers of DME are given operating manuals which describe the type of servicing an owner may perform to properly maintain the equipment. It is reasonable to expect that beneficiaries will perform this maintenance. Thus, hiring a third party to do such work is for the convenience of the beneficiary and is not covered. However, more extensive maintenance which, based on the manufacturers' recommendations, is to be performed by authorized technicians, is covered as repairs for medically necessary equipment which a beneficiary owns. This might include, for example, breaking down sealed components and performing tests which require specialized testing equipment not available to the beneficiary. Do not pay for maintenance of purchased items that require frequent and substantial servicing or oxygen equipment.

Since renters of equipment recover from the rental charge the expenses they incur in maintaining in working order the equipment they rent out, separately itemized charges for maintenance of rented equipment are generally not covered. Payment may not be made for maintenance of rented equipment other than the maintenance and servicing fee established for capped rental items. For capped rental items which have reached the 13-month rental cap, contractors pay claims for maintenance and servicing fees after 6 months have passed from the end of the final paid rental month or from the end of the period the item is no longer covered under the supplier's or manufacturer's warranty, whichever is later. See the Medicare Claims Processing Manual, Chapter 20, "Durable Medical Equipment, Prosthetics and Orthotics, and Supplies (DMEPOS)," for additional instruction and an example.

A new CMN and/or physician's order is not needed for covered maintenance.

In cases where one or more monthly rental payments have been made in accordance with 42 CFR 414.229 for a capped rental DME item, medical necessity for the equipment has been established. In cases where one or more rental payments have been made for an item classified as capped rental DME, and the supplier transfers title to the equipment prior to the end of a 13 month period of continuous use per 42 CFR 414.230, Medicare payment can be made for reasonable and necessary maintenance and servicing of the beneficiary-owned DME. Under the regulations at 42 CFR 414.210(e)(1), reasonable and necessary charges for maintenance and servicing are those made for parts and labor not otherwise covered under a manufacturer's or supplier's warranty. Charges for routine maintenance and servicing would not be covered. Charges for maintenance and servicing that exceed the purchase price of the equipment (i.e., the capped rental monthly fee multiplied by 10) would not be reasonable and necessary and should be denied.

C. Replacement

Replacement refers to the provision of an identical or nearly identical item. Situations involving the provision of a different item because of a change in medical condition are not addressed in this section.

Equipment which the beneficiary owns or is a capped rental item may be replaced in cases of loss or irreparable damage. Irreparable damage refers to a specific accident or to a natural disaster (e.g., fire, flood). A physician's order and/or new

Certificate of Medical Necessity (CMN), when required, is needed to reaffirm the medical necessity of the item.

Irreparable wear refers to deterioration sustained from day-to-day usage over time and a specific event cannot be identified. Replacement of equipment due to irreparable wear takes into consideration the reasonable useful lifetime of the equipment. If the item of equipment has been in continuous use by the patient on either a rental or purchase basis for the equipment's useful lifetime, the beneficiary may elect to obtain a new piece of equipment. Replacement may be reimbursed when a new physician order and/or new CMN, when required, is needed to reaffirm the medical necessity of the item.

The reasonable useful lifetime of durable medical equipment is determined through program instructions. In the absence of program instructions, A/B MACS (B) may determine the reasonable useful lifetime of equipment, but in no case can it be less than 5 years. Computation of the useful lifetime is based on when the equipment is delivered to the beneficiary, not the age of the equipment. Replacement due to wear is not covered during the reasonable useful lifetime of the equipment. During the reasonable useful lifetime, Medicare does cover repair up to the cost of replacement (but not actual replacement) for medically necessary equipment owned by the beneficiary. (See subsection A.)

Charges for the replacement of oxygen equipment, items that require frequent and substantial servicing or inexpensive or routinely purchased items which are being rented are not covered.

Cases suggesting malicious damage, culpable neglect, or wrongful disposition of equipment should be investigated and denied where the DME MACs determines that it is unreasonable to make program payment under the circumstances. DME MACs refer such cases to the program integrity specialist in the RO.

D. Delivery

Payment for delivery of DME whether rented or purchased is generally included in the fee schedule allowance for the item. See Pub. 100-04, Medicare Claims Processing Manual, Chapter 20, "Durable Medical Equipment, Prosthetics and Orthotics, and Supplies (DMEPOS)," for the rules that apply to making reimbursement for exceptional cases.

100-2, Chapter-15, 110.3

Coverage of Supplies and Accessories

Payment may be made for supplies, e.g., oxygen, that are necessary for the effective use of durable medical equipment. Such supplies include those drugs and biologicals which must be put directly into the equipment in order to achieve the therapeutic benefit of the durable medical equipment or to assure the proper functioning of the equipment, e.g., tumor chemotherapy agents used with an infusion pump or heparin used with a home dialysis system. However, the coverage of such drugs or biologicals does not preclude the need for a determination that the drug or biological itself is reasonable and necessary for treatment of the illness or injury or to improve the functioning of a malformed body member.

In the case of prescription drugs, other than oxygen, used in conjunction with durable medical equipment, prosthetic, orthotics, and supplies (DMEPOS) or prosthetic devices, the entity that dispenses the drug must furnish it directly to the patient for whom a prescription is written. The entity that dispenses the drugs must have a Medicare supplier number, must possess a current license to dispense prescription drugs in the State in which the drug is dispensed, and must bill and receive payment in its own name.

A supplier that is not the entity that dispenses the drugs cannot purchase the drugs used in conjunction with DME for resale to the beneficiary. Reimbursement may be made for replacement of essential accessories such as hoses, tubes, mouthpieces, etc., for necessary DME, only if the beneficiary owns or is purchasing the equipment.

100-2, Chapter-15, 120

Prosthetic Devices

A. General

Prosthetic devices (other than dental) which replace all or part of an internal body organ (including contiguous tissue), or replace all or part of the function of a permanently inoperative or malfunctioning internal body organ are covered when furnished on a physician's order. This does not require a determination that there is no possibility that the patient's condition may improve sometime in the future. If the medical record, including the judgment of the attending physician, indicates the condition is of long and indefinite duration, the test of permanence is considered met. (Such a device may also be covered under §60.1 as a supply when furnished incident to a physician's service.)

Examples of prosthetic devices include artificial limbs, parenteral and enteral (PEN) nutrition, cardiac pacemakers, prosthetic lenses (see subsection B), breast prostheses (including a surgical brassiere) for post mastectomy patients, maxillofacial devices, and devices which replace all or part of the ear or nose. A urinary collection and retention system with or without a tube is a prosthetic device replacing bladder function in case of permanent urinary incontinence. The Foley catheter is also considered a prosthetic device when ordered for a patient with permanent urinary incontinence. However, chucks, diapers, rubber sheets, etc., are supplies that are not covered under this provision. Although hemodialysis equipment is a prosthetic device, payment for the rental or purchase of such equipment in the home is made only for use under the provisions for payment applicable to durable medical equipment.

An exception is that if payment cannot be made on an inpatient's behalf under Part A, hemodialysis equipment, supplies, and services required by such patient could be covered under Part B as a prosthetic device, which replaces the function of a kidney. See the Medicare Benefit Policy Manual, Chapter 11, "End Stage Renal Disease," for payment for hemodialysis equipment used in the home. See the Medicare Benefit Policy Manual, Chapter 1, "Inpatient Hospital Services," §10, for additional instructions on hospitalization for renal dialysis.

NOTE: Medicare does not cover a prosthetic device dispensed to a patient prior to the time at which the patient undergoes the procedure that makes necessary the use of the device. For example, the carrier does not make a separate Part B payment for an intraocular lens (IOL) or pacemaker that a physician, during an office visit prior to the actual surgery, dispenses to the patient for his or her use. Dispensing a prosthetic device in this manner raises health and safety issues. Moreover, the need for the device cannot be clearly established until the procedure that makes its use possible is successfully performed. Therefore, dispensing a prosthetic device in this manner is not considered reasonable and necessary for the treatment of the patient's condition.

Colostomy (and other ostomy) bags and necessary accouterments required for attachment are covered as prosthetic devices. This coverage also includes irrigation and flushing equipment and other items and supplies directly related to ostomy care, whether the attachment of a bag is required.

Accessories and/or supplies which are used directly with an enteral or parenteral device to achieve the therapeutic benefit of the prosthesis or to assure the proper functioning of the device may also be covered under the prosthetic device benefit subject to the additional guidelines in the Medicare National Coverage Determinations Manual.

Covered items include catheters, filters, extension tubing, infusion bottles, pumps (either food or infusion), intravenous (I.V.) pole, needles, syringes, dressings, tape, Heparin Sodium (parenteral only), volumetric monitors (parenteral only), and parenteral and enteral nutrient solutions. Baby food and other regular grocery products that can be blenderized and used with the enteral system are not covered. Note that some of these items, e.g., a food pump and an I.V. pole, qualify as DME. Although coverage of the enteral and parenteral nutritional therapy systems is provided on the basis of the prosthetic device benefit, the payment rules relating to lump sum or monthly payment for DME apply to such items.

The coverage of prosthetic devices includes replacement of and repairs to such devices as explained in subsection D.

Finally, the Benefits Improvement and Protection Act of 2000 amended §1834(h)(1) of the Act by adding a provision (1834 (h)(1)(G)(i)) that requires Medicare payment to be made for the replacement of prosthetic devices which are artificial limbs, or for the replacement of any part of such devices, without regard to continuous use or useful lifetime restrictions if an ordering physician determines that the replacement device, or replacement part of such a device, is necessary.

Payment may be made for the replacement of a prosthetic device that is an artificial limb, or replacement part of a device if the ordering physician determines that the replacement device or part is necessary because of any of the following:

1. A change in the physiological condition of the patient;
2. An irreparable change in the condition of the device, or in a part of the device; or
3. The condition of the device, or the part of the device, requires repairs and the cost of such repairs would be more than 60 percent of the cost of a replacement device, or, as the case may be, of the part being replaced.

This provision is effective for items replaced on or after April 1, 2001. It supersedes any rule that that provided a 5-year or other replacement rule with regard to prosthetic devices.

B. Prosthetic Lenses

The term "internal body organ" includes the lens of an eye. Prostheses replacing the lens of an eye include post-surgical lenses customarily used during convalescence from eye surgery in which the lens of the eye was removed. In addition, permanent lenses are also covered when required by an individual lacking the organic lens of the eye because of surgical removal or congenital absence. Prosthetic lenses obtained on or after the beneficiary's date of entitlement to supplementary medical insurance benefits may be covered even though the surgical removal of the crystalline lens occurred before entitlement.

1. Prosthetic Cataract Lenses

One of the following prosthetic lenses or combinations of prosthetic lenses furnished by a physician (see §30.4 for coverage of prosthetic lenses prescribed by a doctor of optometry) may be covered when determined to be reasonable and necessary to restore essentially the vision provided by the crystalline lens of the eye:

- Prosthetic bifocal lenses in frames;
- Prosthetic lenses in frames for far vision, and prosthetic lenses in frames for near vision; or

- When a prosthetic contact lens(es) for far vision is prescribed (including cases of binocular and monocular aphakia), make payment for the contact lens(es) and prosthetic lenses in frames for near vision to be worn at the same time as the contact lens(es), and prosthetic lenses in frames to be worn when the contacts have been removed.

Lenses which have ultraviolet absorbing or reflecting properties may be covered, in lieu of payment for regular (untinted) lenses, if it has been determined that such lenses are medically reasonable and necessary for the individual patient.

Medicare does not cover cataract sunglasses obtained in addition to the regular (untinted) prosthetic lenses since the sunglasses duplicate the restoration of vision function performed by the regular prosthetic lenses.

2. Payment for Intraocular Lenses (IOLs) Furnished in Ambulatory Surgical Centers (ASCs)

Effective for services furnished on or after March 12, 1990, payment for intraocular lenses (IOLs) inserted during or subsequent to cataract surgery in a Medicare certified ASC is included with the payment for facility services that are furnished in connection with the covered surgery.

Refer to the Medicare Claims Processing Manual, Chapter 14, "Ambulatory Surgical Centers," for more information.

3. Limitation on Coverage of Conventional Lenses

One pair of conventional eyeglasses or conventional contact lenses furnished after each cataract surgery with insertion of an IOL is covered.

C. Dentures

Dentures are excluded from coverage. However, when a denture or a portion of the denture is an integral part (built-in) of a covered prosthesis (e.g., an obturator to fill an opening in the palate), it is covered as part of that prosthesis.

D. Supplies, Repairs, Adjustments, and Replacement

Supplies are covered that are necessary for the effective use of a prosthetic device (e.g., the batteries needed to operate an artificial larynx). Adjustment of prosthetic devices required by wear or by a change in the patient's condition is covered when ordered by a physician. General provisions relating to the repair and replacement of durable medical equipment in §110.2 for the repair and replacement of prosthetic devices are applicable. (See the Medicare Benefit Policy Manual, Chapter 16, "General Exclusions from Coverage," §40.4, for payment for devices replaced under a warranty.) Replacement of conventional eyeglasses or contact lenses furnished in accordance with §120.B.3 is not covered.

Necessary supplies, adjustments, repairs, and replacements are covered even when the device had been in use before the user enrolled in Part B of the program, so long as the device continues to be medically required.

100-2, Chapter-15, 130

Leg, Arm, Back, and Neck Braces, Trusses, and Artificial Legs, Arms, and Eyes

These appliances are covered under Part B when furnished incident to physicians' services or on a physician's order. A brace includes rigid and semi-rigid devices which are used for the purpose of supporting a weak or deformed body member or restricting or eliminating motion in a diseased or injured part of the body. Elastic stockings, garter belts, and similar devices do not come within the scope of the definition of a brace. Back braces include, but are not limited to, special corsets, e.g., sacroiliac, sacrolumbar, dorsolumbar corsets, and belts.

A terminal device (e.g., hand or hook) is covered under this provision whether an artificial limb is required by the patient. Stump stockings and harnesses (including replacements) are also covered when these appliances are essential to the effective use of the artificial limb.

Adjustments to an artificial limb or other appliance required by wear or by a change in the patient's condition are covered when ordered by a physician.

Adjustments, repairs and replacements are covered even when the item had been in use before the user enrolled in Part B of the program so long as the device continues to be medically required.

100-2, Chapter-15, 140

Therapeutic Shoes for Individuals with Diabetes

Coverage of therapeutic shoes (depth or custom-molded) along with inserts for individuals with diabetes is available as of May 1, 1993. These diabetic shoes are covered if the requirements as specified in this section concerning certification and prescription are fulfilled. In addition, this benefit provides for a pair of diabetic shoes even if only one foot suffers from diabetic foot disease. Each shoe is equally equipped so that the affected limb, as well as the remaining limb, is protected. Claims for therapeutic shoes for diabetics are processed by the Durable Medical Equipment Medicare Administrative Contractors (DME MACs). Therapeutic shoes for diabetics are not DME and are not considered DME nor orthotics, but a separate category of coverage under Medicare Part B. (See §1861(s)(12) and §1833(o) of the Act.)

A. Definitions

The following items may be covered under the diabetic shoe benefit:

1. Custom-Molded Shoes

Custom-molded shoes are shoes that:

- Are constructed over a positive model of the patient's foot;
- Are made from leather or other suitable material of equal quality;
- Have removable inserts that can be altered or replaced as the patient's condition warrants; and
- Have some form of shoe closure.

2. Depth Shoes

Depth shoes are shoes that:

- Have a full length, heel-to-toe filler that, when removed, provides a minimum of 3/16 inch of additional depth used to accommodate custom-molded or customized inserts;
- Are made from leather or other suitable material of equal quality;
- Have some form of shoe closure; and
- Are available in full and half sizes with a minimum of three widths so that the sole is graded to the size and width of the upper portions of the shoes according to the American standard last sizing schedule or its equivalent. (The American standard last sizing schedule is the numerical shoe sizing system used for shoes sold in the United States.)

3. Inserts

Inserts are total contact, multiple density, removable inlays that are directly molded to the patient's foot or a model of the patient's foot or directly carved from a patient-specific, rectified electronic model and that are made of a suitable material with regard to the patient's condition.

B. Coverage

1. Limitations

For each individual, coverage of the footwear and inserts is limited to one of the following within one calendar year:

- No more than one pair of custom-molded shoes (including inserts provided with such shoes) and two additional pairs of inserts; or
- No more than one pair of depth shoes and three pairs of inserts (not including the noncustomized removable inserts provided with such shoes).

2. Coverage of Diabetic Shoes and Brace

Orthopedic shoes, as stated in the Medicare Claims Processing Manual, Chapter 20, "Durable Medical Equipment, Surgical Dressings and Casts, Orthotics and Artificial Limbs, and Prosthetic Devices," generally are not covered. This exclusion does not apply to orthopedic shoes that are an integral part of a leg brace. In situations in which an individual qualifies for both diabetic shoes and a leg brace, these items are covered separately. Thus, the diabetic shoes may be covered if the requirements for this section are met, while the brace may be covered if the requirements of §130 are met.

3. Substitution of Modifications for Inserts

An individual may substitute modification(s) of custom-molded or depth shoes instead of obtaining a pair(s) of inserts in any combination. Payment for the modification(s) may not exceed the limit set for the inserts for which the individual is entitled. The following is a list of the most common shoe modifications available, but it is not meant as an exhaustive list of the modifications available for diabetic shoes:

- Rigid Rocker Bottoms - These are exterior elevations with apex positions for 51 percent to 75 percent distance measured from the back end of the heel. The apex is a narrowed or pointed end of an anatomical structure. The apex must be positioned behind the metatarsal heads and tapered off sharply to the front tip of the sole. Apex height helps to eliminate pressure at the metatarsal heads. Rigidity is ensured by the steel in the shoe. The heel of the shoe tapers off in the back in order to cause the heel to strike in the middle of the heel;
- *Roller Bottoms (Sole or Bar) -* These are the same as rocker bottoms, but the heel is tapered from the apex to the front tip of the sole;
- *Metatarsal Bars -* An exterior bar is placed behind the metatarsal heads in order to remove pressure from the metatarsal heads. The bars are of various shapes, heights, and construction depending on the exact purpose;
- *Wedges (Posting) -* Wedges are either of hind foot, fore foot, or both and may be in the middle or to the side. The function is to shift or transfer weight bearing upon standing or during ambulation to the opposite side for added support, stabilization, equalized weight distribution, or balance; and
- *Offset Heels -* This is a heel flanged at its base either in the middle, to the side, or a combination, that is then extended upward to the shoe in order to stabilize extreme positions of the hind foot.

Other modifications to diabetic shoes include, but are not limited to flared heels, Velcro closures, and inserts for missing toes.

4. Separate Inserts

Inserts may be covered and dispensed independently of diabetic shoes if the supplier of the shoes verifies in writing that the patient has appropriate footwear into which the insert can be placed. This footwear must meet the definitions found above for depth shoes and custom-molded shoes.

C. Certification

The need for diabetic shoes must be certified by a physician who is a doctor of medicine or a doctor of osteopathy and who is responsible for diagnosing and treating the patient's diabetic systemic condition through a comprehensive plan of care. This managing physician must:

- Document in the patient's medical record that the patient has diabetes;
- Certify that the patient is being treated under a comprehensive plan of care for diabetes, and that the patient needs diabetic shoes; and
- Document in the patient's record that the patient has one or more of the following conditions:
    - Peripheral neuropathy with evidence of callus formation;
    - History of pre-ulcerative calluses;
    - History of previous ulceration;
    - Foot deformity;
    - Previous amputation of the foot or part of the foot; or
    - Poor circulation.

D. Prescription

Following certification by the physician managing the patient's systemic diabetic condition, a podiatrist or other qualified physician who is knowledgeable in the fitting of diabetic shoes and inserts may prescribe the particular type of footwear necessary.

E. Furnishing Footwear

The footwear must be fitted and furnished by a podiatrist or other qualified individual such as a pedorthist, an orthotist, or a prosthetist. The certifying physician may not furnish the diabetic shoes unless the certifying physician is the only qualified individual in the area. It is left to the discretion of each A/B MAC (B) to determine the meaning of "in the area."

100-2, Chapter-15, 150

Dental Services

As indicated under the general exclusions from coverage, items and services in connection with the care, treatment, filling, removal, or replacement of teeth or structures directly supporting the teeth are not covered. "Structures directly supporting the teeth" means the periodontium, which includes the gingivae, dentogingival junction, periodontal membrane, cementum of the teeth, and alveolar process.

In addition to the following, see Pub 100-01, the Medicare General Information, Eligibility, and Entitlement Manual, Chapter 5, Definitions and Pub 3, the Medicare National Coverage Determinations Manual for specific services which may be covered when furnished by a dentist. If an otherwise non covered procedure or service is performed by a dentist as incident to and as an integral part of a covered procedure or service performed by the dentist, the total service performed by the dentist on such an occasion is covered.

EXAMPLE 1:

The reconstruction of a ridge performed primarily to prepare the mouth for dentures is a noncovered procedure. However, when the reconstruction of a ridge is performed as a result of and at the same time as the surgical removal of a tumor (for other than dental purposes), the totality of surgical procedures is a covered service.

EXAMPLE 2:

Medicare makes payment for the wiring of teeth when this is done in connection with the reduction of a jaw fracture.

The extraction of teeth to prepare the jaw for radiation treatment of neoplastic disease is also covered. This is an exception to the requirement that to be covered, a noncovered procedure or service performed by a dentist must be an incident to and an integral part of a covered procedure or service performed by the dentist. Ordinarily, the dentist extracts the patient's teeth, but another physician, e.g., a radiologist, administers the radiation treatments.

When an excluded service is the primary procedure involved, it is not covered, regardless of its complexity or difficulty. For example, the extraction of an impacted tooth is not covered. Similarly, an alveoplasty (the surgical improvement of the shape and condition of the alveolar process) and a frenectomy are excluded from coverage when either of these procedures is performed in connection with an excluded service, e.g., the preparation of the mouth for dentures. In a like manner, the removal of a torus palatinus (a bony protuberance of the hard palate) may be a covered service. However, with rare exception, this surgery is performed in connection with an excluded service, i.e., the preparation of the mouth for dentures. Under such circumstances, Medicare does not pay for this procedure.

Dental splints used to treat a dental condition are excluded from coverage under 1862(a)(12) of the Act. On the other hand, if the treatment is determined to be a covered medical condition (i.e., dislocated upper/lower jaw joints), then the splint can be covered. Whether such services as the administration of anesthesia, diagnostic X-rays, and other related procedures are covered depends upon whether the primary procedure being performed by the dentist is itself covered. Thus, an X-ray taken in connection with the reduction of a fracture of the jaw or facial bone is covered. However, a single X-ray or X-ray survey taken in connection with the care or treatment of teeth or the periodontium is not covered.

Medicare makes payment for a covered dental procedure no matter where the service is performed. The hospitalization or non hospitalization of a patient has no direct bearing on the coverage or exclusion of a given dental procedure.

Payment may also be made for services and supplies furnished incident to covered dental services. For example, the services of a dental technician or nurse who is under the direct supervision of the dentist or physician are covered if the services are included in the dentist's or physician's bill.

100-2, Chapter-15, 150.1

Treatment of Temporomandibular Joint (TMJ) Syndrome

There are a wide variety of conditions that can be characterized as TMJ, and an equally wide variety of methods for treating these conditions. Many of the procedures fall within the Medicare program's statutory exclusion that prohibits payment for items and services that have not been demonstrated to be reasonable and necessary for the diagnosis and treatment of illness or injury (§1862(a)(1) of the Act). Other services and appliances used to treat TMJ fall within the Medicare program's statutory exclusion at 1862(a)(12), which prohibits payment "for services in connection with the care, treatment, filling, removal, or replacement of teeth or structures directly supporting teeth...." For these reasons, a diagnosis of TMJ on a claim is insufficient. The actual condition or symptom must be determined.

100-2, Chapter-15, 230

Practice of Physical Therapy, Occupational Therapy, and Speech-Language Pathology

A. Group Therapy Services. Contractors pay for outpatient physical therapy services (which includes outpatient speech-language pathology services) and outpatient occupational therapy services provided simultaneously to two or more individuals by a practitioner as group therapy services (97150). The individuals can be, but need not be performing the same activity. The physician or therapist involved in group therapy services must be in constant attendance, but one-on-one patient contact is not required.

B. Therapy Students

1. General

Only the services of the therapist can be billed and paid under Medicare Part B. The services performed by a student are not reimbursed even if provided under "line of sight" supervision of the therapist; however, the presence of the student "in the room" does not make the service unbillable. Pay for the direct (one-to-one) patient contact services of the physician or therapist provided to Medicare Part B patients. Group therapy services performed by a therapist or physician may be billed when a student is also present "in the room".

EXAMPLES

Therapists may bill and be paid for the provision of services in the following scenarios:

- The qualified practitioner is present and in the room for the entire session. The student participates in the delivery of services when the qualified practitioner is directing the service, making the skilled judgment, and is responsible for the assessment and treatment.

- The qualified practitioner is present in the room guiding the student in service delivery when the therapy student and the therapy assistant student are participating in the provision of services, and the practitioner is not engaged in treating another patient or doing other tasks at the same time.

- The qualified practitioner is responsible for the services and as such, signs all documentation. (A student may, of course, also sign but it is not necessary since the Part B payment is for the clinician's service, not for the student's services).

2. Therapy Assistants as Clinical Instructors

Physical therapist assistants and occupational therapy assistants are not precluded from serving as clinical instructors for therapy students, while providing services within their scope of work and performed under the direction and supervision of a licensed physical or occupational therapist to a Medicare beneficiary.

3. Services Provided Under Part A and Part B

The payment methodologies for Part A and B therapy services rendered by a student are different. Under the MPFS (Medicare Part B), Medicare pays for services provided by physicians and practitioners that are specifically authorized by statute. Students do not meet the definition of practitioners under Medicare Part B. Under SNF PPS, payments are based upon the case mix or Resource Utilization Group (RUG) category that describes the patient. In the rehabilitation groups, the number of therapy minutes delivered to the patient determines the RUG category. Payment levels for each category are based upon the costs of caring for patients in each group rather than providing specific payment for each therapy service as is done in Medicare Part B.

100-2, Chapter-15, 231

Pulmonary Rehabilitation (PR) Program Services Furnished On or After January 1, 2010

A pulmonary rehabilitation (PR) program is typically a physician-supervised, multidisciplinary program individually tailored and designed to optimize physical and social performance and autonomy of care for patients with chronic respiratory impairment. The main goal is to empower the individuals' ability to exercise independently. Exercise is combined with other training and support mechanisms to encourage long-term adherence to the treatment plan. Effective January 1, 2010, Medicare Part B pays for PR programs and related items and services if specific criteria is met by the Medicare beneficiary, the PR program itself, the setting in which it is administered, and the physician administering the program, as outlined below:

PR Program Beneficiary Requirements:

As specified in 42 CFR 410.47, Medicare covers PR items and services for patients with moderate to very severe chronic obstructive pulmonary disease (COPD) (defined as GOLD classification II, III, and IV), when referred by the physician treating the chronic respiratory disease. Additional medical indications for coverage for PR program services may be established through the national coverage determination process.

PR Program Component Requirements:

- Physician-prescribed exercise. This physical activity includes techniques such as exercise conditioning, breathing retraining, and step and strengthening exercises. Some aerobic exercise must be included in each PR session. Both low-and high-intensity exercise is recommended to produce clinical benefits and a combination of endurance and strength training should be conducted at least twice per week.

- Education or training. This should be closely and clearly related to the individual's care and treatment and tailored to the individual's needs, including information on respiratory problem management and, if appropriate, brief smoking cessation counseling. Any education or training must assist in achievement of individual goals towards independence in activities of daily living, adaptation to limitations, and improved quality of life (QoL).

- Psychosocial assessment. This assessment means a written evaluation of an individual's mental and emotional functioning as it relates to the individual's rehabilitation or respiratory condition. It should include: (1) an assessment of those aspects of the individual's family and home situation that affects the individual's rehabilitation treatment, and, (2) a psychological evaluation of the individual's response to, and rate of progress under, the treatment plan. Periodic re-evaluations are necessary to ensure the individual's psychosocial needs are being met.

- Outcomes assessment. These should include: (1) beginning and end evaluations based on patient-centered outcomes, which are conducted by the physician at the start and end of the program, and, (2) objective clinical measures of the effectiveness of the PR program for the individual patient, including exercise performance and self-reported measures of shortness of breath, and behavior. The assessments should include clinical measures such as the 6-minute walk, weight, exercise performance, self-reported dyspnea, behavioral measures(supplemental oxygen use, smoking status,) and a QoL assessment.

- An individualized treatment plan describing the individual's diagnosis and detailing how components are utilized for each patient. The plan must be established, reviewed, and signed by a physician every 30 days. The plan may initially be developed by the referring physician or the PR physician. If the plan is developed by the referring physician who is not the PR physician, the PR physician must also review and sign the plan prior to imitation of the PR program. It is expected that the supervising physician would have initial, direct contact with the individual prior to subsequent treatment by ancillary personnel, and also have at least one direct contact in each 30-day period. The plan must have written specificity with regards to the type, amount, frequency, and duration of PR items and services furnished to the individual, and specify the appropriate mix of services for the patient's needs. It must include measurable and expected outcomes and estimated timetables to achieve these outcomes.

As specified at 42 CFR 410.47(f), PR program sessions are limited to a maximum of 2 1-hour sessions per day for up to 36 sessions, with the option for an additional 36 sessions if medically necessary.

PR Program Setting Requirements:

PR items and services must be furnished in a physician's office or a hospital outpatient setting. The setting must have the necessary cardio-pulmonary, emergency, diagnostic, and therapeutic life-saving equipment accepted by the medical community as medically necessary (for example, oxygen, cardiopulmonary resuscitation equipment, and a defibrillator) to treat chronic respiratory disease. All settings must have a physician immediately available and accessible for medical consultations and emergencies at all times that the PR items and services are being furnished under the program. This provision is satisfied if the physician meets the requirements for direct supervision of physician office services as specified at 42 CFR 410.26, and for hospital outpatient therapeutic services as specified at 42 CFR 410.27.

PR Program Physician Requirements:

Medicare Part B pays for PR services supervised by a physician only if the physician meets all of the following requirements: (1) expertise in the management of individuals with respiratory pathophysiology, (2) licensed to practice medicine in the state in which the PR program is offered, (3) responsible and accountable for the PR program, and, (4) involved substantially, in consultation with staff, in directing the progress of the individual in the PR program.

(See Publication 100-04, Claims Processing Manual, chapter 32, section 140.4, for specific claims processing, coding, and billing requirements for PR program services.)

100-2, Chapter-15, 232

Cardiac Rehabilitation (CR) and Intensive Cardiac Rehabilitation (ICR) Services Furnished On or After January 1, 2010

Cardiac rehabilitation (CR) services mean a physician-supervised program that furnishes physician prescribed exercise, cardiac risk factor modification, including education, counseling, and behavioral intervention; psychosocial assessment, outcomes assessment, and other items/services as determined by the Secretary under certain conditions. Intensive cardiac rehabilitation (ICR) services mean a physician-supervised program that furnishes the same items/services under the same conditions as a CR program but

must also demonstrate, as shown in peer-reviewed published research, that it improves patients' cardiovascular disease through specific outcome measurements described in 42 CFR 410.49(c). Effective January 1, 2010, Medicare Part B pays for CR/ICR programs and related items/services if specific criteria is met by the Medicare beneficiary, the CR/ICR program itself, the setting in which is it administered, and the physician administering the program, as outlined below:

CR/ICR Program Beneficiary Requirements:

Medicare covers CR/ICR program services for beneficiaries who have experienced one or more of the following:

- Acute myocardial infarction within the preceding 12 months;
- Coronary artery bypass surgery;
- Current stable angina pectoris;
- Heart valve repair or replacement;
- Percutaneous transluminal coronary angioplasty (PTCA) or coronary stenting;
- Heart or heart-lung transplant;

For cardiac rehabilitation only: Stable, chronic heart failure defined as patients with left ventricular ejection fraction of 35% or less and New York Heart Association (NYHA) class II to IV symptoms despite being on optimal heart failure therapy for at least 6 weeks. (Effective February 18, 2014.)

CR/ICR Program Component Requirements:

Physician-prescribed exercise. This physical activity includes aerobic exercise combined with other types of exercise (i.e., strengthening, stretching) as determined to be appropriate for individual patients by a physician each day CR/ICR items/services are furnished.

Cardiac risk factor modification. This includes education, counseling, and behavioral intervention, tailored to the patients' individual needs.

Psychosocial assessment. This assessment means an evaluation of an individual's mental and emotional functioning as it relates to the individual's rehabilitation. It should include: (1) an assessment of those aspects of the individual's family and home situation that affects the individual's rehabilitation treatment, and, (2) a psychosocial evaluation of the individual's response to, and rate of progress under, the treatment plan.

Outcomes assessment. These should include: (i) minimally, assessments from the commencement and conclusion of CR/ICR, based on patient-centered outcomes which must be measured by the physician immediately at the beginning and end of the program, and, (ii) objective clinical measures of the effectiveness of the CR/ICR program for the individual patient, including exercise performance and self-reported measures of exertion and behavior.

Individualized treatment plan. This plan should be written and tailored to each individual patient and include (i) a description of the individual's diagnosis; (ii) the type, amount, frequency, and duration of the CR/ICR items/services furnished; and (iii) the goals set for the individual under the plan. The individualized treatment plan must be established, reviewed, and signed by a physician every 30 days.

As specified at 42 CFR 410.49(f)(1), CR sessions are limited to a maximum of 2 1-hour sessions per day for up to 36 sessions over up to 36 weeks with the option for an additional 36 sessions over an extended period of time if approved by the contractor under section 1862(a)(1)(A) of the Act. ICR sessions are limited to 72 1-hour sessions (as defined in section 1848(b)(5) of the Act), up to 6 sessions per day, over a period of up to 18 weeks.

CR/ICR Program Setting Requirements:

CR/ICR services must be furnished in a physician's office or a hospital outpatient setting (for ICR, the hospital outpatient setting must provide ICR using an approved ICR program). All settings must have a physician immediately available and accessible for medical consultations and emergencies at all times when items/services are being furnished under the program. This provision is satisfied if the physician meets the requirements for direct supervision of physician office services as specified at 42 CFR 410.26, and for hospital outpatient services as specified at 42 CFR 410.27.

ICR Program Approval Requirements:

All prospective ICR programs must be approved through the national coverage determination (NCD) process. To be approved as an ICR program, it must demonstrate through peer-reviewed, published research that it has accomplished one or more of the following for its patients: (i) positively affected the progression of coronary heart disease, (ii) reduced the need for coronary bypass surgery, or, (iii) reduced the need for percutaneous coronary interventions.

An ICR program must also demonstrate through peer-reviewed, published research that it accomplished a statistically significant reduction in five or more of the following measures for patients from their levels before CR services to after CR services: (i) low density lipoprotein, (ii) triglycerides, (iii) body mass index, (iv) systolic blood pressure, (v) diastolic blood pressure, and (vi) the need for cholesterol, blood pressure, and diabetes medications.

A list of approved ICR programs, identified through the NCD process, will be posted to the CMS Web site and listed in the Federal Register.

Once an ICR program is approved through the NCD process, all prospective ICR sites wishing to furnish ICR items/services via an approved ICR program may enroll with their local contractor to become an ICR program supplier using the designated forms as specified at 42 CFR 424.510, and report specialty code 31 to be identified as an enrolled ICR supplier. For purposes of appealing an adverse determination concerning site approval, an ICR site is considered a supplier (or prospective supplier) as defined in 42 CFR 498.2.

CR/ICR Program Physician Requirements:

Physicians responsible for CR/ICR programs are identified as medical directors who oversee or supervise the CR/ICR program at a particular site. The medical director, in consultation with staff, is involved in directing the progress of individuals in the program. The medical director, as well as physicians acting as the supervising physician, must possess all of the following: (1) expertise in the management of individuals with cardiac pathophysiology, (2) cardiopulmonary training in basic life support or advanced cardiac life support, and (3) licensed to practice medicine in the state in which the CR/ICR program is offered. Direct physician supervision may be provided by a supervising physician or the medical director.

(See Pub. 100-03, Medicare National Coverage Determinations Manual, Chapter 1, Part 1, section 20.10.1, Pub. 100-04, Medicare Claims Processing Manual, Chapter 32, section 140, Pub. 100-08, Medicare Program Integrity Manual, Chapter 15, section 15.4.2.8, for specific claims processing, coding, and billing requirements for CR/ICR program services).

100-2, Chapter-15, 270

Telehealth Services

For information on telehealth services, see Pub. 100-04, Medicare Claims Processing Manual, chapter 12, section 190.

Background

Section 223 of the Medicare, Medicaid and SCHIP Benefits Improvement and Protection Act of 2000 (BIPA) -Revision of Medicare Reimbursement for Telehealth Services amended §1834 of the Act to provide for an expansion of Medicare payment for telehealth services.

Effective October 1, 2001, coverage and payment for Medicare telehealth includes consultation, office visits, individual psychotherapy, and pharmacologic management delivered via a telecommunications system. Eligible geographic areas include rural health professional shortage areas (HPSA) and counties not classified as a metropolitan statistical area (MSA). Additionally, Federal telemedicine demonstration projects as of December 31, 2000, may serve as the originating site regardless of geographic location.

An interactive telecommunications system is required as a condition of payment; however, BIPA does allow the use of asynchronous "store and forward" technology in delivering these services when the originating site is a Federal telemedicine demonstration program in Alaska or Hawaii. BIPA does not require that a practitioner present the patient for interactive telehealth services.

With regard to payment amount, BIPA specified that payment for the professional service performed by the distant site practitioner (i.e., where the expert physician or practitioner is physically located at time of telemedicine encounter) is equal to what would have been paid without the use of telemedicine. Distant site practitioners include only a physician as described in §1861(r) of the Act and a medical practitioner as described in §1842(b)(18)(C) of the Act. BIPA also expanded payment under Medicare to include a $20 originating site facility fee (location of beneficiary).

Previously, the Balanced Budget Act of 1997 (BBA) limited the scope of Medicare telehealth coverage to consultation services and the implementing regulation prohibited the use of an asynchronous 'store and forward' telecommunications system. The BBA of 1997 also required the professional fee to be shared between the referring and consulting practitioners, and prohibited Medicare payment for facility fees and line charges associated with the telemedicine encounter.

The BIPA required that Medicare Part B (Supplementary Medical Insurance) pay for this expansion of telehealth services beginning with services furnished on October 1, 2001.

Section 149 of the Medicare Improvements for Patients and Providers Act of 2008 (MIPPA) amended §1834(m) of the Act to add certain entities as originating sites for payment of telehealth services. Effective for services furnished on or after January 1, 2009, eligible originating sites include a hospital-based or critical access hospital-based renal dialysis center (including satellites); a skilled nursing facility (as defined in §1819(a) of the Act); and a community mental health center (as defined in §1861(ff)(3)(B) of the Act). MIPPA also amended§1888(e)(2)(A)(ii) of the Act to exclude telehealth services furnished under §1834(m)(4)(C)(ii)(VII) from the consolidated billing provisions of the skilled nursing facility prospective payment system (SNF PPS).

NOTE: MIPPA did not add independent renal dialysis facilities as originating sites for payment of telehealth services.

The telehealth provisions authorized by §1834(m) of the Act are implemented in 42 CFR 410.78 and 414.65.

100-2, Chapter-15, 280.1

Glaucoma Screening

A. Conditions of Coverage

The regulations implementing the Benefits Improvements and Protection Act of 2000, §102, provide for annual coverage for glaucoma screening for beneficiaries in the following high risk categories:

- Individuals with diabetes mellitus;

- Individuals with a family history of glaucoma; or

- African-Americans age 50 and over.

In addition, beginning with dates of service on or after January 1, 2006, 42 CFR 410.23(a)(2), revised, the definition of an eligible beneficiary in a high-risk category is expanded to include:

- Hispanic-Americans age 65 and over.

Medicare will pay for glaucoma screening examinations where they are furnished by or under the direct supervision in the office setting of an ophthalmologist or optometrist, who is legally authorized to perform the services under State law.

Screening for glaucoma is defined to include:

- A dilated eye examination with an intraocular pressure measurement; and

- A direct ophthalmoscopy examination, or a slit-lamp biomicroscopic examination.

Payment may be made for a glaucoma screening examination that is performed on an eligible beneficiary after at least 11 months have passed following the month in which the last covered glaucoma screening examination was performed.

The following HCPCS codes apply for glaucoma screening:

G0117-Glaucoma screening for high-risk patients furnished by an optometrist or ophthalmologist; and

G0118 -Glaucoma screening for high-risk patients furnished under the direct supervision of an optometrist or ophthalmologist.

The type of service for the above G codes is: TOS Q.

For providers who bill A/B MACs, applicable types of bill for screening glaucoma services are 13X, 22X, 23X, 71X, 73X, 75X, and 85X. The following revenue codes should be reported when billing for screening glaucoma services:

- Comprehensive outpatient rehabilitation facilities (CORFs), critical access hospitals (CAHs), skilled nursing facilities (SNFs), independent and provider-based RHCs and free standing and provider-based FQHCs bill for this service under revenue code 770. CAHs electing the optional method of payment for outpatient services report this service under revenue codes 96X, 97X,or 98X.

- Hospital outpatient departments bill for this service under any valid/appropriate revenue code. They are not required to report revenue code 770.

Calculating the Frequency

- Once a beneficiary has received a covered glaucoma screening procedure, the beneficiary may receive another procedure after 11 full months have passed. To determine the 11-month period, start the count beginning with the month after the month in which the previous covered screening procedure was performed.

Diagnosis Coding Requirements

- Providers bill glaucoma screening using diagnosis codes for screening services. Claims submitted without a screening diagnosis code may be returned to the provider as unprocessable.

Payment Methodology

A/B MACs (B)

- Contractors pay for glaucoma screening based on the Medicare physician fee schedule. Deductible and coinsurance apply. Claims from physicians or other providers where assignment was not taken are subject to the Medicare limiting charge (refer to the Medicare Claims Processing Manual, Chapter 12, "Physician/Non-physician Practitioners," for more information about the Medicare limiting charge).

A/B MACs (A)

- Payment is made for the facility expense as follows:
- Independent and provider-based RHC/free standing and provider-based FQHC -payment is made under the all-inclusive rate for the screening glaucoma service based on the visit furnished to the RHC/FQHC patient;
- CAH -payment is made on a reasonable cost basis unless the CAH has elected the optional method of payment for outpatient services in which case, procedures outlined in the Medicare Claims Processing Manual, Chapter 3, §30.1.1, should be followed;
- CORF -payment is made under the Medicare physician fee schedule;
- Hospital outpatient department -payment is made under outpatient prospective payment system (OPPS);
- Hospital inpatient Part B -payment is made under OPPS;
- SNF outpatient -payment is made under the Medicare physician fee schedule (MPFS); and
- SNF inpatient Part B -payment is made under MPFS

Deductible and coinsurance apply.

E. Special Billing Instructions for RHCs and FQHCs

Screening glaucoma services are considered RHC/FQHC services. RHCs and FQHCs bill the contractor under bill type 71X or 73X along with revenue code 770 and HCPCS codes G0117 or G0118 and RHC/FQHC revenue code 520 or 521 to report the related visit. Reporting of revenue code 770 and HCPCS codes G0117 and G0118 in addition to revenue code 520 or 521 is required for this service in order for CWF to perform frequency editing.

Payment should not be made for a screening glaucoma service unless the claim also contains a visit code for the service. Therefore, the contractor installs an edit in its system to assure payment is not made for revenue code 770 unless the claim also contains a visit revenue code (520 or 521).

100-2, Chapter-15, 280.5

Annual Wellness Visit (AWV) Providing Personalized Prevention Plan Services (PPPS)

A. General

Pursuant to section 4103 of the Affordable Care Act of 2010 (the ACA), the; Centers for Medicare & Medicaid Services (CMS) amended section 42 CFR 411.15(a)(1) and 42 CFR 411.15(k)(15) (list of examples of routine physical examinations excluded from coverage), effective for services furnished on or after January 1, 2011. This expanded coverage, as established at 42 CFR 410.15, is subject to certain eligibility and other limitations that allow payment for an annual wellness visit (AWV) providing personalized prevention plan services (PPPS), when performed by a health professional (as defined in this section), for an individual who is no longer within 12 months after the effective date of his/her first Medicare Part B coverage period, and has not received either an initial preventive physical examination (IPPE) or an AWV within the past 12 months. Medicare coinsurance and Part B deductibles do not apply.

The AWV will include the establishment of, or update to, the individual's medical/family history, measurement of his/her height, weight, body-mass index (BMI) or waist circumference, and blood pressure (BP), with the goal of health promotion and disease detection and encouraging patients to obtain the screening and preventive services that may already be covered and paid for under Medicare Part B. Definitions relative to the AWV are included below.

Coverage is available for an AWV that meets the following requirements:

1. It is performed by a health professional; and,
2. It is furnished to an eligible beneficiary who is no longer within 12 months after the effective date of his/her first Medicare Part B coverage period, and he/she has not received either an IPPE or an AWV providing PPPS within the past 12 months.

Sections 4103 and 4104 of the ACA also provide for a waiver of the Medicare coinsurance and Part B deductible requirements for an AWV effective for services furnished on or after January 1, 2011.

B. Definitions Relative to the AWV:

Detection of any cognitive impairment: The assessment of an individual's cognitive function by direct observation, with due consideration of information obtained by way of patient reports, concerns raised by family members, friends, caretakers, or others.

Eligible beneficiary: An individual who is no longer within 12 months after the effective date of his/her first Medicare Part B coverage period and who has not received either an IPPE or an AWV providing PPPS within the past 12 months.

Establishment of, or an update to, the individual's medical/family history:

At a minimum, the collection and documentation of the following:

a. Past medical and surgical history, including experiences with illnesses, hospital stays, operations, allergies, injuries, and treatments.
b. Use or exposure to medications and supplements, including calcium and vitamins.
c. Medical events in the beneficiary's parents and any siblings and children, including diseases that may be hereditary or place the individual at increased risk.

First AWV providing PPPS: The provision of the following services to an eligible beneficiary by a health professional that include, and take into account the results of, a health risk assessment as those terms are defined in this section:

a. Review (and administration if needed) of a health risk assessment (as defined in this section).
b. Establishment of an individual's medical/family history.
c. Establishment of a list of current providers and suppliers that are regularly involved in providing medical care to the individual.

d. Measurement of an individual's height, weight, BMI (or waist circumference, if appropriate), BP, and other routine measurements as deemed appropriate, based on the beneficiary's medical/family history.
e. Detection of any cognitive impairment that the individual may have as defined in this section.
f. Review of the individual's potential (risk factors) for depression, including current or past experiences with depression or other mood disorders, based on the use of an appropriate screening instrument for persons without a current diagnosis of depression, which the health professional may select from various available standardized screening tests designed for this purpose and recognized by national medical professional organizations.
g. Review of the individual's functional ability and level of safety based on direct observation, or the use of appropriate screening questions or a screening questionnaire, which the health professional may select from various available screening questions or standardized questionnaires designed for this purpose and recognized by national professional medical organizations.
h. Establishment of the following:
   1. A written screening schedule for the individual, such as a checklist for the next 5 to 10 years, as appropriate, based on recommendations of the United States Preventive Services Task Force (USPSTF) and the Advisory Committee on Immunization Practices (ACIP), and the individual's health risk assessment (as that term is defined in this section), the individual's health status, screening history, and age-appropriate preventive services covered by Medicare.
   2. A list of risk factors and conditions for which primary, secondary, or tertiary interventions are recommended or are underway for the individual, including any mental health conditions or any such risk factors or conditions that have been identified through an IPPE, and a list of treatment options and their associated risks and benefits.
i. Furnishing of personalized health advice to the individual and a referral, as appropriate, to health education or preventive counseling services or programs aimed at reducing identified risk factors and improving self-management, or community-based lifestyle interventions to reduce health risks and promote self-management and wellness, including weight loss, physical activity, smoking cessation, fall prevention, and nutrition.
j. Any other element determined appropriate through the National Coverage Determination (NCD) process.

Health professional:

a. A physician who is a doctor of medicine or osteopathy (as defined in section 1861(r)(1) of the Social Security Act (the Act); or,
b. A physician assistant, nurse practitioner, or clinical nurse specialist (as defined in section 1861(aa)(5) of the Act); or,
c. A medical professional (including a health educator, registered dietitian, or nutrition professional or other licensed practitioner) or a team of such medical professionals, working under the direct supervision (as defined in 42CFR 410.32(b)(3)(ii)) of a physician as defined in this section.

Health Risk Assessment means, for the purposes of the annual wellness visit, an evaluation tool that meets the following criteria:

a. collects self-reported information about the beneficiary.

b. can be administered independently by the beneficiary or administered by a health professional prior to or as part of the AWV encounter.

c. is appropriately tailored to and takes into account the communication needs of underserved populations, persons with limited English proficiency, and persons with health literacy needs.

d. takes no more than 20 minutes to complete.

e. addresses, at a minimum, the following topics:

1. demographic data, including but not limited to age, gender, race, and ethnicity.

2. self-assessment of health status, frailty, and physical functioning.

3. psychosocial risks, including but not limited to, depression/life satisfaction, stress, anger, loneliness/social isolation, pain, and fatigue.

4. Behavioral risks, including but not limited to, tobacco use, physical activity, nutrition and oral health, alcohol consumption, sexual health, motor vehicle safety (seat belt use), and home safety.

5. Activities of daily living (ADLs), including but not limited to, dressing, feeding, toileting, grooming, physical ambulation (including balance/risk of falls), and bathing.

6. Instrumental activities of daily living (IADLs), including but not limited to, shopping, food preparation, using the telephone, housekeeping, laundry, mode of transportation, responsibility for own medications, and ability to handle finances.

Review of the individual's functional ability and level of safety: At a minimum, includes assessment of the following topics:

a. Hearing impairment,

b. Ability to successfully perform activities of daily living,

c. Fall risk, and,

d. Home safety.

Subsequent AWV providing PPPS: The provision of the following services to an eligible beneficiary by a health professional that include, and take into account the results of an updated health risk assessment, as those terms are defined in this section:

a. Review (and administration if needed) of an updated health risk assessment (as defined in this section).

b. An update of the individual's medical/family history.

c. An update of the list of current providers and suppliers that are regularly involved in providing medical care to the individual, as that list was developed for the first AWV providing PPPS or the previous subsequent AWV providing PPPS.

d. Measurement of an individual's weight (or waist circumference), BP, and other routine measurements as deemed appropriate, based on the individual's medical/family history.

e. Detection of any cognitive impairment that the individual may have as defined in this section.

f. An update to the following:

1. The written screening schedule for the individual as that schedule is defined in this section, that was developed at the first AWV providing PPPS, and,

2. The list of risk factors and conditions for which primary, secondary, or tertiary interventions are recommended or are under way for the individual, as that list was developed at the first AWV providing PPPS or the previous subsequent AWV providing PPPS.

g. Furnishing of personalized health advice to the individual and a referral, as appropriate, to health education or preventive counseling services or programs as that advice and related services are defined for the first AWV providing PPPS.

h. Any other element determined appropriate by the Secretary through the NCD process.

See Pub. 100-04, Medicare Claims Processing Manual, chapter 18, section 140, for detailed claims processing and billing instructions.

100-2, Chapter-15, 290

Foot Care

A. Treatment of Subluxation of Foot

Subluxations of the foot are defined as partial dislocations or displacements of joint surfaces, tendons ligaments, or muscles of the foot. Surgical or nonsurgical treatments undertaken for the sole purpose of correcting a subluxated structure in the foot as an isolated entity are not covered.

However, medical or surgical treatment of subluxation of the ankle joint (talo-crural joint) is covered. In addition, reasonable and necessary medical or surgical services, diagnosis, or treatment for medical conditions that have resulted from or are associated with partial displacement of structures is covered. For example, if a patient has osteoarthritis that has resulted in a partial displacement of joints in the foot, and the primary treatment is for the osteoarthritis, coverage is provided.

B. Exclusions from Coverage

The following foot care services are generally excluded from coverage under both Part A and Part B. (See §290.Fand §290.Gfor instructions on applying foot care exclusions.)

1. Treatment of Flat Foot

The term "flat foot" is defined as a condition in which one or more arches of the foot have flattened out. Services or devices directed toward the care or correction of such conditions, including the prescription of supportive devices, are not covered.

2. Routine Foot Care

Except as provided above, routine foot care is excluded from coverage. Services that normally are considered routine and not covered by Medicare include the following:

- The cutting or removal of corns and calluses;

- The trimming, cutting, clipping, or debriding of nails; and

- Other hygienic and preventive maintenance care, such as cleaning and soaking the feet, the use of skin creams to maintain skin tone of either ambulatory or bedfast patients, and any other service performed in the absence of localized illness, injury, or symptoms involving the foot.

3. Supportive Devices for Feet

Orthopedic shoes and other supportive devices for the feet generally are not covered. However, this exclusion does not apply to such a shoe if it is an integral part of a leg brace, and its expense is included as part of the cost of the brace. Also, this exclusion does not apply to therapeutic shoes furnished to diabetics.

C. Exceptions to Routine Foot Care Exclusion

1. Necessary and Integral Part of Otherwise Covered Services

In certain circumstances, services ordinarily considered to be routine may be covered if they are performed as a necessary and integral part of otherwise covered services, such as diagnosis and treatment of ulcers, wounds, or infections.

2. Treatment of Warts on Foot

The treatment of warts (including plantar warts) on the foot is covered to the same extent as services provided for the treatment of warts located elsewhere on the body.

3. Presence of Systemic Condition

The presence of a systemic condition such as metabolic, neurologic, or peripheral vascular disease may require scrupulous foot care by a professional that in the absence of such condition(s) would be considered routine (and, therefore, excluded from coverage). Accordingly, foot care that would otherwise be considered routine may be covered when systemic condition(s) result in severe circulatory embarrassment or areas of diminished sensation in the individual's legs or feet. (See subsection A.)

In these instances, certain foot care procedures that otherwise are considered routine (e.g., cutting or removing corns and calluses, or trimming, cutting, clipping, or debriding nails) may pose a hazard when performed by a nonprofessional person on patients with such systemic conditions. (See§290.G for procedural instructions.)

4. Mycotic Nails

In the absence of a systemic condition, treatment of mycotic nails may be covered.

The treatment of mycotic nails for an ambulatory patient is covered only when the physician attending the patient's mycotic condition documents that (1) there is clinical evidence of mycosis of the toenail, and (2) the patient has marked limitation of ambulation, pain, or secondary infection resulting from the thickening and dystrophy of the infected toenail plate.

The treatment of mycotic nails for a nonambulatory patient is covered only when the physician attending the patient's mycotic condition documents that (1) there is clinical evidence of mycosis of the toenail, and (2) the patient suffers from pain or secondary infection resulting from the thickening and dystrophy of the infected toenail plate.

For the purpose of these requirements, documentation means any written information that is required by the carrier in order for services to be covered. Thus, the information submitted with claims must be substantiated by information found in the patient's medical record. Any information, including that contained in a form letter, used for documentation purposes is subject to carrier verification in order to ensure that the information adequately justifies coverage of the treatment of mycotic nails.

D. Systemic Conditions That Might Justify Coverage

Although not intended as a comprehensive list, the following metabolic, neurologic, and peripheral vascular diseases (with synonyms in parentheses) most commonly represent the underlying conditions that might justify coverage for routine foot care.

Diabetes mellitus *

Arteriosclerosis obliterans (A.S.O., arteriosclerosis of the extremities, occlusive peripheral arteriosclerosis)

Buerger's disease (thromboangiitis obliterans)

Chronic thrombophlebitis *

Peripheral neuropathies involving the feet-

Associated with malnutrition and vitamin deficiency *

- Malnutrition (general, pellagra)
- Alcoholism
- Malabsorption (celiac disease, tropical sprue)
- Pernicious anemia

Associated with carcinoma *

Associated with diabetes mellitus *

Associated with drugs and toxins *

Associated with multiple sclerosis *

Associated with uremia (chronic renal disease) *

Associated with traumatic injury

Associated with leprosy or neurosyphilis

Associated with hereditary disorders

- Hereditary sensory radicular neuropathy
- Angiokeratoma corporis diffusum (Fabry's)
- Amyloid neuropathy

When the patient's condition is one of those designated by an asterisk (*), routine procedure s are covered only if the patient is under the active care of a doctor of medicine or osteopathy who documents the condition.

E. Supportive Devices for Feet

Orthopedic shoes and other supportive devices for the feet generally are not covered. However, this exclusion does not apply to such a shoe if it is an integral part of a leg brace, and its expense is included as part of the cost of the brace. Also, this exclusion does not apply to therapeutic shoes furnished to diabetics.

F. Presumption of Coverage

In evaluating whether the routine services can be reimbursed, a presumption of coverage may be made where the evidence available discloses certain physical and/or clinical findings consistent with the diagnosis and indicative of severe peripheral involvement. For purposes of applying this presumption the following findings are pertinent:

Class A Findings

Nontraumatic amputation of foot or integral skeletal portion thereof.

Class B Findings

Absent posterior tibial pulse;

Advanced trophic changes as: hair growth (decrease or absence) nail changes (thickening) pigmentary changes (discoloration) skin texture (thin, shiny) skin color (rubor or redness) (Three required); and

Absent dorsalis pedis pulse.

Class C Findings

Claudication;

Temperature changes (e.g., cold feet);

Edema;

Paresthesias (abnormal spontaneous sensations in the feet); and

Burning.

The presumption of coverage may be applied when the physician rendering the routine foot care has identified:

1. A Class A finding;
2. Two of the Class B findings; or
3. One Class B and two Class C findings

Cases evidencing findings falling short of these alternatives may involve podiatric treatment that may constitute covered care and should be reviewed by the intermediary's medical staff and developed as necessary.

For purposes of applying the coverage presumption where the routine services have been rendered by a podiatrist, the contractor may deem the active care requirement met if the claim or other evidence available discloses that the patient has seen an M.D. or D.O. for treatment and/or evaluation of the complicating disease process during the 6-month period prior to the rendition of the routine-type services. The intermediary may also accept the podiatrist's statement that the diagnosing and treating M.D. or D.O. also concurs with the podiatrist's findings as to the severity of the peripheral involvement indicated.

Services ordinarily considered routine might also be covered if they are performed as a necessary and integral part of otherwise covered services, such as diagnosis and treatment of diabetic ulcers, wounds, and infections.

G. Application of Foot Care Exclusions to Physician's Services

The exclusion of foot care is determined by the nature of the service. Thus, payment for an excluded service should be denied whether performed by a podiatrist, osteopath, or a doctor of medicine, and without regard to the difficulty or complexity of the procedure.

When an itemized bill shows both covered services and noncovered services not integrally related to the covered service, the portion of charges attributable to the noncovered services should be denied. (For example, if an itemized bill shows surgery for an ingrown toenail and also removal of calluses not necessary for the performance of toe surgery, any additional charge attributable to removal of the calluses should be denied.)

In reviewing claims involving foot care, the carrier should be alert to the following exceptional situations:

1. Payment may be made for incidental noncovered services performed as a necessary and integral part of, and secondary to, a covered procedure. For example, if trimming of toenails is required for application of a cast to a fractured foot, the carrier need not allocate and deny a portion of the charge for the trimming of the nails. However, a separately itemized charge for such excluded service should be disallowed. When the primary procedure is covered the administration of anesthesia necessary for the performance of such procedure is also covered.
2. Payment may be made for initial diagnostic services performed in connection with a specific symptom or complaint if it seems likely that its treatment would be covered even though the resulting diagnosis may be one requiring only noncovered care.

The name of the M.D. or D.O. who diagnosed the complicating condition must be submitted with the claim. In those cases, where active care is required, the approximate date the beneficiary was last seen by such physician must also be indicated.

NOTE: Section 939 of P.L. 96-499 removed "warts" from the routine foot care exclusion effective July 1, 1981.

Relatively few claims for routine-type care are anticipated considering the severity of conditions contemplated as the basis for this exception. Claims for this type of foot care should not be paid in the absence of convincing evidence that nonprofessional performance of the service would have been hazardous for the beneficiary because of an underlying systemic disease. The mere statement of a diagnosis such as those mentioned in §D above does not of itself indicate the severity of the condition. Where development is indicated to verify diagnosis and/or severity the carrier should follow existing claims processing practices, which may include review of carrier's history and medical consultation as well as physician contacts.

The rules in §290.F concerning presumption of coverage also apply.

Codes and policies for routine foot care and supportive devices for the feet are not exclusively for the use of podiatrists. These codes must be used to report foot care services regardless of the specialty of the physician who furnishes the services. Carriers must instruct physicians to use the most appropriate code available when billing for routine foot care.

100-2, Chapter-15, 300

Diabetes Self-Management Training Services

Section 4105 of the Balanced Budget Act of 1997 permits Medicare coverage of diabetes self-management training (DSMT) services when these services are furnished by a certified provider who meets certain quality standards. This program is intended to educate beneficiaries in the successful self-management of diabetes. The program includes instructions in self-monitoring of blood glucose; education about diet and exercise; an insulin treatment plan developed specifically for the patient who is insulin-dependent; and motivation for patients to use the skills for self-management.

Diabetes self-management training services may be covered by Medicare only if the treating physician or treating qualified non-physician practitioner who is managing the beneficiary's diabetic condition certifies that such services are needed. The referring physician or qualified non-physician practitioner must maintain the plan of care in the beneficiary's medical record and documentation substantiating the need for training on an individual basis when group training is typically covered, if so ordered. The order must also include a statement signed by the physician that the service is needed as well as the following:

- The number of initial or follow-up hours ordered (the physician can order less than 10 hours of training);
- The topics to be covered in training (initial training hours can be used for the full initial training program or specific areas such as nutrition or insulin training); and
- A determination that the beneficiary should receive individual or group training.

The provider of the service must maintain documentation in a file that includes the original order from the physician and any special conditions noted by the physician.

When the training under the order is changed, the training order/referral must be signed by the physician or qualified non-physician practitioner treating the beneficiary and maintained in the beneficiary's file in the DSMT's program records.

NOTE: All entities billing for DSMT under the fee-for-service payment system or other payment systems must meet all national coverage requirements.

100-2, Chapter-15, 300.2

Certified Providers

A designated certified provider bills for DSMT provided by an accredited DSMT program. Certified providers must submit a copy of their accreditation certificate to the contractor. The statute states that a "certified provider" is a physician or other individual or entity designated by the Secretary that, in addition to providing outpatient self-management training services, provides other items and services for which payment may be made under title XVIII, and meets certain quality standards. The CMS is designating all providers and suppliers that bill Medicare for other individual services such as hospital outpatient departments, renal dialysis facilities, physicians and durable medical equipment suppliers as certified. All suppliers/providers who may bill for other Medicare services or items and who represent a DSMT program that is accredited as meeting quality standards can bill and receive payment for the entire DSMT program. Registered dietitians are eligible to bill on behalf of an entire DSMT program on or after January 1, 2002, as long as the provider has obtained a Medicare provider number. A dietitian may not be the sole provider of the DSMT service. There is an exception for rural areas. In a rural area, an individual who is qualified as a registered dietitian and as a certified diabetic educator who is currently certified by an organization approved by CMS may furnish training and is deemed to meet the multidisciplinary team requirement.

The CMS will not reimburse services on a fee-for-service basis rendered to a beneficiary under Part A.

NOTE: While separate payment is not made for this service to Rural Health Clinics (RHCs), the service is covered but is considered included in the all-inclusive encounter rate. Effective January 1, 2006, payment for DSMT provided in a Federally Qualified Health Clinic (FQHC) that meets all of the requirements identified in Pub. 100-04, chapter 18, section 120 may be made in addition to one other visit the beneficiary had during the same day.

All DSMT programs must be accredited as meeting quality standards by a CMS approved national accreditation organization. Currently, CMS recognizes the American Diabetes Association, American Association of Diabetes Educators and the Indian Health Service as approved national accreditation organizations. Programs without accreditation by a CMS-approved national accreditation organization are not covered. Certified providers may be asked to submit updated accreditation documents at any time or to submit outcome data to an organization designated by CMS.

Enrollment of DMEPOS Suppliers

The DMEPOS suppliers are reimbursed for diabetes training through local carriers. In order to file claims for DSMT, a DMEPOS supplier must be enrolled in the Medicare program with the National Supplier Clearinghouse (NSC). The supplier must also meet the quality standards of a CMS-approved national accreditation organization as stated above. DMEPOS suppliers must obtain a provider number from the local carrier in order to bill for DSMT.

The carrier requires a completed Form CMS-855, along with an accreditation certificate as part of the provider application process. After it has been determined that the quality standards are met, a billing number is assigned to the supplier. Once a supplier has received a National Provider Identification (NPI) number, the supplier can begin receiving reimbursement for this service.

Carriers should contact the National Supplier Clearinghouse (NSC) according to the instruction in Pub 100-08, the Medicare Program Integrity Manual, Chapter 10, "Healthcare Provider/Supplier Enrollment," to verify an applicant is currently enrolled and eligible to receive direct payment from the Medicare program.

The applicant is assigned specialty 87.

Any DMEPOS supplier that has its billing privileges deactivated or revoked by the NSC will also have the billing number deactivated by the carrier.

100-2, Chapter-15, 300.3

Frequency of Training

A -Initial Training

The initial year for DSMT is the 12 month period following the initial date.

Medicare will cover initial training that meets the following conditions:

- Is furnished to a beneficiary who has not previously received initial or follow-up training under HCPCS codes G0108 or G0109;
- Is furnished within a continuous 12-month period;
- Does not exceed a total of 10 hours* (the 10 hours of training can be done in any combination of 1/2 hour increments);
- With the exception of 1 hour of individual training, training is usually furnished in a group setting, which can contain other patients besides Medicare beneficiaries, and;
- One hour of individual training may be used for any part of the training including insulin training.

* When a claim contains a DSMT HCPCS code and the associated units cause the total time for the DSMT initial year to exceed '10' hours, a CWF error will set.

B -Follow-Up Training

Medicare covers follow-up training under the following conditions:

- No more than 2 hours individual or group training per beneficiary per year;
- Group training consists of 2 to 20 individuals who need not all be Medicare beneficiaries;
- Follow-up training for subsequent years is based on a 12 month calendar after completion of the full 10 hours of initial training;
- Follow-up training is furnished in increments of no less than one-half hour*; and
- The physician (or qualified non-physician practitioner) treating the beneficiary must document in the beneficiary's medical record that the beneficiary is a diabetic.

*When a claim contains a DSMT HCPCS code and the associated units cause the total time for any follow-up year to exceed 2 hours, a CWF error will set.

100-2, Chapter-15, 300.4

Coverage Requirements for Individual Training

Medicare covers training on an individual basis for a Medicare beneficiary under any of the following conditions.

- No group session is available within 2 months of the date the training is ordered;

- The beneficiary's physician (or qualified non-physician practitioner) documents in the beneficiary's medical record that the beneficiary has special needs resulting from conditions, such as severe vision, hearing or language limitations or other such special conditions as identified by the treating physician or non-physician practitioner, that will hinder effective participation in a group training session; or
- The physician orders additional insulin training.
- The need for individual training must be identified by the physician or non-physician practitioner in the referral.

NOTE: If individual training has been provided to a Medicare beneficiary and subsequently the carrier or intermediary determines that training should have been provided in a group, carriers and intermediaries down-code the reimbursement from individual to the group level and provider education would be the appropriate actions instead of denying the service as billed.

100-2, Chapter-15, 310

Kidney Disease Patient Education Services

By definition, chronic kidney disease (CKD) is kidney damage for 3 months or longer, regardless of the cause of kidney damage. CKD typically evolves over a long period of time and patients may not have symptoms until significant, possibly irreversible, damage has been done. Complications can develop from kidneys that do not function properly, such as high blood pressure, anemia, and weak bones. When CKD progresses, it may lead to kidney failure, which requires artificial means to perform kidney functions (dialysis) or a kidney transplant to maintain life.

Patients can be classified into 5 stages based on their glomerular filtration rate (GFR, how quickly blood is filtered through the kidneys), with stage I having kidney damage with normal or increased GFR to stage V with kidney failure, also called end-stage renal disease (ESRD). Once patients with CKD are identified, treatment is available to help prevent complications of decreased kidney function, slow the progression of kidney disease, and reduce the risk of other diseases such as heart disease.

Beneficiaries with CKD may benefit from kidney disease education (KDE) interventions due to the large amount of medical information that could affect patient outcomes, including the increasing emphasis on self-care and patients' desire for informed, autonomous decision-making. Pre-dialysis education can help patients achieve better understanding of their illness, dialysis modality options, and may help delay the need for dialysis. Education interventions should be patient-centered, encourage collaboration, offer support to the patient, and be delivered consistently.

Effective for claims with dates of service on and after January 1, 2010, Section 152(b) of the Medicare Improvements for Patients and Providers Act of 2008 (MIPPA) covers KDE services under Medicare Part B. KDE services are designed to provide beneficiaries with Stage IV CKD comprehensive information regarding: the management of comorbidities, including delaying the need for dialysis; prevention of uremic complications; all therapeutic options (each option for renal replacement therapy, dialysis access options, and transplantation); ensuring that the beneficiary has opportunities to actively participate in his/her choice of therapy; and that the services be tailored to meet the beneficiary's needs.

Regulations for KDE services were established at 42 CFR 410.48. Claims processing instructions and billing requirements can be found in Pub. 100-04, Medicare Claims Processing Manual, Chapter 32 –Billing Requirements for Special Services, Section 20.

100-2, Chapter-15, 310.1

Beneficiaries Eligible for Coverage

Medicare Part B covers outpatient, face-to-face KDE services for a beneficiary that:

- is diagnosed with Stage IV CKD, using the Modification of Diet in Renal Disease (MDRD) Study formula (severe decrease in GFR, GFR value of 15-29 mL/min/1.73 m2), and
- obtains a referral from the physician managing the beneficiary's kidney condition. The referral should be documented in the beneficiary's medical records.

100-2, Chapter-15, 310.2

Qualified Person

Medicare Part B covers KDE services provided by a 'qualified person,' meaning a:

- physician (as defined in section 30 of this chapter),
- physician assistant, nurse practitioner, or clinical nurse specialist (as defined in sections 190, 200, and 210 of this chapter),
- hospital, critical access hospital (CAH), skilled nursing facility (SNF), comprehensive outpatient rehabilitation facility (CORF), home health agency (HHA), or hospice, if the KDE services are provided in a rural area (using the actual geographic location core based statistical area (CBSA) to identify facilities located in rural areas), or
- hospital or CAH that is treated as being rural (was reclassified from urban to rural status per 42 CFR 412.103).

NOTE: The "incident to" requirements at section 1861(s)(2)(A) of the Social Security Act (the Act) do not apply to KDE services.

The following providers are not 'qualified persons' and are excluded from furnishing KDE services:

- A hospital, CAH, SNF, CORF, HHA, or hospice located outside of a rural area (using the actual geographic location CBSA to identify facilities located outside of a rural area), unless the services are furnished by a hospital or CAH that is treated as being in a rural area; and
- Renal dialysis facilities.

100-2, Chapter-15, 310.3

Limitations for Coverage

Medicare Part B covers KDE services:

- Up to six (6) sessions as a beneficiary lifetime maximum. A session is 1 hour. In order to bill for a session, a session must be at least 31 minutes in duration. A session that lasts at least 31 minutes, but less than 1 hour still constitutes 1 session.
- On an individual basis or in group settings; if the services are provided in a group setting, a group consists of 2 to 20 individuals who need not all be Medicare beneficiaries.

NOTE: Two HCPCS codes were created for this benefit and one or the other must be present, along with the appropriate ICD diagnosis codes.

The diagnosis codes are:

- ICD-9-CM - code 585.4 (chronic kidney disease, Stage IV (severe)), or

- ICD-10-CM - code N18.4 (chronic kidney disease, Stage IV).

The HCPCS codes are:

- G0420: Face-to-face educational services related to the care of chronic kidney disease; individual, per session, per one hour

- G0421: Face-to-face educational services related to the care of chronic kidney disease; group, per session, per one hour

100-2, Chapter-15, 310.4

Standards for Content

Medicare Part B covers KDE services, provided by a qualified person, which provide comprehensive information regarding:

A. The management of comorbidities, including delaying the need for dialysis, which includes, but is not limited to, the following topics:

- Prevention and treatment of cardiovascular disease,

- Prevention and treatment of diabetes,

- Hypertension management,

- Anemia management,

- Bone disease and disorders of calcium and phosphorus metabolism management,

- Symptomatic neuropathy management, and

- Impairments in functioning and well-being.

B. Prevention of uremic complications, which includes, but is not limited to, the following topics

- Information on how the kidneys work and what happens when the kidneys fail,

- Understanding if remaining kidney function can be protected, preventing disease progression, and realistic chances of survival,

- Diet and fluid restrictions, and

- Medication review, including how each medication works, possible side effects and minimization of side effects, the importance of compliance, and informed decision making if the patient decides not to take a specific drug.

C. Therapeutic options, treatment modalities and settings, advantages and disadvantages of each treatment option, and how the treatments replace the kidney, including, but not limited to, the following topics:

- Hemodialysis, both at home and in-facility;

- Peritoneal dialysis (PD), including intermittent PD, continuous ambulatory PD, and continuous cycling PD, both at home and in-facility;

- All dialysis access options for hemodialysis and peritoneal dialysis; and

- Transplantation.

D. Opportunities for beneficiaries to actively participate in the choice of therapy and be tailored to meet the needs of the individual beneficiary involved, which includes, but is not limited to, the following topics:

- Physical symptoms,

- Impact on family and social life,

- Exercise,

- The right to refuse treatment,

- Impact on work and finances,

- The meaning of test results, and

- Psychological impact.

100-2, Chapter-15, 310.5

Outcomes Assessment

Qualified persons that provide KDE services must develop outcomes assessments that are designed to measure beneficiary knowledge about CKD and its treatment. The assessment must be administered to the beneficiary during a KDE session, and be made available to the Centers for Medicare & Medicaid Services (CMS) upon request. The outcomes assessments serve to assist KDE educators and CMS in improving subsequent KDE programs, patient understanding, and assess program effectiveness of:

- Preparing the beneficiary to make informed decisions about their healthcare options related to CKD, and

- Meeting the communication needs of underserved populations, including persons with disabilities, persons with limited English proficiency, and persons with health literacy needs.

100-2, Chapter-16, 10

General Exclusions From Coverage

No payment can be made under either the hospital insurance or supplementary medical insurance program for certain items and services, when the following conditions exist:

- Not reasonable and necessary (§20);

- No legal obligation to pay for or provide (§40);

- Paid for by a governmental entity (§50);

- Not provided within United States (§60);

- Resulting from war (§70);

- Personal comfort (§80);

- Routine services and appliances (§90);

- Custodial care (§110);

- Cosmetic surgery (§120);

- Charges by immediate relatives or members of household (§130);

- Dental services (§140);

- Paid or expected to be paid under workers' compensation (§150);

- Non-physician services provided to a hospital inpatient that were not provided directly or arranged for by the hospital (§170);

- Services Related to and Required as a Result of Services Which are not Covered Under Medicare (§180);

- Excluded foot care services and supportive devices for feet (§30); or,

- Excluded investigational devices (See Chapter 14).

100-2, Chapter-16, 20

Services Not Reasonable and Necessary

Items and services which are not reasonable and necessary for the diagnosis or treatment of illness or injury or to improve the functioning of a malformed body member are not covered, e.g., payment cannot be made for the rental of a special hospital bed to be used by the patient in their home unless it was a reasonable and necessary part of the patient's treatment. See also §80.

A health care item or service for the purpose of causing, or assisting to cause, the death of any individual (assisted suicide) is not covered. This prohibition does not apply to the provision of an item or service for the purpose of alleviating pain or discomfort, even if such use may increase the risk of death, so long as the item or service is not furnished for the specific purpose of causing death.

100-2, Chapter-16, 90

Routine Services and Appliances

Routine physical checkups; eyeglasses, contact lenses, and eye examinations for the purpose of prescribing, fitting, or changing eyeglasses; eye refractions by whatever practitioner and for whatever purpose performed; hearing aids and examinations for hearing aids; and immunizations are not covered.

The routine physical checkup exclusion applies to (a) examinations performed without relationship to treatment or diagnosis for a specific illness, symptom, complaint, or injury; and (b) examinations required by third parties such as insurance companies, business establishments, or Government agencies.

The routine physical checkup exclusion does not apply to the following services (as noted in section 42 CFR 411.15(a)(1)):

- Screening mammography,
- Colorectal cancer screening tests,
- Screening pelvic exams,
- Prostate cancer screening tests,
- Glaucoma screening exams,
- Ultrasound screening for abdominal aortic aneurysms (AAA),
- cardiovascular disease screening tests,
- diabetes screening tests,
- screening electrocardiogram,
- Initial preventive physical examinations,
- Annual wellness visits providing personalized prevention plan services, and
- Additional preventive services that meet the criteria specified in 42 CFR 410.64.

If the claim is for a diagnostic test or examination performed solely for the purpose of establishing a claim under title IV of Public Law 91-173, "Black Lung Benefits," the service is not covered under Medicare and the claimant should be advised to contact their Social Security office regarding the filing of a claim for reimbursement under the "Black Lung" program.

The exclusions apply to eyeglasses or contact lenses, and eye examinations for the purpose of prescribing, fitting, or changing eyeglasses or contact lenses for refractive errors. The exclusions do not apply to physicians' services (and services incident to a physicians' service) performed in conjunction with an eye disease, as for example, glaucoma or cataracts, or to

post-surgical prosthetic lenses which are customarily used during convalescence from eye surgery in which the lens of the eye was removed, or to permanent prosthetic lenses required by an individual lacking the organic lens of the eye, whether by surgical removal or congenital disease. Such prosthetic lens is a replacement for an internal body organ -the lens of the eye. (See the Medicare Benefit Policy Manual, Chapter 15, "Covered Medical and Other Health Services," §120).

Expenses for all refractive procedures, whether performed by an ophthalmologist (or any other physician) or an optometrist and without regard to the reason for performance of the refraction, are excluded from coverage.

A. Immunizations

Vaccinations or inoculations are excluded as immunizations unless they are either:

- Directly related to the treatment of an injury or direct exposure to a disease or condition, such as antirabies treatment, tetanus antitoxin or booster vaccine, botulin antitoxin, antivenin sera, or immune globulin. (In the absence of injury or direct exposure, preventive immunization (vaccination or inoculation) against such diseases as smallpox, polio, diphtheria, etc., is not covered.); or
- Specifically covered by statute, as described in the Medicare Benefit Policy Manual, Chapter 15, "Covered Medical and Other Health Services," §50.4.4.2.

B. Antigens

Prior to the Omnibus Reconciliation Act of 1980, a physician who prepared an antigen for a patient could not be reimbursed for that service unless the physician also administered the antigen to the patient. Effective January 1, 1981, payment may be made for a reasonable supply of antigens that have been prepared for a particular patient even though they have not been administered to the patient by the same physician who prepared them if:

- The antigens are prepared by a physician who is a doctor of medicine or osteopathy, and
- The physician who prepared the antigens has examined the patient and has determined a plan of treatment and a dosage regimen.

A reasonable supply of antigens is considered to be not more than a 12-month supply of antigens that has been prepared for a particular patient at any one time. The purpose of the reasonable supply limitation is to assure that the antigens retain their potency and effectiveness over the period in which they are to be administered to the patient. (See the Medicare Benefit Policy Manual, Chapter 15, "Covered Medical and Other Health Services," §50.4.4.1)

100-2, Chapter-16, 140

Dental Services Exclusion

Items and services in connection with the care, treatment, filling, removal, or replacement of teeth, or structures directly supporting the teeth are not covered. Structures directly supporting the teeth mean the periodontium, which includes the gingivae, dentogingival junction, periodontal membrane, cementum, and alveolar process. However, payment may be made for certain other services of a dentist. (See the Medicare Benefit Policy Manual, Chapter 15, "Covered Medical and Other Health Services," §150.)

The hospitalization or nonhospitalization of a patient has no direct bearing on the coverage or exclusion of a given dental procedure.

When an excluded service is the primary procedure involved, it is not covered regardless of its complexity or difficulty. For example, the extraction of an impacted tooth is not covered. Similarly, an alveoplasty (the surgical improvement of the shape and condition of the alveolar process) and a frenectomy are excluded from coverage when either of these procedures is performed in connection with an excluded service, e.g., the preparation of the mouth for dentures. In like manner, the removal of the torus palatinus (a bony protuberance of the hard palate) could be a covered service. However, with rare exception, this surgery is performed in connection with an excluded service, i.e., the preparation of the mouth for dentures. Under such circumstances, reimbursement is not made for this purpose.

The extraction of teeth to prepare the jaw for radiation treatments of neoplastic disease is also covered. This is an exception to the requirement that to be covered, a noncovered procedure or service performed by a dentist must be an incident to and an integral part of a covered procedure or service performed by the dentist. Ordinarily, the dentist extracts the patient's teeth, but another physician, e.g., a radiologist, administers the radiation treatments.

Whether such services as the administration of anesthesia, diagnostic X-rays, and other related procedures are covered depends upon whether the primary procedure being performed by the dentist is covered. Thus, an X-ray taken in connection with the reduction of a fracture of the jaw or facial bone is covered. However, a single X-ray or X-ray survey taken in connection with the care or treatment of teeth or the periodontium is not covered.

See also the Medicare Benefit Policy Manual, Chapter 1, "Inpatient Hospital Services," §70, and Chapter 15, "Covered Medical and Other Health Services," §150 for additional information on dental services

100-3, Chapter-1, Part 1, 10.2

Transcutaneous Electrical Nerve Stimulation (TENS) for Acute Post-Operative Pain

The use of transcutaneous electrical nerve stimulation (TENS) for the relief of acute post-operative pain is covered under Medicare. TENS may be covered whether used as an adjunct to the use of drugs, or as an alternative to drugs, in the treatment of acute pain resulting from surgery.

The TENS devices, whether durable or disposable, may be used in furnishing this service. When used for the purpose of treating acute post-operative pain, TENS devices are considered supplies. As such they may be hospital supplies furnished inpatients covered under Part A, or supplies incident to a physician's service when furnished in connection with surgery done on an outpatient basis, and covered under Part B.

It is expected that TENS, when used for acute post-operative pain, will be necessary for relatively short periods of time, usually 30 days or less. In cases when TENS is used for longer periods, contractors should attempt to ascertain whether TENS is no longer being used for acute pain but rather for chronic pain, in which case the TENS device may be covered as durable medical equipment as described in §160.27.

Cross-references:

Medicare Benefit Policy Manual, Chapter 1, "Inpatient Hospital Services," §40;

Medicare Benefit Policy Manual, Chapter 2, "Hospital Services Covered Under Part B," §§20, 20.4, and 80; Medicare Benefit Policy Manual, Chapter 15, "Covered Medical and other Health Services, §110."

100-3, Chapter-1, Part 1, 20.21

Chelation Therapy for Treatment of Atherosclerosis

Chelation therapy is the application of chelation techniques for the therapeutic or preventive effects of removing unwanted metal ions from the body. The application of chelation therapy using ethylenediamine-tetra-acetic acid (EDTA) for the treatment and prevention of atherosclerosis is controversial. There is no widely accepted rationale to explain the beneficial effects attributed to this therapy. Its safety is questioned and its clinical effectiveness has never been established by well-designed, controlled clinical trials. It is not widely accepted and practiced by American physicians. EDTA chelation therapy for atherosclerosis is considered experimental. For these reasons, EDTA chelation therapy for the treatment or prevention of atherosclerosis is not covered. Some practitioners refer to this therapy as chemoendarterectomy and may also show a diagnosis other than atherosclerosis, such as arteriosclerosis or calcinosis. Claims employing such variant terms should also be denied under this section.

Cross-reference: §20.22

100-3, Chapter-1, Part 1, 20.22

Ethylenediamine-Tetra-Acetic (EDTA) Chelation Therapy for Treatment of Atherosclerosis

The use of EDTA as a chelating agent to treat atherosclerosis, arteriosclerosis, calcinosis, or similar generalized condition not listed by the FDA as an approved use is not covered. Any such use of EDTA is considered experimental. See §20.21 for an explanation of this conclusion.

100-3, Chapter-1, Part 1, 40.7

Outpatient Intravenous Insulin Treatment (Effective December 23, 2009)

A. General

The term outpatient intravenous (IV) insulin therapy (OIVIT) refers to an outpatient regimen that integrates pulsatile or continuous intravenous infusion of insulin via any means, guided by the results of measurement of:

- respiratory quotient; and/or
- urine urea nitrogen (UUN); and/or
- arterial, venous, or capillary glucose; and/or
- potassium concentration; and

performed in scheduled recurring periodic intermittent episodes.

This regimen is also sometimes termed Cellular Activation Therapy (CAT), Chronic Intermittent Intravenous Insulin Therapy (CIIT), Hepatic Activation Therapy (HAT), Intercellular Activation Therapy (iCAT), Metabolic Activation Therapy (MAT), Pulsatile Intravenous Insulin Treatment (PIVIT), Pulse Insulin Therapy (PIT), and Pulsatile Therapy (PT).

In OIVIT, insulin is intravenously administered in the outpatient setting for a variety of indications. Most commonly, it is delivered in pulses, but it may be delivered as a more conventional drip solution. The insulin administration is adjunctive to the patient's routine diabetic management regimen (oral agent or insulin-based) or other disease management regimen, typically performed on an intermittent basis (often weekly), and frequently performed chronically without duration limits. Glucose or other carbohydrate is available ad libitum (in accordance with patient desire).

B. Nationally Covered Indications

N/A

C. Nationally Non-Covered Indications

Effective for claims with dates of service on and after December 23, 2009, the Centers for Medicare and Medicaid Services (CMS) determines that the evidence does not support a conclusion that OIVIT improves health outcomes in Medicare beneficiaries. Therefore, CMS has determined that OIVIT is not reasonable and necessary for any indication under section 1862(a)(1)(A) of the Social Security Act. Services comprising an OIVIT regimen are nationally non-covered under Medicare when furnished pursuant to an OIVIT regimen (see subsection A. above).

D. Other

Individual components of OIVIT may have medical uses in conventional treatment regimens for diabetes and other conditions. Coverage for such other uses may be determined by other local or national Medicare determinations, and do not pertain to OIVIT. For example, see Pub. 100-03, NCD Manual, Section 40.2, Home Blood Glucose Monitors, Section 40.3, Closed-loop Blood Glucose Control Devices (CBGCD), Section 190.20, Blood Glucose Testing, and Section 280.14, Infusion Pumps, as well as Pub. 100-04, Claims Processing Manual, Chapter 18, Section 90, Diabetics Screening.

100-3, Chapter-1, Part 1, 80.2

Photodynamic Therapy

Photodynamic therapy is a medical procedure which involves the infusion of a photosensitive (light-activated) drug with a very specific absorption peak. This drug is chemically designed to have a unique affinity for the diseased tissue intended for treatment. Once introduced to the body, the drug accumulates and is retained in diseased tissue to a greater degree than in normal tissue. Infusion is followed by the targeted irradiation of this tissue with a non-thermal laser, calibrated to emit light at a wavelength that corresponds to the drug's absorption peak. The drug then becomes active and locally treats the diseased tissue.

Ocular Photodynamic Therapy (OPT)

Ocular Photodynamic Therapy (OPT) is used in the treatment of ophthalmologic diseases. OPT is only covered when used in conjunction with verteporfin (see section 80.3, "Photosensitive Drugs").

- Classic Subfoveal Choroidal Neovascular (CNV) Lesions -OPT is covered with a diagnosis of neovascular age-related macular degeneration (AMD) with predominately classic subfoveal choroidal neovascular (CNV) lesions (where the area of classic CNV occupies ≥ 50 percent of the area of the entire lesion) at the initial visit as determined by a fluorescein angiogram. Subsequent follow-up visits will require either an optical coherence tomography (OCT) or a fluorescein angiogram (FA) to access treatment response. There are no requirements regarding visual acuity, lesion size, and number of re-treatments.

- Occult Subfoveal Choroidal Neovascular (CNV) Lesions -OPT is noncovered for patients with a diagnosis of age-related macular degeneration (AMD) with occult and no classic CNV lesions.

Other Conditions -Use of OPT with verteporfin for other types of AMD (e.g., patients with minimally classic CNV lesions, atrophic, or dry AMD) is noncovered. OPT with verteporfin for other ocular indications such as pathologic myopia or presumed ocular histoplasmosis syndrome, is eligible for coverage through individual contractor discretion.

100-3, Chapter-1, Part 1, 80.2.1

Ocular Photodynamic Therapy (OPT) - Effective April 3, 2013

A. General

Ocular Photodynamic Therapy (OPT) is used in the treatment of ophthalmologic diseases; specifically, for age-related macular degeneration (AMD), a common eye disease among the elderly. OPT involves the infusion of an intravenous photosensitizing drug called verteporfin followed by exposure to a laser. OPT is only covered when used in conjunction with verteporfin.

Effective July 1, 2001, OPT with verteporfin was approved for a diagnosis of neovascular AMD with predominately classic subfoveal choroidal neovascularization (CNV) lesions (where the area of classic CNV occupies ≥ 50% of the area of the entire lesion) at the initial visit as determined by a fluorescein angiogram (FA).

On October 17, 2001, the Centers for Medicare & Medicaid Services (CMS) announced its "intent to cover" OPT with verteporfin for AMD patients with occult and no classic subfoveal CNV as determined by an FA. The October 17, 2001, decision was never implemented.

On March 28, 2002, after thorough review and reconsideration of the October 17, 2001, intent to cover policy, CMS determined that the current non-coverage policy for OPT for verteporfin for AMD patients with occult and no classic subfoveal CNV as determined by an FA should remain in effect.

Effective August 20, 2002, CMS issued a non-covered instruction for OPT with verteporfin for AMD patients with occult and no classic subfoveal CNV as determined by an FA.

B. Nationally Covered Indications

Effective April 1, 2004, OPT with verteporfin continues to be approved for a diagnosis of neovascular AMD with predominately classic subfoveal CNV lesions (where the area of classic CNV occupies ≥ 50% of the area of the entire lesion) at the initial visit as determined by an FA. (CNV lesions are comprised of classic and/or occult components.) Subsequent follow-up visits require either an optical coherence tomography (OCT) (effective April 3. 2013) or an FA (effective April 1, 2004) to access treatment response. There are no requirements regarding visual acuity, lesion size, and number of re-treatments when treating predominantly classic lesions.

In addition, after thorough review and reconsideration of the August 20, 2002, non-coverage policy, CMS determines that the evidence is adequate to conclude that OPT with verteporfin is reasonable and necessary for treating:

1. Subfoveal occult with no classic CNV associated with AMD; and,

2. Subfoveal minimally classic CNV (where the area of classic CNV occupies <50% of the area of the entire lesion) associated with AMD.

The above 2 indications are considered reasonable and necessary only when:

1. The lesions are small (4 disk areas or less in size)at the time of initial treatment or within the 3 months prior to initial treatment; and,

2. The lesions have shown evidence of progression within the 3 months prior to initial treatment. Evidence of progression must be documented by deterioration of visual acuity (at least 5 letters on a standard eye examination chart), lesion growth (an increase in at least 1 disk area), or the appearance of blood associated with the lesion.

C. Nationally Non-Covered Indications

Other uses of OPT with verteporfin to treat AMD not already addressed by CMS will continue to be non-covered. These include, but are not limited to, the following AMD indications:

- Juxtafoveal or extrafoveal CNV lesions (lesions outside the fovea),
- Inability to obtain a fluorescein angiogram,
- Atrophic or "dry" AMD.

D. Other

The OPT with verteporfin for other ocular indications, such as pathologic myopia or presumed ocular histoplasmosis syndrome, continue to be eligible for local coverage determinations through individual contractor discretion.

100-3, Chapter-1, Part 1, 80.3

Photosensitive Drugs

Photosensitive drugs are the light-sensitive agents used in photodynamic therapy. Once introduced into the body, these drugs selectively identify and adhere to diseased tissue. The drugs remain inactive until they are exposed to a specific wavelength of light, by means of a laser, that corresponds to their absorption peak. The activation of a photosensitive drug results in a photochemical reaction which treats the diseased tissue without affecting surrounding normal tissue.

Verteporfin

Verteporfin, a benzoporphyrin derivative, is an intravenous lipophilic photosensitive drug with an absorption peak of 690 nm. This drug was first approved by the Food and Drug Administration (FDA) on April 12, 2000, and subsequently, approved for inclusion in the United States Pharmacopoeia on July 18, 2000, meeting Medicare's definition of a drug when used in conjunction with ocular photodynamic therapy (OPT) (see section 80.2, "Photodynamic Therapy") when furnished intravenously incident to a physician's service. For patients with age-related macular degeneration (AMD), Verteporfin is only covered with a diagnosis of neovascular age-related macular degeneration with predominately classic subfoveal choroidal neovascular (CNV) lesions (where the area of classic CNV occupies ≥ 50 percent of the area of the entire lesion) at the initial visit as determined by a fluorescein angiogram (FA). Subsequent follow-up visits will require either an optical coherence tomography (OCT) or an FA to access treatment response. OPT with verteporfin is covered for the above indication and will remain non-covered for all other indications related to AMD (see section 80.2). OPT with Verteporfin for use in non-AMD conditions is eligible for coverage through individual contractor discretion.

100-3, Chapter-1, Part 1, 80.3.1

Verteporfin -Effective April 3, 2013

A. General

Verteporfin, a benzoporphyrin derivative, is an intravenous lipophilic photosensitive drug with an absorption peak of 690 nm. Verteporfin was first approved by the Food and Drug Administration on April 12, 2000, and subsequently approved for inclusion in the United States Pharmacopoeia on July 18, 2000, meeting Medicare's definition of a drug as defined under §1861(t)(1) of the Social Security Act. Verteporfin is only covered when used in conjunction with ocular photodynamic therapy OPT) when furnished intravenously incident to a physician's service.

B. Nationally Covered Indications

Effective April 1, 2004, OPT with verteporfin is covered for patients with a diagnosis of neovascular age-related macular degeneration (AMD) with:

- Predominately classic subfoveal choroidal neovascularization (CNV) lesions (where the area of classic CNV occupies ≥ 50% of the area of the entire lesion) at the initial visit as determined by a fluorescein angiogram. (CNV lesions are comprised of classic and/or occult components.) Subsequent follow-up visits require either an optical coherence tomography (OCT) (effective April 3, 2013) or a fluorescein angiogram (FA) (effective April 1, 2004) to access treatment response.

  There are no requirements regarding visual acuity, lesion size, and number of retreatments when treating predominantly classic lesions.

- Subfoveal occult with no classic associated with AMD.

- Subfoveal minimally classic CNV (where the area of classic CNV occupies <50% of the area of the entire lesion) associated with AMD.

- The above 2 indications are considered reasonable and necessary only when:

1. The lesions are small (4 disk areas or less in size) at the time of initial treatment or within the 3 months prior to initial treatment; and,

2. The lesions have shown evidence of progression within the 3 months prior to initial treatment. Evidence of progression must be documented by deterioration of visual acuity (at least 5 letters on a standard eye examination chart), lesion growth (an increase in at least 1 disk area), or the appearance of blood associated with the lesion.

C. Nationally Non-Covered Indications

Other uses of OPT with verteporfin to treat AMD not already addressed by the Centers for Medicare & Medicaid Services will continue to be non-covered. These include, but are not limited to, the following AMD indications: juxtafoveal or extrafoveal CNV lesions (lesions outside the fovea), inability to obtain an FA, or atrophic or "dry" AMD.

D. Other

The OPT with verteporfin for other ocular indications, such as pathologic myopia or presumed ocular histoplasmosis syndrome, continue to be eligible for local coverage determinations through individual contractor discretion.

100-3, Chapter-1, Part 2, 90.1

Pharmacogenomic Testing to Predict Warfarin Responsiveness (Effective August 3, 2009)

A. General

Warfarin sodium is an orally administered anticoagulant drug that is marketed most commonly as Coumadin®. (The Food and Drug Administration (FDA) approved labeling for Coumadin® includes a Black Box Warning dating back to 2007.) Anticoagulant drugs are sometimes referred to as blood thinners by the lay public. Warfarin affects the vitamin K-dependent clotting factors II, VII, IX, and X. Warfarin is thought to interfere with clotting factor synthesis by inhibition of the C1 subunit of the vitamin K epoxide reductase (VKORC1) enzyme complex, thereby reducing the regeneration of vitamin K1 epoxide. The elimination of warfarin is almost entirely by metabolic conversion to inactive metabolites by cytochrome P450 (CYP) enzymes in liver cells. CYP2C9 is the principal cytochrome P450 enzyme that modulates the anticoagulant activity of warfarin. From results of clinical studies, genetic variation in the CYP2C9 and/or VKORC1 genes can, in concert with clinical factors, predict how each individual responds to warfarin.

Pharmacogenomics denotes the study of how an individual's genetic makeup, or genotype, affects the body's response to drugs. Pharmacogenomics as a science examines associations among variations in genes with individual responses to a drug or medication. In application, pharmacogenomic results (i.e., information on the patient's genetic variations) can contribute to predicting a patient's response to a given drug: good, bad, or none at all. Pharmacogenomic testing of CYP2C9 or VKORC1 alleles to predict a patient's response to warfarin occurs ideally prior to initiation of the drug. This would be an once-in-a-lifetime test, absent any reason to believe that the patient's personal genetic characteristics would change over time. Although such pharmacogenomic testing would be used to attempt to better approximate the best starting dose of warfarin, it would not eliminate the need for periodic PT/INR testing, a standard diagnostic test for coagulation activity and for assessing how a patient is reacting to a warfarin dose.

Nationally Covered Indications

Effective August 3, 2009, the Centers for Medicare & Medicaid Services (CMS) believes that the available evidence supports that coverage with evidence development (CED) under §1862(a)(1)(E) of the Social Security Act (the Act) is appropriate for pharmacogenomic testing of CYP2C9 or VKORC1 alleles to predict warfarin responsiveness by any method, and is therefore covered only when provided to Medicare beneficiaries who are candidates for anticoagulation therapy with warfarin who:

1. Have not been previously tested for CYP2C9 or VKORC1 alleles; and

2. Have received fewer than five days of warfarin in the anticoagulation regimen for which the testing is ordered; and

3. Are enrolled in a prospective, randomized, controlled clinical study when that study meets the following standards.

A clinical study seeking Medicare payment for pharmacogenomic testing of CYP2C9 or VKORC1 alleles to predict warfarin responsiveness provided to the Medicare beneficiary who is a candidate for anticoagulation therapy with warfarin pursuant to CED must address one or more aspects of the following question:

Prospectively, in Medicare-aged subjects whose warfarin therapy management includes pharmacogenomic testing of CYP2C9 or VKORC1 alleles to predict warfarin response, what is the frequency and severity of the following outcomes, compared to subjects whose warfarin therapy management does not include pharmacogenomic testing?

- Major hemorrhage
- Minor hemorrhage
- Thromboembolism related to the primary indication for anticoagulation
- Other thromboembolic event
- Mortality

The study must adhere to the following standards of scientific integrity and relevance to the Medicare population:

a. The principal purpose of the research study is to test whether a particular intervention potentially improves the participants' health outcomes.

b. The research study is well-supported by available scientific and medical information or it is intended to clarify or establish the health outcomes of interventions already in common clinical use.

c. The research study does not unjustifiably duplicate existing studies.

d. The research study design is appropriate to answer the research question being asked in the study.

e. The research study is sponsored by an organization or individual capable of executing the proposed study successfully.

f. The research study is in compliance with all applicable Federal regulations concerning the protection of human subjects found in the Code of Federal Regulations (CFR) at 45 CFR Part 46. If a study is regulated by the FDA, it also must be in compliance with 21 CFR Parts 50 and 56.

g. All aspects of the research study are conducted according to the appropriate standards of scientific integrity.

h. The research study has a written protocol that clearly addresses, or incorporates by reference, the Medicare standards.

i. The clinical research study is not designed to exclusively test toxicity or disease pathophysiology in healthy individuals. Trials of all medical technologies measuring therapeutic outcomes as one of the objectives meet this standard only if the disease or condition being studied is life-threatening as defined in 21 CFR § 312.81(a) and the patient has no other viable treatment options.

j. The clinical research study is registered on the www. ClinicalTrials.gov website by the principal sponsor/investigator prior to the enrollment of the first study subject.

k. The research study protocol specifies the method and timing of public release of all pre-specified outcomes to be measured including release of outcomes if outcomes are negative or study is terminated early. The results must be made public within 24 months of the end of data collection. If a report is planned to be published in a peer-reviewed journal, then that initial release may be an abstract that meets the requirements of the International Committee of Medical Journal Editors. However, a full report of the outcomes must be made public no later than 3 years after the end of data collection.

l. The research study protocol must explicitly discuss subpopulations affected by the treatment under investigation, particularly traditionally underrepresented groups in clinical studies, how the inclusion and exclusion criteria affect enrollment of these populations, and a plan for the retention and reporting of said populations on the trial. If the inclusion and exclusion criteria are expected to have a negative effect on the recruitment or retention of underrepresented populations, the protocol must discuss why these criteria are necessary.

m. The research study protocol explicitly discusses how the results are or are not expected to be generalizable to the Medicare population to infer whether Medicare patients may benefit from the intervention. Separate discussions in the protocol may be necessary for populations eligible for Medicare due to age, disability or Medicaid eligibility.

B. Nationally Non-Covered Indications

The CMS believes that the available evidence does not demonstrate that pharmacogenomic testing of CYP2C9 or VKORC1 alleles to predict warfarin responsiveness improves health outcomes in Medicare beneficiaries outside the context of CED, and is therefore not reasonable and necessary under §1862(a)(1)(A) of the Act.

C. Other

This NCD does not determine coverage to identify CYP2C9 or VKORC1 alleles for other purposes, nor does it determine national coverage to identify other alleles to predict warfarin responsiveness.

100-3, Chapter-1, Part 2, 110.22

Autologous Cellular Immunotherapy Treatment (Effective June 30, 2011)

A. General

Prostate cancer is the most common non-cutaneous cancer in men in the United States. In 2009, an estimated 192,280 new cases of prostate cancer were diagnosed and an estimated 27,360 deaths were reported. The National Cancer Institute states that prostate cancer is predominantly a cancer of older men; the median age at diagnosis is 72 years. Once the patient has castration-resistant, metastatic prostate cancer the median survival is generally less than two years.

In 2010 the Food and Drug Administration (FDA) approved sipuleucel-T (PROVENGE®; APC8015), for patients with castration-resistant, metastatic prostate cancer. The posited mechanism of action, immunotherapy, is different from that of anti-cancer chemotherapy such as docetaxel. This is the first immunotherapy for prostate cancer to receive FDA approval.

The goal of immunotherapy is to stimulate the body's natural defenses (such as the white blood cells called dendritic cells, T-lymphocytes and mononuclear cells) in a specific manner so that they attack and destroy, or at least prevent, the proliferation of cancer cells. Specificity is attained by intentionally exposing a patient's white blood cells to a particular protein (called an antigen) associated with the prostate cancer. This exposure "trains" the white blood cells to target and attack the prostate cancer cells. Clinically, this is expected to result in a decrease in the size and/or number of cancer sites, an increase in the time to cancer progression, and/or an increase in survival of the patient.

Sipuleucel-T differs from other infused anti-cancer therapies. Most such anti-cancer therapies are manufactured and sold by a biopharmaceutical company and then purchased by and dispensed from a pharmacy. In contrast, once the decision is made to treat with sipuleucel-T, a multi-step process is used to produce sipuleucel-T. Sipuleucel-T is made individually for each patient with his own white blood cells. The patient's white blood cells are removed via a procedure called leukapheresis. In a laboratory the white blood cells are exposed to PA2024, which is a molecule created by linking prostatic acid phosphatase (PAP) with granulocyte/macrophage-colony stimulating factor (GM-CSF). PAP is an antigen specifically associated with prostate cancer cells; GM-CSF is a protein that targets a receptor on the surface of white blood cells. Hence, PAP serves to externally manipulate the immunological functioning of the patient's white blood cells while GM-CSF serves to stimulate the white blood cells into action. As noted in the FDA's clinical review, each dose of sipuleucel-T contains a minimum of 40 million treated white blood cells, however there is "high inherent variability" in the yield of sipuleucel-T from leukapheresis to leukapheresis in the same patient as well as from patient to patient. The treated white blood cells are then infused back into the same patient. The FDA-approved dosing regimen is three doses with each dose administered two weeks apart.

Indications and Limitations of Coverage

B. Nationally Covered Indications

Effective for services performed on or after June 30, 2011, The Centers for Medicare and Medicaid Services (CMS) proposes that the evidence is adequate to conclude that the use of autologous cellular immunotherapy treatment -sipuleucel-T; PROVENGE® improves health outcomes for Medicare beneficiaries with asymptomatic or minimally symptomatic metastatic castrate-resistant (hormone refractory) prostate cancer, and thus is reasonable and necessary for this on-label indication under 1862(a)(1)(A) of the Social Security Act.

C. Nationally Non-Covered Indications

N/A

D. Other

Effective for services performed on or after June 30, 2011, coverage of all off-label uses of autologous cellular immunotherapy treatment –sipuleucel-T; PROVENGE® for the treatment of pro state cancer is left to the discretion of the local Medicare Administrative Contractors.

(NCD last reviewed June 2011.)

100-3, Chapter-1, Part 2, 150.11

Thermal Intradiscal Procedures (TIPs) (Effective September 29, 2008)

A. General

Percutaneous thermal intradiscal procedures (TIPs) involve the insertion of a catheter(s)/probe(s) in the spinal disc under fluoroscopic guidance for the purpose of producing or applying heat and/or disruption within the disc to relieve low back pain.

The scope of this national coverage determination on TIPs includes percutaneous intradiscal techniques that employ the use of a radiofrequency energy source or electrothermal energy to apply or create heat and/or disruption within the disc for coagulation and/or decompression of disc material to treat symptomatic patients with annular disruption of a contained herniated disc, to seal annular tears or fissures, or destroy nociceptors for the purpose of relieving pain. This includes techniques that use single or multiple probe(s)/catheter(s), which utilize a resistance coil or other delivery system technology, are flexible or rigid, and are placed within the nucleus, the nuclear-annular junction, or the annulus.

Although not intended to be an all-inclusive list, TIPs are commonly identified as intradiscal electrothermal therapy (IDET), intradiscal thermal annuloplasty (IDTA), percutaneous intradiscal radiofrequency thermocoagulation (PIRFT), radiofrequency annuloplasty (RA), intradiscal biacuplasty (IDB), percutaneous (or plasma) disc decompression (PDD) or coblation, or targeted disc decompression (TDD). At times, TIPs are identified or labeled based on the name of the catheter/probe that is used (e.g., SpineCath, discTRODE, SpineWand, Accutherm, or TransDiscal electrodes). Each technique or device has its own protocol for application of the therapy. Percutaneous disc decompression or nucleoplasty procedures that do not utilize a radiofrequency energy procedure) are not within the scope of this NCD.

B. Nationally Covered Indications

N/A

C. Nationally Non-Covered Indications

Effective for services performed on or after September 29, 2008, the Centers for Medicare and Medicaid Services has determined that TIPs are not reasonable and necessary for the treatment of low back pain. Therefore, TIPs, which include procedures that employ the use of a radiofrequency energy source or electrothermal energy to apply or create heat and/or disruption within the disc for the treatment of low back pain, are noncovered.

D. Other

N/A

(This NCD last reviewed September 2008.)

100-3, Chapter-1, Part 2, 150.12

Collagen Meniscus Implant (Effective May 25, 2010)

A. General

The knee menisci are wedge-shaped, semi-lunar discs of fibrous tissue located in the knee joint between the ends of the femur and the tibia and fibula. There is a lateral and medial meniscus in each knee. It is known now that the menisci provide mechanical support, localized pressure distribution, and lubrication of the knee joint. Initially, meniscal tears were treated with total meniscectomy; however, as knowledge of the function of the menisci and the potential long term effects of total meniscectomy on the knee joint evolved, treatment of symptomatic meniscal tears gravitated to repair of the tear, when possible, or partial meniscectomy.

The collagen meniscus implant (also referred to as collagen scaffold (CS), CMI or Menaflex™ meniscus implant throughout the published literature) is used to fill meniscal defects that result from partial meniscectomy. The collagen meniscus implant is not intended to replace the entire meniscus at it requires a meniscal rim for attachment. The literature describes the placement of the collagen meniscus implant through an arthroscopic procedure with an additional incision for capture of the repair needles and tying of the sutures. After debridement of the damaged meniscus, the implant is trimmed to the size of meniscal defect and sutured into place. The collagen meniscus implant is described as a tissue engineered scaffold to support the generation of new meniscus-like tissue. The collagen meniscus implant is manufactured from bovine collagen and should not be confused with the meniscus

transplant which involves the replacement of the meniscus with a transplant meniscus from a cadaver donor. The meniscus transplant is not addressed under this national coverage determination.

B. Nationally Covered Indications

N/A

C. Nationally Non-Covered Indications

Effective for claims with dates of service performed on or after May 25, 2010, the Centers for Medicare & Medicaid Services has determined that the evidence is adequate to conclude that the collagen meniscus implant does not improve health outcomes and, therefore, is not reasonable and necessary for the treatment of meniscal injury/tear under section 1862(a)(1)(A) of the Social Security Act. Thus, the collagen meniscus implant is non-covered by Medicare.

D. Other

N/A

(This NCD last reviewed May 2010.)

100-3, Chapter-1, Part 2, 160.13

Supplies Used in the Delivery of Transcutaneous Electrical Nerve Stimulation (TENS) and Neuromuscular Electrical Stimulation (NMES)

Transcutaneous Electrical Nerve Stimulation (TENS) and/or Neuromuscular Electrical Stimulation (NMES) can ordinarily be delivered to patients through the use of conventional electrodes, adhesive tapes and lead wires. There may be times, however, where it might be medically necessary for certain patients receiving TENS or NMES treatment to use, as an alternative to conventional electrodes, adhesive tapes and lead wires, a form-fitting conductive garment (i.e., a garment with conductive fibers which are separated from the patients' skin by layers of fabric).

A form-fitting conductive garment (and medically necessary related supplies) may be covered under the program only when:

1. It has received permission or approval for marketing by the Food and Drug Administration;

2. It has been prescribed by a physician for use in delivering covered TENS or NMES treatment; and

3. One of the medical indications outlined below is met:

   • The patient cannot manage without the conductive garment because there is such a large area or so many sites to be stimulated and the stimulation would have to be delivered so frequently that it is not feasible to use conventional electrodes, adhesive tapes and lead wires;

   • The patient cannot manage without the conductive garment for the treatment of chronic intractable pain because the areas or sites to be stimulated are inaccessible with the use of conventional electrodes, adhesive tapes and lead wires;

   • The patient has a documented medical condition such as skin problems that preclude the application of conventional electrodes, adhesive tapes and lead wires;

   • The patient requires electrical stimulation beneath a cast either to treat disuse atrophy, where the nerve supply to the muscle is intact, or to treat chronic intractable pain; or

   • The patient has a medical need for rehabilitation strengthening (pursuant to a written plan of rehabilitation) following an injury where the nerve supply to the muscle is intact.

A conductive garment is not covered for use with a TENS device during the trial period specified in §160.3 unless:

4. The patient has a documented skin problem prior to the start of the trial period; and

5. The A/B MAC (B)'s medical consultants are satisfied that use of such an item is medically necessary for the patient.

(See conditions for coverage of the use of TENS in the diagnosis and treatment of chronic intractable pain in §§160.3, 160.13, and 160.27, and the use of NMES in the treatment of disuse atrophy in §150.4.)

100-3, Chapter-1, Part 2, 160.27

Transcutaneous Electrical Nerve Stimulation (TENS) for Chronic Low Back Pain (CLBP)

The TENS is a type of electrical nerve stimulator that is employed to treat chronic intractable pain. This stimulator is attached to the surface of the patient's skin over the peripheral nerve to be stimulated. It may be applied in a variety of settings (in the patient's home, a physician's office, or in an outpatient clinic). Payment for TENS may be made under the durable medical equipment benefit.

A. General

For the purposes of this decision chronic low back pain (CLBP) is defined as:

1. an episode of low back pain that has persisted for three months or longer; and

2. is not a manifestation of a clearly defined and generally recognizable primary disease entity. For example, there are cancers that, through metastatic spread to the spine or pelvis, may elicit pain in the lower back as a symptom; and certain systemic diseases such as rheumatoid arthritis and multiple sclerosis manifest many debilitating symptoms of which low back pain is not the primary focus.

B. Nationally Covered Indications

Effective June 8, 2012, the Centers for Medicare & Medicaid Services (CMS) will allow coverage for Transcutaneous Electrical Nerve Stimulation (TENS) for CLBP only when all of the following conditions are met.

In order to support additional research on the use of TENS for CLBP, we will cover this item under section 1862(a)(1)(E) of the Social Security Act (the Act) subject to all of the following conditions:

1. Coverage under this section expires three years after the publication of this decision on the CMS website.

2. The beneficiary is enrolled in an approved clinical study meeting all of the requirements below. The study must address one or more aspects of the following questions in a randomized, controlled design using validated and reliable instruments. This can include randomized crossover designs when the impact of prior TENS use is appropriately accounted for in the study protocol.

   i. Does the use of TENS provide clinically meaningful reduction in pain in Medicare beneficiaries with CLBP?

   ii. Does the use of TENS provide a clinically meaningful improvement of function in Medicare beneficiaries with CLBP?

   iii. Does the use of TENS impact the utilization of other medical treatments or services used in the medical management of CLBP?

These studies must be designed so that the patients in the control and comparison groups receive the same concurrent treatments and either sham (placebo) TENS or active TENS intervention.

The study must adhere to the following standards of scientific integrity and relevance to the Medicare population:

a. The principal purpose of the research study is to test whether a particular intervention potentially improves the participants' health outcomes.

b. The research study is well supported by available scientific and medical information or it is intended to clarify or establish the health outcomes of interventions already in common clinical use.

c. The research study does not unjustifiably duplicate existing studies.

d. The research study design is appropriate to answer the research question being asked in the study.

e. The research study is sponsored by an organization or individual capable of executing the proposed study successfully.

f. The research study is in compliance with all applicable Federal regulations concerning the protection of human subjects found at 45 CFR Part 46. If a study is regulated by the Food and Drug Administration (FDA), it must be in compliance with 21 CFR parts 50 and 56.

g. All aspects of the research study are conducted according to appropriate standards of scientific integrity (see http://www.icmje.org).

h. The research study has a written protocol that clearly addresses, or incorporates by reference, the standards listed here as Medicare requirements for CED coverage.

i. The clinical research study is not designed to exclusively test toxicity or disease pathophysiology in healthy individuals. Trials of all medical technologies measuring therapeutic outcomes as one of the objectives meet this standard only if the disease or condition being studied is life threatening as defined in 21 CFR §312.81(a) and the patient has no other viable treatment options.

j. The clinical research study is registered on the ClinicalTrials.gov website by the principal sponsor/investigator prior to the enrollment of the first study subject.

k. The research study protocol specifies the method and timing of public release of all prespecified outcomes to be measured including release of outcomes if outcomes are negative or study is terminated early. The results must be made public within 24 months of the end of data collection. If a report is planned to be published in a peer reviewed journal, then that initial release may be an abstract that meets the requirements of the International Committee of Medical Journal Editors (http://www.icmje.org).

l. The research study protocol must explicitly discuss subpopulations affected by the treatment under investigation, particularly traditionally underrepresented groups in clinical studies, how the inclusion and exclusion criteria effect enrollment of these populations, and a plan for the retention and reporting of said populations on the trial. If the inclusion and exclusion criteria are expected to have a negative effect on the recruitment or retention of underrepresented populations, the protocol must discuss why these criteria are necessary.

m. The research study protocol explicitly discusses how the results are or are not expected to be generalizable to the Medicare population to infer whether Medicare patients may benefit from the intervention. Separate discussions in the protocol may be necessary for populations eligible for Medicare due to age, disability or Medicaid eligibility.

C. Nationally Non-Covered Indications

TENS is not reasonable and necessary for the treatment of CLBP under section 1862(a)(1)(A) of the Act.

D. Other

See§160.13 for an explanation of coverage of medically necessary supplies for the effective use of TENS. See §160.7.1 for an explanation of coverage for assessing patients suitability for electrical nerve stimulation therapy. See §10.2 for an explanation of coverage of transcutaneous electrical nerve stimulation (TENS) for acute post-operative pain. Please note, §280.13 Transcutaneous Electrical Nerve Stimulators (TENS) NCD has been removed from the NCD manual and incorporated into NCD 160.27

(This NCD last reviewed June 2012.)

100-3, Chapter-1, Part 2, 160.7.1

Assessing Patients Suitability for Electrical Nerve Stimulation Therapy

Electrical nerve stimulation is an accepted modality for assessing a patient's suitability for ongoing treatment with a transcutaneous or an implanted nerve stimulator.

Accordingly, program payment may be made for the following techniques when used to determine the potential therapeutic usefulness of an electrical nerve stimulator:

A. Transcutaneous Electrical Nerve Stimulation (TENS)

This technique involves attachment of a transcutaneous nerve stimulator to the surface of the skin over the peripheral nerve to be stimulated. It is used by the patient on a trial basis and its effectiveness in modulating pain is monitored by the physician, or physical therapist. Generally, the physician or physical therapist is able to determine whether the patient is likely to derive a significant therapeutic benefit from continuous use of a transcutaneous stimulator within a trial period of one month; in a few cases this determination may take longer to make. Document the medical necessity for such services which are furnished beyond the first month.(See §160.13 for an explanation of coverage of medically necessary supplies for the effective use of TENS.)

If TENS significantly alleviates pain, it may be considered as primary treatment; if it produces no relief or greater discomfort than the original pain electrical nerve stimulation therapy is ruled out. However, where TENS produces incomplete relief, further evaluation with percutaneous electrical nerve stimulation may be considered to determine whether an implanted peripheral nerve stimulator would provide significant relief from pain.

Usually, the physician or physical therapist providing the services will furnish the equipment necessary for assessment. Where the physician or physical therapist advises the patient to rent the TENS from a supplier during the trial period rather than supplying it himself/herself, program payment may be made for rental of the TENS as well as for the services of the physician or physical therapist who is evaluating its use. However, the combined program payment which is made for the physician's or physical therapist's services and the rental of the stimulator from a supplier should not exceed the amount which would be payable for the total service, including the stimulator, furnished by the physician or physical therapist alone.

B. Percutaneous Electrical Nerve Stimulation (PENS)

This diagnostic procedure which involves stimulation of peripheral nerves by a needle electrode inserted through the skin is performed only in a physician's office, clinic, or hospital outpatient department. Therefore, it is covered only when performed by a physician or incident to physician's service. If pain is effectively controlled by percutaneous stimulation, implantation of electrodes is warranted.

As in the case of TENS (described in subsection A), generally the physician should be able to determine whether the patient is likely to derive a significant therapeutic benefit from continuing use of an implanted nerve stimulator within a trial period of 1 month. In a few cases, this determination may take longer to make. The medical necessity for such diagnostic services which are furnished beyond the first month must be documented.

NOTE: Electrical nerve stimulators do not prevent pain but only alleviate pain as it occurs. A patient can be taught how to employ the stimulator, and once this is done, can use it safely and effectively without direct physician supervision. Consequently, it is inappropriate for a patient to visit his/her physician, physical therapist, or an outpatient clinic on a continuing basis for treatment of pain with electrical nerve stimulation. Once it is determined that electrical nerve stimulation should be continued as therapy and the patient has been trained to use the stimulator, it is expected that a stimulator will be implanted or the patient will employ the TENS on a continual basis in his/her home. Electrical nerve stimulation treatments furnished by a physician in his/her office, by a physical therapist or outpatient clinic are excluded from coverage by §1862(a)(1) of the Act. (See §160.7 for an explanation of coverage of the therapeutic use of implanted peripheral nerve stimulators under the prosthetic devices benefit.) See §160.27 for an explanation of coverage of the therapeutic use of TENS under the durable medical equipment benefit.

100-3, Chapter-1, Part 3, 190.11

Home Prothrombin Time/International Normalized Ratio (PT/INR) Monitoring for Anticoagulation Management –Effective March 19, 2008

A. General

Use of the International Normalized Ratio (INR) or prothrombin time (PT) -standard measurement for reporting the blood's clotting time) -allows physicians to determine the level of anticoagulation in a patient independent of the laboratory reagents used. The INR is the ratio of the patient's PT (extrinsic or tissue-factor dependent coagulation pathway) compared to the mean PT for a group of normal individuals. Maintaining patients within his/her prescribed therapeutic range minimizes adverse events associated with inadequate or excessive anticoagulation such as serious bleeding or thromboembolic events. Patient self-testing and self-management through the use of a home INR monitor may be used to improve the time in therapeutic rate (TTR) for select groups of patients. increased TTR leads to improved clinical outcomes and reductions in thromboembolic and hemorrhagic events.

Warfarin (also prescribed under other trade names, e.g., Coumadin®) is a self-administered, oral anticoagulant (blood thinner) medication that affects the vitamin K-dependent clotting factors II, VII, IX and X. It is widely used for various medical conditions, and has a narrow therapeutic index, meaning it is a drug with less than a 2-fold difference between median lethal dose and median effective dose. For this reason, since October 4, 2006, it falls under the category of a Food and Drug Administration (FDA) "black-box" drug whose dosage must be closely monitored to avoid serious complications. A PT/INR monitoring system is a portable testing device that includes a finger-stick and an FDA-cleared meter that measures the time it takes for a person's blood plasma to clot.

B. Nationally Covered Indications

For services furnished on or after March 19, 2008, Medicare will cover the use of home PT/INR monitoring for chronic, oral anticoagulation management for patients with mechanical heart valves, chronic atrial fibrillation, or venous thromboembolism (inclusive of deep venous thrombosis and pulmonary embolism) on warfarin. The monitor and the home testing must be prescribed by a treating physician as provided at 42 CFR 410.32(a), and all of the following requirements must be met:

1. The patient must have been anticoagulated for at least 3 months prior to use of the home INR device; and,

2. The patient must undergo a face-to-face educational program on anticoagulation management and must have demonstrated the correct use of the device prior to its use in the home; and,

3. The patient continues to correctly use the device in the context of the management of the anticoagulation therapy following the initiation of home monitoring; and,

4. Self-testing with the device should not occur more frequently than once a week.

C. Nationally Non-Covered Indications

N/A

D. Other

1. All other indications for home PT/INR monitoring not indicated as nationally covered above remain at local Medicare contractor discretion.

2. This national coverage determination (NCD) is distinct from, and makes no changes to, the PT clinical laboratory NCD at section 190.17 of Publication 100-03 of the NCD Manual.

(This NCD last reviewed March 2008.)

100-3, Chapter-1, Part 3, 190.14

Human Immunodeficiency Virus (HIV) Testing (Diagnosis)

Diagnosis of HIV infection is primarily made through the use of serologic assays. These assays take one of two forms: antibody detection assays and specific HIV antigen (p24) procedures. The antibody assays are usually enzyme immunoassays (EIA), which are used to confirm exposure of an individual's immune system to specific viral antigens. These assays may be formatted to detect HIV-1, HIV-2, or HIV-1 and 2 simultaneously, and to detect both IgM and IgG. When the initial EIA test is repeatedly positive or indeterminant, an alternative test is used to confirm the specificity of the antibodies to individual viral components. The most commonly used method is the Western Blot.

The HIV-1 core antigen (p24) test detects circulating viral antigen which may be found prior to the development of antibodies and may also be present in later stages of illness in the form of recurrent or persistent antigenemia. Its prognostic utility in HIV infection has been diminished as a result of development of sensitive viral RNA assays, and its primary use today is as a routine screening tool in potential blood donors.

In several unique situations, serologic testing alone may not reliably establish an HIV infection. This may occur because the antibody response (particularly the IgG response detected by Western Blot) has not yet developed (that is, acute retroviral syndrome) or is persistently equivocal because of inherent viral antigen variability. It is also an issue in perinatal HIV infection due to transplacental passage of maternal HIV antibody. In these situations, laboratory evidence of HIV in blood by culture, antigen assays, or proviral DNA or viral RNA assays, is required to establish a definitive determination of HIV infection.

Indications

Diagnostic testing to establish HIV infection may be indicated when there is a strong clinical suspicion supported by one or more of the following clinical findings:

1. The patient has a documented, otherwise unexplained, AIDS-defining or AIDS-associated opportunistic infection.

2. The patient has another documented sexually transmitted disease, which identifies significant risk of exposure to HIV and the potential for an early or subclinical infection.

3. The patient has documented acute or chronic Hepatitis B or C infection that identifies a significant risk of exposure to HIV and the potential for an early or subclinical infection.

4. The patient has a documented AIDS-defining or AIDS-associated neoplasm.

5. The patient has a documented AIDS-associated neurologic disorder or otherwise unexplained dementia.

6. The patient has another documented AIDS-defining clinical condition, or a history of other severe, recurrent, or persistent conditions which suggest an underlying immune deficiency (for example, cutaneous or mucosal disorders).

7. The patient has otherwise unexplained generalized signs and symptoms suggestive of a chronic process with an underlying immune deficiency (for example, fever, weight loss, malaise, fatigue, chronic diarrhea, failure to thrive, chronic cough, hemoptysis, shortness of breath, or lymphadenopathy).

8. The patient has otherwise unexplained laboratory evidence of a chronic disease process with an underlying immune deficiency (for example, anemia, leukopenia, pancytopenia, lymphopenia, or low CD4+ lymphocyte count).

9. The patient has signs and symptoms of acute retroviral syndrome with fever, malaise, lymphadenopathy, and skin rash.

10. The patient has documented exposure to blood or body fluids known to be capable of transmitting HIV (for example, needle sticks and other significant blood exposures) and antiviral therapy is initiated or anticipated to be initiated.

11. The patient is undergoing treatment for rape. (HIV testing is part of the rape treatment protocol.)

Limitations

1. HIV antibody testing in the United States is usually performed using HIV-1 or HIV-1/2 combination tests. HIV-2 testing is indicated if clinical circumstances suggest HIV-2 is likely (that is, compatible clinical finding and HIV-1 test negative). HIV-2 testing may also be indicated in areas of the country where there is greater prevalence of HIV-2 infections.

2. The Western Blot test should be performed only after documentation that the initial EIA tests are repeatedly positive or equivocal on a single sample.

3. The HIV antigen tests currently have no defined diagnostic usage.

4. Direct viral RNA detection may be performed in those situations where serologic testing does not establish a diagnosis but strong clinical suspicion persists (for example, acute retroviral syndrome, nonspecific serologic evidence of HIV, or perinatal HIV infection).

5. If initial serologic tests confirm an HIV infection, repeat testing is not indicated.

6. If initial serologic tests are HIV EIA negative and there is no indication for confirmation of infection by viral RNA detection, the interval prior to retesting is 3-6 months.

7. Testing for evidence of HIV infection using serologic methods may be medically appropriate in situations where there is a risk of exposure to HIV.

8. The CPT® Editorial Panel has issued a number of codes for infectious agent detection by direct antigen or nucleic acid probe techniques that have not yet been developed or are only being used on an investigational basis. Laboratory providers are advised to remain current on FDA-approved status for these tests.

100-3, Chapter-1, Part 4, 210.3

Colorectal Cancer Screening Tests

A. General

Sections 1861(s)(2)(R) and 1861(pp) of the Social Security Act (the Act) and regulations at 42 CFR 410.37 authorize Medicare coverage for screening colorectal cancer tests under Medicare Part B. The statute and regulations authorize the Secretary to add other tests and procedures (and modifications to tests and procedures for colorectal cancer screening) as the Secretary finds appropriate based on consultation with appropriate experts and organizations.

B. Nationally Covered Indications

1. Fecal Occult Blood Tests (FOBT) (effective January 1, 2004)

Fecal occult blood tests (FOBTs) are generally divided into two types: immunoassay and guaiac types. Immunoassay (or immunochemical) fecal occult blood tests (iFOBT) use "antibodies directed against human globin epitopes. While most iFOBTs use spatulas to collect stool samples, some use a brush to collect toilet water surrounding the stool. Most iFOBTs require laboratory processing.

Guaiac fecal occult blood tests (gFOBT) use a peroxidase reaction to indicate presence of the heme portion of hemoglobin. Guaiac turns blue after oxidation by oxidants or peroxidases in the presence of an oxygen donor such as hydrogen peroxide. Most FOBTs use sticks to collect stool samples and may be developed in a physician's office or a laboratory. In 1998, Medicare began reimbursement for guaiac FOBTs, but not immunoassay type tests for colorectal cancer screening. Since the undamental process is similar for other iFOBTs, the Centers for Medicare & Medicaid Services evaluated colorectal cancer screening using immunoassay FOBTs in general.

Effective for dates of service on and after January 1, 2004, Medicare covers one screening FOBT per annum for the early detection of colorectal cancer. This means that Medicare will cover one guaiac-based (gFOBT) or one immunoassay-based (iFOBT) at a frequency of every 12 months; i.e., at least 1 months have passed following the month in which the last covered screening FOBT was performed, for beneficiaries aged 50 years and older. The beneficiary completes the existing gFOBT by taking samples from two different sites of three consecutive stools; the beneficiary completes the iFOBT by taking the appropriate number of stool samples according to the specific manufacturer's instructions. This screening requires a written order from the beneficiary's attending physician. ("Attending physician" means a doctor of medicine or osteopathy (as defined in §1861(r)(1) of the Act) who is fully knowledgeable about the beneficiary's medical condition, and who would be responsible for using the results of any examination performed in the overall management of the beneficiary's specific medical problem.)

2. The Cologuard™ - Multitarget Stool DNA (sDNA) Test (effective October 9, 2014)

Screening stool or fecal DNA (deoxyribonucleic acid, sDNA) testing detects molecular markers of altered DNA that are contained in the cells shed by colorectal cancer and pre-malignant colorectal epithelial neoplasia into the lumen of the large bowel. Through the use of selective enrichment and amplification techniques, sDNA tests are designed to detect very small amounts of DNA markers to identify colorectal cancer or pre-malignant colorectal neoplasia. The Cologuard™ - multitarget sDNA test is a proprietary in vitro diagnostic device that incorporates both sDNA and fecal immunochemical test techniques and is designed to analyze patients' stool samples for markers associated with the presence of colorectal cancer and pre-malignant colorectal neoplasia.

Effective for dates of service on or after October 9, 2014, The Cologuard™ test is covered once every three years for Medicare beneficiaries that meet all of the following criteria:

- Age 50 to 85 years, and,
- Asymptomatic (no signs or symptoms of colorectal disease including but not limited to lower gastrointestinal pain, blood in stool, positive guaiac fecal occult blood test (gFOBT) or fecal immunochemical test (iFOBT)), and,
- At average risk of developing colorectal cancer (no personal history of adenomatous polyps, colorectal cancer, or inflammatory bowel disease, including Crohn's Disease and ulcerative colitis; no family history of colorectal cancers or adenomatous polyps, familial adenomatous polyposis, or hereditary nonpolyposis colorectal cancer).

C. Nationally Non-Covered Indications

All other indications for colorectal cancer screening not otherwise specified in the Act and regulations, or otherwise specified above remain nationally non-covered. Noncoverage specifically includes:

1. All screening sDNA tests, effective April 28, 2008, through October 8, 2014. Effective for dates of service on or after October 9, 2014, all other screening sDNA tests not otherwise specified above remain nationally non-covered.

2. Screening computed tomographic colonography (CTC), effective May 12, 2009.

D. Other

N/A

(This NCD last reviewed October 2014.)

100-3, Chapter-1, Part 4, 210.4

Smoking and Tobacco-Use Cessation Counseling

(Rev.202, Issued: 08- 25-17, Effective: 09-26-17, Implementation: 09- 26-17) Effective September 30, 2015 this section is deleted and the remaining NCD entitled Counseling to Prevent Tobacco Use (210.4.1) remains effective.

100-3, Chapter-1, Part-4, 210.7

Screening for the Human Immunodeficiency Virus (HIV)

A. General

Infection with the human immunodeficiency virus (HIV) is a continuing, worldwide pandemic described by the World Health Organization as "the most serious infectious disease challenge to global public health". Acquired immunodeficiency syndrome (AIDS) is diagnosed when a HIV-infected person's immune system becomes severely compromised and/or a person becomes ill with a HIV-related opportunistic infection. Without treatment, AIDS usually develops within 8-10 years after a person's initial HIV infection. While there is presently no cure for HIV, an infected individual can be recognized by screening, and subsequent access to skilled care plus vigilant monitoring and adherence to continuous antiretroviral therapy may delay the onset of AIDS and increase quality of life for many years.

Significantly, more than half of new HIV infections are estimated to be sexually transmitted from infected individuals who are unaware of their HIV status. Consequently, improved secondary disease prevention and wider availability of screening linked to HIV care and treatment would not only delay disease progression and complications in untested or unaware older individuals, but could also decrease the spread of disease to those living with or partnered with HIV-infected individuals.

HIV antibody testing first became available in 1985. These commonly used, Food and Drug Administration (FDA)-approved HIV antibody screening tests –using serum or plasma from a venipuncture or blood draw –are known as EIA (enzyme immunoassay) or ELISA (enzyme-linked immunosorbent assay) tests.

Developed for point-of-care testing using alternative samples, six rapid HIV-1 and/or HIV-2 antibody tests –using fluid obtained from the oral cavity or using whole blood, serum, or plasma from a blood draw or fingerstick –were approved by the FDA from 2002-2006.

Effective January 1, 2009, the Centers for Medicare & Medicaid Services (CMS) is allowed to add coverage of "additional preventive services" through the national coverage determination (NCD) process if certain statutory requirements are met, as provided under section 101(a) of the Medicare Improvements for Patients and Providers Act. One of those requirements is that the service(s) be categorized as a grade A (strongly recommends) or grade B (recommends) rating by the US Preventive Services Task Force (USPSTF). The USPSTF strongly recommends screening for all adolescents and adults at risk for HIV infection, as well as all pregnant women.

B. Nationally Covered Indications

Effective for claims with dates of service on and after December 8, 2009, CMS determines that the evidence is adequate to conclude that screening for HIV infection is reasonable and necessary for early detection of HIV and is appropriate for individuals entitled to benefits under Part A or

enrolled under Part B. Therefore, CMS proposes to cover both standard and FDA-approved HIV rapid screening tests for:

1. A maximum of one, annual voluntary HIV screening of Medicare beneficiaries at increased risk for HIV infection per USPSTF guidelines as follows:

   - Men who have had sex with men after 1975

   - Men and women having unprotected sex with multiple [more than one] partners

   - Past or present injection drug users

   - Men and women who exchange sex for money or drugs, or have sex partners who do

   - Individuals whose past or present sex partners were HIV-infected, bisexual or injection drug users

   - Persons being treated for sexually transmitted diseases

   - Persons with a history of blood transfusion between 1978 and 1985

   - Persons who request an HIV test despite reporting no individual risk factors, since this group is likely to include individuals not willing to disclose high-risk behaviors; and,

2. A maximum of three, voluntary HIV screenings of pregnant Medicare beneficiaries: (1) when the diagnosis of pregnancy is known, (2) during the third trimester, and (3) at labor, if ordered by the woman's clinician.

C. Nationally Non-Covered Indications

Effective for claims with dates of service on and after December 8, 2009, Medicare beneficiaries with any known diagnosis of a HIV-related illness are not eligible for this screening test.

Medicare beneficiaries (other than those who are pregnant) who have had a prior HIV screening test within one year are not eligible (11 full months must have elapsed following the month in which the previous test was performed in order for the subsequent test to be covered).

Pregnant Medicare beneficiaries who have had three screening tests within their respective term of pregnancy are not eligible (beginning with the date of the first test).

D. Other

N/A

(This NCD last reviewed November 2009.)

100-3, Chapter-1, Part-4, 210.8

Screening and Behavioral Counseling Interventions in Primary Care to Reduce Alcohol Misuse(Effective October 14, 2011)

A. General

Based upon authority to cover "additional preventive services" for Medicare beneficiaries if certain statutory requirements are met, the Centers for Medicare & Medicaid Services (CMS) initiated a new national coverage analysis on annual screening and brief behavioral counseling in primary care to reduce alcohol misuse in adults, including pregnant women. Annual screening and behavioural counseling for alcohol misuse in adults is recommended with a grade of B by the U.S. Preventive Services Task Force (USPSTF) and is appropriate for individuals entitled to benefits under Part A and Part B.

CMS will cover annual alcohol screening and up to four, brief face-to-face behavioral counseling in primary care settings to reduce alcohol misuse. CMS does not identify specific alcohol misuse screening tools. Rather, the decision to use a specific tool is at the discretion of the clinician in the primary care setting. Various screening tools are available for screening for alcohol misuse.

B. Nationally Covered Indications

Effective for claims with dates of service on or after October 14, 2011, CMS will cover annual alcohol screening, and for those that screen positive, up to four brief, face-to-face, behavioral counseling interventions per year for Medicare beneficiaries, including pregnant women:

- Who misuse alcohol, but whose levels or patterns of alcohol consumption do not meet criteria for alcohol dependence (defined as at least three of the following: tolerance, withdrawal symptoms, impaired control, preoccupation with acquisition and/or use, persistent desire or unsuccessful efforts to quit, sustains social, occupational, or recreational disability, use continues despite adverse consequences); and

- Who are competent and alert at the time that counseling is provided; and,

- Whose counseling is furnished by qualified primary care physicians or other primary care practitioners in a primary care setting.

Each of the behavioral counseling interventions should be consistent with the 5A's approach that has been adopted by the USPSTF to describe such services. They are:

1. Assess: Ask about/assess behavioral health risk(s) and factors affecting choice of behavior change goals/methods.

2. Advise: Give clear, specific, and personalized behavior change advice, including information about personal health harms and benefits.

3. Agree: Collaboratively select appropriate treatment goals and methods based on the patient's interest in and willingness to change the behavior.

4. Assist: Using behavior change techniques (self-help and/or counseling), aid the patient in achieving agreed upon goals by acquiring the skills, confidence, and social/environmental supports for behavior change, supplemented with adjunctive medical treatments when appropriate.

5. Arrange: Schedule follow-up contacts (in person or by telephone) to provide ongoing assistance/support and to adjust the treatment plan as needed, including referral to more intensive or specialized treatment.

For the purposes of this policy, a primary care setting is defined as one in which there is provision of integrated, accessible health care services by clinicians who are accountable for addressing a large majority of personal health care needs, developing a sustained partnership with patients, and practicing in the context of family and community. Emergency departments, inpatient hospital settings, ambulatory surgical centers, independent diagnostic testing facilities, skilled nursing facilities, inpatient rehabilitation facilities and hospices are not considered primary care settings under this definition.

For the purposes of this policy a "primary care physician" and "primary care practitioner" are to be defined based on two existing sections of the Social Security Act, §1833(u)(6), §1833(x)(2)(A)(i)(I) and §1833(x)(2)(A)(i)(II):

§1833(u)

6. Physician Defined.—For purposes of this paragraph, the term "physician" means a physician described in section 1861(r)(1) and the term "primary care physician" means a physician who is identified in the available data as a general practitioner, family practice practitioner, general internist, or obstetrician or gynecologist.

§1833(x)(2)(A)(i)

i. is a physician (as described in section 1861(r)(1)) who has a primary specialty designation of family medicine, internal medicine, geriatric medicine, or pediatric medicine; or

ii. is a nurse practitioner, clinical nurse specialist, or physician assistant (as those terms are defined in section 1861(aa)(5)).

C. Nationally Non-Covered Indications

1. Alcohol screening is non-covered when performed more than one time in a 12-month period.

2. Brief face-to-face behavioral counseling interventions are non-covered when performed more than once a day; that is, two counseling interventions on the same day are non-covered.

3. Brief face-to-face behavioral counseling interventions are non-covered when performed more than four times in a 12-month period

D. Other

Medicare coinsurance and Part B deductible are waived for this preventive service

(This NCD last reviewed October 2011.)

100-3, Chapter-1, Part-4, 210.10

Screening for Sexually Transmitted Infections (STIs) and High Intensity Behavioral Counseling (HIBC) to Prevent STIs

A. General

Sexually transmitted infections (STIs) are infections that are passed from one person to another through sexual contact. STIs remain an important cause of morbidity in the United States and have both health and economic consequences. Many of the complications of STIs are borne by women and children Often, STIs do not present any symptoms so can go untreated for long periods of time The presence of an STI during pregnancy may result in significant health complications for the woman and infant. In fact, any person who has an STI may develop health complications. Screening tests for the STIs in this national coverage determination (NCD) are laboratory tests.

Under §1861(ddd) of the Social Security Act (the Act), the Centers for Medicare & Medicaid Services (CMS) has the authority to add coverage of additional preventive services if certain statutory requirements are met. The regulations provide:

§410.64 Additional preventive services

a. Medicare Part B pays for additional preventive services not described in paragraph (1) or (3) of the definition of "preventive services" under §410.2, that identify medical conditions or risk factors for individuals if the Secretary determines through the national coverage determination process (as defined in section 1869(f)(1)(B) of the Act) that these services are all of the following: (1) reasonable and necessary for the prevention or early detection of illness or disability.(2)recommended with a grade of A or B by the United States Preventive Services Task Force, (3) appropriate for individuals entitled to benefits under Part A or enrolled under Part B.

b. In making determinations under paragraph (a) of this section regarding the coverage of a new preventive service, the Secretary may conduct an assessment of the relation between predicted outcomes and the expenditures for such services and may take into account the results of such an assessment in making such national coverage determinations.

The scope of the national coverage analysis for this NCD evaluated the evidence for the following STIs and high intensity behavioral counseling (HIBC) to prevent STIs for which the United States Preventive Services Task Force (USPSTF) has issued either an A or B recommendation:

*   Screening for chlamydial infection for all sexually active non-pregnant young women aged 24 and younger and for older non-pregnant women who are at increased risk,
*   Screening for chlamydial infection for all pregnant women aged 24 and younger and for older pregnant women who are at increased risk,
*   Screening for gonorrhea infection in all sexually active women, including those who are pregnant, if they are at increased risk,
*   Screening for syphilis infection for all pregnant women and for all persons at increased risk,
*   Screening for Hepatitis B virus (HBV) infection in pregnant women at their first prenatal visit,
*   HIBC for the prevention of STIs for all sexually active adolescents, and for adults at increased risk for STIs

B. Nationally Covered Indications

CMS has determined that the evidence is adequate to conclude that screening for chlamydia, gonorrhea, syphilis, and Hepatitis B, as well as HIBC to prevent STIs, consistent with the grade A and B recommendations by the USPSTF, is reasonable and necessary for the early detection or prevention of an illness or disability and is appropriate for individuals entitled to benefits under Part A or enrolled under Part B.

Therefore, effective for claims with dates of services on or after November 8, 2011, CMS will cover screening for these USPSTF-indicated STIs with the appropriate Food and Drug Administration (FDA) -approved/cleared laboratory tests, used consistent with FDA-approved labeling, and in compliance with the Clinical Laboratory Improvement Act (CLIA) regulations, when ordered by the primary care physician or practitioner, and performed by an eligible Medicare provider for these services.

Screening for chlamydia and gonorrhea:

*   Pregnant women who are 24 years old or younger when the diagnosis of pregnancy is known, and then repeat screening during the third trimester if high-risk sexual behavior has occurred since the initial screening test.
*   Pregnant women who are at increased risk for STIs when the diagnosis of pregnancy is known, and then repeat screening during the third trimester if high-risk sexual behavior has occurred since the initial screening test.
*   Women at increased risk for STIs annually.

Screening for syphilis:

*   Pregnant women when the diagnosis of pregnancy is known, and then repeat screening during the third

trimester and at delivery if high-risk sexual behaviour has occurred since the previous screening test.
*   Men and women at increased risk for STIs annually.

Screening for Hepatitis B:

*   Pregnant women at the first prenatal visit when the diagnosis of pregnancy is known, and then rescreening at time of delivery for those with new or continuing risk factors.

In addition, effective for claims with dates of service on or after November 8, 2011, CMS will cover up to two individual 20-to 30-minute, face-to-face counseling sessions annually for Medicare beneficiaries for HIBC to prevent STIs, for all sexually active adolescents, and for adults at increased risk for STIs, if referred for this service by a primary care physician or practitioner, and provided by a Medicare eligible primary care provider in a primary care setting. Coverage of HIBC to prevent STIs is consistent with the USPSTF recommendation. HIBC is defined as a program intended to promote sexual risk reduction or risk avoidance, which includes each of these broad topics, allowing flexibility for appropriate patient-focused elements:

*   education,
*   skills training,
*   guidance on how to change sexual behavior.

The high/increased risk individual sexual behaviors, based on the USPSTF guidelines, include any of the following:

*   Multiple sex partners
*   Using barrier protection inconsistently
*   Having sex under the influence of alcohol or drugs
*   Having sex in exchange for money or drugs
*   Age (24 years of age or younger and sexually active for women for chlamydia and gonorrhea)
*   Having an STI within the past year
*   IV drug use (for Hepatitis B only)
*   In addition for men - men having sex with men (MSM) and engaged in high risk sexual behavior, but no regard to age

In addition to individual risk factors, in concurrence with the USPSTF recommendations, community social factors such as high prevalence of STIs in the community populations should be considered in determining high/increased risk for chlamydia, gonorrhea, syphilis, and for recommending HIBC.

High/increased risk sexual behavior for STIs is determined by the primary care provider by assessing the patient's sexual history which is part of any complete medical history, typically part of an annual wellness visit or prenatal visit and considered in the development of a comprehensive prevention plan. The medical record should be a reflection of the service provided.

For the purposes of this NCD, a primary care setting defined as the provision of integrated, accessible health care services by clinicians who are accountable for addressing a large majority of personal health care needs, developing a sustained partnership with patients, and practicing in the context of family and community. Emergency departments, inpatient hospital settings, ambulatory surgical centers, independent diagnostic testing facilities, skilled nursing facilities, inpatient rehabilitation facilities, clinics providing a limited focus of health care services, and hospice are examples of settings not considered primary care settings under this definition.

For the purposes of this NCD, a "primary care physician" and "primary care practitioner" will be defined based on existing sections of the Social Security Act (§1833(u)(6), §1833(x)(2)(A)(i)(I) and §1833(x)(2)(A)(i)(II)).

§1833(u)

(6) Physician Defined.—For purposes of this paragraph, the term "physician" means a

physician described in section 1861(r)(1)and the term "primary care physician" means a physician who is identified in the available data as a general practitioner, family practice practitioner, general internist, or obstetrician or gynecologist.

§1833(x)(2)(A)(i)

i. is a physician (as described in section 1861(r)(1)) who has a primary specialty designation of family medicine, internal medicine, geriatric medicine, or pediatric medicine; or

ii. is a nurse practitioner, clinical nurse specialist, or physician assistant (as those terms are defined in section 1861(aa)(5));

C. Nationally Non-Covered Indications

Unless specifically covered in this NCD, any other NCD, or in statute, preventive services are non-covered by Medicare.

D. Other

Medicare coinsurance and Part B deductible are waived for these preventive services.

HIBC to prevent STIs may be provided on the same date of services as an annual wellness visit, evaluation and management (E&M) service, or during the global billing period for obstetrical car, but only one HIBC may be provided on any one date of service. See the claims processing manual for further instructions on claims processing.

For services provided on an annual basis, this is defined as a 12-Month period.

(This NCD last reviewed November 2011.)

100-3, Chapter-1, Part-4, 210.11

Intensive Behavioral Therapy for Cardiovascular Disease (CVD) (Effective November 8, 2011)

A. General

Cardiovascular disease (CVD) is the leading cause of mortality in the United States. CVD, which is comprised of hypertension, coronary heart disease (such as myocardial infarction and angina pectoris), heart failure and stroke, is also the leading cause of hospitalizations. Although the overall adjusted mortality rate from heart disease has declined over the past decade, opportunities for improvement still exist. Risk factors for CVD include being overweight, obesity, physical inactivity, diabetes, cigarette smoking, high blood pressure, high blood cholesterol, family history of myocardial infarction, and older age.

Under §1861(ddd) of the Social Security Act (the Act), the Centers for Medicare & Medicaid Services (CMS) has the authority to add coverage of additional preventive services through the National Coverage Determination (NCD) process if certain statutory requirements are met. Following its review, CMS has determined that the evidence is adequate to conclude that intensive behavioral therapy for CVD is reasonable and necessary for the prevention or early detection of illness or disability, is appropriate for individuals entitled to benefits under Part A or enrolled under Part B, and is

comprised of components that are recommended with a grade of A or B by the U.S. Preventive Services Task Force (USPSTF).

B. Nationally Covered Indications

Effective for claims with dates of service on or after November 8, 2011, CMS covers intensive behavioral therapy for CVD (referred to below as a CVD risk reduction visit), which consists of the following three components:

- encouraging aspirin use for the primary prevention of CVD when the benefits outweigh the risks for men age 45-79 years and women 55-79 years;

- screening for high blood pressure in adults age 18 years and older; and

- intensive behavioral counseling to promote a healthy diet for adults with hyperlipidemia, hypertension, advancing age, and other known risk factors for cardiovascular-and diet-related chronic disease.

We note that only a small proportion (about 4%) of the Medicare population is under 45 years (men) or 55 years (women), therefore the vast majority of beneficiaries should receive all three components. Intensive behavioral counseling to promote a healthy diet is broadly recommended to cover close to 100% of the population due to the prevalence of known risk factors.

Therefore, CMS covers one, face-to-face CVD risk reduction visit per year for Medicare beneficiaries who are competent and alert at the time that counseling is provided, and whose counseling is furnished by a qualified primary care physician or other primary care practitioner in a primary care setting.

The behavioral counseling intervention for aspirin use and healthy diet should be consistent with the Five As approach that has been adopted by the USPSTF to describe such services:

- **Assess:** Ask about/assess behavioral health risk(s) and factors affecting choice of behavior change goals/methods.

- **Advise:** Give clear, specific, and personalized behavior change advice, including information about personal health harms and benefits.

- **Agree:** Collaboratively select appropriate treatment goals and methods based on the patient's interest in and willingness to change the behavior.

- **Assist:** Using behavior change techniques (self-help and/or counseling), aid the patient in achieving agreed-upon goals by acquiring the skills, confidence, and social/environmental supports for behavior change, supplemented with adjunctive medical treatments when appropriate.

- **Arrange:** Schedule follow-up contacts (in person or by telephone) to provide ongoing assistance/support and to adjust the treatment plan as needed, including referral to more intensive or specialized treatment.

For the purpose of this NCD, a primary care setting is defined as the provision of integrated, accessible health care services by clinicians who are accountable for addressing a large majority of personal health care needs, developing a sustained partnership with patients, and practicing in the context of family and community. Emergency departments, inpatient hospital settings, ambulatory surgical centers, independent diagnostic testing facilities, skilled nursing facilities, inpatient rehabilitation facilities, and hospices are not considered primary care settings under this definition.

For the purpose of this NCD, a "primary care physician" and "primary care practitioner" are defined consistent with existing sections of the Act (§1833(u)(6), §1833(x)(2)(A)(i)(I) and §1833(x)(2)(A)(i)(II)).

§1833(u)

(6) Physician Defined.—For purposes of this paragraph, the term "physician" means a physician described in section 1861(r)(1)and the term "primary care physician" means a physician who is identified in the available data as a general practitioner, family practice practitioner, general internist, or obstetrician or gynecologist.

physician who is identified in the available data as a general practitioner, family practice practitioner, general internist, or obstetrician or gynecologist.

§1833(x)(2) (A) Primary care practitioner.—The term "primary care practitioner" means an individual—

(i) who—

I. is a physician (as described in section 1861(r)(1)) who has a primary specialty designation of family medicine, internal medicine, geriatric medicine, or pediatric medicine; or

II. is a nurse practitioner, clinical nurse specialist, or physician assistant (as those terms are defined in section 1861(aa)(5)).

C. Nationally Non-Covered Indications

Unless specifically covered in this NCD, any other NCD, or in statute, preventive services are non-covered by Medicare.

D. Other

Medicare coinsurance and Part B deductible are waived for this preventive service.

(This NCD last reviewed November 2011.)

100-3, Chapter-1, Part-4, 210.12

Intensive Behavioral Therapy for Obesity (Effective November 29, 2011)

A. General

Based upon authority to cover "additional preventive services" for Medicare beneficiaries if certain statutory requirements are met, the Centers for Medicare & Medicaid Services (CMS) initiated a new national coverage analysis on intensive behavioral therapy for obesity. Screening for obesity in adults is recommended with a grade of B by the U.S. Preventive Services Task Force (USPSTF) and is appropriate for individuals entitled to benefits under Part A and Part B.

The Centers for Disease Control (CDC) reported that "obesity rates in the U.S. have increased dramatically over the last 30 years, and obesity is now epidemic in the United States." In the Medicare population over 30% of men and women are obese. Obesity is directly or indirectly associated with many chronic diseases including cardiovascular disease, musculoskeletal conditions and diabetes.

B. Nationally Covered Indications

Effective for claims with dates of service on or after November 29, 2011, CMS covers intensive behavioral therapy for obesity, defined as a body mass index (BMI) ≥ 30 kg/m2, for the prevention or early detection of illness or disability.

Intensive behavioral therapy for obesity consists of the following:

1. Screening for obesity in adults using measurement of BMI calculated by dividing weight in kilograms by the square of height in meters (expressed kg/m2);

2. Dietary (nutritional) assessment; and Intensive behavioral counseling and behavioral therapy to promote sustained

3. weight loss through high intensity interventions on diet and exercise.

The intensive behavioral intervention for obesity should be consistent with the 5-A

framework that has been highlighted by the USPSTF:

1. **Assess:** Ask about/assess behavioral health risk(s) and factors affecting choice of behavior change goals/ methods.

2. **Advise:** Give clear, specific, and personalized behavior change advice, including information about personal health harms and benefits.

3. **Agree:** Collaboratively select appropriate treatment goals and methods based on the patient's interest in and willingness to change the behavior.

4. **Assist:** Using behavior change techniques (self-help and/or counseling), aid the patient in achieving agreed-upon goals by acquiring the skills, confidence, and social/environmental supports for behavior change, supplemented with adjunctive medical treatments when appropriate.

5. **Arrange:** Schedule follow-up contacts (in person or by telephone) to provide ongoing assistance/support and to adjust the treatment plan as needed, including referral to more intensive or specialized treatment.

For Medicare beneficiaries with obesity, who are competent and alert at the time that counseling is provided and whose counseling is furnished by a qualified primary care physician or other primary care practitioner and in a primary care setting, CMS covers:

- One face-to-face visit every week for the first month;
- One face-to-face visit every other week for months 2-6;
- One face-to-face visit every month for months 7-12, if the beneficiary meets the 3kg weight loss requirement during the first six months as discussed below.

At the six month visit, a reassessment of obesity and a determination of the amount of weight loss must be performed. To be eligible for additional face-to-face visits occurring once a month for an additional six months, beneficiaries must have achieved a reduction in weight of at least 3kg over the course of the first six months of intensive therapy. This determination must be documented in the physician office records for applicable beneficiaries consistent with usual practice. For beneficiaries who do not achieve a weight loss of at least 3kg during the first six months of intensive therapy, a reassessment of their readiness to change and BMI is appropriate after an additional six month period.

For the purposes of this decision memorandum, a primary care setting is defined as one in which there is provision of integrated, accessible health care services by clinicians who are accountable for addressing a large majority of personal health care needs, developing a sustained partnership with patients, and practicing in the context of family and community. Emergency departments, inpatient hospital settings, ambulatory surgical centers, independent diagnostic testing facilities, skilled nursing facilities, inpatient rehabilitation facilities and hospices are not considered primary care settings under this definition.

For the purposes of this decision memorandum a "primary care physician" and "primary care practitioner" will be defined consistent with existing sections of the Social Security Act (§1833(u)(6), §1833(x)(2)(A)(i)(I) and §1833(x)(2)(A)(i)(II)).

§1833(u)

(6) Physician Defined.—For purposes of this paragraph, the term "physician" means a physician described in section 1861(r)(1) and the term "primary care physician" means a physician who is identified in the available data as a general practitioner, family practice practitioner, general internist, or obstetrician or gynecologist.

§1833(x)(2)(A)

Primary care practitioner—The term "primary care practitioner" means an individual—

(i) who—

I. is a physician (as described in section 1861(r)(1)) who has a primary specialty designation of family medicine, internal medicine, geriatric medicine, or pediatric medicine; or

II. is a nurse practitioner, clinical nurse specialist, or physician assistant (as those terms are defined in section 1861(aa)(5))

C. Nationally Non-Covered Indications

All other indications remain non-covered.

D. Other

Medicare coinsurance and Part B deductible are waived for this service

(This NCD last reviewed November 2011)

100-3, Chapter-1, Part-4, 220.6

Positron Emission Tomography (PET) Scans

Positron Emission Tomography (PET) is a minimally invasive diagnostic imaging procedure used to evaluate metabolism in normal tissues as well as in diseased tissues in conditions such as cancer, ischemic heart disease, and some neurologic disorders. A radiopharmaceutical is injected into the patient that gives off sub-atomic particles, known as positrons, as it decays. PET uses a positron camera (tomograph) to measure the decay of the radiopharmaceutical. The rate of decay provides biochemical information to on the metabolism of the tissue being studied.

NOTE: This manual section, 220.6 lists all Medicare–covered uses of PET scans. Except as set forth below in cancer indications listed as "Coverage with Evidence Development," a particular use of PET scans is not covered unless this manual specifically provides that such use is covered. Although this section, 220.6 lists some non-covered uses of PET scans, it does not non-covered uses of PET scans, it does not constitute an exhaustive list of all non- covered uses.

Effective for dates of service on or after March 7, 2013, local Medicare Administrative Contractors (MACs) may determine coverage within their respective jurisdictions for positron emission tomography (PET) using radiopharmaceuticals for their Food and Drug Administration (FDA) approved labeled indications for oncologic imaging.

We emphasize each of the following points:

1. Changing the 'restrictive' language of prior PET decisions will not by itself suffice to expand Medicare coverage to new PET radiopharmaceuticals.

2. The scope of this change extends only to FDA-approved indications for oncologic uses of PET tracers.

3. This change does not include screening uses of PET scanning.

The Centers for Medicare & Medicaid Services (CMS) acknowledges the advances relating to the assessment of diagnostic performance and patient safety, as pioneered by the FDA in its regulatory policies and guidelines for diagnostic PET imaging agents and systems during the past decade. We note for completeness that local coverage cannot be in conflict with NCDs or other national policies. Finally, we note that future CMS NCDs, if any, regarding diagnostic PET imaging would not be precluded by this NCD.

100-3, Chapter-1, Part-4, 220.6.1

PET for Perfusion of the Heart (220.6.1) (Various Effective Dates)

1. Rubidium 82 (Effective March 14, 1995)

Effective for services performed on or after March 14, 1995, PET scans performed at rest or with pharmacological stress used for noninvasive imaging of the perfusion of the heart for the diagnosis and management of patients with known or suspected coronary artery disease using the FDA approved radiopharmaceutical Rubidium 82 (Rb 82) are covered, provided the requirements below are met:

- The PET scan, whether at rest alone, or rest with stress, is performed in place of, but not in addition to, a single photon emission computed tomography (SPECT); or

- The PET scan, whether at rest alone or rest with stress, is used following a SPECT that was found to be inconclusive. In these cases, the PET scan must have been considered necessary in order to determine what medical or surgical intervention is required to treat the patient. (For purposes of this requirement, an inconclusive test is a test(s) whose results are equivocal, technically uninterpretable, or discordant with a patient's other clinical data and must be documented in the beneficiary's file.)

- For any PET scan for which Medicare payment is claimed for dates of services prior to July 1, 2001, the claimant must submit additional specified information on the claim form (including proper codes and/or modifiers), to indicate the results of the PET scan. The claimant must also include information on whether the PET scan was performed after an inconclusive non-invasive cardiac test. The information submitted with respect to the previous noninvasive cardiac test must specify the type of test performed prior to the PET scan and whether it was inconclusive or unsatisfactory. These explanations are in the form of special G codes used for billing PET scans using Rb 82. Beginning July 1, 2001, claims should be submitted with the appropriate codes.

2. Ammonia N-13 (Effective October 1, 2003)

Effective for services performed on or after October 1, 2003, PET scans performed at rest or with pharmacological stress used for noninvasive imaging of the perfusion of the heart for the diagnosis and management of patients with known or suspected coronary artery disease using the FDA approved radiopharmaceutical ammonia N-13 are covered, provided the requirements below are met:

- The PET scan, whether at rest alone, or rest with stress, is performed in place of, but not in addition to, a SPECT; or

- The PET scan, whether at rest alone or rest with stress, is used following a SPECT that was found to be inconclusive. In these cases, the PET scan must have been considered necessary in order to determine what medical or surgical intervention is required to treat the patient. (For purposes of this requirement, an inconclusive test is a test whose results are equivocal, technically uninterpretable, or discordant with a patient's other clinical data and must be documented in the beneficiary's file.)

(This NCD last reviewed March 2005.)

100-3, Chapter-1, Part-4, 220.6.17

Positron Emission Tomography (FDG PET) for Oncologic Conditions (Effective June 11, 2013)

A. General

FDG (2-[F18] fluoro-2-deoxy-D-glucose) Positron Emission Tomography (PET) is a minimally-invasive diagnostic imaging procedure used to evaluate glucose metabolism in normal tissue as well as in diseased tissues in conditions such as cancer, ischemic heart disease, and some neurologic disorders. FDG is an injected radionuclide (or radiopharmaceutical) that emits sub-atomic particles, known as positrons, as it decays. FDG PET uses a positron camera (tomograph) to measure the decay of FDG. The rate of FDG decay provides biochemical information on glucose metabolism in the tissue being studied. As malignancies can cause abnormalities of metabolism and blood flow, FDG PET evaluation may indicate the probable presence or absence of a malignancy based upon observed differences in biologic activity compared to adjacent tissues.

The Centers for Medicare and Medicaid Services (CMS) was asked by the National Oncologic PET Registry (NOPR) to reconsider section 220.6 of the National Coverage Determinations (NCD) Manual to end the prospective data collection requirements under Coverage with Evidence Development (CED) across all oncologic indications of FDG PET imaging. The CMS received public input indicating that the current coverage framework of prospective data collection under CED be ended for all oncologic uses of FDG PET imaging.

1. Framework

Effective for claims with dates of service on and after June 11, 2013, CMS is adopting a coverage framework that ends the prospective data collection requirements by NOPR under CED for all oncologic uses of FDG PET imaging. CMS is making this change for all NCDs that address coverage of FDG PET for oncologic uses addressed in this decision. This decision does not change coverage for any use of PET imaging using radiopharmaceuticals NaF-18 (fluorine-18 labeled sodium fluoride), ammonia N-13, or rubidium-82 (Rb-82).

4. Initial Anti-Tumor Treatment Strategy

CMS continues to believe that the evidence is adequate to determine that the results of FDG PET imaging are useful in determining the appropriate initial anti-tumor treatment strategy for beneficiaries with suspected cancer and improve health outcomes and thus are reasonable and necessary under §1862(a)(1)(A) of the Social Security Act (the Act).

Therefore, CMS continues to nationally cover one FDG PET study for beneficiaries who have cancers that are biopsy proven or strongly suspected based on other diagnostic testing when the beneficiary's treating physician determines that the FDG PET study is needed to determine the location and/or extent of the tumor for the following therapeutic purposes related to the initial anti-tumor treatment strategy:

- To determine whether or not the beneficiary is an appropriate candidate for an invasive diagnostic or therapeutic procedure; or
- To determine the optimal anatomic location for an invasive procedure; or
- To determine the anatomic extent of tumor when the recommended anti-tumor treatment reasonably depends on the extent of the tumor.

See the table at the end of this section for a synopsis of all nationally covered and non-covered oncologic uses of FDG PET imaging.

B.1. Initial Anti-Tumor Treatment Strategy Nationally Covered Indications

a. CMS continues to nationally cover FDG PET imaging for the initial anti-tumor treatment strategy for male and female breast cancer only when used in staging distant metastasis.

b. CMS continues to nationally cover FDG PET to determine initial anti-tumor treatment strategy for melanoma other than for the evaluation of regional lymph Nodes

c. CMS continues to nationally cover FDG PET to determine initial anti-tumor treatment strategy for melanoma other than for the evaluation of regional lymph nodes

C.1 Initial Anti-Tumor Treatment Strategy Nationally Non-Covered Indications

a. CMS continues to nationally non-cover initial anti-tumor treatment strategy in Medicare beneficiaries who have adenocarcinoma of the prostate.

b. CMS continues to nationally non-cover FDG PET imaging for diagnosis of breast cancer and initial staging of axillary nodes.

c. CMS continues to nationally non-cover FDG PET imaging for initial anti-tumor treatment strategy for the evaluation of regional lymph nodes in melanoma.

d. CMS continues to nationally non-cover FDG PET imaging for the diagnosis of cervical cancer related to initial anti-tumor treatment strategy.

3. Subsequent Anti-Tumor Treatment Strategy

B.2. Subsequent Anti-Tumor Treatment Strategy Nationally Covered Indications

Three FDG PET scans are nationally covered when used to guide subsequent management of anti-tumor treatment strategy after completion of initial anti-cancer therapy. Coverage of more than three FDG PET scans to guide subsequent management of anti-tumor treatment strategy after completion of initial anti-cancer therapy shall be determined by the local Medicare Administrative Contractors.

4. Synopsis of Coverage of FDG PET for Oncologic Conditions

Effective for claims with dates of service on and after June 11, 2013, the chart below summarizes national FDG PET coverage for oncologic conditions:

FDG PET for Cancers Tumor Type	Initial Treatment Strategy (formerly "diagnosis" & "staging"	Subsequent Treatment Strategy (formerly "restaging" & "monitoring response to treatment"
Colorectal	Cover	Cover
Esophagus	Cover	Cover

FDG PET for Cancers Tumor Type	Initial Treatment Strategy (formerly "diagnosis" & "staging"	Subsequent Treatment Strategy (formerly "restaging" & "monitoring response to treatment"
Head and Neck (not thyroid, CNS)	Cover	Cover
Lymphoma	Cover	Cover
Non-small cell lung	Cover	Cover
Ovary	Cover	Cover
Brain	Cover	Cover
Cervix	Cover with exceptions *	Cover
Small cell lung	Cover	Cover
Soft tissue sarcoma	Cover	Cover
Pancreas	Cover	Cover
Testes	Cover	Cover
Prostate	Non-cover	Cover
Thyroid	Cover	Cover
Breast (male and female)	Cover with exceptions *	Cover
Melanoma	Cover with exceptions *	Cover
All other solid tumors	Cover	Cover
Myeloma	Cover	Cover
All other cancers not listed	Cover	Cover

*Cervix: Nationally non-covered for the initial diagnosis of cervical cancer related to initial anti-tumor treatment strategy. All other indications for initial anti-tumor treatment strategy for cervical cancer are nationally covered.

*Breast: Nationally non-covered for initial diagnosis and/or staging of axillary lymph nodes. Nationally covered for initial staging of metastatic disease. All other indications for initial anti-tumor treatment strategy for breast cancer are nationally covered.

*Melanoma: Nationally non-covered for initial staging of regional lymph nodes. All other indications for initial anti-tumor treatment strategy for melanoma are nationally covered.

D. Other

N/A

100-3, Chapter-1, Part-4, 220.6.19

Positron Emission Tomography NaF-18 (NaF-18 PET) to Identify Bone Metastasis of Cancer (Effective February 26, 2010)

A. General

Positron Emission Tomography (PET) is a non-invasive, diagnostic imaging procedure that assesses the level of metabolic activity and perfusion in various organ systems of the body. A positron camera (tomograph) is used to produce cross-sectional tomographic images, which are obtained from positron-emitting radioactive tracer substances (radiopharmaceuticals) such as F-18 sodium fluoride. NaF-

18 PET has been recognized as an excellent technique for imaging areas of altered osteogenic activity in bone. The clinical value of detecting and assessing the initial extent of metastatic cancer in bone is attested by a number of professional guidelines for oncology. Imaging to detect bone metastases is also recommended when a patient, following completion of initial treatment, is symptomatic with bone pain suspicious for metastases from a known primary tumor.

B. Nationally Covered Indications

Effective February 26, 2010, the Centers for Medicare & Medicaid Services (CMS) will cover NaF-18 PET imaging when the beneficiary's treating physician determines that the NaF-18 PET study is needed to inform to inform the initial antitumor treatment strategy or to guide subsequent antitumor treatment strategy after the completion of initial treatment, and when the beneficiary is enrolled in, and the NaF-18 PET provider is participating in, the following type of prospective clinical study:

A NaF-18 PET clinical study that is designed to collect additional information at the time of the scan to assist in initial antitumor treatment planning or to guide subsequent treatment strategy by the identification, location and quantification of bone metastases in beneficiaries in whom bone metastases are strongly suspected based on clinical symptoms or the results of other diagnostic studies. Qualifying clinical studies must ensure that specific hypotheses are addressed; appropriate data elements are collected; hospitals and providers are qualified to provide the PET scan and interpret the results; participating hospitals and providers accurately report data on all enrolled patients not included in other qualifying trials through adequate auditing mechanisms; and all patient confidentiality, privacy, and other Federal laws must be followed.

The clinical studies for which Medicare will provide coverage must answer one or more of the following questions:

Prospectively, in Medicare beneficiaries whose treating physician determines that the NaF-18 PET study results are needed to inform the initial antitumor treatment strategy or to guide subsequent antitumor treatment strategy after the completion of initial treatment, does the addition of NaF-18 PET imaging lead to:

- A change in patient management to more appropriate palliative care; or
- A change in patient management to more appropriate curative care; or
- Improved quality of life; or
- Improved survival?

The study must adhere to the following standards of scientific integrity and relevance to the Medicare population:

a. The principal purpose of the research study is to test whether a particular intervention potentially improves the participants' health outcomes.

b. The research study is well-supported by available scientific and medical information or it is intended to clarify or establish the health outcomes of interventions already in common clinical use.

c. The research study does not unjustifiably duplicate existing studies.

d. The research study design is appropriate to answer the research question being asked in the study

e. The research study is sponsored by an organization or individual capable of executing the proposed study successfully.

f. The research study is in compliance with all applicable Federal regulations concerning the protection of human subjects found in the Code of Federal Regulations (CFR) at 45 CFR Part 46. If a study is regulated by the Food and Drug Administration (FDA), it also must be in compliance with 21 CFR Parts 50 and 56.

g. All aspects of the research study are conducted according to the appropriate standards of scientific integrity.

h. The research study has a written protocol that clearly addresses, or incorporates by reference, the Medicare standards.

i. The clinical research study is not designed to exclusively test toxicity or disease pathophysiology in healthy individuals. Trials of all medical technologies measuring therapeutic outcomes as one of the objectives meet this standard only if the disease or condition being studied is life-threatening as defined in 21 CFR §312.81(a) and the patient has no other viable treatment options.

j. The clinical research study is registered on the www.ClinicalTrials.gov Web site by the principal sponsor/investigator prior to the enrollment of the first study subject.

k. The research study protocol specifies the method and timing of public release of all pre-specified outcomes to be measured including release of outcomes if outcomes are negative or study is terminated early. The results must be made public within 24 months of the end of data collection. If a report is planned to be published in a peer-reviewed journal, then that initial release may be an abstract that meets the requirements of the International Committee of Medical Journal Editors. However, a full report of the outcomes must be made public no later than three (3) years after the end of data collection.

l. The research study protocol must explicitly discuss subpopulations affected by the treatment under investigation, particularly traditionally underrepresented groups in clinical studies, how the inclusion and exclusion criteria affect enrollment of these populations, and a plan for the retention and reporting of said populations on the trial. If the inclusion an exclusion criteria are expected to have a negative effect on the recruitment or retention of underrepresented populations, the protocol must discuss why these criteria are necessary.

m. The research study protocol explicitly discusses how the results are or are not expected to be generalizable to the Medicare population to infer whether Medicare patients may benefit from the intervention. Separate discussions in the protocol may be necessary for populations eligible for Medicare due to age, disability or Medicaid eligibility.

Consistent with section 1142 of the Social Security Act (the Act), the Agency for Healthcare Research and Quality (AHRQ) supports clinical research studies that the Centers for Medicare and Medicaid Services (CMS) determines meet the above-listed standards and address the above-listed research questions.

C. Nationally Non-Covered Indications

Effective February 26, 2010, CMS determines that the evidence is not sufficient to determine that the results of NaF-18 PET imaging to identify bone metastases improve health outcomes of beneficiaries with cancer and is not reasonable and necessary under §1862(a)(1)(A) of the Act unless it is to inform initial antitumor treatment strategy or to guide subsequent antitumor treatment strategy after completion of initial treatment, and then only under CED. All other uses and clinical indications of NaF-18 PET are nationally non-covered.

D. Other

The only radiopharmaceutical diagnostic imaging agents covered by Medicare for PET cancer imaging are 2-[F-18] Fluoro-D-Glucose (FDG) and NaF-18 (sodium fluoride-18). All other PET radiopharmaceutical diagnostic imaging agents are non-covered for this indication.

(This NCD was last reviewed in February 2010.)

100-3, Chapter-1, Part-4, 240.4

Continuous Positive Airway Pressure (CPAP) Therapy For Obstructive Sleep Apnea (OSA) (Effective April 4, 2005) (Effective March 13, 2008)

A. General

Continuous Positive Airway Pressure (CPAP) is a non-invasive technique for providing single levels of air pressure from a flow generator, via a nose mask, through the nares. The purpose is to prevent the collapse of the oropharyngeal walls and the obstruction of airflow during sleep, which occurs in obstructive sleep apnea (OSA).

The apnea hypopnea index (AHI) is equal to the average number of episodes of apnea and hypopnea per hour. The respiratory disturbance index (RDI) is equal to the average number of respiratory disturbances per hour.

Apnea is defined as a cessation of airflow for at least 10 seconds. Hypopnea is defined as an abnormal respiratory event lasting at least 10 seconds with at least a 30% reduction in thoracoabdominal movement or airflow as compared to baseline, and with at least a 4% oxygen desaturation.

The AHI and/or RDI may be measured by polysomnography (PSG) in a facility-based sleep study laboratory, or by a Type II home sleep test (HST) monitor, a Type III HST monitor, or a Type IV HST monitor measuring at least 3 channels.

B. Nationally Covered Indications

Effective for claims with dates of service on and after March 13, 2008, the Centers for Medicare & Medicaid Services (CMS) determines that CPAP therapy when used in adult patients with OSA is considered reasonable and necessary under the following situations:

1. The use of CPAP is covered under Medicare when used in adult patients with OSA. Coverage of CPAP is initially limited to a 12-week period to identify beneficiaries diagnosed with OSA as subsequently described who benefit from CPAP. CPAP is subsequently covered only for those beneficiaries diagnosed with OSA who benefit from CPAP during this 12-week period.

2. The provider of CPAP must conduct education of the beneficiary prior to the use of the CPAP device to ensure that the beneficiary has been educated in the proper use of the device. A caregiver, for example a family member, may be compensatory, if consistently available in the beneficiary's home and willing and able to safely operate the CPAP device.

3. A positive diagnosis of OSA for the coverage of CPAP must include a clinical evaluation and a positive:

    a. attended PSG performed in a sleep laboratory; or

    b. unattended HST with a Type II home sleep monitoring device; or

    c. unattended HST with a Type III home sleep monitoring device; or

    d. unattended HST with a Type IV home sleep monitoring device that measures at least 3 channels.

4. The sleep test must have been previously ordered by the beneficiary's treating physician and furnished under appropriate physician supervision.

5. An initial 12-week period of CPAP is covered in adult patients with OSA if either of the following criterion using the AHI or RDI are met:

   a. AHI or RDI greater than or equal to 15 events per hour, or

   b. AHI or RDI greater than or equal to 5 events and less than or equal to 14 events per hour with documented symptoms of excessive daytime sleepiness, impaired cognition, mood disorders or insomnia, or documented hypertension, ischemic heart disease, or history of stroke.

6. The AHI or RDI is calculated on the average number of events of per hour. If the AHI or RDI is calculated based on less than 2 hours of continuous recorded sleep, the total number of recorded events to calculate the AHI or RDI during sleep testing must be at a minimum the number of events that would have been required in a 2-hour period.

7. Apnea is defined as a cessation of airflow for at least 10 seconds. Hypopnea is defined as an abnormal respiratory event lasting at least 10 seconds with at least a 30% reduction in thoracoabdominal movement or airflow as compared to baseline, and with at least a 4% oxygen desaturation.

8. Coverage with Evidence Development (CED): Medicare provides the following limited coverage for CPAP in adult beneficiaries who do not qualify for CPAP coverage based on criteria 1-7 above. A clinical study seeking Medicare payment for CPAP provided to a beneficiary who is an enrolled subject in that study must address one or more of the following questions:

   a. In Medicare-aged subjects with clinically identified risk factors for OSA, how does the diagnostic accuracy of a clinical trial of CPAP compare with PSG and Type II, III & IV HST in identifying subjects with OSA who will respond to CPAP?

   b. In Medicare-aged subjects with clinically identified risk factors for OSA who have not undergone confirmatory testing with PSG or Type II, III & IV HST, does CPAP cause clinically meaningful harm?

   c. The study must meet the following additional standards:

   d. The principal purpose of the research study is to test whether a particular intervention potentially improves the participants' health outcomes.

   e. The research study is well-supported by available scientific and medical information or it is intended to clarify or establish the health outcomes of interventions already in common clinical use.

   f. The research study does not unjustifiably duplicate existing studies.

   g. The research study design is appropriate to answer the research question being asked in the study.

   h. The research study is sponsored by an organization or individual capable of executing the proposed study successfully.

   i. The research study is in compliance with all applicable Federal regulations concerning the protection of human subjects found at 45 CFR Part 46. If a study is Food and Drug Administration-regulated, it also must be in compliance with 21 CFR Parts 50 and 56.

   j. All aspects of the research study are conducted according to the appropriate standards of scientific integrity.

   k. The research study has a written protocol that clearly addresses, or incorporates by reference, the Medicare standards.

   l. The clinical research study is not designed to exclusively test toxicity or disease pathophysiology in healthy individuals. Trials of all medical technologies measuring therapeutic outcomes as one of the objectives meet this standard only if the disease or condition being studied is life-threatening as defined in 21 CFR §312.81(a) and the patient has no other viable treatment options.

   m. The clinical research study is registered on the ClinicalTrials.gov Web site by the principal sponsor/investigator prior to the enrollment of the first study subject.

   n. The research study protocol specifies the method and timing of public release of all pre-specified outcomes to be measured, including release of outcomes if outcomes are negative or study is terminated early. The results must be made public within 24 months of the end of data collection. If a report is planned for publication in a peer-reviewed journal, then that initial release may be an abstract that meets the requirements of the International Committee of Medical Journal Editors. However, a full report of the outcomes must be made public no later than 3 years after the end of data collection.

   o. The research study protocol must explicitly discuss subpopulations affected by the treatment under investigation, particularly traditionally underrepresented groups in clinical studies, how the inclusion and exclusion criteria affect enrollment of these populations, and a plan for the retention and reporting of said populations in the trial. If the inclusion and exclusion criteria are expected to have a negative effect on the recruitment or retention of underrepresented populations, the protocol must discuss why these criteria are necessary.

   p. The research study protocol explicitly discusses how the results are or are not expected to be generalizable to the Medicare population to infer whether Medicare patients may benefit from the intervention. Separate discussions in the protocol may be necessary for populations eligible for Medicare due to age, disability, or Medicaid eligibility.

C. Nationally Non-covered Indications

Effective for claims with dates of services on and after March 13, 2008, other diagnostic tests for the diagnosis of OSA, other than those noted above for prescribing CPAP, are not sufficient for the coverage of CPAP.

D. Other

N/A

(This NCD last reviewed March 2008.)

100-3, Chapter-1, Part-4, 240.4.1

Sleep Testing for Obstructive Sleep Apnea (OSA) (Effective March 3, 2009)

A. General

Obstructive sleep apnea (OSA) is the collapse of the oropharyngeal walls and the obstruction of airflow occurring during sleep. Diagnostic tests for OSA have historically been classified into four types. The most comprehensive is designated Type I attended facility based polysomnography (PSG), which is considered the reference standard for diagnosing OSA. Attended facility based polysomnogram is a comprehensive diagnostic sleep test including at least electroencephalography (EEG), electro-oculography (EOG), electromyography (EMG), heart rate or electrocardiography (ECG), airflow, breathing/respiratory effort, and arterial oxygen saturation (SaO2) furnished in a sleep laboratory facility in which a technologist supervises the recording during sleep time and has the ability to intervene if needed. Overnight PSG is the conventional diagnostic test for OSA. The American Thoracic Society and the American Academy of Sleep Medicine have recommended supervised PSG in the sleep laboratory over 2 nights for the diagnosis of OSA and the initiation of continuous positive airway pressure (CPAP).

Three categories of portable monitors (used both in attended and unattended settings) have been developed for the diagnosis of OSA. Type II monitors have a minimum of 7 channels (e.g., EEG, EOG, EMG, ECG-heart rate, airflow, breathing/respiratory effort, SaO2)-this type of device monitors sleep staging, so AHI can be calculated). Type III monitors have a minimum of 4 monitored channels including ventilation or airflow (at least two channels of respiratory movement or respiratory movement and airflow), heart rate or ECG, and oxygen saturation. Type IV devices may measure one, two, three or more parameters but do not meet all the criteria of a higher category device. Some monitors use an actigraphy algorithm to identify periods of sleep and wakefulness.

B. Nationally Covered Indications

Effective for claims with dates of service on and after March 3, 2009, the Centers for Medicare & Medicaid Services finds that the evidence is sufficient to determine that the results of the sleep tests identified below can be used by a beneficiary's treating physician to diagnose OSA, that the use of such sleep testing technologies demonstrates improved health outcomes in Medicare beneficiaries who have OSA and receive the appropriate treatment, and that these tests are thus reasonable and necessary under section 1862(a)(1)(A) of the Social Security Act.

1. Type I PSG is covered when used to aid the diagnosis of OSA in beneficiaries who have clinical signs and symptoms indicative of OSA if performed attended in a sleep lab facility.

2. Type II or Type III sleep testing devices are covered when used to aid the diagnosis of OSA in beneficiaries who have clinical signs and symptoms indicative of OSA if performed unattended in or out of a sleep lab facility or attended in a sleep lab facility.

3. Type IV sleep testing devices measuring three or more channels, one of which is airflow, are covered when used to aid the diagnosis of OSA in beneficiaries who have signs and symptoms indicative of OSA if performed unattended in or out of a sleep lab facility or attended in a sleep lab facility.

4. Sleep testing devices measuring three or more channels that include actigraphy, oximetry, and peripheral arterial tone, are covered when used to aid the diagnosis of OSA in beneficiaries who have signs and symptoms indicative of OSA if performed unattended in or out of a sleep lab facility or attended in a sleep lab facility.

C. Nationally Non-Covered Indications

Effective for claims with dates of services on and after March 3, 2009, other diagnostic sleep tests for the diagnosis of OSA, other than those noted above for prescribing CPAP, are not sufficient for the coverage of CPAP and are not covered.

D. Other

N/A

(This NCD last reviewed March 2009.)

100-3, Chapter-1, Part-4, 250.5

Dermal Injections for the Treatment of Facial Lipodystrophy Syndrome (LDS) - Effective March 23, 2010

A. General

Treatment of persons infected with the human immunodeficiency virus (HIV) or persons who have Acquired Immune Deficiency Syndrome (AIDS) may include highly active antiretroviral therapy (HAART). Drug reactions commonly associated with long-term use of HAART include metabolic complications such as, lipid abnormalities, e.g., hyperlipidemia, hyperglycemia, diabetes, lipodystrophy, and heart disease. Lipodystrophy is characterized by abnormal fat distribution in the body.

The LDS is often characterized by a loss of fat that results in a facial abnormality such as severely sunken cheeks. The patient's physical appearance may contribute to psychological conditions (e.g., depression) or adversely impact a patient's adherence to antiretroviral regimens (therefore jeopardizing their health) and both of these are important health-related outcomes of interest in this population. Therefore, improving a patient's physical appearance through the use of dermal injections could improve these health-related outcomes.

B. Nationally Covered Indications

Effective for claims with dates of service on and after March 23, 2010, dermal injections for LDS are only reasonable and necessary using dermal fillers approved by the Food and Drug Administration (FDA) for this purpose, and then only in HIV-infected beneficiaries when LDS caused by antiretroviral HIV treatment is a significant contributor to their depression.

C. Nationally Non-Covered Indications

1. Dermal fillers that are not approved by the FDA for the treatment of LDS.

2. Dermal fillers that are used for any indication other than LDS in HIV-infected individuals who manifest depression as a result of their antiretroviral HIV treatments.

D. Other

N/A

(This NCD last reviewed March 2010.)

100-3, Chapter-1, Part-4, 260.6

Dental Examination Prior to Kidney Transplantation

Despite the "dental services exclusion" in §1862(a)(12) of the Act (see the Medicare Benefit Policy Manual, Chapter 16, "General Exclusions From Coverage," §140;), an oral or dental examination performed on an inpatient basis as part of a comprehensive workup prior to renal transplant surgery is a covered service. This is because the purpose of the examination is not for the care of the teeth or structures directly supporting the teeth. Rather, the examination is for the identification, prior to a complex surgical procedure, of existing medical problems where the increased possibility of infection would not only reduce the chances for successful surgery but would also expose the patient to additional risks in undergoing such surgery.

Such a dental or oral examination would be covered under Part A of the program if performed by a dentist on the hospital's staff, or under Part B if performed by a physician. (When performing a dental or oral examination, a dentist is not recognized as a physician under §1861(r) of the Act.) (See the Medicare General Information, Eligibility, and Entitlement Manual, Chapter 5, "Definitions," §70.2, and the Medicare Benefit Policy Manual, Chapter 15, "Covered Medical and Other Health Services," §150.)

100-3, Chapter-1, Part-4, 270.3

Blood-Derived Products for Chronic Non-Healing Wounds

A. General

Wound healing is a dynamic, interactive process that involves multiple cells and proteins. There are three progressive stages of normal wound healing, and the typical wound healing duration is about 4 weeks. While cutaneous wounds are a disruption of the normal, anatomic structure and function of the skin, subcutaneous wounds involve tissue below the skin's surface. Wounds are categorized as either acute, in where the normal wound healing stages are not yet completed but it is presumed they will be, resulting in orderly and timely wound repair, or chronic, in where a wound has failed to progress through the normal wound healing stages and repair itself within a sufficient time period.

Platelet-rich plasma (PRP) is produced in an autologous or homologous manner. Autologous PRP is comprised of blood from the patient who will ultimately receive the PRP. Alternatively, homologous PRP is derived from blood from multiple donors.

Blood is donated by the patient and centrifuged to produce an autologous gel for treatment of chronic, non-healing cutaneous wounds that persists for 30 days or longer and fail to properly complete the healing process. Autologous blood derived products for chronic, non-healing wounds includes both: (1) platelet derived growth factor (PDGF) products (such as Procuren), and (2) PRP (such as AutoloGel).

The PRP is different from previous products in that it contains whole cells including white cells, red cells, plasma, platelets, fibrinogen, stem cells, macrophages, and fibroblasts.

The PRP is used by physicians in clinical settings in treating chronic, non-healing wounds, open, cutaneous wounds, soft tissue, and bone. Alternatively, PDGF does not contain cells and was previously marketed as a product to be used by patients at home.

B. Nationally Covered Indications

Effective August 2, 2012, upon reconsideration, The Centers for Medicare and Medicaid Services (CMS) has determined that platelet-rich plasma (PRP) – an autologous blood-derived product, will be covered only for the treatment of chronic non-healing diabetic, venous and/or pressure wounds and only when the following conditions are met:

The patient is enrolled in a clinical trial that addresses the following questions using validated and reliable methods of evaluation. Clinical study applications for coverage pursuant to this National coverage Determination (NCD) must be received by August 2, 2014.

The clinical research study must meet the requirements specified below to assess the effect of PRP for the treatment of chronic non-healing diabetic, venous and/or pressure wounds. The clinical study must address:

Prospectively, do Medicare beneficiaries that have chronic non-healing diabetic, venous and/or pressure wounds who receive well-defined optimal usual care along with PRP therapy, experience clinically significant health outcomes compared to patients who receive well-defined optimal usual care for chronic non-healing diabetic, venous and/or pressure wounds as indicated by addressing at least one of the following:

a. Complete wound healing?

b. Ability to return to previous function and resumption of normal activities?

c. Reduction of wound size or healing trajectory which results in the patient's ability to return to previous function and resumption of normal activities?

The required clinical trial of PRP must adhere to the following standards of scientific integrity and relevance to the Medicare population:

a. The principal purpose of the CLINICAL STUDY is to test whether PRP improves the participants' health outcomes.

b. The CLINICAL STUDY is well supported by available scientific and medical information or it is intended to clarify or establish the health outcomes of interventions already in common clinical use.

c. The CLINICAL STUDY does not unjustifiably duplicate existing studies.

d. The CLINICAL STUDY design is appropriate to answer the research question being asked in the study.

e. The CLINICAL STUDY is sponsored by an organization or individual capable of executing the proposed study successfully.

f. The CLINICAL STUDY is in compliance with all applicable Federal regulations concerning the protection of human subjects found at 45 CFR Part 46.

g. All aspects of the CLINICAL STUDY are conducted according to appropriate standards of scientific integrity set by the International Committee of Medical Journal Editors (http://www.icmje.org).

h. The CLINICAL STUDY has a written protocol that clearly addresses, or incorporates by reference, the standards listed here as Medicare requirements for coverage with evidence development (CED).

i. The CLINICAL STUDY is not designed to exclusively test toxicity or disease pathophysiology in healthy individuals. Trials of all medical technologies measuring therapeutic outcomes as one of the objectives meet this standard only if the disease or condition being studied is life threatening as defined in 21 CFR §312.81(a) and the patient has no other viable treatment options.

j. The CLINICAL STUDY is registered on the ClinicalTrials.gov website by the principal sponsor/investigator prior to the enrollment of the first study subject.

k. The CLINICAL STUDY protocol specifies the method and timing of public release of all pre-specified outcomes to be measured including release of outcomes if outcomes are negative or study is terminated early. The results must be made public within 24 months of the end of data collection. If a report is planned to be published in a peer reviewed journal, then that initial release may be an abstract that meets the requirements of the International Committee of Medical Journal Editors (http://www.icmje.org). However a full report of the outcomes must be made public no later than three (3) years after the end of data collection.

l. The CLINICAL STUDY protocol must explicitly discuss subpopulations affected by the treatment under investigation, particularly traditionally underrepresented groups in clinical studies, how the inclusion and exclusion criteria effect enrollment of these populations, and a plan for the retention and reporting of said populations on the trial. If the inclusion and exclusion criteria are expected to have a negative effect on the recruitment or retention of underrepresented populations, the protocol must discuss why these criteria are necessary.

m. The CLINICAL STUDY protocol explicitly discusses how the results are or are not expected to be generalizable to the Medicare population to infer whether Medicare patients may benefit from the intervention. Separate discussions in the protocol may be necessary for populations eligible for Medicare due to age, disability or Medicaid eligibility.

Consistent with §1142 of the Social Security Act (the Act), the Agency for Healthcare Research and Quality (AHRQ) supports clinical research studies that CMS determines meet the above-listed standards and address the above-listed research questions.

Any clinical study undertaken pursuant to this NCD must be approved no later than August 2, 2014. If there are no approved clinical studies on or before August 2, 2014, this CED will expire. Any clinical study approved will adhere to the timeframe designated in the approved clinical study protocol.

C. Nationally Non-Covered Indications

1. Effective December 28, 1992, the Centers for Medicare & Medicaid Services (CMS) issued a national non-coverage determination for platelet-derived wound-healing formulas intended to treat patients with chronic, non-healing wounds. This decision was based on a lack of sufficient published data to determine safety and efficacy, and a public health service technology assessment.

2. Effective July 23, 2004, upon reconsideration, the clinical effectiveness of autologous PDGF products continues to not be adequately proven in scientific literature. As the evidence is insufficient to conclude that autologous PDGF in a platelet-poor plasma is reasonable and necessary, it remains non-covered for treatment of chronic, non-healing cutaneous wounds. Also, the clinical evidence does not support a benefit in the application of autologous PRP for the treatment of chronic, non-healing, cutaneous wounds. Therefore, CMS determines it is not reasonable and necessary and is nationally non-covered.

3. Effective April 27, 2006, coverage for treatments utilizing coverage for treatments utilizing becaplermin,

a non-autologous growth factor for chronic, non-healing subcutaneous wounds, remains nationally non-covered under Part B based on section 1861(s)(2)(A) and (B) of the Social Security Act because this product is usually administered by the patient.

4. Effective March 19, 2008, upon reconsideration, the evidence is not adequate to conclude that autologous PRP is reasonable and necessary and remains non-covered for the treatment of chronic non-healing, cutaneous wounds. Additionally, upon reconsideration, the evidence is not adequate to conclude that autologous PRP is reasonable and necessary for the treatment of acute surgical wounds when the autologous PRP is applied directly to the closed incision, or for dehiscent wounds.

D. Other

In accordance with section 310.1 of the National Coverage Determinations Manual, the routine costs in Federally sponsored or approved clinical trials assessing the efficacy of autologous PRP in treating chronic, non-healing cutaneous wounds are covered by Medicare.

100-4, Chapter-1, 30.3.1

Mandatory Assignment on Carrier Claims

The following practitioners who provide services under the Medicare program are required to accept assignment for all Medicare claims for their services. This means that they must accept the Medicare allowed amount as payment in full for their practitioner services. The beneficiary's liability is limited to any applicable deductible plus the 20 percent coinsurance.

Assignment is mandated for the following claims:

- Clinical diagnostic laboratory services and physician lab services;
- Physician services to individuals dually entitled to Medicare and Medicaid;

Services of physician assistants, nurse practitioners, clinical nurse specialists, nurse midwives, certified registered nurse anesthetists, clinical psychologists, clinical social workers, registered dietitians/nutritionists, anesthesiologist assistants, and mass immunization roster billers.

NOTE: The provider type Mass Immunization Roster Biller can only bill for influenza and pneumococcal vaccinations and administrations. These services are not subject to the deductible or the 20 percent coinsurance.

- Ambulatory surgical center services; (No deductible and 25% coinsurance for colorectal cancer screening colonoscopies (G0105 and G0121) and effective for dates of service on or after January 1, 2008 G0104 also applies);
- Home dialysis supplies and equipment paid under Method II for dates of service prior to January 1, 2011. Refer to Section 30.3.8 for information regarding the elimination of Method II home dialysis for dates of service on and after January 1, 2011;
- Drugs and biologicals; and,
- Ambulance services

When these claims are inadvertently submitted as unassigned, carriers process them as assigned.

Note that, unlike physicians, practitioners, or suppliers bound by a participation agreement, practitioners/entities providing the services/supplies identified above are required to accept assignment only with respect to these services/supplies (unless they have signed participation agreements which blanket the full range of their services).

The carrier system must be able to identify (and update) the codes for those services subject to the assignment mandate.

For the practitioner services of physicians and independently practicing physical and occupational therapists, the acceptance of assignment is not mandatory. Nor is the acceptance of assignment mandatory for the suppliers of radiology services or diagnostic tests. However, these practitioners and suppliers may nevertheless voluntarily agree to participate to take advantage of the higher payment rate, in which case the participation status makes assignment mandatory for the term of the agreement. Such an agreement is known as the Medicare Participating Physician or Supplier Agreement. (See §30.3.12.2 Carrier Participation Agreement.) Physicians, practitioners, and suppliers who sign this agreement to participate are agreeing to accept assignment on all Medicare claims. The Medicare Participation Agreement and general instructions are on the CMS Web site.

Future updates to this section will be communicated in a Recurring Update Notification.

100-4, Chapter-1, 30.3.5

Effect of Assignment Upon Purchase of Cataract Glasses From Participating Physician or Supplier on Claims Submitted to Carriers

A pair of cataract glasses is comprised of two distinct products: a professional product (the prescribed lenses) and a retail commercial product (the frames). The frames serve not only as a holder of lenses but also as an article of personal apparel. As such, they are usually selected on the basis of personal taste and style. Although Medicare will pay only for standard frames, most patients want deluxe frames. Participating physicians and suppliers cannot profitably furnish such deluxe frames unless they can make an extra (noncovered) charge for the frames even though they accept assignment.

Therefore, a participating physician or supplier (whether an ophthalmologist, optometrist, or optician) who accepts assignment on cataract glasses with deluxe frames may charge the Medicare patient the difference between his/her usual charge to private pay patients for glasses with standard frames and his/her usual charge to such patients for glasses with deluxe frames, in addition to the applicable deductible and coinsurance on glasses with standard frames, if all of the following requirements are met:

A. The participating physician or supplier has standard frames available, offers them for sale to the patient, and issues and ABN to the patient that explains the price and other differences between standard and deluxe frames. Refer to Chapter 30.

B. The participating physician or supplier obtains from the patient (or his/her representative) and keeps on file the following signed and dated statement:

Name of Patient	Medicare Claim Number

Having been informed that an extra charge is being made by the physician or supplier for deluxe frames, that this extra charge is not covered by Medicare, and that standard frames are available for purchase from the physician or supplier at no extra charge, I have chosen to purchase deluxe frames.

Signature Date

C. The participating physician or supplier itemizes on his/her claim his/her actual charge for the lenses, his/her actual charge for the standard frames, and his/her actual extra charge for the deluxe frames (charge differential).

Once the assigned claim for deluxe frames has been processed, the carrier will follow the ABN instructions as described in §60.

100-4, Chapter-1, 50.3.2

Policy and Billing Instructions for Condition Code 44

In cases where a hospital or a CAH's UR committee determines that an inpatient admission does not meet the hospital's inpatient criteria, the hospital or CAH may change the beneficiary's status from inpatient to outpatient and submit an outpatient claim (bill type 13x or 85x) for medically necessary Medicare Part B services that were furnished to the beneficiary, provided all of the following conditions are met:

1. The change in patient status from inpatient to outpatient is made prior to discharge or release, while the beneficiary is still a patient of the hospital;

2. The hospital has not submitted a claim to Medicare for the inpatient admission;

3. The practitioner responsible for the care of the patient and the UR committee concur with the decision; and

4. The concurrence of the practitioner responsible for the care of the patient and the UR committee is documented in the patient's medical record.

While typically the full UR committee makes the decision for the committee that a change in patient status under Condition Code 44 is warranted, in accordance with §482.30(d)(1) one physician member of the UR committee may make the decision for the committee, provided he or she is a different person from the concurring practitioner who is responsible for the care of the patient.

When the hospital has determined that it may submit an outpatient claim according to the conditions described above, the entire episode of care should be billed as an outpatient episode of care on a 13x or 85x bill type and outpatient services that were ordered and furnished should be billed as appropriate.

Refer to Pub. 100-04, Medicare Claims Processing Manual; Chapter 30, Financial Liability Protections; Section 20, Limitation On Liability (LOL) Under §1879 Where Medicare Claims Are Disallowed, for information regarding financial liability protections.

When the hospital submits a 13x or 85x bill for services furnished to a beneficiary whose status was changed from inpatient to outpatient, the hospital is required to report Condition Code 44 on the outpatient claim in one of Form Locators 24-30, or in the ASC X12N 837 institutional claim in loop 2300, HI segment, with qualifier BG, on the outpatient claim. Additional information may be found in Chapter 25 of this manual, (Completing and Processing the Form CMS-1450 Data Set). Condition Code 44 is used by CMS and QIOs to track and monitor these occurrences. The reporting of Condition Code 44 on a claim does not affect the amount of hospital outpatient payment that would otherwise be made for a hospital outpatient claim that did not require the reporting Condition Code 44.

One of the requirements for the use of Condition Code 44 is concurrence by the practitioner who is responsible for the care of the patient with the determination that an inpatient admission does not meet the hospital's admission criteria and that the patient should have been registered as an outpatient. This prerequisite for use of Condition Code 44 is consistent with the requirements in the CoP in §482.30 (d) of the regulations. This paragraph provides that the practitioner or practitioners responsible for the care of the patient must be consulted and allowed to present their views before the UR committee or QIO makes its determination that an admission is not medically necessary. It may also be appropriate to include the practitioner who admitted the patient if this is a different person than the practitioner responsible for the care of the patient.

If the conditions for use of Condition Code 44 are not met, the hospital may submit a 12x bill type for covered "Part B Only" services that were furnished to the inpatient. Medicare may still make payment for certain Part B services furnished to an inpatient of a hospital when payment cannot be made under Part A because an inpatient admission is determined not to be medically necessary. Information about "Part B Only" services is located in Pub. 100-02, Medicare Benefit Policy Manual, chapter 6, section 10. Examples of such services include, but are not limited to, diagnostic X-ray tests, diagnostic laboratory tests, surgical dressings and splints, prosthetic devices, and certain other services. The Medicare Benefit Policy Manual includes a complete list of the payable "Part B Only" services. See Pub. 100-04, Medicare Claims Processing Manual, chapter 4, section 10.12 for a discussion of the billing and payment rules regarding services furnished within the payment window for outpatient services treated as inpatient services.

Entries in the medical record cannot be expunged or deleted and must be retained in their original form. Therefore, all orders and all entries related to the inpatient admission must be retained in the record in their original form. If a patient's status changes in accordance with the requirements for use of Condition Code 44, the change must be fully documented in the medical record, complete with orders and notes that indicate why the change was made, the care that was furnished to the beneficiary, and the participants in making the decision to change the patient's status.

When Condition Code 44 is appropriately used, the hospital reports on the outpatient bill the services that were ordered and provided to the patient for the entire patient encounter. However, in accordance with the general Medicare requirements for services furnished to beneficiaries and billed to Medicare, even in Condition Code 44 situations, hospitals may not report observation services using HCPCS code G0378 (Hospital observation service, per hour) for observation services furnished during a hospital encounter prior to a physician's order for observation services. Medicare does not permit retroactive orders or the inference of physician orders. Like all hospital outpatient services, observation services must be ordered by a physician. The clock time begins at the time that observation services are initiated in accordance with a physician's order.

While hospitals may not report observation services under HCPCS code G0378 for the time period during the hospital encounter prior to a physician's order for observation services, in Condition Code 44 situations, as for all other hospital outpatient encounters, hospitals may include charges on the outpatient claim for the costs of all hospital resources utilized in the care of the patient during the entire encounter. For example, a beneficiary is admitted as an inpatient and receives 12 hours of monitoring and nursing care, at which point the hospital changes the status of the beneficiary from inpatient to outpatient and the physician orders observation services, with all criteria for billing under Condition Code 44 being met. On the outpatient claim on an uncoded line with revenue code 0762, the hospital could bill for the 12 hours of monitoring and

nursing care that were provided prior to the change in status and the physician order for observation services, in addition to billing HCPCS code G0378 for the observation services that followed the change in status and physician order for observation services. For other rules related to billing and payment of observation services, see chapter 4, section 290 of this manual, and Pub.100-02, Medicare Benefit Policy Manual, chapter 6, Section 20.6.

100-4, Chapter-3, 10.4

Payment of Nonphysician Services for Inpatients

All items and nonphysician services furnished to inpatients must be furnished directly by the hospital or billed through the hospital under arrangements. This provision applies to all hospitals, regardless of whether they are subject to PPS.

A. Other Medical Items, Supplies, and Services

The following medical items, supplies, and services furnished to inpatients are covered under Part A. Consequently, they are covered by the prospective payment rate or reimbursed as reasonable costs under Part A to hospitals excluded from PPS.

- Laboratory services (excluding anatomic pathology services and certain clinical pathology services);
- Pacemakers and other prosthetic devices including lenses, and artificial limbs, knees, and hips;
- Radiology services including computed tomography (CT) scans furnished to inpatients by a physician's office, other hospital, or radiology clinic;
- Total parenteral nutrition (TPN) services; and
- Transportation, including transportation by ambulance, to and from another hospital or freestanding facility to receive specialized diagnostic or therapeutic services not available at the facility where the patient is an inpatient.

The hospital must include the cost of these services in the appropriate ancillary service cost center, i.e., in the cost of the diagnostic or therapeutic service. It must not show them separately under revenue code 0540.

EXCEPTIONS:

- **Pneumococcal Vaccine** - is payable under Part B only and is billed by the hospital on the Form CMS-1450.
- **Ambulance Service** - For purposes of this section "hospital inpatient" means a beneficiary who has been formally admitted it does not include a beneficiary who is in the process of being transferred from one hospital to another. Where the patient is transferred from one hospital to another, and is admitted as an inpatient to the second, the ambulance service is payable under only Part B. If transportation is by a hospital owned and operated ambulance, the hospital bills separately on Form CMS-1450 as appropriate. Similarly, if the hospital arranges for the ambulance transportation with an ambulance operator, including paying the ambulance operator, it bills separately. However, if the hospital does not assume any financial responsibility, the billing is to the carrier by the ambulance operator or beneficiary, as appropriate, if an ambulance is used for the transportation of a hospital inpatient to another facility for diagnostic tests or special treatment the ambulance trip is considered part of the DRG, and not separately billable, if the resident hospital is under PPS.
- **Part B Inpatient Services** - Where Part A benefits are not payable, payment may be made to the hospital under

Part B for certain medical and other health services. See Chapter 4 for a description of Part B inpatient services.

- **Anesthetist Services "Incident to" Physician Services** - If a physician's practice was to employ anesthetists and to bill on a reasonable charge basis for these services and that practice was in effect as of the last day of the hospital's most recent 12-month cost reporting period ending before September 30, 1983, the physician may continue that practice through cost reporting periods beginning October 1, 1984. However, if the physician chooses to continue this practice, the hospital may not add costs of the anesthetist's service to its base period costs for purposes of its transition payment rates. If it is the existing or new practice of the physician to employ certified registered nurse anesthetists (CRNAs) and other qualified anesthetists and include charges for their services in the physician bills for anesthesiology services for the hospital's cost report periods beginning on or after October 1, 1984, and before October 1, 1987, the physician may continue to do so.

B. Exceptions/Waivers

These provisions were waived before cost reporting periods beginning on or after October 1, 1986, under certain circumstances. The basic criteria for waiver was that services furnished by outside suppliers are so extensive that a sudden change in billing practices would threaten the stability of patient care. Specific criteria for waiver and processing procedures are in §2804 of the Provider Reimbursement Manual (CMS Pub. 15-1).

100-4, Chapter-3, 20.7.3

Payment for Blood Clotting Factor Administered to Hemophilia Inpatients

Section 6011 of Public Law (P.L.) 101-239 amended §1886(a)(4) of the Social Security Act (the Act) to provide that prospective payment system (PPS) hospitals receive an additional payment for the costs of administering blood clotting factor to Medicare hemophiliacs who are hospital inpatients. Section 6011(b) of P.L. 101.239 specified that the payment be based on a predetermined price per unit of clotting factor multiplied by the number of units provided. This add-on payment originally was effective for blood clotting factors furnished on or after June 19, 1990, and before December 19, 1991. Section 13505 of P. L. 103-66 amended §6011 (d) of P.L. 101-239 to extend the period covered by the add-on payment for blood clotting factors administered to Medicare inpatients with hemophilia through September 30, 1994 Section 4452 of P.L. 105-33 amended §6011(d) of P.L. 101-239 to reinstate the add-on payment for the costs of administering blood-clotting factor to Medicare beneficiaries who have hemophilia and who are hospital inpatients for discharges occurring on or after October 1, 1998.

A/B MACs (B) shall process non-institutional blood clotting factor claims.

The A/B MACs (A) shall process institutional blood clotting factor claims payable under either Part A or Part B.

A. Inpatient Bills

Under the Inpatient Prospective Payment System (IPPS), hospitals receive a special add-on payment for the costs of furnishing blood clotting factors to Medicare beneficiaries with hemophilia, admitted as inpatients of PPS hospitals. The clotting factor add-on payment is calculated using the number of units (as defined in the HCPCS code long descriptor) billed by the provider under special instructions for units of service.

The PPS Pricer software does not calculate the payment amount. The Fiscal Intermediary Shared System (FISS) calculates the payment amount and subtracts the charges from those submitted to Pricer so that the clotting factor charges are not included in cost outlier computations.

Blood clotting factors not paid on a cost or PPS basis are priced as a drug/biological under the Medicare Part B Drug Pricing File effective for the specific date of service. As of January 1, 2005, the average sales price (ASP) plus 6 percent shall be used.

If a beneficiary is in a covered Part A stay in a PPS hospital, the clotting factors are paid in addition to the DRG/HIPPS payment (For FY 2004, this payment is based on 95 percent of average wholesale price.) For a SNF subject to SNF/PPS, the payment is bundled into the SNF/PPS rate.

For SNF inpatient Part A, there is no add-on payment for blood clotting factors.

The codes for blood-clotting factors are found on the Medicare Part B Drug Pricing File. This file is distributed on a quarterly basis.

For discharges occurring on or after October 1, 2000, and before December 31, 2005, report HCPCS Q0187 based on 1 billing unit per 1.2 mg. Effective January 1, 2006, HCPCS code J7189 replaces Q0187 and is defined as 1 billing unit per 1 microgram (mcg).

The examples below include the HCPCS code and indicate the dosage amount specified in the descriptor of that code. Facilities use the units field as a multiplier to arrive at the dosage amount.

EXAMPLE 1

HCPCS	Drug	Dosage
J7189	Factor VIIa	1 mcg

Actual dosage: 13,365 mcg

On the bill, the facility shows J7189 and 13,365 in the units field (13,365 mcg divided by 1 mcg = 13,365 units).

NOTE: The process for dealing with one international unit (IU) is the same as the process of dealing with one microgram.

EXAMPLE 2

HCPCS	Drug	Dosage
J9355	Trastuzumab	10 mg

Actual dosage: 140 mg

On the bill, the facility shows J9355 and 14 in the units field (140 mg divided by 10mg = 14 units).

When the dosage amount is greater than the amount indicated for the HCPCS code, the facility rounds up to determine units. When the dosage amount is less than the amount indicated for the HCPCS code, use 1 as the unit of measure.

EXAMPLE 3

HCPCS	Drug	Dosage
J9355	Tenecteplase	50 mg

Actual Dosage: 40 mg

The provider would bill for 1 unit, even though less than 1 full unit was furnished.

At times, the facility provides less than the amount provided in a single use vial and there is waste, i.e.; some drugs may be available only in packaged amounts that exceed the needs of an individual patient. Once the drug is reconstituted in the hospital's pharmacy, it may have a limited shelf life. Since an individual patient may receive less than the fully reconstituted amount, we encourage hospitals to schedule patients in such a way that the hospital can use the drug most efficiently. However, if the hospital must discard the remainder of a vial after administering part of it to a Medicare patient, the provider may bill for the amount of drug discarded plus the amount administered.

Example 1:

Drug X is available only in a 100-unit size. A hospital schedules three Medicare patients to receive drug X on the same day within the designated shelf life of the product. An appropriate hospital staff member administers 30 units to each patient. The remaining 10 units are billed to Medicare on the account of the last patient. Therefore, 30 units are billed on behalf of the first patient seen and 30 units are billed on behalf of the second patient seen. Forty units are billed on behalf of the last patient seen because the hospital had to discard 10 units at that point.

Example 2:

An appropriate hospital staff member must administer 30 units of drug X to a Medicare patient, and it is not practical to schedule another patient who requires the same drug. For example, the hospital has only one patient who requires drug X, or the hospital sees the patient for the first time and did not know the patient's condition. The hospital bills for 100 units on behalf of the patient, and Medicare pays for 100 units.

When the number of units of blood clotting factor administered to hemophiliac inpatients exceeds 99,999, the hospital reports the excess as a second line for revenue code 0636 and repeats the HCPCS code. One hundred thousand fifty (100,050) units are reported on one line as 99,999, and another line shows 1,051.

Revenue Code 0636 is used. It requires HCPCS. Some other inpatient drugs continue to be billed without HCPCS codes under pharmacy.

No changes in beneficiary notices are required. Coverage is applicable to hospital Part A claims only. Coverage is also applicable to inpatient Part B services in SNFs and all types of hospitals, including CAHs. Separate payment is not made to SNFs for beneficiaries in an inpatient Part A stay.

B. -A/B MAC (A) Action

The contractor is responsible for the following:

- It accepts HCPCS codes for inpatient services;
- It edits to require HCPCS codes with Revenue Code 0636. Multiple iterations of the revenue code are possible with the same or different HCPCS codes. It does not edit units except to ensure a numeric value;
- It reduces charges forwarded to Pricer by the charges for hemophilia clotting factors in revenue code 0636. It retains the charges and revenue and HCPCS codes for CWF; and
- It modifies data entry screens to accept HCPCS codes for hospital (including CAH) swing bed, and SNF inpatient claims (bill types 11X, 12X, 18x, 21x and, 22x).

The September 1, 1993, IPPS final rule (58 FR 46304) states that payment will be made for the blood clotting factor only if an ICD-9-CM diagnosis code for hemophilia is included on the bill.

Inpatient blood-clotting factors are covered only for beneficiaries with hemophilia. One of the following hemophilia diagnosis codes must be reported on the claim for payment to be made for blood clotting factors.

100-4, Chapter-3, 40.2.2

Charges to Beneficiaries for Part A Services

The hospital submits a bill even where the patient is responsible for a deductible which covers the entire amount of the charges for non-PPS hospitals, or in PPS hospitals, where the DRG payment amount will be less than the deductible.

A hospital receiving payment for a covered hospital stay (or PPS hospital that includes at least one covered day, or one treated as covered under guarantee of payment or limitation on liability) may charge the beneficiary, or other person, for items and services furnished during the stay only as described in subsections A through H. If limitation of liability applies, a beneficiary's liability for payment is governed by the limitation on liability notification rules in Chapter 30 of this manual. For related notices for inpatient hospitals, see CMS Transmittal 594, Change Request 3903, dated June 24, 2005.

A. Deductible and Coinsurance

The hospital may charge the beneficiary or other person for applicable deductible and coinsurance amounts. The deductible is satisfied only by charges for covered services. The FI deducts the deductible and coinsurance first from the PPS payment. Where the deductible exceeds the PPS amount, the excess will be applied to a subsequent payment to the hospital. (See Chapter 3 of the Medicare General Information, Eligibility, and Entitlement Manual for specific policies.)

B. Blood Deductible

The Part A blood deductible provision applies to whole blood and red blood cells, and reporting of the number of pints is applicable to both PPS and non-PPS hospitals. (See Chapter 3 of the Medicare General Information, Eligibility, and Entitlement Manual for specific policies.) Hospitals shall report charges for red blood cells using revenue code 381, and charges for whole blood using revenue code 382.

C. Inpatient Care No Longer Required

The hospital may charge for services that are not reasonable and necessary or that constitute custodial care. Notification may be required under limitation of liability. See CMS Transmittal 594, Change Request 3903, dated June 24, 2005, section V. of the attachment, for specific notification requirements. Note this transmittal will be placed in Chapter 30 of this manual at a future point. Chapter 1, section 150 of this manual also contains related billing information in addition to that provided below.

In general, after proper notification has occurred, and assuming an expedited decision is received from a Quality Improvement Organization (QIO), the following entries are required on the bill the hospital prepares:

- Occurrence code 31 (and date) to indicate the date the hospital notified the patient in accordance with the first bullet above;
- Occurrence span code 76 (and dates) to indicate the period of noncovered care for which it is charging the beneficiary;
- Occurrence span code 77 (and dates) to indicate the period of noncovered care for which the provider is liable, when it is aware of this prior to billing; and

- Value code 31 (and amount) to indicate the amount of charges it may bill the beneficiary for days for which inpatient care was no longer required. They are included as noncovered charges on the bill.

D. Change in the Beneficiary's Condition

If the beneficiary remains in the hospital after receiving notice as described in subsection C, and the hospital, the physician who concurred in the hospital's determination, or the QIO, subsequently determines that the beneficiary again requires inpatient hospital care, the hospital may not charge the beneficiary or other person for services furnished after the beneficiary again required inpatient hospital care until proper notification occurs (see subsection C).

If a patient who needs only a SNF level of care remains in the hospital after the SNF bed becomes available, and the bed ceases to be available, the hospital may continue to charge the beneficiary. It need not provide the beneficiary with another notice when the patient chose not to be discharged to the SNF bed.

E. Admission Denied

If the entire hospital admission is determined to be not reasonable or necessary, limitation of liability may apply. See 2005 CMS transmittal 594, section V. of the attachment, for specific notification requirements.

NOTE: This transmittal will be placed in Chapter 30 of this manual at a future point.

In such cases the following entries are required on the bill:

- Occurrence code 31 (and date) to indicate the date the hospital notified the beneficiary.
- Occurrence span code 76 (and dates) to indicate the period of noncovered care for which the hospital is charging the beneficiary.
- Occurrence span code 77 (and dates) to indicate any period of noncovered care for which the provider is liable (e.g., the period between issuing the notice and the time it may charge the beneficiary) when the provider is aware of this prior to billing.
- Value code 31 (and amount) to indicate the amount of charges the hospital may bill the beneficiary for hospitalization that was not necessary or reasonable. They are included as noncovered charges on the bill.

F. Procedures, Studies and Courses of Treatment That Are Not Reasonable or Necessary

If diagnostic procedures, studies, therapeutic studies and courses of treatment are excluded from coverage as not reasonable and necessary (even though the beneficiary requires inpatient hospital care) the hospital may charge the beneficiary or other person for the services or care according the procedures given in CMS Transmittal 594, Change Request 3903, dated June 24, 2005.

The following bill entries apply to these circumstances:

- Occurrence code 32 (and date) to indicate the date the hospital provided the notice to the beneficiary.
- Value code 31 (and amount) to indicate the amount of such charges to be billed to the beneficiary. They are included as noncovered charges on the bill.

G. Nonentitlement Days and Days after Benefits Exhausted

If a hospital stay exceeds the day outlier threshold, the hospital may charge for some, or all, of the days on which the patient is not entitled to Medicare Part A, or after the Part A benefits are exhausted (i.e., the hospital may charge its customary charges for services furnished on those days). It may charge the beneficiary for the lesser of:

- The number of days on which the patient was not entitled to benefits or after the benefits were exhausted; or
- The number of outlier days. (Day outliers were discontinued at the end of FY 1997.)

If the number of outlier days exceeds the number of days on which the patient was not entitled to benefits, or after benefits were exhausted, the hospital may charge for all days on which the patient was not entitled to benefits or after benefits were exhausted. If the number of days on which the beneficiary was not entitled to benefits, or after benefits were exhausted, exceeds the number of outlier days, the hospital determines the days for which it may charge by starting with the last day of the stay (i.e., the day before the day of discharge) and identifying and counting off in reverse order, days on which the patient was not entitled to benefits or after the benefits were exhausted, until the number of days counted off equals the number of outlier days. The days counted off are the days for which the hospital may charge.

H. Contractual Exclusions

In addition to receiving the basic prospective payment, the hospital may charge the beneficiary for any services that are excluded from coverage for reasons other than, or in addition to, absence of medical necessity, provision of custodial care, non-entitlement to Part A, or exhaustion of benefits. For example, it may charge for most cosmetic and dental surgery.

I. Private Room Care

Payment for medically necessary private room care is included in the prospective payment. Where the beneficiary requests private room accommodations, the hospital must inform the beneficiary of the additional charge. (See the Medicare Benefit Policy Manual, Chapter 1.) When the beneficiary accepts the liability, the hospital will supply the service, and bill the beneficiary directly. If the beneficiary believes the private room was medically necessary, the beneficiary has a right to a determination and may initiate a Part A appeal.

J. Deluxe Item or Service

Where a beneficiary requests a deluxe item or service, i.e., an item or service which is more expensive than is medically required for the beneficiary's condition, the hospital may collect the additional charge if it informs the beneficiary of the additional charge. That charge is the difference between the customary charge for the item or service most commonly furnished by the hospital to private pay patients with the beneficiary's condition, and the charge for the more expensive item or service requested. If the beneficiary believes that the more expensive item or service was medically necessary, the beneficiary has a right to a determination and may initiate a Part A appeal.

K. Inpatient Acute Care Hospital Admission Followed By a Death or Discharge Prior To Room Assignment

A patient of an acute care hospital is considered an inpatient upon issuance of written doctor's orders to that effect. If a patient either dies or is discharged prior to being assigned and/or occupying a room, a hospital may enter an appropriate room and board charge on the claim. If a patient leaves of their own volition prior to being assigned and/or occupying a room, a hospital may enter an appropriate room and board charge on the claim as well as a patient status code 07 which indicates they left against medical advice. A hospital is not required to enter a room and board charge, but failure to do so may have a minimal impact on future DRG weight calculations.

100-4, Chapter-4, 10.4

Packaging

Under the OPPS, packaged services are items and services that are considered to be an integral part of another service that is paid under the OPPS. No separate payment is made for packaged services, because the cost of these items and services is included in the APC payment for the service of which they are an integral part. For example, routine supplies, anesthesia, recovery room use, and most drugs are considered to be an integral part of a surgical procedure so payment for these items is packaged into the APC payment for the surgical procedure.

A. Packaging for Claims Resulting in APC Payments

If a claim contains services that result in an APC payment but also contains packaged services, separate payment for the packaged services is not made since payment is included in the APC. However, charges related to the packaged services are used for outlier and Transitional Corridor Payments (TOPs) as well as for future rate setting. Therefore, it is extremely important that hospitals report all HCPCS codes consistent with their descriptors; CPT® and/or CMS instructions and correct coding principles, and all charges for all services they furnish, whether payment for the services is made separately paid or is packaged.

B. Packaging for Claims Resulting in No APC Payments

If the claim contains only services payable under cost reimbursement, such as corneal tissue, and services that would be packaged services if an APC were payable, then the packaged services are not separately payable. In addition, these charges for the packaged services are not used to calculate TOPs.

If the claim contains only services payable under a fee schedule, such as clinical diagnostic laboratory tests, and also contains services that would be packaged services if an APC were payable, the packaged services are not separately payable. In addition, the charges are not used to calculate TOPs.

If a claim contains services payable under cost reimbursement, services payable under a fee schedule, and services that would be packaged services if an APC were payable, the packaged services are not separately payable. In addition, the charges are not used to calculate TOPs payments.

C. Packaging Types Under the OPPS

1. Unconditionally packaged services are services for which separate payment is never made because the payment for the service is always packaged into the payment for other services. Unconditionally packaged services are identified in the OPPS Addendum B with status indictor of N. See the OPPS Web site at http://www.cms.hhs.gov/HospitalOutpatientPPS/ for the most recent Addendum B (HCPCS codes with status indicators). In general, the charges for unconditionally packaged services are used to calculate outlier and TOPS payments when they appear on a claim with a service that is separately paid under the OPPS because the packaged service is considered to be part of the package of services for which payment is being made through the APC payment for the separately paid service.

2. STV-packaged services are services for which separate payment is made only if there is no service with status indicator S, T, or V reported on the same claim. If a claim includes a service that is assigned status indicator S, T,

or V reported on the same claim as the STV- packaged service, the payment for the STV-packaged service is packaged into the payment for the service(s) with status indicator S, T, V and no separate payment is made for the STV-packaged service. STV-packaged services are assigned status indicator Q1. See the OPPS Webpage at http://www.cms.hhs.gov/HospitalOutpatientPPS/ for identification of STV-packaged codes.

3. T-packaged services are services for which separate payment is made only if there is no service with status indicator T reported on the same claim. When there is a claim that includes a service that is assigned status indicator T reported on the same claim as the T-packaged service, the payment for the T-packaged service is packaged into the payment for the service(s) with status indicator T and no separate payment is made for the T-packaged service. T-packaged services are assigned status indicator Q2. See the OPPS Web site at http://www.cms.hhs.gov/HospitalOutpatientPPS/ for identification of T-packaged codes.

4. A service that is assigned to a composite APC is a major component of a single episode of care. The hospital receives one payment through a composite APC for multiple major separately identifiable services. Services mapped to composite APCs are assigned status indicator Q3. See the discussion of composite APCs in section 10.2.1.

5. Q4 services are assigned to laboratory HCPCS codes that appear on the Clinical Laboratory Fee Schedule (CLFS). Status indicator Q4 designates packaged APC payment if billed on the same claim as a HCPCS code assigned status indicator "J1," "J2," "S," "T," "V," "Q1," "Q2," or "Q3." When a Q4 service is not billed on the same claim as another separately payable service then the IOCE automatically changes their status indicator to "A" and separate payment is made at the CLFS payment rate.

6. J1 services are assigned to comprehensive APCs. Payment for all adjunctive services reported on the same claim as a J1 service is packaged into payment for the primary J1 service. See the discussion of comprehensive APCs in section 10.2.3.

7. J2 services are assigned to comprehensive APCs when a specific combination of services are reported on the claim. Payment for all adjunctive services reported on the same claim as a J2 service is packaged into payment for the J2 service when certain conditions are met. See the discussion of comprehensive APCs in section 10.2.3.

100-4, Chapter-4, 160

Clinic and Emergency Visits

CMS has acknowledged from the beginning of the OPPS that CMS believes that CPT® Evaluation and Management (E/M) codes were designed to reflect the activities of physicians and do not describe well the range and mix of services provided by hospitals during visits of clinic and emergency department patients. While awaiting the development of a national set of facility-specific codes and guidelines, providers should continue to apply their current internal guidelines to the existing CPT® codes. Each hospital's internal guidelines should follow the intent of the CPT® code descriptors, in that the guidelines should be designed to reasonably relate the intensity of hospital resources to the different levels of effort represented by the codes. Hospitals should ensure that their guidelines accurately reflect resource distinctions between the five levels of codes.

Effective January 1, 2007, CMS is distinguishing between two types of emergency departments: Type A emergency departments and Type B emergency departments.

A Type A emergency department is defined as an emergency department that is available 24 hours a day, 7 days a week and is either licensed by the State in which it is located under applicable State law as an emergency room or emergency department or it is held out to the public (by name, posted signs, advertising, or other means) as a place that provides care for emergency medical conditions on an urgent basis without requiring a previously scheduled appointment.

A Type B emergency department is defined as an emergency department that meets the definition of a "dedicated emergency department" as defined in 42 CFR 489.24 under the EMTALA regulations. It must meet at least one of the following requirements:

(1) It is licensed by the State in which it is located under applicable State law as an emergency room or emergency department;

(2) It is held out to the public (by name, posted signs, advertising, or other means) as a place that provides care for emergency medical conditions on an urgent basis without requiring a previously scheduled appointment; or

(3) During the calendar year immediately preceding the calendar year in which a determination under 42 CFR 489.24 is being made, based on a representative sample of patient visits that occurred during that calendar year, it provides at least one-third of all of its outpatient visits for the treatment of emergency medical conditions on an urgent basis without requiring a previously scheduled appointment.

Hospitals must bill for visits provided in Type A emergency departments using CPT® emergency department E/M codes. Hospitals must bill for visits provided in Type B emergency departments using the G-codes that describe visits provided in Type B emergency departments.

Hospitals that will be billing the new Type B ED visit codes may need to update their internal guidelines to report these codes.

Emergency department and clinic visits are paid in some cases separately and in other cases as part of a composite APC payment.

100-4, Chapter-4, 160.1

Critical Care Services

Hospitals should separately report all HCPCS codes in accordance with correct coding principles, CPT® code descriptions, and any additional CMS guidance, when available. Specifically with respect to CPT® code 99291 (Critical care, evaluation and management of the critically ill or critically injured patient; first 30-74 minutes), hospitals must follow the CPT® instructions related to reporting that CPT® code. Prior to January 1, 2011, any services that CPT® indicates are included in the reporting of CPT® code 99291 (including those services that would otherwise be reported by and paid to hospitals using any of the CPT® codes specified by CPT®) should not be billed separately by the hospital. Instead, hospitals should report charges for any services provided as part of the critical care services. In establishing payment rates for critical care services, and other services, CMS packages the costs of certain items and services separately reported by HCPCS codes into payment for critical care services and other services, according to the standard OPPS methodology for packaging costs.

Beginning January 1, 2011, in accordance with revised CPT® guidance, hospitals that report in accordance with the CPT® guidelines will begin reporting all of the ancillary services and their associated charges separately when they are provided in conjunction with critical care. CMS will continue to recognize the existing CPT® codes for critical care services and will establish payment rates based on historical data, into which the cost of the ancillary services is intrinsically packaged. The I/OCE conditionally packages payment for the ancillary services that are reported on the same date of service as critical care services in order to avoid overpayment. The payment status of the ancillary services does not change when they are not provided in conjunction with critical care services. Hospitals may use HCPCS modifier -59 to indicate when an ancillary procedure or service is distinct or independent from critical care when performed on the same day but in a different encounter.

Beginning January 1, 2007, critical care services will be paid at two levels, depending on the presence or absence of trauma activation. Providers will receive one payment rate for critical care without trauma activation and will receive additional payment when critical care is associated with trauma activation.

To determine whether trauma activation occurs, follow the National Uniform Billing Committee (NUBC) guidelines in the Claims Processing Manual, Pub 100-04, Chapter 25, §75.4 related to the reporting of the trauma revenue codes in the 68x series. The revenue code series 68x can be used only by trauma centers/hospitals as licensed or designated by the state or local government authority authorized to do so, or as verified by the American College of Surgeons. Different subcategory revenue codes are reported by designated Level 1-4 hospital trauma centers. Only patients for whom there has been prehospital notification based on triage information from prehospital caregivers, who meet either local, state or American College of Surgeons field triage criteria, or are delivered by inter-hospital transfers, and are given the appropriate team response can be billed a trauma activation charge.

When critical care services are provided without trauma activation, the hospital may bill CPT® code 99291, Critical care, evaluation and management of the critically ill or critically injured patient; first 30-74 minutes (and 99292, if appropriate). If trauma activation occurs under the circumstances described by the NUBC guidelines that would permit reporting a charge under 68x, the hospital may also bill one unit of code G0390, which describes trauma activation associated with hospital critical care services. Revenue code 68x must be reported on the same date of service. The OCE will edit to ensure that G0390 appears with revenue code 68x on the same date of service and that only one unit of G0390 is billed. CMS believes that trauma activation is a one-time occurrence in association with critical care services, and therefore, CMS will only pay for one unit of G0390 per day.

The CPT® code 99291 is defined by CPT® as the first 30-74 minutes of critical care. This 30 minute minimum has always applied under the OPPS. The CPT® code 99292, Critical care, evaluation and management of the critically ill or critically injured patient; each additional 30 minutes, remains a packaged service under the OPPS, so that hospitals do not have the ongoing administrative burden of reporting precisely the time for each critical service provided. As the CPT® guidelines indicate, hospitals that provide less than 30 minutes of critical care should bill for a visit, typically an emergency department visit, at a level consistent with their own internal guidelines.

Under the OPPS, the time that can be reported as critical care is the time spent by a physician and/or hospital staff engaged in active face-to-face critical care of a critically ill or critically injured patient. If the physician and hospital staff or multiple hospital staff members are simultaneously engaged in this active face-to-face care, the time involved can only be counted once.

- Beginning in CY 2007 hospitals may continue to report a charge with RC 68x without any HCPCS code when trauma team activation occurs. In order to receive additional payment when critical care services are associated with trauma activation, the hospital must report G0390 on the same date of service as RC 68x, in addition to CPT® code 99291 (or 99292, if appropriate.)
- Beginning in CY 2007 hospitals should continue to report 99291 (and 99292 as appropriate) for critical care services furnished without trauma team activation. CPT® 99291 maps to APC 0617 (Critical Care). (CPT® 99292 is packaged and not paid separately, but should be reported if provided.)

Critical care services are paid in some cases separately and in other cases as part of a composite APC payment.

Future updates will be issued in a Recurring Update Notification.

100-4, Chapter-4, 200.1

Billing for Corneal Tissue

Corneal tissue will be paid on a cost basis, not under OPPS. To receive cost based reimbursement hospitals must bill charges for corneal tissue using HCPCS code V2785.

100-4, Chapter-4, 200.2

Hospital Dialysis Services For Patients With and Without End Stage Renal Disease (ESRD)

Effective with claims with dates of service on or after August 1, 2000, hospital-based End Stage Renal Disease (ESRD) facilities must submit services covered under the ESRD benefit in 42 CFR 413.174 (maintenance dialysis and those items and services directly related to dialysis such as drugs, supplies) on a separate claim from services not covered under the ESRD benefit. Items and services not covered under the ESRD benefit must be billed by the hospital using the hospital bill type and be paid under the Outpatient Prospective Payment System (OPPS) (or to a CAH at reasonable cost). Services covered under the ESRD benefit in 42 CFR 413.174 must be billed on the ESRD bill type and must be paid under the ESRD PPS. This requirement is necessary to properly pay only unrelated ESRD services (those not covered under the ESRD benefit) under OPPS (or to a CAH at reasonable cost).

Medicare does not allow payment for routine or related dialysis treatments, which are covered and paid under the ESRD PPS, when furnished to ESRD patients in the outpatient department of a hospital. However, in certain medical situations in which the ESRD outpatient cannot obtain her or his regularly scheduled dialysis treatment at a certified ESRD facility, the OPPS rule for 2003 allows payment for non-routine dialysis treatments (which are not covered under the ESRD benefit) furnished to ESRD outpatients in the outpatient department of a hospital. Payment for unscheduled dialysis furnished to ESRD outpatients and paid under the OPPS is limited to the following circumstances:

- Dialysis performed following or in connection with a dialysis-related procedure such as vascular access procedure or blood transfusions;

- Dialysis performed following treatment for an unrelated medical emergency; e.g., if a patient goes to the emergency room for chest pains and misses a regularly scheduled dialysis treatment that cannot be rescheduled, CMS allows the hospital to provide and bill Medicare for the dialysis treatment; or

- Emergency dialysis for ESRD patients who would otherwise have to be admitted as inpatients in order for the hospital to receive payment.

In these situations, non-ESRD certified hospital outpatient facilities are to bill Medicare using the Healthcare Common Procedure Coding System (HCPCS) code G0257 (Unscheduled or emergency dialysis treatment for an ESRD patient in a hospital outpatient department that is not certified as an ESRD facility).

HCPCS code G0257 may only be reported on type of bill 13X (hospital outpatient service) or type of bill 85X (critical access hospital) because HCPCS code G0257 only reports services for hospital outpatients with ESRD and only these bill types are used to report services to hospital outpatients. Effective for services on and after October 1, 2012, claims containing HCPCS code G0257 will be returned to the provider for correction if G0257 is reported with a type of bill other than 13X or 85X (such as a 12x inpatient claim).

HCPCS code 90935 (Hemodialysis procedure with single physician evaluation) may be reported and paid only if one of the following two conditions is met:

1. The patient is a hospital inpatient with or without ESRD and has no coverage under Part A, but has Part B coverage. The charge for hemodialysis is a charge for the use of a prosthetic device. See Benefits Policy Manual 100-02 Chapter 15 section 120. A. The service must be reported on a type of bill 12X or type of bill 85X. See the Benefits Policy Manual 100-02 Chapter 6 section 10 (Medical and Other Health Services Furnished to Inpatients of Participating Hospitals) for the criteria that must be met for services to be paid when a hospital inpatient has Part B coverage but does not have coverage under Part A; or

2. A hospital outpatient does not have ESRD and is receiving hemodialysis in the hospital outpatient department. The service is reported on a type of bill 13X or type of bill 85X.

CPT® code 90945 (Dialysis procedure other than hemodialysis (e.g. peritoneal dialysis, hemofiltration, or other continuous replacement therapies)), with single physician evaluation, may be reported by a hospital paid under the OPPS or CAH method I or method II on type of bill 12X, 13X or 85X.

100-4, Chapter-4, 200.4

Billing for Amniotic Membrane

Hospitals should report HCPCS code V2790 (Amniotic membrane for surgical reconstruction, per procedure) to report amniotic membrane tissue when the tissue is used. A specific procedure code associated with use of amniotic membrane tissue is CPT® code 65780 (Ocular surface reconstruction; amniotic membrane transplantation). Payment for the amniotic membrane tissue is packaged into payment for CPT® code 65780 or other procedures with which the amniotic membrane is used.

100-4, Chapter-4, 200.6

Billing and Payment for Alcohol and/or Substance Abuse Assessment and Intervention Services

For CY 2008, the CPT® Editorial Panel has created two new Category I CPT® codes for reporting alcohol and/or substance abuse screening and intervention services. They are CPT® code 99408 (Alcohol and/or substance (other than tobacco) abuse structured screening (e.g., AUDIT, DAST), and brief intervention (SBI) services; 15 to 30 minutes); and CPT® code 99409 (Alcohol and/or substance (other than tobacco) abuse structured screening (e.g., AUDIT, DAST), and brief intervention (SBI) services; greater than 30 minutes). However, screening services are not covered by Medicare without specific statutory authority, such as has been provided for mammography, diabetes, and colorectal cancer screening. Therefore, beginning January 1, 2008, the OPPS recognizes two parallel G-codes (HCPCS codes G0396 and G0397) to allow for appropriate reporting and payment of alcohol and substance abuse structured assessment and intervention services that are not provided as screening services, but that are performed in the context of the diagnosis or treatment of illness or injury.

Contractors shall make payment under the OPPS for HCPCS code G0396 (Alcohol and/or substance (other than tobacco) abuse structured assessment (e.g., AUDIT, DAST) and brief intervention, 15 to 30 minutes) and HCPCS code G0397, (Alcohol and/or substance (other than tobacco) abuse structured assessment (e.g., AUDIT, DAST) and intervention greater than 30 minutes), only when reasonable and necessary (i.e., when the service is provided to evaluate patients with signs/symptoms of illness or injury) as per section 1862(a)(1)(A) of the Act.

HCPCS codes G0396 and G0397 are to be used for structured alcohol and/or substance (other than tobacco) abuse assessment and intervention services that are distinct from other clinic and emergency department visit services performed during the same encounter. Hospital resources expended performing services described by HCPCS codes G0396 and G0397 may not be counted as resources for determining the level of a visit service and vice versa (i.e., hospitals may not double count the same facility resources in order to reach a higher level clinic or emergency department visit). However, alcohol and/or substance structured assessment or intervention services lasting less than 15 minutes should not be reported using these HCPCS codes, but the hospital resources expended should be included in determining the level of the visit service reported.

100-4, Chapter-4, 200.7.2

Cardiac Echocardiography With Contrast

Hospitals are instructed to bill for echocardiograms with contrast using the applicable HCPCS code(s) included in Table 200.7.2 below. Hospitals should also report the appropriate units of the HCPCS codes for the contrast agents used in the performance of the echocardiograms.

Table 200.7.2 – HCPCS Codes For Echocardiograms With Contrast

HCPCS	Long Descriptor
C8921	Transthoracic echocardiography with contrast, or without contrast followed by with contrast, for congenital cardiac anomalies; complete
C8922	Transthoracic echocardiography with contrast, or without contrast followed by with contrast, for congenital cardiac anomalies; follow-up or limited study
C8923	Transthoracic echocardiography with contrast, or without contrast followed by with contrast, real-Time with image documentation (2D), includes M-mode recording, when performed, complete, without spectral or color Doppler echocardiography
C8924	Transthoracic echocardiography with contrast, or without contrast followed by with contrast, real-time with image documentation (2D), includes M-mode recording, when performed, follow-up or limited study
C8925	Transesophageal echocardiography (TEE) with contrast, or without contrast followed by with contrast, real time with image documentation (2D) (with or without M-mode recording); including probe placement, image acquisition, interpretation and report
C8926	Transesophageal echocardiography (TEE) with contrast, or without contrast followed by with contrast, for congenital cardiac anomalies; including probe placement, image acquisition, interpretation and report
C8927	Transesophageal echocardiography (TEE) with contrast, or without contrast followed by with contrast, for monitoring purposes, including probe placement, real time 2-dimensional image acquisition and interpretation leading to ongoing (continuous) assessment of (dynamically changing) cardiac pumping function and to therapeutic measures on an immediate time basis
C8928	Transthoracic echocardiography with contrast, or without contrast followed by with contrast, real-time with image documentation (2D), includes M-mode recording, when performed, during rest and cardiovascular stress test using treadmill, bicycle exercise and/or pharmacologically induced stress, with interpretation and report
C8929	Transthoracic echocardiography with contrast, or without contrast followed by with contrast, real-time with image documentation (2D), includes M-mode recording, when performed, complete, with spectral Doppler echocardiography, and with color flow Doppler echocardiography
C8930	Transthoracic echocardiography, with contrast, or without contrast followed by with contrast, real-time with image documentation (2D), includes M-mode recording, when performed, during rest and cardiovascular stress test using treadmill, bicycle exercise and/or pharmacologically induced stress, with interpretation and report; including performance of continuous electrocardiographic monitoring, with physician supervision

100-4, Chapter-4, 230.2

Coding and Payment for Drug Administration

A. Overview

Drug administration services furnished under the Hospital Outpatient Prospective Payment System (OPPS) during CY 2005 were reported using CPT® codes 90780, 90781, and 96400-96459.

Effective January 1, 2006, some of these CPT® codes were replaced with more detailed CPT® codes incorporating specific procedural concepts, as defined and described by the CPT® manual, such as initial, concurrent, and sequential.

Hospitals are instructed to use the full set of CPT® codes, including those codes referencing concepts of initial, concurrent, and sequential, to bill for drug administration services furnished in the hospital outpatient department beginning January 1, 2007. In addition, hospitals are instructed to continue billing the HCPCS codes that most accurately describe the service(s) provided.

Hospitals are reminded to bill a separate Evaluation and Management code (with modifier 25) only if a significant, separately identifiable E/M service is performed in the same encounter with OPPS drug administration services.

B. Billing for Infusions and Injections

Beginning in CY 2007, hospitals were instructed to use the full set of drug administration CPT® codes (90760-90779; 96401-96549), (96413-96523 beginning in CY 2008) (96360-96549 beginning in CY 2009) when billing for drug administration services provided in the hospital outpatient department. In addition, hospitals are to continue to bill HCPCS code C8957 (Intravenous infusion for therapy/diagnosis; initiation of prolonged infusion (more than 8 hours), requiring use of portable or implantable pump) when appropriate. Hospitals are expected to report all drug administration CPT® codes in a manner consistent with their descriptors, CPT® instructions, and correct coding principles. Hospitals should note the conceptual changes between CY 2006 drug administration codes effective under the OPPS and the CPT® codes in effect beginning January 1, 2007, in order to ensure accurate billing under the OPPS. Hospitals should report all HCPCS codes that describe the drug administration services provided, regardless of whether or not those services are separately paid or their payment is packaged.

Medicare's general policy regarding physician supervision within hospital outpatient departments meets the physician supervision requirements for use of CPT® codes 90760-90779, 96401-96549, (96413-96523 beginning in CY 2008). (Reference: Pub.100-02, Medicare Benefit Policy Manual, Chapter 6, §20.4.)

Drug administration services are to be reported with a line item date of service on the day they are provided. In addition, only one initial drug administration service is to be reported per vascular access site per encounter, including during an encounter where observation services span more than 1 calendar day.

C. Payments For Drug Administration Services

For CY 2007, OPPS drug administration APCs were restructured, resulting in a six-level hierarchy where active HCPCS codes have been assigned according to their clinical coherence and resource use. Contrary to the CY 2006 payment structure that bundled payment for several instances of a type of service (non-chemotherapy, chemotherapy by infusion, non-infusion chemotherapy) into a per-encounter APC payment, structure introduced in CY 2007 provides a separate APC payment for each reported unit of a separately payable HCPCS code.

Hospitals should note that the transition to the full set of CPT® drug administration codes provides for conceptual differences when reporting, such as those noted below.

- In CY 2006, hospitals were instructed to bill for the first hour (and any additional hours) by each type of infusion service (non-chemotherapy, chemotherapy by infusion, non-infusion chemotherapy). Beginning in CY 2007, the first hour concept no longer exists. CPT® codes in CY 2007 and beyond allow for only one initial service per encounter, for each vascular access site, no matter how many types of infusion services are provided; however,

hospitals will receive an APC payment for the initial service and separate APC payment(s) for additional hours of infusion or other drug administration services provided that are separately payable.

- In CY 2006, hospitals were instructed to bill for the first hour (and any additional hours) by each type of infusion service (non-chemotherapy, chemotherapy by infusion, non-infusion chemotherapy). Beginning in CY 2007, the first hour concept no longer exists. CPT® codes in CY 2007 and beyond allow for only one initial service per encounter, for each vascular access site, no matter how many types of infusion services are provided; however, hospitals will receive an APC payment for the initial service and separate APC payment(s) for additional hours of infusion or other drug administration services provided that are separately payable.

(**NOTE:** This list above provides a brief overview of a limited number of the conceptual changes between CY 2006 OPPS drug administration codes and CY 2007 OPPS drug administration codes - this list is not comprehensive and does not include all items hospitals will need to consider during this transition)

For APC payment rates, refer to the most current quarterly version of Addendum B on the CMS Web site at http://www.cms.hhs.gov/HospitalOutpatientPPS/.

D. Infusions Started Outside the Hospital

Hospitals may receive Medicare beneficiaries for outpatient services who are in the process of receiving an infusion at their time of arrival at the hospital (e.g., a patient who arrives via ambulance with an ongoing intravenous infusion initiated by paramedics during transport). Hospitals are reminded to bill for all services provided using the HCPCS code(s) that most accurately describe the service(s) they provided. This includes hospitals reporting an initial hour of infusion, even if the hospital did not initiate the infusion, and additional HCPCS codes for additional or sequential infusion services if needed.

100-4, Chapter-4, 231.4

Billing for Split Unit of Blood

HCPCS code P9011 was created to identify situations where one unit of blood or a blood product is split and some portion of the unit is transfused to one patient and the other portions are transfused to other patients or to the same patient at other times. When a patient receives a transfusion of a split unit of blood or blood product, OPPS providers should bill P9011 for the blood product transfused, as well as CPT® 86985 (Splitting, blood products) for each splitting procedure performed to prepare the blood product for a specific patient.

Providers should bill split units of packed red cells and whole blood using Revenue Code 389 (Other blood), and should not use Revenue Codes 381 (Packed red cells) or 382 (Whole blood). Providers should bill split units of other blood products using the applicable revenue codes for the blood product type, such as 383 (Plasma) or 384 (Platelets), rather than 389. Reporting revenue codes according to these specifications will ensure the Medicare beneficiary's blood deductible is applied correctly

EXAMPLE: OPPS provider splits off a 100cc aliquot from a 250 cc unit of leukocyte-reduced red blood cells for a transfusion to Patient X. The hospital then splits off an 80cc aliquot of the remaining unit for a transfusion to Patient Y. At a later time, the remaining 70cc from the unit is transfused to Patient Z.

In billing for the services for Patient X and Patient Y, the OPPS provider should report the charges by billing P9011 and 86985 in addition to the CPT® code for the transfusion service, because a specific splitting service was required to prepare a split unit for transfusion to each of those patients. However, the OPPS provider should report only P9011 and the CPT® code for the transfusion service for Patient Z because no additional splitting was necessary to prepare the split unit for transfusion to Patient Z. The OPPS provider should bill Revenue Code 0389 for each split unit of the leukocyte-reduced red blood cells that was transfused.

100-4, Chapter-4, 240

Inpatient Part B Hospital Services

Medicare pays for hospital (including CAH) inpatient Part B services in the circumstances provided in Pub. 100-02, Medicare Benefit Policy Manual, Chapter 6, § 10 ("Medical and Other Health Services Furnished to Inpatients of Participating Hospitals"). Hospitals must bill Part B inpatient services on a 12x Type of Bill. This Part B inpatient claim is subject to the statutory time limit for filing Part B claims described in chapter 1, §70 of this manual.

Inpatient Part B services include inpatient ancillary services that do not require an outpatient status and are not strictly provided in an outpatient setting. Services that require an outpatient status and are provided only in an outpatient setting are not payable inpatient Part B services, including Clinic Visits, Emergency Department Visits, and Observation Services (this is not a complete listing).

Inpatient routine services in a hospital generally are those services included by the provider in a daily service charge— sometimes referred to as the "Room and Board" charge. They include the regular room, dietary and nursing services, minor medical and surgical supplies, medical social services, psychiatric social services, and the use of certain equipment and facilities for which a separate charge is not customarily made to Medicare Part A. Many nursing services provided by the floor nurse (such as IV infusions and injections, blood administration, and nebulizer treatments, etc.) may or may not have a separate charge established depending upon the classification of an item or service as routine or ancillary among providers of the same class in the same State. Some provider's customary charging practice has established separate charges for these services following the PRM–1 instructions, however, in order for a provider's customary charging practice to be recognized it must be consistently followed for all patients and this must not result in an inequitable apportionment of cost to the program. If the PRM–1 instructions have not been followed, a provider cannot bill these services as separate charges. Additionally, it is important that the charges for service rendered and documentation meet the definition of the HCPCS in order to separately bill.

100-4, Chapter-4, 290.1

Observation Services Overview

Observation care is a well-defined set of specific, clinically appropriate services, which include ongoing short term treatment, assessment, and reassessment, that are furnished while a decision is being made regarding whether patients will require further treatment as hospital inpatients or if they are able to be discharged from the hospital. Observation services are commonly ordered for patients who present to the emergency department and who then require a significant period of treatment or monitoring in order to make a decision concerning their admission or discharge. Observation services

are covered only when provided by the order of a physician or another individual authorized by State licensure law and hospital staff bylaws to admit patients to the hospital or to order outpatient services.

Observation services must also be reasonable and necessary to be covered by Medicare. In only rare and exceptional cases do reasonable and necessary outpatient observation services span more than 48 hours. In the majority of cases, the decision whether to discharge a patient from the hospital following resolution of the reason for the observation care or to admit the patient as an inpatient can be made in less than 48 hours, usually in less than 24 hours.

100-4, Chapter-4, 290.2.2

Reporting Hours of Observation

Observation time begins at the clock time documented in the patient's medical record, which coincides with the time that observation care is initiated in accordance with a physician's order. Hospitals should round to the nearest hour. For example, a patient who began receiving observation services at 3:03 p.m. according to the nurses' notes and was discharged to home at 9:45 p.m. when observation care and other outpatient services were completed, should have a "7" placed in the units field of the reported observation HCPCS code.

General standing orders for observation services following all outpatient surgery are not recognized. Hospitals should not report as observation care, services that are part of another Part B service, such as postoperative monitoring during a standard recovery period (e.g., 4-6 hours), which should be billed as recovery room services. Similarly, in the case of patients who undergo diagnostic testing in a hospital outpatient department, routine preparation services furnished prior to the testing and recovery afterwards are included in the payments for those diagnostic services.

Observation services should not be billed concurrently with diagnostic or therapeutic services for which active monitoring is a part of the procedure (e.g., colonoscopy, chemotherapy). In situations where such a procedure interrupts observation services, hospitals may determine the most appropriate way to account for this time. For example, a hospital may record for each period of observation services the beginning and ending times during the hospital outpatient encounter and add the length of time for the periods of observation services together to reach the total number of units reported on the claim for the hourly observation services HCPCS code G0378 (Hospital observation service, per hour). A hospital may also deduct the average length of time of the interrupting procedure, from the total duration of time that the patient receives observation services.

Observation time ends when all medically necessary services related to observation care are completed. For example, this could be before discharge when the need for observation has ended, but other medically necessary services not meeting the definition of observation care are provided (in which case, the additional medically necessary services would be billed separately or included as part of the emergency department or clinic visit). Alternatively, the end time of observation services may coincide with the time the patient is actually discharged from the hospital or admitted as an inpatient. Observation time may include medically necessary services and follow-up care provided after the time that the physician writes the discharge order, but before the patient is discharged. However, reported observation time would not include the time patients remain in the hospital after treatment is finished for reasons such as waiting for transportation home.

If a period of observation spans more than 1 calendar day, all of the hours for the entire period of observation must be included on a single line and the date of service for that line is the date that observation care begins.

100-4, Chapter-4, 290.4.1

Billing and Payment for All Hospital Observation Services Furnished Between January 1, 2006 and December 31, 2007

Since January 1, 2006, two G-codes have been used to report observation services and direct referral for observation care. For claims for dates of service January 1, 2006 through December 31, 2007, the Integrated Outpatient Code Editor (I/OCE) determines whether the observation care or direct referral services are packaged or separately payable. Thus, hospitals provide consistent coding and billing under all circumstances in which they deliver observation care.

Beginning January 1, 2006, hospitals should not report CPT® codes 99217-99220 or 99234-99236 for observation services. In addition, the following HCPCS codes were discontinued as of January 1, 2006: G0244 (Observation care by facility to patient), G0263 (Direct Admission with congestive heart failure, chest pain or asthma), and G0264 (Assessment other than congestive heart failure, chest pain, or asthma).

The three discontinued G-codes and the CPT® codes that were no longer recognized were replaced by two new G-codes to be used by hospitals to report all observation services, whether separately payable or packaged, and direct referral for observation care, whether separately payable or packaged:

• G0378- Hospital observation service, per hour; and
• G0379- Direct admission of patient for hospital observation care.

The I/OCE determines whether observation services billed as units of G0378 are separately payable under APC 0339 (Observation) or whether payment for observation services will be packaged into the payment for other services provided by the hospital in the same encounter. Therefore, hospitals should bill HCPCS code G0378 when observation services are ordered and provided to any patient regardless of the patient's condition. The units of service should equal the number of hours the patient receives observation services.

Hospitals should report G0379 when observation services are the result of a direct referral for observation care without an associated emergency room visit, hospital outpatient clinic visit, critical care service, or hospital outpatient surgical procedure (status indicator T procedure) on the day of initiation of observation services. Hospitals should only report HCPCS code G0379 when a patient is referred directly for observation care after being seen by a physician in the community (see §290.4.2 below)

Some non-repetitive OPPS services provided on the same day by a hospital may be billed on different claims, provided that all charges associated with each procedure or service being reported are billed on the same claim with the HCPCS code which describes that service. See chapter 1, section 50.2.2 of this manual. It is vitally important that all of the charges that pertain to a non-repetitive, separately paid procedure or service be reported on the same claim with that procedure or service. It should also be emphasized that this relaxation of same day billing requirements for some non-repetitive services does not apply to non-repetitive services provided on the same day as either direct referral to observation care or observation services because the OCE claim-by-claim logic cannot function properly unless

all services related to the episode of observation care, including diagnostic tests, lab services, hospital clinic visits, emergency department visits, critical care services, and status indicator T procedures, are reported on the same claim. Additional guidance can be found in chapter 1, section 50.2.2 of this manual.

100-4, Chapter-4, 290.4.2

Separate and Packaged Payment for Direct Referral for Observation Services Furnished Between January 1, 2006 and December 31, 2007

In order to receive separate payment for a direct referral for observation care (APC 0604), the claim must show:

1. Both HCPCS codes G0378 (Hourly Observation) and G0379 (Direct Admit to Observation) with the same date of service;
2. That no services with a status indicator T or V or Critical care (APC 0617) were provided on the same day of service as HCPCS code G0379; and
3. The observation care does not qualify for separate payment under APC 0339.

Only a direct referral for observation services billed on a 13X bill type may be considered for a separate APC payment.

Separate payment is not allowed for HCPCS code G0379, direct admission to observation care, when billed with the same date of service as a hospital clinic visit, emergency room visit, critical care service, or "T" status procedure.

If a bill for the direct referral for observation services does not meet the three requirements listed above, then payment for the direct referral service will be packaged into payments for other separately payable services provided to the beneficiary in the same encounter.

100-4, Chapter-4, 290.4.3

Separate and Packaged Payment for Observation Services Furnished Between January 1, 2006 and December 31, 2007

Separate payment may be made for observation services provided to a patient with congestive heart failure, chest pain, or asthma. The list of ICD-9-CM diagnosis codes eligible for separate payment is reviewed annually. Any changes in applicable ICD-9-CM diagnosis codes are included in the October quarterly update of the OPPS and also published in the annual OPPS Final Rule. The list of qualifying ICD-9-CM diagnosis codes is also published on the OPPS Web page.

All of the following requirements must be met in order for a hospital to receive a separate APC payment for observation services through APC 0339:

1. Diagnosis Requirements
   a. The beneficiary must have one of three medical conditions: congestive heart failure, chest pain, or asthma.
   b. Qualifying ICD-9-CM diagnosis codes must be reported in Form Locator (FL) 76, Patient Reason for Visit, or FL 67, principal diagnosis, or both in order for the hospital to receive separate payment for APC 0339. If a qualifying ICD-9-CM diagnosis code(s) is reported in the secondary diagnosis field, but is not reported in either the Patient Reason for Visit field (FL 76) or in the principal diagnosis field (FL 67), separate payment for APC 0339 is not allowed.

2. Observation Time

  a. Observation time must be documented in the medical record.

  b. Hospital billing for observation services begins at the clock time documented in the patient's medical record, which coincides with the time that observation services are initiated in accordance with a physician's order for observation services.

  c. A beneficiary's time receiving observation services (and hospital billing) ends when all clinical or medical interventions have been completed, including follow-up care furnished by hospital staff and physicians that may take place after a physician has ordered the patient be released or admitted as an inpatient.

  d. The number of units reported with HCPCS code G0378 must equal or exceed 8 hours.

3. Additional Hospital Services

  a. The claim for observation services must include one of the following services in addition to the reported observation services. The additional services listed below must have a line item date of service on the same day or the day before the date reported for observation:

   • An emergency department visit (APC 0609, 0613, 0614, 0615, 0616) or

   • A clinic visit (APC 0604, 0605, 0606, 0607, 0608); or

   • Critical care (APC 0617); or

   • Direct referral for observation care reported with HCPCS code G0379 (APC 0604); must be reported on the same date of service as the date reported for observation services.

  b. No procedure with a T status indicator can be reported on the same day or day before observation care is provided.

4. Physician Evaluation

  a. The beneficiary must be in the care of a physician during the period of observation, as documented in the medical record by outpatient registration, discharge, and other appropriate progress notes that are timed, written, and signed by the physician.

  b. The medical record must include documentation that the physician explicitly assessed patient risk to determine that the beneficiary would benefit from observation care.

Only observation services that are billed on a 13X bill type may be considered for a separate APC payment.

Hospitals should bill all of the other services associated with the observation care, including direct referral for observation, hospital clinic visits, emergency room visits, critical care services, and T status procedures, on the same claim so that the claims processing logic may appropriately determine the payment status (either packaged or separately payable) of HCPCS codes G0378 and G0379.

If a bill for observation care does not meet all of the requirements listed above, then payment for the observation care will be packaged into payments for other separately payable services provided to the beneficiary in the same encounter.

100-4, Chapter-4, 290.5.1

Billing and Payment for Observation Services Beginning January 1, 2008 and December 31, 2015

Observation services are reported using HCPCS code G0378 (Hospital observation service, per hour). Beginning January 1, 2008, HCPCS code G0378 for hourly observation services is assigned status indicator N, signifying that its payment is always packaged. No separate payment is made for observation services reported with HCPCS code G0378, and APC 0339 is deleted as of January 1, 2008. In most circumstances, observation services are supportive and ancillary to the other services provided to a patient. Beginning January 1, 2014, in certain circumstances when observation care is billed in conjunction with a clinic visit, high level Type A emergency department visit (Level 4 or 5), high level Type B emergency department visit (Level 5), critical care services, or a direct referral as an integral part of a patient's extended encounter of care, payment may be made for the entire extended care encounter through APC 8009 (Extended Assessment and Management Composite) when certain criteria are met. Prior to January 1, 2014, in certain circumstances when observation care was billed in conjunction with a high level clinic visit (Level 5), high level Type A emergency department visit (Level 4 or 5), high level Type B emergency department visit (Level 5), critical care services, or a direct referral as an integral part of a patient's extended encounter of care, payment could be made for the entire extended care encounter through one of two composite APCs (APCs 8002 and 8003) when certain criteria were met. APCs 8002 and 8003 are deleted as of January 1, 2014. For information about payment for extended assessment and management composite APC, see §10.2.1 (Composite APCs) of this chapter.

There is no limitation on diagnosis for payment of APC 8009; however, composite APC payment will not be made when observation services are reported in association with a surgical procedure (T status procedure) or the hours of observation care reported are less than 8. The I/OCE evaluates every claim received to determine if payment through a composite APC is appropriate. If payment through a composite APC is inappropriate, the I/OCE, in conjunction with the Pricer, determines the appropriate status indicator, APC, and payment for every code on a claim.

All of the following requirements must be met in order for a hospital to receive an APC payment for an extended assessment and management composite APC:

1. Observation Time

  a. Observation time must be documented in the medical record.

  b. Hospital billing for observation services begins at the clock time documented in the patient's medical record, which coincides with the time that observation services are initiated in accordance with a physician's order for observation services.

  c. A beneficiary's time receiving observation services (and hospital billing) ends when all clinical or medical interventions have been completed, including follow-up care furnished by hospital staff and physicians that may take place after a physician has ordered the patient be released or admitted as an inpatient.

  d. The number of units reported with HCPCS code G0378 must equal or exceed 8 hours.

2. Additional Hospital Services

  a. The claim for observation services must include one of the following services in addition to the reported observation services. The additional services listed below must have a line item date of service on the same day or the day before the date reported for observation:

- A Type A or B emergency department visit (CPT® codes 99284 or 99285 or HCPCS code G0384); or

- A clinic visit (HCPCS code G0463 beginning January 1, 2014; CPT® code 99205 or 99215 prior to January 1, 2014); or

- Critical care (CPT® code 99291); or

- Direct referral for observation care reported with HCPCS code G0379 (APC 0633) must be reported on the same date of service as the date reported for observation services.

b. No procedure with a T status indicator can be reported on the same day or day before observation care is provided.

3. Physician Evaluation.

a. The beneficiary must be in the care of a physician during the period of observation, as documented in the medical record by outpatient registration, discharge, and other appropriate progress notes that are timed, written, and signed by the physician.

b. The medical record must include documentation that the physician explicitly assessed patient risk to determine that the beneficiary would benefit from observation care.

Criteria 1 and 3 related to observation care beginning and ending time and physician evaluation apply regardless of whether the hospital believes that the criteria will be met for payment of the extended encounter through extended assessment and management composite payment.

Only visits, critical care and observation services that are billed on a 13X bill type may be considered for a composite APC payment.

Non-repetitive services provided on the same day as either direct referral for observation care or observation services must be reported on the same claim because the OCE claim-by-claim logic cannot function properly unless all services related to the episode of observation care, including hospital clinic visits, emergency department visits, critical care services, and T status procedures, are reported on the same claim. Additional guidance can be found in chapter 1, section 50.2.2 of this manual.

If a claim for services provided during an extended assessment and management encounter including observation care does not meet all of the requirements listed above, then the usual APC logic will apply to separately payable items and services on the claim; the special logic for direct admission will apply, and payment for the observation care will be packaged into payments for other separately payable services provided to the beneficiary in the same encounter.

100-4, Chapter-4, 290.5.2

Billing and Payment for Direct Referral for Observation Care Furnished Beginning January 1, 2008

Direct referral for observation is reported using HCPCS code G0379 (Direct referral for hospital observation care). : Prior to January 1, 2010, the code descriptor for HCPCS code G0379 was (Direct admission of patient for hospital observation care). Hospitals should report G0379 when observation services are the result of a direct referral for observation care without

an associated emergency room visit, hospital outpatient clinic visit, or critical care service on the day of initiation of observation services. Hospitals should only report HCPCS code G0379 when a patient is referred directly to observation care after being seen by a physician in the community.

Payment for direct referral for observation care will be made either separately as a low level hospital clinic visit under APC 0633 (Level 3 Examinations & Related Services) or packaged into payment for composite APC 8009 (Extended Assessment and Management Composite) or packaged into the payment for other separately payable services provided in the same encounter. For information about payment for extended assessment and management composite APCs, see, §10.2.1 (Composite APCs) of this chapter.

The criteria for payment of HCPCS code G0379 under either APC 0633 or APC 8009 include:

1. Both HCPCS codes G0378 (Hospital observation services, per hr.) and G0379 (Direct referral for hospital observation care) are reported with the same date of service.

2. No service with a status indicator of T or V or Critical Care (APC 0617) is provided on the same day of service as HCPCS code G0379.

If either of the above criteria is not met, HCPCS code G0379 will be assigned status indicator N and will be packaged into payment for other separately payable services provided in the same encounter.

Only a direct referral for observation services billed on a 13X bill type may be considered for a composite APC payment.

100-4, Chapter-4, 300.6

Common Working File (CWF) Edits

The CWF edit will allow 3 hours of therapy for MNT in the initial calendar year. The edit will allow more than 3 hours of therapy if there is a change in the beneficiary's medical condition, diagnosis, or treatment regimen and this change must be documented in the beneficiary's medical record. Two new G codes have been created for use when a beneficiary receives a second referral in a calendar year that allows the beneficiary to receive more than 3 hours of therapy. Another edit will allow 2 hours of follow-up MNT with another referral in subsequent years.

Advance Beneficiary Notice (ABN)

The beneficiary is liable for services denied over the limited number of hours with referrals for MNT. An ABN should be issued in these situations. In absence of evidence of a valid ABN, the provider will be held liable.

An ABN should not be issued for Medicare-covered services such as those provided by hospital dietitians or nutrition professionals who are qualified to render the service in their state but who have not obtained Medicare provider numbers.

Duplicate Edits

Although beneficiaries are allowed to receive training and therapy during the same time period Diabetes Self-Management and Training (DSMT) and Medical Nutrition Therapy (MNT) services may not be provided on the same day to the same beneficiary. Effective April 1, 2010 CWF shall implement a new duplicate crossover edit to identify and prevent claims for DSMT/MNT services from being billed with the same dates of services for the same beneficiaries submitted from institutional providers and from a professional provider.

100-4, Chapter-4, 320

Outpatient Intravenous Insulin Treatment (OIVIT)

Effective for claims with dates of service on and after December 23, 2009, the Centers for Medicare and Medicaid Services (CMS) determines that the evidence does not support a conclusion that OIVIT improves health outcomes in Medicare beneficiaries. Therefore, CMS has determined that OIVIT is not reasonable and necessary for any indication under section 1862(a)(1)(A) of the Social Security Act. Services comprising an OIVIT regimen are nationally non-covered under Medicare when furnished pursuant to an OIVIT regimen.

See Pub. 100-03, Medicare National Coverage Determinations Manual, Section 40.7, Outpatient Intravenous Insulin Treatment (Effective December 23, 2009), for general information and coverage indications.

100-4, Chapter-4, 320.1

HCPCS Coding for OIVIT

HCPCS code G9147, effective with the April IOCE and MPFSDB updates, is to be used on claims with dates of service on and after December 23, 2009, billing for non-covered OIVIT and any services comprising an OIVIT regimen.

NOTE: HCPCS codes 99199 or 94681(with or without diabetes related conditions 250.00-250.93) are not to be used on claims billing for non-covered OIVIT and any services comprising an OIVIT regimen when furnished pursuant to an OIVIT regimen. Claims billing for HCPCS codes 99199 and 94681 for non-covered OIVIT are to be returned to provider/returned as unprocessable.

100-4, Chapter-4, 320.2

Medicare Summary Notices (MSN), Reason Codes, and Remark Codes

Contractors shall return non-covered OIVIT claims billed with HCPCS 99199 to provider/return as unprocessable.

The contractor shall use the following remittance advice messages and associated codes when rejecting/denying claims under this policy. This CARC/RARC combination is compliant with CAQH CORE Business Scenario Two.

Group Code: CO

CARC: 16

RARC: MA66, N56

MSN: N/A

Contractors shall return non-covered OIVIT claims billed with HCPCS 94681 with or without diabetes-related conditions 250-00-250.93 to provider/return as unprocessable.

The contractor shall use the following remittance advice messages and associated codes when rejecting/denying claims under this policy. This CARC/RARC combination is compliant with CAQH CORE Business Scenario Three.

Group Code: CO

CARC: 16

RARC: MA66, N56

MSN: N/A

Contractors shall deny claims for non-covered OIVIT and any services comprising an OIVIT regimen billed with HCPCS code G9147.

The contractor shall use the following remittance advice messages and associated codes when rejecting/denying claims under this policy. This CARC/RARC combination is compliant with CAQH CORE Business Scenario Three.

Group Code: CO

CARC: 96

RARC: N386

MSN: 16.10

100-4, Chapter-5, 10.2

The Financial Limitation Legislation

A. Legislation on Limitations

The dollar amount of the limitations (caps) on outpatient therapy services is established by statute. The updated amount of the caps is released annually via Recurring Update Notifications and posted on the CMS Website www.cms.gov/TherapyServices, on contractor Websites, and on each beneficiary's Medicare Summary Notice. Medicare contractors shall publish the financial limitation amount in educational articles. It is also available at 1-800-Medicare.

Section 4541(a)(2) of the Balanced Budget Act (BBA) (P.L. 105-33) of 1997, which added §1834(k)(5) to the Act, required payment under a prospective payment system (PPS) for outpatient rehabilitation services (except those furnished by or under arrangements with a hospital). Outpatient rehabilitation services include the following services:

- Physical therapy
- Speech-language pathology; and
- Occupational therapy.

Section 4541(c) of the BBA required application of financial limitations to all outpatient rehabilitation services (except those furnished by or under arrangements with a hospital). In 1999, an annual per beneficiary limit of $1,500 was applied, including all outpatient physical therapy services and speech-language pathology services. A separate limit applied to all occupational therapy services. The limits were based on incurred expenses and included applicable deductible and coinsurance. The BBA provided that the limits be indexed by the Medicare Economic Index (MEI) each year beginning in 2002.

Since the limitations apply to outpatient services, they do not apply to skilled nursing facility (SNF) residents in a covered Part A stay, including patients occupying swing beds. Rehabilitation services are included within the global Part A per diem payment that the SNF receives under the prospective payment system (PPS) for the covered stay. Also, limitations do not apply to any therapy services covered under prospective payment systems for home health or inpatient hospitals, including critical access hospitals.

The limitation is based on therapy services the Medicare beneficiary receives, not the type of practitioner who provides the service. Physical therapists, speech-language pathologists, and occupational therapists, as well as physicians and certain nonphysician practitioners, could render a therapy service.

B. Moratoria and Exceptions for Therapy Claims

Since the creation of therapy caps, Congress has enacted several moratoria. The Deficit Reduction Act of 2005 directed CMS to develop exceptions to therapy caps for calendar year 2006 and the exceptions have been extended periodically. The cap exception for therapy services billed by outpatient hospitals was part of the original legislation and applies as long as caps are in effect. Exceptions to caps based on the medical necessity of the service are in effect only when Congress legislates the exceptions.

100-4, Chapter-5, 10.6

Functional Reporting

A. General

Section 3005(g) of the Middle Class Tax Relief and Jobs Creation Act (MCTRJCA) amended Section 1833(g) of the Act to require a claims-based data collection system for outpatient therapy services, including physical therapy (PT), occupational therapy (OT) and speech-language pathology (SLP) services. 42 CFR 410.59, 410.60, 410.61, 410.62 and 410.105 implement this requirement. The system will collect data on beneficiary function during the course of therapy services in order to better understand beneficiary conditions, outcomes, and expenditures.

Beneficiary unction information is reported using 42 nonpayable functional G-codes and seven severity/complexity modifiers on claims for PT, OT, and SLP services. Functional reporting on one functional limitation at a time is required periodically throughout an entire PT, OT, or SLP therapy episode of care.

The nonpayable G-codes and severity modifiers provide information about the beneficiary's functional status at the outset of the therapy episode of care, including projected goal status, at specified points during treatment, and at the time of discharge. These G-codes, along with the associated modifiers, are required at specified intervals on all claims for outpatient therapy services – not just those over the cap.

B. Application of New Coding Requirements

This functional data reporting and collection system is effective for therapy services with dates of service on and after January 1, 2013. A testing period will be in effect from January 1, 2013, until July 1, 2013, to allow providers and practitioners to use the new coding requirements to assure that systems work. Claims for therapy services furnished on and after July 1, 2013, that do not contain the required functional G-code/modifier information will be returned or rejected, as applicable.

C. Services Affected

These requirements apply to all claims for services furnished under the Medicare Part B outpatient therapy benefit and the PT, OT, and SLP services furnished under the CORF benefit. They also apply to the therapy services furnished personally by and incident to the service of a physician or a nonphysician practitioner (NPP), including a nurse practitioner (NP), a certified nurse specialist (CNS), or a physician assistant (PA), as applicable.

D. Providers and Practitioners Affected.

The functional reporting requirements apply to the therapy services furnished by the following providers: hospitals, CAHs, SNFs, CORFs, rehabilitation agencies, and HHAs (when the beneficiary is not under a home health plan of care). It applies to the following practitioners: physical therapists, occupational therapists, and speech-language pathologists in private practice (TPPs), physicians, and NPPs as noted above. The term "clinician" is applied to these practitioners throughout this manual section. (See definition section of Pub. 100-02, Chapter 15, section 220.)

E. Function-related G-codes

There are 42 functional G-codes, 14 sets of three codes each. Six of the G-code sets are generally for PT and OT functional

limitations and eight sets of G-codes are for SLP functional limitations.

The following G-codes are for functional limitations typically seen in beneficiaries receiving PT or OT services. The first four of these sets describe categories of functional limitations and the final two sets describe "other" functional limitations, which are to be used for functional limitations not described by one of the four categories.

NONPAYABLE G-CODES FOR FUNCTIONAL LIMITATIONS		
Code	Long Descriptor	Short Descriptor
Mobility G-code Set		
G8978	Mobility: walking & moving around functional limitation, current status, at therapy episode outset and at reporting intervals	Mobility current status
G8979	Mobility: walking & moving around functional limitation, projected goal status, at therapy episode outset, at reporting intervals, and at discharge or to end reporting	Mobility goal status
G8980	Mobility: walking & moving around functional limitation, discharge status, at discharge from therapy or to end reporting	Mobility D/C status
Changing & Maintaining Body Position G-code Set		
G8981	Changing & maintaining body position functional limitation, current status, at therapy episode outset and at reporting intervals	Body pos current status
G8982	Changing & maintaining body position functional limitation, projected goal status, at therapy episode outset, at reporting intervals, and at discharge or to end reporting	Body pos goal status
G8983	Changing & maintaining body position functional limitation, discharge status, at discharge from therapy or to end reporting	Body pos D/C status
Carrying, Moving & Handling Objects G-code Set		
G8984	Carrying, moving & handling objects functional limitation, current status, at therapy episode outset and at reporting intervals	Carry current status
G8985	Carrying, moving & handling objects functional limitation, projected goal status, at therapy episode outset, at reporting intervals, and at discharge or to end reporting	Carry goal status
G8986	Carrying, moving & handling objects functional limitation, discharge status, at discharge from therapy or to end reporting	Carry D/C status
Self-Care G-code Set		
G8987	Self-care functional limitation, current status, at therapy episode outset and at reporting intervals	Self-care current status
G8988	Self-care functional limitation, projected goal status, at therapy episode outset, at reporting intervals, and at discharge or to end reporting	Self-care goal status
G8989	Self-care functional limitation, discharge status, at discharge from therapy or to end reporting	Self-care D/C status

The following "other PT/OT" functional G-codes are used to report:

- a beneficiary's functional limitation that is not defined by one of the above four categories;

- a beneficiary whose therapy services are not intended to treat a functional limitation;

- or a beneficiary's functional limitation when an overall, composite or other score from a functional assessment too is used and it does not clearly represent a functional limitation defined by one of the above four code sets.

Code	Long Descriptor	Short Descriptor
Other PT/OT Primary G-code Set		
G8990	Other physical or occupational therapy primary functional limitation, current status, at therapy episode outset and at reporting intervals	Other PT/OT current status
G8991	Other physical or occupational therapy primary functional limitation, projected goal status, at therapy episode outset, at reporting intervals, and at discharge or to end reporting	Other PT/OT goal status
G8992	Other physical or occupational therapy primary functional limitation, discharge status, at discharge from therapy or to end reporting	Other PT/OT D/C status
Other PT/OT Subsequent G-code Set		
G8993	Other physical or occupational therapy subsequent functional limitation, current status, at therapy episode outset and at reporting intervals	Sub PT/OT current status
G8994	Other physical or occupational therapy subsequent functional limitation, projected goal status, at therapy episode outset, at reporting intervals, and at discharge or to end reporting	Sub PT/OT goal status

The following G-codes are for functional limitations typically seen in beneficiaries receiving SLP services. Seven are for specific functional communication measures, which are modeled after the National Outcomes Measurement System (NOMS), and one is for any "other" measure not described by one of the other seven.

Code	Long Descriptor	Short Descriptor
Swallowing G-code Set		
G8996	Swallowing functional limitation, current status, at therapy episode outset and at reporting intervals	Swallow current status
G8997	Swallowing functional limitation, projected goal status, at therapy episode outset, at reporting intervals, and at discharge or to end reporting	Swallow goal status
G8998	Swallowing functional limitation, discharge status, at discharge from therapy or to end reporting	Swallow D/C status
Motor Speech G-code Set (***NOTE:*** These codes are not sequentially numbered)		
G8999	Motor speech functional limitation, current status, at therapy episode outset and at reporting intervals	Motor speech current status
G9186	Motor speech functional limitation, projected goal status at therapy episode outset, at reporting intervals, and at discharge or to end reporting	Motor speech goal status
G9158	Motor speech functional limitation, discharge status, at discharge from therapy or to end reporting	Motor speech D/C status

Code	Long Descriptor	Short Descriptor
Spoken Language Comprehension G-code Set		
G9159	Spoken language comprehension functional limitation, current status, at therapy episode outset and at reporting intervals	Lang comp current status
G9160	Spoken language comprehension functional limitation, projected goal status, at therapy episode outset, at reporting intervals, and at discharge or to end reporting	Lang comp goal status
G9161	Spoken language comprehension functional limitation, discharge status, at discharge from therapy or to end reporting	Lang comp D/C status
Spoken Language Expressive G-code Set		
G9162	Spoken language expression functional limitation, current status, at therapy episode outset and at reporting intervals	Lang express current status
G9163	Spoken language expression functional limitation, projected goal status, at therapy episode outset, at reporting intervals, and at discharge or to end reporting	Lang press goal status
G9164	Spoken language expression functional limitation, discharge status, at discharge from therapy or to end reporting	Lang express D/C status
Attention G-code Set		
G9165	Attention functional limitation, current status, at therapy episode outset and at reporting intervals	Atten current status
G9166	Attention functional limitation, projected goal status, at therapy episode outset, at reporting intervals, and at discharge or to end reporting	Atten goal status
G9167	Attention functional limitation, discharge status, at discharge from therapy or to end reporting	Atten D/C status
Memory G-code Set		
G9168	Memory functional limitation, current status, at therapy episode outset and at reporting intervals	Memory current status
G9169	Memory functional limitation, projected goal status, at therapy episode outset, at reporting intervals, and at discharge or to end reporting	Memory goal status
G9170	Memory functional limitation, discharge status, at discharge from therapy or to end reporting	Memory D/C status
Voice G-code Set		
G9171	Voice functional limitation, current status, at therapy episode outset and at reporting intervals	Voice current status
G9172	Voice functional limitation, projected goal status, at therapy episode outset, at reporting intervals, and at discharge or to end reporting	Voice goal status
G9173	Voice functional limitation, discharge status, at discharge from therapy or to end reporting	Voice D/C status

The following "other SLP" G-code set is used to report:

- on one of the other eight NOMS-defined functional measures not described by the above code sets; or

- to report an overall, composite or other score from assessment tool that does not clearly represent one of the above seven categorical SLP functional measures.

Code	Long Descriptor	Short Descriptor
Other Speech Language Pathology G-code Set		
G9174	Other speech language pathology functional limitation, current status, at therapy episode outset and at reporting intervals	Speech lang current status
G9175	Other speech language pathology functional limitation, projected goal status, at therapy episode outset, at reporting intervals, and at discharge or to end reporting	Speech lang goal status
G9176	Other speech language pathology functional limitation, discharge status, at discharge from therapy or to end reporting	Speech lang D/C status

F. Severity/Complexity Modifiers

For each nonpayable functional G-code, one of the modifiers listed below must be used to report the severity/complexity for that functional limitation.

Modifier	Impairment Limitation Restriction
CH	0 percent impaired, limited or restricted
CI	At least 1 percent but less than 20 percent impaired, limited or restricted
CJ	At least 20 percent but less than 40 percent impaired, limited or restricted
CK	At least 40 percent but less than 60 percent impaired, limited or restricted
CL	At least 60 percent but less than 80 percent impaired, limited or restricted
CM	At least 80 percent but less than 100 percent impaired, limited or restricted
CN	100 percent impaired, limited or restricted

The severity modifiers reflect the beneficiary's percentage of functional impairment as determined by the clinician furnishing the therapy services.

G. Required Reporting of Functional G-codes and Severity Modifiers

The functional G-codes and severity modifiers listed above are used in the required reporting on therapy claims at certain specified points during therapy episodes of care. Claims containing these functional G-codes must also contain another billable and separately payable (non-bundled) service. Only one functional limitation shall be reported at a given time for each related therapy plan of care (POC).

Functional reporting using the G-codes and corresponding severity modifiers is required reporting on specified therapy claims. Specifically, they are required on claims:

- At the outset of a therapy episode of care (i.e., on the claim for the date of service (DOS) of the initial therapy service);

- At least once every 10 treatment days, which corresponds with the progress reporting period;

- When an evaluative procedure, including a re-evaluative one, (HCPCS/CPT® codes 92521, 92522, 92523, 92524, 92597, 92607, 92608, 92610, 92611, 92612, 92614, 92616, 96105, 96125, 97001, 97002, 97003, 97004) is furnished and billed;

- At the time of discharge from the therapy episode of care— (i.e., on the date services related to the discharge [progress] report are furnished); and

- At the time reporting of a particular functional limitation is ended in cases where the need for further therapy is necessary.

- At the time reporting is begun for a new or different functional limitation within the same episode of care (i.e., after the reporting of the prior functional limitation is ended)

Functional reporting is required on claims throughout the entire episode of care. When the beneficiary has reached his or her goal or progress has been maximized on the initially selected functional limitation, but the need for treatment continues, reporting is required for a second functional limitation using another set of G-codes. In these situations two or more functional limitations will be reported for a beneficiary during the therapy episode of care. Thus, reporting on more than one functional limitation may be required for some beneficiaries but not simultaneously.

When the beneficiary stops coming to therapy prior to discharge, the clinician should report the functional information on the last claim. If the clinician is unaware that the beneficiary is not returning for therapy until after the last claim is submitted, the clinician cannot report the discharge status.

When functional reporting is required on a claim for therapy services, two G-codes will generally be required.

Two exceptions exist:

1. Therapy services under more than one therapy POC — Claims may contain more than two nonpayable functional G-codes when in cases where a beneficiary receives therapy services under multiple POCs (PT, OT, and/or SLP) from the same therapy provider.

2. One-Time Therapy Visit — When a beneficiary is seen and future therapy services are either not medically indicated or are going to be furnished by another provider, the clinician reports on the claim for the DOS of the visit, all three G-codes in the appropriate code set (current status, goal status and discharge status), along with corresponding severity modifiers.

Each reported functional G-code must also contain the following line of service information:

- Functional severity modifier

- Therapy modifier indicating the related discipline/POC — GP, GO or GN — for PT, OT, and SLP services, respectively

- Date of the related therapy service

- Nominal charge, e.g., a penny, for institutional claims submitted to the A/B MACs (A). For professional claims, a zero charge is acceptable for the service line. If provider billing software requires an amount for professional claims, a nominal charge, e.g., a penny, may be included.

NOTE: The KX modifier is not required on the claim line for nonpayable G-codes, but would be required with the procedure code for medically necessary therapy services furnished once the beneficiary's annual cap has been reached.

The following example demonstrates how the G-codes and modifiers are used. In this example, the clinician determines that the beneficiary's mobility restriction is the most clinically relevant functional limitation and selects the Mobility G-code set (G8978 – G8980) to represent the beneficiary's functional limitation. The clinician also determines the severity/complexity of the beneficiary's functional limitation and selects the appropriate modifier. In this example, the clinician determines that the beneficiary has a 75 percent mobility restriction for which the CL modifier is applicable. The clinician expects that at the end of therapy the beneficiaries will have only a 15 percent mobility restriction for which the CI modifier is applicable. When the beneficiary attains the mobility goal, therapy continues to be medically necessary to address a functional limitation for which there is no categorical G-code. The clinician reports this using (G8990 – G8992).

At the outset of therapy — On the DOS for which the initial evaluative procedure is furnished or the initial treatment day of a therapy POC, the claim for the service will also include two G-codes as shown below.

- G8978-CL to report the functional limitation (Mobility with current mobility limitation of "at least 60 percent but less than 80 percent impaired, limited or restricted")

- G8979-CI to report the projected goal for a mobility restriction of "at least 1 percent but less than 20 percent impaired, limited or restricted."

At the end of each progress reporting period — On the claim for the DOS when the services related to the progress report (which must be done at least once each 10 treatment days) are furnished, the clinician will report the same two G-codes but the modifier for the current status may be different.

- G8978 with the appropriate modifier are reported to show the beneficiary's current status as of this DOS. So if the beneficiary has made no progress, this claim will include G8978-CL. If the beneficiary made progress and now has a mobility restriction of 65 percent CL would still be the appropriate modifier for 65 percent, and G8978-CL would be reported in this case. If the beneficiary now has a mobility restriction of 45 percent, G8978-CK would be reported.

- G8979-CI would be reported to show the projected goal. This severity modifier would not change unless the clinician adjusts the beneficiary's goal.

This step is repeated as necessary and clinically appropriate, adjusting the current status modifier used as the beneficiary progresses through therapy.

At the time the beneficiary is discharged from the therapy episode. The final claim for therapy episode will include two G-codes.

- G8979-CI would be reported to show the projected goal. G8980-CI would be reported if the beneficiary attained the 15 percent mobility goal. Alternatively, if the beneficiary's mobility restriction only reached 25 percent; G8980-CJ would be reported.

To end reporting of one functional limitation — As noted above, functional reporting is required to continue throughout the entire episode of care. Accordingly, when further therapy is medically necessary after the beneficiary attains the goal for the first reported functional limitation, the clinician would end reporting of the first functional limitation by using the same G-codes and modifiers that would be used at the time of discharge. Using the mobility example, to end reporting of the mobility functional limitation, G8979-CI and G8980-CI would be reported on the same DOS that coincides with end of that progress reporting period.

To begin reporting of a second functional limitation. At the time reporting is begun for a new and different functional limitation, within the same episode of care (i.e., after the reporting of the prior functional limitation is ended). Reporting on the second functional limitation, however, is not begun until the DOS of the next treatment day — which is day one of the new progress reporting period. When the next functional limitation to be reported is NOT defined by one of the other three PT/OT categorical codes, the G-code set (G8990 - G8992) for the "other PT/OT primary" functional limitation is used, rather than the G-code set for the "other PT/OT subsequent" because it is the first reported "other PT/OT" functional limitation. This reporting begins on the DOS of the first treatment day

following the mobility "discharge" reporting, which is counted as the initial service for the "other PT/OT primary" functional limitation and the first treatment day of the new progress reporting period. In this case, G8990 and G8991, along with the corresponding modifiers, are reported on the claim for therapy services.

The table below illustrates when reporting is required using this example and what G-codes would be used.

Example of Required Reporting

Key: Reporting Period (RP)	Begin RP #1 for Mobility at Episode Outset	End RP#1for Mobility at Progress Report	Mobility RP #2 Begins Next Treatment Day	End RP #2 for Mobility at Progress Report	Mobility RP #3 Begins Next Treatment Day	D/C or End Reporting for Mobility	Begin RP #1 for Other PT/OT Primary
Mobility: Walking & Moving Around							
G8978 – Current Status	X	X		X			
G 8979– Goal Status	X	X		X		X	
G8980 – Discharge Status						X	
Other PT/OT Primary							
G8990 – Current Status							X
G8991 – Goal Status							X
G8992 – Discharge Status							
No Functional Reporting Required			X		X		

H. Required Tracking and Documentation of Functional G-codes and Severity Modifiers

The clinician who furnishes the services must not only report the functional information on the therapy claim, but, he/she must track and document the G-codes and severity modifiers used for this reporting in the beneficiary's medical record of therapy services.

For details related to the documentation requirements, refer to, Medicare Benefit Policy Manual, Pub. 100-02, Chapter 15, section 220.4 - Functional Reporting. For coverage rules related to MCTRJCA and therapy goals, refer to Pub. 100-02: a) for outpatient therapy services, see Chapter 15, section 220.1.2 B and b) for instructions specific to PT, OT, and SLP services in the CORF, see Chapter 12, section 10.

100-4, Chapter-5, 20

HCPCS Coding Requirement

A. Uniform Coding

Section 1834(k)(5) of the Act requires that all claims for outpatient rehabilitation therapy services and all comprehensive outpatient rehabilitation facility (CORF) services be reported using a uniform coding system. The current Healthcare Common Procedure Coding System/Current Procedural Terminology is used for the reporting of these services. The uniform coding requirement in the Act is specific to payment for all CORF services and outpatient rehabilitation therapy services - including physical therapy, occupational therapy, and speech-language pathology - that is provided and billed to Medicare contractors. The Medicare physician fee schedule (MPFS) is used to make payment for these therapy services at the non facility rate.

Effective for claims submitted on or after April 1, 1998, providers that had not previously reported HCPCS/CPT® for outpatient rehabilitation and CORF services began using HCPCS to report these services. This requirement does not apply to outpatient rehabilitation services provided by:

- Critical access hospitals, which are paid on a cost basis, not MPFS;

- RHCs, and FQHCs for which therapy is included in the all-inclusive rate; or

- Providers that do not furnish therapy services.

The following "providers of services" must bill the A/B MAC (A) for outpatient rehabilitation services using HCPCS codes:

- Hospitals (to outpatients and inpatients who are not in a covered Part A stay);
- Skilled nursing facilities (SNFs) (to residents not in a covered Part A stay and to nonresidents who receive outpatient rehabilitation services from the SNF);
- Home health agencies (HHAs) (to individuals who are not homebound or otherwise are not receiving services under a home health plan of care (POC).
- Comprehensive outpatient rehabilitation facilities (CORFs); and
- Providers of outpatient physical therapy and speech-language pathology services (OPTs), also known as rehabilitation agencies (previously termed outpatient physical therapy facilities in this instruction).

Note 1. The requirements for hospitals and SNFs apply to inpatient Part B and outpatient services only. Inpatient Part A services are bundled into the respective prospective payment system payment; no separate payment is made.

Note 2. For HHAs, HCPCS/CPT® coding for outpatient rehabilitation services is required only when the HHA provides such service to individuals that are not homebound and, therefore, not under a home health plan of care.

The following practitioners must bill the A/B MAC (B) for outpatient rehabilitation therapy services using HCPCS/CPT® codes:

- Physical therapists in private practice (PTPPs),

- Occupational therapists in private practice (OTPPs),

- Speech-language pathologists in private practice (SLPPs),

- Physicians, including MDs, DOs, podiatrists and optometrists, and

- Certain nonphysician practitioners (NPPs), acting within their State scope of practice, e.g., nurse practitioners and clinical nurse specialists.

Providers billing to intermediaries shall report:

- The date the therapy plan of care was either established or last reviewed (see §220.1.3B) in Occurrence Code 17, 29, or 30.

- The first day of treatment in Occurrence Code 35, 44, or 45.

B. Applicable Outpatient Rehabilitation HCPCS Codes

The CMS identifies the codes listed at:

http://www.cms.hhs.gov/TherapyServices/05_Annual_ Therapy_Update.asp#TopOfPage as therapy services, regardless of the presence of a financial limitation. Therapy services include only physical therapy, occupational therapy and speech-language pathology services. Therapist means only a physical therapist, occupational therapist or speech language pathologist. Therapy modifiers are GP for physical therapy, GO for occupational therapy, and GN for speech-language pathology.

When in effect, any financial limitation will also apply to services represented unless otherwise noted on the therapy page on the CMS Web site.

C. Additional HCPCS Codes

Some HCPCS/CPT® codes that are not on the list of therapy services should not be billed with a modifier. For example, outpatient non-rehabilitation HCPCS codes G0237, G0238, and G0239 should be billed without therapy modifiers. These HCPCS codes describe services for the improvement of respiratory function and may represent either "incident to" services or respiratory therapy services that may be appropriately billed in the CORF setting. When the services described by these G-codes are provided by physical therapists (PTs) or occupational therapists (OTs) treating respiratory conditions, they are considered therapy services and must meet the other conditions for physical and occupational therapy. The PT or OT would use the appropriate HCPCS/CPT® code(s) in the 97000 - 97799 series and the corresponding therapy modifier, GP or GO, must be used.

Another example of codes that are not on the list of therapy services and should not be billed with a therapy modifier includes the following HCPCS codes: 95860, 95861, 95863, 95864, 95867, 95869, 95870, 95900, 95903, 95904, and 95934. These services represent diagnostic services - not therapy services; they must be appropriately billed and shall not include therapy modifiers.

Other codes not on the therapy code list, and not paid under another fee schedule, are appropriately billed with therapy modifiers when the services are furnished by therapists or provided under a therapy plan of care and where the services are covered and appropriately delivered (e.g., the therapist is qualified to provide the service). One example of non-listed codes where a therapy modifier is indicated regards the provision of services described in the CPT® code series, 29000 through 29590, for the application of casts and strapping. Some of these codes previously appeared on the therapy code list, but were deleted because we determined that they represented services that are most often performed outside a therapy plan of care. However, when these services are provided by therapists or as an integral part of a therapy plan of care, the CPT® code must be accompanied with the appropriate therapy modifier.

NOTE: The above lists of HCPCS/CPT® codes are intended to facilitate the contractor's ability to pay claims under the MPFS. It is not intended to be an exhaustive list of covered services, imply applicability to provider settings, and does not assure coverage of these services.

100-4, Chapter-5, 20.4

Coding Guidance for Certain CPT® Codes - All Claims

The following provides guidance about the use of codes 96105, 97026, 97150, 97545, 97546, and G0128.

- CPT® Codes 96105, 97545, and 97546.

Providers report code 96105, assessment of aphasia with interpretation and report in 1- hour units. This code represents formal evaluation of aphasia with an instrument such as the Boston Diagnostic Aphasia Examination. If this formal assessment is performed during treatment, it is typically performed only once during treatment and its medical necessity should be documented. If the test is repeated during treatment, the medical necessity of the repeat administration of the test must also be documented. It is common practice for regular assessment of a patient's progress in therapy to be documented in the chart, and this may be done using test items taken from the formal examinations. This is considered to be part of the treatment and should not be billed as 96105 unless a full, formal assessment is completed. Other timed physical medicine codes are 97545 and 97546. The interval for code 97545 is 2 hours and for code 97546, 1 hour. These are specialized codes to be used in the context of rehabilitating a worker to return to a job. The expectation is that the entire time period specified in the codes 97545 or 97546 would be the treatment period, since a shorter period of treatment could be coded with another code such as codes 97110, 97112, or 97537. (Codes 97545 and 97546 were developed for reporting services to persons in the worker's compensation program, thus CMS does not expect to see them reported for Medicare patients except under very unusual circumstances. Further, CMS would not expect to see code 97546 without also seeing code 97545 on the same claim. Code 97546, when used, is used in conjunction with 97545.)

- CPT® Code 97026

Effective for services performed on or after October 24, 2006, the Centers for Medicare & Medicaid Services announce a NCD stating the use of infrared and/or near-infrared light and/or heat, including monochromatic infrared energy (MIRE), is non-covered for the treatment, including symptoms such as pain arising from these conditions, of diabetic and/or non-diabetic peripheral sensory neuropathy, wounds and/or ulcers of the skin and/or subcutaneous tissues in Medicare beneficiaries. Further coverage guidelines can be found in the National Coverage Determination Manual (Pub. 100-03), section 270.6.

Contractors shall deny claims with CPT® 97026 (infrared therapy incident to or as a PT/OT benefit) and HCPCS E0221 or A4639, if the claim contains any of the following diagnosis codes:

ICD-9-CM

250.60 - 250.63

354.4, 354.5, 354.9

355.1 - 355.4

355.6 - 355.9

356.0, 356.2-356.4, 356.8-356.9

357.0 - 357.7

674.10, 674.12, 674.14, 674.20, 674.22, 674.24

707.00 -707.07, 707.09-707.15, 707.19

870.0 - 879.9

880.00 - 887.7

890.0 - 897.7

998.31 - 998.32

ICD-10-CM

See Addendum A Chapter 5, Section 20.4 (at end of this chapter) for the list of ICD 10-CM diagnosis codes that require denial with the above HCPCD codes.

Contractors can use the following messages when denying the service:

- Medicare Summary Notice # 21.11 "This service was not covered by Medicare at the time you received it."

- Reason Claim Adjustment Code #50 "These are non covered services because this is not deemed a medical necessity by the payer."

Advanced Beneficiary Notice (ABN):

Physicians, physical therapists, occupational therapists, outpatient rehabilitation facilities (ORFs), comprehensive outpatient rehabilitation facilities (CORFs), home health agencies (HHA), and hospital outpatient departments are liable if the service is performed, unless the beneficiary signs an ABN.

Similarly, DME suppliers and HHA are liable for the devices when they are supplied, unless the beneficiary signs an ABN.

100-4, Chapter-5, 100.4

Outpatient Mental Health Treatment Limitation

The Outpatient Mental Health Treatment Limitation (the limitation) is not applicable to CORF services because CORFs do not provide services to treat mental, psychoneurotic and personality disorders that are subject to the limitation in section 1833(c) of the Act. For dates of service on or after October 1, 2012, HCPCS code G0409 is the only code allowed for social work and psychological services furnished in a CORF. This service is not subject to the limitation because it is not a psychiatric mental health treatment service.

For additional information on the limitation, see Publication 100-01, Chapter 3, section 30 and Publication 100-02, Chapter 12, sections 50-50.5.

100-4, Chapter-5, 100.11

Billing for Social Work and Psychological Services in a CORF

The CORF providers shall only bill social work and psychological services with the following HCPCS code:

G0409 –Social work and psychological services, directly relating to and/or the patient's rehabilitation goals, each 15 minutes, face-to-face; individual (services provided by a CORF-qualified social worker or psychologist in a CORF)

In addition, HCPCS code G0409 shall only be billed with revenue code 0569 or 0911.

100-4, Chapter-8, 60.2.1.1

Separately Billable ESRD Drugs

The following categories of drugs (including but not limited to) are separately billable when used to treat the patient's renal condition:

- Antibiotics;
- Analgesics;
- Anabolics;
- Hematinics;
- Muscle relaxants;

- Sedatives;
- Tranquilizers; and
- Thrombolytics: used to declot central venous catheters. **NOTE:** Thrombolytics were removed from the separately billable drugs for claims with dates of service on or after January 1, 2013.

For claims with dates of service on or after July 1, 2013, when these drugs are administered through the dialysate the provider must append the modifier JE (Administered via Dialysate).

These separately billable drugs may only be billed by an ESRD facility if they are actually administered in the facility by the facility staff. Staff time used to administer separately billable drugs is covered under the composite rate and may not be billed separately. However, the supplies used to administer these drugs may be billed in addition to the composite rate.

Effective January 1, 2011, section 153b of the MIPPA requires that all ESRD-related drugs and biologicals be billed by the renal dialysis facility. When a drug or biological is billed by providers other than the ESRD facility and the drug or biological furnished is designated as a drug or biological that is included in the ESRD PPS (ESRD-related), the claim will be rejected or denied. In the event that an ESRD-related drug or biological was furnished to an ESRD beneficiary for reasons other than for the treatment of ESRD, the provider may submit a claim for separate payment using modifier AY.

All drugs reported on the renal dialysis facility claim are considered included in the ESRD PPS. The list of drugs and biologicals for consolidated billing are designated as always ESRD-related and therefore not allowing separate payment to be made to ESRD facilities. However, CMS has determined that some of these drugs may warrant separate payment.

Exceptions to "Always ESRD Related" Drugs:

The following drugs have been approved for separate payment consideration when billed with the AY modifier attesting to the drug not being used for the treatment of ESRD. The ESRD facility is required to indicate (in accordance with ICD-coding guidelines) the diagnosis code for which the drug is indicated.

- Vancomycin, effective January 1, 2012
- Daptomycin, effective January 1, 2013

Items and services subject to the consolidated billing requirements for the ESRD PPS can be found on the CMS website at:

http://www.cms.gov/ESRDPayment/50_Consolidated_Billing.asp# TopOfPage.

Other drugs and biologicals may be considered separately payable to the dialysis facility if the drug was not for the treatment of ESRD. The facility must include the modifier AY to indicate it was not for the treatment of ESRD.

Drugs are assigned HCPCS codes. If no HCPCS code is listed for a drug (e.g., a new drug) the facility bills using HCPCS code J3490, "Unclassified Drugs," and submits documentation identifying the drug. To establish a code for the drug, the FI checks HCPCS to verify that there is no acceptable HCPCS code for billing and if a code is not found checks with the local carrier, which may have a code and price that is appropriate.

If no code is found the drug is processed under HCPCS code J3490. See Chapter 17 for a complete description of drug pricing.

100-4, Chapter-8, 60.4

Erythropoietin Stimulating Agents (ESAs)

Coverage rules for ESAs are explained in the Medicare Benefit Policy Manual, Publication 100-02, chapter 11.

Fiscal intermediaries (FIs) pay for ESAs, to end-stage renal disease (ESRD) facilities as separately billable drugs to the composite rate. No additional payment is made to administer an ESA, whether in a facility or a home. Effective January 1, 2005, the cost of supplies to administer EPO may be billed to the FI. HCPCS A4657 and Revenue Code 270 should be used to capture the charges for syringes used in the administration of EPO.

ESAs and their administration supplies are included in the payment for the ESRD Prospective Payment System effective January 1, 2011. Providers must continue to report ESAs on the claim as ESAs are subject to a national claims monitoring program and are entitled to outlier payment consideration. The Medicare allowed payment (MAP) amount for outlier includes the ESA rate provided on the Average Sale Price (ASP) list, subject to reduction based on the ESA monitoring policy.

Medicare has an established national claims monitoring policy for erythropoietin stimulating agents for the in-facility dialysis population as outlined in the sections below.

100-4, Chapter-8, 60.4.1

ESA Claims Monitoring Policy

Effective for services provided on or after April 1, 2006, Medicare has implemented a national claims monitoring policy for ESAs administered in Medicare renal dialysis facilities. This policy does not apply to claims for ESAs for patients who receive their dialysis at home and self-administer their ESA.

While Medicare is not changing its coverage policy on erythropoietin use to maintain a target hematocrit level between 30% and 36%, we believe the variability in response to ESAs warrants postponing requiring monitoring until the hematocrit reaches higher levels. For dates of services April 1, 2006, and later, the Centers for Medicare & Medicaid Services (CMS) claims monitoring policy applies when the hematocrit level exceeds 39.0% or the hemoglobin level exceeds 13.0g/dL. This does not preclude the contractors from performing medical review at lower levels.

Effective for services provided on or after April 1, 2006, for claims reporting hematocrit or hemoglobin levels exceeding the monitoring threshold, the dose shall be reduced by 25% over the preceding month. Providers may report that a dose reduction did occur in response to the reported elevated hematocrit or hemoglobin level by adding a GS modifier on the claim. The definition of the GS modifier is defined as: "Dosage of ESA has been reduced and maintained in response to hematocrit or hemoglobin level." Thus, for claims reporting a hematocrit level or hemoglobin level exceeding the monitoring threshold without the GS modifier, CMS will reduce the covered dosage reported on the claim by 25%. The excess dosage is considered to be not reasonable and necessary. Providers are reminded that the patient's medical records should reflect hematocrit/hemoglobin levels and any dosage reduction reported on the claim during the same time period for which the claim is submitted.

Effective for dates of service provided on and after January 1, 2008, requests for payments or claims for ESAs for ESRD patients receiving dialysis in renal dialysis facilities reporting a hematocrit level exceeding 39.0% (or hemoglobin exceeding 13.0g/dL) shall also include modifier ED or EE. Claims reporting neither modifier or both modifiers will be returned to the provider for correction.

The definition of modifier ED is "The hematocrit level has exceeded 39.0% (or hemoglobin level has exceeded 13.0g/dL) 3 or more consecutive billing cycles immediately prior to and including the current billing cycle." The definition of modifier EE is "The hematocrit level has exceeded 39.0% (or hemoglobin level has exceeded 13.0g/dL) less than 3 consecutive billing cycles immediately prior to and including the current billing cycle." The GS modifier continues to be defined as stated above.

Providers may continue to report the GS modifier when the reported hematocrit or hemoglobin levels exceed the monitoring threshold for less than 3 months and a dose reduction has occurred. When both modifiers GS and EE are included, no reduction in the covered dose will occur. Claims reporting a hematocrit or hemoglobin level exceeding the monitoring threshold and the ED modifier shall have an automatic 50% reduction in the covered dose applied, even if the claim also reports the GS modifier.

Below is a chart illustrating the resultant claim actions under all possible reporting scenarios:

Hct Exceeds 39.0% or Hgb Exceeds 13.0g/dL	ED Modifier? (Hct >39% or Hgb >13g/dL ≥3 cycles)	EE Modifier? (Hct >39% or Hgb >13g/dL <3 cycles)	GS Modifier? (Dosage reduced and maintained)	Claim Action
No	N/A	N/A	N/A	Do not reduce reported dose.
Yes	No	No	No	Return to provider for correction. Claim must report either modifier ED or EE.
Yes	No	No	Yes	Return to provider for correction. Claim must report either modifier ED or EE.
Yes	No	Yes	Yes	Do not reduce reported dose.
Yes	No	Yes	No	Reduce reported dose 25%.
Yes	Yes	No	Yes	Reduce reported dose 50%.
Yes	Yes	No	No	Reduce reported dose 50%.

In some cases, physicians may believe there is medical justification to maintain a hematocrit above 39.0% or hemoglobin above 13.0g/dL. Beneficiaries, physicians, and/or renal facilities may submit additional medical documentation to justify this belief under the routine appeal process. You may reinstate any covered dosage reduction amounts under this first level appeal process when you believe the documentation supports a higher hematocrit/hemoglobin level.

Providers are reminded that, in accordance with FDA labeling, CMS expects that as the hematocrit approaches 36.0% (hemoglobin 12.0g/dL), a dosage reduction occurs. Providers are expected to maintain hematocrit levels between 30.0 to 36.0% (hemoglobin 10.0-12.0g/dL). Hematocrit levels that remain below 30.0% (hemoglobin levels below 10.0g/dL)) despite dosage increases, should have causative factors evaluated. The patient's medical record should reflect the clinical reason for dose changes and hematocrit levels outside the range of 30.0-36.0% (hemoglobin

levels 10.0-12.0g/dL). Medicare contractors may review medical records to assure appropriate dose reductions are applied and maintained and hematological target ranges are maintained.

These hematocrit requirements apply only to ESAs furnished as an ESRD benefit under §1881(b) of the Social Security Act.

Medically Unlikely Edits (MUE)

For dates of service on and after January 1, 2008, the MUE for claims billing for Epogen® is reduced to 400,000 units from 500,000. The MUE for claims for Aranesp® is reduced to 1200 mcg from 1500 mcg.

For dates of service on and after April 1, 2013, the MUE for claims billing for peginesatide is applicable when units billed are equal to or greater than 26 mg.

It is likely that claims reporting doses exceeding the threshold reflect typographical errors and will be returned to providers for correction.

100-4, Chapter-8, 60.4.4.1

Payment for Epoetin Alfa (EPO) in Other Settings

With the implementation of the ESRD PPS, ESRD-related EPO is included in ESRD PPS payment amount and is not separately payable on Part B claims with dates of service on or after January 1, 2011 for other providers with the exception of a hospital billing for an emergency or unscheduled dialysis session.

In the hospital inpatient setting, payment under Part A is included in the DRG.

In the hospital inpatient setting, payment under Part B is made on bill type 12x. Hospitals report the drug units based on the units defined in the HCPCS description. Hospitals do not report value code 68 for units of EPO. For dates of service prior to April 1, 2006, report EPO under revenue code 0636. For dates of service from April 1, 2006 report EPO under the respective revenue code 0634 for EPO less than 10,000 units and revenue code 0635 for EPO over 10,000 units. Payment will be based on the ASP Pricing File.

In a skilled nursing facility (SNF), payment for EPO covered under the Part B EPO benefit is not included in the prospective payment rate for the resident's Medicare-covered SNF stay.

In a hospice, payment is included in the hospice per diem rate.

For a service furnished by a physician or incident to a physician's service, payment is made to the physician by the carrier in accordance with the rules for 'incident to" services. When EPO is administered in the renal facility, the service is not an "incident to" service and not under the "incident to" provision.

100-4, Chapter-8, 60.4.4.2

Epoetin Alfa (EPO) Provided in the Hospital Outpatient Departments

When ESRD patients come to the hospital for an unscheduled or emergency dialysis treatment they may also require the administration of EPO. Effective January 1, 2005, EPO will be paid based on the ASP Pricing File.

Hospitals use type of bill 13X (or 85X for Critical Access Hospitals) and report charges under the respective revenue code 0634 for EPO less than 10,000 units and revenue code 0635 for EPO over 10,000 units. Hospitals report the drug units based on the units defined in the HCPCS description. Hospitals do not report value code 68 for units of EPO. Value code 49 must be reported with the hematocrit value for the hospital outpatient visits prior to January 1, 2006, and for all claims with dates of service on or after January 1, 2008.

100-4, Chapter-8, 60.4.5.1

Self-Administered ESA Supply

Initially, facilities may bill for up to a 2-month supply of an ESA for Method I beneficiaries who meet the criteria for selection for self-administration. After the initial two months' supply, the facility will bill for one month's supply at a time. Condition code 70 is used to indicate payment requested for a supply of an ESA furnished a beneficiary. Usually, revenue code 0635 would apply to EPO since the supply would be over 10,000 units. Facilities leave FL 46, Units of Service, blank since they are not administering the drug.

For claims with dates of service on or after January 1, 2008, supplies of an ESA for self administration should be billed according to the pre-determined plan of care schedule provided to the beneficiary. Submit a separate line item for each date an administration is expected to be performed with the expected dosage. In the event that the schedule was changed, the provider should note the changes in the medical record and bill according to the revised schedule. For patients beginning to self administer an ESA at home receiving an extra month supply of the drug, bill the one month reserve supply on one claim line and include modifier EM defined as "Emergency Reserve Supply (for ESRD benefit only)".

When billing for drug wastage in accordance with the policy in chapter 17 of this manual, section 40.1 the provider must show the wastage on a separate line item with the modifier JW. The line item date of service should be the date of the last covered administration according to the plan of care or if the patient dies use the date of death.

Condition code 70 should be reported on claims billing for home dialysis patients that self administer anemia management drugs including ESAs.

100-4, Chapter-8, 60.4.6.3

Payment Amount for Darbepoetin Alfa (Aranesp)

For Method I patients, the FI pays the facility per one mcg of Aranesp administered, in accordance with the MMA Drug Payment Limits Pricing File rounded up to the next highest whole mcg. Effective January 1, 2005, Aranesp will be paid based on the ASP Pricing File. Effective January 1, 2005, the cost of supplies to administer Aranesp may be billed to the FI. HCPCS A4657 and Revenue Code 270 should be used to capture the charges for syringes used in the administration of Aranesp.

Physician payment is calculated through the drug payment methodology described in Chapter 17, of the Claims Processing Manual.

The coinsurance and deductible are based on the Medicare allowance payable, not on the provider's charges. The provider may not charge the beneficiary more than 20 percent of the Medicare Aranesp allowance. This rule applies to independent and hospital based renal facilities.

Payment for ESRD-related Aranesp is included in the ESRD PPS for claims with dates of service on or after January 1, 2011.

100-4, Chapter-8, 60.4.6.4

Payment for Darbepoetin Alfa (Aranesp) in Other Settings

In the hospital inpatient setting, payment under Part A for Aranesp is included in the DRG.

In the hospital inpatient setting, payment under Part B is made on bill type 12x when billed with revenue code 0636. The total number of units as a multiple of 1mcg is placed in the unit field. Reimbursement is based on the payment allowance limit for Medicare Part B drugs as found in the ASP pricing file.

In a skilled nursing facility (SNF), payment for Aranesp covered under the Part B EPO benefit is not included in the prospective payment rate for the resident's Medicare-covered SNF stay.

In a hospice, payment is included in the hospice per diem rate.

For a service furnished by a physician or incident to a physician's service, payment is made to the physician by the carrier in accordance with the rules for 'incident to" services. When Aranesp is administered in the renal facility, the service is not an "incident to" service and not under the "incident to" provision.

With the implementation of the ESRD PPS, ESRD-related Aranesp is included in the ESRD PPS payment amount and is not separately payable on Part B claims with dates of service on or after January 1,2011 for other providers, with the exception of a hospital billing for an emergency or unscheduled dialysis session.

100-4, Chapter-8, 60.4.6.5

Payment for Darbepoetin Alfa (Aranesp) in the Hospital Outpatient Department

When ESRD patients come to the hospital for an unscheduled or emergency dialysis treatment they may also require the administration of Aranesp. For patients with ESRD who are on a regular course of dialysis, Aranesp administered in a hospital outpatient department is paid the MMA Drug Pricing File rate. Effective January 1, 2005, Aranesp will be paid based on the ASP Pricing File.

Hospitals use bill type 13X (or 85X for Critical Access Hospitals) and report charges under revenue code 0636. The total number of units as a multiple of 1mcg is placed in the unit field. Value code 49 must be reported with the hematocrit value for the hospital outpatient visits prior to January 1, 2006, and for all claims with dates of service on or after January 1, 2008.

100-4, Chapter-8, 60.4.7

Payment for Peginesatide in the Hospital Outpatient Department

When ESRD patients come to the hospital for an unscheduled or emergency dialysis treatment they may also require the administration of an ESA, such as peginesatide. When hospitals bill for an unscheduled or emergency outpatient dialysis session (G0257) they may include the administration of an ESA.

100-4, Chapter-8, 60.6

Vaccines Furnished to ESRD Patients

The Medicare program covers Hepatitis B, influenza virus and Pneumococcal pneumonia virus (PPV) vaccines and their administration when furnished to eligible beneficiaries in accordance with coverage rules. Payment may be made for both the vaccine and the administration. The costs associated with the syringe and supplies are included in the administration fee: HCPCS code A4657 should not be billed for these vaccines.

Vaccines and their administration are reported using separate codes. See Chapter 18 of this manual for the codes required for billing vaccines and the administration of the vaccine.

Payment for vaccine administration (PPV, Influenza Virus, and Hepatitis B Virus) to freestanding RDFs is based on the Medicare Physician Fee Schedule (MPFS) according to the rate in the MPFS associated with code 90782 for services provided prior to March 1, 2003 and code 90471 for services provided March 1, 2005 and later and on reasonable cost for provider-based RDFs.

Vaccines remain separately payable under the ESRD PPS.

100-4, Chapter-9, 70.5

Diabetes Self-Management Training (DSMT) and Medical Nutrition Services (MNT)

FQHCs billing under the AIR system

Payment is made at the all-inclusive encounter rate to the FQHC for DSMT or MNT. This payment can be in addition to payment for another qualifying visit on the same date of service as the beneficiary received qualifying DSMT services.

For FQHCs to qualify for a separate visit payment for DSMT or MNT services, the services must be a one-on-one face-to-face encounter. Group sessions do not constitute a billable visit for any FQHC services. To receive separate payment for DSMT or MNT services, the services must be billed on TOB 77x with HCPCS code G0108 (DSMT) or HCPCS code 97802, 97803, or G0270 (MNT) and the appropriate site of service revenue code in the 052X revenue code series. This payment can be in addition to payment for any other qualifying visit on the same date of service that the beneficiary received qualifying DSMT/MNT services as long as the claim for DSMT/MNT services contains the appropriate coding specified above. Additional information on DSMT can be found in Chapter 18, section 120 of Pub. 100-04.

Additional information on MNT can be found in Chapter 4, section 300 of Pub. 100-04.

Group services (G0109, 97804 and G0271) do not meet the criteria for a separate qualifying encounter. All line items billed on TOBs 77x with group services will be denied.

DSMT and MNT services are subject to the frequency edits described in Pub. 100-04, Chapter 18, and should not be reported on the same day.

FQHCs billing under the PPS

DSMT and MNT are qualifying visits when billed under G0466 or G0467. For additional information on the payment specific codes and qualifying visits, see section 60.2 of this manual. Under the FQHC PPS, DSMT and MNT do not qualify for a separate payment when billed on the same day with another qualified visit.

RHCs

RHCs are not paid separately for DSMT and MNT services. All line items billed on TOB 71x with HCPCS codes for DSMT and MNT services will be denied.

100-4, Chapter-9, 70.6

Initial Preventive Physical Examination (IPPE)

FQHCs and RHCs billing under the AIR system

Medicare provides for coverage for one IPPE for new beneficiaries only, subject to certain eligibility and other limitations.

Payment for the professional services will be made under the AIR. However, RHCs/FQHCs can receive a separate payment for an encounter in addition to the payment for the IPPE when they are performed on the same day.

When IPPE is provided in an RHC or FQHC, the professional portion of the service is billed on TOBs 71X and 77X, respectively, and the appropriate site of service revenue code in the 052X revenue code series, and must include HCPCS code G0402. Additional information on IPPE can be found in Chapter 18, section 80 of Pub. 100-04.

EKGs

The professional component is included in the AIR or FQHC PPS and is not separately billable.

The technical component of an EKG performed at a RHC/FQHC billed to Medicare on professional claims (Form CMS-1500 or 837P) under the practitioner's ID following instructions for submitting practitioner claims for independent/freestanding clinics. Practitioners at provider-based clinics bill the applicable TOB to the A/B MAC using the base provider's ID.

FQHCs billing under the PPS:

IPPE is qualifying visits when billed under G0468, for additional information on the payment specific codes and qualifying visits, please refer to section 60.2 of this manual. Under the FQHC PPS, IPPE does not qualify for a separate payment when billed on the same day with another encounter/visit.

100-4, Chapter-10, 40.2

HH PPS Claims

The following data elements are required to submit a claim under home health PPS. For billing of home health claims not under an HH plan of care (not under HH PPS), see §90. Home health services under a plan of care are paid based on a 60-day episode of care (before January 1, 2020) or a 30-day period of care (on or after January 1, 2020). Payment for this episode or period will usually be made in two parts. After a RAP has been paid and an episode or period has been completed, or the patient has been discharged, the HHA submits a claim to receive the balance of payment due.

HH PPS claims will be processed in Medicare claims processing systems as debit/credit adjustments against the record created by the RAP, except in the case of "No-RAP" LUPA claims (see §40.3). As the claim is processed the payment on the RAP will be reversed in full and the full payment due for the episode will be made on the claim. Both the debit and credit actions will be reflected on the RA so the net payment on the claim can be easily understood. Detailed RA information is contained in chapter 22 of this manual.

Billing Provider Name, Address, and Telephone Number

Required - The HHA's minimum entry is the agency's name, city, state, and ZIP Code. The post office box number or street name and number may be included. The state may be abbreviated using standard post office abbreviations. Five or nine-digit ZIP Codes are acceptable. A/B MACs (HHH) use this information in connection with the provider identifier to verify provider identity.

Patient Control Number and Medical/Health Record Number

Required - The patient's control number may be shown if the patient is assigned one and the number is needed for association and reference purposes.

The HHA may enter the number assigned to the patient's medical/health record. If this number is entered, the A/B MAC (HHH) must carry it through their system and return it on the remittance record.

Type of Bill

Required - This 4-digit alphanumeric code gives two pieces of information. The first three digits indicate the base type of bill. The fourth digit indicates the sequence of this bill in this particular episode of care. The types of bill accepted for HH PPS claims are:

032x - Home Health Services under a Plan of Treatment

4th Digit - Definition

7 - Replacement of Prior Claim - HHAs use to correct a previously submitted bill. Apply this code for the corrected or "new" bill. These adjustment claims must be accepted at any point within the timely filing period after the payment of the original claim.

8 - Void/Cancel of a Prior Claim - HHAs use this code to indicate this bill is an exact duplicate of an incorrect bill previously submitted. A replacement RAP or claim must be submitted for the episode to be paid.

9 - Final Claim for an HH PPS Episode - This code indicates the HH bill should be processed as a debit/credit adjustment to the RAP. This code is specific to home health and does not replace codes 7, or 8.

HHAs must submit HH PPS claims with the 4th digit of "9." These claims may be adjusted with code "7" or cancelled with code "8." A/B MACs (HHH) do not accept late charge bills, submitted with code "5," on HH PPS claims. To add services within the period of a paid HH claim, the HHA must submit an adjustment.

NOTE: Type of bill 033x is no longer valid, effective October 1, 2013.

Statement Covers Period

The Patient-Driven Groupings Model is effective for periods of care beginning January 1, 2020. The HHA should follow all prior claims submission instructions for claims with "From" dates before January 1, 2020, including episodes that span into 2020. The HHA should follow PDGM instructions for claims with "From" dates on or after January 1, 2020.

Required - The beginning and ending dates of the period covered by this claim. The "from" date must match the date submitted on the RAP for the episode. For continuous care episodes, the "through" date must be 59 days after the "from" date for a 60-day episode or 29 days after the "From" date for a 30-day period of care

In cases where the beneficiary has been discharged or transferred within the episode or period, HHAs will report the date of discharge in accordance with internal discharge procedures as the "through" date. If the beneficiary has died, the HHA reports the date of death in the "through date."

The HHA may submit claims for payment immediately after the claim "through" date. It is not required to hold claims until the end of the episode or period unless the beneficiary continues under care.

Patient Name/Identifier

Required - The HHA enters the patient's last name, first name, and middle initial

Patient Address

Required - The HHA enters the patient's full mailing address, including street number and name, post office box number or RFD, City, State, and ZIP Code.

Patient Birth Date

Required - The HHA enters the month, day, and year of birth of patient. If the full correct date is not known, leave blank.

Patient Sex

Required - "M" for male or "F" for female must be present. This item is used in conjunction with diagnoses and surgical procedures to identify inconsistencies.

Admission/Start of Care Date

Required - The HHA enters the same date of admission that was submitted on the RAP for the episode.

Point of Origin for Admission or Visit

Required - The HHA enters the same point of origin code that was submitted on the RAP for the episode.

Patient Discharge Status

Required - The HHA enters the code that most accurately describes the patient's status as of the "Through" date of the billing period. Any applicable NUBC approved code may be used.

Patient status code 06 should be reported in all cases where the HHA is aware that the episode will be paid as a PEP adjustment. These are cases in which the agency is aware that the beneficiary has transferred to another HHA within the 60-day episode or 30-day period, or the agency is aware that the beneficiary was discharged with the goals of the original plan of care met and has been readmitted within the episode or period. Situations may occur in which the HHA is unaware at the time of billing the discharge that these circumstances exist. In these situations, Medicare claims processing systems will adjust the discharge claim automatically to reflect the PEP adjustment, changing the patient status code on the paid claims record to 06.

In cases where an HHA is changing the A/B MAC (HHH) to which they submit claims, the service dates on the claims must fall within the provider's effective dates at each A/B MAC (HHH). To ensure this, RAPs for all episodes with "from" dates before the provider's termination date must be submitted to the A/B MAC (HHH) the provider is leaving. The resulting episode must be resolved by the provider submitting claims for shortened periods, with "through" dates on or before the termination date. The provider must indicate that these claims will be PEP adjustments by using patient status code 06. Billing for the beneficiary is being "transferred" to the new A/B MAC (HHH).

In cases where the ownership of an HHA is changing and the CMS certification number (CCN) also changes, the service dates on the claims must fall within the effective dates of the terminating CCN. To ensure this, RAPs for all episodes with "from" dates before the termination date of the CCN must be resolved by the provider submitting claims for shortened periods, with "through" dates on or before the termination date. The provider must indicate that these claims will be PEP adjustments by using patient status 06. Billing for the beneficiary is being "transferred" to the new agency ownership. In changes of ownership which do not affect the CCN, billing for episodes is also unaffected.

In cases where an HHA is aware in advance that a beneficiary will become enrolled in a Medicare Advantage (MA) Organization as of a certain date, the provider should submit a claim for the shortened period prior to the MA Organization enrollment date. The claim should be coded with patient status 06. Payment responsibility for the beneficiary is being "transferred" from Medicare fee-for-service to MA Organization, since HH PPS applies only to Medicare fee-for-service.

If HHAs require guidance on OASIS assessment procedures in these cases, they should contact the appropriate state OASIS education coordinator.

Condition Codes

Conditional - The HHA enters any NUBC approved code to describe conditions that apply to the claim.

If the RAP is for an episode in which the patient has transferred from another HHA, the HHA enters condition code 47.

If the claim is for an episode in which there are no skilled HH visits in billing period, but a policy exception that allows billing for covered services is documented at the HHA, the HHA enters condition code 54.

HHAs that are adjusting previously paid claims enter one of the condition codes representing Claim Change Reasons (code values D0 through E0). If adjusting the claim to correct a HIPPS code, HHAs use condition code D2 and enter "Remarks" indicating the reason for the HIPPS code change. HHAs use D9 if multiple changes are necessary.

When submitting an HH PPS claim as a demand bill, HHAs use condition code 20. See §50 for more detailed instructions regarding demand billing.

When submitting an HH PPS claim for a denial notice, HHAs use condition code 21. See §60 for more detailed instructions regarding no-payment billing.

Required - If canceling the claim (TOB 0328), HHAs report the condition codes D5 or D6 and enter "Remarks" indicating the reason for cancellation of the claim.

Occurrence Codes and Dates

Required – On claims with "From" dates on or after January 1, 2020, the HHA enters occurrence code 50 and the date the OASIS assessment corresponding to the period of care was completed (OASIS item M0090). If occurrence code 50 is not reported on a claim or adjustment, the claim will be returned to the provider for correction.

On claims for initial periods of care (i.e. when the From and Admission dates match), the HHA reports an inpatient admission that ended within 14 days of the "From" date by using one of the following codes.

Code	Short Descriptor	Long Descriptor
61	Hospital Discharge Date	The Through date of a hospital stay that ended within 14 days prior to the From date this HHA claim.
62	Other Institutional Discharge Date	The Through date of skilled nursing facility (SNF), inpatient rehabilitation facility (IRF), long term care hospital (LTCH) or inpatient psychiatric facility (IPF) stay that ended within 14 days prior to this HHA admission.

On claims for continuing periods of care, the HHA reports an inpatient hospital admission that ended within 14 days of the "From" date by using occurrence code 61.

If more than one inpatient discharge occurs during the 14 day period, the HHA reports only the most recent discharge date. Claims reporting more than one of any combination of occurrence codes 61 and 62 will be returned to the provider for correction.

Conditional - The HHA enters any other NUBC approved code to describe occurrences that apply to the claim.

Occurrence Span Code and Dates

Conditional - The HHA enters any NUBC approved Occurrence Span code to describe occurrences that apply to the claim. Reporting of occurrence span code 74 is not required to show the dates of an inpatient admission during an episode.

Value Codes and Amounts

Required - Home health episode payments must be based upon the site at which the beneficiary is served. For certain dates of service when required by law, payments may be further adjusted if the site is in a rural CBSA or rural county. For episodes in which the beneficiary's site of service changes from one CBSA or county to another within the episode period, HHAs should submit the CBSA code or State and County code corresponding to the site of service at the end of the episode on the claim.

Provider-submitted codes:

Code	Title	Definition
61	Location Where Service is Furnished (HHA and Hospice)	HHAs report the MSA number or Core Based Statistical Area (CBSA) number (or rural state code) of the location where the home health or hospice service is delivered. The HHA reports the number in dollar portion of the form locator right justified to the left of the dollar/cents delimiter, add two zeros to the cents field if no cents.
85	County Where Service is Rendered	Where required by law or regulation, report the Federal Information Processing Standards (FIPS) State and County Code of the place of residence where the home health service is delivered.

Medicare-applied codes: The following codes are added during processing and may be visible in the A/B MAC (HHH)'s online claim history. They are never submitted by the HHA.

Code	Title	Definition
17	Outlier Amount	The amount of any outlier payment returned by the Pricer with this code. (Contractors always place condition code 61 on the claim along with this value code.)
61	Location Where Service is Furnished (HHA and Hospice)	HHAs report the MSA number or Core Based Statistical Area (CBSA) number (or rural state code) of the location where the home health or hospice service is delivered. The HHA reports the number in dollar portion of the form locator right justified to the left of the dollar/cents delimiter, add two zeros to the cents field if no cents.
62	HH Visits - Part A	The number of visits determined by Medicare to be payable from the Part A trust fund to reflect the shift of payments from the Part A to the Part B trust fund as mandated by §1812 (a) (3) of the Social Security Act.

Code	Title	Definition
63	HH Visits - Part B	The number of visits determined by Medicare to be payable from the Part B trust fund to reflect the shift of payments from the Part A to the Part B trust fund as mandated by §1812 (a)(3) of the Social Security Act.
64	HH Reimbursement - Part A	The dollar amounts determined to be associated with the HH visits identified in a value code 62 amount. This Part A payment reflects the shift of payments from the Part A to the Part B trust fund as mandated by §1812 (a)(3) of the Social Security Act.
65	HH Reimbursement - Part B	The dollar amounts determined to be associated with the HH visits identified in a value code 63 amount. This Part B payment reflects the shift of payments from the Part A to the Part B trust fund as mandated by §1812 (a)(3) of the Social Security Act.

If information returned from the CWF indicates all visits on the claim are Part A, the shared system must place value codes 62 and 64 on the claim record, showing the total visits and total PPS payment amount as the values, and send the claim to CWF with RIC code V.

If information returned from CWF indicates all visits on the claim are Part B, the shared system must place value codes 63 and 65 on the claim record, showing the total visits and total PPS payment amount as the values, and send the claim to CWF with RIC code W.

If information returned from CWF indicates certain visits on the claim are payable from both Part A and Part B, the shared system must place value codes 62, 63, 64, and 65 on the claim record. The shared system also must populate the values for code 62 and 63 based on the numbers of visits returned from CWF and prorate the total PPS reimbursement amount based on the numbers of visits to determine the dollars amounts to be associated with value codes 64 and 65. The shared system will return the claim to CWF with RIC code U.

Revenue Code and Revenue Description Required

HH PPS claims must report a 0023 revenue code line on which the first four positions of the HIPPS code match the code submitted on the RAP. This HIPPS code is used to match the claim to the corresponding RAP that was previously paid. After this match is completed, grouping to determine the HIPPS code used for final payment of the period of care will occur in Medicare systems. At that time, the submitted HIPPS code on the claim will be replaced with the system-calculated code.

For claims with "From" dates before January 1, 2020, the fifth position of the code represents the NRS severity level. This fifth position may differ to allow the HHA to change a code that represents that supplies were provided to a code that represents that supplies were not provided, or vice versa. However, the fifth position may only change between the two values that represent the same NRS severity level. Section 10.1.9 of this chapter contains the pairs of corresponding values. If these criteria are not met, Medicare claims processing systems will return the claim.

HHAs enter only one 0023 revenue code per claim in all cases.

Unlike RAPs, claims must also report all services provided to the beneficiary within the episode/period. All services must be billed on one claim for the entire episode/period. The A/B MAC (HHH) will return to the provider TOB 0329 when submitted without any visit charges.

Each service must be reported in line item detail. Each service visit (revenue codes 042x, 043x, 044x, 055x, 056x and 057x) must be reported as a separate line. Any of the following revenue codes may be used:

027x	Medical/Surgical Supplies (Also see 062x, an extension of 027x) Required detail: With the exception of revenue code 0274 (prosthetic and orthotic devices), only service units and a charge must be reported with this revenue code. If also reporting revenue code 0623 to separately identify specific wound care supplies, not just supplies for wound care patients, ensure that the charge amounts for revenue code 0623 lines are mutually exclusive from other lines for supply revenue codes reported on the claim. Report only nonroutine supply items in this revenue code or in 0623. Revenue code 0274 requires an HCPCS code, the date of service units and a charge amount. **NOTE:** Revenue Codes 0275 through 0278 are not used for Medicare billing on HH PPS types of bills
042x	Physical Therapy Required detail: One of the physical therapy HCPCS codes defined below in the instructions for the HCPCS code field, the date of service, service units which represent the number of 15 minute increments that comprised the visit, and a charge amount.
043x	Occupational Therapy Required detail: One of the occupational therapy HCPCS codes defined below in the instructions for the HCPCS code field, the date of service, service units which represent the number of 15 minute increments that comprised the visit, and a charge amount.
044x	Speech-Language Pathology Required detail: One of the speech-language pathology HCPCS codes defined below in the instructions for the HCPCS code field, the date of service, service units which represent the number of 15 minute increments that comprised the visit, and a charge amount.
055x	Skilled Nursing Required detail: One of the skilled nursing HCPCS codes defined below in the instructions for the HCPCS code field, the date of service, service units which represent the number of 15 minute increments that comprised the visit, and a charge amount.
056x	Medical Social Services Required detail: The medical social services HCPCS code defined below in the instructions for the HCPCS code field, the date of service, service units which represent the number of 15 minute increments that comprised the visit, and a charge amount.
057x	Home Health Aide (Home Health) Required detail: The home health aide HCPCS code defined below in the instructions for the HCPCS code field, the date of service, service units which represent the number of 15 minute increments that comprised the visit, and a charge amount.

NOTE: A/B MACs (HHH) do not accept revenue codes 058x or 059x when submitted with covered charges on Medicare home health claims under HH PPS. They also do not accept revenue code 0624, investigational devices, on HH claims under HH PPS.

Revenue Codes for Optional Billing of DME

Billing of DME provided in the episode is not required on the HH PPS claim. Home health agencies retain the option to bill these services to their A/B MAC (HHH) processing home health claims or to have the services provided under arrangement with a supplier that bills these services to the DME MAC. Agencies that choose to bill DME services on their HH PPS claims must use the revenue codes below. These services will be paid separately in addition to the HH PPS amount, based on the applicable Medicare fee schedule. For additional instructions for billing DME services see chapter 20 of this manual.

0274	Prosthetic/Orthotic Devices Required detail: The applicable HCPCS code for the item, a date of service, a number of service units, and a charge amount.
029x	Durable Medical Equipment (DME) (Other Than Renal) Required detail: The applicable HCPCS code for the item, a date of service indicating the purchase date or the beginning date of a monthly rental, a number of service units, and a charge amount. Monthly rental items should be reported with a separate line for each month's rental and service units of one. Revenue code 0294 is used to bill drugs/supplies for the effective use of DME.
060x	Oxygen (Home Health) Required detail: The applicable HCPCS code for the item, a date of service, a number of service units, and a charge amount.

Revenue Code for Optional Reporting of Wound Care Supplies

0623	Medical/Surgical Supplies - Extension of 027x Required detail: Only service units and a charge must be reported with this revenue code. If also reporting revenue code 027x to identify nonroutine supplies other than those used for wound care, the HHA must ensure that the charge amounts for the two revenue code lines are mutually exclusive.

HHAs may voluntarily report a separate revenue code line for charges for nonroutine wound care supplies, using revenue code 0623. Notwithstanding the standard abbreviation "surg dressings," HHAs use this code to report charges for ALL nonroutine wound care supplies, including but not limited to surgical dressings.

Pub. 100-02, Medicare Benefit Policy Manual, chapter 7, defines routine vs. nonroutine supplies. HHAs use that definition to determine whether any wound care supply item should be reported in this line because it is nonroutine.

HHAs can assist Medicare's future refinement of payment rates if they consistently and accurately report their charges for nonroutine wound care supplies under revenue center code 0623. HHAs should ensure that charges reported under revenue code 027x for nonroutine supplies are also complete and accurate.

Validating Required Reporting of Supply Revenue Code

For claims with "From" dates before January 1, 2020, the HH PPS includes a separate case-mix adjustment for non-routine supplies. Non-routine supply severity levels are indicated on HH PPS claims through a code value in the fifth position of the HIPPS code. The fifth position of the HIPPS code can contain two sets of values. One set of codes (the letters S through X) indicate that supplies were provided. The second set of codes (the numbers 1 through 6) indicate the HHA is intentionally reporting that they did not provide supplies during the episode. See section 10.1.9 for the complete composition of HIPPS under the HH PPS.

HHAs must ensure that if they are submitting a HIPPS code with a fifth position containing the letters S through X, the claim must also report a non-routine supply revenue code with covered charges. This revenue code may be either revenue code 27x, excluding 274, or revenue code 623, consistent with the instructions for optional separate reporting of wound care supplies.

Medicare systems will return the claim to the HHA if the HIPPS code indicates nonroutine supplies were provided and supply charges are not reported on the claim. When the HHA receives a claim returned for this reason, the HHA must review their records regarding the supplies provided to the beneficiary. The HHA may take one of the following actions, based on the review of their records:

- If non-routine supplies were provided, the supply charges must be added to the claim using the appropriate supply revenue code.
- If non-routine supplies were not provided, the HHA must indicate that on the claim by changing the fifth position of the HIPPS code to the appropriate numeric value in the range 1 through 6.

After completing one of these actions, the HHA may return the claim to the A/B MAC (HHH) for continued adjudication.

HCPCS/Accommodation Rates/HIPPS Rate Codes

Required - On the 0023 revenue code line, the HHA must report the HIPPS code that was reported on the RAP. The first four positions of the code must be identical to the value reported on the RAP. For claims with "From" dates before January 1, 2020, the fifth position may vary from the letter value reported on the RAP to the corresponding number which represents the same non-routine supply severity level but which reports that nonroutine supplies were not provided.

HHAs enter only one HIPPS code per claim in all cases. Claims submitted with additional HIPPS codes will be returned to the provider.

For episodes with "From" dates before January 1, 2020, Medicare may change the HIPPS used for payment of the claim in the course of claims processing, but the HIPPS code submitted by the provider in this field is never changed or replaced. If the HIPPS code is changed, the code used for payment is recorded in the APC-HIPPS field of the electronic claim record.

For episodes with "From" dates on or after January 1, 2020, Medicare will determine the appropriate HIPPS code for payment based on claims and OASIS data and will replace the provider-submitted HIPPS code as necessary. If the HIPPS code further changed based on medical review or other processes, the code used for payment is recorded in the APC-HIPPS field of the electronic claim record.

For revenue code lines other than 0023, the HHA reports HCPCS codes as appropriate to that revenue code.

To report HH visits, the HHA reports one of the following HCPCS codes to represent a visit by each HH care discipline:

Physical Therapy (revenue code 042x)

G0151 Services performed by a qualified physical therapist in the home health or hospice setting, each 15 minutes.

G0157 Services performed by a qualified physical therapist assistant in the home health or hospice setting, each 15 minutes.

G0159 Services performed by a qualified physical therapist, in the home health setting, in the establishment or delivery of a safe and effective physical therapy maintenance program, each 15 minutes.

Occupational Therapy (revenue code 043x)

G0152 Services performed by a qualified occupational therapist in the home health or hospice setting, each 15 minutes.

G0158 Services performed by a qualified occupational therapist assistant in the home health or hospice setting, each 15 minutes.

G0160 Services performed by a qualified occupational therapist, in the home health setting, in the establishment or delivery of a safe and effective occupational therapy maintenance program, each 15 minutes.

Speech-Language Pathology (revenue code 044x)

G0153 Services performed by a qualified speech-language pathologist in the home health or hospice setting, each 15 minutes.

G0161 Services performed by a qualified speech-language pathologist, in the home health setting, in the establishment or delivery of a safe and effective speech-language pathology maintenance program, each 15 minutes.

Note that modifiers indicating services delivered under a therapy plan of care (modifiers GN, GO or GP) are not required on HH PPS claims.

Skilled Nursing (revenue code 055x)

General skilled nursing:

For dates of service before January 1, 2016: G0154 Direct skilled services of a licensed nurse (LPN or RN) in the home health or hospice setting, each 15 minutes.

For dates of service on or after January 1, 2016: Visits previously reported with G0154 are reported with one of the following codes:

G0299 Direct skilled nursing services of a registered nurse (RN) in the home health or hospice setting

G0300 Direct skilled nursing of a licensed practical nurse (LPN) in the home health or hospice setting.

Care plan oversight:

For dates of service before January 1, 2017:

G0162 Skilled services by a licensed nurse (RN only) for management and evaluation of the plan of care, each 15 minutes (the patient's underlying condition or complication requires an RN to ensure that essential non-skilled care achieves its purpose in the home health or hospice setting).

G0163 Skilled services of a licensed nurse (LPN or RN) for the observation and assessment of the patient's condition, each 15 minutes (the change in the patient's condition requires skilled nursing personnel to identify and evaluate the patient's need for possible modification of treatment in the home health or hospice setting).

For dates of service on or after January 1, 2017, HHAs report visits previously reported with G0163 with one of the following codes:

G0493 Skilled services of a registered nurse (RN) for the observation and assessment of the patient's condition, each 15 minutes (the change in the patient's condition requires skilled nursing personnel to identify and evaluate the patient's need for possible modification of treatment in the home health or hospice setting).

G0494 Skilled services of a licensed practical nurse (LPN) for the observation and assessment of the patient's condition, each 15 minutes (the change in the patient's condition requires skilled nursing personnel to identify and evaluate the patient's need for possible modification of treatment in the home health or hospice setting).

Training:

For dates of service before January 1, 2017: G0164 Skilled services of a licensed nurse (LPN or RN), in the training and/or education of a patient or family member, in the home health or hospice setting, each 15 minutes.

For dates of service on or after January 1, 2017, HHAs report visits previously reported with G0164 with one of the following codes:

G0495 Skilled services of a registered nurse (RN), in the training and/or education of a patient or family member, in the home health or hospice setting, each 15 minutes.

G0496 Skilled services of a licensed practical nurse (LPN), in the training and/or education of a patient or family member, in the home health or hospice setting, each 15 minutes.

Medical Social Services (revenue code 056x)

G0155 Services of a clinical social worker under a home health plan of care, each 15 minutes.

Home Health Aide (revenue code 057x)

G0156 Services of a home health aide under a home health plan of care, each 15 minutes.

Regarding all skilled nursing and skilled therapy visits

In the course of a single visit, a nurse or qualified therapist may provide more than one of the nursing or therapy services reflected in the codes above. HHAs must not report more than one G-code for each visit regardless of the variety of services provided during the visit. In cases where more than one nursing or therapy service is provided in a visit, the HHA must report the G-code which reflects the service for which the clinician spent most of his/her time.

For instance, if direct skilled nursing services are provided, and the nurse also provides training/education of a patient or family member during that same visit, Medicare would expect the HHA to report the G-code which reflects the service for which most of the time was spent during that visit. Similarly, if a qualified therapist is performing a therapy service and also establishes a maintenance program during the same visit, the HHA should report the G-code that reflects the service for which most of the time was spent during that visit. In all cases, however, the number of 15-minute increments reported for the visit should reflect the total time of the visit

For episodes beginning on or after July 1, 2013, HHAs must report where home health services were provided. The following codes are used for this reporting:

Q5001: Hospice or home health care provided in patient's home/residence

Q5002: Hospice or home health care provided in assisted living facility

Q5009: Hospice or home health care provided in place not otherwise specified

The location where services were provided must always be reported along with the first visit reported on the claim. In addition to reporting a visit line using the G codes as described above, HHAs must report an additional line item with the same revenue code and date of service, reporting one of the three Q codes (Q5001, Q5002, and Q5009), one unit and a nominal covered charge (e.g., a penny). If the location where services were provided changes during the episode, the new location should be reported with an additional line corresponding to the first visit provided in the new location.

Service Date

Required - For initial episodes/periods of care, the HHA reports on the 0023 revenue code line the date of the first covered visit provided during the episode/period. For subsequent episodes, the HHA reports on the 0023 revenue code the date of the first visit provided during the episode/period, regardless of whether the visit was covered or non-covered.

For other line items detailing all services within the episode period, it reports service dates as appropriate to that revenue code. For service visits that begin in 1 calendar day and span into the next calendar day, report one visit using the date the visit ended as the service date.

When the claim Admission Date matches the Statement Covers "From" Date, Medicare systems ensure that the Service Date on the 0023 revenue code line also matches these dates.

Service Units

Required - Transaction standards require the reporting of a number greater than zero as the units on the 0023 revenue code line. However, Medicare systems will disregard the submitted units in processing the claim. For line items detailing all services within the episode period, the HHA reports units of service as appropriate to that revenue code. Coding detail for each revenue code under HH PPS is defined above under Revenue Codes.

For the revenue codes that represent home health visits (042x, 043x, 044x, 055x, 056x, and 057x), the HHA reports as service units a number of 15 minute increments that comprise the time spent treating the beneficiary. Time spent completing the OASIS assessment in the home as part of an otherwise covered and billable visit and time spent updating medical records in the home as part of such a visit may also be reported.

Visits of any length are to be reported, rounding the time to the nearest 15-minute increment. If any visits report over 96 units (over 24 hours) on a single line item, Medicare systems return the claim returned to the provider.

Effective January 1, 2017, covered and noncovered increments of the same visit must be reported on separate lines. This is to ensure that only covered increments are included in the per-unit based calculation of outlier payments.

Total Charges

Required - The HHA must report zero charges on the 0023 revenue code line (the field must contain zero).

For line items detailing all services within the episode period, the HHA reports charges as appropriate to that revenue code. Coding detail for each revenue code under HH PPS is defined above under Revenue Codes. Charges may be reported in dollars and cents (i.e., charges are not required to be rounded to dollars and zero cents). Medicare claims processing systems will not make any payments based upon submitted charge amounts.

Non-covered Charges

Required - The HHA reports the total non-covered charges pertaining to the related revenue code here. Examples of non-covered charges on HH PPS claims may include:

- Visits provided exclusively to perform OASIS assessments
- Visits provided exclusively for supervisory or administrative purposes
- Therapy visits provided prior to the required re-assessments

Payer Name

Required - See chapter 25.

Release of Information Certification Indicator

Required - See chapter 25.

National Provider Identifier – Billing Provider

Required - The HHA enters their provider identifier.

Insured's Name

Required only if MSP involved. See Pub. 100-05, Medicare Secondary Payer Manual.

Patient's Relationship To Insured

Required only if MSP involved. See Pub. 100-05, Medicare Secondary Payer Manual.

Insured's Unique Identifier

Required only if MSP involved. See Pub. 100-05, Medicare Secondary Payer Manual.

Insured's Group Name

Required only if MSP involved. See Pub. 100-05, Medicare Secondary Payer Manual.

Insured's Group Number

Required only if MSP involved. See Pub. 100-05, Medicare Secondary Payer Manual.

Treatment Authorization Code

Required - On claims with "From" dates before January 1, 2020, the code on the claim will match that submitted on the RAP.

In cases of billing for denial notice, using condition code 21, this code may be filled with a placeholder value as defined in section 60.

The investigational device (IDE) revenue code, 0624, is not allowed on HH PPS claims. Therefore, treatment authorization codes associated with IDE items must never be submitted in this field.

Medicare systems validate the length or the treatment authorization code and ensure that each position is in the correct format. If the format is incorrect, the contractor returns the claim to the provider

On claims with "From" dates on of after January 1, 2020, treatment authorization codes are no longer required on all claims. The HHA submits a code in this field only if the period is subject to Pre-Claim Review. In that case, the required tracking number is submitted in the first position of the field in all submission formats.

Document Control Number (DCN)

Required - If submitting an adjustment (TOB 0327) to a previously paid HH PPS claim, the HHA enters the control number assigned to the original HH PPS claim here.

Since HH PPS claims are processed as adjustments to the RAP, Medicare claims processing systems will match all HH PPS claims to their corresponding RAP and populate this field on the electronic claim record automatically. Providers do not need to submit a DCN on all HH PPS claims, only on adjustments to paid claims.

Required only if MSP involved. See Pub. 100-05, Medicare Secondary Payer Manual.

Principal Diagnosis Code

Required - The HHA enters the ICD code for the principal diagnosis. The code must be reported according to Official ICD Guidelines for Coding and Reporting, as required by the HIPAA. The code must be the full diagnosis code, including all five digits for ICD-9- CM or all seven digits for ICD-10 CM where applicable. Where the proper code has fewer than the maximum number of digits, the HHA does not fill it with zeros.

Medicare systems may return claims to the provider when the principal diagnosis code is not sufficient to determine the HHRG assignment under the PDGM.

For claim "From" dates before January 1, 2020, the ICD code and principle diagnosis reported must match the primary diagnosis code reported on the OASIS form item M1020 (Primary Diagnosis).

For claim "From" dates on or after January 1, 2020, the ICD code and principle diagnosis used for payment grouping will be claim coding rather than the OASIS item. As a result, the claim and OASIS diagnosis codes will no longer be expected to match in all cases.

Typically, the codes will match between the first claim in an admission and the start of care (Reason for Assessment –RFA 01) assessment and claims corresponding to recertification (RFA 04) assessments. Second 30-day claims in any 60-day period will not necessarily match the OASIS assessment. When diagnosis codes change between one 30-day claim and the next, there is no absolute requirement for the HHA to complete an 'other follow-up' (RFA 05) assessment to ensure that diagnosis coding on the claim matches to the assessment. However, the HHA would be required to complete an 'other follow-up' (RFA 05) assessment when such a change would be considered a major decline or improvement in the patient's health status.

Other Diagnosis Codes

Required - The HHA enters the full diagnosis codes for additional conditions if they coexisted at the time of the establishment of the plan of care. These codes may not duplicate the principal diagnosis as an additional or secondary diagnosis.

In listing the diagnoses, the HHA places them in order to best reflect the seriousness of the patient's condition and to justify the disciplines and services provided in accordance with the Official ICD Guidelines for Coding and Reporting. The sequence of codes should follow ICD guidelines for reporting manifestation codes. Medicare does not have any additional requirements regarding the reporting or sequence of the codes beyond those contained in ICD guidelines.

For claim "From" dates before January 1, 2020, the other diagnoses and ICD codes reported on the claim must match the additional diagnoses reported on the OASIS, form item M1022 (Other Diagnoses).

For claim "From" dates on or after January 1, 2020, claim and OASIS diagnosis codes may vary as described under Principal Diagnosis.

Attending Provider Name and Identifiers

Required - The HHA enters the name and national provider identifier (NPI) of the attending physician who signed the plan of care.

Other Provider (Individual) Names and Identifiers

Required - The HHA enters the name and NPI of the physician who certified/re-certified the patient's eligibility for home health services.

NOTE: Both the attending physician and other provider fields should be completed unless the patient's designated attending physician is the same as the physician who certified/re-certified the patient's eligibility. When the attending physician is also the certifying/re-certifying physician, only the attending physician is required to be reported.

Remarks

Conditional - Remarks are required only in cases where the claim is cancelled or adjusted.

100-4, Chapter-10, 90.1

Osteoporosis Injections as HHA Benefit

A -Billing Requirements

The administration of the drug is included in the charge for the skilled nursing visit billed using type of bill 32X. The cost of the drug is billed using type of bill 34X, using revenue code 0636. Drugs that have the ingredient calcitonin are billed using HCPCS code J0630. Drugs that have the ingredient teriparatide may be billed using HCPCS code J3110, if all existing guidelines for coverage under the home health benefit are met. All other osteoporosis drugs that are FDA approved and are awaiting an HCPCS code must use the miscellaneous code of J3490 until a specific HCPCS code is approved for use.

HCPCS code J0630 is defined as up to 400 units. Therefore, the provider must calculate units for the bill as follows:

Units Furnished During Billing Period	Units of Service Entry on Bill
100-400	1
401-800	2
801-1200	3
1201-1600	4
1601-2000	5
2001-2400	6

HCPCS code J3110 is defined as 10 mcg. Providers should report 1 unit for each 10 mcg dose provided during the billing period. These codes are paid on a reasonable cost basis, using the provider's submitted charges to make initial payments, which are subject to annual cost settlement. Coverage requirements for osteoporosis drugs are found in Pub. 100-02, Medicare Benefit Policy Manual, chapter 7, section 50.4.3. Coverage requirements for the home health benefit in general are found in Pub. 100-02, Medicare Benefit Policy Manual, chapter 7, section 30.

B -Edits

Medicare system edits require that the date of service on a 34Xclaim for covered osteoporosis drugs falls within the start and end dates of an existing home health PPS episode. Once the system ensures the service dates on the 34X claim fall within an HH PPS episode that is open for the beneficiary on CWF, CWF edits to assure that the provider number on the 34X claim matches the provider number on the episode file. This is to reflect that although the osteoporosis drug is paid separately from the HH PPS episode rate it is included in consolidated billing requirements(see §10.1.25 regarding consolidated billing).

Claims are also edited to assure that the claim is an HH claim (type of bill 34X), the beneficiary is female and that the diagnosis code 733.01 (post-menopausal osteoporosis) is present.

100-4, Chapter-11, 10.1

Hospice Pre-Election Evaluation and Counseling Services

Effective January 1, 2005, Medicare allows payment to a hospice for specified hospice pre-election evaluation and counseling services when furnished by a physician who is either the medical director of or employee of the hospice.

Medicare covers a one-time only payment on behalf of a beneficiary who is terminally ill, (defined as having a prognosis of 6 months or less if the disease follows its normal course), has no previous hospice elections, and has not previously received hospice pre-election evaluation and counseling services.

HCPCS code G0337 "Hospice Pre-Election Evaluation and Counseling Services" is used to designate that these services have been provided by the medical director or a physician employed by the ho spice. Hospice agencies bill their Medicare contractor with home health and hospice jurisdiction directly using HCPCS G0337 with Revenue Code 0657. No other revenue codes may appear on the claim.

Claims for "Hospice Pre-Election and Counseling Services", HCPCS code G0337, are not subject to the editing usually required on hospice claims to match the claim to an established hospice period. Further, contractors do not apply payments for hospice pre-election evaluation and counseling consultation services to the overall hospice cap amount.

Medicare must ensure that this counseling service occurs only one time per beneficiary by imposing safeguards to detect and prevent duplicate billing for similar services. If "new patient" physician services (HCPCS codes 99201-99205) are submitted by a Medicare contractor to CWF for payment authorization but HCPCS code G0337 (Hospice Pre-Election Evaluation and Counseling Services) has already been approved for a hospice claim for the same beneficiary, for the same date of service, by the same physician, the physician service will be rejected by CWF and the service shall be denied as a duplicate. Medicare contractors use the following messages in this case:

HCPCS code G0337 is only payable when billed on a hospice claim. Contractors shall not make payment for HCPCS code G0337 on professional claims. Contractors shall deny line items on professional claims for HCPCS code G0337 and use the following messages:

MSN message 17.9: "Medicare (Part A/Part B) pays for this service. The provider must bill the correct Medicare contractor."

CARC 109: "Claim not covered by this payer/contractor. You must send the claim to the correct payer/contractor ."

100-4, Chapter-11, 30.3

Data Required on the Institutional Claim to A/B MAC (HHH)

See Pub. 100-02, Medicare Benefit Policy Manual, chapter 9, for coverage requirements for Hospice benefits. This section addresses only claims submission. Before submitting claims, the hospice must submit a Notice of Election (NOE) to the A/B MAC (HHH).

See section 20, of this chapter for information on NOE transaction types.

The Social Security Act at §1862 (a)(22) requires that all claims for Medicare payment must be submitted in an electronic form specified by the Secretary of Health and Human Services, unless an exception described at §1862 (h) applies. The electronic format required for billing hospice services is the ASC X12 837 institutional claim transaction. Since the data structure of this transaction is difficult to express in narrative form and to provide assistance to small providers excepted from the electronic claim requirement, the instructions below are given relative to the data element names on the Form CMS-1450 hardcopy form. Each data element name is shown in bold type. Information regarding the form locator numbers that correspond to these data element names is found in Chapter 25.

Because claim formats serve the needs of many payers, some data elements may not be needed by a particular payer. Detailed information is given only for items required for Medicare hospice claims. Items not listed need not be completed although hospices may complete them when billing multiple payers.

Provider Name, Address, and Telephone Number

The hospice enters this information for their agency.

Type of Bill

The hospice enters on of the following Type of Bill codes:

081x – Hospice (non-hospital based) 082x – Hospice (hospital based)

4th Digit – Frequency	Definition
0 - Nonpayment/Zero Claims	Used when no payment from Medicare is anticipated.
I - Admit Through Discharge Claim	This code is used for a bill encompassing an entire course of hospice treatment for which the provider expects payment from the payer, i.e., no further bills will be submitted for this patient.
2 - Interim – First Claim	This code is used for the first of an expected series of payment bills for a hospice course of treatment.
3 - Interim - Continuing Claim	This code is used when a payment bill for a hospice course of treatment has already been submitted and further bills are expected to be submitted.
4 - Interim - Last Claim	This code is used for a payment bill that is the last of a series for a hospice course of treatment. The "Through" date of this bill is the discharge date, transfer date, or date of death.
7 - Replacement of Prior Claim	This code is used by the provider when it wants to correct a previously submitted bill. This is the code used on the corrected or "new" bill.
8 - Void/Cancel of a Prior Claim	This code is used to cancel a previously processed claim.

Statement Covers Period (From-Through)

The hospice shows the beginning and ending dates of the period covered by this bill in numeric fields (MM-DD-YY). The hospice does not show days before the patient's entitlement began.

Statement periods should follow the frequency of billing instructions in section 90.

Patient Name/Identifier

The hospice enters the beneficiary's name exactly as it appears on the Medicare card.

Patient Address Patient Birth date Patient Sex

The hospice enters the appropriate address, date of birth and gender information describing the beneficiary.

Admission/Start of Care Date

The hospice enters the admission date, which must be the same date as the effective date of the hospice election or change of election. The date of admission may not precede the physician's certification by more than 2 calendar days.

The admission date stays the same on all continuing claims for the same hospice election.

Patient Discharge Status

This code indicates the patient's status as of the "Through" date of the billing period. The hospice enters the most appropriate National Uniform Billing Committee (NUBC) approved code. Valid values most commonly used on hospice claims include:

Code	Description
01	Discharged to home or self-care
30	Still patient
40	Expired at home
41	Expired in a medical facility
42	Expired- place unknown
50	Discharged/transferred to hospice- home
51	Discharged/transferred to hospice- medical facility

NOTE: that patient discharge status code 20 is not used on hospice claims. If the patient has died during the billing period, use codes 40, 41 or 42 as appropriate.

Medicare regulations at 42 CFR 418.26 define three reasons for discharge from hospice care:

1. The beneficiary moves out of the hospice's service area or transfers to another hospice,
2. The hospice determines that the beneficiary is no longer terminally ill or
3. The hospice determines the beneficiary meets their internal policy regarding discharge for cause.

Each of these discharge situations requires different coding on Medicare claims.

Reason 1: A beneficiary may move out of the hospice's service area either with, or without, a transfer to another hospice. In the case of a discharge when the beneficiary moves out of the hospice's service area without a transfer, the hospice uses the NUBC approved discharge status code that best describes the beneficiary's situation and appends condition code 52. The hospice does not report occurrence code 42 on their claim. This discharge claim will terminate the beneficiary's current hospice benefit period as of the "Through" date on the claim. The beneficiary may re-elect the hospice benefit at any time as long they remain eligible for the benefit.

In the case of a discharge when the beneficiary moves out of the hospice's service area and transfers to another hospice, the hospice uses discharge status code 50 or 51, depending on whether the beneficiary is transferring to home hospice or hospice in a medical facility.

The hospice does not report occurrence code 42 on their claim. This discharge claim does not terminate the beneficiary's current hospice benefit period. The admitting hospice submits a transfer Notice of Election (type of bill 8xC) after the transfer has occurred and the beneficiary's hospice benefit is not affected.

Reason 2: In the case of a discharge when the hospice determines the beneficiary is no longer terminally ill, the hospice uses the NUBC approved discharge status code that best describes the beneficiary's situation. The hospice does not report occurrence code 42 on their claim. This discharge claim will terminate the beneficiary's current hospice benefit period as of the "Through" date on the claim.

Reason 3: In the case of a discharge for cause, the hospice uses the NUBC approved discharge status code that best describes the beneficiary's situation. The hospice does not report occurrence code 42 on their claim. Instead, the hospice reports condition code H2 to indicate a discharge for cause. The effect of this discharge claim on the beneficiary's current hospice benefit period depends on the discharge status.

If the beneficiary is transferred to another hospice (discharge status codes 50 or 51) the claim does not terminate the beneficiary's current hospice benefit period. The admitting hospice submits a transfer Notice of Election (type of bill 8xC) after the transfer has occurred and the beneficiary's hospice benefit is not affected. If any other appropriate discharge status code is used, this discharge claim will terminate the beneficiary's current hospice benefit period as of the "Through" date on the claim. The beneficiary may re- elect the hospice benefit if they are certified as terminally ill and eligible for the benefit again in the future and are willing to be compliant with care.

If the beneficiary has chosen to revoke their hospice election, the provider uses the NUBC approved discharge patient status code and the occurrence code 42 indicating the date the beneficiary revoked the benefit. The beneficiary may re-elect the hospice benefit if they are certified as terminally ill and eligible for the benefit again in the future.

Discharge Reason	Coding Required in Addition to Patient Status Code
Beneficiary Moves Out of Service Area	Condition Code 52
Beneficiary Transfers Hospices	Patient Status Code 50 or 51; no other indicator
Beneficiary No Longer Terminally Ill	No other indicator
Beneficiary Discharged for Cause	Condition code H2
Beneficiary Revokes	Occurrence code 42

If a hospice beneficiary is discharged alive or if a hospice beneficiary revokes the election of hospice care, the hospice shall file a timely-filed Notice of Election Termination / Revocation (NOTR) using type of bill 8xB, unless it has already filed a final claim. A timely-filed NOTR is a NOTR that is submitted to the A/B MAC (HHH) and accepted by the A/B MAC (HHH) within 5 calendar days after the effective date of discharge or revocation. While a timely-filed NOTR is one that is submitted to and accepted by the A/B MAC (HHH) within 5 calendar days after the hospice election, posting to the CWF may not occur within that same timeframe. The date of posting to the CWF is not a reflection of whether the NOTR is considered timely-filed. A NOTR (type of bill 8xB) is entered via Direct Data Entry in the same way as an NOE (type of bill 8xA). Hospices continue to have 12 months from the date of service in which to file their claims timely.

A patient can also be admitted and discharged on the same day. They would submit an 8x1 Type of Bill ("Admission through Discharge Claim"), matching "From" and "Through" dates, and whatever the appropriate level of care the revenue code was, with 1 unit. A patient cannot be discharged and re-admitted to the same hospice on the same day.

85	Delayed recertification of hospice terminal illness	Code indicates the hospice received the recertification of terminal illness later than 2 days after the first day of a new benefit period. This code is reported with occurrence span code 77, which reports the provider liable days associated with the untimely recertification.

Untimely Face-to-Face Encounters and Discharge

When a required face-to-face encounter occurs prior to, but no more than 30 calendar days prior to, the third benefit period recertification and every benefit period recertification thereafter, it is considered timely. A timely face-to-face encounter would be evident when examining the face-to-face attestation, which is part of the recertification, as that attestation includes the date of the encounter. While the face-to-face encounter itself must occur no more than 30 calendar days prior to the start of the third benefit period recertification and each subsequent recertification, its accompanying attestation must be completed before the claim is submitted.

If the required face-to-face encounter is not timely, the hospice would be unable to recertify the patient as being terminally ill, and the patient would cease to be eligible for the Medicare hospice benefit. In such instances, the hospice must discharge the patient from the Medicare hospice benefit because he or she is not considered terminally ill for Medicare purposes.

When a discharge from the Medicare hospice benefit occurs due to failure to perform a required face-to-face encounter timely, the claim should include the most appropriate patient discharge status code. Occurrence span code 77 does not apply when the face-to-face encounter has not occurred timely.

The hospice can re-admit the patient to the Medicare hospice benefit once the required encounter occurs, provided the patient continues to meet all of the eligibility requirements and the patient (or representative) files an election statement in accordance with CMS regulations. Where the only reason the patient ceases to be eligible for the Medicare hospice benefit is the hospice's failure to meet the face-to-face requirement, CMS would expect the hospice to continue to care for the patient at its own expense until the required encounter occurs, enabling the hospice to re-establish Medicare eligibility.

Condition Codes

The hospice enters any appropriate NUBC approved code(s) identifying conditions related to this bill that may affect processing.

Codes listed below are only those most frequently applicable to hospice claims. For a complete list of codes, see the NUBC manual.

07	Treatment of Non-terminal Condition for Hospice	Code indicates the patient has elected hospice care but the provider is not treating the terminal condition, and is, therefore, requesting regular Medicare payment.
20	Beneficiary Requested Billing	Code indicates the provider realizes the services on this bill are at a noncovered level of care or otherwise excluded from coverage, but the beneficiary has requested a formal determination.
21	Billing for Denial Notice	Code indicates the provider realizes services are at a noncovered level of care or excluded, but requests a denial notice from Medicare in order to bill Medicaid or other insurers.
H2	Discharge by a Hospice Provider for Cause	Discharge by a Hospice Provider for Cause. **NOTE:** Used by the provider to indicate the patient meets the hospice's documented policy addressing discharges for cause.
52	Out of Hospice Service Area	Code indicates the patient is discharged for moving out of the hospice service area. This can include patients who relocate or who go on vacation outside of the hospice's service area, or patients who are admitted to a hospital or SNF that does not have contractual arrangements with the hospice.

Occurrence Codes and Dates

The hospice enters any appropriate NUBC approved code(s) and associated date(s) defining specific event(s) relating to this billing period. Event codes are two numeric digits, and dates are six numeric digits (MM-DD-YY). If there are more occurrences than there are spaces on the form, use the occurrence span code fields to record additional occurrences and dates.

Codes listed below are only those most frequently applicable to hospice claims. For a complete list of codes, see the NUBC manual.

Code	Title	Definition
23	Cancellation of Hospice Election Period (A/B MAC (HHH) USE ONLY)	Code indicates date on which a hospice period of election is cancelled by an A/B MAC (HHH) as opposed to revocation by the beneficiary.
24	Date Insurance Denied	Code indicates the date of receipt of a denial of coverage by a higher priority payer.
27	Date of Hospice Certification or Re-Certification	Code indicates the date of certification or re-certification of the hospice benefit period, beginning with the first 2 initial benefit periods of 90 days each and the subsequent 60-day benefit periods. **NOTE:** regarding transfers from one hospice to another hospice: If a patient is in the first certification period when they transfer to another hospice, the receiving hospice would use the same certification date as the previous hospice until the next certification period. However, if they were in the next certification at the time of transfer, then they would enter that date in the Occurrence Code 27 and date.
42	Date of Termination of Hospice Benefit	Enter code to indicate the date on which beneficiary terminated his/her election to receive hospice benefits. This code can be used only when the beneficiary has revoked the benefit. It is not used in transfer situations. **NOTE:** Occurrence code 42 is not required on the NOTR, since the through date represents the revocation date. Occurrence codes are only necessary on NOTRs when carrying the original revocation date on a correction.
55	Beneficiary is Deceased	Report the appropriate NUBC discharge status code that best describes the place in which the beneficiary died (40, 41, or 42). Discharge status code 20 is not used on hospice claims.

Occurrence code 27 is reported on the claim for the billing period in which the certification or re-certification was obtained. When the re-certification is late and not obtained during the month it was due, the occurrence span code 77 should be reported with the through date of the span code equal to the through date of the claim.

Occurrence Span Code and Dates

The hospice enters any appropriate NUBC approved code(s) and associated beginning and ending date(s) defining a specific event relating to this billing period are shown.

Event codes are two alphanumeric digits and dates are shown numerically as MM-DD-YY.

Codes listed below are only those most frequently applicable to hospice claims. For a complete list of codes, see the NUBC manual.

Code	Title	Definition
M2	Dates of Inpatient Respite Care	Code indicates From/Through dates of a period of inpatient respite care for hospice patients to differentiate separate respite periods of less than 5 days each. M2 is used when respite care is provided more than once during a benefit period.
77	Provider Liability – Utilization Charged	Code indicates From/Through dates for a period of non-covered hospice care for which the provider accepts payment liability (other than for medical necessity or custodial care).

Respite care is payable only for periods of respite up to 5 consecutive days. Claims reporting respite periods greater than 5 consecutive days will be returned to the provider. Days of respite care beyond 5 days must be billed at the appropriate home care rate for payment consideration.

For example: If the patient enters a respite period on July 1 and is returned to routine home care on July 6, the units of respite reported on the line item would be 5 representing July 1 through July 5, July 6 is reported as a day of routine home care regardless of the time of day entering respite or returning to routine home care.

When there is more than one respite period in the billing period, the provider must include the M2 occurrence span code for all periods of respite. The individual respite periods reported shall not exceed 5 days, including consecutive respite periods.

For example: If the patient enters a respite period on July 1 and is returned to routine home care on July 6 and later returns to respite care from July 15 to July 18, and completes the month on routine home care, the provider must report two separate line items for the respite periods and two occurrence span code M2, as follows:

Revenue Line items:

- Revenue code 0655 with line item date of service 07/01/XX (for respite period July 1 through July 5) and line item units reported as 5
- Revenue code 0651 with line item date of service 07/06/XX (for routine home care July 6 through July 14) and line item units reported as 9
- Revenue code 0655 with line item date of service 07/15/XX (for respite period July 15 through 17th) and line item units reported as 3
- Revenue code 0651 with line item date of service 07/18/XX (for routine home care on date of discharge from respite through July 31 and line item units reported as 14.

Occurrence Span Codes:

- M2 0701XX – 07/05/XX
- M2 0715XX – 07/17/XX

Provider Liability Periods Using Occurrence Span Code 77: Hospices must use occurrence span code 77 to identify days of care that are not covered by Medicare due to:

- Untimely physician recertification. This is particularly important when the non- covered days fall at the beginning of a billing period other than the initial certification period.

- Late-filing of a Notice of Election (NOE). A timely-filed NOE is a NOE that is submitted to the A/B MAC (HHH) and accepted by the A/B MAC (HHH) within 5 calendar days after the hospice admission date. When the hospice files a NOE late, Medicare shall not cover and pay for the days of hospice care from the hospice admission date to the date the NOE is submitted to and accepted by the A/B MAC (HHH). The date the NOE is submitted to and accepted by the A/B MAC (HHH) is an allowable day for payment.

Example:

Admission date is 10/10/20XX (Fri).

Day 1 = Sat. 10/11/20XX

Day 2 = Sun. 10/12/20XX

Day 3 = Mon. 10/13/20XX

Day 4 = Tues. 10/14/20XX

Day 5 = Weds. 10/15/20XX 10/15/20XX is the NOE Due Date.

IF NOE Receipt date is 10/16/20XX, the hospice reports 10/10- 10/15 as non- covered days using occurrence span code 77 or Medicare systems return the claim to the provider for correction.

Value Codes and Amounts

The hospice enters any appropriate NUBC approved code(s) and the associated value amounts identifying numeric information related to this bill that may affect processing.

Provider-submitted codes:

The most commonly used value codes on hospice claims are value codes 61 and G8, which are used to report the location of the site of hospice services. Otherwise, value codes are commonly used only to indicate Medicare is secondary to another payer. For detailed information on reporting Medicare secondary payer information, see the Medicare Secondary Payer Manual.

Code	Title	Definition
61	Place of Residence where Service is Furnished (Routine Home Care and Continuous Home Care)	MSA or Core-Based Statistical Area (CBSA) number (or rural State code) of the location where the hospice service is delivered. A residence can be an inpatient facility if an individual uses that facility as a place of residence. It is the level of care that is required and not the location where hospice services are provided that determines payment. In other words, if an individual resides in a freestanding hospice facility and requires routine home care, then claims are submitted for routine home care. Hospices must report value code 61 when billing revenue codes 0651 and 0652.
G8	Facility where Inpatient Hospice Service is Delivered (General Inpatient and Inpatient Respite Care).	MSA or Core Based Statistical Area (CBSA) number (or rural State code) of the facility where inpatient hospice services are delivered. Hospices must report value code G8 when billing revenue codes 0655 and 0656.

If hospice services are provided to the beneficiary in more than one CBSA area during the billing period, the hospice reports the CBSA that applies at the end of the billing period.

For routine home care and continuous home care (e.g., the beneficiary's residence changes between locations in different CBSAs), report the CBSA of the beneficiary's residence at the end of the billing period. For general inpatient and inpatient respite care (e.g., the beneficiary is served in inpatient facilities in different CBSAs), report the CBSA of the latest facility that served the beneficiary. If the beneficiary receives both home and inpatient care during the billing period, the latest home CBSA is reported with value code 61 and the latest facility CBSA is reported with value code G8.

Medicare-applied codes: The following codes are added during processing and may be visible in the A/B MAC (HHH)'s online claim history. They are never submitted by the hospice.

Code	Title	Definition
62	Number of High Routine Home Care Days	Days that fall within the first 60 days of a routine home care hospice claim. The Medicare system puts the high days returned by Pricer on the claim as a value code 62 amount.
63	Number of Low Routine Home Care Days	Days that come after the first 60 days of a routine home care hospice claim. The Medicare system puts the low days returned by Pricer on the claim as a value code 63 amount.

Revenue Codes

The hospice assigns a revenue code for each type of service provided and enters the appropriate four-digit numeric revenue code to explain each charge.

Hospice claims are required to report separate line items for the level of care each time the level of care changes. This includes revenue codes 0651, 0655 and 0656. For example, if a patient begins the month receiving routine home care followed by a period of general inpatient care and then later returns to routine home care all in the same month, in addition to the one line reporting the general inpatient care days, there should be two separate line items for routine home care. Each routine home care line reports a line item date of service to indicate the first date that level of care began for that consecutive period.

Code	Description	Standard Abbreviation
0651	Routine Home Care	RTN Home
0652	Continuous Home Care	CTNS Home A minimum of 8 hours of primarily nursing care within a 24-hour period. The 8-hours of care do not need to be continuous within the 24-hour period, but a need for an aggregate of 8 hours of primarily nursing care is required. Nursing care must be provided by a registered nurse or a licensed practical nurse. If skilled intervention is required for less than 8 aggregate hours (or less than 32 units) within a 24 hour period, then the care rendered would be covered as a routine home care day. Services provided by a nurse practitioner as the attending physician are not included in the CHC computation nor is care that is not directly related to the crisis included in the computation. CHC billing should reflect direct patient care during a period of crisis and should not reflect time related to staff working hours, time taken for meal breaks, time used for educating staff, time used to report etc.
0655**	Inpatient Respite Care	IP Respite

Code	Description	Standard Abbreviation
0656**	General Inpatient Care	GNL IP
0657	Physician Services	PHY SER (must be accompanied by a physician procedure code)

** The date of discharge from general inpatient or inpatient respite care is paid at the appropriate home care rate and must be billed with the appropriate home care revenue code unless the patient is deceased at time of discharge in which case, the appropriate inpatient respite or general inpatient care revenue code should be used.

NOTE: Hospices use revenue code 0657 to identify hospice charges for services furnished to patients by physicians, nurse practitioners, or physician assistants employed by the hospice; or physicians, nurse practitioners or physician assistants receiving compensation from the hospice. Procedure codes are required in order for the A/B MAC (HHH) to determine the reimbursement rate for the physician services. Appropriate procedure codes are available from the A/B MAC (HHH).

Additional revenue codes are reported describing the visits provided under each level of care.

To constitute a visit, the discipline, (as defined above) must have provided care to the beneficiary. Services provided by a social worker to the beneficiary's family also constitute a visit. For example, documentation in the medical/clinical record, interdisciplinary group meetings, obtaining physician orders, rounds in a facility or any other activity that is not related to the provision of items or services to a beneficiary, do not count towards a visit to be placed on the claim. During an initial or comprehensive assessment, it would not be best practice to wait until later (after the clinician has left the home) to document the findings of an assessment or the interventions provided during a patient visit. It is recommended that this information be documented as close to the time of the assessment or intervention as possible. In addition, the visit must be reasonable and necessary for the palliation and management of the terminal illness and related conditions as described in the patient's plan of care.

If a hospice patient is receiving routine home care while residing in a nursing home, the hospice would record visits for all of its physicians, nurses, social workers, and home health aides who visit the patient to provide care for the palliation and management of the terminal illness and related conditions, as described in the patient's plan of care. In this example the nursing home is acting as the patient's home. Only the patient care provided by the hospice staff constitutes a visit.

When making the determination as to whether or not a particular visit should be reported, a hospice should consider whether the visit would have been reported, and how it would have been reported, if the patient were receiving RHC in his or her private home. If a group of tasks would normally be performed in a single visit to a patient living in his or her private home, then the hospice should count the tasks as a single visit for the patient residing in a facility. Hospices should not record a visit every time a staff member enters the patient's room. Hospices should use clinical judgment in counting visits and summing time.

Hospices report social worker phone calls and all visits performed by hospice staff in 15 minute increments using the following revenue codes and associated HCPCS. This includes visits by hospice nurses, aides, social workers, physical therapists, occupational therapists, and speech-language pathologists.

All visits to provide care related to the palliation and management of the terminal illness or related conditions, whether provided by hospice employees or provided under arrangement, must be reported. The two exceptions are related to General Inpatient Care and Respite care. CMS is not requiring hospices to report visit data at this time for visits made by non-hospice staff providing General Inpatient Care or respite care in contract facilities. However, General Inpatient Care or respite care visits related to the palliation and management of the terminal illness or related conditions provided by hospice staff in contract facilities must be reported, and all General Inpatient Care and respite care visits related to the palliation and management of the terminal illness or related conditions provided in hospice-owned facilities must be reported.

Social worker phone calls made to the patient or the patient's family should be reported using revenue code 0569, and HCPCS G-code G0155 for the length of the call, with each call being a separate line item. Only phone calls that are necessary for the palliation and management of the terminal illness and related conditions as described in the patient's plan of care (such as counseling or speaking with a patient's family or arranging for a placement) should be reported. Report only social worker phone calls related to providing and or coordinating care to the patient and family and documented as such in the clinical records.

When recording any visit or social worker phone call time, providers should sum the time for each visit or call, rounding to the nearest 15 minute increment. Providers should not include travel time or documentation time in the time recorded for any visit or call.

Additionally, hospices may not include interdisciplinary group time in time and visit reporting.

Hospice agencies shall report injectable and non-injectable prescription drugs for the palliation and management of the terminal illness and related conditions on their claims. Both injectable and non-injectable prescription drugs shall be reported on claims on a line-item basis per fill, based on the amount dispensed by the pharmacy.

When a facility (hospital, SNF, NF, or hospice inpatient facility) uses a medication management system where each administration of a hospice medication is considered a fill for hospice patients receiving care, the hospice shall report a monthly total for each drug (i.e., report a total for the period covered by the claim), along with the total dispensed.

For dates of service before October 1, 2018, Hospices shall report multi-ingredient compound prescription drugs (non-injectable) using revenue code 0250. The hospice shall specify the same prescription number for each ingredient of a compound drug according to the 837i guidelines in loop 2410. In addition, the hospice shall provide the NDC for each ingredient in the compound; the NDC qualifier represents the quantity of the drug filled (meaning the amount dispensed) and shall be reported as the unit measure.

When reporting prescription drugs in a comfort kit/pack, the hospice shall report the NDC of each prescription drug within the package, in accordance with the procedures for non-injectable prescriptions.

Hospice agencies shall report infusion pumps (a type of DME) on a line-item basis for each pump and for each medication fill and refill. The hospice claim shall reflect the total charge for the infusion pump for the period covered by the claim, whether the hospice is billed for it daily, weekly, biweekly, with each medication refill, or in some other fashion. The hospice shall include on the claim the infusion pump charges on whatever basis is easiest for its billing systems, so long as in total, the claim reflects the charges for the pump for the time period of that claim.

Effective for dates of service on and after 10/1/2018, hospices are no longer required to report drugs using line item detail. Hospices may report summary charges for drugs as shown in the table below.

Hospices must enter the following visit revenue codes, when applicable:

Revenue Code	Required HCPCS	Required Detail
0250 Non-injectable Prescription Drugs	N/A	Required detail: Report on a line-item basis per fill, using revenue code 0250 and the National Drug Code (NDC). The NDC qualifier represents the quantity of the drug filled, and should be reported as the unit measure. For dates of service on and after 10/1/2018: Report a monthly charge total for all drugs (i.e., report a total charge amount for the period covered by the claim) using revenue code 0250.
029X Infusion pumps	Applicable HCPCS	Required detail: Report on the claim on a line-item basis per pump order and per medication refill, using revenue code 029X for the equipment and 0294 for the drugs along with the appropriate HCPCS.
	N/A	For dates of service on and after 10/1/18: Report a monthly charge total for DME (i.e., report a total charge amount for the period covered by the claim), including DME infusion drugs, using revenue center 029X for the item of DME and 0294 for DME infusion drugs.
042x Physical Therapy	G0151	Required detail: Each visit is identified on a separate line item with the appropriate line item date of service and a charge amount. The units reported on the claim are the multiplier for the total time of the visit defined in the HCPCS description.
043x Occupational Therapy	G0152	Required detail: Each visit is identified on a separate line item with the appropriate line item date of service and a charge amount. The units reported on the claim are the multiplier for the total time of the visit defined in the HCPCS description.
044x Speech Therapy – Language Pathology	G0153	Required detail: Each visit is identified on a separate line item with the appropriate line item date of service and a charge amount. The units reported on the claim are the multiplier for the total time of the visit defined in the HCPCS description.
055x Skilled Nursing	G0154 (before 01/01/2016)) G0299 or G0300 (on or after 01/01/2016)	Required detail: Each visit is identified on a separate line item with the appropriate line item date of service and a charge amount. The units reported on the claim are the multiplier for the total time of the visit defined in the HCPCS description.

Revenue Code	Required HCPCS	Required Detail
056x Medical Social Services	G0155	Required detail: Each visit is identified on a separate line item with the appropriate line item date of service and a charge amount. The units reported on the claim are the multiplier for the total time of the visit defined in the HCPCS description.
0569 Other Medical Social Services	G0155	Required detail: Each social service phone call is identified on a separate line item with the appropriate line item date of service and a charge amount. The units reported on the claim are the multiplier for the total time of the call defined in the HCPCS description.
057x Aide	G0156	Required detail: Each visit is identified on a separate line item with the appropriate line item date of service and a charge amount. The units reported on the claim are the multiplier the total time of the visit defined in the HCPCS description.
0636 Injectable Drugs	Applicable HCPCS	Required detail: Report on a line item basis per fill with units representing the amount filled. (i.e., Q1234 Drug 100mg and the fill was for 200 mg, units reported = 2). For dates of service on and after 10/1/2018: Revenue code 0636 is not required.

Visits by registered nurses, licensed vocational nurses and nurse practitioners (unless the nurse practitioner is acting as the beneficiary's attending physician) are reported under revenue code 055x.

Charges associated with the reported visits are covered under the hospice bundled payment and reflected in the payment for the level of care billed on the claim. No additional payment is made on the visit revenue lines.

The contractor shall use the following remittance advice messages and associated codes when bundling line items under this policy. This CARC/RARC combination is compliant with CAQH CORE Business Scenario Four.

Group Code: CO CARC: 97 RARC: N/A MSN: N/A

Effective January 1, 2016, Medicare requires hospices to use G0299 for "direct skilled nursing services of a registered nurse (RN) in the home health or hospice setting" and G0300 "direct skilled nursing of a licensed practical nurse (LPN) in the home health or hospice setting." G0154 is retired as of 12/31/2015

Hospices should report in the unit field on the line level the units as a multiplier of the visit time defined in the HCPCS description.

HCPCS/Accommodation Rates/HIPPS Rate Codes

Hospices must report a HCPCS code along with each level of care revenue code (651, 652, 655 and 656) to identify the type of service location where that level of care was provided.

The following HCPCS codes will be used to report the type of service location for hospice services:

HCPCS Code	Definition
Q5001	HOSPICE CARE PROVIDED IN PATIENT'S HOME/RESIDENCE
Q5002	HOSPICE CARE PROVIDED IN ASSISTED LIVING FACILITY

HCPCS Code	Definition
Q5003	HOSPICE CARE PROVIDED IN NURSING LONG TERM CARE FACILITY (LTC) OR NON-SKILLED NURSING FACILITY (NF)
Q5004	HOSPICE CARE PROVIDED IN SKILLED NURSING FACILITY (SNF)
Q5005	HOSPICE CARE PROVIDED IN INPATIENT HOSPITAL
Q5006	HOSPICE CARE PROVIDED IN INPATIENT HOSPICE FACILITY
Q5007	HOSPICE CARE PROVIDED IN LONG TERM CARE HOSPITAL (LTCH)
Q5008	HOSPICE CARE PROVIDED IN INPATIENT PSYCHIATRIC FACILITY
Q5009	HOSPICE CARE PROVIDED IN PLACE NOT OTHERWISE SPECIFIED (NOS)
Q5010	Hospice home care provided in a hospice facility

If care is rendered at multiple locations, each location is to be identified on the claim with a corresponding HCPCS code. For example, routine home care may be provided for a portion of the billing period in the patient's residence and another portion in an assisted living facility. In this case, report one revenue code 651 line with HCPCS code Q5001 and the number of days of routine home care provided in the residence and another revenue code 651 line with HCPCS code Q5002 and the number of days of routine home care provided in the assisted living facility.

Q5004 shall be used for hospice patients in a skilled nursing facility (SNF), or hospice patients in the SNF portion of a dually-certified nursing facility. There are 4 situations where this would occur:

1. If the beneficiary is receiving hospice care in a solely-certified SNF.
2. If the beneficiary is receiving general inpatient care in the SNF.
3. If the beneficiary is in a SNF receiving SNF care under the Medicare SNF benefit for a condition unrelated to the terminal illness and related conditions, and is receiving hospice routine home care; this is uncommon.
4. If the beneficiary is receiving inpatient respite care in a SNF.

If a beneficiary is in a nursing facility but doesn't meet the criteria above for Q5004, the site shall be coded as Q5003, for a long term care nursing facility.

General inpatient care provided by hospice staff requires line item visit reporting in units of 15 minute increments when provided in the following sites of service: Skilled Nursing Facility (Q5004), Inpatient Hospital (Q5005), Long Term Care Hospital (Q5007), Inpatient Psychiatric Facility (Q5008).

These service location HCPCS codes are not required on revenue code lines describing the visits provided under each level of care. These lines report the HCPCS codes shown in the table under Revenue Codes.

Modifiers

The following modifier is required reporting for claims:

PM – Post-mortem visits. Hospices shall report visits and length of visits (rounded to the nearest 15 minute increment), for nurses, aides, social workers, and therapists who are employed by the hospice, that occur on the date of death, after the patient has passed away. Post mortem visits occurring on a date subsequent to the date of death are not to be reported. The reporting of post-mortem visits, on the date of death, should occur regardless of the patient's level of care or site of service. Date of death is defined as the date of death reported on the death certificate. Hospices shall report hospice visits that occur before death on a separate line from those which occur after death.

For example, assume that a nurse arrives at the home at 9 pm to provide routine home care (RHC) to a dying patient, and that the patient passes away at 11 pm. The nurse stays with the family until 1:30 am. The hospice should report a nursing visit with eight 15- minute time units for the visit from 9 pm to 11 pm. On a separate line, the hospice should report a nursing visit with a PM modifier with four 15-minute time units for the portion of the visit from 11 pm to midnight to account for the 1 hour post mortem visit.

If the patient passes away suddenly, and the hospice nurse does not arrive until after his death at 11:00 pm, and remains with the family until 1:30 am, then the hospice should report a line item nursing visit with a PM modifier and four 15-minute increments of time as the units to account for the 1 hour post mortem visit from 11:00 pm to midnight.

The following modifier may be used to identify requests for an exception to the consequences of not filing the NOE timely:

KX - Even if a hospice believes that exceptional circumstances beyond its control are the cause of its late-filed NOE, the hospice shall file the associated claim with occurrence span code 77 used to identify the non-covered, provider liable days. The hospice shall also report a KX modifier with the Q HCPCS code reported on the earliest dated level of care line on the claim. The KX modifier shall prompt the A/B MAC (HHH) to request the documentation supporting the request for an exception.

Based on that documentation, the A/B MAC (HHH) shall determine if a circumstance encountered by a hospice qualifies for an exception.

If the request for an exception is approved by the A/B MAC (HHH), the A/B MAC (HHH) shall process the claim with the CWF override code and remove the submitted provider liable days, which will allow payment for the days associated with the late-filed NOE. If the A/B MAC (HHH) finds that the documentation does not support allowing an exceptional circumstance, the A/B MAC (HHH) shall process the claim as submitted.

The contractor shall use the following remittance advice messages and associated codes under this policy. This CARC/RARC combination is compliant with CAQH CORE Business Scenario Three

Group Code: CO

CARC: 96 RARC: MA54

MSN: N/A

Hospices may appeal the contractor's determination that an exceptional circumstance did not apply.

Modifier GV may be used to identify attending physician services performed by a doctor of medicine, doctor of osteopathy, nurse practitioner or physician assistant.

Service Date

The HIPAA standard 837 Institutional claim format requires line item dates of service for all outpatient claims. Medicare classifies hospice claims as outpatient claims (see Chapter 1, §60.4).

Service date reporting requirements will vary between continuous home care lines (revenue code 652) and other revenue code lines.

Revenue code 652 – report a separately dated line item for each day that continuous home care is provided, reporting the number of hours, or parts of hours rounded to 15- minute increments, of continuous home care that was provided on that date.

Other level of care revenue codes – report a separate line for each level of care provided at each service location type, as described in the instructions for HCPCS coding reported above. Hospices report the earliest date that each level of care was provided at each service location. Attending physician services should be individually dated, reporting the date that each HCPCS code billed was delivered.

Service reporting revenue codes – report dates as described in the table above under Revenue Codes.

For service visits that begin in one calendar day and span into the next calendar day, report one visit using the date the visit ended as the service date.

Service Units

The hospice enters the number of units for each type of service. Units are measured in days for revenue codes 651, 655, and 656., Units for revenue code 652 are reported in 15-minute increments.

When days are non-covered due to not filing a timely NOE, the hospice reports two lines for the affected level of care. For example, if a billing period contains 31 days of routine home care and the first 5 days are non-covered due to not filing a timely NOE:

- The hospice reports one revenue code 0651 line containing the earliest non- covered date of service, 5 units and all non-covered charge
- The hospice reports a second revenue code 0651 line containing the first covered date of service, 26 units and all covered charges.

Report units for service reporting lines as a multiplier of the visit time defined in the HCPCS description.

For dates of service on and after 10/1/2018, units for summary drug charges lines may be reported using '1' to satisfy the required field or using a number of drugs provided during the billing period, at the option of the hospice. Service unit data will not be used by Medicare for payment or data analysis.

Total Charges

The hospice enters the total charge for the service described on each revenue code line. This information is being collected for purposes of research and will not affect the amount of reimbursement.

Non-Covered Charges

The hospice enters a charge amount equal to the Total Charges for any revenue code line with a Service Date within a non-covered period (e.g., an occurrence span code 77 period).

Payer Name

The hospice identifies the appropriate payer(s) for the claim.

National Provider Identifier – Billing Provider

The hospice enters its own National Provider Identifier (NPI).

Principal Diagnosis Code

The hospice enters diagnosis coding as required by ICD-9-CM/ICD-10-CM Coding Guidelines.

CMS accepts only HIPAA approved ICD-9-CM or ICD-10-CM/ICD-10-PCS codes, depending on the date of service. The official ICD-9-CM codes, which were updated annually through October 1, 2013, are posted at http://www.cms.gov/Medicare/Coding/ICD9ProviderDiagnosticCodes/codes.html

The official annual updates to ICD-10-CM and ICD-10-PCS codes are posted at http://www.cms.gov/Medicare/Coding/ICD10/index.html.

Use full diagnosis codes including all applicable digits, up to five digits for ICD-9- CM and up to seven digits for ICD-10-CM.

The principal diagnosis listed is the diagnosis most contributory to the terminal prognosis.

Non-reportable Principal Diagnosis Codes to be returned to the provider for correction:

- Hospices may not report ICD-9CM v-codes and ICD-10-CM z-codes as the principal diagnosis on hospice claims.
- Hospices may not report debility, failure to thrive, or dementia codes classified as unspecified as principal hospice diagnoses on the hospice claim.
- Hospices may not report diagnosis codes that cannot be used as the principal diagnosis according to ICD-9-CM or ICD-10-CM Coding Guidelines or require further compliance with various ICD-9-CM or ICD-10-CM coding conventions, such as those that have principal diagnosis code sequencing guidelines.

Other Diagnosis Codes

The hospice enters diagnosis coding as required by ICD-9-CM and ICD-10-CM Coding Guidelines. All of a patient's coexisting or additional diagnoses that are related to the terminal illness and related conditions should be reported on the hospice claim.

Attending Provider Name and Identifiers

The hospice enters the National Provider Identifier (NPI) and name of the physician currently responsible for certifying the terminal illness, and signing the individual's plan of care for medical care and treatment.

The hospice shall enter the NPI and name of the attending physician designated by the patient as having the most significant role in the determination and delivery of the patient's medical care.

Other Provider Name and Identifiers

If the attending physician is a nurse practitioner or physician assistant, the hospice enters the NPI and name of the nurse practitioner or physician assistant.

The hospice enters the NPI and name of the hospice physician responsible for certifying that the patient is terminally ill, with a life expectancy of 6 months or less if the disease runs its normal course. **NOTE:** Both the attending physician and other physician fields should be completed unless the patient's designated attending physician is the same as the physician certifying the terminal illness. When the attending physician is also the physician certifying the terminal illness, only the attending physician is required to be reported.

NOTE: For electronic claims, this information is reported in Loop ID 2310F – Referring Provider Name.

Hospices shall report the NPI of any nursing facility, hospital, or hospice inpatient facility where the patient is receiving hospice services, regardless of the level of care provided when the site of service is not the billing hospice. The billing hospice shall obtain the NPI for the facility where the patient is receiving care and report the facility's name, address and NPI on the 837 Institutional claim format in loop 2310 E Service Facility Location. When the patient has received care in more than one facility during the billing month, the hospice shall report the NPI of the facility where the patient was last treated. Failure to report this information for claims reporting place of service HCPCS Q5003 (long term care nursing facility), Q5004 (skilled nursing facility), Q5005 (inpatient hospital), Q5007 (long term care hospital) and Q50 8 (inpatient psychiatric facility) will result in the claim being returned to the provider.

100-4, Chapter-11, 40.1.3.1

Care Plan Oversight

Care plan oversight (CPO) exists where there is physician supervision of patients under care of hospices that require complex and multidisciplinary care modalities involving regular physician development and/or revision of care plans. Implicit in the concept of CPO is the expectation that the physician has coordinated an aspect of the patient's care with the hospice during the month for which CPO services were billed.

For a physician or NP employed by or under arrangement with a hospice agency, CPO functions are incorporated and are part of the hospice per diem payment and as such may not be separately billed.

For information on separately billable CPO services by the attending physician, or nurse practitioner, or physician assistant see Chapter 12, §180 of this manual.

100-4, Chapter-11, 100.1

Billing for Denial of Hospice Room and Board Charges

Hospice providers wishing to receive a line item denial for room and board charges may submit the charges as non-covered using revenue code 0659 with HCPCS A9270 and modifier GY on an otherwise covered hospice claim.

100-4, Chapter-12, 30.4

Cardiovascular System (Codes 92950-93799)

A. Echocardiography Contrast Agents

Effective October 1, 2000, physicians may separately bill for contrast agents used in echocardiography. Physicians should use HCPCS Code A9700 (Supply of Injectable Contrast Material for Use in Echocardiography, per study). The type of service code is 9. This code will be carrier-priced.

B. Electronic Analyses of Implantable Cardioverter-defibrillators and Pacemakers

The CPT® codes 93731, 93734, 93741 and 93743 are used to report electronic analyses of single or dual chamber pacemakers and single or dual chamber implantable cardioverter-defibrillators. In the office, a physician uses a device called a programmer to obtain information about the status and performance of the device and to evaluate the patient's cardiac rhythm and response to the implanted device.

Advances in information technology now enable physicians to evaluate patients with implanted cardiac devices without requiring the patient to be present in the physician's office. Using a manufacturer's specific monitor/transmitter, a patient can send complete device data and specific cardiac data to a distant receiving station or secure Internet server. The electronic analysis of cardiac device data that is remotely obtained provides immediate and long-term data on the device and clinical data on the patient's cardiac functioning equivalent to that obtained during an in-office evaluation. Physicians should report the electronic analysis of an implanted cardiac device using remotely obtained data as described above with CPT® code 93731, 93734, 93741 or 93743, depending on the type of cardiac device implanted in the patient.

100-4, Chapter-12, 30.6.15.4

Power Mobility Devices (PMDs) (Code G0372)

Section 302(a)(2)(E)(iv) of the Medicare Prescription Drug, Improvement, and Modernization Act of 2003 (MMA) sets forth revised conditions for Medicare payment of Power Mobility Devices (PMDs). This section of the MMA states that payment for motorized or power wheelchairs may not be made unless a physician (as defined in §1861(r)(1) of the Act), a physician assistant, nurse practitioner, or a clinical nurse specialist (as those terms are defined in §1861(aa)(5)) has conducted a face-to-face examination of the beneficiary and written a prescription for the PMD.

Payment for the history and physical examination will be made through the appropriate evaluation and management (E&M) code corresponding to the history and physical examination of the patient. Due to the MMA requirement that the physician or treating practitioner create a written prescription and a regulatory requirement that the physician or treating practitioner prepare pertinent parts of the medical record for submission to the durable medical equipment supplier, code G0372 (physician service required to establish and document the need for a power mobility device)has been established to recognize additional physician services and resources required to establish and document the need for the PMD.

The G code indicates that all of the information necessary to document the PMD prescription is included in the medical record, and the prescription and supporting documentation is delivered to the PMD supplier within 30 days after the face-to-face examination.

Effective October 25, 2005, G0372 will be used to recognize additional physician services and resources required to establish and document the need for the PMD and will be added to the Medicare physician fee schedule.

100-4, Chapter-12,80.1

Coverage of Physicians' Services Provided in Comprehensive Outpatient Rehabilitation Facility
B3-2220

Rehabilitation services furnished by comprehensive outpatient rehabilitation facilities (CORFs) are covered by Medicare Part B.

Under §1832(a)(2)(E), §1861(cc)(2), and related provisions of the Act, a CORF is recognized as a provider of services on the basis of its reasonable costs. Except for diagnostic and therapeutic services provided by physicians to individual patients, payment is made to the CORF by intermediaries (acting in the role of the Part B carrier.)

Physicians' diagnostic and therapeutic services furnished to a CORF patient are not considered CORF physician's services. Instead they are services that the physician must bill to the Part B carrier. If covered services, payment is made according to the

Medicare Physician Fee Schedule. When physician's diagnostic and therapeutic services are furnished in a CORF, the claim must be annotated to show the CORF as the place of treatment.

Services considered administrative services provided by the physician associated with the CORF are considered CORF services reimbursable to the CORF by the FI. Administrative services include consultation with and medical supervision of nonphysician staff, establishing and reviewing the plan of treatment, and other medical and facility administration activities.

100-4, Chapter-12, 100.1.1

Evaluation and Management (E/M) Services
A. General Documentation Requirements

Evaluation and Management (E/M) Services -- For a given encounter, the selection of the appropriate level of E/M service should be determined according to the code definitions in the American Medical Association's Current Procedural Terminology (CPT®) book and any applicable documentation guidelines.

For purposes of payment, E/M services billed by teaching physicians require that the medical records must demonstrate:

- That the teaching physician performed the service or was physically present during the key or critical portions of the service when performed by the resident; and
- The participation of the teaching physician in the management of the patient.

The presence of the teaching physician during E/M services may be demonstrated by the notes in the medical records made by physicians, residents, or nurses.

B. E/M Service Documentation Provided By Students

Any contribution and participation of students to the performance of a billable service (other than the review of systems and/or past family/social history which are not separately billable, but are taken as part of an E/M service) must be performed in the physical presence of a teaching physician or physical presence of a resident in a service meeting the requirements set forth in this section for teaching physician billing.

Students may document services in the medical record. However, the teaching physician must verify in the medical record all student documentation or findings, including history, physical exam and/or medical decision making. The teaching physician must personally perform (or re-perform) the physical exam and medical decision making activities of the E/M service being billed, but may verify any student documentation of them in the medical record, rather than re-documenting this work.

C. Exception for E/M Services Furnished in Certain Primary Care Centers

Teaching physicians providing E/M services with a GME program granted a primary care exception may bill Medicare for lower and mid-level E/M services provided by residents. For the E/M codes listed below, teaching physicians may submit claims for services furnished by residents in the absence of a teaching physician:

New Patient	Established Patient
99201	99211
99202	99212
99203	99213

Effective January 1, 2005, the following code is included under the primary care exception: HCPCS code G0402 (Initial preventive physical examination; face-to-face visit services limited to new beneficiary during the first 12 months of Medicare enrollment).

Effective January 1, 2011, the following codes are included under the primary care exception: HCPCS codes G0438 (Annual wellness visit, including personal preventive plan service, first visit) and G0439 (Annual wellness visit, including personal preventive plan service, subsequent visit).

If a service other than those listed above needs to be furnished, then the general teaching physician policy set forth in §100.1 applies. For this exception to apply, a center must attest in writing that all the following conditions are met for a particular residency program. Prior approval is not necessary, but centers exercising the primary care exception must maintain records demonstrating that they qualify for the exception. The services must be furnished in a center located in the outpatient department of a hospital or another ambulatory care entity in which the time spent by residents in patient care activities is included in determining direct GME payments to a teaching hospital by the hospital's A/B MAC (A). This requirement is not met when the resident is assigned to a physician's office away from the center or makes home visits. In the case of a nonhospital entity, verify with the A/B MAC (A) that the entity meets the requirements of a written agreement between the hospital and the entity set forth at 42 CFR 413.78(e)(3)(ii).

Under this exception, residents providing the billable patient care service without the physical presence of a teaching physician must have completed at least 6 months of a GME approved residency program. Centers must maintain information under the provisions at 42 CFR 413.79(a)(6).

Teaching physicians submitting claims under this exception may not supervise more than four residents at any given time and must direct the care from such proximity as to constitute immediate availability. Teaching physicians may include residents with less than 6 months in a GME approved residency program in the mix of four residents under the teaching physician's supervision. However, the teaching physician must be physically present for the critical or key portions of services furnished by the residents with less than 6 months in a GME approved residency program. That is, the primary care exception does not apply in the case of residents with less than 6 months in a GME approved residency program.

Teaching physicians submitting claims under this exception must:

- Not have other responsibilities (including the supervision of other personnel) at the time the service was provided by the residents;
- Have the primary medical responsibility for patients cared for by the residents;
- Ensure that the care provided was reasonable and necessary;
- Review the care provided by the residents during or immediately after each visit. This must include a review of the patient's medical history, the resident's findings on physical examination, the patient's diagnosis, and treatment plan (i.e., record of tests and therapies); and

Patients under this exception should consider the center to be their primary location for health care services. The residents must be expected to generally provide care to the same group of established patients during their residency training. The

types of services furnished by residents under this exception include:

- Acute care for undifferentiated problems or chronic care for ongoing conditions including chronic mental illness;
- Coordination of care furnished by other physicians and providers; and,
- Comprehensive care not limited by organ system or diagnosis.

Residency programs most likely qualifying for this exception include family practice, general internal medicine, geriatric medicine, pediatrics, and obstetrics/gynecology.

Certain GME programs in psychiatry may qualify in special situations such as when the program furnishes comprehensive care for chronically mentally ill patients. These would be centers in which the range of services the residents are trained to furnish, and actually do furnish, include comprehensive medical care as well as psychiatric care. For example, antibiotics are being prescribed as well as psychotropic drugs.

The patient medical record must document the extent of the teaching physician's participation in the review and direction of the services furnished to each beneficiary. The extent of the teaching physician's participation may be demonstrated by the notes in the medical records made by physicians, residents, or nurses.

100-4, Chapter-12, 180

Care Plan Oversight Services

The Medicare Benefit Policy Manual, Chapter 15, contains requirements for coverage for medical and other health services including those of physicians and non-physician practitioners.

Care plan oversight (CPO)is the physician supervision of a patient receiving complex and/or multidisciplinary care as part of Medicare-covered services provided by a participating home health agency or Medicare approved hospice. CPO services require complex or multidisciplinary care modalities involving:

- Regular physician development and/or revision of care plans;
- Review of subsequent reports of patient status;
- Review of related laboratory and other studies;
- Communication with other health professionals not employed in the same practice who are involved in the patient's care;
- Integration of new information into the medical treatment plan; and/or
- Adjustment of medical therapy.

The CPO services require recurrent physician supervision of a patient involving 30 or more minutes of the physician's time per month. Services not countable toward the 30 minutes threshold that must be provided in order to bill for CPO include, but are not limited to:

- Time associated with discussions with the patient, his or her family or friends to adjust medication or treatment;
- Time spent by staff getting or filing charts;
- Travel time; and/or
- Physician's time spent telephoning prescriptions into the pharmacist unless the telephone conversation involves discussions of pharmaceutical therapies.

Implicit in the concept of CPO is the expectation that the physician has coordinated an aspect of the patient's care with the home health agency or hospice during the month for which CPO services were billed. The physician who bills for CPO must be the same physician who signs the plan of care.

Nurse practitioners, physician assistants, and clinical nurse specialists, practicing within the scope of State law, may bill for care plan oversight. These non-physician practitioners must have been providing ongoing care for the beneficiary through evaluation and management services. These non-physician practitioners may not bill for CPO if they have been involved only with the delivery of the Medicare-covered home health or hospice service.

A. Home Health CPO

Non-physician practitioners can perform CPO only if the physician signing the plan of care provides regular ongoing care under the same plan of care as does the NPP billing for CPO and either:

- The physician and NPP are part of the same group practice; or
- If the NPP is a nurse practitioner or clinical nurse specialist, the physician signing the plan of care also has a collaborative agreement with the NPP; or
- If the NPP is a physician assistant, the physician signing the plan of care is also the physician who provides general supervision of physician assistant services for the practice. Billing may be made for care plan oversight services furnished by an NPP when:
- The NPP providing the care plan oversight has seen and examined the patient;
- The NPP providing care plan oversight is not functioning as a consultant whose participation is limited to a single medical condition rather than multidisciplinary coordination of care; and
- The NPP providing care plan oversight integrates his or her care with that of the physician who signed the plan of care. NPPs may not certify the beneficiary for home health care.

NPPs may not certify the beneficiary for home health care.

B. Hospice CPO

The attending physician or nurse practitioner (who has been designated as the attending physician) may bill for hospice CPO when they are acting as an "attending physician". An "attending physician" is one who has been identified by the individual, at the time he/she elects hospice coverage, as having the most significant role in the determination and delivery of their medical care. They are not employed nor paid by the hospice. The care plan oversight services are billed using Form CMS-1500 or electronic equivalent. For additional information on hospice CPO, see Chapter 11, §40.1.3.1 of this manual.

100-4, Chapter-12, 180.1

Care Plan Oversight Billing Requirements

A. Codes for Which Separate Payment May Be Made

Effective January 1, 1995, separate payment may be made for CPO oversight services for 30 minutes or more if the requirements specified in the Medicare Benefits Policy Manual, Chapter 15 are met.

Providers billing for CPO must submit the claim with no other services billed on that claim and may bill only after the end of the month in which the CPO services were rendered. CPO services may not be billed across calendar months and should be submitted (and paid) only for one unit of service.

Physicians may bill and be paid separately for CPO services only if all the criteria in the Medicare Benefit Policy Manual, Chapter 15 are met.

B. Physician Certification and Recertification of Home Health Plans of Care

Effective 2001, two new HCPCS codes for the certification and recertification and development of plans of care for Medicare-covered home health services were created.

See the Medicare General Information, Eligibility, and Entitlement Manual, Pub. 100-01, Chapter 4, "Physician Certification and Recertification of Services," §10-60, and the Medicare Benefit Policy Manual, Pub. 100-02, Chapter 7, "Home Health Services", §30.

The home health agency certification code can be billed only when the patient has not received Medicare-covered home health services for at least 60 days. The home health agency recertification code is used after a patient has received services for at least 60 days (or one certification period) when the physician signs the certification after the initial certification period. The home health agency recertification code will be reported only once every 60 days, except in the rare situation when the patient starts a new episode before 60 days elapses and requires a new plan of care to start a new episode.

C. Provider Number of Home Health Agency (HHA) or Hospice

For claims for CPO submitted on or after January 1, 1997, physicians must enter on the Medicare claim form the 6-character Medicare provider number of the HHA or hospice providing Medicare-covered services to the beneficiary for the period during which CPO services was furnished and for which the physician signed the plan of care. Physicians are responsible for obtaining the HHA or hospice Medicare provider numbers.

Additionally, physicians should provide their UPIN to the HHA or hospice furnishing services to their patient.

NOTE: There is currently no place on the HIPAA standard ASC X12N 837 professional format to specifically include the HHA or hospice provider number required for a care plan oversight claim. For this reason, the requirement to include the HHA or hospice provider number on a care plan oversight claim is temporarily waived until a new version of this electronic standard format is adopted under HIPAA and includes a place to provide the HHA and hospice provider numbers for care plan oversight claims.

100-4, Chapter-12, 190.3

List of Medicare Telehealth Services

The use of a telecommunications system may substitute for an in-person encounter for professional consultations, office visits, office psychiatry services, and a limited number of other physician fee schedule (PFS) services. The various services and corresponding current procedure terminology (CPT®) or Healthcare Common Procedure Coding System (HCPCS) codes are listed on the CMS website at www.cms.gov/Medicare/Medicare-General-Information/Telehealth/

NOTE: Beginning January 1, 2010, CMS eliminated the use of all consultation codes, except for inpatient telehealth consultation G-codes. CMS no longer recognizes office/outpatient or inpatient consultation CPT® codes for payment of office/outpatient or inpatient visits. Instead, physicians and practitioners are instructed to bill a new or established patient office/outpatient visit CPT® code or appropriate hospital or nursing facility care code, as appropriate to the particular patient, for all office/outpatient or inpatient visits.

100-4, Chapter-12, 190.3.1

Telehealth Consultation Services, Emergency Department or Initial Inpatient versus Inpatient Evaluation and Management (E/M) Visits

A consultation service is an evaluation and management (E/M) service furnished to evaluate and possibly treat a patient's problem(s). It can involve an opinion, advice, recommendation, suggestion, direction, or counsel from a physician or qualified nonphysician practitioner (NPP) at the request of another physician or appropriate source.

Section 1834(m) of the Social Security Act includes "professional consultations" in the definition of telehealth services. Inpatient or emergency department consultations furnished via telehealth can facilitate the provision of certain services and/or medical expertise that might not otherwise be available to a patient located at an originating site.

The use of a telecommunications system may substitute for an in-person encounter for emergency department or initial and follow-up inpatient consultations.

Medicare contractors pay for reasonable and medically necessary inpatient or emergency department telehealth consultation services furnished to beneficiaries in hospitals or SNFs when all of the following criteria for the use of a consultation code are met:

- An inpatient or emergency department consultation service is distinguished from other inpatient or emergency department evaluation and management (E/M) visits because it is provided by a physician or qualified nonphysician practitioner (NPP) whose opinion or advice regarding evaluation and/or management of a specific problem is requested by another physician or other appropriate source. The qualified NPP may perform consultation services within the scope of practice and licensure requirements for NPPs in the State in which he/she practices;

- A request for an inpatient or emergency department telehealth consultation from an appropriate source and the need for an inpatient or emergency department telehealth consultation (i.e., the reason for a consultation service) shall be documented by the consultant in the patient's medical record and included in the requesting physician or qualified NPP's plan of care in the patient's medical record; and

- After the inpatient or emergency department telehealth consultation is provided, the consultant shall prepare a written report of his/her findings and recommendations, which shall be provided to the referring physician.

The intent of an inpatient or emergency department telehealth consultation service is that a physician or qualified NPP or other appropriate source is asking another physician or qualified NPP for advice, opinion, a recommendation, suggestion, direction, or counsel, etc. in evaluating or treating a patient because that individual has expertise in a specific medical area beyond the requesting professional's knowledge.

Unlike inpatient or emergency department telehealth consultations, the majority of subsequent inpatient hospital, emergency department and nursing facility care services require in-person visits to facilitate the comprehensive, coordinated, and personal care that medically volatile, acutely ill patients require on an ongoing basis.

Subsequent hospital care services are limited to one telehealth visit every 3 days. Subsequent nursing facility care services are limited to one telehealth visit every 30 days.

100-4, Chapter-12, 190.3.2

Telehealth Consultation Services, Emergency Department or Initial Inpatient Defined

Emergency department or initial inpatient telehealth consultations are furnished to beneficiaries in hospitals or SNFs via telehealth at the request of the physician of record, the attending physician, or another appropriate source. The physician or practitioner who furnishes the emergency department or initial inpatient consultation via telehealth cannot be the physician of record or the attending physician, and the emergency department or initial inpatient telehealth consultation would be distinct from the care provided by the physician of record or the attending physician. Counseling and coordination of care with other providers or agencies is included as well, consistent with the nature of the problem(s) and the patient's needs. Emergency department or initial inpatient telehealth consultations are subject to the criteria for emergency department or initial inpatient telehealth consultation services, as described in section 190.3.1 of this chapter.

Payment for emergency department or initial inpatient telehealth consultations includes all consultation related services furnished before, during, and after communicating with the patient via telehealth. Pre-service activities would include, but would not be limited to, reviewing patient data (for example, diagnostic and imaging studies, interim labwork) and communicating with other professionals or family members. Intra-service activities must include the three key elements described below for each procedure code. Post-service activities would include, but would not be limited to, completing medical records or other documentation and communicating results of the consultation and further care plans to other health care professionals. No additional E/M service could be billed for work related to an emergency department or initial inpatient telehealth consultation.

Emergency department or initial inpatient telehealth consultations could be provided at various levels of complexity:

- Practitioners taking a problem focused history, conducting a problem focused examination, and engaging in medical decision making that is straightforward, would bill HCPCS code G0425 (Telehealth consultation, emergency department or initial inpatient, typically 30 minutes communicating with the patient via telehealth).

- Practitioners taking a detailed history, conducting a detailed examination, and engaging in medical decision making that is of moderate complexity, would bill HCPCS code G0426 (Telehealth consultation, emergency department or initial inpatient, typically 50 minutes communicating with the patient via telehealth).

- Practitioners taking a comprehensive history, conducting a comprehensive examination, and engaging in medical decision making that is of high complexity, would bill HCPCS code G0427 (Telehealth consultation, emergency department or initial inpatient, typically 70 minutes or more communicating with the patient via telehealth).

Although emergency department or initial inpatient telehealth consultations are specific to telehealth, these services must be billed with either the -GT or -GQ modifier to identify the telehealth technology used to provide the service.

100-4, Chapter-12, 190.3.3

Follow-Up Inpatient Telehealth Consultations Defined

Follow-up inpatient telehealth consultations are furnished to beneficiaries in hospitals or SNFs via telehealth to follow-up on an initial consultation, or subsequent consultative visits requested by the attending physician. The initial inpatient consultation may have been provided in-person or via telehealth.

Follow-up inpatient telehealth consultations include monitoring progress, recommending management modifications, or advising on a new plan of care in response to changes in the patient's status or no changes on the consulted health issue. Counseling and coordination of care with other providers or agencies is included as well, consistent with the nature of the problem(s) and the patient's needs.

The physician or practitioner who furnishes the inpatient follow-up consultation via telehealth cannot be the physician of record or the attending physician, and the follow-up inpatient consultation would be distinct from the follow-up care provided by the physician of record or the attending physician. If a physician consultant has initiated treatment at an initial consultation and participates thereafter in the patient's ongoing care management, such care would not be included in the definition of a follow-up inpatient consultation. Follow-up inpatient telehealth consultations are subject to the criteria for inpatient telehealth consultation services, as described in section 190.3.1 of this chapter.

Payment for follow-up inpatient telehealth consultations includes all consultation related services furnished before, during, and after communicating with the patient via telehealth. Pre-service activities would include, but would not be limited to, reviewing patient data (for example, diagnostic and imaging studies, interim labwork) and communicating with other professionals or family members. Intra-service activities must include at least two of the three key elements described below for each procedure code. Post-service activities would include, but would not be limited to, completing medical records or other documentation and communicating results of the consultation and further care plans to other health care professionals. No additional evaluation and management service could be billed for work related to a follow-up inpatient telehealth consultation.

Follow-up inpatient telehealth consultations could be provided at various levels of complexity:

- Practitioners taking a problem focused interval history, conducting a problem focused examination, and engaging in medical decision making that is straightforward or of low complexity, would bill a limited service, using HCPCS code G0406 (Follow-up inpatient telehealth consultation, limited, physicians typically spend 15 minutes communicating with the patient via telehealth).
- Practitioners taking an expanded focused interval history, conducting an expanded problem focused examination, and engaging in medical decision making that is of moderate complexity, would bill an intermediate service using HCPCS code G0407(Follow-up inpatient telehealth consultation, intermediate, physicians typically spend 25 minutes communicating with the patient via telehealth).
- Practitioners taking a detailed interval history, conducting a detailed examination, and engaging in medical decision making that is of high complexity, would bill a complex service, using HCPCS code G0408 (Follow-up

inpatient telehealth consultation, complex, physicians typically spend 35 minutes or more communicating with the patient via telehealth).Although follow-up inpatient telehealth consultations are specific to telehealth, these services must be billed with either the -GT or –GQ modifier to identify the telehealth technology used to provide the service.

100-4, Chapter-12, 190.3.4

Payment for ESRD-Related Services as a Telehealth Service

The ESRD-related services included in the monthly capitation payment (MCP) with 2 or 3 visits per month and ESRD-related services with 4 or more visits per month may be paid as Medicare telehealth services. However, at least 1 visit must be furnished face-to-face "hands on" to examine the vascular access site by a physician, clinical nurse specialist, nurse practitioner, or physician assistant. An interactive audio and video telecommunications system may be used for providing additional visits required under the 2-to-3 visit MCP and the 4-or-more visit MCP. The medical record must indicate that at least one of the visits was furnished face-to-face "hands on" by a physician, clinical nurse specialist, nurse practitioner, or physician assistant.

The MCP physician, for example, the physician or practitioner who is responsible for the complete monthly assessment of the patient and establishes the patient's plan of care, may use other physicians and practitioners to furnish ESRD-related visits through an interactive audio and video telecommunications system. The non-MCP physician or practitioner must have a relationship with the billing physician or practitioner such as a partner, employees of the same group practice or an employee of the MCP physician, for example, the non MCP physician or practitioner is either a W-2 employee or 1099 independent contractor. However, the physician or practitioner who is responsible for the complete monthly assessment and establishes the ESRD beneficiary's plan of care should bill for the MCP in any given month.

Clinical Criteria

The visit, including a clinical examination of the vascular access site, must be conducted face-to-face "hands on" by a physician, clinical nurse specialist, nurse practitioner or physician's assistant. For additional visits, the physician or practitioner at the distant site is required, at a minimum, to use an interactive audio and video telecommunications system that allows the physician or practitioner to provide medical management services for a maintenance dialysis beneficiary. For example, an ESRD-related visit conducted via telecommunications system must permit the physician or practitioner at the distant site to perform an assessment of whether the dialysis is working effectively and whether the patient is tolerating the procedure well (physiologically and psychologically). During this assessment, the physician or practitioner at the distant site must be able to determine whether alteration in any aspect of the beneficiary's prescription is indicated, due to such changes as the estimate of the patient's dry weight.

100-4, Chapter-12, 190.3.5

Payment for Subsequent Hospital Care Services and Subsequent Nursing Facility Care Services as Telehealth Services

(Rev. 3476, Issued: 03-11-16, Effective: 01-01-15, Effective: 04-11-16)

Subsequent hospital care services are limited to one telehealth visit every 3 days. The frequency limit of the benefit is not intended to apply to consulting physicians or practitioners, who should continue to report initial or follow-up inpatient telehealth consultations using the applicable HCPCS G-codes.

Similarly, subsequent nursing facility care services are limited to one telehealth visit every 30 days. Furthermore, subsequent nursing facility care services reported for a Federally-mandated periodic visit under 42 CFR 483.40(c) may not be furnished through telehealth. The frequency limit of the benefit is not intended to apply to consulting physicians or practitioners, who should continue to report initial or follow-up inpatient telehealth consultations using the applicable HCPCS G-codes.

Inpatient telehealth consultations are furnished to beneficiaries in hospitals or skilled nursing facilities via telehealth at the request of the physician of record, the attending physician, or another appropriate source. The physician or practitioner who furnishes the initial inpatient consultation via telehealth cannot be the physician or practitioner of record or the attending physician or practitioner, and the initial inpatient telehealth consultation would be distinct from the care provided by the physician or practitioner of record or the attending physician or practitioner. Counseling and coordination of care with other providers or agencies is included as well, consistent with the nature of the problem(s) and the patient's needs. Initial and follow-up inpatient telehealth consultations are subject to the criteria for inpatient telehealth consultation services, as described in section 190.3 of this chapter.

100-4, Chapter-12, 190.3.6

Payment for Diabetes Self-Management Training (DSMT) as a Telehealth Service

Individual and group DSMT services may be paid as a Medicare telehealth service; however, at least 1 hour of the 10 hour benefit in the year following the initial DSMT service must be furnished in-person to allow for effective injection training. The injection training may be furnished through either individual or group DSMT services. By reporting POS 02 with HCPCS code G0108 (Diabetes outpatient self-management training services, individual, per 30 minutes) or G0109 (Diabetes outpatient self-management training services, group session (2 or more), per 30 minutes), the distant site practitioner certifies that the beneficiary has received or will receive 1 hour of in-person DSMT services for purposes of injection training during the year following the initial DSMT service.

As specified in 42 CFR 410.141(e) and stated in Pub. 100-02, Medicare Benefit Policy Manual, chapter 15, section 300.2, individual DSMT services may be furnished by a physician, individual, or entity that furnishes other services for which direct Medicare payment may be made and that submits necessary documentation to, and is accredited by, an accreditation organization approved by CMS. However, consistent with the statutory requirements of section 1834(m)(1) of the Act, as provided in 42 CFR 410.78(b)(1) and (b)(2)

and stated in section 190.6 of this chapter, Medicare telehealth services, including individual DSMT services furnished as a telehealth service, could only be furnished by a licensed PA, NP, CNS, CNM, clinical psychologist, clinical social worker, or registered dietitian or nutrition professional.

100-4, Chapter-12, 190.5

Originating Site Facility Fee Payment Methodology

1. Originating site defined

The term originating site means the location of an eligible Medicare beneficiary at the time the service being furnished via a telecommunications system occurs. For asynchronous, store and forward telecommunications technologies, an originating site is only a Federal telemedicine demonstration program conducted in Alaska or Hawaii.

2. Facility fee for originating site

The originating site facility fee is a separately billable Part B payment. The contractor pays it outside of other payment methodologies. This fee is subject to post payment verification.

For telehealth services furnished from October 1, 2001, through December 31, 2002, the originating site facility fee is the lesser of $20 or the actual charge. For services furnished on or after January 1 of each subsequent year, the originating site facility fee is updated by the Medicare Economic Index. The updated fee is included in the Medicare Physician Fee Schedule (MPFS) Final Rule, which is published by November 1 prior to the start of the calendar year for which it is effective. The updated fee for each calendar year is also issued annually in a Recurring Update Notification instruction for January of each year.

3. Payment amount:

The originating site facility fee is a separately billable Part B payment. The payment amount to the originating site is the lesser of 80 percent of the actual charge or 80 percent of the originating site facility fee, except CAHs. The beneficiary is responsible for any unmet deductible amount and Medicare coinsurance.

The originating site facility fee payment methodology for each type of facility is clarified below.

Hospital outpatient department. When the originating site is a hospital outpatient department, payment for the originating site facility fee must be made as described above and not under the outpatient prospective payment system (OPPS). Payment is not based on the OPPS payment methodology.

Hospital inpatient. For hospital inpatients, payment for the originating site facility fee must be made outside the diagnostic related group (DRG) payment, since this is a Part B benefit, similar to other services paid separately from the DRG payment, (e.g., hemophilia blood clotting factor).

Critical access hospitals. When the originating site is a critical access hospital, make payment separately from the cost-based reimbursement methodology. For CAH's, the payment amount is 80 percent of the originating site facility fee.

Federally qualified health centers (FQHCs) and rural health clinics (RHCs). The originating site facility fee for telehealth services is not an FQHC or RHC service. When an FQHC or RHC serves as the originating site, the originating site facility fee must be paid separately from the center or clinic all-inclusive rate.

Physicians' and practitioners' offices. When the originating site is a physician's or practitioner's office, the payment amount, in accordance with the law, is the lesser of 80 percent of the actual charge or 80 percent of the originating site facility fee, regardless of geographic location. The carrier shall not apply the geographic practice cost index (GPCI) to the originating site facility fee. This fee is statutorily set and is not subject to the geographic payment adjustments authorized under the MPFS.

Hospital-based or critical access-hospital based renal dialysis center (or their satellites). When a hospital-based or critical access hospital-based renal dialysis center (or their satellites) serves as the originating site, the originating site facility fee is covered in addition to any composite rate or MCP amount.

Skilled nursing facility (SNF). The originating site facility fee is outside the SNF prospective payment system bundle and, as such, is not subject to SNF consolidated billing. The originating site facility fee is a separately billable Part B payment.

Community Mental Health Center (CMHC). The originating site facility fee is not a partial hospitalization service. The originating site facility fee does not count towards the number of services used to determine payment for partial hospitalization services. The originating site facility fee is not bundled in the per diem payment for partial hospitalization. The originating site facility fee is a separately billable Part B payment.

To receive the originating facility site fee, the provider submits claims with HCPCS code "Q3014, telehealth originating site facility fee"; short description "telehealth facility fee." The type of service for the telehealth originating site facility fee is "9, other items and services." For carrier-processed claims, the "office" place of service (code 11) is the only payable setting for code Q3014. There is no participation payment differential for code Q3014. Deductible and coinsurance rules apply to Q3014. By submitting Q3014 HCPCS code, the originating site authenticates they are located in either a rural HPSA or non-MSA county.

This benefit may be billed on bill types 12X, 13X, 22X, 23X, 71X, 72X, 73X, 76X, and 85X. Unless otherwise applicable, report the originating site facility fee under revenue code 078X and include HCPCS code "Q3014, telehealth originating site facility fee."

Hospitals and critical access hospitals bill their intermediary for the originating site facility fee. Telehealth bills originating in inpatient hospitals must be submitted on a 12X TOB using the date of discharge as the line item date of service.

Independent and provider-based RHCs and FQHCs bill the appropriate intermediary using the RHC or FQHC bill type and billing number. HCPCS code Q3014 is the only non-RHC/FQHC service that is billed using the clinic/center bill type and provider number. All RHCs and FQHCs must use revenue code 078X when billing for the originating site facility fee. For all other non-RHC/FQHC services, provider based RHCs and FQHCs must bill using the base provider's bill type and billing number. Independent RHCs and FQHCs must bill the carrier for all other non-RHC/FQHC services. If an RHC/FQHC visit occurs on the same day as a telehealth service, the RHC/FQHC serving as an originating site must bill for HCPCS code Q3014 telehealth originating site facility fee on a separate revenue line from the RHC/FQHC visit using revenue code 078X.

Hospital-based or CAH-based renal dialysis centers (including satellites) bill their local FIs and/or Part A MACs for the originating site facility fee. Telehealth bills originating in renal dialysis centers must be submitted on a 72X TOB. All hospital-based or CAH-based renal dialysis centers (including satellites) must use revenue code 078X when billing for the

originating site facility fee. The renal dialysis center serving as an originating site must bill for HCPCS code Q3014, telehealth originating site facility fee, on a separate revenue line from any other services provided to the beneficiary.

Skilled nursing facilities (SNFs) bill their local FIs and/or Part A MACs for the originating site facility fee. Telehealth bills originating in SNFs must be submitted on TOB 22X or 23X. For SNF inpatients in a covered Part A stay, the originating site facility fee must be submitted on a 22X TOB. All SNFs must use revenue code 078X when billing for the originating site facility fee. The SNF serving as an originating site must bill for HCPCS code Q3014, telehealth originating site facility fee, on a separate revenue line from any other services provided to the beneficiary.

Community mental health centers (CMHCs) bill their local FIs and/or Part A MACs for the originating site facility fee. Telehealth bills originating in CMHCs must be submitted on a 76X TOB. All CMHCs must use revenue code 078X when billing for the originating site facility fee. The CMHC serving as an originating site must bill for HCPCS code Q3014, telehealth originating site facility fee, on a separate revenue line from any other services provided to the beneficiary. Note that Q3014 does not count towards the number of services used to determine per diem payments for partial hospitalization services.

The beneficiary is responsible for any unmet deductible amount and Medicare coinsurance.

100-4, Chapter-12, 190.7

A/B MAC (B) Editing of Telehealth Claims

Medicare telehealth services (as listed in section 190.3) are billed with POS 02. The contractor shall approve covered telehealth services if the physician or practitioner is licensed under State law to provide the service. Contractors must familiarize themselves with licensure provisions of States for which they process claims and disallow telehealth services furnished by physicians or practitioners who are not authorized to furnish the applicable telehealth service under State law. For example, if a nurse practitioner is not licensed to provide individual psychotherapy under State law, he or she would not be permitted to receive payment for individual psychotherapy under Medicare. The contractor shall install edits to ensure that only properly licensed physicians and practitioners are paid for covered telehealth services.

If a contractor receives claims for professional telehealth services coded with the "GQ" modifier (representing "via asynchronous telecommunications system"), it shall approve/pay for these services only if the physician or practitioner is affiliated with a Federal telemedicine demonstration conducted in Alaska or Hawaii. The contractor may require the physician or practitioner at the distant site to document his or her participation in a Federal telemedicine demonstration program conducted in Alaska or Hawaii prior to paying for telehealth services provided via asynchronous, store and forward technologies. Contractors shall deny telehealth services if the physician or practitioner is not eligible to bill for them.

> The following reflects the remittance advice messages and associated codes that will appear when rejecting/denying claims under this policy. This CARC/RARC combination is compliant with CAQH CORE Business Scenario 3.
>
> Group Code: CO
>
> CARC: 185

RARC: N/A

MSN: 21.18

If a service is billed with POS 02 and the procedure code is not designated as a covered telehealth service, the contractor denies the service.

> The following reflects the remittance advice messages and associated codes that will appear when rejecting/denying claims under this policy. This CARC/RARC combination is compliant with CAQH CORE Business Scenario 3.

> Group Code: CO

> CARC: 96

> RARC: N776

> MSN: 9.4

The only claims from institutional facilities that FIs shall pay for telehealth services at the distant site, except for MNT services, are for physician or practitioner services when the distant site is located in a CAH that has elected Method II, and the physician or practitioner has reassigned his/her benefits to the CAH. The CAH bills its regular FI for the professional services provided at the distant site via a telecommunications system, in any of the revenue codes 096x, 097x or 098x. All requirements for billing distant site telehealth services apply. Claims from hospitals or CAHs for MNT services are submitted to the hospital's or CAH's regular FI. Payment is based on the non-facility amount on the Medicare Physician Fee Schedule for the particular HCPCS codes.

100-4, Chapter-12, 210

Outpatient Mental Health Treatment Limitation

Regardless of the actual expenses a beneficiary incurs in connection with the treatment of mental, psychoneurotic, and personality disorders while the beneficiary is not an inpatient of a hospital at the time such expenses are incurred, the amount of those expenses that may be recognized for Part B deductible and payment purposes is limited to 62.5 percent of the Medicare approved amount for those services. This limitation is called the outpatient mental health treatment limitation (the limitation). The 62.5 percent limitation has been in place since the inception of the Medicare Part B program and it will remain effective at this percentage amount until January 1, 2010. However, effective January 1, 2010, through January 1, 2014, the limitation will be phased out as follows:

- January 1, 2010 –December 31, 2011, the limitation percentage is 68.75%.
  (Medicare pays 55% and the patient pays 45%).

- January 1, 2012 –December 31, 2012, the limitation percentage is 75%.
  (Medicare pays 60% and the patient pays 40%).

- January 1, 2013 –December 31, 2013, the limitation percentage is 81.25%.
  (Medicare pays 65% and the patient pays 35%).

- January 1, 2014 –onward, the limitation percentage is 100%.
  (Medicare pays 80% and the patient pays 20%).

For additional details concerning computation of the limitation, please see the examples under section 210.1 E.

100-4, Chapter-12, 210.1

Application of the Limitation

A. Status of Patient

The limitation is applicable to expenses incurred in connection with the treatment of an individual who is not an inpatient of a hospital. Thus, the limitation applies to mental health services furnished to a person in a physician's office, in the patient's home, in a skilled nursing facility, as an outpatient, and so forth. The term "hospital" in this context means an institution, which is primarily engaged in providing to inpatients, by or under the supervision of a physician(s):

- Diagnostic and therapeutic services for medical diagnosis, treatment and care of injured, disabled, or sick persons;
- Rehabilitation services for injured, disabled, or sick persons; or
- Psychiatric services for the diagnosis and treatment of mentally ill patients.

B. Disorders Subject to the Limitation

The term "mental, psychoneurotic, and personality disorders" is defined as the specific psychiatric diagnoses described in the International Classification of Diseases, 9th Revision (ICD-9), under the code range 290-319.When the treatment services rendered are both for a psychiatric diagnosis as defined in the ICD-9 and one or more nonpsychiatric conditions, separate the expenses for the psychiatric aspects of treatment from the expenses for the nonpsychiatric aspects of treatment. However, in any case in which the psychiatric treatment component is not readily distinguishable from the nonpsychiatric treatment component, all of the expenses are allocated to whichever component constitutes the primary diagnosis.

1. Diagnosis Clearly Meets Definition –If the primary diagnosis reported for a particular service is the same as or equivalent to a condition described in the ICD-9 under the code range 290-319 that represents mental, psychoneurotic and personality disorders, the expense for the service is subject to the limitation except as described in subsection

2. Diagnosis Does Not Clearly Meet Definition -When it is not clear whether the primary diagnosis reported meets the definition of mental, psychoneurotic, and personality disorders, it may be necessary to contact the practitioner to clarify the diagnosis. In deciding whether contact is necessary in a given case, give consideration to such factors as the type of services rendered, the diagnosis, and the individual's previous utilization history.

C. Services Subject to the Limitation

Medicare Contractors must apply the limitation to claims for professional services that represent mental health treatment furnished to individuals who are not hospital inpatients by physicians, clinical psychologists, clinical social workers, nurse practitioners, clinical nurse specialists and physician assistants. Items and supplies furnished by physicians or other mental health practitioners in connection with treatment are also subject to the limitation.

Generally, Medicare Contractors must apply the limitation only to treatment services. However, diagnostic psychological and neuropsychological testing services performed to evaluate a patient's progress during treatment are considered part of treatment and are subject to the limitation.

D. Services Not Subject to the Limitation

1. Diagnosis of Alzheimer's Disease or Related Disorder -When the primary diagnosis reported for a particular service is Alzheimer's Disease or an Alzheimer's related disorder, Medicare Contractors must look to the nature of the service that has been rendered in determining whether it is subject to the limitation. Alzheimer's disease is coded 331.0 in the "International Classification of Diseases, 9th Revision", which is outside the code range 290-319 that represents mental, psychoneurotic and personality disorders. Additionally, Alzheimer's related disorders are identified by contractors under ICD-9 codes that are within the 290-319 code range (290.XX or others as contractors determine appropriate) or outside the 290-319 code range as determined appropriate by contractors. When the primary treatment rendered to a patient with a diagnosis of Alzheimer's disease or a related disorder is psychotherapy, it is subject to the limitation. However, typically, treatment provided to a patient with a diagnosis of Alzheimer's Disease or a related disorder represents medical management of the patient's condition (such as described under CPT® code 90862 or any successor code) and is not subject to the limitation. CPT® code 90862 describes pharmacologic management, including prescription, use, and review of medication with no more than minimal medical psychotherapy.

2. Brief Office Visits for Monitoring or Changing Drug Prescriptions -Brief office visits for the sole purpose of monitoring or changing drug prescriptions used in the treatment of mental, psychoneurotic and personality disorders are not subject to the limitation. These visits are reported using HCPCS code M0064 or any successor code (brief office visit for the sole purpose of monitoring or changing drug prescriptions used in the treatment of mental, psychoneurotic, and personality disorders). Claims where the diagnosis reported is a mental, psychoneurotic, or personality disorder (other than a diagnosis specified in subsection A) are subject to the limitation except for the procedure identified by HCPCS code M0064 or any successor code.

3. Diagnostic Services –Medicare Contractors do not apply the limitation to psychiatric diagnostic evaluations and diagnostic psychological and neuropsychological tests performed to establish or confirm the patient's diagnosis. Diagnostic services include psychiatric diagnostic evaluations billed under CPT® codes 90801 or 90802 (or any successor codes) and, psychological and neuropsychological tests billed under CPT® code range 96101-96118 (or any successor code range).

An initial visit to a practitioner for professional services often combines diagnostic evaluation and the start of therapy. Such a visit is neither solely diagnostic nor solely therapeutic. Therefore, contractors must deem the initial visit to be diagnostic so that the limitation does not apply. Separating diagnostic and therapeutic components of a visit is not administratively feasible, unless the practitioner already has separately identified them on the bill. Determining the entire visit to be therapeutic is not justifiable since some diagnostic work must be done before even a tentative diagnosis can be made and certainly before therapy can be instituted. Moreover, the patient should not be disadvantaged because therapeutic as well as diagnostic services were provided in the initial visit. In the rare cases where a practitioner's diagnostic services take more than one visit, Medicare contractors must not apply the limitation to the additional visits. However, it is expected such cases are few. Therefore, when a practitioner bills for more than one visit for professional diagnostic services, Medicare contractors may find it necessary to request documentation to justify the reason for more than one diagnostic visit.

4. Partial Hospitalization Services Not Directly Provided by a Physician or a Practitioner -The limitation does not apply to partial hospitalization services that are not directly provided by a physician, clinical psychologist, nurse practitioner, clinical nurse specialist or a physician assistant. Partial hospitalization services are billed by hospital outpatient departments and community mental health centers (CMHCs) to Medicare Contractors. However, services furnished by physicians, clinical psychologists, nurse practitioners, clinical nurse specialists, and physician assistants to partial hospitalization patients are billed separately from the partial hospitalization program of services. Accordingly, these professional's mental health services to partial hospitalization patients are paid under the physician fee schedule by Medicare Contractors and may be subject to the limitation. (See chapter 4, section 260.1C).

E. Computation of Limitation

Medicare Contractors determine the Medicare approved payment amount for services subject to the limitation. They:

- Multiply the approved amount by the limitation percentage amount;
- Subtract any unsatisfied deductible; and,
- Multiply the remainder by 0.8 to obtain the amount of Medicare payment.

The beneficiary is responsible for the difference between the amount paid by Medicare and the full Medicare approved amount.

The following examples illustrate the application of the limitation in various circumstances as it is gradually reduced under section 102 of the Medicare Improvements for Patients and Providers Act (MIPPA). Please note that although the calendar year 2009 Part B deductible of $135 is used under these examples, the actual deductible amount for calendar year 2010 and future years is unknown and will be subject to change.

Example #1: In 2010, a clinical psychologist submits a claim for $200 for outpatient treatment of a patient's mental disorder. The Medicare-approved amount is $180. Since clinical psychologists must accept assignment, the patient is not liable for the $20 in excess charges. The patient previously satisfied the $135 annual Part B deductible. The limitation reduces the amount of incurred expenses to 68 ¾ percent of the approved amount. Medicare pays 80 percent of the remaining incurred expenses. The Medicare payment and patient liability are computed as follows:

1. Actual charges $200.00
2. Medicare-approved amount.. $180.00
3. Medicare incurred expenses (0.6875 x line 2............................ $123.75
4. Unmet deductible.. $0.00
5. Remainder after subtracting deductible
   (line 3 minus line 4)... $123.75
6. Medicare payment (0.80 x line 5) $99.00
7. Patient liability (line 2 minus line 6) $81.00

Example #2: In 2012, a clinical social worker submits a claim for $135 for outpatient treatment of a patient's mental disorder. The Medicare-approved amount is $120. Since clinical social workers must accept assignment, the patient is not liable for the $15 in excess charges. The limitation reduces the amount of incurred expenses to 75 percent of the approved amount. The patient previously satisfied $70 of the $135 annual Part

B deductible, leaving $65 unmet. The Medicare payment and patient liability are computed as follows:

1. Actual charges...$135.00
2. Medicare-approved amount...$120.00
3. Medicare incurred expenses (0.75 x line 2).................$90.00
4. Unmet deductible..$65.00
5. Remainder after subtracting deductible
   (line 3 minus line 4)..$25.00
6. Medicare payment (0.80 x line 5)................................$20.00
7. Patient liability (line 2 minus line 6)..........................$100.00

Example #3: In calendar year 2013, a physician who does not accept assignment submits a claim for $780 for services in connection with the treatment of a mental disorder that did not require inpatient hospitalization. The Medicare-approved amount is $750. Because the physician does not accept assignment, the patient is liable for the $30 in excess charges. The patient has not satisfied any of the $135 Part B annual deductible. The Medicare payment and patient liability are computed as follows:

1. Actual charges...$780.00
2. Medicare-approved amount...$750.00
3. Medicare incurred expenses (0.8125 x line 2)............$609.38
4. Unmet deductible..$135.00
5. Remainder after subtracting deductible
   (line 3 minus line 4)..$474.38
6. Medicare payment (0.80 x line 5)................................$379.50
7. Patient liability (line 1 minus line 6)..........................$400.50

Example #4: A patient's Part B expenses during calendar year 2014 are for a physician's services in connection with the treatment of a mental disorder that initially required inpatient hospitalization, with subsequent physician services furnished on an outpatient basis. The patient has not satisfied any of the $135 Part B deductible. The physician accepts assignment and submits a claim for $780. The Medicare-approved amount is $750. Since the limitation will be completely phased out as of January 1, 2014, the entire $750 Medicare-approved amount is recognized as the total incurred expenses because such expenses are no longer reduced. Also, there is no longer any distinction between mental health services the patient receives as an inpatient or outpatient. The Medicare payment and patient liability are computed as follows:

1. Actual charges...$780.00
2. Medicare-approved amount...$750.00
3. Medicare incurred expenses (1.00 x line 2).................$750.00
4. Unmet deductible..$135.00
5. Remainder after subtracting deductible
   (line 3 minus line 4)..$615.00
6. Medicare payment (0.80 x line 5)................................$492.00
   Beneficiary liability (line 2 minus line 6)....................$258.00

100-4, Chapter-13, 40

Magnetic Resonance Imaging (MRI) Procedures

Effective September 28, 2009

The Centers for Medicare & Medicaid Services (CMS) finds that the non-coverage of magnetic resonance imaging (MRI) for blood flow determination is no longer supported by the available evidence. CMS is removing the phrase "blood flow measurement" and local Medicare contractors will have the discretion to cover (or not cover).

Consult Publication (Pub.) 100-03, National Coverage Determinations (NCD) Manual, chapter 1, section 220.2, for specific coverage and non-coverage indications associated with MRI and MRA (Magnetic Resonance Angiography).

Prior to January 1, 2007

Carriers do not make additional payments for three or more MRI sequences. The relative value units (RVUs) reflect payment levels for two sequences.

The technical component (TC) RVUs for MRI procedures that specify "with contrast" include payment for paramagnetic contrast media. Carriers do not make separate payment under code A4647.

A diagnostic technique has been developed under which an MRI of the brain or spine is first performed without contrast material, then another MRI is performed with a standard (0.1mmol/kg) dose of contrast material and, based on the need to achieve a better image, a third MRI is performed with an additional double dosage (0.2mmol/kg) of contrast material. When the high-dose contrast technique is utilized, carriers:

- Do not pay separately for the contrast material used in the second MRI procedure;

- Pay for the contrast material given for the third MRI procedure through supply code Q9952, the replacement code for A4643, when billed with Current Procedural Terminology (CPT®) codes 70553, 72156, 72157, and 72158;

- Do not pay for the third MRI procedure. For example, in the case of an MRI of the brain, if CPT® code 70553 (without contrast material, followed by with contrast material(s) and further sequences) is billed, make no payment for CPT® code 70551 (without contrast material(s)), the additional procedure given for the purpose of administering the double dosage, furnished during the same session. Medicare does not pay for the third procedure (as distinguished from the contrast material) because the CPT® definition of code 70553 includes all further sequences; and

- Do not apply the payment criteria for low osmolar contrast media in §30.1.2 to billings for code Q9952, the replacement code for A4643.

Effective January 1, 2007

With the implementation for calendar year 2007 of a bottom-up methodology, which utilizes the direct inputs to determine the practice expense (PE) relative value units (RVUs), the cost of the contrast media is not included in the PE RVUs. Therefore, a separate payment for the contrast media used in various imaging procedures is paid. In addition to the CPT® code representing the imaging procedure, separately bill the appropriate HCPCS "Q" code (Q9945 –Q9954; Q9958-Q9964) for the contrast medium utilized in performing the service.

Effective February 24, 2011

Medicare will allow for coverage of MRI for beneficiaries with implanted PMs or cardioverter defibrillators (ICDs) for use in an MRI environment in a Medicare-approved clinical study as described in section 220.C.1 of the NCD manual.

Effective July 7, 2011

Medicare will allow for coverage of MRI for beneficiaries with implanted pacemakers (PMs) when the PMs are used according to the Food and Drug Administration (FDA)-approved labeling for use in an MRI environment as described in section 220.2.C.1 of the NCD Manual.

100-4, Chapter-13, 40.1.2

HCPCS Coding Requirements

Providers must report HCPCS codes when submitting claims for MRA of the chest, abdomen, head, neck or peripheral vessels of lower extremities. The following HCPCS codes should be used to report these services:

MRA of head	70544, 70544-26, 70544-TC
MRA of head	70545, 70545-26, 70545-TC
MRA of head	70546, 70546-26, 70546-TC
MRA of neck	70547, 70547-26, 70547-TC
MRA of neck	70548, 70548-26, 70548-TC
MRA of neck	70549, 70549-26, 70549-TC
MRA of chest	71555, 71555-26, 71555-TC
MRA of pelvis	72198, 72198-26, 72198-TC
MRA of abdomen (dates of service on or after July 1, 2003) –see below.	74185, 74185-26, 74185-TC
MRA of peripheral vessels of lower extremities	73725, 73725-26, 73725-TC

Hospitals subject to OPPS should report the following C codes in place of the above HCPCS codes as follows:

- MRA of chest 71555: C8909 – C8911
- MRA of abdomen 74185: C8900 – C8902
- MRA of peripheral vessels of lower extremities 73725: C8912 – C8914

For claims with dates of service on or after July 1, 2003, coverage under this benefit has been expanded for the use of MRA for diagnosing pathology in the renal or aortoiliac arteries. The following HCPCS code should be used to report this expanded coverage of MRA:

- MRA, pelvis, with or without contrast material(s) 72198, 72198-26, 72198-TC

Hospitals subject to OPPS report the following C codes in place of HCPCS code 72198:

- MRA, pelvis, with or without contrast material(s) 72198: C8918 - C8920

NOTE: Information regarding the claim form locator that corresponds to the HCPCS code and a table to crosswalk its CMS-1450 form locator to the 837 transaction is found in Chapter 25.

100-4, Chapter-13, 60

Positron Emission Tomography (PET) Scans – General Information

Positron emission tomography (PET) is a noninvasive imaging procedure that assesses perfusion and the level of metabolic activity in various organ systems of the human body. A positron camera (tomograph) is used to produce cross-sectional tomographic images which are obtained by detecting radioactivity from a radioactive tracer substance (radiopharmaceutical) that emits a radioactive tracer substance (radiopharmaceutical FDG) such as 2 –[F-18] flouro-D-glucose FDG, that is administered intravenously to the patient.

The Medicare National Coverage Determinations (NCD) Manual, chapter 1, §220.6, contains additional coverage instructions to indicate the conditions under which a PET scan is performed.

A. Definitions

For all uses of PET, excluding Rubidium 82 for perfusion of the heart, myocardial viability and refractory seizures, the following definitions apply:

Diagnosis: PET is covered only in clinical situations in which the PET results may assist in avoiding an invasive diagnostic procedure, or in which the PET results may assist in determining the optimal anatomical location to perform an invasive diagnostic procedure. In general, for most solid tumors, a tissue diagnosis is made prior to the performance of PET scanning. PET scans following a tissue diagnosis are generally performed for the purpose of staging, rather than diagnosis. Therefore, the use of PET in the diagnosis of lymphoma, esophageal and colorectal cancers, as well as in melanoma, should be rare. PET is not covered for other diagnostic uses, and is not covered for screening (testing of patients without specific signs and symptoms of disease).

Staging: PET is covered in clinical situations in which (1) (a) the stage of the cancer remains in doubt after completion of a standard diagnostic workup, including conventional imaging (computed tomography, magnetic resonance imaging, or ultrasound) or, (b) the use of PET would also be considered reasonable and necessary if it could potentially replace one or more conventional imaging studies when it is expected that conventional study information is insufficient for the clinical management of the patient and, (2) clinical management of the patient would differ depending on the stage of the cancer identified.

NOTE: Effective for services on or after April 3, 2009, the terms "diagnosis" and "staging" will be replaced with "Initial Treatment Strategy." For further information on this new term, refer to Pub. 100-03, NCD Manual, section 220.6.17.

Restaging: PET will be covered for restaging: (1) after the completion of treatment for the purpose of detecting residual disease, (2) for detecting suspected recurrence, or metastasis, (3) to determine the extent of a known recurrence, or (4) if it could potentially replace one or more conventional imaging studies when it is expected that conventional study information is to determine the extent of a known recurrence, or if study information is insufficient for the clinical management of the patient. Restaging applies to testing after a course of treatment is completed and is covered subject to the conditions above.

Monitoring: Use of PET to monitor tumor response to treatment during the planned course of therapy (i.e., when a change in therapy is anticipated).

NOTE: Effective for services on or after April 3, 2009, the terms "restaging" and "monitoring" will be replaced with "Subsequent Treatment Strategy." For further information on this new term, refer to Pub. 100-03, NCD Manual, section 220.6.17.

B. Limitations

For staging and restaging: PET is covered in either/or both of the following circumstances:

- The stage of the cancer remains in doubt after completion of a standard diagnostic workup, including conventional imaging (computed tomography, magnetic resonance imaging, or ultrasound); and/or

- The clinical management of the patient would differ depending on the stage of the cancer identified. PET will be covered for restaging after the completion of treatment for the purpose of detecting residual disease, for detecting suspected recurrence, or to determine the extent of a known recurrence. Use of PET would also be considered reasonable and necessary if it could potentially replace one or more conventional imaging studies when it is expected that conventional study information is insufficient for the clinical management of the patient.

The PET is not covered for other diagnostic uses, and is not covered for screening (testing of patients without specific symptoms). Use of PET to monitor tumor response during the planned course of therapy (i.e., when no change in therapy is being contemplated) is not covered.

100-4, Chapter-13, 60.3

PET Scan Qualifying Conditions and HCPCS Code Chart

Below is a summary of all covered PET scan conditions, with effective dates.

NOTE: The G codes below except those a # can be used to bill for PET Scan services through January 27, 2005. Effective for dates of service on or after January 28, 2005, providers must bill for PET Scan services using the appropriate CPT® codes. See section 60.3.1. The G codes with a # can continue to be used for billing after January 28, 2005 and these remain non-covered by Medicare. (**NOTE:** PET Scanners must be FDA-approved.)

Conditions	Coverage Effective Date	****HCPCS/ CPT®
*Myocardial perfusion imaging (following previous PET G0030-G0047) single study, rest or stress (exercise and/or pharmacologic)	3/14/95	G0030
*Myocardial perfusion imaging (following previous PET G0030-G0047) multiple studies, rest or stress (exercise and/or pharmacologic)	3/14/95	G0031
*Myocardial perfusion imaging (following rest SPECT, 78464); single study, rest or stress (exercise and/or pharmacologic)	3/14/95	G0032
*Myocardial perfusion imaging (following rest SPECT 78464); multiple studies, rest or stress (exercise and/or pharmacologic)	3/14/95	G0033
*Myocardial perfusion (following stress SPECT 78465); single study, rest or stress (exercise and/or pharmacologic)	3/14/95	G0034
*Myocardial Perfusion Imaging (following stress SPECT 78465); multiple studies, rest or stress (exercise and/or pharmacologic)	3/14/95	G0035
*Myocardial Perfusion Imaging (following coronary angiography 93510-93529); single study, rest or stress (exercise and/or pharmacologic)	3/14/95	G0036
*Myocardial Perfusion Imaging, (following coronary angiography), 93510-93529; multiple studies, rest or stress (exercise and/or pharmacologic)	3/14/95	G0037

Conditions	Coverage Effective Date	****HCPCS/ CPT®
*Myocardial Perfusion Imaging (following stress planar myocardial perfusion, 78460); single study, rest or stress (exercise and/or pharmacologic)	3/14/95	G0038
*Myocardial Perfusion Imaging (following stress planar myocardial perfusion, 78460); multiple studies, rest or stress (exercise and/or pharmacologic)	3/14/95	G0039
*Myocardial Perfusion Imaging (following stress echocardiogram 93350); single study, rest or stress (exercise and/or pharmacologic)	3/14/95	G0040
*Myocardial Perfusion Imaging (following stress echocardiogram, 93350); multiple studies, rest or stress (exercise and/or pharmacologic)	3/14/95	G0041
*Myocardial Perfusion Imaging (following stress nuclear ventriculogram 78481 or 78483); single study, rest or stress (exercise and/or pharmacologic)	3/14/95	G0042
*Myocardial Perfusion Imaging (following stress nuclear ventriculogram 78481 or 78483); multiple studies, rest or stress (exercise and/or pharmacologic)	3/14/95	G0043
*Myocardial Perfusion Imaging (following stress ECG, 93000); single study, rest or stress (exercise and/or pharmacologic)	3/14/95	G0044
*Myocardial perfusion (following stress ECG, 93000), multiple studies; rest or stress (exercise and/or pharmacologic)	3/14/95	G0045
*Myocardial perfusion (following stress ECG, 93015), single study; rest or stress (exercise and/or pharmacologic)	3/14/95	G0046
*Myocardial perfusion (following stress ECG, 93015); multiple studies, rest or stress (exercise and/or pharmacologic)	3/14/95	G0047
PET imaging regional or whole body; single pulmonary nodule	1/1/98	G0125
Lung cancer, non-small cell (PET imaging whole body) Diagnosis, Initial Staging, Restaging	7/1/01	G0210 G0211 G0212
Colorectal cancer (PET imaging whole body) Diagnosis, Initial Staging, Restaging	7/1/01	G0213 G0214 G0215
Melanoma (PET imaging whole body) Diagnosis, Initial Staging, Restaging	7/1/01	G0216 G0217 G0218
Melanoma for non-covered indications	7/1/01	#G0219
Lymphoma (PET imaging whole body) Diagnosis, Initial Staging, Restaging	7/1/01	G0220 G0221 G0222
Head and neck cancer; excluding thyroid and CNS cancers (PET imaging whole body or regional) Diagnosis, Initial Staging, Restaging	7/1/01	G0223 G0224 G0225
Esophageal cancer (PET imaging whole body) Diagnosis, Initial Staging, Restaging	7/1/01	G0226 G0227 G0228
Metabolic brain imaging for pre-surgical evaluation of refractory seizures	7/1/01	G0229

Conditions	Coverage Effective Date	****HCPCS/ CPT®
Metabolic assessment for myocardial viability following inconclusive SPECT study	7/1/01	G0230
Recurrence of colorectal or colorectal metastatic cancer (PET whole body, gamma cameras only)	1/1/02	G0231
Staging and characterization of lymphoma (PET whole body, gamma cameras only)	1/1/02	G0232
Recurrence of melanoma or melanoma metastatic cancer (PET whole body, gamma cameras only)	1/1/02	G0233
Regional or whole body, for solitary pulmonary nodule following CT, or for initial staging of non-small cell lung cancer (gamma cameras only)	1/1/02	G0234
Non-Covered Service PET imaging, any site not otherwise specified	1/28/05	#G0235
Non-Covered Service Initial diagnosis of breast cancer and/or surgical planning for breast cancer (e.g., initial staging of axillary lymph nodes), not covered (full- and partial-ring PET scanners only)	10/1/02	#G0252
Breast cancer, staging/restaging of local regional recurrence or distant metastases, i.e., staging/restaging after or prior to course of treatment (full- and partial-ring PET scanners only)	10/1/02	G0253
Breast cancer, evaluation of responses to treatment, performed during course of treatment (full- and partial-ring PET scanners only)	10/1/02	G0254
Myocardial imaging, positron emission tomography (PET), metabolic evaluation)	10/1/02	78459
Restaging or previously treated thyroid cancer of follicular cell origin following negative I-131 whole body scan (full- and partial-ring PET scanner only)	10/1/03	G0296
Tracer Rubidium**82 (Supply of Radiopharmaceutical Diagnostic Imaging Agent) (This is only billed through Outpatient Perspective Payment System, OPPS.) (Carriers must use HCPCS Code A4641).	10/1/03	Q3000
Supply of Radiopharmaceutical Diagnostic Imaging Agent, Ammonia N-13	01/1/04	A9526
PET imaging, brain imaging for the differential diagnosis of Alzheimer's disease with aberrant features vs. fronto-temporal dementia	09/15/04	Appropriate CPT® Code from section 60.3.1
PET Cervical Cancer Staging as adjunct to conventional imaging, other staging, diagnosis, restaging, monitoring	1/28/05	Appropriate CPT® Code from section 60.3.1

NOTE: A/B MACs (B) must report A4641 for the tracer Rubidium 82 when used with PET scan codes G0030 through G0047 for services performed on or before January 27, 2005.

**NOTE:* Not FDG PET

***NOTE:* For dates of service October 1, 2003, through December 31, 2003, use temporary code Q4078 for billing this radiopharmaceutical.

100-4, Chapter-13, 60.3.1

Appropriate CPT® Codes Effective for PET Scans for Services Performed on or After January 28, 2005

NOTE: All PET scan services require the use of a radiopharmaceutical diagnostic imaging agent (tracer). The applicable tracer code should be billed when billing for a PET scan service. See section 60.3.2 below for applicable tracer codes.

CPT® Code	Description
78459	Myocardial imaging, positron emission tomography (PET), metabolic evaluation
78491	Myocardial imaging, positron emission tomography (PET), perfusion, single study at rest or stress
78492	Myocardial imaging, positron emission tomography (PET), perfusion, multiple studies at rest and/or stress
78608	Brain imaging, positron emission tomography (PET); metabolic evaluation
78811	Tumor imaging, positron emission tomography (PET); limited area (eg, chest, head/neck)
78812	Tumor imaging, positron emission tomography (PET); skull base to mid-thigh
78813	Tumor imaging, positron emission tomography (PET); whole body
78814	Tumor imaging, positron emission tomography (PET) with concurrently acquired computed tomography (CT) for attenuation correction and anatomical localization; limited area (e.g., chest, head/neck)
78815	Tumor imaging, positron emission tomography (PET) with concurrently acquired computed tomography (CT) for attenuation correction and anatomical localization; skull base to mid-thigh
78816	Tumor imaging, positron emission tomography (PET) with concurrently acquired computed tomography (CT) for attenuation correction and anatomical localization; whole body

100-4, Chapter-13, 60.3.2

Tracer Codes Required for Positron Emission Tomography (PET) Scans

An applicable tracer/radiopharmaceutical code, along with an applicable Current Procedural Technology (CPT®) code, is necessary for claims processing of any Positron Emission Tomography (PET) scan services. While there are a number of PET tracers already billable for a diverse number of medical indications, there have been, and may be in the future, additional PET indications that might require a new PET tracer. Under those circumstances, the process to request/approve/implement a new code could be time-intensive. To help alleviate inordinate spans of time between when a national coverage determination is made, or when the Food and Drug Administration (FDA) approves a particular radiopharmaceutical for an oncologic indication already approved by the Centers for Medicare & Medicaid Services (CMS), and when it can be fully implemented via valid claims processing, CMS has created two new PET radiopharmaceutical unclassified tracer codes that can be used temporarily. This time period would be pending the creation/approval/implementation of permanent CPT® codes that would later specifically define their function by CMS in official instructions.

Effective with dates of service on or after January 1, 2018, the following Healthcare Common Procedure Coding System

(HCPCS) codes shall be used ONLY AS NECESSARY FOR AN INTERIM PERIOD OF TIME under the circumstances explained here. Specifically, there are two circumstances that would warrant use of the below codes: (1) After FDA approval of a PET oncologic indication, or, (2) after CMS approves coverage of a new PET indication, and ONLY if either of those situations requires the use of a dedicated PET radiopharmaceutical/tracer that is currently non-existent. Once permanent replacement codes are officially implemented by CMS, use of the temporary code for that particular indication will simultaneously be discontinued.

NOTE: The following two codes were effective as of January 1, 2017, with the January 2017 quarterly HCPCS update.

A9597 - Positron emission tomography radiopharmaceutical, diagnostic, for tumor identification, not otherwise classified

A9598 - Positron emission tomography radiopharmaceutical, diagnostic, for non-tumor identification, not otherwise classified

Effective for claims with dates of service on and after January 1, 2018, when PET tracer code A9597 or A9598 are present on a claim, that claim must also include:

-an appropriate PET HCPCS code, either 78459, 78491, 78492, 78608, 78811, 78812, 78813, 78814, 78815, or 78816,

-if tumor-related, either the -PI or -PS modifier as appropriate,

-if clinical trial, registry, or study-related outside of NCD220.6.17, PET for Solid Tumors, clinical trial modifier –Q0,

-if clinical trial, registry, or study-related, all claims require the 8-digit clinical trial number,

-if Part A OP and clinical trial, registry, or study-related outside of NCD220.6.17, PET for Solid Tumors, also include condition code 30 and ICD-10 diagnosis Z00.6.

Effective for claims with dates of service on and after January 1, 2018, A/Medicare Administrative Contractors (MACs) shall line-item deny, and B/MACs shall line-item reject, PET claims for A9597 or A9598 that don't include the elements noted above as appropriate.

Contractors shall use the following messaging when line-item denying (Part A) or line item rejecting (Part B) PET claims containing HCPCS A9597 or A9598:

Remittance Advice Remark Codes (RARC) N386

Claim Adjustment Reason Code (CARC) 50, 96, and/or 119.

Group Code CO (Contractual Obligation) assigning financial liability to the provider (if a claim is received with a GZ modifier indicating no signed ABN is on file).

(The above new verbiage will supersede any existing verbiage in chapter 13, section 60.3.2.)

100-4, Chapter-13, 60.13

Billing Requirements for PET Scans for Specific Indications of Cervical Cancer for Services Performed on or After January 28, 2005

Contractors shall accept claims for these services with the appropriate CPT® code listed in section 60.3.1. Refer to Pub. 100-03, section 220.6.17, for complete coverage guidelines for this new PET oncology indication. The implementation date for these CPT® codes will be April 18, 2005. Also see section 60.17, of this chapter for further claims processing instructions for cervical cancer indications.

100-4, Chapter-13, 60.14

Billing Requirements for PET Scans for Non-Covered Indications

For services performed on or after January 28, 2005, contractors shall accept claims with the following HCPCS code for non-covered PET indications:

-G0235: PET imaging, any site not otherwise specified Short Descriptor: PET not otherwise specified Type of Service:4

NOTE: This code is for a non-covered service.

100-4, Chapter-13, 60.15

Billing Requirements for CMS - Approved Clinical Trials and Coverage With Evidence Development Claims for PET Scans for Neurodegenerative Diseases, Previously Specified Cancer Indications, and All Other Cancer Indications Not Previously Specified

A/B MACs (A and B)

Effective for services on or after January 28, 2005, contractors shall accept and pay for claims for Positron Emission Tomography (PET) scans for lung cancer, esophageal cancer, colorectal cancer, lymphoma, melanoma, head & neck cancer, breast cancer, thyroid cancer, soft tissue sarcoma, brain cancer, ovarian cancer, pancreatic cancer, small cell lung cancer, and testicular cancer, as well as for neurodegenerative diseases and all other cancer indications not previously mentioned in this chapter, if these scans were performed as part of a Centers for Medicare & Medicaid (CMS)-approved clinical trial. (See Pub. 100-03, National Coverage Determinations (NCD) Manual, sections 220.6.13 and 220.6.17.)

Contractors shall also be aware that PET scans for all cancers not previously specified at Pub. 100-03, NCD Manual, section 220.6.17, remain nationally non-covered unless performed in conjunction with a CMS-approved clinical trial.

Effective for dates of service on or after June 11, 2013, Medicare has ended the coverage with evidence development (CED) requirement for FDG (2-[F18] fluoro-2-deoxy-Dglucose) PET and PET/computed tomography (CT) and PET/magnetic resonance imaging (MRI) for all oncologic indications contained in section 220.6.17 of the NCD Manual. Modifier -Q0 (Investigational clinical service provided in a clinical research study that is in an approved clinical research study) or -Q1 (routine clinical service provided in a clinical research study that is in an approved clinical research study) is no longer mandatory for these services when performed on or after June 11, 2013.

A/B MACs (B) Only

A/B MACs (B) shall pay claims for PET scans for beneficiaries participating in a CMS approved clinical trial submitted with an appropriate current procedural terminology (CPT®) code from section 60.3.1 of this chapter and modifier Q0/Q1 for services performed on or after January 1, 2008, through June 10, 2013. (**NOTE:** Modifier QR (Item or service provided in a Medicare specified study) and QA (FDA investigational device exemption) were replaced by modifier Q0 effective January 1, 2008.) Modifier QV (item or service provided as routine care in a Medicare qualifying clinical trial) was replaced by modifier Q1 effective January 1, 2008.) Beginning with services performed on or after June 11, 2013, modifier Q0/Q1 is no longer required for PET FDG services.

A/B MACs (A) Only

In order to pay claims for PET scans on behalf of beneficiaries participating in a CMS approved clinical trial, A/B MACs (A) require providers to submit claims with, if ICD-9- CM is applicable, ICD-9 code V70.7; if ICD-10-CM is applicable, ICD-10 code Z00.6 in the primary/secondary diagnosis position using the ASC X12 837 institutional claim format or on Form CMS-1450, with the appropriate principal diagnosis code and an appropriate CPT® code from section 60.3.1. Effective for PET scan claims for dates of service on or after January 28, 2005, through December 31, 2007, A/B MACs (A) shall accept claims with the QR, QV, or QA modifier on other than inpatient claims. Effective for services on or after January 1, 2008, through June 10, 2013, modifier Q0 replaced the QR and QA modifier, modifier Q1 replaced the QV modifier. Modifier Q0/Q1 is no longer required for services performed on or after June 11, 2013

100-4, Chapter-13, 60.16

Billing and Coverage Changes for PET Scans Effective for Services on or After April 3, 2009

A. Summary of Changes

Effective for services on or after April 3, 2009, Medicare will not cover the use of FDG PET imaging to determine initial treatment strategy in patients with adenocarcinoma of the prostate.

Medicare will also not cover FDG PET imaging for subsequent treatment strategy for tumor types other than breast, cervical, colorectal, esophagus, head and neck (non-CNS/thyroid), lymphoma, melanoma, myeloma, non-small cell lung, and ovarian, unless the FDG PET is provided under the coverage with evidence development (CED) paradigm (billed with modifier -Q0/-Q1, see section 60.15 of this chapter).

Medicare will cover FDG PET imaging for initial treatment strategy for myeloma.

Effective for services performed on or after June 11, 2013, Medicare has ended the CED requirement for FDG PET and PET/CT and PET/MRI for all oncologic indications contained in section 220.6.17 of the NCD Manual. Effective for services on or after June 11, 2013, the Q0/Q1 modifier is no longer required.

Beginning with services performed on or after June 11, 2013, contractors shall pay for up to three (3) FDG PET scans when used to guide subsequent management of anti-tumor treatment strategy (modifier PS) after completion of initial anti-cancer therapy (modifier PI) for the exact same cancer diagnosis.

Coverage of any additional FDG PET scans (that is, beyond 3) used to guide subsequent management of anti-tumor treatment strategy after completion of initial anti-tumor therapy for the same cancer diagnosis will be determined by the A/B MACs (A or B). Claims will include the KX modifier indicating the coverage criteria is met for coverage of four or more FDG PET scans for subsequent treatment strategy for the same cancer diagnosis under this NCD.

A different cancer diagnosis whether submitted with a PI or a PS modifier will begin the count of one initial and three subsequent FDG PET scans not requiring the KX modifier and four or more FDG PET scans for subsequent treatment strategy for the same cancer diagnosis requiring the KX modifier.

NOTE: The presence or absence of an initial treatment strategy claim in a beneficiary's record does not impact the frequency criteria for subsequent treatment strategy claims for the same cancer diagnosis.

NOTE: Providers please refer to the following link for a list of appropriate diagnosis codes, http://cms.gov/medicare/coverage/determinationprocess/downloads/petforsolidtumorsonc ologicdxcodesattachment_NCD220_6_17.pdf

For further information regarding the changes in coverage, refer to Pub.100-03, NCD Manual, section 220.6.17.

B. Modifiers for PET Scans

Effective for claims with dates of service on or after April 3, 2009, the following modifiers have been created for use to inform for the initial treatment strategy of biopsy-proven or strongly suspected tumors or subsequent treatment strategy of cancerous tumors:

PI Positron Emission Tomography (PET) or PET/Computed Tomography (CT) to inform the initial treatment strategy of tumors that are biopsy proven or strongly suspected of being cancerous based on other diagnostic testing.

Short descriptor: PET tumor init tx strat

PS Positron Emission Tomography (PET) or PET/Computed Tomography (CT) to inform the subsequent treatment strategy of cancerous tumors when the beneficiary's treatment physician determines that the PET study is needed to inform subsequent anti-tumor strategy.

Short descriptor: PS - PET tumor subsq tx strategy

C. Billing for A/B MACs (A and B)

Effective for claims with dates of service on or after April 3, 2009, contractors shall accept FDG PET claims billed to inform initial treatment strategy with the following CPT® codes AND modifier PI: 78608, 78811, 78812, 78813, 78814, 78815, 78816.

Effective for claims with dates of service on or after April 3, 2009, contractors shall accept FDG PET claims with modifier PS for the subsequent treatment strategy for solid tumors using a CPT® code above AND a cancer diagnosis code.

Contractors shall also accept FDG PET claims billed to inform initial treatment strategy or subsequent treatment strategy when performed under CED with one of the PET or PET/CT CPT® codes above AND modifier PI OR modifier PS AND a cancer diagnosis code AND modifier Q0/Q1. Effective for services performed on or after June 11, 2013, the CED requirement has ended and modifier Q0/Q1, along with condition code 30 (institutional claims only), or ICD-9 code V70.7, (both institutional and practitioner claims) are no longer required.

D. Medicare Summary Notices, Remittance Advice Remark Codes, and Claim Adjustment Reason Codes

Effective for dates of service on or after April 3, 2009, contractors shall return as unprocessable/return to provider claims that do not include the PI modifier with one of the PET/PET/CT CPT® codes listed in subsection C. above when billing for the initial treatment strategy for solid tumors in accordance with Pub.100-03, NCD Manual, section 220.6.17.

In addition, contractors shall return as unprocessable/return to provider claims that do not include the PS modifier with one of the CPT® codes listed in subsection C. above when billing for the subsequent treatment strategy for solid tumors in accordance with Pub.100-03, NCD Manual, section 220.6.17.

The contractor shall use the following remittance advice messages and associated codes when returning claims under this policy. This CARC/RARC combination is compliant with CAQH CORE Business Scenario Two.

Group Code: CO

CARC: 4

RARC: MA130

MSN: N/A

Effective for claims with dates of service on or after April 3, 2009, through June 10, 2013, contractors shall return as unprocessable/return to provider FDG PET claims billed to inform initial treatment strategy or subsequent treatment strategy when performed under CED without one of the PET/ PET/CT CPT® codes listed in subsection C. above AND modifier PI OR modifier PS AND a cancer diagnosis code AND modifier Q0/Q1.

The contractor shall use the following remittance advice messages and associated codes when returning claims under this policy. This CARC/RARC combination is compliant with CAQH CORE Business Scenario Two.

Group Code: CO

CARC: 4

RARC: MA130

MSN: N/A

Effective April 3, 2009, contractors shall deny claims with ICD-9/ICD-10 diagnosis code 185/C61 for FDG PET imaging for the initial treatment strategy of patients with adenocarcinoma of the prostate.

For dates of service prior to June 11, 2013, contractors shall also deny claims for FDG PET imaging for subsequent treatment strategy for tumor types other than breast, cervical, colorectal, esophagus, head and neck (non-CNS/thyroid), lymphoma, melanoma, myeloma, non-small cell lung, and ovarian, unless the FDG PET is provided under CED (submitted with the Q0/Q1 modifier) and use the following messages:

The contractor shall use the following remittance advice messages and associated codes when rejecting/denying claims under this policy. This CARC/RARC combination is compliant with CAQH CORE Business Scenario Three.

Group Code: PR (if claim is received with a GA modifier) otherwise CO

CARC: 50

RARC: N/A

MSN: 15.4

Effective for dates of service on or after June 11, 2013, contractors shall use the following messages when denying claims in excess of three for PET FDG scans for subsequent treatment strategy when the KX modifier is not included, identified by CPT® codes 78608, 78811, 78812, 78813, 78814, 78815, or 78816, modifier PS, HCPCS A9552, and the same cancer diagnosis code.

The contractor shall use the following remittance advice messages and associated codes when rejecting/denying claims under this policy. This CARC/RARC combination is compliant with CAQH CORE Business Scenario Three.

Group Code: PR (if claim is received with a GA modifier) otherwise CO

CARC: 96

RARC: N435

MSN: 23.17

100-4, Chapter-13, 60.17

Billing and Coverage Changes for PET Scans for Cervical

A. Billing Changes for A/B MACs (A and B)

Effective for claims with dates of service on or after November 10, 2009, contractors shall accept FDG PET oncologic claims billed to inform initial treatment strategy; specifically for staging in beneficiaries who have biopsy-proven cervical cancer when the beneficiary's treating physician determines the FDG PET study is needed to determine the location and/or extent of the tumor as specified in Pub. 100-03, section 220.6.17.

EXCEPTION: CMS continues to non-cover FDG PET for initial diagnosis of cervical cancer related to initial treatment strategy.

NOTE: Effective for claims with dates of service on and after November 10, 2009, the – Q0 modifier is no longer necessary for FDG PET for cervical cancer.

B. Medicare Summary Notices, Remittance Advice Remark Codes, and Claim

Adjustment Reason Codes

Additionally, contractors shall return as unprocessable / return to provider for FDG PET for cervical cancer for initial treatment strategy billed without the following: one of the PET/PET/CT CPT® codes listed in 60.16 C above AND modifier PI AND a cervical cancer diagnosis code.

The contractor shall use the following remittance advice messages and associated codes when returning claims under this policy. This CARC/RARC combination is compliant with CAQH CORE Business Scenario Two.

Group Code: CO

CARC: 4

RARC: MA130

MSN: N/A

100-4, Chapter-13, 60.18

Billing and Coverage Changes for PET (NaF-18) Scans to Identify Bone Metastasis of Cancer Effective for Claims With Dates of Services on or After February 26, 2010

A. Billing Changes for A/B MACs (A and B)

Effective for claims with dates of service on and after February 26, 2010, contractors shall pay for NaF-18 PET oncologic claims to inform of initial treatment strategy (PI) or subsequent treatment strategy (PS) for suspected or biopsy proven bone metastasis ONLY in the context of a clinical study and as specified in Pub. 100-03, section 220.6. All other claims for NaF-18 PET oncology claims remain non-covered.

B. Medicare Summary Notices, Remittance Advice Remark Codes, and Claim Adjustment Reason Codes

Effective for claims with dates of service on or after February 26, 2010, contractors shall return as unprocessable NaF-18 PET oncologic claims billed with modifier TC or globally (for A/B MACs (A) modifier TC or globally does not apply)

and HCPCS A9580 to inform the initial treatment strategy or subsequent treatment strategy for bone metastasis that do not include ALL of the following:

- PI or PS modifier AND
- PET or PET/CT CPT® code (78811, 78812, 78813, 78814, 78815, 78816) AND
- Cancer diagnosis code AND
- Q0 modifier - Investigational clinical service provided in a clinical research study, are present on the claim.

NOTE: For institutional claims, continue to include ICD-9 diagnosis code V70.7 or ICD-10 diagnosis code Z00.6 and condition code 30 to denote a clinical study.

The contractor shall use the following remittance advice messages and associated codes when returning claims under this policy. This CARC/RARC combination is compliant with CAQH CORE Business Scenario Two

Group Code: CO

CARC: 4

RARC: MA130

MSN: N/A

Effective for claims with dates of service on or after February 26, 2010, contractors shall accept PET oncologic claims billed with modifier 26 and modifier KX to inform the initial treatment strategy or subsequent treatment strategy for bone metastasis that include the following:

- PI or PS modifier AND
- PET or PET/CT CPT® code (78811, 78812, 78813, 78814, 78815, 78816) AND • Cancer diagnosis code AND
- Q0 modifier - Investigational clinical service provided in a clinical research study, are present on the claim.

NOTE: If modifier KX is present on the professional component service, Contractors shall process the service as PET NaF-18 rather than PET with FDG.

Contractors shall also return as unprocessable NaF-18 PET oncologic professional component claims (i.e., claims billed with modifiers 26 and KX) to inform the initial treatment strategy or subsequent treatment strategy for bone metastasis billed with HCPCS A9580.

The contractor shall use the following remittance advice messages and associated codes when returning claims under this policy. This CARC/RARC combination is compliant with CAQH CORE Business Scenario Two.

Group Code: CO

CARC: 4

RARC: MA130

MSN: N/A

100-4, Chapter-13, 140

Bone Mass Measurements (BMMs)

Sections 1861(s)(15)and (rr)(1)of the Social Security Act (the Act) (as added by §4106 of the Balanced Budget Act (BBA) of 1997) standardize Medicare coverage of medically necessary bone mass measurements by providing for uniform coverage under Medicare Part B. This coverage is effective for claims with dates of service furnished on or after July 1, 1998.

Effective for dates of service on and after January 1, 2007, the CY 2007 Physician Fee Schedule final rule expanded the number of beneficiaries qualifying for BMM by reducing the dosage requirement for glucocorticoid (steroid) therapy from 7.5 mg of prednisone per day to 5.0 mg. It also changed the definition of BMM by removing coverage for a single-photon absorptiometry as it is not considered reasonable and necessary under section 1862 (a)(1)(A) of the Act. Finally, it required that in the case of monitoring and confirmatory baseline BMMs, they be performed with a dual-energy X-ray absorptiometry (axial) test.

Conditions of Coverage for BMMs are located in Pub.100-02, Medicare Benefit Policy Manual, chapter 15.

100-4, Chapter-14, 40.3

Payment for Intraocular Lens (IOL)

Prior to January 1, 2008, payment for facility services furnished by an ASC for IOL insertion during or subsequent to cataract surgery includes an allowance for the lens. The procedures that include insertion of an IOL are:

Payment Group 6: CPT®-4 Codes 66985 and 66986

Payment Group 8: CPT®-4 Codes 66982, 66983 and 66984

Physicians or suppliers are not paid for an IOL furnished to a beneficiary in an ASC after July 1, 1988. Separate claims for IOLs furnished to ASC patients beginning March 12, 1990 are denied. Also, effective March 12, 1990, procedures 66983 and 66984 are treated as single procedures for payment purposes.

Beginning January 1, 2008, the Medicare payment for the IOL is included in the Medicare ASC payment for the associated surgical procedure. Consequently, no separate payment for the IOL is made, except for a payment adjustment for NTIOLs established according to the process outlined in 42 CFR 416.185. ASCs should not report separate charges for conventional IOLs because their payment is included in the Medicare payment for the associated surgical procedure. The ASC payment system logic that excluded $150 for IOLs for purposes of the multiple surgery reduction in cases of cataract surgery prior to January 1, 2008 no longer applies, effective for dates of service on or after January 1, 2008.

Effective for dates of service on and after February 27, 2006, through February 26, 2011, Medicare pays an additional $50 for specified Category 3 NTIOLs that are provided in association with a covered ASC surgical procedure. The list of Category 3 NTIOLS is available at: https://www.cms.gov/Medicare/Medicare-Fee-for-ServicePayment/ASCPayment/NTIOLs.html

ASCs should use HCPCS code Q1003 to bill for a Category 3 NTIOL. HCPCS code Q1003, along with one of the approved surgical procedure codes (CPT® codes 66982, 66983, 66984, 66985, 66986) are to be used on all NTIOL Category 3 claims associated with reduced spherical aberration from February 27, 2006, through February 26, 2011. The payment adjustment for the NTIOL is subject to beneficiary coinsurance but is not wage-adjusted.

Any subsequent IOL recognized by CMS as having the same characteristics as the first NTIOL recognized by CMS for a payment adjustment as a Category III NTIOL (those of reduced spherical aberration) will receive the same adjustment for the remainder of the 5- year period established by the first recognized IOL.

100-4, Chapter-14, 40.8

Payment When a Device is Furnished With No Cost or With Full or Partial Credit Beginning January 1, 2008

Contractors pay ASCs a reduced amount for certain specified procedures when a specified device is furnished without cost or for which either a partial or full credit is received (e.g., device recall). For specified procedure codes that include payment for a device, ASCs are required to include modifier –FB on the procedure code when a specified device is furnished without cost or for which full credit is received. If the ASC receives a partial credit of 50 percent or more of the cost of a specified device, the ASC is required to include modifier –FC on the procedure code if the procedure is on the list of specified procedures to which the -FC reduction applies. A single procedure code should not be submitted with both modifiers –FB and -FC. The pricing determination related to modifiers –FB and -FC is made prior to the application of multiple procedure payment reductions. Contractors adjust beneficiary coinsurance to reflect the reduced payment amount. Tables listing the procedures and devices to which the payment adjustments apply, and the full and partial adjustment amounts, are available on the CMS Web site.

In order to report that the receipt of a partial credit of 50 percent or more of the cost of a device, ASCs have the option of either: 1) Submitting the claim for the procedure to their Medicare contractor after the procedure's performance but prior to manufacturer acknowledgement of credit for a specified device, and subsequently contacting the contractor regarding a claims adjustment once the credit determination is made; or 2) holding the claim for the procedure until a determination is made by the manufacturer on the partial credit and submitting the claim with modifier –FC appended to the implantation procedure HCPCS code if the partial credit is 50 percent or more of the cost of the device. If choosing the first billing option, to request a claims adjustment once the credit determination is made, ASCs should keep in mind that the initial Medicare payment for the procedure involving the device is conditional and subject to adjustment.

100-4, Chapter-14, 40.9

Payment and Coding for Presbyopia Correcting IOLs (P-C IOLs) and Astigmatism Correcting IOLs (A-C IOLs)

CMS payment policies and recognition of P-C IOLs and A-C IOLs are contained in Transmittal 636 (CR3927) and Transmittal 1228 (CR5527) respectively.

Effective for dates of service on and after January 1, 2008, when inserting an approved A-C IOL in an ASC concurrent with cataract extraction, HCPCS code V2787 (Astigmatism-correcting function of intraocular lens) should be billed to report the non-covered charges for the A-C IOL functionality of the inserted intraocular lens. Additionally, note that HCPCS code V2788 (Presbyopia-correcting function of intraocular lens) is no longer valid to report non-covered charges associated with the A-C IOL. However, this code continues to be valid to report non-covered charges for a P-C IOL. The payment for the conventional lens portion of the A-C IOL and P-C IOL continues to be bundled with the ASC procedure payment.

Effective for services on and after January 1, 2010, ASCs are to bill for insertion of a Category 3 new technology intraocular lens (NTIOL) that is also an approved A-C IOL or P-C IOL, concurrent with cataract extraction, using three separate codes.

ASCs shall use HCPCS code V2787 or V2788, as appropriate, to report charges associated with the non-covered functionality of the A-C IOL or P-C IOL, the appropriate HCPCS code 66982 (Extracapsular cataract removal with insertion of intraocular lens prosthesis (one stage procedure), manual or mechanical technique (e.g., irrigation and aspiration or phacoemulsification), complex, requiring devices or techniques not generally used in routine cataract surgery (e.g., iris expansion device, suture support for intraocular lens, or primary posterior capsulorrhexis) or performed on patients in the amblyogenic developmental stage); 66983 (Intracapsular cataract extraction with insertion of intraocular lens prosthesis (1 stage procedure)); or 66984 (Extracapsular cataract removal with insertion of intraocular lens prosthesis (1 stage procedure), manual or mechanical technique (e.g., irrigation and aspiration or phacoemulsification)), to report the covered cataract extraction and insertion procedure; and Q1003 (New technology, intraocular lens, category 3 (reduced spherical aberration) as defined in Federal Register notice, Vol. 65, dated May 3, 2000) to report the covered NTIOL aspect of the lens on claims for insertion of an A-C IOL or P-C IOL that is also designated as an NTIOL. Listings of the CMS-approved Category 3 NTIOLs, A-C IOLs, and P-C IOLs are available on the CMS Web site.

100-4, Chapter-14, 60.1

Applicable Messages for NTIOLs

Contractors shall return as unprocessable any claims for NTIOLs containing Q1003 alone or with a code other than one of the procedure codes listed in 40.3.

The contractor shall use the following remittance advice messages and associated codes when returning claims under this policy. This CARC/RARC combination is compliant with CAQH CORE Business Scenario Three.

Group Code: CO

CARC: 16

RARC: M67

MSN: N/A

Contractors shall deny payment for Q1003 if services are furnished in a facility other than a Medicare-approved ASC.

The contractor shall use the following remittance advice messages and associated codes when denying claims under this policy. This CARC/RARC combination is compliant with CAQH CORE Business Scenario Three.

Group Code: CO

CARC: 58

RARC: N/A

MSN: 16.2

Contractors shall deny payment for Q1003 if billed by an entity other than a Medicare approved ASC.

The contractor shall use the following remittance advice messages and associated codes when denying claims under this policy. This CARC/RARC combination is compliant with CAQH CORE Business Scenario Three.

Group Code: CO

CARC: 170

RARC: N/A

MSN: 33.1

Contractors shall deny payment for Q1003 if submitted for payment past the discontinued date (after the 5-year period, or after February 26, 2011).

The contractor shall use the following remittance advice messages and associated codes when rejecting/denying claims under this policy. This CARC/RARC combination is compliant with CAQH CORE Business Scenario Three.

Group Code: CO

CARC: 27

RARC: N/A

MSN: 21.11

A/B MACs (B) shall deny payment for Q1003 if services are furnished in a facility other than a Medicare-approved ASC.

The contractor shall use the following remittance advice messages and associated codes when denying claims under this policy. This CARC/RARC combination is compliant with CAQH CORE Business Scenario Three.

Group Code: CO

CARC: 58

RARC: N/A

MSN: 16.2

100-4, Chapter-15, 10.4

Additional Introductory Guidelines

Since April 1, 2002 (the beginning of the transition to the full implementation of the ambulance fee schedule), payment for a medically necessary ambulance service is based on the level of service provided, not on the vehicle used.

Ambulance services are separately reimbursable only under Part B. Once a beneficiary is admitted to a hospital, Critical Access Hospitals (CAH), or Skilled Nursing Facility (SNF), it may be necessary to transport the beneficiary to another hospital or other site temporarily for specialized care while the beneficiary maintains inpatient status with the original provider. This movement of the patient is considered "patient transportation" and is covered as an inpatient hospital or CAH service under Part A and as a SNF service when the SNF is furnishing it as a covered SNF service and Part A payment is made for that service. Because the service is covered and payable as a beneficiary transportation service under Part A, the service cannot be classified and paid for as an ambulance service under Part B. This includes intra-campus transfers between different departments of the same hospital, even where the departments are located in separate buildings. Such intra-campus transfers are not separately payable under the Part B ambulance benefit. Such costs are accounted for in the same manner as the costs of such a transfer within a single building. See IOM Pub. 100-02, Medicare Benefit Policy Manual, chapter 10 - Ambulance Services, section 10.3.3 - Separately Payable Ambulance Transport Under Part B Versus Patient Transportation that is Covered Under a Packaged Institutional Service for further details. Refer to IOM Pub. 100-04, Medicare Claims Processing Manual, chapter 3 - Inpatient Hospital Billing, section 10.5 - Hospital Inpatient Bundling for additional information on hospital inpatient bundling of ambulance services. Refer to IOM Pub. 100-04, Medicare Claims Processing Manual, chapter 3 - Inpatient Hospital Billing for the definitions of an inpatient for the various inpatient facility types. All Prospective Payment Systems (PPS) have a different criteria for determining when ambulance services are payable (i.e., during an interrupted stay, on date of admission and date of discharge).

NOTE: The cost of oxygen and its administration in connection with and as part of the ambulance service is covered. Under the ambulance FS, oxygen and other items and services provided as part of the transport are included in the FS base payment rate and are NOT separately payable.

The A/B MAC (A) is responsible for the processing of claims for ambulance services furnished by a hospital based ambulance or for ambulance services provided by a supplier if provided under arrangements for an inpatient. The A/B MAC (B) is responsible for processing claims from suppliers; i.e., those entities that are not owned and operated by a provider. See section 10.2 below for further clarification of the definition of Providers and Suppliers of ambulance services.

Effective December 21, 2000, ambulance services furnished by a CAH or an entity that is owned and operated by a CAH are paid on a reasonable cost basis, but only if the CAH or entity is the only provider or supplier of ambulance services located within a 35-mile drive of such CAH or entity. Beginning February 24, 1999, ambulance transports to or from a non-hospital-based dialysis facility, origin and destination modifier "J," satisfy the program's origin and destination requirements for coverage.

Ambulance supplier services furnished under arrangements with a provider, e.g., hospital or SNF are typically not billed by the supplier to its A/B MAC (B), but are billed by the provider to its A/B MAC (A). The A/B MAC (A) is responsible for determining whether the conditions described below are met. In cases where all or part of the ambulance services are billed to the A/B MAC (B), the A/B MAC (B) has this responsibility, and the A/B MAC (A) shall contact the A/B MAC (B) to ascertain whether it has already determined if the crew and ambulance requirements are met. In such a situation, the A/B MAC (A) should accept the A/B MAC (B)'s determination without pursuing its own investigation.

Where a provider furnishes ambulance services under arrangements with a supplier of ambulance services, such services can be covered only if the supplier's vehicles and crew meet the certification requirements applicable for independent ambulance suppliers.

Effective January 1, 2006, items and services which include but are not limited to oxygen, drugs, extra attendants, supplies, EKG, and night differential are no longer paid separately for ambulance services. This occurred when CMS fully implemented the Ambulance Fee Schedule, and therefore, payment is based solely on the ambulance fee schedule.

Effective for claims on or after October 1, 2007, if ambulance claims submitted with a code(s) that is/are not separately billable the payment for the code(s) is included in the base rate.

Contractors shall use the following remittance advice messages and associated codes when rejecting/denying claims under this policy. This CARC/RARC combination is compliant with CAQH CORE Business Scenario Four.

Group Code: CO

CARC: 97

RARC: N390

MSN: 1.6

This is true whether the primary transportation service is allowed or denied. When the service is denied, the services are not separately billable to the beneficiaries as they are already part of the base rate.

Payment for ambulance services may be made only on an assignment related basis.

Prospective payment systems, including the Ambulance Fee Schedule, are exempt from Inherent Reasonableness provisions.

100-4, Chapter-15, 20.1.4

Components of the Ambulance Fee Schedule

The mileage rates provided in this section are the base rates that are adjusted by the yearly ambulance inflation factor (AIF). The payment amount under the fee schedule is determined as follows:

- **For ground ambulance services,** the fee schedule amount includes:
    1. A money amount that serves as a nationally uniform base rate, called a "conversion factor" (CF), for all ground ambulance services;
    2. A relative value unit (RVU) assigned to each type of ground ambulance service;
    3. A geographic adjustment factor (GAF) for each ambulance fee schedule locality area (geographic practice cost index (GPCI));
    4. A nationally uniform loaded mileage rate;
    5. An additional amount for certain mileage for a rural point-of-pickup; and
    6. For specified temporary periods, certain additional payment amounts as described in section 20.1.4A, below.

- **For air ambulance services**, the fee schedule amount includes:
    1. A nationally uniform base rate for fixed wing and a nationally uniform base rate for rotary wing;
    2. A geographic adjustment factor (GAF) for each ambulance fee schedule locality area (GPCI);
    3. A nationally uniform loaded mileage rate for each type of air service; and
    4. A rural adjustment to the base rate and mileage for services furnished for a rural point-of-pickup

A. Ground Ambulance Services
1. Conversion Factor

The conversion factor (CF) is a money amount used to develop a base rate for each category of ground ambulance service. The CF is updated annually by the ambulance inflation factor and for other reasons as necessary.

2. Relative Value Units

Relative value units (RVUs) set a numeric value for ambulance services relative to the value of a base level ambulance service. Since there are marked differences in resources necessary to furnish the various levels of ground ambulance services, different levels of payment are appropriate for the various levels of service. The different payment amounts are based on level of service. An RVU expresses the constant multiplier for a particular type of service (including, where appropriate, an emergency response). An RVU of 1.00 is assigned to the BLS of ground service, e.g., BLS has an RVU of 1; higher RVU values are assigned to the other types of ground ambulance services, which require more service than BLS.

The RVUs are as follows:

Service Level	RVU
BLS	1.00
BLS - Emergency	1.60
ALS1	1.20
ALS1- Emergency	1.90
ALS2	2.75
SCT	3.25
PI	1.75

3. Geographic Adjustment Factor (GAF)

The GAF is one of two factors intended to address regional differences in the cost of furnishing ambulance services. The GAF for the ambulance FS uses the non-facility practice expense (PE) of the geographic practice cost index (GPCI) of the Medicare physician fee schedule to adjust payment to account for regional differences. Thus, the geographic areas applicable to the ambulance FS are the same as those used for the physician fee schedule.

The location where the beneficiary was put into the ambulance (POP) establishes which GPCI applies. For multiple vehicle transports, each leg of the transport is separately evaluated for the applicable GPCI. Thus, for the second (or any subsequent) leg of a transport, the POP establishes the applicable GPCI for that portion of the ambulance transport.

For ground ambulance services, the applicable GPCI is multiplied by 70 percent of the base rate. Again, the base rate for each category of ground ambulance services is the CF multiplied by the applicable RVU. The GPCI is not applied to the ground mileage rate.

4. Mileage

In the context of all payment instructions, the term "mileage" refers to loaded mileage. The ambulance FS provides a separate payment amount for mileage. The mileage rate per statute mile applies for all types of ground ambulance services, except Paramedic Intercept, and is provided to all Medicare contractors electronically by CMS as part of the ambulance FS. Providers and suppliers must report all medically necessary mileage, including the mileage subject to a rural adjustment, in a single line item.

5. Adjustment for Certain Ground Mileage for Rural Points of Pickup (POP)

The payment rate is greater for certain mileage where the POP is in a rural area to account for the higher costs per ambulance trip that are typical of rural operations where fewer trips are made in any given period.

If the POP is a rural ZIP Code, the following calculations should be used to determine the rural adjustment portion of the payment allowance. For loaded miles 1-17, the rural adjustment for ground mileage is 1.5 times the rural mileage allowance.

For services furnished during the period July 1, 2004 through December 31, 2008, a 25 percent increase is applied to the appropriate ambulance FS mileage rate to each mile of a transport (both urban and rural POP) that exceeds 50 miles (i.e., mile 51 and greater).

The following chart summarizes the above information:

Service	Dates of Service	Bonus	Calculation
Loaded miles 1-17, Rural POP	Beginning 4/1/02	50%	FS Rural mileage * 1.5
Loaded miles 18-50, Rural POP	4/1/02 – 12/31/03	25%	FS Rural mileage * 1.25
All loaded miles (Urban or Rural POP) 51+	7/1/04 – 12/31/08	25%	FS Urban or Rural mileage * 1.25

The POP, as identified by ZIP Code, establishes whether a rural adjustment applies to a particular service. Each leg of a multi-leg transport is separately evaluated for a rural adjustment application. Thus, for the second (or any subsequent) leg of a transport, the ZIP Code of the POP establishes whether a rural adjustment applies to such second (or subsequent) transport.

For the purpose of all categories of ground ambulance services except paramedic intercept, a rural area is defined as a U.S. Postal Service (USPS) ZIP Code that is located, in whole or in part, outside of either a Metropolitan Statistical Area (MSA) or in New England, a New England County Metropolitan Area (NECMA), or is an area wholly within an MSA or NECMA that has been identified as rural under the "Goldsmith modification." (The Goldsmith modification establishes an operational definition of rural areas within large counties that contain one or more metropolitan areas. The Goldsmith areas are so isolated by distance or physical features that they are more rural than urban in character and lack easy geographic access to health services.)

For Paramedic Intercept, an area is a rural area if:

- It is designated as a rural area by any law or regulation of a State;
- It is located outside of an MSA or NECMA; or
- It is located in a rural census tract of an MSA as determined under the most recent Goldsmith modification.

See IOM Pub. 100-02, Medicare Benefit Policy Manual, chapter 10 –Ambulance Services, section 30.1.1 –Ground Ambulance Services for coverage requirements for the Paramedic Intercept benefit. Presently, only the State of New York meets these requirements.

Although a transport with a POP located in a rural area is subject to a rural adjustment for mileage, Medicare still pays the lesser of the billed charge or the applicable FS amount for mileage. Thus, when rural mileage is involved, the contractor compares the calculated FS rural mileage payment rate to the provider's/supplier's actual charge for mileage and pays the lesser amount.

The CMS furnishes the ambulance FS files to claims processing contractors electronically. A version of the Ambulance Fee Schedule is also posted to the CMS website (http://www.cms.hhs.gov/AmbulanceFeeSchedule/02_afspuf.asp) for public consumption. To clarify whether a particular ZIP Code is rural or urban, please refer to the most recent version of the Medicare supplied ZIP Code file.

6. Regional Ambulance FS Payment Rate Floor for Ground Ambulance Transports

For services furnished during the period July 1, 2004 through December 31, 2009, the base rate portion of the payment under the ambulance FS for ground ambulance transports is subject to a minimum amount. This minimum amount depends upon the area of the country in which the service is furnished. The country is divided into 9 census divisions and each of the census divisions has a regional FS that is constructed using the same methodology as the national FS. Where the regional FS is greater than the national FS, the base rates for ground ambulance transports are determined by a blend of the national rate and the regional rate in accordance with the following schedule:

Year	National FS Percentage	Regional FS Percentage
7/1/04 - 12/31/04	20%	80%
CY 2005	40%	60%
CY 2006	60%	40%
CY 2007 – CY 2009	80%	20%
CY 2010 and thereafter	100%	0%

Where the regional FS is not greater than the national FS, there is no blending and only the national FS applies. Note that this provision affects only the FS portion of the blended transition payment rate. This floor amount is calculated by CMS centrally and is incorporated into the FS amount that appears in the FS file maintained by CMS and downloaded by CMS contractors. There is no calculation to be done by the Medicare B/MAC or A/MAC in order to implement this provision.

7. Adjustments for FS Payment Rate for Certain Rural Ground Ambulance Transports

For services furnished during the period July 1, 2004 through December 31, 2010, the base rate portion of the payment under the FS for ground ambulance transports furnished in certain rural areas is increased by a percentage amount determined by CMS. Section 3105 (c) and 10311 (c) of the Affordable Care Act amended section 1834 (1) (13) (A) of the Act to extend this rural bonus for an additional year through December 31, 2010. This increase applies if the POP is in a rural county (or Goldsmith area) that is comprised by the lowest quartile by population of all such rural areas arrayed by population density. CMS will determine this bonus amount and the designated POP rural ZIP Codes in which the bonus applies. Beginning on July 1, 2004, rural areas qualifying for the additional bonus amount will be identified with a "B" indicator on the national ZIP Code file. Contractors must apply the additional rural bonus amount as a multiplier to the base rate portion of the FS payment for all ground transports originating in the designated POP ZIP Codes.

Subsequently, section of 106 (c) of the MMEA again amended section 1843 (l) (13) (A) of the Act to extend the rural bonus an additional year, through December 31, 2011

8. Adjustments for FS Payment Rates for Ground Ambulance Transports

The payment rates under the FS for ground ambulance transports (both the fee schedule base rates and the mileage amounts) are increased for services furnished during the period July 1, 2004 through December 31, 2006 as well as July 1, 2008 through December 31, 2010. For ground ambulance transport services furnished where the POP is urban, the rates are increased by 1 percent for claims with dates of service July 1, 2004 through December 31, 2006 in accordance with Section 414 of the Medicare Modernization Act (MMA) of 2004 and by 2 percent for claims with dates of service July 1, 2008 through December 31, 2010 in accordance with Section 146(a) of the Medicare Improvements for Patients and Providers Act of 2008 and Sections 3105(a) and 10311(a) of the Patient Protection and Affordable Care Act (ACA) of 2010. For ground ambulance transport services furnished where the POP is rural, the rates are increased by 2 percent for claims with dates of service July 1, 2004 through December 31, 2006 in accordance with Section 414 of the Medicare Modernization Act (MMA) of 2004 and by 3 percent for claims with dates of service July 1, 2008 through December 31, 2010 in accordance with Section 146(a) of the Medicare Improvements for Patients and Providers Act of 2008 and Sections 3105(a) and 10311(a) of the Patient Protection and Affordable Care Act (ACA) of 2010. Subsequently, section 106 (a) of the Medicare and Medicaid Extenders Act of 2010 (MMEA) again amended section 1834 (1) (12) (A) of the Act to extend the payment increases for an additional year, through December 31, 2011. These amounts are incorporated into the fee schedule amounts that appear in the Ambulance FS file maintained by CMS and downloaded by CMS contractors. There is no calculation to be done by the Medicare carrier or intermediary in order to implement this provision.

The following chart summarizes the Medicare Prescription Drug, Improvement, and Modernization Act (MMA) of 2003 payment changes for ground ambulance services that became effective on July 1, 2004 as well as the Medicare Improvement for Patients and Providers Act (MIPPA) of 2008 changes that became effective July 1, 2008 and were extended by the Patient Protection and Affordable Care Act of 2010 and the Medicare and Medicaid Extenders Act of 2010 (MMEA).

Summary Chart of Additional Payments for Ground Ambulance Services Provided by MMA, MIPPA and MMEA

Service	Effective Dates	Payment Increase*
All rural miles	7/1/04 - 12/31/06	2%
All rural miles	7/1/08 – 12/31/11	3%
Rural miles 51+	7/1/04 - 12/31/08	25% **
All urban miles	7/1/04 - 12/31/06	1%
All urban miles	7/1/08 – 12/31/11	2%
Urban miles 51+	7/1/04 - 12/31/08	25% **
All rural base rates	7/1/04 - 12/31/06	2%
All rural base rates	7/1/08 – 12/31/11	3%
Rural base rates (lowest quartile)	7/1/04 - 12/31/11	22.6 %**
All urban base rates	7/1/04 - 12/31/06	1%
All urban base rates	7/1/08 – 12/31/11	2%
All base rates (regional fee schedule blend)	7/1/04 - 12/31/09	Floor

NOTES: *All payments are percentage increases and all are cumulative.

**Contractor systems perform this calculation. All other increases are incorporated into the CMS Medicare Ambulance FS file.

B. Air Ambulance Services

1. Base Rates

Each type of air ambulance service has a base rate. There is no conversion factor (CF) applicable to air ambulance services.

2. Geographic Adjustment Factor (GAF)

The GAF, as described above for ground ambulance services, is also used for air ambulance services. However, for air ambulance services, the applicable GPCI is applied to 50 percent of each of the base rates (fixed and rotary wing).

3. Mileage

The FS for air ambulance services provides a separate payment for mileage.

4. Adjustment for Services Furnished in Rural Areas

The payment rates for air ambulance services where the POP is in a rural area are greater than in an urban area. For air ambulance services (fixed or rotary wing), the rural adjustment

is an increase of 50 percent to the unadjusted FS amount, e.g., the applicable air service base rate multiplied by the GAF plus the mileage amount or, in other words, 1.5 times both the applicable air service base rate and the total mileage amount.

The basis for a rural adjustment for air ambulance services is determined in the same manner as for ground services. That is, whether the POP is within a rural ZIP Code as described above for ground services.

100-4, Chapter-15, 20.2

Payment for Mileage Charges

Charges for mileage must be based on loaded mileage only, e.g., from the pickup of a patient to his/her arrival at destination. It is presumed that all unloaded mileage costs are taken into account when a supplier establishes his basic charge for ambulance services and his rate for loaded mileage. Suppliers should be notified that separate charges for unloaded mileage will be denied.

Instructions on billing mileage are found in §30.

100-4, Chapter-15, 20.3

Air Ambulance

Refer to IOM Pub. 100-02, Medicare Benefit Policy Manual, chapter 10 -Ambulance Services, section 10.4 –Air Ambulance Services, for additional information on the coverage of air ambulance services. Under certain circumstances, transportation by airplane or helicopter may qualify as covered ambulance services. If the conditions of coverage are met, payment may be made for the air ambulance services.

Air ambulance services are paid at different rates according to two air ambulance categories:

- AIR ambulance service, conventional air services, transport, one way, fixed wing (FW) (HCPCS code A0430)
- AIR ambulance service, conventional air services, transport, one way, rotary wing(RW) (HCPCS code A0431)

Covered air ambulance mileage services are paid when the appropriate HCPCS code is reported on the claim:

- HCPCS code A0435 identifies FIXED WING AIR MILEAGE
- HCPCS code A0436 identifies ROTARY WING AIR MILEAGE

Air mileage must be reported in whole numbers of loaded statute miles flown. Contractors must ensure that the appropriate air transport code is used with the appropriate mileage code.

Air ambulance services may be paid only for ambulance services to a hospital. Other destinations e.g., skilled nursing facility, a physician's office, or a patient's home may not be paid air ambulance. The destination is identified by the use of an appropriate modifier As defined in Section 30(A) of this chapter.

Claims for air transports may account for all mileage from the point of pickup, including where applicable: ramp to taxiway, taxiway to runway, takeoff run, air miles, roll out upon landing, and taxiing after landing. Additional air mileage may be allowed by the contractor in situations where additional mileage is incurred, due to circumstances beyond the pilot's control. These circumstances include, but are not limited to, the following:

- Military base and other restricted zones, air-defense zones, and similar FAA restrictions and prohibitions;
- Hazardous weather; or
- Variances in departure patterns and clearance routes required by an air traffic controller.

If the air transport meets the criteria for medical necessity, Medicare pays the actual miles flown for legitimate reasons as determined by the Medicare contractor, once the Medicare beneficiary is loaded onto the air ambulance.

IOM Pub. 100-08, Medicare Program Integrity Manual, chapter 6 –Intermediary MR Guidelines for Specific Services contains instructions for Medical Review of Air Ambulance Services.

100-4, Chapter-15, 20.6

Payment for Non-Emergency Trips to/from ESRD Facilities

Section 637 of the American Taxpayer Relief Act of 2012 requires that, effective for transports occurring on and after October 1, 2013, fee schedule payments for non-emergency basic life support (BLS) transports of individuals with end-stage renal disease (ESRD) to and from renal dialysis treatment be reduced by 10%. The payment reduction affects transports (base rate and mileage) to and from hospital-based and freestanding renal dialysis treatment facilities for dialysis services provided on a non-emergency basis. Non-emergency BLS ground transports are identified by Healthcare Common Procedure Code System (HCPCS) code A0428. Ambulance transports to and from renal dialysis treatment are identified by modifier codes "G" (hospital-based ESRD) and "J" (freestanding ESRD facility) in either the first position (origin code) or second position (destination code) within the two-digit ambulance modifier. (See Section 30 (A) for information regarding modifiers specific to ambulance.)

Effective for claims with dates of service on and after October 1, 2013, the 10% reduction will be calculated and applied to HCPCS code A0428 when billed with modifier code "G" or "J". The reduction will also be applied to any mileage billed in association with a non-emergency transport of a beneficiary with ESRD to and from renal dialysis treatment. BLS mileage is identified by HCPCS code A0425.

The 10% reduction will be taken after calculation of the normal fee schedule payment amount, including any add-on or bonus payments, and will apply to transports in rural and urban areas as well as areas designated as "super rural".

Payment for emergency transports is not affected by this reduction. Payment for non-emergency BLS transports to other destinations is also not affected. This reduction does not affect or change the Ambulance Fee Schedule.

NOTE: The 10% reduction applies to beneficiaries with ESRD that are receiving non-emergency BLS transport to and from renal dialysis treatment. While it is possible that a beneficiary who is not diagnosed with ESRD will require routine transport to and from renal dialysis treatment, it is highly unlikely. However, contractors have discretion to override or reverse the reduction on appeal if they deem it appropriate based on supporting documentation.

100-4, Chapter-15, 30.1.2

Coding Instructions for Paper and Electronic Claim Forms

The term Medicare beneficiary identifier (MBI) is a general term describing a beneficiary's Medicare identification number. For purposes of this manual, Medicare beneficiary identifier references both the Health Insurance Claim Number (HICN) and the Medicare Beneficiary Identifier (MBI) during the new Medicare card transition period and after for certain business areas that will continue to use the HICN as part of their processes.

Except as otherwise noted, beginning with dates of service on or after January 1, 2001, the following coding instructions must be used.

Origin

Electronic billers should refer to the Implementation Guide to determine how to report the origin information (e.g., the ZIP Code of the point of pickup). Beginning with the early implementation of version 5010 of the ASC X12 837 professional claim format on January 1, 2011, electronic billers are required to submit, in addition to the loaded ambulance trip's origin information (e.g., the ZIP Code of the point of pickup), the loaded ambulance trip's destination information (e.g., the ZIP code of the point of drop-off). Refer to the appropriate Implementation Guide to determine how to report the destination information. Only the ZIP Code of the point of pickup will be used to adjudicate and price the ambulance claim, not the point of drop-off. However, the point of drop-off is an additional reporting requirement on version 5010 of the ASC X12 837 professional claim format.

Where the CMS-1500 Form is used the ZIP code is reported in item 23. Since the ZIP Code is used for pricing, more than one ambulance service may be reported on the same paper claim for a beneficiary if all points of pickup have the same ZIP Code. Suppliers must prepare a separate paper claim for each trip if the points of pickup are located in different ZIP Codes.

Claims without a ZIP Code in item 23 on the CMS-1500 Form item 23, or with multiple ZIP Codes in item 23, must be returned as unprocessable.

The contractor shall use the following remittance advice messages and associated codes when rejecting/denying claims under this policy. This CARC/RARC combination is compliant with CAQH CORE Business Scenario Two.

Group Code: CO

CARC: 16

RARC: N53

MSN: N/A

ZIP Codes must be edited for validity.

The format for a ZIP Code is five numerics. If a nine-digit ZIP Code is submitted, the last four digits are ignored. If the data submitted in the required field does not match that format, the claim is rejected.

Mileage

Generally, each ambulance trip will require two lines of coding, e.g., one line for the service and one line for the mileage. Suppliers who do not bill mileage would have one line of code for the service.

Beginning with dates of service on or after January 1, 2011, mileage billed must be reported as fractional units in the following situations:

- Where billing is by ASC X12 claims transaction (professional or institutional), and
- Where billing is by CMS-1500 paper form.

Electronic billers should see the appropriate Implementation Guide to determine where to report the fractional units. Item 24G of the Form CMS-1500 paper claim is used.

Fractional units are not required on Form CMS-1450

For trips totaling up to 100 covered miles suppliers must round the total miles up to the nearest tenth of a mile and report the resulting number with the appropriate HCPCS code for ambulance mileage. The decimal must be used in the appropriate place (e.g., 99.9).

For trips totaling 100 covered miles and greater, suppliers must report mileage rounded up to the next whole number mile without the use of a decimal (e.g., 998.5 miles should be reported as 999).

For trips totaling less than 1 mile, enter a "0" before the decimal (e.g., 0.9).

For mileage HCPCS billed on the ASC X12 837 professional transaction or the CMS-1500 paper form only, contractors shall automatically default to "0.1" units when the total mileage units are missing.

Multiple Patients on One Trip

Ambulance suppliers submitting a claim using the ASC X12 professional format or the CMS1500 paper form for an ambulance transport with more than one patient onboard must use the "GM" modifier ("Multiple Patients on One Ambulance Trip") for each service line item. In addition, suppliers are required to submit documentation to A/B MACs (Part B) to specify the particulars of a multiple patient transport. The documentation must include the total number of patients transported in the vehicle at the same time and the Medicare beneficiary identifiers for each Medicare beneficiary. A/B/MACs (Part B) shall calculate payment amounts based on policy instructions found in Pub.100-02, Medicare Benefit Policy Manual, Chapter 10 – Ambulance Services, Section 10.3.10 – Multiple Patient Ambulance Transport.

Ambulance claims submitted on or after January 1, 2011, in version 5010 of the ASC X12 837 professional claim format require the presence of a diagnosis code and the absence of diagnosis code will cause the ambulance claim to not be accepted into the claims processing system. The presence of a diagnosis code on an ambulance claim is not required as a condition of ambulance payment policy. The adjudicative process does not take into account the presence (or absence) of a diagnosis code, but a diagnosis code is required on the ASC X12 837 professional claim format.

100-4, Chapter-15, 30.2

Fiscal Intermediary Shared System (FISS) Guidelines

For SNF Part A, the cost of medically necessary ambulance transportation to receive most services included in the RUG rate is included in the cost for the service. Payment for the SNF claim is based on the RUGs, which takes into account the cost of such transportation to receive the ancillary services.

Refer to Pub. 100-04, Medicare Claims Processing Manual, chapter 6 – SNF Inpatient Part A Billing, Section 20.3.1 – Ambulance Services, for additional information on SNF consolidated billing and ambulance transportation.

Refer to Pub. 100-04, Medicare Claims Processing Manual, chapter 3 – Inpatient Hospital Billing, section 10.5 – Hospital Inpatient Bundling, for additional information on hospital inpatient bundling of ambulance services.

In general, the A/B MAC (A) processes claims for Part B ambulance services provided by an ambulance supplier under arrangements with hospitals or SNFs. These providers bill A/B MACs (A) using only Method 2.

The provider must furnish the following data in accordance with A/B MAC (A) instructions. The A/B MAC (A) will make arrangements for the method and media for submitting the data:

- A detailed statement of the condition necessitating the ambulance service;
- A statement indicating whether the patient was admitted as an inpatient. If yes the name and address of the facility must be shown;
- Name and address of certifying physician;
- Name and address of physician ordering service if other than certifying physician;
- Point of pickup (identify place and completed address);
- Destination (identify place and complete address);
- Number of loaded miles (the number of miles traveled when the beneficiary was in the ambulance);
- Cost per mile;
- Mileage charge;
- Minimum or base charge; and
- Charge for special items or services. Explain.

A. General

The reasonable cost per trip of ambulance services furnished by a provider of services may not exceed the prior year's reasonable cost per trip updated by the ambulance inflation factor. This determination is effective with services furnished during Federal Fiscal Year (FFY) 1998 (between October 1, 1997, and September 30, 1998). Providers are to bill for Part B ambulance services using the billing method of base rate including supplies, with mileage billed separately as described below.

The following instructions provide billing procedures implementing the above provisions.

B. Applicable Bill Types

The appropriate type of bill (13X, 22X, 23X, 83X, and 85X) must be reported. For SNFs, ambulance cannot be reported on a 21X type of bill.

C. Value Code Reporting

For claims with dates of service on or after January 1, 2001, providers must report on every Part B ambulance claim value code A0 (zero) and the related ZIP Code of the geographic location from which the beneficiary was placed on board the ambulance in the Value Code field. The value code is defined as "ZIP Code of the location from which the beneficiary is initially placed on board the ambulance." Providers report the number in dollar portion of the form location right justified to the left of the dollar/cents delimiter.

More than one ambulance trip may be reported on the same claim if the ZIP Codes of all points of pickup are the same. However, since billing requirements do not allow for value codes (ZIP Codes) to be line item specific and only one ZIP Code may be reported per claim, providers must prepare a separate claim for a beneficiary for each trip if the points of pickup are located in different ZIP Codes.

For claims with dates of service on or after April 1, 2002, providers must report value code 32 (multiple patient ambulance transport) when an ambulance transports more than one patient at a time to the same destination. Providers must report value code 32 and the number of patients transported in the amount field as a whole number to the left of the delimiter.

NOTE: Information regarding the claim form locator that corresponds to the Value Code field is found in Pub.100-04, Medicare Claims Processing Manual, chapter 25 – Completing and Processing the Form CMS-1450 Data Set.

D. Revenue Code/HCPCS Code Reporting

Providers must report revenue code 054X and, for services provided before January 1, 2001, one of the following CMS HCPCS codes for each ambulance trip provided during the billing period:

A0030 (discontinued 12/31/2000); A0040 (discontinued 12/31/2000); A0050 (discontinued 12/31/2000); A0320 (discontinued 12/31/2000); A0322 (discontinued 12/31/2000); A0324 (discontinued 12/31/2000); A0326 (discontinued 12/31/2000); A0328, (discontinued 12/31/2000); or A0330 (discontinued 12/31/2000).

In addition, providers report one of A0380 or A0390 for mileage HCPCS codes. No other HCPCS codes are acceptable for reporting ambulance services and mileage. Providers report one of the following revenue codes:

0540;

0542;

0543;

0545;

0546; or

0548.

Do not report revenue codes 0541, 0544, or 0547.

For claims with dates of service on or after January 1, 2001, providers must report revenue code 540 and one of the following HCPCS codes for each ambulance trip provided during the billing period:

A0426; A0427;

A0428; A0429; A0430; A0431; A0432; A0433; or

A0434.

Providers using an ALS vehicle to furnish a BLS level of service report HCPCS code, A0426 (ALS1) or A0427 (ALS1 emergency), and are paid accordingly. In addition, all providers report one of the following mileage HCPCS codes: A0380; A0390; A0435; or A0436.

Since billing requirements do not allow for more than one HCPCS code to be reported for per revenue code line, providers must report revenue code 0540 (ambulance) on two separate and consecutive lines to accommodate both the Part B ambulance service and the mileage HCPCS codes for each ambulance trip provided during the billing period. Each loaded (e.g., a patient is onboard) 1-way ambulance trip must be reported with a unique pair of revenue code lines on the claim. Unloaded trips and mileage are NOT reported.

However, in the case where the beneficiary was pronounced dead after the ambulance is called but before the ambulance arrives at the scene: Payment may be made for a BLS service if a ground vehicle is dispatched or at the fixed wing or rotary wing base rate, as applicable, if an air ambulance is dispatched. Neither mileage nor a rural adjustment would be paid. The blended rate amount will otherwise apply. Providers report the A0428 (BLS) HCPCS code. Providers report modifier QL (Patient pronounced dead after ambulance

called) in Form Locator (FL) 44 "HCPCS/Rates" instead of the origin and destination modifier. In addition to the QL modifier, providers report modifier QM or QN.

NOTE: Information regarding the claim form locator that corresponds to the HCPCS code is found in Pub. 100-04, Medicare Claims Processing Manual, Chapter 25 – Completing and Processing the Form CMS-1450 Data Set.

E. Modifier Reporting

See the above Section 30 (A) (Modifiers Specific to Ambulance Service Claims) for instructions regarding the usage of modifiers.

F. Line-Item Dates of Service Reporting

Providers are required to report line-item dates of service per revenue code line. This means that they must report two separate revenue code lines for every ambulance trip provided during the billing period along with the date of each trip. This includes situations in which more than one ambulance service is provided to the same beneficiary on the same day. Line-item dates of service are reported in the Service Date field.

NOTE: Information regarding the claim form locator that corresponds to the Service Date is found in Pub. 100-04, Medicare Claims Processing Manual, Chapter 25 – Completing and Processing the Form CMS-1450 Data Set.

G. Service Units Reporting

For line items reflecting HCPCS code A0030, A0040, A0050, A0320, A0322, A0324, A0326, A0328, or A0330 (services before January 1, 2001) or code A0426, A0427, A0428, A0429, A0430, A0431, A0432, A0433, or A0434 (services on and after January 1, 2001), providers are required to report in Service Units each ambulance trip provided during the billing period. Therefore, the service units for each occurrence of these HCPCS codes are always equal to one. In addition, for line items reflecting HCPCS code A0380 or A0390, the number of loaded miles must be reported. (See examples below.)

Therefore, the service units for each occurrence of these HCPCS codes are always equal to one. In addition, for line items reflecting HCPCS code A0380, A0390, A0435, or A0436, the number of loaded miles must be reported.

H. Total Charges Reporting

For line items reflecting HCPCS codes A0426, A0427, A0428, A0429, A0430, A0431, A0432, A0433, or A0434;

Providers are required to report in Total Charges the actual charge for the ambulance service including all supplies used for the ambulance trip but excluding the charge for mileage. For line items reflecting HCPCS code A0380, A0390, A0435, or A0436, report the actual charge for mileage.

NOTE: There are instances where the provider does not incur any cost for mileage, e.g., if the beneficiary is pronounced dead after the ambulance is called but before the ambulance arrives at the scene. In these situations, providers report the base rate ambulance trip and mileage as separate revenue code lines. Providers report the base rate ambulance trip in accordance with current billing requirements. For purposes of reporting mileage, they must report the appropriate HCPCS code, modifiers, and units as a separate line item. For the related charges, providers report $1.00 in FL48 for non-covered charges. A/B MACs (A) should assign remittance adjustment Group Code OA to the $1.00 non- covered mileage line, which in turn informs the beneficiaries and providers that they each have no liability.

Prior to submitting the claim to CWF, the A/B MAC (A) will remove the entire revenue code line containing the mileage amount reported in Non-covered Charges to avoid non-acceptance of the claim.

NOTE: Information regarding the claim form locator that corresponds to the Charges fields is found in Pub. 100-04, Medicare Claims Processing Manual, Chapter 25 – Completing and Processing the Form CMS-1450 Data Set.

EXAMPLES: The following provides examples of how bills for Part B ambulance services should be completed based on the reporting requirements above. These examples reflect ambulance services furnished directly by providers. Ambulance services provided under arrangement between the provider and an ambulance company are reported in the same manner except providers report a QM modifier instead of a QN modifier.

EXAMPLE 1: Claim containing only one ambulance trip:

Revenue Code	HCPCS/ Modifiers	Date of Service	Units	Total Charges
0540	A0428RHQN	082701	1 (trip)	100.00
0540	A0380RHQN	082701	4 (mileage)	8.00

EXAMPLE 2: Claim containing multiple ambulance trips:

For the hard copy Form CMS-1450, providers report as follows:

Revenue Code	HCPCS	Modifiers		Date of Service	Units	Total Charges
		#1	#2			
0540	A0429	RH	QN	082801	1 (trip)	100.00
0540	A0380	RH	QN	082801	2 (mileage)	4.00
0540	A0330	RH	QN	082901	1 (trip)	400.00
0540	A0390	RH	QN	082901	3 (mileage)	6.00

EXAMPLE 3: Claim containing more than one ambulance trip provided on the same day:

For the hard copy CMS-1450, providers report as follows:

Revenue Code	HCPCS	Modifiers		Date of Service	Units	Total Charges
0540	A0429	RH	QN	090201	1 (trip)	100.00
0540	A0380	RH	QN	090201	2 (mileage)	4.00
0540	A0429	HR	QN	090201	1 (trip)	100.00
0540	A0380	HR	QN	090201	2 (mileage)	4.00

I. Edits

FISS edits to assure proper reporting as follows:

For claims with dates of service on or after January 1, 2001, each pair of revenue codes 0540 must have one of the following ambulance HCPCS codes - A0426, A0427, A0428, A0429, A0430, A0431, A0432, A0433, or A0434; and one of the following mileage HCPCS codes – A0435, A0436 or for claims with dates of service on or after April 1, 2002, A0425;

- For claims with dates of service on or after January 1, 2001, the presence of an origin and destination modifier and a QM or QN modifier for every line item containing revenue code 0540;

- The units field is completed for every line item containing revenue code 0540;

- For claims with dates of service on or after January 1, 2001, the units field is completed for every line item containing revenue code 0540;

- Service units for line items containing HCPCS codes A0426, A0427, A0428, A0429, A0430, A0431, A0432, A0433, or A0434 always equal "1"

For claims with dates of service on or after July 1, 2001, each 1-way ambulance trip, line- item dates of service for the ambulance service, and corresponding mileage are equal.

100-4, Chapter-15, 30.2.1

A/B MAC (A) Bill Processing Guidelines Effective April 1, 2002, as a Result of Fee Schedule Implementation

For SNF Part A, the cost of medically necessary ambulance transportation to receive most services included in the RUG rate is included in the cost for the service. Payment for the SNF claim is based on the RUGs, which takes into account the cost of such transportation to receive the ancillary services.

Refer to IOM Pub. 100-04, Medicare Claims Processing Manual, chapter 6 – SNF Inpatient Part A Billing, Section 20.3.1 – Ambulance Services for additional information on SNF consolidated billing and ambulance transportation.

Refer to IOM Pub. 100-04, Medicare Claims Processing Manual, chapter 3 – Inpatient Hospital Billing, section 10.5 – Hospital Inpatient Bundling, for additional information on hospital inpatient bundling of ambulance services.

In general, the A/B MAC (A) processes claims for Part B ambulance services provided by an ambulance supplier under arrangements with hospitals or SNFs. These providers bill A/B MACs (A) using only Method 2.

The provider must furnish the following data in accordance with A/B MAC (A) instructions. The A/B MAC (A) will make arrangements for the method and media for submitting the data:

A detailed statement of the condition necessitating the ambulance service;

- A statement indicating whether the patient was admitted as an inpatient. If yes the name and address of the facility must be shown;
- Name and address of certifying physician;
- Name and address of physician ordering service if other than certifying physician;
- Point of pickup (identify place and completed address);
- Destination (identify place and complete address);
- Number of loaded miles (the number of miles traveled when the beneficiary was in the ambulance);
- Cost per mile;
- Mileage charge;
- Minimum or base charge; and
- Charge for special items or services. Explain.

A. Revenue Code Reporting on Form CMS-1450

Providers report ambulance services under revenue code 540 in FL 42 "Revenue Code."

B. HCPCS Codes Reporting on Form CMS-1450

Providers report the HCPCS codes established for the ambulance fee schedule. No other HCPCS codes are acceptable for the reporting of ambulance services and mileage. The HCPCS code must be used to reflect the type of service the beneficiary received, not the type of vehicle used.

Providers must report one of the following HCPCS codes in FL 44 "HCPCS/Rates" for each base rate ambulance trip provided during the billing period:

A0426;

A0427;

A0428;

A0429;

A0430;

A0431;

A0432;

A0433; or

A0434.

These are the same codes required effective for services January 1, 2001.

In addition, providers must report one of HCPCS mileage codes:

A0425;

A0435; or

A0436.

Since billing requirements do not allow for more than one HCPCS code to be reported per revenue code line, providers must report revenue code 540 (ambulance) on two separate and consecutive line items to accommodate both the ambulance service and the mileage HCPCS codes for each ambulance trip provided during the billing period. Each loaded (e.g., a patient is onboard) 1-way ambulance trip must be reported with a unique pair of revenue code lines on the claim. Unloaded trips and mileage are NOT reported.

For Form CMS-1450 claims submission prior to August 1, 2011, providers code one mile for trips less than a mile. Miles must be entered as whole numbers. If a trip has a fraction of a mile, round up to the nearest whole number.

Beginning with dates of service on or after January 1, 2011, for Form CMS-1450 hard copy claims submissions August 1, 2011 and after, mileage must be reported as fractional units. When reporting fractional mileage, providers must round the total miles up to the nearest tenth of a mile and the decimal must be used in the appropriate place (e.g., 99.9).

For trips totaling less than 1 mile, enter a "0" before the decimal (e.g., 0.9).

100-4, Chapter-15, 30.2.4

Non-covered Charges on Institutional Ambulance Claims

Medicare law contains a restriction that miles beyond the closest available facility cannot be billed to Medicare. Non-covered miles beyond the closest facility are billed with HCPCS procedure code A0888 ("non-covered ambulance mileage per mile, e.g., for miles traveled beyond the closest appropriate facility"). These non-covered line items can be billed on claims also containing covered charges. Ambulance claims may use the –GY modifier on line items for such non-covered mileage, and liability for the service will be assigned correctly to the beneficiary.

The method of billing all miles for the same trip, with covered and non-covered portions, on the same claim is preferable in this scenario. However, billing the non-covered mileage

using condition code 21 claims is also permitted, if desired, as long as all line items on the claims are non-covered and the beneficiary is liable. Additionally, unless requested by the beneficiary or required by specific Medicare policy, services excluded by statute do not have to be billed to Medicare.

When the scenario is point of pick up outside the United States, including U.S. territories but excepting some points in Canada and Mexico in some cases, mileage is also statutorily excluded from Medicare coverage. Such billings are more likely to be submitted on entirely non-covered claims using condition code 21. This scenario requires the use of a different message on the Medicare Summary Notice (MSN) sent to beneficiaries.

Another scenario in which billing non-covered mileage to Medicare may occur is when the beneficiary dies after the ambulance has been called but before the ambulance arrives. The –QL modifier should be used on the base rate line in this scenario, in place of origin and destination modifiers, and the line is submitted with covered charges. The –QL modifier should also be used on the accompanying mileage line, if submitted, with non-covered charges. Submitting this non-covered mileage line is optional for providers.

Non-covered charges may also apply is if there is a subsidy of mileage charges that are never charged to Medicare. Because there are no charges for Medicare to share in, the only billing option is to submit non-covered charges, if the provider bills Medicare at all (it is not required in such cases). These non-covered charges are unallowable, and should not be considered in settlement of cost reports. However, there is a difference in billing if such charges are subsidized, but otherwise would normally be charged to Medicare as the primary payer. In this latter case, CMS examination of existing rules relating to grants policy since October 1983, supported by Federal regulations (42CFR 405.423), generally requires providers to reduce their costs by the amount of grants and gifts restricted to pay for such costs. Thereafter, section 405.423 was deleted from the regulations.

Thus, providers were no longer required to reduce their costs for restricted grants and gifts, and charges tied to such grants/gifts/subsidies should be submitted as covered charges. This is in keeping with Congress's intent to encourage hospital philanthropy, allowing the provider receiving the subsidy to use it, and also requiring Medicare to share in the unreduced cost. Treatment of subsidized charges as non-covered Medicare charges serves to reduce Medicare payment on the Medicare cost report contrary to the 1983 change in policy.

Medicare requires the use of the –TQ modifier so that CMS can track the instances of the subsidy scenario for non-covered charges. The –TQ should be used whether the subsidizing entity is governmental or voluntary. The -TQ modifier is not required in the case of covered charges submitted when a subsidy has been made, but charges are still normally made to Medicare as the primary payer.

If providers believe they have been significantly or materially penalized in the past by the failure of their cost reports to consider covered charges occurring in the subsidy case, since Medicare had previous billing instructions that stated all charges in the case of a subsidy, not just charges when the entity providing the subsidy never charges another entity/primary payer, should be submitted as non-covered charges, they may contact their FI about reopening the reports in question for which the time period in 42 CFR 405.1885 has not expired. FIs have the discretion to determine if the amount in question warrants reopening. The CMS does not expect many such cases to occur.

Billing requirements for all these situations, including the use of modifiers, are presented in the chart below:

Mileage Scenario	HCPCS	Modifiers*	Liability	Billing	Remit. Requirements	MSN Message
STATUTE: Miles beyond closest facility, OR **Pick up point outside of U.S.	A0888 on line item for the non-covered mileage	-QM or –QN, origin/destination modifier, and –GY unless condition code 21 claim used	Beneficiary	Bill mileage line item with A0888 –GY and other modifiers as needed to establish liability, line item will be denied; OR bill service on condition code 21 claim, no –GY required, claim will be denied	Group code PR, reason code 96	16.10 "Medicare does not pay for this item or service"; OR, "Medicare no paga por este artículo o servicio"
Beneficiary dies after ambulance is called	Most appropriate ambulance HCPCS mileage code (i.e., ground, air)	–QL unless condition code –21 claim	Provider	Bill mileage line item with –QL as non-covered, line item will be denied	Group Code CO, reason code 96	16.58 "The provider billed this charge as non-covered. You do not have to pay this amount."; OR, "El proveedor facuró este cargo como no cubierto. Usted no tiene que pagar ests cantidad."
Subsidy or government owned Ambulance, Medicare NEVER billed***	A0888 on line item for the non-covered mileage	-QM or –QN, origin/destination modifier, and -TQ must be used for policy purposes	Provider	Bill mileage line item with A0888, and modifiers as non-covered, line item will be denied	Group Code CO, reason code 96	16.58 "The provider billed this charge as non-covered. You do not have to pay this amount."; OR, "El proveedor facuró este cargo como no cubierto. Usted no tiene que pagar ests cantidad."

*Current ambulance billing requirements state that either the –QM or –QN modifier must be used on services. The –QM is used when the "ambulance service is provided under arrangement by a provider of services," and the –QN when the "ambulance service is provided directly by a provider of services." Line items using either the –QM or –QN modifiers are not subject to the FISS edit associated with FISS reason code 31322 so that these lines items will process to completion. Origin/destination modifiers, also required by current instruction, combine two alpha characters: one for origin, one for destination, and are not non-covered by definition.

** This is the one scenario where the base rate is not paid in addition to mileage, and there are certain exceptions in Canada and Mexico where mileage is covered as described in existing ambulance instructions.

***If Medicare would normally have been billed, submit mileage charges as covered charges despite subsidies.

Medicare systems may return claims to the provider if they do not comply with the requirements in the table.

100-4, Chapter-15, 40

Medical Conditions List and Instructions

See http://www.cms.gov/Center/Provider-Type/Ambulances-Services-Center.html for a medical conditions list and instructions to assist ambulance providers and suppliers to communicate the patient's condition to Medicare contractors, as reported by the dispatch center and as observed by the ambulance crew. Use of the medical conditions list does not guarantee payment of the claim or payment for a certain level of service.

In addition to reporting one of the medical conditions on the claim, one of the transportation indicators may be included on the claim to indicate why it was necessary for the patient to be transported in a particular way or circumstance. The provider or supplier will place the transportation indicator in the "narrative" field on the claim. Information on the appropriate use of transportation indicators is also available at http://www.cms.gov/Center/ProviderType/Ambulances-Services-Center.html.

100-4, Chapter-16, 60.1.4

Coding Requirements for Specimen Collection

The following HCPCS codes and terminology must be used:

- 36415 - Collection of venous blood by venipuncture.
- G0471 - Collection of venous blood by venipuncture or urine sample by catheterization from an individual in a skilled nursing facility (SNF) or by a laboratory on behalf of a home health agency (HHA)
- P9615 - Catheterization for collection of specimen(s).

The allowed amount for specimen collection in each of the above circumstances is included in the laboratory fee schedule distributed annually by CMS.

100-4, Chapter-16, 60.2

Travel Allowance

In addition to a specimen collection fee allowed under §60.1, Medicare, under Part B, covers a specimen collection fee and travel allowance for a laboratory technician to draw a specimen from either a nursing home patient or homebound patient under §1833(h)(3) of the Act and payment is made based on the clinical laboratory fee schedule. The travel allowance is intended to cover the estimated travel costs of collecting a specimen and to reflect the technician's salary and travel costs.

The additional allowance can be made only where a specimen collection fee is also payable, i.e., no travel allowance is made where the technician merely performs a messenger service to pick up a specimen drawn by a physician or nursing home personnel. The travel allowance may not be paid to a physician unless the trip to the home, or to the nursing home was solely for the purpose of drawing a specimen. Otherwise travel costs are considered to be associated with the other purposes of the trip.

The travel allowance is not distributed by CMS. Instead, the carrier must calculate the travel allowance for each claim using the following rules for the particular Code. The following HCPCS codes are used for travel allowances:

Per Mile Travel Allowance (P9603)

- The minimum "per mile travel allowance" is $1.03. The per mile travel allowance is to be used in situations where the average trip to patients' homes is longer than 20 miles round trip, and is to be pro-rated in situations where specimens are drawn or picked up from non-Medicare patients in the same trip. - one way, in connection with medically necessary laboratory specimen collection drawn from homebound or nursing home bound patient; prorated miles actually traveled (carrier allowance on per mile basis); or

- The per mile allowance was computed using the Federal mileage rate plus an additional 45 cents a mile to cover the technician's time and travel costs (57.5 cents plus 45 cents equals 1.025 cents and is rounded up to 1.03 cents per mile to reflect system capabilities). Contractors have the option of establishing a higher per mile rate in excess of the minimum ($1.03 a mile in CY 2020) if local conditions warrant it. The minimum mileage rate will be reviewed and updated in conjunction with the clinical lab fee schedule as needed. At no time will the laboratory be allowed to bill for more miles than are reasonable or for miles not actually traveled by the laboratory technician.

Example 1: In CY 2020, a laboratory technician travels 60 miles round trip from a lab in a city to a remote rural location, and back to the lab to draw a single Medicare patient's blood. The total reimbursement would be $61.80 (60 miles x $1.03 a mile), plus the specimen collection fee.

Example 2: In CY 2020, a laboratory technician travels 40 miles from the lab to a Medicare patient's home to draw blood, and then travels an additional 10 miles to a nonMedicare patient's home and then travels 30 miles to return to the lab. The total miles traveled would be 80 miles. The claim submitted would be for one half of the miles traveled or $41.20 (40 x $1.03), plus the specimen collection fee.

Flat Rate (P9604)

The CMS will pay a minimum of $10.30 (based on CY 2020) one way flat rate travel allowance. The flat rate travel allowance is to be used in areas where average trips are less than 20 miles round trip. The flat rate travel fee is to be pro-rated for more than one blood drawn at the same address, and for stops at the homes of Medicare and nonMedicare patients. The laboratory does the pro-ration when the claim is submitted based on the number of patients seen on that trip. The specimen collection fee will be paid for each patient encounter.

This rate is based on an assumption that a trip is an average of 15 minutes and up to 10 miles one way. It uses the Federal mileage rate and a laboratory technician's time of $17.66 an hour, including overhead. Contractors have the option of establishing a flat rate in excess of the minimum of $10.00, if local conditions warrant it. The minimum national flat rate will be reviewed and updated in conjunction with the clinical laboratory fee schedule, as necessitated by adjustments in the Federal travel allowance and salaries.

The claimant identifies round trip travel by use of the LR modifier

Example 3: A laboratory technician travels from the laboratory to a single Medicare patient's home and returns to the laboratory without making any other stops. The flat rate would be calculated as follows: 2 x $10.30 for a total trip reimbursement of $20.60, plus the specimen collection fee.

Example 4: A laboratory technician travels from the laboratory to the homes of five patients to draw blood, four of the patients are Medicare patients and one is not. An additional flat rate would be charged to cover the 5 stops and the return trip to the lab (6 x $10.30 = $61.80). Each of the claims submitted would be for $12.36 ($61.80/5 = $12.36). Since one of the patients is non-Medicare, four claims would be submitted for $12.36 each, plus the specimen collection fee for each.

Example 5: A laboratory technician travels from a laboratory to a nursing home and draws blood from 5 patients and returns to the laboratory. Four of the patients are on Medicare and one is not. The $10.30 flat rate is multiplied by two to cover the return trip to the laboratory (2 x $10.30 = $20.60) and then divided by five (1/5 of $20.60 = $4.12). Since one of the patients is non-Medicare, four claims would be submitted for $4.12 each, plus the specimen collection fee.

If a carrier determines that it results in equitable payment, the carrier may extend the former payment allowances for additional travel (such as to a distant rural nursing home) to all circumstances where travel is required. This might be appropriate, for example, if the carrier's former payment allowance was on a per mile basis. Otherwise, it should establish an appropriate allowance and inform the suppliers in its service area. If a carrier decides to establish a new allowance, one method is to consider developing a travel allowance consisting of:

- The current Federal mileage allowance for operating personal automobiles, plus a personnel allowance per mile to cover personnel costs based upon an estimate of average hourly wages and average driving speed.

Carriers must prorate travel allowance amounts claimed by suppliers by the number of patients (including Medicare and non-Medicare patients) from whom specimens were drawn on a given trip.

The carrier may determine that payment in addition to the routine travel allowance determined under this section is appropriate if:

- The patient from whom the specimen must be collected is in a nursing home or is homebound; and.

- The clinical laboratory tests are needed on an emergency basis outside the general business hours of the laboratory making the collection.

- Subsequent updated travel allowance amounts will be issued by CMS via Recurring Update Notification (RUN) on an annual basis.

100-4, Chapter-16, 70.8

Certificate of Waiver

Effective September 1, 1992, all laboratory testing sites (except as provided in 42CFR 493.3(b)) must have either a CLIA certificate of waiver, certificate for provider-performed microscopy procedures, certificate of registration, certificate of compliance, or certificate of accreditation to legally perform clinical laboratory testing on specimens from individuals in the United States.

The Food and Drug Administration approves CLIA waived tests on a flow basis. The CMS identifies CLIA waived tests by providing an updated list of waived tests to the Medicare contractors on a quarterly basis via a Recurring Update Notification. To be recognized as a waived test, some CLIA waived tests have unique HCPCS procedure codes and some must have a QW modifier included with the HCPCS code.

For a list of specific HCPCS codes subject to CLIA see

http://www.cms.hhs.gov/CLIA/downloads/waivetbl.pdf

100-4, Chapter-17, 80.4.1

Clotting Factor Furnishing Fee

The Medicare Modernization Act section 303(e)(1) added section 1842(o)(5)(C) of the Social Security Act which requires that, beginning January 1, 2005, a furnishing fee will be paid for items and services associated with clotting factor.

Beginning January 1, 2005, a clotting factor furnishing fee is separately payable to entities that furnish clotting factor unless the costs associated with furnishing the clotting factor is paid through another payment system.

The clotting factor furnishing fee is updated each calendar year based on the percentage increase in the consumer price index (CPI) for medical care for the 12-month period ending with June of the previous year. The clotting factor furnishing fees applicable for dates of service in each calendar year (CY) are listed below:

CY 2005 - 0.140 per unit

CY 2006 - 0.146 per unit

CY 2007 - 0.152 per unit

CY 2008 - 0.158 per unit

CY 2009 - 0.164 per unit

CY 2010 - 0.170 per unit

CY 2011 - 0.176 per unit

CY 2012 - 0.181 per unit

CY 2013 - 0.188 per unit

CY 2014 - 0.192 per unit

CY 2015 - 0.197 per unit

Annual updates to the clotting factor furnishing fee are subsequently communicated by a Recurring Update Notification.

CMS includes this clotting factor furnishing fee in the nationally published payment limit for clotting factor billing codes. When the clotting factor is not included on the Average Sales Price (ASP) Medicare Part B Drug Pricing File or Not Otherwise Classified (NOC) Pricing File, the contractor must make payment for the clotting factor as well as make payment for the furnishing fee.

100-4, Chapter-17, 90.3

Hospital Outpatient Payment Under OPPS for New, Unclassified Drugs and Biologicals After FDA Approval But Before Assignment of a Product-Specific Drug or Biological HCPCS Code

Section 621(a) of the MMA amends Section 1833(t) of the Social Security Act by adding paragraph (15), Payment for New Drugs and Biologicals Until HCPCS Code Assigned. Under this provision, payment for an outpatient drug or biological that is furnished as part of covered outpatient department services for which a product-specific HCPCS code has not been assigned shall be paid an amount equal to 95 percent of average wholesale price (AWP). This provision applies only to payments under the hospital outpatient prospective payment system (OPPS).

Beginning January 1, 2004, hospital outpatient departments may bill for new drugs and biologicals that are approved by the FDA on or after January 1, 2004, for which a product-specific HCPCS code has not been assigned. Beginning on or after the date of FDA approval, hospitals may bill for the drug or biological using HCPCS code C9399, Unclassified drug or biological.

Hospitals report in the ASC X12 837 institutional claim format in specific locations, or in the "Remarks" section of Form CMS-1450):

- the National Drug Code (NDC),

- the quantity of the drug that was administered, expressed in the unit of measure applicable to the drug or biological, and

- the date the drug was furnished to the beneficiary.

Contractors shall manually price the drug or biological at 95 percent of AWP. They shall pay hospitals 80 percent of the calculated price and shall bill beneficiaries 20 percent of the calculated price, after the deductible is met. Drugs and biologicals that are manually priced at 95 percent of AWP are not eligible for outlier payment.

HCPCS code C9399 is only to be reported for new drugs and biologicals that are approved by FDA on or after January 1, 2004, for which there is no HCPCS code that describes the drug.

100-4, Chapter-18, 10.1.2

Influenza Virus Vaccine

Effective for services furnished on or after May 1, 1993, the influenza virus vaccine and its administration is covered when furnished in compliance with any applicable State law. Typically, this vaccine is administered once a flu season. Medicare does not require for coverage purposes that a doctor of medicine or osteopathy order the vaccine. Therefore, the beneficiary may receive the vaccine upon request without a physician's order and without physician supervision. Since there is no yearly limit, contractors determine whether such services are reasonable and allow payment if appropriate.

See Pub. 100-02, Medicare Benefit Policy Manual, Chapter 15, Section 50.4.4.2 for additional coverage requirements for influenza virus vaccine.

100-4, Chapter-18, 10.2.1

Healthcare Common Procedure Coding System (HCPCS) and Diagnosis Codes

Vaccines and their administration are reported using separate codes. The following codes are for reporting the vaccines only.

HCPCS **Definition**

90630 Influenza virus vaccine, quadrivalent (IIV4), split virus, preservative free, for intradermal use

90653 Influenza virus vaccine, inactivated, subunit, adjuvanted, for intramuscular use

90654 Influenza virus vaccine, split virus, preservative-free, for intradermal use, for adults ages 18 – 64;

90655 Influenza virus vaccine, split virus, preservative free, for children 6- 35 months of age, for intramuscular use;

90656 Influenza virus vaccine, split virus, preservative free, for use in individuals 3 years and above, for intramuscular use;

90657 Influenza virus vaccine, split virus, for children 6-35 months of age, for intramuscular use;

90658 Influenza virus vaccine, trivalent (IIV3), split virus, 0.5 mL dosage, for intramuscular use

90660 Influenza virus vaccine, live, for intranasal use;

90661 Influenza virus vaccine, derived from cell cultures, subunit, preservative and antibiotic free, for intramuscular use

90662 Influenza virus vaccine, split virus, preservative free, enhanced immunogenicity via increased antigen content, for intramuscular use

90670 Pneumococcal conjugate vaccine, 13 valent, for intramuscular use

90672 Influenza virus vaccine, live, quadrivalent, for intranasal use

90673 Influenza virus vaccine, trivalent, derived from recombinant DNA

(RIV3), hemagglutinin (HA) protein only, preservative and antibiotic free, for intramuscular use

90674 Influenza virus vaccine, quadrivalent (ccIIV4), derived from cell cultures, subunit, preservative and antibiotic free, 0.5 mL dosage, for intramuscular use

90682 Influenza virus vaccine, quadrivalent (RIV4), derived from recombinant DNA, hemagglutinin (HA) protein only, preservative and antibiotic free, for intramuscular use

90685 Influenza virus vaccine, quadrivalent, split virus, preservative free, when administered to children 6-35 months of age, for intramuscular use

90686 Influenza virus vaccine, quadrivalent, split virus, preservative free, when administered to individuals 3 years of age and older, for intramuscular use

90687 Influenza virus vaccine, quadrivalent, split virus, when administered to children 6-35 months of age, for intramuscular use

90688 Influenza virus vaccine, quadrivalent, split virus, when administered to individuals 3 years of age and older, for intramuscular use

90694 Influenza virus vaccine, quadrivalent (aIIV4), inactivated, adjuvanted, preservative free, 0.5 mL dosage, for intramuscular use

90732 Pneumococcal polysaccharide vaccine, 23-valent, adult or immunosuppressed patient dosage, for us in individuals 2 years or older, for subcutaneous or intramuscular use;

90739 Hepatitis B vaccine, adult dosage (2 dose schedule), for intramuscular use

90740 Hepatitis B vaccine, dialysis or immunosuppressed patient dosage (3 dose schedule), for intramuscular use;

90743 Hepatitis B vaccine, adolescent (2 dose schedule), for intramuscular use;

90744 Hepatitis B vaccine, pediatric/adolescent dosage (3 dose schedule), for intramuscular use;

90746 Hepatitis B vaccine, adult dosage, for intramuscular use; and

90747 Hepatitis B vaccine, dialysis or immunosuppressed patient dosage (4 dose schedule), for intramuscular use.

90756 Influenza virus vaccine, quadrivalent (ccIIV4), derived from cell cultures, subunit, antibiotic free, 0.5mL dosage, for intramuscular use

The following codes are for reporting administration of the vaccines only. The administration of the vaccines is billed using:

HCPCS **Definition**

G0008 Administration of influenza virus vaccine; G0009 Administration of pneumococcal vaccine; and

*G0010 Administration of Hepatitis B vaccine.

*90471 Immunization administration. (For OPPS hospitals billing for the Hepatitis B vaccine administration)

*90472 Each additional vaccine. (For OPPS hospitals billing for the Hepatitis B vaccine administration)

* **NOTE:** For claims with dates of service prior to January 1, 2006, OPPS and non- OPPS hospitals report G0010 for Hepatitis B vaccine administration. For claims with dates of service January 1, 2006 until December 31, 2010, OPPS hospitals report 90471 or 90472 for Hepatitis B vaccine administration as appropriate in place of G0010. Beginning January 1, 2011, providers should report G0010 for billing under the OPPS rather than 90471 or 90472 to ensure correct waiver of coinsurance and deductible for the administration of Hepatitis B vaccine.

One of the following diagnosis codes must be reported as appropriate. If the sole purpose for the visit is to receive a vaccine or if a vaccine is the only service billed on a claim, the applicable following diagnosis code may be used.

ICD-9-CM Diagnosis Code	Description
V03.82	Pneumococcus
V04.81**	Influenza
V06.6***	Pneumococcus and Influenza
V05.3	Hepatitis B

*Effective for influenza virus claims with dates of service October 1, 2003 and later.

***Effective October 1, 2006, providers may report ICD-9-CM diagnosis code V06.6 on claims for pneumococcus and/or influenza virus vaccines when the purpose of the visit was to receive both vaccines.

NOTE: ICD-10-CM diagnosis code Z23 may be used for an encounter for immunizations effective October 15, 2015, when ICD-10 was implemented. If a diagnosis code for pneumococcus, Hepatitis B, or influenza virus vaccination is not reported on a claim, contractors may not enter the diagnosis on the claim. Contractors must follow current resolution processes for claims with missing diagnosis codes.

If the diagnosis code and the narrative description are correct, but the HCPCS code is incorrect, the A/B MAC (A or B) may correct the HCPCS code and pay the claim. For example, if the reported diagnosis code is V04.81 and the narrative description (if annotated on the claim) says "flu shot" but the HCPCS code is incorrect, contractors may change the HCPCS code and pay for the flu vaccine. Effective October 1, 2006, A/B MACs (B) should follow the instructions in Pub. 100-04, Chapter 1, Section

- (A/B MAC (B) Data Element Requirements) for claims submitted without a HCPCS code.

Claims for Hepatitis B vaccinations must report the I.D. Number of the referring physician. In addition, if a doctor of medicine or osteopathy does not order the influenza virus vaccine, the A/B MACs (A) claims require:

- UPIN code SLF000 to be reported on claims submitted prior to May 23, 2008, when Medicare began accepting NPIs, only
- The provider's own NPI to be reported in the NPI field for the attending physician on claims submitted on or after May 23, 2008, when NPI requirements were implemented.

100-4, Chapter-18, 10.2.2.1

Payment for Pneumococcal Pneumonia Virus, Influenza Virus, and Hepatitis B Virus Vaccines and Their Administration on Institutional Claims

Payment for Vaccines

Payment for these vaccines is as follows:

Facility	Type of Bill	Payment
Hospitals, other than Indian Health Service (IHS) Hospitals and Critical Access Hospitals (CAHs)	012x, 013x	Reasonable cost
IHS Hospitals	012x, 013x, 083x	95% of AWP
IHS CAHs	085x	95% of AWP
CAHs		
Method I and Method II	085x	Reasonable cost
Skilled Nursing Facilities	022x, 023x	Reasonable cost
Home Health Agencies	034x	Reasonable cost
Hospices	081x, 082x	95% of AWP
Comprehensive Outpatient Rehabilitation Facilities	075x	95% of the AWP
Independent Renal Dialysis Facilities	072x	95% of the AWP
Hospital-based Renal Dialysis Facilities	072x	Reasonable cost

Payment for Vaccine Administration

Payment for the administration of influenza virus and pneumococcal vaccines is as follows:

Facility	Type of Bill	Payment
Hospitals, other than IHS Hospitals and CAHs	012x, 013x	Outpatient Prospective Payment System (OPPS) for hospitals subject to OPPS Reasonable cost for hospitals not subject to OPPS
IHS Hospitals	012x, 013x, 083x	MPFS
IHS CAHs	085x	MPFS
CAHs Method I and II	085x	Reasonable cost
Skilled Nursing Facilities	022x, 023x	MPFS
Home Health Agencies	034x	OPPS
Hospices	081x, 082x	MPFS
Comprehensive Outpatient Rehabilitation Facilities	075x	MPFS
Independent RDFs	072x	MPFS
Hospital-based RDFs	072x	Reasonable cost
Payment for the administration of Hepatitis B vaccine is as follows: Facility	Type of Bill	Payment
Hospitals other than IHS hospitals and CAHs	012x, 013x	Outpatient Prospective Payment System (OPPS) for hospitals subject to OPPS Reasonable cost for hospitals not subject to OPPS
IHS Hospitals	012x, 013x, 083x	MPFS
CAHs Method I and II	085x	Reasonable cost
IHS CAHs	085x	MPFS
Skilled Nursing Facilities	022x, 023x	MPFS
Home Health Agencies	034x	OPPS
Hospices	081x, 082x	MPFS
Comprehensive Outpatient Rehabilitation Facilities	075x	MPFS
Independent RDFs	072x	MPFS
Hospital-based RDFs	072x	Reasonable cost

100-4, Chapter-18, 10.2.5.2

A/B MAC Payment Requirements

Payment for pneumococcal, influenza virus, and Hepatitis B vaccines follows the same standard rules that are applicable to any injectable drug or biological. (See chapter 17 for procedures for determining the payment rates for pneumococcal and influenza virus vaccines.)

Effective for claims with dates of service on or after February 1, 2001, §114, of the Benefits Improvement and Protection Act of 2000 mandated that all drugs and biologicals be paid based on mandatory assignment. Therefore, all providers of influenza virus and pneumococcal vaccines must accept assignment for the vaccine.

Prior to March 1, 2003, the administration of pneumococcal, influenza virus, and Hepatitis B vaccines, (HCPCS codes G0008, G0009, and G0010), though not reimbursed directly through the MPFS, were reimbursed at the same rate as HCPCS code 90782 on the MPFS for the year that corresponded to the date of service of the claim.

Prior to March 1, 2003, HCPCS codes G0008, G0009, and G0010 are reimbursed at the same rate as HCPCS code 90471. Assignment for the administration is not mandatory, but is applicable should the provider be enrolled as a provider type "Mass Immunization Roster Biller," submits roster bills, or participates in the centralized billing program.

Carriers/AB MACs may not apply the limiting charge provision for pneumococcal, influenza virus vaccine, or Hepatitis B vaccine and their administration in accordance with §§1833(a)(1) and 1833(a)(10)(A) of the Social Security Act (the Act.) The administration of the influenza virus vaccine is covered in the influenza virus vaccine benefit under §1861(s)(10)(A) of the Act, rather than under the physicians' services benefit. Therefore, it is not eligible for the 10 percent Health Professional Shortage Area (HPSA) incentive payment or the 5 percent Physician Scarcity Area (PSA) incentive payment.

No Legal Obligation to Pay

Nongovernmental entities that provide immunizations free of charge to all patients, regardless of their ability to pay, must provide the immunizations free of charge to Medicare beneficiaries and may not bill Medicare. (See Pub. 100-02, Medicare Benefit Policy Manual, chapter 16.) Thus, for example, Medicare may not pay for influenza virus vaccinations administered to Medicare beneficiaries if a physician provides free vaccinations to all non-Medicare patients or where an employer offers free vaccinations to its employees. Physicians also may not charge Medicare beneficiaries more for a vaccine than they would charge non-Medicare patients. (See §1128(b)(6)(A) of the Act.) When an employer offers free vaccinations to its employees, it must also offer the free vaccination to an employee who is also a Medicare beneficiary. It does not have to offer free vaccinations to its non-Medicare employees.

Nongovernmental entities that do not charge patients who are unable to pay or reduce their charges for patients of limited means, yet expect to be paid if the patient has health insurance coverage for the services provided, may bill Medicare and expect payment.

Governmental entities (such as PHCs) may bill Medicare for pneumococcal, Hepatitis B, and influenza virus vaccines administered to Medicare beneficiaries when services are rendered free of charge to non-Medicare beneficiaries.

100-4, Chapter-18, 10.3.1.1

Centralized Billing for Influenza Virus and Pneumococcal Vaccines to A/B MACs (B)

The CMS currently authorizes a limited number of providers to centrally bill for influenza virus and pneumococcal immunization claims. Centralized billing is an optional program available to providers who qualify to enroll with Medicare as the provider type "Mass Immunization Roster Biller," as well as to other individuals and entities that qualify to enroll as regular Medicare providers. Centralized billers must roster bill, must accept assignment, and must bill electronically.

To qualify for centralized billing, a mass immunizer must be operating in at least three payment localities for which there are three different contractors processing claims. Individuals and entities providing the vaccine and administration must be properly licensed in the State in which the immunizations are given and the contractor must verify this through the enrollment process.

Centralized billers must send all claims for influenza virus and pneumococcal immunizations to a single contractor for payment, regardless of the jurisdiction in which the vaccination was administered. (This does not include claims for the Railroad Retirement Board, United Mine Workers or Indian Health Services. These claims must continue to go to the appropriate processing entity.) Payment is made based on the payment locality where the service was provided. This process is only available for claims for the influenza virus and pneumococcal vaccines and their administration. The general coverage and coding rules still apply to these claims.

This section applies only to those individuals and entities that provide mass immunization services for influenza virus and pneumococcal vaccinations and that have been authorized by CMS to centrally bill. All other providers, including those individuals and entities that provide mass immunization services that are not authorized to centrally bill, must continue to bill for these claims to their regular A/B MAC (B) per the instructions in §10.3.1 of this chapter.

The claims processing instructions in this section apply only to the designated processing contractor. However, all A/B MACs (B) must follow the instructions in §10.3.1.1.J, below, "Provider Education Instructions for All A/B MACs (B)."

A. Processing Contractor

The CMS central office will notify centralized billers of the appropriate contractor to bill when they receive their notification of acceptance into the centralized billing program.

B. Request for Approval

Approval to participate in the CMS centralized billing program is a two part approval process. Individuals and corporations who wish to enroll as a CMS mass immunizer centralized biller must send their request in writing. CMS will complete Part 1 of the approval process by reviewing preliminary demographic information included in the request for participation letter. Completion of Part 1 is not approval to set up vaccination clinics, vaccinate beneficiaries, and bill Medicare for reimbursement. All new participants must complete Part 2 of the approval process (Form CMS-855 Application) before they may set up vaccination clinics, vaccinate Medicare beneficiaries, and bill Medicare for reimbursement. If an individual or entity's request is approved for centralized billing, the approval is limited to 12 months from September to August 31 of the next year. It is the responsibility of the centralized biller to reapply for approval each year. The designated contractor shall provide in writing to CMS and approved centralized billers notification of completion and approval of Part 2 of the approval process. The designated contractor may not process claims for any centralized biller who has not completed Parts 1 and 2 of the approval process. If claims are submitted by a provider who has not received approval of Parts 1 and 2 of the approval process to participate as a centralized biller, the contractor must return the claims to the provider to submit to the A/B MAC (B) for payment.

C. Notification of Provider Participation to the Processing Contractor

Before September 1 of every year, CMS will provide the designated contractor with the names of the entities that are authorized to participate in centralized billing for the 12 month period beginning September 1 and ending August 31 of the next year.

D. Enrollment

Though centralized billers may already have a Medicare provider number, for purposes of centralized billing, they must also obtain a provider number from the processing contractor for centralized billing through completion of the Form CMS-855 (Provider Enrollment Application). Providers/suppliers are encouraged to apply to enroll as a centralized biller early as possible. Applicants who have not completed the entire enrollment process and received approval from CMS and the designated contractor to participate as a Medicare mass immunizer centralized biller will not be allowed to submit claims to Medicare for reimbursement.

Whether an entity enrolls as a provider type "Mass Immunization Roster Biller" or some other type of provider, all normal enrollment processes and procedures must be followed. Authorization from CMS to participate in centralized billing is dependent upon the entity's ability to qualify as some type of Medicare provider. In addition, as under normal enrollment procedures, the contractor must verify that the entity is fully qualified and certified per state requirements in each state in which they plan to operate.

The contractor will activate the provider number for the 12-month period from September 1 through August 31 of the following year. If the provider is authorized to participate in the centralized billing program the next year, the contractor will extend the activation of the provider number for another year. The entity need not re-enroll with the contractor every year. However, should there be changes in the states in which the entity plans to operate, the contractor will need to verify that the entity meets all state certification and licensure requirements in those new states.

E. Electronic Submission of Claims on Roster Bills

Centralized billers must agree to submit their claims on roster bills in an electronic media claims format. The processing contractor must provide instructions on acceptable roster billing formats to the approved centralized billers. Paper claims will not be accepted.

F. Required Information on Roster Bills for Centralized Billing

In addition to the roster billing instructions found in §10.3.1 of this chapter, centralized billers must provide on the claim the ZIP code (to determine the payment locality for the claim), and the provider of service/supplier's billing name, address, ZIP code, and telephone number. In addition, the NPI of the billing provider or group must be appropriately reported.

G. Payment Rates and Mandatory Assignment

The payment rates for the administration of the vaccinations are based on the Medicare Physician Fee Schedule (MPFS) for the appropriate year. Payment made through the MPFS is based on geographic locality. Therefore, payments vary based on the geographic locality where the service was performed.

The HCPCS codes G0008 and G0009 for the administration of the vaccines are not paid on the MPFS. However, prior to March 1, 2003, they must be paid at the same rate as HCPCS code 90782, which is on the MPFS. The designated contractor

must pay per the correct MPFS file for each calendar year based on the date of service of the claim. Beginning March 1, 2003, HCPCS codes G0008, G0009, and G0010 are to be reimbursed at the same rate as HCPCS code 90471.

In order to pay claims correctly for centralized billers, the designated contractor must have the correct name and address, including ZIP code, of the entity where the service was provided.

The following remittance advice and Medicare Summary Notice (MSN) messages apply:

Claim adjustment reason code 16, "Claim/service lacks information which is needed for adjudication. At least one Remark Code must be provided (may be comprised of either the Remittance Advice Remark Code or NCPDP Reject Reason Code,

Remittance advice remark code MA114, "Missing/incomplete/invalid information on where the services were furnished."

MSN 9.4 - "This item or service was denied because information required to make payment was incorrect."

The payment rates for the vaccines must be determined by the standard method used by Medicare for reimbursement of drugs and biologicals. (See chapter 17 for procedures for determining the payment rates for vaccines.)

Effective for claims with dates of service on or after February 1, 2001, §114, of the Benefits Improvement and Protection Act of 2000 mandated that all drugs and biologicals be paid based on mandatory assignment. Therefore, all providers of influenza virus and pneumococcal vaccines must accept assignment for the vaccine. In addition, as a requirement for both centralized billing and roster billing, providers must agree to accept assignment for the administration of the vaccines as well. This means that they must agree to accept the amount that Medicare pays for the vaccine and the administration. Also, since there is no coinsurance or deductible for the influenza virus and pneumococcal benefit, accepting assignment means that Medicare beneficiaries cannot be charged for the vaccination.

H. Common Working File Information

To identify these claims and to enable central office data collection on the project, special processing number 39 has been assigned. The number should be entered on the HUBC claim record to CWF in the field titled Demonstration Number.

I. Provider Education Instructions for the Processing Contractor

The processing contractor must fully educate the centralized billers on the processes for centralized billing as well as for roster billing. General information on influenza virus and pneumococcal coverage and billing instructions is available on the CMS Web site for providers.

J. Provider Education Instructions for All A/B MACs (B)

By April 1 of every year, all A/B MACs (B) must publish in their bulletins and put on their Web sites the following notification to providers. Questions from interested providers should be forwarded to the central office address below. A/B MACs (B) must enter the name of the assigned processing contractor where noted before sending.

NOTIFICATION TO PROVIDERS

Centralized billing is a process in which a provider, who provides mass immunization services for influenza virus and pneumococcal pneumonia virus (PPV) immunizations, can send all claims to a single contractor for payment regardless of the geographic locality in which the vaccination was administered. (This does not include claims for the Railroad Retirement Board, United Mine Workers or Indian Health Services. These claims must continue to go to the appropriate processing entity.) This process is only available for claims for the influenza virus and pneumococcal vaccines and their administration. The administration of the vaccinations is reimbursed at the assigned rate based on the Medicare physician fee schedule for the appropriate locality. The vaccines are reimbursed at the assigned rate using the Medicare standard method for reimbursement of drugs and biologicals.

Individuals and entities interested in centralized billing must contact CMS central office, in writing, at the following address by June 1 of the year they wish to begin centrally billing.

Center for Medicare & Medicaid Services

Division of Practitioner Claims Processing

Provider Billing Group

7500 Security Boulevard

Mail Stop C4-10-07

Baltimore, Maryland 21244

By agreeing to participate in the centralized billing program, providers agree to abide by the following criteria.

CRITERIA FOR CENTRALIZED BILLING

- To qualify for centralized billing, an individual or entity providing mass immunization services for influenza virus and pneumococcal vaccinations must provide these services in at least three payment localities for which there are at least three different contractors processing claims.
- Individuals and entities providing the vaccine and administration must be properly licensed in the state in which the immunizations are given.
- Centralized billers must agree to accept assignment (i.e., they must agree to accept the amount that Medicare pays for the vaccine and the administration). Since there is no coinsurance or deductible for the influenza virus and pneumococcal benefit, accepting assignment means that Medicare beneficiaries cannot be charged for the vaccination, i.e., beneficiaries may not incur any out-of-pocket expense. For example, a drugstore may not charge a Medicare beneficiary $10 for an influenza virus vaccination and give the beneficiary a coupon for $10 to be used in the drugstore.

NOTE: The practice of requiring a beneficiary to pay for the vaccination upfront and to file their own claim for reimbursement is inappropriate. All Medicare providers are required to file claims on behalf of the beneficiary per §1848(g)(4)(A) of the Social Security Act and centralized billers may not collect any payment.

- The contractor assigned to process the claims for centralized billing is chosen at the discretion of CMS based on such considerations as workload, user-friendly software developed by the contractor for billing claims, and overall performance. The assigned contractor for this year is [Fill in name of contractor.]
- The payment rates for the administration of the vaccinations are based on the Medicare physician fee schedule (MPFS) for the appropriate year. Payment

made through the MPFS is based on geographic locality. Therefore, payments received may vary based on the geographic locality where the service was performed. Payment is made at the assigned rate.

- The payment rates for the vaccines are determined by the standard method used by Medicare for reimbursement of drugs and biologicals. Payment is made at the assigned rate.
- Centralized billers must submit their claims on roster bills in an approved electronic format. Paper claims will not be accepted.
- Centralized billers must obtain certain information for each beneficiary including name, health insurance number, date of birth, sex, and signature. [Fill in name of contractor] must be contacted prior to the season for exact requirements. The responsibility lies with the centralized biller to submit correct beneficiary Medicare information (including the beneficiary's Medicare Health Insurance Claim Number) as the contractor will not be able to process incomplete or incorrect claims.
- Centralized billers must obtain an address for each beneficiary so that a Medicare Summary Notice (MSN) can be sent to the beneficiary by the contractor. Beneficiaries are sometimes confused when they receive an MSN from a contractor other than the contractor that normally processes their claims which results in unnecessary beneficiary inquiries to the Medicare contractor. Therefore, centralized billers must provide every beneficiary receiving an influenza virus or pneumococcal vaccination with the name of the processing contractor. This notification must be in writing, in the form of a brochure or handout, and must be provided to each beneficiary at the time he or she receives the vaccination.
- Centralized billers must retain roster bills with beneficiary signatures at their permanent location for a time period consistent with Medicare regulations. [Fill in name of contractor] can provide this information.
- Though centralized billers may already have a Medicare provider number, for purposes of centralized billing, they must also obtain a provider number from [Fill in name of contractor]. This can be done by completing the Form CMS-855 (Provider Enrollment Application), which can be obtained from [Fill in name of contractor].
- If an individual or entity's request for centralized billing is approved, the approval is limited to the 12 month period from September 1 through August 31 of the following year. It is the responsibility of the centralized biller to reapply to CMS CO for approval each year by June 1. Claims will not be processed for any centralized biller without permission from CMS.
- Each year the centralized biller must contact [Fill in name of contractor] to verify understanding of the coverage policy for the administration of the pneumococcal vaccine, and for a copy of the warning language that is required on the roster bill.
- The centralized biller is responsible for providing the beneficiary with a record of the pneumococcal vaccination.
- The information in items 1 through 8 below must be included with the individual or entity's annual request to participate in centralized billing:

    1. Estimates for the number of beneficiaries who will receive influenza virus vaccinations;

2. Estimates for the number of beneficiaries who will receive pneumococcal vaccinations;

3. The approximate dates for when the vaccinations will be given;

4. A list of the states in which influenza virus and pneumococcal clinics will be held;

5. The type of services generally provided by the corporation (e.g., ambulance, home health, or visiting nurse);

6. Whether the nurses who will administer the influenza virus and pneumococcal vaccinations are employees of the corporation or will be hired by the corporation specifically for the purpose of administering influenza virus and pneumococcal vaccinations;

7. Names and addresses of all entities operating under the corporation's application;

8. Contact information for designated contact person for centralized billing program.

100-4, Chapter-18, 10.4.1

CWF Edits on A/B MAC (A) Claims

In order to prevent duplicate payment by the same A/B MAC (A), CWF edits by line item on the A/B MAC (A) number, the beneficiary Health Insurance Claim (HIC) number, and the date of service, the influenza virus procedure codes 90630, 90653, 90654, 90655, 90656, 90657, 90658, 90660, 90661, 90662, 90672, 90673, 90674, 90682, 90685, 90686, 90687, 90688, 90694, or 90756 and the pneumococcal procedure codes 90670 or 90732, and the administration codes G0008 or G0009.

If CWF receives a claim with either HCPCS codes 90630, 90653, 90654, 90655, 90656, 90657, 90658, 90660, 90661, 90662, 90672, 90673, 90674, 90685, 90686, 90687, 90688, 90694, or 90756 and it already has on record a claim with the same HIC number, same A/B MAC (A) number, same date of service, and any one of those HCPCS codes, the second claim submitted to CWF rejects.

If CWF receives a claim with HCPCS codes 90670 or 90732 and it already has on record a claim with the same HIC number, same A/B MAC (A) number, same date of service, and the same HCPCS code, the second claim submitted to CWF rejects when all four items match.

If CWF receives a claim with HCPCS administration codes G0008 or G0009 and it already has on record a claim with the same HIC number, same A/B MAC (A) number, same date of service, and same procedure code, CWF rejects the second claim submitted when all four items match.

CWF returns to the A/B MAC (A) a reject code "7262" for this edit. A/B MACs (A) must deny the second claim and use the same messages they currently use for the denial of duplicate claims.

100-4, Chapter-18, 10.4.2

CWF Edits on A/B MAC (B) Claims

In order to prevent duplicate payment by the same A/B MAC (B), CWF will edit by line item on the A/B MAC (B) number, the HIC number, the date of service, the influenza virus procedure codes 90630, 90653, 90654, 90655, 90656, 90657, 90658, 90660, 90661, 90662, 90672, 90673, 90674, 90682, 90685, 90686, 90687, 90688, 90694, or 90756; the pneumococcal procedure codes 90670 or 90732; and the administration code G0008 or G0009.

If CWF receives a claim with either HCPCS codes 90630, 90653, 90654, 90655, 90656, 90657, 90658, 90660, 90661, 90662, 90672, 90673, 90674, 90682, 90685, 90686, 90687, 90688, 90694, or 90756 and it already has on record a claim with the same HIC number, same A/B MAC (B) number, same date of service, and any one of those HCPCS codes, the second claim submitted to CWF will reject.

If CWF receives a claim with HCPCS codes 90670 or 90732 and it already has on record a claim with the same HIC number, same A/B MAC (B) number, same date of service, and the same HCPCS code, the second claim submitted to CWF will reject when all four items match.

If CWF receives a claim with HCPCS administration codes G0008 or G0009 and it already has on record a claim with the same HIC number, same A/B MAC (B) number, same date of service, and same procedure code, CWF will reject the second claim submitted.

CWF will return to the A/B MAC (B) a specific reject code for this edit. A/B MACs (B) must deny the second claim and use the same messages they currently use for the denial of duplicate claims.

In order to prevent duplicate payment by the centralized billing contractor and local A/B MAC (B), CWF will edit by line item for A/B MAC (B) number, same HIC number, same date of service, the influenza virus procedure codes 90630, 90653, 90654, 90655, 90656, 90657, 90658, 90660, 90661, 90662, 90672, 90673, 90674, 90685, 90686, 90687, 90688, 90694, or 90756; the pneumococcal procedure codes 90670 or 90732; and the administration code G0008 or G0009.

If CWF receives a claim with either HCPCS codes 90630, 90653, 90654, 90655, 90656, 90657, 90658, 90660, 90661, 90662, 90672, 90673, 90674, 90682, 90685, 90686, 90687, 90688, 90694, or 90756 and it already has on record a claim with a different A/B MAC (B) number, but same HIC number, same date of service, and any one of those same HCPCS codes, the second claim submitted to CWF will reject.

If CWF receives a claim with HCPCS codes 90670 or 90732 and it already has on record a claim with the same HIC number, different A/B MAC (B) number, same date of service, and the same HCPCS code, the second claim submitted to CWF will reject.

If CWF receives a claim with HCPCS administration codes G0008 or G0009 and it already has on record a claim with a different A/B MAC (B) number, but the same HIC number, same date of service, and same procedure code, CWF will reject the second claim submitted.

CWF will return a specific reject code for this edit. A/B MACs (B) must deny the second claim. For the second edit, the reject code should automatically trigger the following Medicare Summary Notice (MSN) and Remittance Advice (RA) messages.

MSN: 7.2 – "This is a duplicate of a claim processed by another contractor. You should receive a Medicare Summary Notice from them."

Claim Adjustment Reason Code 18 – Exact duplicate claim/ service

100-4, Chapter-18, 10.4.3

CWF Crossover Edits for A/B MAC (B) Claims

When CWF receives a claim from the A/B MAC (B), it will review Part B outpatient claims history to verify that a duplicate claim has not already been posted.

CWF will edit on the beneficiary HIC number; the date of service; the influenza virus procedure codes 90630, 90653, 90654, 90655, 90656, 90657, 90658, 90660, 90661, 90662, 90672, 90673, 90674, 90682, 90685, 90686, 90687, 90688, 90694, or 90756; the pneumococcal procedure codes 90670 or 90732; and the administration code G0008 or G0009.

CWF will return a specific reject code for this edit. A/B MACs (B) must deny the second claim and use the same messages they currently use for the denial of duplicate claims.

100-4, Chapter-18, 20

Mammography Services (Screening and Diagnostic)

A. Screening Mammography

Beginning January 1, 1991, Medicare provides Part B coverage of screening mammographies for women. Screening mammographies are radiologic procedures for early detection of breast cancer and include a physician's interpretation of the results. A doctor's prescription or referral is not necessary for the procedure to be covered. Whether payment can be made is determined by a woman's age and statutory frequency parameter. See Pub. 100-02, Medicare Benefit Policy Manual, chapter 15, section 280.3 for additional coverage information for a screening mammography.

Section 4101 of the Balanced Budget Act (BBA) of 1997 provides for annual screening mammographies for women over age 39 and waives the Part B deductible. Coverage applies as follows:

Age Groups	Screening Period
Under age 35	No payment allowed for screening mammography.
35-39	Baseline (pay for only one screening mammography performed on a woman between her 35th and 40th birthday)
Over age 39	Annual (11 full months have elapsed following the month of last screening

NOTE: Count months between screening mammographies beginning the month after the date of the examination. For example, if Mrs. Smith received a screening mammography examination in January 2005, begin counting the next month (February 2005) until 11 months have elapsed. Payment can be made for another screening mammography in January 2006.

B. Diagnostic Mammography

A diagnostic mammography is a radiological mammogram and is a covered diagnostic test under the following conditions:

- A patient has distinct signs and symptoms for which a mammogram is indicated;
- A patient has a history of breast cancer; or
- A patient is asymptomatic, but based on the patient's history and other factors the physician considers significant, the physician's judgment is that a mammogram is appropriate.
- Beginning January 1, 2005, Medicare Prescription Drug, Improvement, and Modernization Act (MMA) of

2003, §644, Public Law 108-173 has changed the way Medicare pays for diagnostic mammography. Medicare will pay based on the MPFS in lieu of OPPS or the lower of the actual change.

100-4, Chapter-18, 20.4

Billing Requirements - A/B MAC (A) Claims

A/B MACs use the weekly-updated MQSA file to verify that the billing facility is certified by the FDA to perform mammography services, and has the appropriate certification to perform the type of mammogram billed (film and/or digital). (See §20.1.) A/B MACs (A) use the provider number submitted on the claim to identify the facility and use the MQSA data file to verify the facility's certification(s). A/B MAC (A) complete the following activities in processing mammography claims:

- If the provider number on the claim does not correspond with a certified mammography facility on the MQSA file, then A/B MACs (A) deny the claim.
- When a film mammography HCPCS code is on a claim, the claim is checked for a "1" film indicator.
- If a film mammography HCPCS code comes in on a claim and the facility is certified for film mammography, the claim is paid if all other relevant Medicare criteria are met.
- If a film mammography HCPCS code is on a claim and the facility is certified for digital mammography only, the claim is denied.
- When a digital mammography HCPCS code is on a claim, the claim is checked for "2" digital indicator.
- If a digital mammography HCPCS code is on a claim and the facility is certified for digital mammography, the claim is paid if all other relevant Medicare criteria are met.
- If a digital mammography HCPCS code is on a claim and the facility is certified for film mammography only, the claim is denied.

NOTE: The Common Working File (CWF) no longer receives the mammography file for editing purposes.

Except as provided in the following sections for RHCs and FQHCs, the following procedures apply to billing for screening mammographies:

The technical component portion of the screening mammography is billed on Form CMS-1450 under bill type 12X, 13X, 14X** , 22X, 23X or 85X using revenue code 0403 and HCPCS code 77067* (G0202*).

The technical component portion of the diagnostic mammography is billed on Form CMS-1450 under bill type 12X, 13X, 14X** , 22X, 23X or 85X using revenue code 0401 and HCPCS code 77065* (G0206*),* 77066*(G0204).

Separate bills are required for claims for screening mammographies with dates of service prior to January 1, 2002. Providers include on the bill only charges for the screening mammography.

Separate bills are not required for claims for screening mammographies with dates of service on or after January 1, 2002.

See separate instructions below for rural health clinics (RHCs) and federally qualified health centers (FQHCs).

* For claims with dates of service January 1, 2017 through December 31, 2017, providers report CPT® codes G0202, G0204, and G0206. For claims with dates of service January

1, 2018 and later, providers report CPT® codes 77067, 77066, and 77065 respectively.

** For claims with dates of service April 1, 2005 and later, hospitals bill for all mammography services under the 13X type of bill or for dates of service April 1, 2007 and later, 12X or 13X as appropriate. The 14X type of bill is no longer applicable. Appropriate bill types for providers other than hospitals are 22X, 23X, and 85X.

In cases where screening mammography services are self-referred and as a result an attending physician NPI is not available, the provider shall duplicate their facility NPI in the attending physician identifier field on the claim.

100-4, Chapter-18, 60.1

Payment

Payment is under the Medicare Physician Fee Schedule (MPFS) except as follows:

- FOBTs [CPT® 82270* (HCPCS G0107*) and HCPCS G0328] are paid under the clinical laboratory fee schedule (CLFS) except reasonable cost is paid to all non-outpatient prospective payment system (OPPS) hospitals, including Critical Access Hospitals (CAHs), but not Indian Health Service (IHS) hospitals billing on type of bill (TOB) 83X. IHS hospitals billing on TOB 83X are paid the Ambulatory Surgery Center (ASC) payment amount. Other IHS hospitals (billing on TOB 13X) are paid the Office of Management and Budget (OMB)-approved all-inclusive rate (AIR), or the facility specific per visit amount as applicable. Deductible and coinsurance do not apply for these tests. See section A below for payment to Maryland waiver hospitals on TOB 13X. Payment to all hospitals for non-patient laboratory specimens on TOB 14X will be based on the CLFS, including CAHs and Maryland waiver hospitals.

- For claims with dates of service on or after January 1, 2015 through December 31, 2015, the Cologuard™ multitarget sDNA test (HCPCS G0464) is paid under the CLFS.

  NOTE: For claims with dates of service October 9, 2014 thru December 31, 2014, HCPCS code G0464 is paid under local contractor pricing.

- For claims with dates of service on or after January 1, 2016, CPT® code 81528 replaces G0464 on the CLFS.

- Flexible sigmoidoscopy (code G0104) is paid under OPPS for hospital outpatient departments and on a reasonable cost basis for CAHs; or current payment methodologies for hospitals not subject to OPPS.

- Colonoscopies (HCPCS G0105 and G0121) and barium enemas (HCPCS G0106 and G0120) are paid under OPPS for hospital outpatient departments and on a reasonable cost basis for CAHs or current payment methodologies for hospitals not subject to OPPS. Also colonoscopies may be performed in an ASC and when done in an ASC, the ASC rate applies. The ASC rate is the same for diagnostic and screening colonoscopies. The ASC rate is paid to IHS hospitals when the service is billed on TOB 83X.

The following screening codes must be paid at rates consistent with the rates of the diagnostic codes indicated. Coinsurance and deductible apply to diagnostic codes.

HCPCS Screening Code	HCPCS Diagnostic Code
G0104	45330
G0105 and G0121	45378
G0106 and G0120	74280

A. Special Payment Instructions for TOB 13X Maryland Waiver Hospitals

For hospitals in Maryland under the jurisdiction of the Health Services Cost Review Commission, screening colorectal services HCPCS G0104, G0105, G0106, 82270* (G0107*), G0120, G0121, G0328, G0464 and 81528 are paid according to the terms of the waiver, that is 94% of submitted charges minus any unmet existing deductible, co-insurance and non-covered charges. Maryland Hospitals bill TOB 13X for outpatient colorectal cancer screenings.

B. Special Payment Instructions for Non-Patient Laboratory Specimen (TOB 14X) for All Hospitals

Payment for colorectal cancer screenings (CPT® 82270* (HCPCS G0107*), HCPCS G0328, and G0464 (Effective January 1, 2016, HCPCS G0464 is discontinued and replaced with CPT® 81528) to a hospital for a non-patient laboratory specimen (TOB 14X), is the lesser of the actual charge, the fee schedule amount, or the National Limitation Amount (NLA), (including CAHs and Maryland Waiver hospitals). Part B deductible and coinsurance do not apply.

- *NOTE: For claims with dates of service prior to January 1, 2007, physicians, suppliers, and providers report HCPCS G0107. Effective January 1, 2007, HCPCS G0107 was discontinued and replaced with CPT® 82270.

100-4, Chapter-18, 60.2

HCPCS Codes, Frequency Requirements, and Age Requirements (If Applicable)

Effective for services furnished on or after January 1, 1998, the following codes are used for colorectal cancer screening services:

- CPT® 82270* (HCPCS G0107*) - Colorectal cancer screening; fecal-occult blood tests, 1-3 simultaneous determinations;
- HCPCS G0104 - Colorectal cancer screening; flexible sigmoidoscopy;
- HCPCS G0105 - Colorectal cancer screening; colonoscopy on individual at high risk;
- HCPCS G0106 - Colorectal cancer screening; barium enema; as an alternative to HCPCS G0104, screening sigmoidoscopy;
- HCPCS G0120 - Colorectal cancer screening; barium enema; as an alternative to HCPCS G0105, screening colonoscopy.

Effective for services furnished on or after July 1, 2001, the following codes are added for colorectal cancer screening services:

- HCPCS G0121 - Colorectal cancer screening; colonoscopy on individual not meeting criteria for high risk.
- HCPCS G0122 - Colorectal cancer screening; barium enema (noncovered).

Effective for services furnished on or after January 1, 2004, the following code is added for colorectal cancer screening services as an alternative to CPT® 82270* (HCPCS G0107*):

- HCPCS G0328 - Colorectal cancer screening; immunoassay, fecal-occult blood test, 1-3 simultaneous determinations.

Effective for services furnished on or after October 9, 2014, the following code is added for colorectal cancer screening services:

- HCPCS G0464 – (this code has been deleted in 2017) Colorectal cancer screening; stool-based DNA and fecal occult hemoglobin (e.g., KRAS, NDRG4 and BMP3). Effective January 1, 2016, HCPCS G0464 is discontinued and replaced with CPT® 81528.

NOTE: For claims with dates of service prior to January 1, 2007, physicians, suppliers, and providers report HCPCS G0107. Effective January 1, 2007, HCPCS G0107 is discontinued and replaced with CPT® 82270.

G0104 - Colorectal Cancer Screening; Flexible Sigmoidoscopy

Screening flexible sigmoidoscopies (HCPCS G0104) may be paid for beneficiaries who have attained age 50, when performed by a doctor of medicine or osteopathy at the frequencies noted below.

For claims with dates of service on or after January 1, 2002, contractors pay for screening flexible sigmoidoscopies (HCPCS G0104) for beneficiaries who have attained age 50 when these services were performed by a doctor of medicine or osteopathy, or by a physician assistant, nurse practitioner, or clinical nurse specialist (as defined in §1861(aa)(5) of the Social Security Act (the Act) and in the Code of Federal Regulations (CFR) at 42 CFR 410.74, 410.75, and 410.76) at the frequencies noted above. For claims with dates of service prior to January 1, 2002, Medicare Administrative Contractors (MACs) pay for these services under the conditions noted only when a doctor of medicine or osteopathy performs them.

For services furnished from January 1, 1998, through June 30, 2001, inclusive:

- Once every 48 months (i.e., at least 47 months have passed following the month in which the last covered screening flexible sigmoidoscopy was performed).

For services furnished on or after July 1, 2001:

- Once every 48 months as calculated above unless the beneficiary does not meet the criteria for high risk of developing colorectal cancer (refer to §60.3 of this chapter) and he/she has had a screening colonoscopy (HCPCS G0121) within the preceding 10 years. If such a beneficiary has had a screening colonoscopy within the preceding 10 years, then he or she can have covered a screening flexible sigmoidoscopy only after at least 119 months have passed following the month that he/she received the screening colonoscopy (HCPCS G0121).

NOTE: If during the course of a screening flexible sigmoidoscopy a lesion or growth is detected which results in a biopsy or removal of the growth; the appropriate diagnostic procedure classified as a flexible sigmoidoscopy with biopsy or removal along with modifier –PT should be billed and paid rather than HCPCS G0104.

HCPCS G0105 - Colorectal Cancer Screening; Colonoscopy on Individual at High Risk

Screening colonoscopies (HCPCS G0105) may be paid when performed by a doctor of medicine or osteopathy at a frequency of once every 24 months for beneficiaries at high risk for developing colorectal cancer (i.e., at least 23 months have passed following the month in which the last covered HCPCS G0105 screening colonoscopy was performed). Refer to §60.3

of this chapter for the criteria to use in determining whether or not an individual is at high risk for developing colorectal cancer.

NOTE: If during the course of the screening colonoscopy, a lesion or growth is detected which results in a biopsy or removal of the growth, the appropriate diagnostic procedure classified as a colonoscopy with biopsy or removal along with modifier –PT should be billed and paid rather than HCPCS G0105.

A. Colonoscopy Cannot be Completed Because of Extenuating Circumstances

1. A/B MACs (A)

When a covered colonoscopy is attempted but cannot be completed because of extenuating circumstances, Medicare will pay for the interrupted colonoscopy as long as the coverage conditions are met for the incomplete procedure. However, the frequency standards associated with screening colonoscopies will not be applied by the common working file (CWF). When a covered colonoscopy is next attempted and completed, Medicare will pay for that colonoscopy according to its payment methodology for this procedure as long as coverage conditions are met, and the frequency standards will be applied by CWF. This policy is applied to both screening and diagnostic colonoscopies. When submitting a facility claim for the interrupted colonoscopy, providers are to suffix the colonoscopy

Use of HCPCS codes with a modifier of –73 or –74 is appropriate to indicate that the procedure was interrupted. Payment for covered incomplete screening colonoscopies shall be consistent with payment methodologies currently in place for complete screening colonoscopies, including those contained in 42 CFR 419.44(b). In situations where a CAH has elected payment Method II for CAH patients, payment shall be consistent with payment methodologies currently in place as outlined in chapter 3 of this manual. As such, instruct CAHs that elect Method II payment to use modifier –53 to identify an incomplete screening colonoscopy (physician professional service(s) billed in revenue code 096X, 097X, and/or 098X). Such CAHs will also bill the technical or facility component of the interrupted colonoscopy in revenue code 075X (or other appropriate revenue code) using the -73 or -74 modifier as appropriate.

Note that Medicare would expect the provider to maintain adequate information in the patient's medical record in case it is needed by the contractor to document the incomplete procedure.

2. A/B MACs (B)

When a covered colonoscopy is attempted but cannot be completed because of extenuating circumstances (see chapter 12), Medicare will pay for the interrupted colonoscopy at a rate consistent with that of a flexible sigmoidoscopy as long as coverage conditions are met for the incomplete procedure. When a covered colonoscopy is next attempted and completed, Medicare will pay for that colonoscopy according to its payment methodology for this procedure as long as coverage conditions are met. This policy is applied to both screening and diagnostic colonoscopies. When submitting a claim for the interrupted colonoscopy, professional providers are to suffix the colonoscopy code with modifier of –53 to indicate that the procedure was interrupted. When submitting a claim for the facility fee associated with this procedure, ASCs are to suffix the colonoscopy code with modifier –73 or –74 as appropriate. Payment for covered screening colonoscopies, including that for the associated ASC facility fee when applicable, shall be consistent with payment for diagnostic colonoscopies, whether the procedure is complete or incomplete.

Note that Medicare would expect the provider to maintain adequate information in the patient's medical record in case it is needed by the contractor to document the incomplete procedure.

HCPCS G0106 - Colorectal Cancer Screening; Barium Enema; as an Alternative to HCPCS G0104, Screening Sigmoidoscopy

Screening barium enema examinations may be paid as an alternative to a screening sigmoidoscopy (HCPCS G0104). The same frequency parameters for screening sigmoidoscopies (see those codes above) apply. In the case of an individual aged 50 or over, payment may be made for a screening barium enema examination (HCPCS G0106) performed after at least 47 months have passed following the month in which the last screening barium enema or screening flexible sigmoidoscopy was performed. For example, the beneficiary received a screening barium enema examination as an alternative to a screening flexible sigmoidoscopy in January 1999. Start count beginning February 1999. The beneficiary is eligible for another screening barium enema in January 2003.

The screening barium enema must be ordered in writing after a determination that the test is the appropriate screening test. Generally, it is expected that this will be a screening double contrast enema unless the individual is unable to withstand such an exam. This means that in the case of a particular individual, the attending physician must determine that the estimated screening potential for the barium enema is equal to or greater than the screening potential that has been estimated for a screening flexible sigmoidoscopy for the same individual. The screening single contrast barium enema also requires a written order from the beneficiary's attending physician in the same manner as described above for the screening double contrast barium enema examination.

CPT® 82270* (HCPCS G0107*) - Colorectal Cancer Screening; Fecal-Occult Blood Test, 1-3 Simultaneous Determinations

Effective for services furnished on or after January 1, 1998, screening FOBT (CPT® 82270* (HCPCS G0107*) may be paid for beneficiaries who have attained age 50, and at a frequency of once every 12 months (i.e., at least 11 months have passed following the month in which the last covered screening FOBT was performed). This screening FOBT means a guaiac-based test for peroxidase activity, in which the beneficiary completes it by taking samples from two different sites of three consecutive stools. This screening requires a written order from the beneficiary's attending physician, or additionally, effective for dates of service on or after January 27, 2014, the beneficiary's attending physician assistant, nurse practitioner, or clinical nurse specialist. (The term "attending physician" is defined to mean a doctor of medicine or osteopathy (as defined in §1861(r)(1) of the Act) who is fully knowledgeable about the beneficiary's medical condition, and who would be responsible for using the results of any examination performed in the overall management of the beneficiary's specific medical problem.)

Effective for services furnished on or after January 1, 2004, payment may be made for an immunoassay-based FOBT (HCPCS G0328, described below) as an alternative to the guaiac-based FOBT, CPT® 82270* (HCPCS G0107*). Medicare will pay for only one covered FOBT per year, either CPT® 82270* (HCPCS G0107*) or HCPCS G0328, but not both.

*NOTE: For claims with dates of service prior to January 1, 2007, physicians, suppliers, and providers report HCPCS G0107. Effective January 1, 2007, HCPCS G0107 is discontinued and replaced with CPT® 82270.

HCPCS G0328 - Colorectal Cancer Screening; Immunoassay, Fecal-Occult Blood Test, 1-3 Simultaneous Determinations

Effective for services furnished on or after January 1, 2004, screening FOBT, (HCPCS G0328) may be paid as an alternative to CPT® 82270* (HCPCS G0107*) for beneficiaries who have attained age 50. Medicare will pay for a covered FOBT (either CPT® 82270* (HCPCS G0107*) or HCPCS G0328, but not both) at a frequency of once every 12 months (i.e., at least 11 months have passed following the month in which the last covered screening FOBT was performed).

Screening FOBT, immunoassay, includes the use of a spatula to collect the appropriate number of samples or the use of a special brush for the collection of samples, as determined by the individual manufacturer's instructions. This screening requires a written order from the beneficiary's attending physician, or, additionally, effective for claims with dates of service on or after January 27, 2014, the beneficiary's attending physician assistant, nurse practitioner, or clinical nurse specialist. (The term "attending physician" is defined to mean a doctor of medicine or osteopathy (as defined in §1861(r)(1) of the Act) who is fully knowledgeable about the beneficiary's medical condition, and who would be responsible for using the results of any examination performed in the overall management of the beneficiary's specific medical problem.)

HCPCS G0120 - Colorectal Cancer Screening; Barium Enema; as an Alternative to HCPCS G0105, Screening Colonoscopy

Screening barium enema examinations may be paid as an alternative to a screening colonoscopy (HCPCS G0105) examination. The same frequency parameters for screening colonoscopies (see those codes above) apply.

In the case of an individual who is at high risk for colorectal cancer, payment may be made for a screening barium enema examination (HCPCS G0120) performed after at least 23 months have passed following the month in which the last screening barium enema or the last screening colonoscopy was performed. For example, a beneficiary at high risk for developing colorectal cancer received a screening barium enema examination (HCPCS G0120) as an alternative to a screening colonoscopy (HCPCS G0105) in January 2000. Start counts beginning February 2000. The beneficiary is eligible for another screening barium enema examination (HCPCS G0120) in January 2002.

The screening barium enema must be ordered in writing after a determination that the test is the appropriate screening test. Generally, it is expected that this will be a screening double contrast enema unless the individual is unable to withstand such an exam. This means that in the case of a particular individual, the attending physician must determine that the estimated screening potential for the barium enema is equal to or greater than the screening potential that has been estimated for a screening colonoscopy, for the same individual. The screening single contrast barium enema also requires a written order from the beneficiary's attending physician in the same manner as described above for the screening double contrast barium enema examination.

HCPCS G0121 - Colorectal Screening; Colonoscopy on Individual Not Meeting Criteria for High Risk - Applicable On and After July 1, 2001

Effective for services furnished on or after July 1, 2001, screening colonoscopies (HCPCS G0121) performed on individuals not meeting the criteria for being at high risk for developing colorectal cancer (refer to §60.3 of this chapter) may be paid under the following conditions:

- At a frequency of once every 10 years (i.e., at least 119 months have passed following the month in which the last covered HCPCS G0121 screening colonoscopy was performed.)
- If the individual would otherwise qualify to have covered a HCPCS G0121 screening colonoscopy based on the above but has had a covered screening flexible sigmoidoscopy (HCPCS G0104), then he or she may have covered a HCPCS G0121 screening colonoscopy only after at least 47 months have passed following the month in which the last covered HCPCS G0104 flexible sigmoidoscopy was performed.

NOTE: If during the course of the screening colonoscopy, a lesion or growth is detected which results in a biopsy or removal of the growth, the appropriate diagnostic procedure classified as a colonoscopy with biopsy or removal along with modifier –PT should be billed and paid rather than HCPCS G0121.

HCPCS G0464 (Replaced with CPT® 81528) - Multitarget Stool DNA (sDNA) Colorectal Cancer Screening Test - Cologuard™

Effective for dates of service on or after October 9, 2014, colorectal cancer screening using the Cologuard™ multitarget sDNA test (G0464/81528) is covered once every 3 years for Medicare beneficiaries that meet all of the following criteria:

- Ages 50 to 85 years,
- Asymptomatic (no signs or symptoms of colorectal disease including but not limited to lower gastrointestinal pain, blood in stool, positive guaiac fecal occult blood test or fecal immunochemical test), and,
- At average risk of developing colorectal cancer (no personal history of adenomatous polyps, colorectal cancer, or inflammatory bowel disease, including Crohn's Disease and ulcerative colitis; no family history of colorectal cancers or adenomatous polyps, familial adenomatous polyposis, or hereditary nonpolyposis colorectal cancer).

See Pub. 100-03, Medicare National Coverage Determinations Manual, Chapter 1, Section 210.3, for complete coverage requirements.

Effective for claims with dates of service on or after October 9, 2014, providers shall report the following diagnosis codes when submitting claims for the Cologuard™ multitarget sDNA test:

ICD-9: V76.41 and V76.51, or,

ICD-10: Z12.11 and Z12.12

NOTE: Effective January 1, 2016, HCPCS G0464 is discontinued and replaced with CPT® 81528

HCPCS G0122 - Colorectal Cancer Screening; Barium Enema

The code is not covered by Medicare.

100-4, Chapter-18, 60.6

Billing Requirements for Claims Submitted to A/B MACs (A)

Follow the general bill review instructions in chapter 25. Hospitals use the ASC X12 837 institutional claim format to bill the A/B MAC (A) or the hardcopy Form CMS-1450 (UB-04). Hospitals bill revenue codes and HCPCS codes as follows:

Screening Test/ Procedure	Revenue Code	HCPCS Code	TOBs
FOBT	030X	82270*** (G0107***), G0328	12X, 13X, 14X**, 22X, 23X, 83X, 85X
Barium enema	032X	G0106, G0120, G0122	12X, 13X, 22X, 23X, 85X****
Flexible Sigmoidoscopy	*	G0104	12X, 13X, 22X, 23X, 85X****
Colonoscopy-high risk	*	G0105, G0121	12X, 13X, 22X, 23X, 85X****
Multitarget sDNA - Cologuard™	030X	(G0464*****), 81528*****	13X, 14X**, 85X

* The appropriate revenue code when reporting any other surgical procedure.

** 14X is only applicable for non-patient laboratory specimens.

*** For claims with dates of service prior to January 1, 2007, physicians, suppliers, and providers report HCPCS code G0107.

Effective January 1, 2007, HCPCS G0107, was discontinued and replaced with CPT® 82270.

**** CAHs that elect Method II bill revenue code 096X, 097X, and/or 098X for professional services and 075X (or other appropriate revenue code) for the technical or facility component.

***** *Effective January 1, 2016, HCPCS G0464 is discontinued and replaced with CPT® 81528*

Special Billing Instructions for Hospital Inpatients

When these tests/procedures are provided to inpatients of a hospital or when Part A benefits have been exhausted, they are covered under this benefit. However, the provider bills on TOB 12X using the discharge date of the hospital stay to avoid editing in the Common Working File (CWF) as a result of the hospital bundling rules.

100-4, Chapter-18, 80

Initial Preventive Physical Examination (IPPE)

(**NOTE:** For billing and payment requirements for the Annual Wellness Visit, see chapter 18, section 140, of this chapter.)

Background: Sections 1861(s)(2)(w) and 1861(ww) of the Social Security Act (and implementing regulations at 42 CFR 410.16, 411.15(a)(1), and 411.15(k)(11)) authorize coverage under Part B for a one-time initial preventive physical examination (IPPE) for new Medicare beneficiaries that meet certain eligibility requirements.

Coverage: As described in implementing regulations at 42 CFR 410.16, 411.15(a)(1), and 411.15(k)(11), the IPPE may be performed by a doctor of medicine or osteopathy as defined in section 1861 (r)(1) of the Social Security Act (the Act) or by a qualified nonphysician practitioner (NPP) (physician assistant, nurse practitioner, or clinical nurse specialist), not later than

12 months after the date the individual's first coverage begins under Medicare Part B. (See section 80.3 for a list of bill types of facilities that can bill A/B MACs for this service.)

The IPPE includes:

1. review of the individual's medical and social history with attention to modifiable risk factors for disease detection,

2. review of the individual's potential (risk factors) for depression or other mood disorders,

3. review of the individual's functional ability and level of safety;

4. an examination to include measurement of the individual's height, weight, body mass index, blood pressure, a visual acuity screen, and other factors as deemed appropriate, based on the beneficiary's medical and social history;

5. end-of-life planning, upon agreement of the individual.

6. education, counseling, and referral, as deemed appropriate, based on the results of the review and evaluation services described in the previous 5 elements, and

7. education, counseling, and referral including a brief written plan (e.g., a checklist or alternative) provided to the individual for obtaining appropriate screening and other preventive services, which are separately covered under Medicare Part B.

Medicare will pay for only one IPPE per beneficiary per lifetime. The Common Working File (CWF) will edit for this benefit.

The IPPE does not include other preventive services that are currently separately covered and paid under Medicare Part B. (That is: pneumococcal, influenza and Hepatitis B vaccines and their administration, screening mammography, screening pap smear and screening pelvic examinations, prostate cancer screening tests, colorectal cancer screening tests, diabetes outpatient self-management training services, bone mass measurements, glaucoma screening, medical nutrition therapy for individuals with diabetes or renal disease, cardiovascular screening blood tests, diabetes screening tests, screening ultrasound for abdominal aortic aneurysms, an electrocardiogram, and additional preventive services covered under Medicare Part B through the Medicare national coverage determination process.)

For the physician/practitioner billing correct coding and payment policy, refer to chapter 12, section 30.6.1.1, of this manual.

100-4, Chapter-18, 80.1

Healthcare Common Procedure Coding System (HCPCS) Coding for the IPPE

The HCPCS codes listed below were developed for the IPPE benefit effective January 1, 2005, for individuals whose initial enrollment is on or after January 1, 2005.

G0344: Initial preventive physical examination; face-to-face visit, services limited to new beneficiary during the first 6 months of Medicare enrollment

> *Short Descriptor:* Initial Preventive Exam

G0366: Electrocardiogram, routine ECG with 12 leads; performed as a component of the initial preventive examination with interpretation and report

> *Short Descriptor:* EKG for initial prevent exam

G0367: tracing only, without interpretation and report, performed as a component of the initial preventive examination

> *Short Descriptor:* EKG tracing for initial prev

G0368: interpretation and report only, performed as a component of the initial preventive examination

> *Short Descriptor:* EKG interpret & report preve

The following new HCPCS codes were developed for the IPPE benefit effective January 1, 2009, and replaced codes G0344, G0366, G0367, and G0368 shown above beginning with dates of service on or after January 1, 2009:

G0402: Initial preventive physical examination; face-to-face visit, services limited to new beneficiary during the first 12 months of Medicare enrollment

> *Short Descriptor:* Initial Preventive exam

G0403: Electrocardiogram, routine ECG with 12 leads; performed as a screening for the initial preventive physical examination with interpretation and report

> *Short Descriptor:* EKG for initial prevent exam

G0404: Electrocardiogram, routine ECG with 12 leads; tracing only, without interpretation and report, performed as a screening for the initial preventive physical examination

> *Short Descriptor:* EKG tracing for initial prev

G0405: Electrocardiogram, routine ECG with 12 leads; interpretation and report only, performed as a screening for the initial preventive physical examination

> *Short Descriptor:* EKG interpret & report preve

100-4, Chapter-18, 80.2

A/B Medicare Administrative Contractor (MAC) (B)and Contractor Billing Requirements

Effective for dates of service on and after January 1, 2005, through December 31, 2008, contractors shall recognize the HCPCS codes G0344, G0366, G0367, and G0368 shown above in §80.1 for an IPPE. The type of service (TOS) for each of these codes is as follows:

G0344: TOS = 1

G0366: TOS = 5

G0367: TOS = 5

G0368: TOS = 5

Contractors shall pay physicians or qualified nonphysician practitioners for only one IPPE performed not later than 6 months after the date the individual's first coverage begins under Medicare Part B, but only if that coverage period begins on or after January 1, 2005.

Effective for dates of service on and after January 1, 2009, contractors shall recognize the HCPCS codes G0402, G0403, G0404, and G0405 shown above in §80.1 for an IPPE. The TOS for each of these codes is as follows:

G0402: TOS = 1

G0403: TOS = 5

G0404: TOS = 5

G0405: TOS = 5

Under the MIPPA of 2008, contractors shall pay physicians or qualified nonphysician practitioners for only one IPPE performed not later than 12 months after the date the individual's first coverage begins under Medicare Part B only if that coverage period begins on or after January 1, 2009.

Contractors shall allow payment for a medically necessary Evaluation and Management (E/M) service at the same visit as the IPPE when it is clinically appropriate. Physicians and qualified nonphysician practitioners shall use CPT® codes 99201-99215 to report an E/M with CPT® modifier 25 to indicate that the E/M is a significant, separately identifiable service from the IPPE code reported (G0344 or G0402, whichever applies based on the date the IPPE is performed). Refer to chapter 12, §30.6.1.1, of this manual for the physician/practitioner billing correct coding and payment policy regarding E/M services.

If the EKG performed as a component of the IPPE is not performed by the primary physician or qualified NPP during the IPPE visit, another physician or entity may perform and/or interpret the EKG. The referring physician or qualified NPP needs to make sure that the performing physician or entity bills the appropriate G code for the screening EKG, and not a CPT® code in the 93000 series. **Both the IPPE and the EKG should be billed in order for the beneficiary to receive the complete IPPE service.** Effective for dates of service on and after January 1, 2009, the screening EKG is optional and is no longer a mandated service of an IPPE if performed as a result of a referral from an IPPE.

Should the same physician or NPP need to perform an additional medically necessary EKG in the 93000 series on the same day as the IPPE, report the appropriate EKG CPT® code(s) with modifier 59, indicating that the EKG is a distinct procedural service.

Physicians or qualified nonphysician practitioners shall bill the contractor the appropriate HCPCS codes for IPPE. The HCPCS codes for an IPPE and screening EKG are paid under the Medicare Physician Fee Schedule (MPFS). See §1.3 of this chapter for waiver of cost sharing requirements of coinsurance, copayment and deductible for furnished preventive services available in Medicare.

100-4, Chapter-18, 80.3.3

Outpatient Prospective Payment System (OPPS) Hospital Billing

Hospitals subject to OPPS (TOBs 12X and 13X) must use modifier -25 when billing the IPPE G0344 along with the technical component of the EKG, G0367, on the same claim. The same is true when billing IPPE code G0402 along with the technical component of the screening EKG, code G0404. This is due to an OPPS Outpatient Code Editor (OCE) which contains an edit that requires a modifier -25 on any evaluation and management (E/M) HCPCS code if there is also a status "S" or "T" HCPCS procedure code on the claim.

100-4, Chapter-18, 80.4

Coinsurance and Deductible

The Medicare deductible and coinsurance apply for the IPPE provided before January 1, 2009.

The Medicare deductible is waived effective for the IPPE provided on or after January 1, 2009. Coinsurance continues to apply for the IPPE provided on or after January 1, 2009.

As a result of the Affordable Care Act, effective for the IPPE provided on or after January 1, 2011, the Medicare deductible and coinsurance (for HCPCS code G0402 only) are waived.

100-4, Chapter-18, 120.1

Coding and Payment of DSMT Services

The following HCPCS codes are used to report DSMT:

- G0108-Diabetes outpatient self-management training services, individual, per 30 minutes.
- G0109 -Diabetes outpatient self-management training services, group session (2 or more), per 30 minutes.

The type of service for these codes is 1.

Payment to physicians and providers for outpatient DSMT is made as follows:

Type of Facility	Payment Method	Type of Bill
Physician (billed to the carrier)	MPFS	NA
Hospitals subject to OPPS	MPFS	12X, 13X
Method I and Method II Critical Access Hospitals (CAHs) (technical services)	101% of reasonable cost	12X and 85X
Indian Health Service (IHS) providers billing hospital outpatient Part B	OMB-approved outpatient per visit all-inclusive rate (AIR)	13X
IHS providers billing inpatient Part B	All-inclusive inpatient ancillary per diem rate	12X
IHS CAHs billing outpatient Part B	101% of the all-inclusive facility specific per visit rate	85X
IHS CAHs billing inpatient Part B	101% of the all-inclusive facility specific per diem rate	12X
FQHCs*	All-inclusive encounter rate with other qualified services. Separate visit payment available with HCPCS.	73X
Skilled Nursing Facilities **	MPFS non-facility rate	22X, 23X
Maryland Hospitals under jurisdiction of the Health Services Cost Review Commission (HSCRC)	94% of provider submitted charges in accordance with the terms of the Maryland Waiver	12X, 13X
Home Health Agencies (can be billed only if the service is provided outside of the treatment plan)	MPFS non-facility rate	34X

* Effective January 1, 2006, payment for DSMT provided in an FQHC that meets all of the requirements as above, may be made in addition to one other visit the beneficiary had during the same day, if this qualifying visit is billed on TOB 73X, with HCPCS G0108 or G0109, and revenue codes 0520, 0521, 0522, 0524, 0525, 0527, 0528, or 0900.

** The SNF consolidated billing provision allows separate part B payment for training services for beneficiaries that are in skilled Part A SNF stays, however, the SNF must submit these services on a 22 bill type. Training services provided by other provider types must be reimbursed by X the SNF.

NOTE: An ESRD facility is a reasonable site for this service, however, because it is required to provide dietician and nutritional services as part of the care covered in the composite rate, ESRD facilities are not allowed to bill for it separately and do not receive separate reimbursement. Likewise, an RHC is a reasonable site for this service, however it must be provided in an RHC with other qualifying services and paid at the all-inclusive encounter rate.

Deductible and co-insurance apply.

100-4, Chapter-18, 130.1

Healthcare Common Procedure Coding System (HCPCS) for HIV Screening Tests

Effective for claims with dates of service on and after December 8, 2009, implemented with the April 5, 2010, IOCE, the following HCPCS codes are to be billed for HIV screening:

- G0432- Infectious agent antibody detection by enzyme immunoassay (EIA) technique, HIV-1 and/or HIV-2, screening,

- G0433 - Infectious agent antibody detection by enzyme-linked immunosorbent assay (ELISA) technique, HIV-1 and/or HIV-2, screening, and,

- G0435 -Infectious agent antibody detection by rapid antibody test, HIV-1 and/or HIV-2, screening.

100-4, Chapter-18, 130.2

Billing Requirements

Medicare Administrative Contractors (MACs) shall recognize the above HCPCS codes for HIV screening in accordance with Publication 100-03, Medicare National Coverage Determinations Manual, section 210.7.

Effective for claims with dates of service on and after December 8, 2009, MACs shall pay for voluntary HIV screening as follows:

- A maximum of once annually for beneficiaries at increased risk for HIV infection (11 full months must elapse following the month the previous test was performed in order for the subsequent test to be covered), and,

- A maximum of three times per term of pregnancy for pregnant Medicare beneficiaries beginning with the date of the first test when ordered by the woman's clinician.

Claims that are submitted for HIV screening shall be submitted in the following manner:

For beneficiaries reporting increased risk factors, claims shall contain HCPCS code G0432, G0433, or G0435 with diagnosis code V73.89 (Special screening for other specified viral disease) as primary, and V69.8 (Other problems related to lifestyle), as secondary.

For beneficiaries not reporting increased risk factors, claims shall contain HCPCS code G0432, G0433, or G0435 with diagnosis code V73.89 only.

For pregnant Medicare beneficiaries, claims shall contain HCPCS code G0432, G0433, or G0435 with diagnosis code V73.89 as primary, and one of the following ICD-9 diagnosis codes: V22.0 (Supervision of normal first pregnancy), V22.1 (Supervision of other normal pregnancy), or V23.9 (Supervision of unspecified high-risk pregnancy), as secondary.

Effective for claims with dates of service on or after April 13, 2015, MACs shall also pay for voluntary, HIV screening as follows (replacing ICD-9 with ICD-10 beginning October 1, 2015):

For pregnant Medicare beneficiaries, claims shall contain HCPCS code G0432, G0433, G0435, G0475 or CPT®-80081 with primary ICD-9/ICD-10 diagnosis code V73.89/Z11.4, along with one of the following ICD-9/ICD-10 diagnosis codes as secondary listed below, and allow no more than 3 HIV screening tests during each term of pregnancy beginning with the date of the 1st test:

ICD-9:	V22.0	Supervision of normal first pregnancy
ICD-10:	Z34.00	Encounter for supervision of normal first pregnancy, unspecified trimester
	Z34.01	Encounter for supervision of normal first pregnancy, first trimester
	Z34.02	Encounter for supervision of normal first pregnancy, second trimester
	Z34.03	Encounter for supervision of normal first pregnancy, third trimester
ICD-9:	V22.1	Supervision of other normal pregnancy
ICD-10:	Z34.80	Encounter for supervision of other normal pregnancy, unspecified trimester
	Z34.81	Encounter for supervision of other normal pregnancy, first trimester
	Z34.82	Encounter for supervision of other normal pregnancy, second trimester
	Z34.83	Encounter for supervision of other normal pregnancy, third trimester
	Z34.90	Encounter for supervision of normal pregnancy, unspecified, unspecified trimester
	Z34.91	Encounter for supervision of normal pregnancy, unspecified, first trimester
	Z34.92	Encounter for supervision of normal pregnancy, unspecified, second trimester
	Z34.93	Encounter for supervision of normal pregnancy, unspecified, third trimester
ICD-9:	V23.9	Supervision of unspecified high-risk pregnancy
ICD-10:	O09.90	Supervision of high risk pregnancy, unspecified, unspecified trimester
	O09.91	Supervision of high risk pregnancy, unspecified, first trimester
	O09.92	Supervision of high risk pregnancy, unspecified, second trimester
	O09.93	Supervision of high risk pregnancy, unspecified, third trimester

For non-pregnant Medicare beneficiaries, claims shall contain HCPCS code G0432, G0433, G0435, or G0475 for beneficiaries between 15 and 65 years of age one time per annum with ICD-9/ICD-10 diagnosis code V73.89/Z11.4 as primary regardless of risk factors. If primary ICD-9/ICD-10 diagnosis code V73.89/Z11.4 is not present and the beneficiary is between 15 and 65 years of age, or the service is billed more than one time per annum, the detail line shall be denied.

For non-pregnant Medicare beneficiaries, claims shall contain HCPCS code G0432, G0433, G0435, or G0475 for beneficiaries less than 15 and greater than 65 years of age one time per annum with ICD-9/ICD-10 diagnosis code V73.89/ Z11.4 as primary, and one of the following secondary ICD-9/ICD-10 diagnosis codes:

V69.8 (Other problems related to lifestyle)/Z72.89 (Other problems related to lifestyle)

Z72.51 (High risk heterosexual behavior)

Z72.52 (High risk homosexual behavior)

Z72.53 (High risk bisexual behavior)

If ICD-9/ICD-10 diagnosis code V73.89/Z11.4 is not present as primary and one of the ICD-9/ICD-10 secondary codes listed above is not present and the beneficiary is less than 15 or greater than 65 years of age, or the service is billed more than one time per annum, the detail line shall be denied.

100-4, Chapter-18, 130.3

Payment Method

Payment for HIV screening, HCPCS codes G0432, G0433, G0435, is under the Medicare Clinical Laboratory Fee Schedule (CLFS) for Types of Bill (TOB) 12X, 13X, 14X, 22X, and 23X beginning January 1, 2011. For TOB 85X payment is based on reasonable cost. Deductible and coinsurance do not apply. Between December 8, 2009, and April 4, 2010, these services can be billed with unlisted procedure code 87999. Between April 5, 2010, and January 1, 2011, HCPCS codes G0432, G0433, and G0435 will be contractor priced.

Payment for HIV screening, HCPCS code G0475, for institutional claims will be under the Medicare CLFS for TOB 12X, 13X, 14X, 22X, and 23X for claims on or after January 1, 2017. For TOB 85X payment is based on reasonable cost.

Effective for claims with date of service from April 13, 2015 through December 31, 2016, HCPCS code G0475 will be contractor priced. Beginning with date of service January 1, 2017 and after, HCPCS code G0475 will be priced and paid according to the CLFS.

HCPCS code G0475 will be included in the January 2017 CLFS, January 1, 2016 IOCE, the January 2016 OPPS and January 1, 2016 MPFSD. HCPCS code G0475 will be effective retroactive to April 13, 2015 in the IOCE & OPPS.

A/B MACs (B) shall only accept claims submitted with a G0475, G0432, G0433, or G0435 with a Place of Service (POS) Code equal to 81 Independent Lab, and 11, Office.

Deductible and coinsurance do not apply.

100-4, Chapter-18, 130.4

Types of Bill (TOBs) and Revenue Codes

The applicable bill types for HIV screening, HCPCS codes G0432, G0433, G0435, and G0475 are: 12X, 13X, 14X, 22X, 23X, and 85X. (Effective April 1, 2006, TOB 14X is for non-patient laboratory specimens.) Use revenue code 030X (laboratory, clinical diagnostic).

A/B MACs (A) shall apply contractor pricing for HCPCS code G0475, HIV screening, for claims with dates of service on and after April 13, 2015 through December 31, 2016.

100-4, Chapter-18, 130, 130.5

Diagnosis Code Reporting

A claim that is submitted for HIV screening shall be submitted with one or more of the following diagnosis codes in the header and pointed to the line item:

a. For claims where increased risk factors are reported: ICD-9/ICD-10 diagnosis code V73.89/Z11.4 as primary and ICD-9/ICD-10 diagnosis code V69.8/Z72.89, Z72.51, Z72.52, or Z72.53, as secondary.

b. For claims where increased risk factors are NOT reported: ICD-9/ICD-10 diagnosis code V73.89/Z11.4 as primary only.

c. For claims for pregnant Medicare beneficiaries, the following secondary diagnosis codes shall be submitted in addition to primary ICD-9/ICD-10 diagnosis code V73.89/Z11.4 to allow for more frequent screening than once per 12-month period:

ICD-9:	V22.0	Supervision of normal first pregnancy
ICD-10:	Z34.00	Encounter for supervision of normal first pregnancy, unspecified trimester
	Z34.01	Encounter for supervision of normal first pregnancy, first trimester
	Z34.02	Encounter for supervision of normal first pregnancy, second trimester
	Z34.03	Encounter for supervision of normal first pregnancy, third trimester
ICD-9:	V22.1	Supervision of other normal pregnancy
ICD-10:	Z34.80	Encounter for supervision of other normal pregnancy, unspecified trimester
	Z34.81	Encounter for supervision of other normal pregnancy, first trimester
	Z34.82	Encounter for supervision of other normal pregnancy, second trimester
	Z34.83	Encounter for supervision of other normal pregnancy, third trimester
	Z34.90	Encounter for supervision of normal pregnancy, unspecified, unspecified trimester
	Z34.91	Encounter for supervision of normal pregnancy, unspecified, first trimester
	Z34.92	Encounter for supervision of normal pregnancy, unspecified, second trimester
	Z34.93	Encounter for supervision of normal pregnancy, unspecified, third trimester
ICD-9:	V23.9	Supervision of unspecified high-risk pregnancy
ICD-10:	O09.90	Supervision of high risk pregnancy, unspecified, unspecified trimester
	O09.91	Supervision of high risk pregnancy, unspecified, first trimester
	O09.92	Supervision of high risk pregnancy, unspecified, second trimester
	O09.93	Supervision of high risk pregnancy, unspecified, third trimester

100-4, Chapter-18, 140

Annual Wellness Visit (AWV)

Pursuant to section 4103 of the Affordable Care Act of 2010, the Centers for Medicare & Medicaid Services (CMS) amended section 411.15(a)(1) and 411.15(k)(15) of 42 CFR (list of examples of routine physical examinations excluded from coverage) effective for services furnished on or after January 1, 2011. This expanded coverage is subject to certain eligibility and other limitations that allow payment for an annual wellness visit (AWV), including personalized prevention plan services (PPPS), for an individual who is no longer within 12 months after the effective date of his or her first Medicare Part B coverage period, and has not received either an initial preventive physical examination (IPPE) or an AWV within the past 12 months.

The AWV will include the establishment of, or update to, the individual's medical/family history, measurement of his/her height, weight, body-mass index (BMI) or waist circumference, and blood pressure (BP), with the goal of health promotion and disease detection and encouraging patients to obtain the screening and preventive services that may already be covered and paid for under Medicare Part B. CMS amended

42 CFR §§411.15(a)(1) and 411.15(k)(15) to allow payment on or after January 1, 2011, for an AWV (as established at 42 CFR 410.15) when performed by qualified health professionals.

Coverage is available for an AWV that meets the following requirements:

1. It is performed by a health professional;
2. It is furnished to an eligible beneficiary who is no longer within 12 months after the effective date of his/her first Medicare Part B coverage period, and he/she has not received either an IPPE or an AWV providing PPPS within the past 12 months.

See Pub. 100-02,Medicare Benefit Policy Manual, chapter 15, section 280.5, for detailed policy regarding the AWV, including definitions of: (1) detection of cognitive impairment, (2) eligible beneficiary, (3) establishment of, or an update to, an individual's medical/family history, (4&5) first and subsequent AWVs providing PPPS, (6) health professional, and, (7) review of an individual's functional ability/level of safety.

100-4, Chapter-18, 140.1

Healthcare Common Procedure Coding System (HCPCS) Coding for the AWV

The HCPCS codes listed below were developed for the AWV benefit effective January 1, 2011, for individuals whose initial enrollment is on or after January 1, 2011.

G0438 -Annual wellness visit; includes a personalized prevention plan of service (PPPS); first visit

G0439 –Annual wellness visit; includes a personalized prevention plan of service (PPPS); subsequent visit

100-4, Chapter-18, 140.5

Coinsurance and Deductible

Sections 4103 and 4104 of the Affordable Care Act provide for a waiver of Medicare coinsurance/copayment and Part B deductible requirements for the AWV effective for services furnished on or after January 1, 2011.

100-4, Chapter-18, 140.6

Common Working File (CWF) Edits

Effective for claims with dates of service on and after January 1,2011, CWF shall reject:

- AWV claims for G0438 when a previous (first) AWV, HCPCS code G0438, is paid in history regardless of when it occurred.
- AWV claims when a previous AWV, G0438 or G0439, is paid in history within the previous 12 months.
- Beginning January 1, 2011, AWV claims when a previous IPPE, HCPCS code G0402, is paid in history within the previous 12 months.
- AWV claims (G0438 and G0439) billed for a date of service within 12 months after the effective date of a beneficiary's first Medicare Part B coverage period.

The following change shall be effective for claims processed on or after April 1, 2013. Typically, when a preventive service is posted to a beneficiary's utilization history, separate entries are posted for a "professional" service (the professional claim for the delivery of the service itself) and a "technical" service (the institutional claims for a facility fee). However, in the case of AWV services, since

there is no separate payment for a facility fee, the AWV claim will be posted as the "professional" service only, regardless of whether it is paid on a professional claim or an institutional claim.

100-4, Chapter-18, 150

Counseling to Prevent Tobacco Use

Effective September 30, 2016, HCPCS codes G0436 and G0437 are no longer valid. The services previously represented by G0436 and G0437 should be billed under existing CPT® codes 99406 (Smoking and tobacco use cessation counseling visit; intermediate, greater than 3 minutes up to 10 minutes) and 99407 (Smoking and tobacco use cessation counseling visit; intensive, greater 10 minutes) respectively. See Chapter 32 section 12 for coverage and billing requirements for smoking cessation services.

NOTE: Instructions in sections 150 thru 150.4 are no longer valid.

Effective for claims with dates of service on and after August 25, 2010, the Centers for Medicare & Medicaid Services (CMS) will cover counseling to prevent tobacco use services for outpatient and hospitalized Medicare beneficiaries:

1. Who use tobacco, regardless of whether they have signs or symptoms of tobacco-related disease;
2. Who are competent and alert at the time that counseling is provided; and,
3. Whose counseling is furnished by a qualified physician or other Medicare-recognized practitioner.

These individuals who do not have signs or symptoms of tobacco-related disease will be covered under Medicare Part B when the above conditions of coverage are met, subject to certain frequency and other limitations.

Conditions of Medicare Part A and Medicare Part B coverage for counseling to prevent tobacco use are located in the Medicare National Coverage Determinations (NCD) Manual, Publication 100-3, chapter1, section 210.4.1.

100-4, Chapter-18, 150.1

Healthcare Common Procedure Coding System (HCPCS) and Diagnosis Coding

The CMS has created two new G codes for billing for tobacco cessation counseling services to prevent tobacco use for those individuals who use tobacco but do not have signs or symptoms of tobacco-related disease. These are in addition to the two CPT® codes 99406 and 99407 that currently are used for smoking and tobacco-use cessation counseling for symptomatic individuals.

The following HCPCS codes should be reported when billing for counseling to prevent tobacco use effective January 1, 2011:

G0436 (this code has been deleted in 2017)- Smoking and tobacco cessation counseling visit for the asymptomatic patient; intermediate, greater than 3 minutes, up to 10 minutes

Short descriptor: Tobacco-use counsel 3-10 min

G0437 (this code has been deleted in 2017)- Smoking and tobacco cessation counseling visit for the asymptomatic patient; intensive, greater than 10 minutes

Short descriptor: Tobacco-use counsel >10min

NOTE: The above G codes will not be active in contractors' systems until January 1, 2011. Therefore, contractors shall advise non-outpatient perspective payment system (OPPS) providers to use unlisted code 99199 to bill for counseling to prevent tobacco use and tobacco-related disease services during the interim period of August 25, 2010, through December 31, 2010.

On January 3, 2011, contractor's systems will accept the new G codes for services performed on or after August 25, 2010.

Two new C codes have been created for facilities paid under OPPS when billing for counseling to prevent tobacco use and tobacco-related disease services during the interim period of August 25, 2010, through December 31, 2010:

C9801 - Smoking and tobacco cessation counseling visit for the asymptomatic patient, intermediate, greater than 3 minutes, up to 10 minutes

Short descriptor: Tobacco-use counsel 3-10 min

C9802 - Smoking and tobacco cessation counseling visit for the asymptomatic patient, intensive, greater than 10 minutes

Short descriptor: Tobacco-use counsel >10min

Claims for smoking and tobacco use cessation counseling services G0436 (this code has been deleted in 2017) and G0437 (this code has been deleted in 2017) shall be submitted with the applicable diagnosis codes:

ICD-9-CM

V15.82, history of tobacco use, or

305.1, non-dependent tobacco use disorder

ICD-10-CM

F17.200, nicotine dependence, unspecified, uncomplicated,

F17.201, nicotine dependence, unspecified, in remission,

F17.210, nicotine dependence, cigarettes, uncomplicated,

F17.211, nicotine dependence, cigarettes, in remission,

F17.220, nicotine dependence, chewing tobacco, uncomplicated,

F17.221, nicotine dependence, chewing tobacco, in remission,

F17.290, nicotine dependence, other tobacco product, uncomplicated,

F17.291, nicotine dependence, other tobacco product, in remission, or

Z87.891, personal history of nicotine dependence, unspecified, uncomplicated.

Contractors shall allow payment for a medically necessary E/M service on the same day as the smoking and tobacco-use cessation counseling service when it is clinically appropriate. Physicians and qualified non-physician practitioners shall use an appropriate HCPCS code to report an E/M service with modifier -25 to indicate that the E/M service is a separately identifiable service from G0436 (this code has been deleted in 2017) or G0437 (this code has been deleted in 2017).

100-4, Chapter-18, 150.2

A/B MACs (B) Billing Requirements

A/B MACs (B) shall pay for counseling to prevent tobacco use services billed with code G0436 or G0437 for dates of service on or after January 1, 2011. A/B MACs (B) shall pay for counseling services billed with code 99199 for dates of service performed on or after August 25, 2010 through December 31, 2010. The type of service (TOS) for each of the new codes is 1.

A/B MACs (B) pay for counseling services billed based on the Medicare Physician Fee Schedule (MPFS). Deductible and coinsurance apply for services performed on August 25, 2010,

through December 31, 2010. For claims with dates of service on and after January 1, 2011, coinsurance and deductible do not apply on G0436 and G0437.

Physicians or qualified non-physician practitioners shall bill the A/B MACs (B) for counseling to prevent tobacco use services on Form CMS-1500 or an approved electronic format.

NOTE: The above G codes will not be active in MACs' systems until January 1, 2011. Therefore, MACs shall advise providers to use unlisted code 99199 to bill for counseling to prevent tobacco use services during the interim period of August 25, 2010, through December 31, 2010.

100-4, Chapter-18, 150.2.1

A/B MAC (A) and (HHH) Billing Requirements

The A/B MACs (A) and (HHH) shall pay for counseling to prevent tobacco use services with codes G0436 and G0437 for dates of service on or after January 1, 2011. A/B MACs (A) and (HHH) shall pay for counseling services billed with code 99199 for dates of service performed on or after August 25, 2010, through December 31, 2010. For facilities paid under OPPS, A/B MACs (A) shall pay for counseling services billed with codes C9801 and C9802 for dates of service performed on or after August 25, 2010, through December 31, 2010.

Claims for counseling to prevent tobacco use services should be submitted on Form CMS-1450 or its electronic equivalent.

The applicable bill types are 12X, 13X, 22X, 23X, 34X, 71X, 77X, and 85X.

Payment for outpatient services is as follows:

Type of Facility	Method of Payment
Rural Health Centers (RHCs) TOB 71X/Federally Qualified Health Centers (FQHCs)TOB 77X	All-inclusive rate (AIR) for the encounter
Hospitals TOBs 12X and 13X	OPPS for hospitals subject to OPPS MPFS for hospitals not subject to OPPS
Indian Health Services (IHS) Hospitals TOB 13X	AIR for the encounter
Skilled Nursing Facilities (SNFs) TOBs 22X and 23X	Medicare Physician Fee Schedule (MPFS)
Home Health Agencies (HHAs) TOB 34X	MPFS
Critical Access Hospitals (CAHs) TOB 85X	Method I: Technical services are paid at 101% of reasonable cost. Method II: technical services are paid at 101% of reasonable cost, and Professional services are paid at 115% of the MPFS Data Base
IHS CAHs TOB 85X	Based on specific rate
Maryland Hospitals	Payment is based according to the Health Services Cost Review Commission (HSCRC). That is 94% of submitted charges subject to any unmet deductible, coinsurance, and non-covered charges policies.

Deductible and coinsurance apply for services performed on August 25, 2010, through December 31, 2010. For claims with dates of service on and after January 1, 2011, coinsurance and deductible do not apply for G0436 and G0437.

100-4, Chapter-18, 150.4

Common Working File (CWF)

The Common Working File (CWF) shall edit for the frequency of service limitations of counseling to prevent tobacco use sessions and smoking and tobacco-use cessation counseling services (G0436 (this code has been deleted in 2017), G0437 (this code has been deleted in 2017), 99406, 99407) rendered to a beneficiary for a combined total of 8 sessions within a 12-month period. The beneficiary may receive another 8 sessions during a second or subsequent year after 11 full months have passed since the first Medicare covered counseling session was performed. To start the count for the second or subsequent 12-month period, begin with the month after the month in which the first Medicare covered counseling session was performed and count until 11 full months have elapsed.

By entering the beneficiary's health insurance claim number (HICN), providers have the capability to view the number of sessions a beneficiary has received for this service via inquiry through CWF.

100-4, Chapter-18, 160

Intensive Behavioral Therapy (IBT) for Cardiovascular Disease (CVD)

For services furnished on or after November 8, 2011, the Centers for Medicare & Medicaid Services (CMS) covers intensive behavioral therapy (IBT) for cardiovascular disease (CVD). See National Coverage Determinations (NCD) Manual (Pub. 100-03) §210.11 for complete coverage guidelines.

100-4, Chapter-18, 160.1

Coding Requirements for IBT for CVD Furnished on or After November 8, 2011

The following is the applicable Healthcare Procedural Coding System (HCPCS) code for IBT for CVD:

G0446: Annual, face-to-face intensive behavioral therapy for cardiovascular disease, individual, 15 minutes

Contractors shall not apply deductibles or coinsurance to claim lines containing HCPCS code G0446.

100-4, Chapter-18, 160.2.1

Correct Place of Service (POS) Codes for IBT for CVD on Professional Claims

Contractors shall pay for IBT CVD, G0446 only when services are provided at the following POS:

11- Physician's Office

22- Outpatient Hospital

49- Independent Clinic

72- Rural Health Clinic

Claims not submitted with one of the POS codes above will be denied.

The following messages shall be used when Medicare contractors deny professional claims for incorrect POS:

Claim Adjustment Reason Code (CARC) 58: "Treatment was deemed by the payer to have been rendered in an inappropriate or invalid place of service." **NOTE:** Refer to the 835 Healthcare Policy Identification Segment (loop 2110 Service Payment Information REF), if present.

Remittance Advice Remark Code (RARC) N428: "Not covered when performed in this place of service."

Medicare Summary Notice (MSN) 21.25: "This service was denied because Medicare only covers this service in certain settings."

Spanish Version: El servicio fue denegado porque Medicare solamente lo cubre en ciertas situaciones."

Group Code PR (Patient Responsibility) assigning financial liability to the beneficiary, if a claim is received with a GA modifier indicating a signed ABN is on file.

Group Code CO (Contractual Obligation) assigning financial liability to the provider, if a claim is received with a GZ modifier indicating no signed ABN is on file.

100-4, Chapter-18, 160.2.2

Provider Specialty Edits for IBT for CVD on Professional Claims

Contractors shall pay claims for HCPCS code G0446 only when services are submitted by the following provider specialty types found on the provider's enrollment record:

01= General Practice

08 = Family Practice

11= Internal Medicine

16 = Obstetrics/Gynecology

37= Pediatric Medicine

38 = Geriatric Medicine

42= Certified Nurse Midwife

50 = Nurse Practitioner

89 = Certified Clinical Nurse Specialist

97= Physician Assistant

Contractors shall deny claim lines for HCPCS code G0446 performed by any other provider specialty type other than those listed above.

The following messages shall be used when Medicare contractors deny IBT for CVD claims billed with invalid provider specialty types:

CARC 185: "The rendering provider is not eligible to perform the service billed."

NOTE: Refer to the 835 Healthcare Policy Identification Segment (loop 2110 Service Payment Information REF), if present.

RARC N95: "This provider type/provider specialty may not bill this service."

MSN 21.18: "This item or service is not covered when performed or ordered by this provider."

Spanish version: "Este servicio no esta cubierto cuando es ordenado o rendido por este proveedor."

Group Code PR (Patient Responsibility) assigning financial liability to the beneficiary, if a claim is received with a GA modifier indicating a signed ABN is on file.

Group Code CO (Contractual Obligation) assigning financial liability to the provider, if a claim is received with a GZ modifier indicating no signed ABN is on file.

100-4, Chapter-18, 160.3

Correct Types of Bill (TOB) for IBT for CVD on Institutional Claims

Effective for claims with dates of service on and after November 8, 2011, the following types of bill (TOB) may be used for IBT for CVD: 13X, 71X, 77X, or 85X. All other TOB codes shall be denied.

The following messages shall be used when Medicare contractors deny claims for G0446 when submitted on a TOB other than those listed above:

CARC 170: Payment is denied when performed/billed by this type of provider. **NOTE:** Refer to the 835 Healthcare Policy Identification Segment (loop 2110 Service Payment Information REF), if present.

RARC N428: Not covered when performed in this place of service."

MSN 21.25: "This service was denied because Medicare only covers this service in certain settings."

Spanish Version: El servicio fue denegado porque Medicare solamente lo cubre en ciertas situaciones."

Group Code PR (Patient Responsibility) assigning financial liability to the beneficiary, if a claim is received with a GA modifier indicating a signed ABN is on file.

Group Code CO (Contractual Obligation) assigning financial liability to the provider, if a claim is received with a GZ modifier indicating no signed ABN is on file.

100-4, Chapter-18, 160.4

Frequency Edits for IBT for CVD Claims

Contractors shall allow claims for G0446 no more than once in a 12-month period.

NOTE: 11 full months must elapse following the month in which the last G0446 IBT for CVD took place.

Contractors shall deny claims IBT for CVD claims that exceed one (1) visit every 12 months.

Contractors shall allow one professional service and one facility fee claim for each visit.

The following messages shall be used when Medicare contractors deny IBT for CVD claims that exceed the frequency limit:

CARC 119: "Benefit maximum for this time period or occurrence has been reached."

RARC N362: "The number of days or units of service exceeds our acceptable maximum."

MSN 20.5: "These services cannot be paid because your benefits are exhausted at this time."

Spanish Version: "Estos servicios no pueden ser pagados porque sus beneficios se hanagotado."

Group Code PR (Patient Responsibility) assigning financial liability to the beneficiary, if a claim is received with a GA modifier indicating a signed ABN is on file.

Group Code CO (Contractual Obligation) assigning financial liability to the provider, if a claim is received with a GZ modifier indicating no signed ABN is on file.

100-4, Chapter-18, 160.5

Common Working File (CWF) Edits for IBT for CVD Claims

When applying frequency, CWF shall count 11 full months following the month of the last IBT for CVD, G0446 before allowing subsequent payment of another G0446 screening.

When applying frequency limitations to G0446, CWF shall allow both a claim for the professional service and a claim for the facility fee. CWF shall identify the following institutional claims as facility fee claims for screening services: TOB 13X, TOB85X when the revenue code is not 096X, 097X, or 098X. CWF shall identify all other claims as professional service claims for screening services. **NOTE:** This does not apply to RHCs and FQHCs.

100-4, Chapter-18, 170.1

Healthcare Common Procedure Coding System (HCPCS) Codes for Screening for STIs and HIBC to Prevent STIs

Effective for claims with dates of service on and after November 8, 2011, the claims processing instructions for payment of screening tests for STI will apply to the following HCPCS codes:

- Chlamydia: 86631, 86632, 87110, 87270, 87320, 87490, 87491, 87810, 87800 (used for combined chlamydia and gonorrhea testing)
- Gonorrhea: 87590, 87591, 87850, 87800 (used for combined chlamydia and gonorrhea testing)
- Syphilis: 86592, 86593, 86780
- Hepatitis B: (Hepatitis B surface antigen): 87340, 87341

Effective for claims with dates of service on and after November 8, 2011, implemented with the January 2, 2012, IOCE, the following HCPCS code is to be billed for HIBC to prevent STIs

- G0445 –high-intensity behavioral counseling to prevent sexually transmitted infections, face-to-face, individual, includes: education, skills training, and guidance on how to change sexual behavior, performed semi-annually, 30minutes.

100-4, Chapter-18, 170.2

Diagnosis Code Reporting

A claim that is submitted for screening chlamydia, gonorrhea, syphilis, and/or Hepatitis B shall be submitted with one or more of the following diagnosis codes in the header and pointed to the line item:

a. For claims for screening for chlamydia, gonorrhea, and syphilis in women at increased risk who are not pregnant use the following ICD-9-CM diagnosis codes:

- V74.5 - Screening, bacterial - sexually transmitted; and
- V69.8 - Other problems related to lifestyle as secondary. (This diagnosis code is used to indicate high/increased risk for STIs).

Effective with the implementation of ICD-10, use the following ICD-10-CM diagnosis codes:

- Z11.3 - Encounter for screening for infections with a predominantly sexual mode of transmission; and
- any of o Z72.89 - Other problems related to lifestyle,

- Z72.51 - High risk heterosexual behavior,
- Z72.52 - High risk homosexual behavior, or
- Z72.53 - High risk bisexual behavior. (These diagnosis codes are used to indicate high/increased risk for STIs).

b. For claims for screening for syphilis in men at increased risk use the following ICD-9-CM diagnosis codes:

- V74.5 - Screening, bacterial - sexually transmitted; and
- V69.8 - Other problems related to lifestyle as secondary.

Effective with the implementation of ICD-10, use the following ICD-10-CM diagnosis codes:

- Z11.3 - Encounter for screening for infections with a predominantly sexual mode of transmission; and
- any of
  - Z72.89 - Other problems related to lifestyle,
  - Z72.51 - High risk heterosexual behavior,
  - Z72.52 - High risk homosexual behavior, or
  - Z72.53 - High risk bisexual behavior.

c. For claims for screening for chlamydia and gonorrhea in pregnant women at increased risk for STIs use the following ICD-9-CM diagnosis codes, if applicable:

- V74.5 - Screening, bacterial - sexually transmitted; and
- V69.8 - Other problems related to lifestyle, and
- one of,
  - V22.0 - Supervision of normal first pregnancy, or
  - V22.1 - Supervision of other normal pregnancy, or,
  - V23.9 - Supervision of unspecified high-risk pregnancy.

Effective with the implementation of ICD-10, use ICD-10-CM diagnosis code Z11.3 - Encounter for screening for infections with a predominantly sexual mode of transmission; and one of:

- Z72.89 - Other problems related to lifestyle,
- Z72.51 - High risk heterosexual behavior,
- Z72.52 - High risk homosexual behavior, or
- Z72.53 - High risk bisexual behavior.

and also one of the following.

Code	Description
Z34.00	Encounter for supervision of normal first pregnancy, unspecified trimester
Z34.01	Encounter for supervision of normal first pregnancy, first trimester
Z34.02	Encounter for supervision of normal first pregnancy, second trimester
Z34.03	Encounter for supervision of normal first pregnancy, third trimester
Z34.80	Encounter for supervision of other normal pregnancy, unspecified trimester
Z34.81	Encounter for supervision of other normal pregnancy, first trimester
Z34.82	Encounter for supervision of other normal pregnancy, second trimester
Z34.83	Encounter for supervision of other normal pregnancy, third trimester

Code	Description
Z34.90	Encounter for supervision of normal pregnancy, unspecified, unspecified trimester
Z34.91	Encounter for supervision of normal pregnancy, unspecified, first trimester
Z34.92	Encounter for supervision of normal pregnancy, unspecified, second trimester
Z34.93	Encounter for supervision of normal pregnancy, unspecified, third trimester
O09.90	Supervision of high risk pregnancy, unspecified, unspecified trimester
O09.91	Supervision of high risk pregnancy, unspecified, first trimester
O09.92	Supervision of high risk pregnancy, unspecified, second trimester
O09.93	Supervision of high risk pregnancy, unspecified, third trimester

d. For claims for screening for syphilis in pregnant women use the following ICD-9-CM diagnosis codes:

- V74.5 - Screening, bacterial - sexually transmitted; and
- V22.0 - Supervision of normal first pregnancy, or,
- V22.1 - Supervision of other normal pregnancy, or,
- V23.9 - Supervision of unspecified high-risk pregnancy.

Effective with the implementation of ICD-10, use the following ICD-10-CM diagnosis codes:

- Z11.3 - Encounter for screening for infections with a predominantly sexual mode of transmission;
- and one of

Code	Description
Z34.00	Encounter for supervision of normal first pregnancy, unspecified trimester
Z34.01	Encounter for supervision of normal first pregnancy, first trimester
Z34.02	Encounter for supervision of normal first pregnancy, second trimester
Z34.03	Encounter for supervision of normal first pregnancy, third trimester
Z34.80	Encounter for supervision of other normal pregnancy, unspecified trimester
Z34.81	Encounter for supervision of other normal pregnancy, first trimester
Z34.82	Encounter for supervision of other normal pregnancy, second trimester
Z34.83	Encounter for supervision of other normal pregnancy, third trimester
Z34.90	Encounter for supervision of normal pregnancy, unspecified, unspecified trimester
Z34.91	Encounter for supervision of normal pregnancy, unspecified, first trimester
Z34.92	Encounter for supervision of normal pregnancy, unspecified, second trimester
Z34.93	Encounter for supervision of normal pregnancy, unspecified, third trimester
O09.90	Supervision of high risk pregnancy, unspecified, unspecified trimester
O09.91	Supervision of high risk pregnancy, unspecified, first trimester
O09.92	Supervision of high risk pregnancy, unspecified, second trimester
O09.93	Supervision of high risk pregnancy, unspecified, third trimester

e. For claims for screening for syphilis in pregnant women at increased risk for STIs use the following ICD-9-CM diagnosis codes:

- V74.5 - Screening, bacterial - sexually transmitted; and
- V69.8 - Other problems related to lifestyle, and,

- V22.0 - Supervision of normal first pregnancy, or
- V22.1 - Supervision of other normal pregnancy, or,
- V23.9 - Supervision of unspecified high-risk pregnancy.

Effective with the implementation of ICD-10, use the following ICD-10-CM diagnosis codes:

- Z11.3 - Encounter for screening for infections with a predominantly sexual mode of transmission;
- and any of:
  - Z72.89 - Other problems related to lifestyle, or
  - Z72.51 - High risk heterosexual behavior, or
  - Z72.52 - High risk homosexual behavior, or
  - Z72.53 - High risk bisexual behavior

and also one of the following:

Code	Description
Z34.00	Encounter for supervision of normal first pregnancy, unspecified trimester
Z34.01	Encounter for supervision of normal first pregnancy, first trimester
Z34.02	Encounter for supervision of normal first pregnancy, second trimester
Z34.03	Encounter for supervision of normal first pregnancy, third trimester
Z34.80	Encounter for supervision of other normal pregnancy, unspecified trimester
Z34.81	Encounter for supervision of other normal pregnancy, first trimester
Z34.82	Encounter for supervision of other normal pregnancy, second trimester
Z34.83	Encounter for supervision of other normal pregnancy, third trimester
Z34.90	Encounter for supervision of normal pregnancy, unspecified, unspecified trimester
Z34.91	Encounter for supervision of normal pregnancy, unspecified, first trimester
Z34.92	Encounter for supervision of normal pregnancy, unspecified, second trimester
Z34.93	Encounter for supervision of normal pregnancy, unspecified, third trimester
O09.90	Supervision of high risk pregnancy, unspecified, unspecified trimester
O09.91	Supervision of high risk pregnancy, unspecified, first trimester
O09.92	Supervision of high risk pregnancy, unspecified, second trimester
O09.93	Supervision of high risk pregnancy, unspecified, third trimester

f. CM diagnosis codes:
- V73.89 - Screening, disease or disorder, viral, specified type NEC; and
- V22.0 - Supervision of normal first pregnancy, or,
- V22.1 - Supervision of other normal pregnancy, or,
- V23.9 - Supervision of unspecified high-risk pregnancy.

Effective with the implementation of ICD-10, use the following ICD-10-CM diagnosis codes:

- Z11.59 - Encounter for screening for other viral diseases, and any of
- Z34.00 - Encounter for supervision of normal first pregnancy, unspecified trimester, or
- Z34.80 - Encounter for supervision of other normal pregnancy, unspecified trimester, or
- Z34.90 - Encounter for supervision of normal pregnancy, unspecified, unspecified trimester, or

- O09.90 - Supervision of high risk pregnancy, unspecified, unspecified trimester.

g. For claims for screening for Hepatitis B in pregnant women at increased risk for STIs use the following ICD-9-CM diagnosis codes:
- V73.89 - Screening, disease or disorder, viral, specified type NEC; and
- V 69.8 - Other problems related to lifestyle, and,
- V22.0 - Supervision of normal first pregnancy, or,
- V22.1 - Supervision of other normal pregnancy, or,
- V23.9 - Supervision of unspecified high-risk pregnancy.

Effective with the implementation of ICD-10, use the following ICD-10-CM diagnosis codes:

- Z11.59 - Encounter for screening for other viral diseases, and
- Z72.89 - Other problems related to lifestyle, and
- any of
  - Z72.51 - High risk heterosexual behavior, or
  - Z72.52 - High risk homosexual behavior, or
  - Z72.53 - High risk bisexual behavior;
- and also one of the following:

Code	Description
Z34.00	Encounter for supervision of normal first pregnancy, unspecified trimester
Z34.01	Encounter for supervision of normal first pregnancy, first trimester
Z34.02	Encounter for supervision of normal first pregnancy, second trimester
Z34.03	Encounter for supervision of normal first pregnancy, third trimester
Z34.80	Encounter for supervision of other normal pregnancy, unspecified trimester
Z34.81	Encounter for supervision of other normal pregnancy, first trimester
Z34.82	Encounter for supervision of other normal pregnancy, second trimester
Z34.83	Encounter for supervision of other normal pregnancy, third trimester
Z34.90	Encounter for supervision of normal pregnancy, unspecified, unspecified trimester
Z34.91	Encounter for supervision of normal pregnancy, unspecified, first trimester
Z34.92	Encounter for supervision of normal pregnancy, unspecified, second trimester
Z34.93	Encounter for supervision of normal pregnancy, unspecified, third trimester
O09.90	Supervision of high risk pregnancy, unspecified, unspecified trimester
O09.91	Supervision of high risk pregnancy, unspecified, first trimester
O09.92	Supervision of high risk pregnancy, unspecified, second trimester
O09.93	Supervision of high risk pregnancy, unspecified, third trimester

100-4, Chapter-18, 170.3

Billing Requirements

- Effective for dates of service November 8, 2011, and later, A/B MACs (A) and (B) shall recognize HCPCS code G0445 for HIBC. Medicare shall cover up to two occurrences of G0445 when billed for IBC to prevent STIs. A claim that is submitted with HCPCS code G0445 for HIBC shall be submitted with ICD-9-CM diagnosis code V69.8 or ICD-10-CM diagnosis code Z72.89.

- A/B MACs (A) and (B) shall pay for screening for chlamydia, gonorrhea, and syphilis (as indicated by the presence of ICD-9-CM diagnosis code V74.5 or if ICD-10 is applicable, ICD-10-CM diagnosis code Z11.3); and/or Hepatitis B (as indicated by the presence of ICD-9-CM diagnosis code V73.89 or ICD-10-CM diagnosis code Z11.59) as follows:
- One annual occurrence of screening for chlamydia, gonorrhea, and syphilis (i.e., 1 per 12-month period) in women at increased risk who are not pregnant,
- One annual occurrence of screening for syphilis (i.e., 1 per 12-month period) in men at increased risk,
- Up to two occurrences per pregnancy of screening for chlamydia and gonorrhea in pregnant women who are at increased risk for STIs and continued increased risk for the second screening,
- One occurrence per pregnancy of screening for syphilis in pregnant women,
- Up to an additional two occurrences per pregnancy of screening for syphilis in pregnant women if the beneficiary is at continued increased risk for STIs,
- One occurrence per pregnancy of screening for Hepatitis B in pregnant women, and,
- One additional occurrence per pregnancy of screening for Hepatitis B in pregnant women who are at continued increased risk for STIs.

100-4, Chapter-18, 170.4

Types of Bill (TOBs) and Revenue Codes

The applicable types of bill (TOBs) for HIBC screening, HCPCS code G0445, are: 13X, 71X, 77X, and 85X.

On institutional claims, TOBs 71X and 77X, use revenue code 052X to ensure coinsurance and deductible are not applied.

Critical access hospitals (CAHs) electing the optional method of payment for outpatient services report this service under revenue codes 096X, 097X, or 098X.

100-4, Chapter-18, 170.4.1

Payment Method

Payment for HIBC is based on the all-inclusive payment rate for rural health clinics (TOBs 71X) and federally qualified health centers (TOB 77X). Hospital outpatient departments (TOB 13X) are paid based on the outpatient prospective payment system and CAHs (TOB 85X) are paid based on reasonable cost. CAHs electing the optional method of payment for outpatient services are paid based on 115% of the lesser of the Medicare Physician Fee Schedule (MPFS) amount or submitted charge.

Effective for dates of service on and after November 8, 2011, deductible and coinsurance do not apply to claim lines with G0445.

HCPCS code G0445 may be paid on the same date of service as an annual wellness visit, evaluation and management (E&M) code, or during the global billing period for obstetrical care, but only one G0445 may be paid on any one date of service. If billed on the same date of service with an E&M code, the E&M code should have a distinct diagnosis code other than the diagnosis code used to indicate high/increased risk for STIs for the G0445 service. An E&M code should not be billed when the sole reason for the visit is HIBC to prevent STIs.

For Medicare Part B physician and non-practitioner claims, payment for HIBC to prevent STIs is based on the MPFS amount for G0445.

100-4, Chapter-18, 170.5

Specialty Codes and Place of Service (POS)

Medicare provides coverage for screening for chlamydia, gonorrhea, syphilis, and/or Hepatitis B and HIBC to prevent STIs only when ordered by a primary care practitioner (physician or non-physician) with any of the following specialty codes:

- 01 –General Practice
- 08 –Family Practice
- 11 –Internal Medicine
- 16 –Obstetrics/Gynecology
- 37 –Pediatric Medicine
- 38 –Geriatric Medicine
- 42 –Certified Nurse Midwife
- 50 –Nurse Practitioner
- 89 –Certified Clinical Nurse Specialist
- 97 –Physician Assistant

Medicare provides coverage for HIBC to prevent STIs only when provided by a primary care practitioner (physician or non-physician) with any of the specialty codes identified above.

Medicare provides coverage for HIBC to prevent STIs only when the POS billed is 11, 22, 49, or 71.

100-4, Chapter-18, 180

Alcohol Screening and Behavioral Counseling Interventions in Primary Care to Reduce Alcohol Misuse

The United States Preventive Services Task Force (USPSTF) defines alcohol misuse as risky, hazardous, or harmful drinking which places an individual at risk for future problems with alcohol consumption. In the general adult population, alcohol consumption becomes risky or hazardous when consuming:

- Greater than 7 drinks per week or greater than 3 drinks per occasion for women and persons greater than 65 years old.
- Greater than 14 drinks per week or greater than 4 drinks per occasion for men 65 years old and younger.

100-4, Chapter-18, 180.1

Policy

Claims with dates of service on and after October 14, 2011, the Centers for Medicare & Medicaid Services (CMS) will cover annual alcohol misuse screening (HCPCS code G0442) consisting of 1 screening session, and for those that screen positive, upto 4 brief, face-to-face behavioral counseling sessions (HCPCS code G0443) per 12-month period for Medicare beneficiaries, including pregnant women.

Medicare beneficiaries that may be identified as having a need for behavioral counseling sessions include those:

- Who misuse alcohol, but whose levels or patterns of alcohol consumption do not meet criteria for alcohol dependence (defined as at least three of the following: tolerance, withdrawal symptoms, impaired control, preoccupation with acquisition and/or use, persistent desire or unsuccessful efforts to quit, sustains social, occupational, or recreational disability, use continues despite adverse consequences); and,

- Who are competent and alert at the time that counseling is provided; and,
- Whose counseling is furnished by qualified primary care physicians or other primary care practitioners in a primary care setting.

Once a Medicare beneficiary has agreed to behavioral counseling sessions, the counseling sessions are to be completed based on the 5As approach adopted by the United States Preventive Services Task Force (USPSTF.) The steps to the 5As approach are listed below.

1. *Assess:* Ask about/assess behavioral health risk(s) and factors affecting choice of behavior change goals/methods.
2. *Advise:* Give clear, specific, and personalized behavior change advice, including information about personal health harms and benefits.
3. *Agree:* Collaboratively select appropriate treatment goals and methods based on the patient's interest in and willingness to change the behavior.
4. *Assist:* Using behavior change techniques (self-help and/or counseling), aid the patient in achieving agreed-upon goals by acquiring the skills, confidence, and social/environmental supports for behavior change, supplemented with adjunctive medical treatments when appropriate.
5. *Arrange:* Schedule follow-up contacts (in person or by telephone) to provide ongoing assistance/support and to adjust the treatment plan as needed, including referral to more intensive or specialized treatment.

100-4, Chapter18, 180.2

Institutional Billing Requirements

For claims with dates of service on and after October 14, 2011, Medicare will allow coverage for annual alcohol misuse screening, 15 minutes, G0442, and brief, face-to-face behavioral counseling for alcohol misuse, 15 minutes, G0443 for:

- Rural Health Clinics (RHCs) -type of bill (TOB) 71X only –based on the all-inclusive payment rate
- Federally Qualified Health Centers (FQHCs) -TOB 77X only –based on the all-inclusive payment rate
- Outpatient hospitals –TOB 13X -based on Outpatient Prospective Payment System (OPPS)
- Critical Access Hospitals (CAHs) -TOB 85X–based on reasonable cost
- CAH Method II –TOB 85X -based on 115% of the lesser of the Medicare Physician Fee Schedule (MPFS) amount or actual charge as applicable with revenue codes 096X, 097X, or 098X.

For RHCs and FQHCs the alcohol screening/counseling is not separately payable with another face-to-face encounter on the same day. This does not apply to the Initial Preventive Physical Examination (IPPE), unrelated services denoted with modifier 59, and 77X claims containing Diabetes Self-Management Training (DSMT) and Medical Nutrition Therapy (MNT) services. DSMT and MNT apply to FQHCs only. However, the screening/counseling sessions alone when rendered as a face-to-face visit with a core practitioner do constitute an encounter and is paid based on the all-inclusive payment rate.

NOTE: For outpatient hospital settings, as in any other setting, services covered under this NCD must be provided by a primary care provider.

Claims submitted with alcohol misuse screening and behavioral counseling HCPCS codes G0442 and G0443 on a TOB other than 13X, 71X, 77X, and 85X will be denied.

Effective October 14, 2011, deductible and co-insurance should not be applied for line items on claims billed for alcohol misuse screening G0442 and behavioral counseling for alcohol misuse G0443.

100-4, Chapter-18, 180.3

Professional Billing Requirements

For claims with dates of service on and after October 14, 2011, CMS will allow coverage for annual alcohol misuse screening, 15 minutes, G0442, and behavioral counseling for alcohol misuse, 15 minutes, G0443, only when services are submitted by the following provider specialties found on the provider's enrollment record:

01 -General Practice

08 -Family Practice

11 -Internal Medicine

16 -Obstetrics/Gynecology

37 -Pediatric Medicine

38 -Geriatric Medicine

42 –Certified Nurse-Midwife

50 -Nurse Practitioner

89 -Certified Clinical Nurse Specialist

97 -Physician Assistant

Any claims that are not submitted from one of the provider specialty types noted above will be denied.

For claims with dates of service on and after October 14, 2011, CMS will allow coverage for annual alcohol misuse screening, 15 minutes, G0442, and behavioral counseling for alcohol misuse, 15 minutes, G0443, only when submitted with one of the following place of service (POS) codes:

11 -Physician's Office

22 -Outpatient Hospital

49 -Independent Clinic

71 -State or local public health clinic or

Any claims that are not submitted with one of the POS codes noted above will be denied.

The alcohol screening/counseling services are payable with another encounter/visit on the same day. This does not apply for IPPE.

100-4, Chapter-18, 180.4

Claim Adjustment Reason Codes, Remittance Advice Remark Codes, Group Codes, and Medicare Summary Notice Messages

Contractors shall use the appropriate claim adjustment reason codes (CARCs), remittance advice remark codes (RARCs), group codes, or Medicare summary notice (MSN) messages when denying payment for alcohol misuse screening and alcohol misuse behavioral counseling sessions:

- For RHC and FQHC claims that contain screening for alcohol misuse HCPCS code G0442 and alcohol misuse counseling HCPCS code G0443 with another encounter/visit with the same line item date of service, use group code CO and reason code:
  - Claim Adjustment Reason Code (CARC) 97 –The benefit for this service is included in the payment/allowance for another service/procedure that has already been adjudicated. *NOTE:* Refer to the 835 Healthcare Policy Identification Segment (loop 2110 Service Payment Information REF) if present
- Denying claims containing HCPCS code G0442 and HCPCS code G0443 submitted on a TOB other than 13X, 71X, 77X, and 85X:
  - Claim Adjustment Reason Code (CARC) 5 -The procedure code/bill type is inconsistent with the place of service. *NOTE:* Refer to the 835 Healthcare Policy Identification Segment (loop 2110 Service Payment Information REF) if present
  - Remittance Advice Remark Code (RARC) M77 – Missing/incomplete/invalid place of service
  - Group Code PR (Patient Responsibility) assigning financial liability to the beneficiary, if a claim is received with a GA modifier indicating a signed ABN is on file.
  - Group Code CO (Contractual Obligation) assigning financial liability to the provider, if a claim is received with a GZ modifier indicating no signed ABN is on file.
- Denying claims that contains more than one alcohol misuse behavioral counseling session G0443 on the same date of service:
  - Medicare Summary Notice (MSN) 15.6 –The information provided does not support the need for this many services or items within this period of time.
  - Claim Adjustment Reason Code (CARC) 151 – Payment adjusted because the payer deems the information submitted does not support this many/frequency of services.
  - Remittance Advice Remark Code (RARC) M86 – Service denied because payment already made for same/similar procedure within set time frame.
  - Group Code PR (Patient Responsibility) assigning financial liability to the beneficiary, if a claim is received with a GA modifier indicating a signed ABN is on file.
  - Group Code CO (Contractual Obligation) assigning financial liability to the provider, if a claim is received with a GZ modifier indicating no signed ABN is on file.
- Denying claims that are not submitted from the appropriate provider specialties:
  - Medicare Summary Notice (MSN) 21.18 –This item or service is not covered when performed or ordered by this provider.
  - Claim Adjustment Reason Code (CARC) 185 -The rendering provider is not eligible to perform the service billed. *NOTE:* Refer to the 835 Healthcare Policy Identification Segment (loop 2110 Service Payment Information REF), if present.
  - Remittance Advice Remark Code (RARC) N95 -This provider type/provider specialty may not bill this service.

- Group Code PR (Patient Responsibility) assigning financial liability to the beneficiary, if a claim is received with a GA modifier indicating a signed ABN is on file.
- Group Code CO (Contractual Obligation) assigning financial liability to the provider, if a claim is received with a GZ modifier indicating no signed ABN is on file.
- Denying claims without the appropriate POS code:
  - Medicare Summary Notice (MSN) 21.25 –This service was denied because Medicare only covers this service in certain settings.
  - Claim Adjustment Reason Code (CARC) 58 – Treatment was deemed by the payer to have been rendered in an inappropriate or invalid place of service. *NOTE:* Refer to the 835 Healthcare Policy Identification Segment (loop 2110 Service Payment Information REF) if present.
  - Remittance Advice Remark Code (RARC) N428 –Not covered when performed in this place of service.
  - Group Code PR (Patient Responsibility) assigning financial liability to the beneficiary, if a claim is received with a GA modifier indicating a signed ABN is on file.
  - Group Code CO (Contractual Obligation) assigning financial liability to the provider, if a claim is received with a GZ modifier indicating no signed ABN is on file.
- Denying claims for alcohol misuse screening HCPCS code G0442 more than once in a 12-month period, and denying alcohol misuse counseling sessions HCPCS code G0443 more than four times in the same 12-month period:
  - Medicare Summary Notice (MSN) 20.5 –These services cannot be paid because your benefits are exhausted at this time.
  - Claim Adjustment Reason Code (CARC) 119 –Benefit maximum for this time period or occurrence has been reached.
  - Remittance Advice Remark Code (RARC) N362 – The number of Days or Units of service exceeds our acceptable maximum.
  - Group Code PR (Patient Responsibility) assigning financial liability to the beneficiary, if a claim is received with a GA modifier indicating a signed ABN is on file.
  - Group Code CO (Contractual Obligation) assigning financial liability to the provider, if a claim is received with a GZ modifier indicating no signed ABN is on file.

100-4, Chapter-18, 180.5

CWF Requirements

When applying frequency, CWF shall count 11 full months following the month of the last alcohol misuse screening visit, G0442, before allowing subsequent payment of another G0442 screening. Additionally, CWF shall create an edit to allow alcohol misuse brief behavioral counseling, HCPCS G0443, no more than 4 times in a 12-month period and make this edit overridable. CWF shall also count four alcohol misuse counseling sessions HCPCS G0443 in the same 12-month period used for G0442 counting from the date the G0442 screening session was billed.

When applying frequency limitations to G0442 screening on the same date of service as G0443 counseling, CWF shall allow both a claim for the professional service and a claim for a facility fee. CWF shall identify the following institutional claims as facility fee claims for screening services: TOB 13X, TOB 85X when the revenue code is not 096X, 097X, or 098X. CWF shall identify all other claims as professional service claims for screening services. *NOTE:* This does not apply to RHCs and FQHCs.

100-4, Chapter-18, 190

Screening for Depression in Adults (Effective October 14, 2011)

A. Coverage Requirements

Effective October 14, 2011, the Centers for Medicare & Medicaid Services (CMS) will cover annual screening up to 15 minutes for Medicare beneficiaries in primary care settings that have staff-assisted depression care supports in place to assure accurate diagnosis, effective treatment, and follow-up. Various screening tools are available for screening for depression. CMS does not identify specific depression screening tools. Rather, the decision to use a specific tool is at the discretion of the clinician in the primary care setting. Screening for depression is non-covered when performed more than one time in a 12-month period. The Medicare coinsurance and Part B deductible are waived for this preventive service.

Additional information on this National Coverage Determination (NCD) for Screening for Depression in Adults can be found in Publication 100-03, NCD Manual, Section 210.9.

100-4, Chapter-18, 190.1

A/B MAC (B) Billing Requirements

Effective October 14, 2011, contractors shall recognize new HCPCS G0444, annual depression screening, 15 minutes.

100-4, Chapter-18, 190.2

Frequency

A/B MACs (B) shall pay for annual depression screening, G0444, no more than once in a 12-month period.

NOTE: 11 full months must elapse following the month in which the last annual depression screening took place.

100-4, Chapter-18, 190.3

Place of Service (POS)

A/B MACs (B) shall pay for annual depression screening claims, G0444, only when services are provided at the following places of service (POS):

11 –Office

22 –Outpatient Hospital

49 –Independent Clinic

71 –State or Local Public Health Clinic

100-4, Chapter-18, 200

Intensive Behavioral Therapy for Obesity (Effective November 29, 2011)

The United States Preventive Services Task Force (USPSTF) found good evidence that body mass index (BMI) is a reliable and valid indicator for identifying adults at increased risk for mortality and morbidity due to overweight and obesity. It also good evidence that high intensity counseling combined with

behavioral interventions in obese adults (as defined by a BMI ≥30 kg/m2) produces modest, sustained weight loss.

100-4, Chapter-18, 200.1

Policy

For services furnished on or after November 29, 2011, Medicare will cover Intensive Behavioral Therapy for Obesity. Medicare beneficiaries with obesity (BMI ≥30 kg/m2) who are competent and alert at the time that counseling is provided and whose counseling is furnished by a qualified primary care physician or other primary care practitioner in a primary care setting are eligible for:

- One face-to-face visit every week for the first month;
- One face-to-face visit every other week for months 2-6;
- One face-to-face visit every month for months 7-12, if the beneficiary meets the 3kg (6.6 lbs.) weight loss requirement during the first 6 months as discussed below.

The counseling sessions are to be completed based on the 5As approach adopted by the United States Preventive Services Task Force (USPSTF.) The steps to the 5As approach are listed below:

1. **Assess:** Ask about/assess behavioral health risk(s) and factors affecting choice of behavior change goals/methods.
2. **Advise:** Give clear, specific, and personalized behavior change advice, including information about personal health harms and benefits.
3. **Agree:** Collaboratively select appropriate treatment goals and methods based on the patient's interest in and willingness to change the behavior.
4. **Assist:** Using behavior change techniques (self-help and/or counseling), aid the patient in achieving agreed-upon goals by acquiring the skills, confidence, and social/environmental supports for behavior change, supplemented with adjunctive medical treatments when appropriate.
5. **Arrange:** Schedule follow-up contacts (in person or by telephone) to provide ongoing assistance/support and to adjust the treatment plan as needed, including referral to more intensive or specialized treatment.

Medicare will cover Face-to-Face Behavioral Counseling for Obesity, 15 minutes (G0447), Face-to-face behavioral counseling for obesity, group (2-10), 30 minute(s) (G0473), along with 1 of the ICD-9-CM codes for BMI 30.0-BMI 70 (V85.30-V85.39 and V85.41-V85.45), up to 22 sessions in a 12-month period for Medicare beneficiaries. The Medicare coinsurance and Part B deductible are waived for this preventive service.

NOTE: Effective for claims with dates of service on or after January 1, 2015, codes G0473 and G0447 can be billed for a total of no more than 22 sessions in a 12-month period.

Contractors shall note the appropriate ICD-10-CM code(s) that are listed below for future implementation. Contractors shall track the ICD-10-CM codes and ensure that the updated edit is turned on when ICD-10 is implemented.

ICD-10-CM	Description
Z68.30	BMI 30.0-30.9, adult
Z68.31	BMI 31.0-31.9, adult
Z68.32	BMI 32.0-32.9, adult
Z68.33	BMI 33.0-33.9, adult

ICD-10-CM	Description
Z68.34	BMI 34.0-34.9, adult
Z68.35	BMI 35.0-35.9, adult
Z68.36	BMI 36.0-36.9, adult
Z68.37	BMI 37.0-37.9, adult
Z68.38	BMI 38.0-38.9, adult
Z68.39	BMI 39.0-39.9, adult
Z68.41	BMI 40.0-44.9, adult
Z68.42	BMI 45.0-49.9, adult
Z68.43	BMI 50.0-59.9, adult
Z68.44	BMI 60.0-69.9, adult
Z68.45	BMI 70 or greater, adult

See Pub. 100-03, Medicare National Coverage Determinations Manual, §210.12 for complete coverage guidelines.

100-4, Chapter-18, 200.2

Institutional Billing Requirements

Effective for claims with dates of service on and after November 29, 2011, providers may use the following types of bill (TOB) when submitting HCPCS code G0447: 13x, 71X, 77X, or 85X. Service line items on other TOBs shall be denied.

Effective for claims with dates of service on and after January 1, 2015, providers may use the following types of bill (TOB) when submitting HCPCS code G0473: 13x or 85X. Service line items on other TOBs shall be denied.

The service shall be paid on the basis shown below:

* Outpatient hospitals – TOB 13X - based on Outpatient Prospective Payment System (OPPS)
* Critical Access Hospitals (CAHs) - TOB 85X – based on reasonable cost
* CAH Method II – TOB 85X - based on 115% of the lesser of the Medicare Physician Fee Schedule (MPFS) amount or actual charge as applicable with revenue codes 096X, 097X, or 098X.

NOTE: For outpatient hospital settings, as in any other setting, services covered under this NCD must be provided by a primary care provider.

100-4, Chapter-18, 200.3

Professional Billing Requirements

CMS will allow coverage for Face-to-Face Behavioral Counseling for Obesity, 15 minutes, (G0447), Face-to-face behavioral counseling for obesity, group (2-10), 30 minute(s) (G0473), along with 1 of the ICD-9-CM codes for BMI 30.0-BMI 70 (V85.30-V85.39 and V85.41-V85.45), or 1 of the ICD-10-CM codes for BMI 30.0-BMI 70 (Z68.30-Z68.39 and Z68.41-Z68.45) only when services are submitted by the following provider specialties found on the provider's enrollment record:

01 - General Practice

08 - Family Practice

11 - Internal Medicine

16 - Obstetrics/Gynecology

37 - Pediatric Medicine

38 - Geriatric Medicine

50 - Nurse Practitioner

89 - Certified Clinical Nurse Specialist

97 - Physician Assistant

Any claims that are not submitted from one of the provider specialty types noted above will be denied.

CMS will allow coverage for Face-to-Face Behavioral Counseling for Obesity, 15 minutes, (G0447), Face-to-face behavioral counseling for obesity, group (2-10), 30 minute(s) (G0473), along with 1 of the ICD-9-CM codes for BMI 30.0-BMI 70 (V85.30-V85.39 and V85.41-V85.45), or with 1 of the ICD-10-CM codes for BMI 30.0-BMI 70 (Z68.30-Z68.39 and Z68.41-Z68.45) only when submitted with one of the following place of service (POS) codes:

11 - Physician's Office

22 - Outpatient Hospital

49 - Independent Clinic

71 - State or Local Public Health Clinic

Any claims that are not submitted with one of the POS codes noted above will be denied.

NOTE: HCPCS Code G0447 is effective November 29, 2011. HCPCS Code G0473 is effective January 1, 2015.

100-4, Chapter-18, 200.4

Claim Adjustment Reason Codes (CARCs), Remittance Advice Remark Codes (RARCs), Group Codes, and Medicare Summary Notice (MSN) Messages

A/B MACs (A) and (B) shall use the appropriate claim adjustment reason codes (CARCs), remittance advice remark codes (RARCs), group codes, or Medicare summary notice (MSN) messages when denying payment for obesity counseling sessions:

* Denying services submitted on a TOB other than 13X and 85X:

    CARC 171 - Payment is denied when performed by this type of provider on this type of facility. **NOTE:** Refer to the 835 Healthcare Policy Identification Segment (loop 2110 Service Payment Information REF), if present.

    RARC N428 - Not covered when performed in this place of service.

    MSN 16.2 - This service cannot be paid when provided in this location/facility.

    Group Code PR (Patient Responsibility) assigning financial responsibility to the beneficiary (if a claim is received with a GA modifier indicating a signed ABN is on file).

    Group Code CO (Contractual Obligation) assigning financial liability to the provider (if a claim is received with a GZ modifier indicating no signed ABN is on file).

    NOTE: For modifier GZ, use CARC 50 and MSN 8.81.

* Denying services for obesity counseling sessions HCPCS code G0473 or G0447 with 1 of the ICD-9-CM codes (V85.30-V85.39 or V85.41-V85.45) or with one of the ICD-10-CM codes (Z68.30-Z68.39 or Z68.41-Z68.45) when billed for a total of more than 22 sessions in the same 12-month period:

CARC 119 - Benefit maximum for this time period or occurrence has been reached.

RARC N362 - The number of days or units of service exceeds our acceptable maximum.

MSN 20.5 - These services cannot be paid because your benefits are exhausted at this time.

Spanish Version: "Estos servicios no pueden ser pagados porque sus beneficios se han agotado."

Group Code PR (Patient Responsibility) assigning financial responsibility to the beneficiary (if a claim is received with a GA modifier indicating a signed ABN is on file).

Group Code CO (Contractual Obligation) assigning financial liability to the provider (if a claim is received with a GZ modifier indicating no signed ABN is on file).

NOTE: For modifier GZ, use CARC 50 and MSN 8.81.

- Denying claim lines for obesity counseling sessions HCPCS code G0473 or G0447 without 1 of the appropriate ICD-9-CM codes (V85.30-V85.39 or V85.41-V85.45) or 1 of the ICD-10-CM codes (Z68.30-Z68.39 or Z68.41-Z68.45):

    CARC 167 - "This (these) diagnosis(es) is (are) not covered. *NOTE:* Refer to the ASC X12 835 Healthcare Policy Identification Segment (loop 2110 Service Payment Information REF), if present."

    RARC N386 - This decision was based on a National Coverage Determination (NCD). An NCD provides a coverage determination as to whether a particular item or service is covered. A copy of this policy is available at www.cms.gov/mcd/search.asp. If you do not have web access, you may contact the contractor to request a copy of the NCD.

    MSN 14.9 - "Medicare cannot pay for this service for the diagnosis shown on the claim."

    Group Code PR (Patient Responsibility) assigning financial responsibility to the beneficiary (if a claim is received with a GA modifier indicating a signed ABN is on file).

    Group Code CO (Contractual Obligation) assigning financial liability to the provider (if a claim is received with a GZ modifier indicating no signed ABN is on file).

    NOTE: For modifier GZ, use CARC 50 and MSN 8.81.

- Denying claim lines without the appropriate POS code:

    CARC 5 - The procedure code/bill type is inconsistent with the place of service. *NOTE:* Refer to the 835 Healthcare Policy Identification Segment (loop 2110 Service Payment Information REF), if present.

    RARC M77 - Missing/incomplete/invalid place of service.

    MSN 21.25 - This service was denied because Medicare only covers this service in certain settings.

    Group Code CO (Contractual Obligation) assigning financial liability to the provider (if a claim is received with a GZ modifier indicating no signed ABN is on file).

    NOTE: For modifier GZ, use CARC 50 and MSN 8.81.

- Denying claim lines that are not submitted from the appropriate provider specialties:

    CARC 8 - "The procedure code is inconsistent with the provider type/specialty (taxonomy). *NOTE:* Refer to the 835 Healthcare Policy Identification Segment (loop 2110 Service Payment Information REF), if present."

    RARC N95 - "This provider type/provider specialty may not bill this service."

    MSN 21.18 - "This item or service is not covered when performed or ordered by this provider."

    Group Code CO (Contractual Obligation) assigning financial liability to the provider (if a claim is received with a GZ modifier indicating no signed ABN is on file).

    NOTE: For modifier GZ, use CARC 50 and MSN 8.81.

100-4, Chapter-18, 200.5

Common Working File (CWF) Edits

When applying frequency, CWF shall count 22 counseling sessions of any of G0473 and/or G0447 (for a total of no more than 22 sessions in the same 12-month period) along with 1 ICD-9-CM code from V85.30-V85.39 or V85.41-V85.45 in a 12-month period, or if ICD-10 is applicable with 1 ICD-10-CM code from Z68.30-Z68.39 or Z68.41-Z68.45. When applying frequency limitations to G0473 or G0447 counseling CWF shall allow both a claim for the professional service and a claim for a facility fee. CWF shall identify the following institutional claims as facility fee claims for this service: TOB 13X, TOB 85X when the revenue code is not 096X, 097X, or 098X. CWF shall identify all other claims as professional service claims.

100-4, Chapter-20, 30.1.2

Transcutaneous Electrical Nerve Stimulator (TENS)

In order to permit an attending physician time to determine whether the purchase of a TENS is medically appropriate for a particular patient, contractors pay 10 percent of the purchase price of the item for each of 2 months. The purchase price and payment for maintenance and servicing are determined under the same rules as any other frequently purchased item, except that there is no reduction in the allowed amount for purchase due to the two months rental.

Effective June 8, 2012, CMS will allow coverage for TENS use in the treatment of chronic low back pain (CLBP) only under specific conditions which are described in the NCD Manual, Pub. 100-03, chapter 1 Section 160.27.

100-4, Chapter-20, 100.2.2

Evidence of Medical Necessity for Parenteral and Enteral Nutrition (PEN) Therapy

The PEN coverage is determined by information provided by the treating physician and the PEN supplier. A completed certification of medical necessity (CMN) must accompany and support initial claims for PEN to establish whether coverage criteria are met and to ensure that the PEN therapy provided is consistent with the attending or ordering physician's prescription. DME MACs ensure that the CMN contains pertinent information from the treating physician. Uniform specific medical data facilitate the review and promote consistency in coverage determinations and timelier claims processing.

The medical and prescription information on a PEN CMN can be most appropriately completed by the treating physician or from information in the patient's records by an employee of the physician for the physician's review and signature. Although PEN suppliers sometimes may assist in providing the PEN services, they cannot complete the CMN since they do not have the same access to patient information needed to properly enter medical or prescription information. A/B MACs (B) and DME MACs use appropriate professional relations issuances, training sessions, and meetings to ensure that all persons and PEN suppliers are aware of this limitation of their role.

When properly completed, the PEN CMN includes the elements of a prescription as well as other data needed to determine whether Medicare coverage is possible. This practice will facilitate prompt delivery of PEN services and timely submittal of the related claim.

100-4, Chapter-20, 160.1

Billing for Total Parenteral Nutrition and Enteral Nutrition Furnished to Part B Inpatients

Inpatient Part A hospital or SNF care includes total parenteral nutrition (TPN) systems and enteral nutrition (EN).

For inpatients for whom Part A benefits are not payable (e.g., benefits are exhausted or the beneficiary is entitled to Part B only), total parenteral nutrition (TPN) systems and enteral nutrition (EN) delivery systems are covered by Medicare as prosthetic devices when the coverage criteria are met. When these criteria are met, the medical equipment and medical supplies (together with nutrients) being used comprise covered prosthetic devices for coverage purposes rather than durable medical equipment. However, reimbursement rules relating to DME continue to apply to such items.

When a facility supplies TPN or EN systems that meet the criteria for coverage as a prosthetic device to an inpatient whose care is not covered under Part A, the facility must bill one of the DME MACs. Additionally, HHAs, SNFs, and hospitals that provide PEN supplies, equipment and nutrients as a prosthetic device under Part B must use the ASC X12 837 professional claim format or if permissible the Form CMS-1500 paper form to bill the appropriate DME MAC. The DME MAC is determined according to the residence of the beneficiary. Refer to §10 for jurisdiction descriptions.

A/B MACs (A and HHH) return claims containing PEN charges for Part B services where the bill type is 12x, 13x, 22x, 23x, 32x, 33x, or 34x with instructions to the provider to bill the DME MAC.

100-4, Chapter-23, 60.3

Gap-filling DMEPOS Fees

The DME MACs and Part B MACs must gap-fill the DMEPOS fee schedule for items for which charge data were unavailable during the fee schedule data base year using the fee schedule amounts for comparable equipment, using properly calculated fee schedule amounts from a neighboring DME MAC or Part B give space. before MAC area, or using supplier price lists

with prices in effect during the fee schedule data base year. Data base "year" refers to the time period mandated by the statute and/or regulations from which Medicare allowed charge data is to be extracted in order to compute the fee schedule amounts for the various DMEPOS payment categories. For example, the fee schedule base year for inexpensive or routinely purchased durable medical equipment is the 12

month period ending June 30, 1987. Supplier price lists include catalogues and other retail price lists (such as internet retail prices) that provide information on commercial pricing for the item. Potential appropriate sources for such commercial pricing information can also include verifiable information from supplier invoices and non-Medicare payer data (e.g., fee schedule amounts comprised of the median of the commercial pricing information adjusted as described below). Mail order catalogs are particularly suitable sources of price information for items such as urological and ostomy supplies which require constant replacement. DME MACs will gap-fill based on current instructions released each year for implementing and updating the new year's payment amounts.

If the only available price information is from a period other than the base period, apply the deflation factors that are included in the current year implementation instructions against current pricing in order to approximate the base year price for gap-filling purposes.

The deflation factors for gap-filling purposes are:

Year*	OX	CR	PO	SD	PE	SC	IL
1987	0.965	0.971	0.974	n/a	n/a	n/a	n/a
1988	0.928	0.934	0.936	n/a	n/a	n/a	n/a
1989	0.882	0.888	0.890	n/a	n/a	n/a	n/a
1990	0.843	0.848	0.851	n/a	n/a	n/a	n/a
1991	0.805	0.810	0.813	n/a	n/a	n/a	n/a
1992	0.781	0.786	0.788	n/a	n/a	n/a	n/a
1993	0.758	0.763	0.765	0.971	n/a	n/a	n/a
1994	0.740	0.745	0.747	0.947	n/a	n/a	n/a
1995	0.718	0.723	0.725	0.919	n/a	n/a	n/a
1996	0.699	0.703	0.705	0.895	0.973	n/a	n/a
1997	0.683	0.687	0.689	0.875	0.951	n/a	n/a
1998	0.672	0.676	0.678	0.860	0.936	n/a	n/a
1999	0.659	0.663	0.665	0.844	0.918	n/a	n/a
2000	0.635	0.639	0.641	0.813	0.885	n/a	n/a
2001	0.615	0.619	0.621	0.788	0.857	n/a	n/a
2002	0.609	0.613	0.614	0.779	0.848	n/a	n/a
2003	0.596	0.600	0.602	0.763	0.830	n/a	n/a
2004	0.577	0.581	0.582	0.739	0.804	n/a	n/a
2005	0.563	0.567	0.568	0.721	0.784	n/a	n/a
2006	0.540	0.543	0.545	0.691	0.752	n/a	n/a
2007	0.525	0.529	0.530	0.673	0.732	n/a	n/a
2008	0.500	0.504	0.505	0.641	0.697	n/a	n/a
2009	0.508	0.511	0.512	0.650	0.707	n/a	n/a
2010	0.502	0.506	0.507	0.643	0.700	n/a	n/a
2011	0.485	0.488	0.490	0.621	0.676	n/a	n/a
2012	0.477	0.480	0.482	0.611	0.665	n/a	n/a
2013	0.469	0.472	0.473	0.600	0.653	n/a	0.983
2014	0.459	0.462	0.464	0.588	0.640	0.980	0.963
2015	0.459	0.462	0.463	0.588	0.639	0.978	0.962
2016	0.454	0.457	0.458	0.582	0.633	0.969	0.952
2017	0.447	0.450	0.451	0.572	0.623	0.953	0.937
2018	0.435	0.437	0.439	0.556	0.605	0.927	0. 911

* Year price in effect

Payment Category Key:

OX	Oxygen & oxygen equipment (DME)
CR	Capped rental (DME)
IN	Inexpensive/routinely purchased (DME)
FS	Frequently serviced (DME)
SU	DME supplies
PO	Prosthetics & orthotics
SD	Surgical dressings
OS	Ostomy, tracheostomy, and urological supplies
PE	Parental and enteral nutrition
TS	Therapeutic Shoes
SC	Splints and Casts
IL	Intraocular Lenses inserted in a physician's office IN, FS, OS and SU category deflation factors=PO deflation factors

After deflation, the result must be increased by 1.7 percent and by the cumulative covered item update to complete the gap-filling (e.g., an additional .6 percent for a 2002 DME fee).

Note that when gap-filling for capped rental items, it is necessary to first gap-fill the purchase price then compute the base period fee schedule at 10 percent of the base period purchase price.

For used equipment, establish fee schedule amounts at 75 percent of the fee schedule amount for new equipment.

When gap-filling, for those DME MAC or Part B MAC areas where a sales tax was imposed in the base period, add the applicable sales tax, e.g., five percent, to the gap-filled amount where the gap-filled amount does not take into account the sales tax, e.g., where the gap-filled amount is computed from pre-tax price lists or from another DME MAC or Part B MAC area without a sales tax. Likewise, if the gap-filled amount is calculated from another DME MAC's or Part B MAC's fees where a sales tax is imposed, adjust the gap-filled amount to reflect the applicable local sales tax circumstances.

Contractors send their gap-fill information to CMS. After receiving the gap-filled base fees each year, CMS develops national fee schedule floors and ceilings and new fee schedule amounts for these codes and releases them as part of the July update file each year and during the quarterly updates.

100-4, Chapter-32, 11.1

Electrical Stimulation

A. Coding Applicable to Carriers & Fiscal Intermediaries (FIs)

Effective April 1, 2003, a National Coverage Decision was made to allow for Medicare coverage of Electrical Stimulation for the treatment of certain types of wounds. The type of wounds covered are chronic Stage III or Stage IV pressure ulcers, arterial ulcers, diabetic ulcers and venous stasis ulcers. All other uses of electrical stimulation for the treatment of wounds are not covered by Medicare. Electrical stimulation will not be covered as an initial treatment modality.

The use of electrical stimulation will only be covered after appropriate standard wound care has been tried for at least 30 days and there are no measurable signs of healing. If electrical stimulation is being used, wounds must be evaluated periodically by the treating physician but no less than every 30 days by a physician. Continued treatment with electrical stimulation is not covered if measurable signs of healing have

not been demonstrated within any 30-day period of treatment. Additionally, electrical stimulation must be discontinued when the wound demonstrates a 100% epithelialized wound bed.

Coverage policy can be found in Pub. 100-03, Medicare National Coverage Determinations

Manual, Chapter 1, Section 270.1

(http://www.cms.hhs.gov/manuals/103_cov_determ/ncd103index.asp)

The applicable Healthcare Common Procedure Coding System (HCPCS) code for Electrical Stimulation and the covered effective date is as follows:

HCPSC	Definition	Effective Date
G0281	Electrical Stimulation, (unattended), to one or more areas for chronic Stage III and Stage IV pressure ulcers, arterial ulcers, diabetic ulcers and venous stasis ulcers not demonstrating measurable signs of healing after 30 days of conventional care as part of a therapy plan of care.	04/01/2003

B. FI Billing Instructions

The applicable types of bills acceptable when billing for electrical stimulation services are 12X, 13X, 22X, 23X, 71X, 73X, 74X, 75X, and 85X. Chapter 25 of this manual provides general billing instructions that must be followed for bills submitted to FIs. FIs pay for electrical stimulation services under the Medicare Physician Fee Schedule for a hospital, Comprehensive Outpatient Rehabilitation Facility (CORF), Outpatient Rehabilitation Facility (ORF), Outpatient Physical Therapy (OPT) and Skilled Nursing Facility (SNF). Payment methodology for independent Rural Health Clinic (RHC), provider-based RHCs, free-standing Federally Qualified Health Center (FQHC)and provider based FQHCs is made under the all-inclusive rate for the visit furnished to the RHC/FQHC patient to obtain the therapy service. Only one payment will be made for the visit furnished to the RHC/FQHC patient to obtain the therapy service. As of April 1, 2005, RHCs/FQHCs are no longer required to report HCPCS codes when billing for these therapy services.

Payment Methodology for a Critical Access Hospital (CAH) is on a reasonable cost basis unless the CAH has elected the Optional Method and then the FI pays 115% of the MPFS amount for the professional component of the HCPCS code in addition to the technical component.

In addition, the following revenues code must be used in conjunction with the HCPCS code identified:

Revenue Code	Description
420	Physical Therapy
430	Occupational Therapy
520	Federal Qualified Health Center *
521	Rural Health Center *
977,978	Critical Access Hospital-method II CAH professional services only

* **NOTE:** As of April 1, 2005, RHCs/FQHCs are no longer required to report HCPCS codes when billing for these therapy services.

C. Carrier Claims

Carriers pay for Electrical Stimulation services billed with HCPCS codes G0281 based on the MPFS. Claims for

Electrical Stimulation services must be billed on Form CMS-1500 or the electronic equivalent following instructions in chapter 12 of this manual

(http://www.cms.hhs.gov/manuals/104_claims/clm104c12.pdf).

D. Coinsurance and Deductible

The Medicare contractor shall apply coinsurance and deductible to payments for these therapy services except for services billed to the FI by FQHCs. For FQHCs, only co-insurance applies.

100-4, Chapter-32, 11.2

Electromagnetic Therapy

A. HCPCS Coding Applicable to A/B MACs (A and B)

Effective July 1, 2004, a National Coverage Decision was made to allow for Medicare coverage of electromagnetic therapy for the treatment of certain types of wounds. The type of wounds covered are chronic Stage III or Stage IV pressure ulcers, arterial ulcers, diabetic ulcers and venous stasis ulcers. All other uses of electromagnetic therapy for the treatment of wounds are not covered by Medicare. Electromagnetic therapy will not be covered as an initial treatment modality.

The use of electromagnetic therapy will only be covered after appropriate standard wound care has been tried for at least 30 days and there are no measurable signs of healing. If electromagnetic therapy is being used, wounds must be evaluated periodically by the treating physician but no less than every 30 days. Continued treatment with electromagnetic therapy is not covered if measurable signs of healing have not been demonstrated within any 30-day period of treatment. Additionally, electromagnetic therapy must be discontinued when the wound demonstrates a 100% epithelialized wound bed.

Coverage policy can be found in Pub. 100-03, Medicare National Coverage Determinations Manual, Chapter 1 section 270.1.

(http://www.cms.hhs.gov/manuals/103_cov_determ/ncd103index.asp)

The applicable Healthcare Common Procedure Coding System (HCPCS) code for Electrical Stimulation and the covered effective date is as follows:

HCPCS	Definition	Effective Date
G0329	Electromagnetic Therapy, to one or more areas for chronic Stage III and Stage IV pressure ulcers, arterial ulcers, diabetic ulcers and venous stasis ulcers not demonstrating measurable signs of healing after 30 days of conventional care as part of a therapy plan of care.	07/01/2004

Medicare will not cover the device used for the electromagnetic therapy for the treatment of wounds. However, Medicare will cover the service. Unsupervised home use of electromagnetic therapy will not be covered.

B. A/B MAC (A) Billing Instructions

The applicable types of bills acceptable when billing for electromagnetic therapy services are 2X, 13X, 22X, 23X, 71X, 73X, 74X, 75X, and 85X. Chapter 25 of this manual provides general billing instructions that must be followed for bills submitted to A/B MACs (A). A/B MACs (A) pay for electromagnetic therapy services under the Medicare Physician Fee Schedule for a hospital, CORF, ORF, and SNF.

Payment methodology for independent (RHC), provider-based RHCs, free-standing FQHC and provider based FQHCs is made under the all-inclusive rate for the visit furnished to the RHC/FQHC patient to obtain the therapy service. Only one payment will be made for the visit furnished to the RHC/FQHC patient to obtain the therapy service. As of April 1, 2005, RHCs/FQHCs are no longer required to report HCPCS codes when billing for the therapy service.

Payment Methodology for a CAH is payment on a reasonable cost basis unless the CAH has elected the Optional Method and then the A/B MAC (A) pays pay 115% of the MPFS amount for the professional component of the HCPCS code in addition to the technical component.

In addition, the following revenues code must be used in conjunction with the HCPCS code identified:

Revenue Code	Description
420	Physical Therapy
430	Occupational Therapy
520	Federal Qualified Health Center *
521	Rural Health Center *
977,978	Critical Access Hospital-method II CAH professional services only

* NOTE: As of April 1, 2005, RHCs/FQHCs are no longer required to report HCPCS codes when billing for the therapy service.

C. A/B MAC (B) Claims

A/B MACs (B) pay for Electromagnetic Therapy services billed with HCPCS codes G0329 based on the MPFS. Claims for electromagnetic therapy services must be billed using the ASC X12 837 professional claim format or Form CMS-1500 following instructions in chapter 12 of this manual (www.cms.hhs.gov/manuals/104_claims/clm104index.asp).

Payment information for HCPCS code G0329 will be added to the July 2004 update of the Medicare Physician Fee Schedule Database (MPFSD).

D. Coinsurance and Deductible

The Medicare contractor shall apply coinsurance and deductible to payments for electromagnetic therapy services except for services billed to the A/B MAC (A) by FQHCs.

For FQHCs only co-insurance applies.

100-4, Chapter-32, 11.3.1

Policy

Effective for claims with dates of service on or after August 2, 2012, contractors shall accept and pay for autologous platelet-rich plasma (PRP) only for the treatment of chronic non-healing diabetic, venous and/or pressure wounds only in the context of an approved clinical study in accordance with the coverage criteria outlined in Pub. 100-03, chapter 1, section 270.3, of the NCD Manual.

100-4, Chapter-32, 11.3.2

Healthcare Common Procedure Coding System (HCPCS) Codes and Diagnosis Coding

HCPCS Code

Effective for claims with dates of service on or after August 2, 2012 Medicare providers shall report HCPCS code G0460 for PRP services.

If ICD-9 Diagnosis coding is applicable

For claims with dates of service on or after August 2, 2012, PRP, for the treatment of chronic non-healing diabetic, venous and/or pressure wounds only in the context of an approved clinical study must be billed using the following ICD codes:

- V70.7
- ICD-9 code from the approved list of diagnosis codes maintained by the Medicare contractor.

If ICD-10 Diagnosis coding is applicable

For claims with dates of service on or after the implementation of ICD-10, ICD-10 CM diagnosis coding is applicable.

- Z00.6
- ICD-10 code from the approved list of diagnosis codes maintained by the Medicare contractor.

Additional billing requirement:

The following modifier and condition code shall be reported when billing for PRP services only in the context of an approved clinical study:

- Q0 modifier
- Condition code 30 (for institutional claims only)
- Value Code D4 with an 8-digit clinical trial number. **NOTE:** This is optional and only applies to Institutional claims.

100-4, Chapter-32, 11.3.3

Types of Bill (TOB)

The applicable TOBs for PRP services are: 12X, 13X, 22X, 23X, 71X, 75X, 77X, and 85X.

100-4, Chapter-32, 11.3.4

Payment Method

Payment for PRP services is as follows:

- Hospital outpatient departments TOBs 12X and 13X – based on OPPS
- SNFs TOBs 22X and 23X –based on MPFS
- TOB 71X –based on all-inclusive rate
- TOB 75X –based on MPFS
- TOB 77X –based on all-inclusive rate
- TOB 85X –based on reasonable cost
- CAHs TOB 85X and revenue codes 096X, 097X, or 098X –based on MPFS

Contractors shall pay for PRP services for hospitals in Maryland under the jurisdiction of the Health Services Cost Review Commission (HSCRC) on an outpatient basis, TOB 13X, in accordance with the terms of the Maryland waiver.

100-4, Chapter-32, 11.3.5

Place of Service (POS) for Professional Claims

Effective for claims with dates of service on or after August 2, 2012, place of service codes 11, 22, and 49 shall be used for PRP services.

100-4, Chapter-32, 11.3.6

Medicare Summary Notices (MSNs), Remittance Advice Remark Codes (RARCs), Claim Adjustment Reason Codes (CARCs) and Group Codes

Contractors shall use the following messages when returning to provider/returning as unprocessable claims when required information is not included on claims for autologous platelet-rich plasma (PRP) for the treatment of chronic non-healing diabetic, venous and/or pressure wounds only in the context of an approved clinical study:

CARC 16 -Claim/service lacks information or has submission/billing error(s) which is (are) needed for adjudication. At least one Remark Code must be provided (may be comprised of either the NCPDP Reject Reason Code, or Remittance Advice Remark Code that is not an ALERT.)

NOTE: Refer to the 835 Healthcare Policy Identification Segment (loop 2110 Service Payment Information REF), if present.

RARC MA130 – Your claim contains incomplete and/or invalid information, and no appeal rights are afforded because the claim is unprocessable. Please submit a new claim with the complete/correct information.

Contractors shall deny claims for RPR services, HCPCS code G0460, when services are provided on other than TOBs 12X, 13X, 22X, 23X, 71X, 75X, 77X, and 85X using:

MSN 21.25: "This service was denied because Medicare only covers this service in certain settings."

Spanish Version: "El servicio fue denegado porque Medicare solamente lo cubre en ciertas situaciones."

CARC 58: "Treatment was deemed by the payer to have been rendered in an inappropriate or invalid place of service.

NOTE: Refer to the 832 Healthcare Policy Identification Segment (loop 2110 Service payment Information REF), if present.

RARC N428: "Service/procedure not covered when performed in this place of service."

Group Code –CO (Contractual Obligation)

Contractors shall deny claims for PRP services for POS other than 11, 22, or 49 using the following:

MSN 21.25: "This service was denied because Medicare only covers this service in certain settings."

Spanish Version: "El servicio fue denegado porque Medicare solamente lo cubre en ciertas situaciones."

CARC 58: "Treatment was deemed by the payer to have been rendered in an inappropriate or invalid place of service. NOTE; Refer to the 835 Healthcare Policy Identification Segment (loop 2110 Service payment Information REF), if present.

RARC N428: "Service/procedure not covered when performed in this place of service."

Group Code –CO (Contractual Obligation)

100-4, Chapter-32, 30.1

Billing Requirements for HBO Therapy for the Treatment of Diabetic Wounds of the Lower Extremities

Hyperbaric Oxygen Therapy is a modality in which the entire body is exposed to oxygen under increased atmospheric pressure.

Effective April 1, 2003, a National Coverage Decision expanded the use of HBO therapy to include coverage for the treatment of diabetic wounds of the lower extremities. For specific coverage criteria for HBO Therapy, refer to the National Coverage Determinations Manual, Chapter 1, section 20.29.

NOTE: Topical application of oxygen does not meet the definition of HBO therapy as stated above. Also, its clinical efficacy has not been established. Therefore, no Medicare reimbursement may be made for the topical application of oxygen.

I. Billing Requirements for A/B MACs (A)

Claims for HBO therapy should be submitted using the ASC X12 837 institutional claim format or, in rare cases, on Form CMS-1450.

a. Applicable Bill Types

The applicable hospital bill types are 11X, 13X and 85X.

b. Procedural Coding

- 99183 – Physician attendance and supervision of hyperbaric oxygen therapy, per session.
- C1300 – Hyperbaric oxygen under pressure, full body chamber, per 30-minute interval.

NOTE: Code C1300 is not available for use other than in a hospital outpatient department.

In skilled nursing facilities (SNFs), HBO therapy is part of the SNF PPS payment for beneficiaries in covered Part A stays.

For hospital inpatients and critical access hospitals (CAHs) not electing Method I, HBO therapy is reported under revenue code 940 without any HCPCS code. For inpatient services, if ICD-9-is applicable, show ICD-9-CM procedure code 93.59. If ICD-10 is applicable, show ICD-10-PCS code 5A05121.

For CAHs electing Method I, HBO therapy is reported under revenue code 940 along with HCPCS code 99183.

c. Payment Requirements for A/B MACs (A)

Payment is as follows:

A/B MAC (A) payment is allowed for HBO therapy for diabetic wounds of the lower extremities when performed as a physician service in a hospital outpatient setting and for inpatients. Payment is allowed for claims with valid diagnosis codes as shown above with dates of service on or after April 1, 2003. Those claims with invalid codes should be denied as not medically necessary.

For hospitals, payment will be based upon the Ambulatory Payment Classification (APC) or the inpatient Diagnosis Related Group (DRG). Deductible and coinsurance apply.

Payment to Critical Access Hospitals (electing Method I) is made under cost reimbursement. For Critical Access Hospitals electing Method II, the technical component is paid under cost reimbursement and the professional component is paid under the Physician Fee Schedule.

II. A/B MAC (B) Billing Requirements

Claims for this service should be submitted using the ASC X12 837 professional claim format or

Form CMS-1500.

The following HCPCS code applies:

- 99183 –Physician attendance and supervision of hyperbaric oxygen therapy, per session.

a. Payment Requirements for A/B MACs (B)

Payment and pricing information will occur through updates to the Medicare Physician Fee

Schedule Database (MPFSDB). Pay for this service on the basis of the MPFSDB.

Deductible and coinsurance apply. Claims from physicians or other practitioners where assignment was not taken, are subject to the Medicare limiting charge.

III. Medicare Summary Notices (MSNs)

Use the following MSN Messages where appropriate:

In situations where the claim is being denied on the basis that the condition does not meet our coverage requirements, use one of the following MSN Messages:

"Medicare does not pay for this item or service for this condition." (MSN Message 16.48)

The Spanish version of the MSN message should read:

"Medicare no paga por este articulo o servicio para esta afeccion."

In situations where, based on the above utilization policy, medical review of the claim results in a determination that the service is not medically necessary, use the following MSN message:

"The information provided does not support the need for this service or item." (MSN Message 15.4)

The Spanish version of the MSN message should read:

"La informacion proporcionada no confirma la necesidad para este servicio o articulo."

IV. Remittance Advice Notices

Use appropriate existing remittance advice remark codes and claim adjustment reason codes at the line level to express the specific reason if you deny payment for HBO therapy for the treatment of diabetic wounds of lower extremities.

100-4, Chapter-32, 40.1

Coverage Requirements

Effective January 1, 2002, sacral nerve stimulation is covered for the treatment of urinary urge incontinence, urgency-frequency syndrome and urinary retention. Sacral nerve stimulation involves both a temporary test stimulation to determine if an implantable stimulator would be effective and a permanent implantation in appropriate candidates. Both the test and the permanent implantation are covered.

The following limitations for coverage apply to all indications:

- Patient must be refractory to conventional therapy (documented behavioral, pharmacologic and/or surgical corrective therapy) and be an appropriate surgical candidate such that implantation with anesthesia can occur.
- Patients with stress incontinence, urinary obstruction, and specific neurologic diseases (e.g., diabetes with peripheral nerve involvement) that are associated with secondary manifestations of the above three indications are excluded.
- Patient must have had a successful test stimulation in order to support subsequent implantation. Before a patient is eligible for permanent implantation, he/she must demonstrate a 50% or greater improvement through test stimulation. Improvement is measured through voiding diaries.

- Patient must be able to demonstrate adequate ability to record voiding diary data such that clinical results of the implant procedure can be properly evaluated.

100-4, Chapter-32, 50

Deep Brain Stimulation for Essential Tremor and Parkinson's Disease

Deep brain stimulation (DBS) refers to high-frequency electrical stimulation of anatomic regions deep within the brain utilizing neurosurgically implanted electrodes. These DBS electrodes are stereotactically placed within targeted nuclei on one (unilateral) or both (bilateral) sides of the brain. There are currently three targets for DBS —the thalamic ventralis intermedius nucleus (VIM), subthalamic nucleus (STN) and globus pallidus interna (GPi).

Essential tremor (ET) is a progressive, disabling tremor most often affecting the hands. ET may also affect the head, voice and legs. The precise pathogenesis of ET is unknown. While it may start at any age, ET usually peaks within the second and sixth decades. Beta-adrenergic blockers and anticonvulsant medications are usually the first line treatments for reducing the severity of tremor. Many patients, however, do not adequately respond or cannot tolerate these medications. In these medically refractory ET patients, thalamic VIM DBS may be helpful for symptomatic relief of tremor.

Parkinson's disease (PD) is an age-related progressive neurodegenerative disorder involving the loss of dopaminergic cells in the substantia nigra of the midbrain. The disease is characterized by tremor, rigidity, bradykinesia and progressive postural instability. Dopaminergic medication is typically used as a first line treatment for reducing the primary symptoms of PD. However, after prolonged use, medication can become less effective and can produce significant adverse events such as dyskinesias and other motor function complications. For patients who become unresponsive to medical treatments and/or have intolerable side effects from medications, DBS for symptom relief may be considered.

100-4, Chapter-32, 60.4.1

Allowable Covered Diagnosis Codes

For services furnished on or after July 1, 2002, the applicable ICD-9-CM diagnosis code for this benefit is V43.3, organ or tissue replaced by other means; heart valve.

For services furnished on or after March 19, 2008, the applicable ICD-9-CM diagnosis codes for this benefit are:

- V43.3 (organ or tissue replaced by other means; heart valve),
- 289.81 (primary hypercoagulable state),
- 451.0-451.9 (includes 451.11, 451.19, 451.2, 451.80-451.84, 451.89) (phlebitis & thrombophlebitis),
- 453.0-453.3 (other venous embolism & thrombosis),
- 453.40-453.49 (includes 453.40-453.42, 453.6,453.8-453.9) (venous embolism and thrombosis of the deep vessels of the lower extremity, and other specified veins/unspecified sites),
- 415.11-415.12, 415.19 (pulmonary embolism & infarction),or,
- 427.31 (atrial fibrillation (established) (paroxysmal)).

For services furnished on or after the implementation of ICD-10 the applicable ICD-10-CM diagnosis codes for this benefit are:

Heart Valve Replacement

- Z95.2 - Presence of prosthetic heart valve

Primary Hypercoagulable State

ICD-10-CM Code	Code Description
D68.51	Activated protein C resistance
D68.52	Prothrombin gene mutation
D68.59	Other primary thrombophilia
D68.61	Antiphospholipid syndrome
D68.62	Lupus anticoagulant syndrome

Phlebitis & Thrombophlebitis

ICD-10-CM Code	Code Description
I80.00	Phlebitis and thrombophlebitis of superficial vessels of unspecified lower extremity
I80.01	Phlebitis and thrombophlebitis of superficial vessels of right lower extremity
I80.02	Phlebitis and thrombophlebitis of superficial vessels of left lower extremity
I80.03	Phlebitis and thrombophlebitis of superficial vessels of lower extremities, bilateral
I80.10	Phlebitis and thrombophlebitis of unspecified femoral vein
I80.11	Phlebitis and thrombophlebitis of right femoral vein
I80.12	Phlebitis and thrombophlebitis of left femoral vein
I80.13	Phlebitis and thrombophlebitis of femoral vein, bilateral
I80.201	Phlebitis and thrombophlebitis of unspecified deep vessels of right lower extremity
I80.202	Phlebitis and thrombophlebitis of unspecified deep vessels of left lower extremity
I80.203	Phlebitis and thrombophlebitis of unspecified deep vessels of lower extremities, bilateral
I80.209	Phlebitis and thrombophlebitis of unspecified deep vessels of unspecified lower extremity
I80.221	Phlebitis and thrombophlebitis of right popliteal vein
I80.222	Phlebitis and thrombophlebitis of left popliteal vein
I80.223	Phlebitis and thrombophlebitis of popliteal vein, bilateral
I80.229	Phlebitis and thrombophlebitis of unspecified popliteal vein
I80.231	Phlebitis and thrombophlebitis of right tibial vein
I80.232	Phlebitis and thrombophlebitis of left tibial vein
I80.233	Phlebitis and thrombophlebitis of tibial vein, bilateral
I80.239	Phlebitis and thrombophlebitis of unspecified tibial vein
I80.291	Phlebitis and thrombophlebitis of other deep vessels of right lower extremity
I80.292	Phlebitis and thrombophlebitis of other deep vessels of left lower extremity
I80.293	Phlebitis and thrombophlebitis of other deep vessels of lower extremity, bilateral
I80.299	Phlebitis and thrombophlebitis of other deep vessels of unspecified lower extremity
I80.3	Phlebitis and thrombophlebitis of lower extremities, unspecified
I80.211	Phlebitis and thrombophlebitis of right iliac vein
I80.212	Phlebitis and thrombophlebitis of left iliac vein
I80.213	Phlebitis and thrombophlebitis of iliac vein, bilateral
I80.219	Phlebitis and thrombophlebitis of unspecified iliac vein
I80.8	Phlebitis and thrombophlebitis of other sites
I80.9	Phlebitis and thrombophlebitis of unspecified site

Other Venous Embolism & Thrombosis

ICD-10-CM Code	Code Description
I82.0	Budd- Chiari syndrome
I82.1	Thrombophlebitis migrans
I82.211	Chronic embolism and thrombosis of superior vena cava
I82.220	Acute embolism and thrombosis of inferior vena cava
I82.221	Chronic embolism and thrombosis of inferior vena cava
I82.291	Chronic embolism and thrombosis of other thoracic veins
I82.3	Embolism and thrombosis of renal vein

Venous Embolism and thrombosis of the deep vessels of the lower extremity, and other specified veins/unspecified sites

ICD-10-CM Code	Code Description
I82.401	Acute embolism and thrombosis of unspecified deep veins of right lower extremity
I82.402	Acute embolism and thrombosis of unspecified deep veins of left lower extremity
I82.403	Acute embolism and thrombosis of unspecified deep veins of lower extremity, bilateral
I82.409	Acute embolism and thrombosis of unspecified deep veins of unspecified lower extremity
I82.411	Acute embolism and thrombosis of right femoral vein
I82.412	Acute embolism and thrombosis of left femoral vein
I82.413	Acute embolism and thrombosis of femoral vein, bilateral
I82.419	Acute embolism and thrombosis of unspecified femoral vein
I82.421	Acute embolism and thrombosis of right iliac vein
I82.422	Acute embolism and thrombosis of left iliac vein
I82.423	Acute embolism and thrombosis of iliac vein, bilateral
I82.429	Acute embolism and thrombosis of unspecified iliac vein
I82.431	Acute embolism and thrombosis of right popliteal vein
I82.432	Acute embolism and thrombosis of left popliteal vein
I82.433	Acute embolism and thrombosis of popliteal vein, bilateral
I82.439	Acute embolism and thrombosis of unspecified popliteal vein
I82.4Y1	Acute embolism and thrombosis of unspecified deep veins of right proximal lower extremity
I82.4Y2	Acute embolism and thrombosis of unspecified deep veins of left proximal lower extremity
I82.4Y3	Acute embolism and thrombosis of unspecified deep veins of proximal lower extremity, bilateral
I82.4Y9	Acute embolism and thrombosis of unspecified deep veins of unspecified proximal lower extremity
I82.441	Acute embolism and thrombosis of right tibial vein
I82.442	Acute embolism and thrombosis of left tibial vein
I82.443	Acute embolism and thrombosis of tibial vein, bilateral
I82.449	Acute embolism and thrombosis of unspecified tibial vein
I82.491	Acute embolism and thrombosis of other specified deep vein of right lower extremity
I82.492	Acute embolism and thrombosis of other specified deep vein of left lower extremity
I82.493	Acute embolism and thrombosis of other specified deep vein of lower extremity, bilateral

ICD-10-CM Code	Code Description
I82.499	Acute embolism and thrombosis of other specified deep vein of unspecified lower extremity
I82.4Z1	Acute embolism and thrombosis of unspecified deep veins of right distal lower extremity
I82.4Z2	Acute embolism and thrombosis of unspecified deep veins of left distal lower extremity
I82.4Z3	Acute embolism and thrombosis of unspecified deep veins of distal lower extremity, bilateral
I82.4Z9	Acute embolism and thrombosis of unspecified deep veins of unspecified distal lower extremity
I82.501	Chronic embolism and thrombosis of unspecified deep veins of right lower extremity
I82.502	Chronic embolism and thrombosis of unspecified deep veins of left lower extremity
I82.503	Chronic embolism and thrombosis of unspecified deep veins of lower extremity, bilateral
I82.509	Chronic embolism and thrombosis of unspecified deep veins of unspecified lower extremity
I82.591	Chronic embolism and thrombosis of other specified deep vein of right lower extremity
I82.592	Chronic embolism and thrombosis of other specified deep vein of left lower extremity
I82.593	Chronic embolism and thrombosis of other specified deep vein of lower extremity, bilateral
I82.599	Chronic embolism and thrombosis of other specified deep vein of unspecified lower extremity
I82.511	Chronic embolism and thrombosis of right femoral vein
I82.512	Chronic embolism and thrombosis of left femoral vein
I82.513	Chronic embolism and thrombosis of femoral vein, bilateral
I82.519	Chronic embolism and thrombosis of unspecified femoral vein
I82.521	Chronic embolism and thrombosis of right iliac vein
I82.522	Chronic embolism and thrombosis of left iliac vein
I82.523	Chronic embolism and thrombosis of iliac vein, bilateral
I82.529	Chronic embolism and thrombosis of unspecified iliac vein
I82.531	Chronic embolism and thrombosis of right popliteal vein
I82.532	Chronic embolism and thrombosis of left popliteal vein
I82.533	Chronic embolism and thrombosis of popliteal vein, bilateral
I82.539	Chronic embolism and thrombosis of unspecified popliteal vein
I82.5Y1	Chronic embolism and thrombosis of unspecified deep veins of right proximal lower extremity
I82.5Y2	Chronic embolism and thrombosis of unspecified deep veins of left proximal lower extremity
I82.5Y3	Chronic embolism and thrombosis of unspecified deep veins of proximal lower extremity, bilateral
I82.5Y9	Chronic embolism and thrombosis of unspecified deep veins of unspecified proximal lower extremity
I82.541	Chronic embolism and thrombosis of right tibial vein
I82.542	Chronic embolism and thrombosis of left tibial vein
I82.543	Chronic embolism and thrombosis of tibial vein, bilateral
I82.549	Chronic embolism and thrombosis of unspecified tibial vein

ICD-10-CM Code	Code Description
I82.5Z1	Chronic embolism and thrombosis of unspecified deep veins of right distal lower extremity
I82.5Z2	Chronic embolism and thrombosis of unspecified deep veins of left distal lower extremity
I82.5Z3	Chronic embolism and thrombosis of unspecified deep veins of distal lower extremity, bilateral
I82.5Z9	Chronic embolism and thrombosis of unspecified deep veins of unspecified distal lower extremity
I82.611	Acute embolism and thrombosis of superficial veins of right upper extremity
I82.612	Acute embolism and thrombosis of superficial veins of left upper extremity
I82.613	Acute embolism and thrombosis of superficial veins of upper extremity, bilateral
I82.619	Acute embolism and thrombosis of superficial veins of unspecified upper extremity
I82.621	Acute embolism and thrombosis of deep veins of right upper extremity
I82.622	Acute embolism and thrombosis of deep veins of left upper extremity
I82.623	Acute embolism and thrombosis of deep veins of upper extremity, bilateral
I82.629	Acute embolism and thrombosis of deep veins of unspecified upper extremity
I82.601	Acute embolism and thrombosis of unspecified veins of right upper extremity
I82.602	Acute embolism and thrombosis of unspecified veins of left upper extremity
I82.603	Acute embolism and thrombosis of unspecified veins of upper extremity, bilateral
I82.609	Acute embolism and thrombosis of unspecified veins of unspecified upper extremity
I82.A11	Acute embolism and thrombosis of right axillary vein
I82.A12	Acute embolism and thrombosis of left axillary vein
I82.A13	Acute embolism and thrombosis of axillary vein, bilateral
I82.A19	Acute embolism and thrombosis of unspecified axillary vein
I82.A21	Chronic embolism and thrombosis of right axillary vein
I82.A22	Chronic embolism and thrombosis of left axillary vein
I82.A23	Chronic embolism and thrombosis of axillary vein, bilateral
I82.A29	Chronic embolism and thrombosis of unspecified axillary vein
I82.B11	Acute embolism and thrombosis of right subclavian vein
I82.B12	Acute embolism and thrombosis of left subclavian vein
I82.B13	Acute embolism and thrombosis of subclavian vein, bilateral
I82.B19	Acute embolism and thrombosis of unspecified subclavian vein
I82.B21	Chronic embolism and thrombosis of right subclavian vein
I82.B22	Chronic embolism and thrombosis of left subclavian vein
I82.B23	Chronic embolism and thrombosis of subclavian vein, bilateral
I82.B29	Chronic embolism and thrombosis of unspecified subclavian vein

ICD-10-CM Code	Code Description
I82.C11	Acute embolism and thrombosis of right internal jugular vein
I82.C12	Acute embolism and thrombosis of left internal jugular vein
I82.C13	Acute embolism and thrombosis of internal jugular vein, bilateral
I82.C19	Acute embolism and thrombosis of unspecified internal jugular vein
I82.C21	Chronic embolism and thrombosis of right internal jugular vein
I82.C22	Chronic embolism and thrombosis of left internal jugular vein
I82.C23	Chronic embolism and thrombosis of internal jugular vein, bilateral
I82.C29	Chronic embolism and thrombosis of unspecified internal jugular vein
I82.210	Acute embolism and thrombosis of superior vena cava
I82.290	Acute embolism and thrombosis of other thoracic veins
I82.701	Chronic embolism and thrombosis of unspecified veins of right upper extremity
I82.702	Chronic embolism and thrombosis of unspecified veins of left upper extremity
I82.703	Chronic embolism and thrombosis of unspecified veins of upper extremity, bilateral
I82.709	Chronic embolism and thrombosis of unspecified veins of unspecified upper extremity
I82.711	Chronic embolism and thrombosis of superficial veins of right upper extremity
I82.712	Chronic embolism and thrombosis of superficial veins of left upper extremity
I82.713	Chronic embolism and thrombosis of superficial veins of upper extremity, bilateral
I82.719	Chronic embolism and thrombosis of superficial veins of unspecified upper extremity
I82.721	Chronic embolism and thrombosis of deep veins of right upper extremity
I82.722	Chronic embolism and thrombosis of deep veins of left upper extremity
I82.723	Chronic embolism and thrombosis of deep veins of upper extremity, bilateral
I82.729	Chronic embolism and thrombosis of deep veins of unspecified upper extremity
I82.811	Embolism and thrombosis of superficial veins of right lower extremities
I82.812	Embolism and thrombosis of superficial veins of left lower extremities
I82.813	Embolism and thrombosis of superficial veins of lower extremities, bilateral
I82.819	Embolism and thrombosis of superficial veins of unspecified lower extremities
I82.890	Acute embolism and thrombosis of other specified veins
I82.891	Chronic embolism and thrombosis of other specified veins
I82.90	Acute embolism and thrombosis of unspecified vein
I82.91	Chronic embolism and thrombosis of unspecified vein

Pulmonary Embolism & Infarction

ICD-10- CM Code	Code Description
I26.90	Septic pulmonary embolism without acute cor pulmonale
I26.99	Other pulmonary embolism without acute cor pulmonale
I26.01	Septic pulmonary embolism with acute cor pulmonale
I26.90	Septic pulmonary embolism without acute cor pulmonale
I26.09	Other pulmonary embolism with acute cor pulmonale
I26.99	Other pulmonary embolism without acute cor pulmonale

Atrial Fibrillation

ICD-10-CM Code	Code Description
I48.0	Paroxysmal atrial fibrillation
I48.2	Chronic atrial fibrillation
I48	-91 Unspecified atrial fibrillation Other
I23.6	Thrombosis of atrium, auricular appendage, and ventricle as current complications following acute myocardial infarction
I27.82	Chronic pulmonary embolism
I67.6	Nonpyogenic thrombosis of intracranial venous system
O22.50	Cerebral venous thrombosis in pregnancy, unspecified trimester
O22.51	Cerebral venous thrombosis in pregnancy, first trimester
O22.52	Cerebral venous thrombosis in pregnancy, second trimester
O22.53	Cerebral venous thrombosis in pregnancy, third trimester
O87.3	Cerebral venous thrombosis in the puerperium
Z79.01	Long term (current) use of anticoagulants

100-4, Chapter-32, 80

Billing of the Diagnosis and Treatment of Peripheral Neuropathy with Loss of Protective Sensation in People with Diabetes

Coverage Requirements -Peripheral neuropathy is the most common factor leading to amputation in people with diabetes. In diabetes, peripheral neuropathy is an anatomically diffuse process primarily affecting sensory and autonomic fibers; however, distal motor findings may be present in advanced cases. Long nerves are affected first, with symptoms typically beginning insidiously in the toes and then advancing proximally. This leads to loss of protective sensation (LOPS), whereby a person is unable to feel minor trauma from mechanical, thermal, or chemical sources. When foot lesions are present, the reduction in autonomic nerve functions may also inhibit wound healing.

Peripheral neuropathy with LOPS, secondary to diabetes, is a localized illness of the feet and falls within the regulation's exception to the general exclusionary rule (see 42 C.F.R. §411.15(l)(l)(i)). Foot exams for people with diabetic peripheral neuropathy with LOPS are reasonable and necessary to allow for early intervention in serious complications that typically afflict diabetics with the disease.

Effective for services furnished on or after July 1, 2002, Medicare covers, as a physician service, an evaluation (examination and treatment) of the feet no more often than every 6 months for individuals with a documented diagnosis of diabetic sensory neuropathy and LOPS, as long as the beneficiary has not seen a foot care specialist for some other reason in the interim. LOPS shall be diagnosed through

sensory testing with the 5.07 monofilament using established guidelines, such as those developed by the National Institute of Diabetes and Digestive and Kidney Diseases guidelines. Five sites should be tested on the plantar surface of each foot, according to the National Institute of Diabetes and Digestive and Kidney Diseases guidelines. The areas must be tested randomly since the loss of protective sensation may be patchy in distribution, and the patient may get clues if the test is done rhythmically. Heavily callused areas should be avoided. As suggested by the American Podiatric Medicine Association, an absence of sensation at two or more sites out of 5 tested on either foot when tested with the 5.07 Semmes-Weinstein monofilament must be present and documented to diagnose peripheral neuropathy with loss of protective sensation.

100-4, Chapter-32, 80.2

Applicable HCPCS Codes

G0245 - Initial physician evaluation and management of a diabetic patient with diabetic sensory neuropathy resulting in a loss of protective sensation (LOPS) which must include:

1. The diagnosis of LOPS;
2. A patient history;
3. A physical examination that consists of at least the following elements:
    a. visual inspection of the forefoot, hindfoot, and toe web spaces,
    b. evaluation of a protective sensation,
    c. evaluation of foot structure and biomechanics,
    d. evaluation of vascular status and skin integrity,
    e. evaluation and recommendation of footwear, and
4.   Patient education.

G0246 -Follow-up physician evaluation and management of a diabetic patient with diabetic sensory neuropathy resulting in a loss of protective sensation (LOPS) to include at least the following:

1. a patient history;
2. a physical examination that includes:
    a. (a) visual inspection of the forefoot, hindfoot, and toe web spaces,
    b. evaluation of protective sensation,
    c. evaluation of foot structure and biomechanics,
    d. evaluation of vascular status and skin integrity,
    e. evaluation and recommendation of footwear, and 3.patient education.

G0247 -Routine foot care by a physician of a diabetic patient with diabetic sensory neuropathy resulting in a LOPS to include if present, at least the following:

1. local care of superficial (i.e., superficial to muscle and fascia) wounds;
2. debridement of corns and calluses; and
3. trimming and debridement of nails.

NOTE: Code G0247 must be billed on the same date of service with either G0245 or G0246 in order to be considered for payment.

The short descriptors for the above HCPCS codes are as follows:

G0245 – INITIAL FOOT EXAM PTLOPS

G0246 – FOLLOW-UP EVAL OF FOOT PT LOP

G0247 – ROUTINE FOOTCARE PT W LOPS

100-4, Chapter-32, 80.8

CWF Utilization Edits

Edit 1- Should CWF receive a claim from an FI for G0245 or G0246 and a second claim from a contractor for either G0245 or G0246 (or vice versa) and they are different dates of service and less than 6 months apart, the second claim will reject. CWF will edit to allow G0245 or G0246 to be paid no more than every 6 months for a particular beneficiary, regardless of who furnished the service. If G0245 has been paid, regardless of whether it was posted as a facility or professional claim, it must be 6 months before G0245 can be paid again or G0246 can be paid. If G0246 has been paid, regardless of whether it was posted as a facility or professional claim, it must be 6 months before G0246 can be paid again or G0245 can be paid. CWF will not impose limits on how many times each code can be paid for a beneficiary as long as there has been 6 months between each service.

The CWF will return a specific reject code for this edit to the contractors and FIs that will be identified in the CWF documentation. Based on the CWF reject code, the contractors and FIs must deny the claims and return the following messages:

MSN 18.4 — This service is being denied because it has not been ___ months since your last examination of this kind (**NOTE:** Insert 6 as the appropriate number of months.)

RA claim adjustment reason code 96 – Non-covered charges, along with remark code M86 – Service denied because payment already made for same/similar procedure within set time frame.

Edit 2

The CWF will edit to allow G0247 to pay only if either G0245 or G0246 has been submitted <u>and accepted as payable</u> on the same date of service. CWF will return a specific reject code for this edit to the contractors and FIs that will be identified in the CWF documentation. Based on this reject code, contractors and FIs will deny the claims and return the following messages:

MSN 21.21 - This service was denied because Medicare only covers this service under certain circumstances.

RA claim adjustment reason code 107 – The related or qualifying claim/service was not identified on this claim.

Edit 3

Once a beneficiary's condition has progressed to the point where routine foot care becomes a covered service, payment will no longer be made for LOPS evaluation and management services. Those services would be considered to be included in the regular exams and treatments afforded to the beneficiary on a routine basis. The physician or provider must then just bill the routine foot care codes, per Pub 100-02, Chapter 15, §290.

The CWF will edit to reject LOPS codes G0245, G0246, and/or G0247 when on the beneficiary's record it shows that one of the following routine foot care codes were billed and paid within the prior 6 months: 11055, 11056, 11057, 11719, 11720, and/or 11721.

The CWF will return a specific reject code for this edit to the contractors and FIs that will be identified in the CWF documentation. Based on the CWF reject code, the contractors and FIs must deny the claims and return the following messages:

MSN 21.21 - This service was denied because Medicare only covers this service under certain circumstances.

The RA claim adjustment reason code 96 –Non-covered charges, along with remark code M86 –Service denied because payment already made for same/similar procedure within set time frame.

100-4, Chapter-32, 100

Billing Requirements for Expanded Coverage of Cochlear Implantation

Effective for dates of services on and after April 4, 2005, the Centers for Medicare & Medicaid Services (CMS) has expanded the coverage for cochlear implantation to cover moderate-to-profound hearing loss in individuals with hearing test scores equal to or less than 40% correct in the best aided listening condition on tape-recorded tests of open-set sentence recognition and who demonstrate limited benefit from amplification. (See Publication 100-03, chapter 1, section 50.3, for specific coverage criteria).

In addition CMS is covering cochlear implantation for individuals with open-set sentence recognition test scores of greater than 40% to less than or equal to 60% correct but only when the provider is participating in, and patients are enrolled in, either:

- A Food and Drug Administration (FDA)-approved category B investigational device exemption (IDE) clinical trial; or

- A trial under the CMS clinical trial policy (see Pub. 100-03, section 310.1); or

A prospective, controlled comparative trial approved by CMS as consistent with the evidentiary requirements for national coverage analyses and meeting specific quality standards.

100-4, Chapter-32, 110.5

DMERC Billing Instructions

Effective for dates of service on or after April 27, 2005, DMERCs shall allow payment for ultrasonic osteogenic stimulators with the following HCPCS codes:

E0760 for low intensity ultrasound (include modifier "KF"), or;

E1399 for other ultrasound stimulation (include modifier "KF")

100-4, Chapter-32, 120.1

Payment for Services and Supplies

For an IOL inserted following removal of a cataract in a hospital, on either an outpatient or inpatient basis, that is paid under the hospital Outpatient Prospective Payment System (OPPS) or the Inpatient Prospective Payment System (IPPS), respectively; or in a Medicare-approved ambulatory surgical center (ASC) that is paid under the ASC fee schedule:

- Medicare does not make separate payment to the hospital or ASC for an IOL inserted subsequent to extraction of a cataract. Payment for the IOL is packaged into the payment for the surgical cataract extraction/lens replacement procedure.

- Any person or ASC, who presents or causes to be presented a bill or request for payment for an IOL inserted during or subsequent to cataract surgery for which payment is made under the ASC fee schedule, is subject to a civil money penalty.

- For a P-C IOL or A-C IOL inserted subsequent to removal of a cataract in a hospital, on either an outpatient or inpatient basis, that is paid under the OPPS or the IPPS, respectively; or in a Medicare-approved ASC that is paid under the ASC fee schedule:

- The facility shall bill for the removal of a cataract with insertion of a conventional IOL, regardless of whether a conventional, P-C IOL, or A-C IOL is inserted. When a beneficiary receives a P-C or A-C IOL following removal of a cataract, hospitals and ASCs shall report the same CPT® code that is used to report removal of a cataract with insertion of a conventional IOL. Physicians, hospitals and ASCs may also report an additional HCPCS code, V2788, to indicate any additional charges that accrue when a P-C IOL or A-C IOL is inserted in lieu of a conventional IOL until January 1, 2008. Effective for A-C IOL insertion services on or after January 1, 2008, physicians, hospitals and ASCs should use V2787 to report any additional charges that accrue. On or after January 1, 2008, physicians, hospitals, and ASCs should continue to report HCPCS code V2788 to indicate any additional charges that accrue for insertion of a P-C IOL. See Section 120.2 for coding guidelines.

- There is no Medicare benefit category that allows payment of facility charges for services and supplies required to insert and adjust a P-C or A-C IOL following removal of a cataract that exceed the facility charges for services and supplies required for the insertion and adjustment of a conventional IOL.

- There is no Medicare benefit category that allows payment of facility charges for subsequent treatments, services and supplies required to examine and monitor the beneficiary who receives a P-C or A-C IOL following removal of a cataract that exceeds the facility charges for subsequent treatments, services and supplies required to examine and monitor a beneficiary after cataract surgery followed by insertion of a conventional IOL.

A -For a P-C IOL or A-C IOL inserted in a physician's office

-A physician shall bill for a conventional IOL, regardless of a whether a conventional, P-C IOL, or A-C IOL is inserted (see section 120.2, General Billing Requirements)

-There is no Medicare benefit category that allows payment of physician charges for services and supplies required to insert and adjust a P-C or A-C IOL following removal of a cataract that exceed the physician charges for services and supplies for the insertion and adjustment of a conventional IOL.

-There is no Medicare benefit category that allows payment of physician charges for subsequent treatments, service and supplies required to examine and monitor a beneficiary following removal of a cataract with insertion of a P-C or A-C IOL that exceed physician charges for services and supplies to examine and monitor a beneficiary following removal of a cataract with insertion of a conventional IOL.

B - For a P-C IOL or A-C IOL inserted in a hospital

-A physician may not bill Medicare for a P-C or A-C IOL inserted during a cataract procedure performed in a hospital setting because the payment for the lens is included in the payment made to the facility for the surgical procedure.

-There is no Medicare benefit category that allows payment of physician charges for services and supplies required to insert and adjust a P-C or A-C IOL following removal of a cataract that exceed the physician charges for services and supplies required for the insertion of a conventional IOL.

C - For a P-C IOL or A-C IOL inserted in an Ambulatory Surgical Center

-Refer to Chapter 14, Section 40.3 for complete guidance on payment for P-C IOL or A-C IOL in Ambulatory Surgical Centers.

100-4, Chapter-32, 120.2

Coding and General Billing Requirements

Physicians and hospitals must report one of the following Current Procedural Terminology (CPT®) codes on the claim:

- 66982 - Extracapsular cataract removal with insertion of intraocular lens prosthesis (one stage procedure), manual or mechanical technique (e.g., irrigation and aspiration or phacoemulsification), complex requiring devices or techniques not generally used in routine cataract surgery (e.g., iris expansion device, suture support for intraocular lens, or primary posterior capsulorrhexis) or performed on patients in the amblyogenic development stage.

- 66983- Intracapsular cataract with insertion of intraocular lens prosthesis (one stage procedure)

- 66984 - Extracapsular cataract removal with insertion of intraocular lens prosthesis (one stage procedure), manual or mechanical technique (e.g., irrigation and aspiration or phacoemulsification)

- 66985 - Insertion of intraocular lens prosthesis (secondary implant), not associated with concurrent cataract extraction

- 66986 - Exchange of intraocular lens

In addition, physicians inserting a P-C IOL or A-C IOL in an office setting may bill code V2632 (posterior chamber intraocular lens) for the IOL. Medicare will make payment for the lens based on reasonable cost for a conventional IOL. Place of Service (POS) = 11.

Effective for dates of service on and after January 1, 2006, physician, hospitals and ASCs may also bill the non-covered charges related to the P-C function of the IOL using HCPCS code V2788. Effective for dates of service on and after January 22, 2007 through January 1, 2008, non-covered charges related to A-C function of the IOL can be billed using HCPCS code V2788. The type of service indicator for the non-covered billed charges is Q. (The type of service is applied by the Medicare carrier and not the provider). Effective for A-C IOL insertion services on or after January 1, 2008, physicians, hospitals and ASCs should use V2787 rather than V2788 to report any additional charges that accrue.

When denying the non-payable charges submitted with V2787 or V2788, contractors shall use an appropriate Medical Summary Notice (MSN) such as 16.10 (Medicare does not pay for this item or service) and an appropriate claim adjustment reason code such as 96 (non-covered charges) for claims submitted with the non-payable charges.

Hospitals and physicians may use the proper CPT® code(s) to bill Medicare for evaluation and management services usually associated with services following cataract extraction surgery, if appropriate.

A - Applicable Bill Types

The hospital applicable bill types are 12X, 13X, 83X and 85X.

B - Other Special Requirements for Hospitals

Hospitals shall continue to pay CAHs method 2 claims under current payment methodologies for conditional IOLs.

100-4, Chapter-32, 130

External Counterpulsation (ECP) Therapy

Commonly referred to as enhanced external counterpulsation, is a non-invasive outpatient treatment for coronary artery disease refractory medical and/or surgical therapy. Effective for dates of service July 1, 1999, and after, Medicare will cover ECP when its use is in patients with stable angina (Class III or Class IV, Canadian Cardiovascular Society Classification or equivalent classification) who, in the opinion of a cardiologist or cardiothoracic surgeon, are not readily amenable to surgical intervention, such as PTCA or cardiac bypass, because:

- Their condition is inoperable, or at high risk of operative complications or post-operative failure;
- Their coronary anatomy is not readily amenable to such procedures; or
- They have co-morbid states that create excessive risk.

(Refer to Publication 100-03, section 20.20 for further coverage criteria.)

100-4, Chapter-32, 130.1

Billing and Payment Requirements

Effective for dates of service on or after January 1, 2000, use HCPCS code G0166 (External counterpulsation, per session) to report ECP services. The codes for external cardiac assist (92971), ECG rhythm strip and report (93040 or 93041), pulse oximetry (94760 or 94761) and plethysmography (93922 or 93923) or other monitoring tests for examining the effects of this treatment are not clinically necessary with this service and should not be paid on the same day, unless they occur in a clinical setting not connected with the delivery of the ECP. Daily evaluation and management service, e.g., 99201-99205, 99211-99215, 99217-99220, 99241-99245, cannot be billed with the ECP treatments. Any evaluation and management service must be justified with adequate documentation of the medical necessity of the visit. Deductible and coinsurance apply.

100-4, Chapter-32, 140.2.2.1

Correct Place of Service (POS) Code for CR and ICR Services on Professional Claims

Effective for claims with dates of service on and after January 1, 2010, place of service (POS) code 11 shall be used for CR and ICR services provided in a physician's office and POS 22 shall be used for services provided in a hospital outpatient setting. All other POS codes shall be denied. Contractors shall adjust their prepayment procedure edits as appropriate.

The following messages shall be used when contractors deny CR and ICR claims for POS:

Claim Adjustment Reason Code (CARC) 171 –Payment is denied when performed/billed by this type of provider in this type of facility.

NOTE: Refer to the 832 Healthcare Policy Identification Segment (loop 2110 Service payment Information REF), if present.

Remittance Advice Remark Code (RARC) N428 - Service/procedure not covered when performed in this place of service.

Medicare Summary Notice (MSN) 21.25 -This service was denied because Medicare only covers this service in certain settings.

Group Code PR (Patient Responsibility) -Where a claim is received with the GA modifier indicating that a signed ABN is on file.

Group Code CO (Contractor Responsibility) –Where a claim is received with the GZ modifier indicating that no signed ABN is on file.

100-4, Chapter-32, 140.3

Intensive Cardiac Rehabilitation Program Services Furnished On or After January 1, 2010

As specified at 42 CFR 410.49, Medicare covers intensive cardiac rehabilitation items and services for patients who have experienced one or more of the following:

- An acute myocardial infarction within the preceding 12 months; or
- A coronary artery bypass surgery; or
- Current stable angina pectoris; or
- Heart valve repair or replacement; or
- Percutaneous transluminal coronary angioplasty (PTCA) or coronary stenting; or
- A heart or heart-lung transplant; or
- A stable, chronic heart failure defined as patients with left ventricular ejection fraction of 35% or less and New York Heart Association (NYHA) class II to IV symptoms despite being on optimal heart failure therapy for at least 6 weeks(effective February 18, 2014).

Intensive cardiac rehabilitation programs must include the following components:

- Physician-prescribed exercise each day cardiac rehabilitation items and services are furnished;
- Cardiac risk factor modification, including education, counseling, and behavioral intervention at least once during the program, tailored to patients' individual needs;
- Psychosocial assessment;
- Outcomes assessment; and
- An individualized treatment plan detailing how components are utilized for each patient.

Intensive cardiac rehabilitation programs must be approved by Medicare. In order to be approved, a program must demonstrate through peer-reviewed published research that it has accomplished one or more of the following for its patients:

- Positively affected the progression of coronary heart disease;
- Reduced the need for coronary bypass surgery; and
- Reduced the need for percutaneous coronary interventions.

An intensive cardiac rehabilitation program must also demonstrate through peer- reviewed published research that it accomplished a statistically significant reduction in five or more of the following measures for patients from their levels before cardiac rehabilitation services to after cardiac rehabilitation services:

- Low density lipoprotein;
- Triglycerides;
- Body mass index;
- Systolic blood pressure;
- Diastolic blood pressure; and
- The need for cholesterol, blood pressure, and diabetes medications.

Intensive cardiac rehabilitation items and services must be furnished in a physician's office or a hospital outpatient setting. All settings must have a physician immediately available and accessible for medical consultations and emergencies at all times items and services are being furnished under the program. This provision is satisfied if the physician meets the requirements for direct supervision of physician office services as specified at 42 CFR 410.26 and for hospital outpatient therapeutic services as specified at 42 CFR 410.27.

As specified at 42 CFR 410.49(f)(2), intensive cardiac rehabilitation program sessions are limited to 72 1-hour sessions, up to 6 sessions per day, over a period of up to 18 weeks.

100-4, Chapter-32, 140.3.1

Coding Requirements for Intensive Cardiac Rehabilitation Services Furnished On or After January 1, 2010

The following are the applicable HCPCS codes for intensive cardiac rehabilitation services:

G0422 (Intensive cardiac rehabilitation; with or without continuous ECG monitoring, with exercise, per hour, per session)

G0423 (Intensive cardiac rehabilitation; with or without continuous ECG monitoring, without exercise, per hour, per session)

Effective for dates of service on or after January 1, 2010, hospitals and practitioners may report a maximum of 6 1-hour sessions per day. In order to report one session of cardiac rehabilitation services in a day, the duration of treatment must be at least 31 minutes.

Additional sessions of intensive cardiac rehabilitation services beyond the first session may only be reported in the same day if the duration of treatment is 31 minutes or greater beyond the hour increment. In other words, in order to report 6 sessions of intensive cardiac rehabilitation services on a given date of service, the first five sessions would account for 60 minutes each and the sixth session would account for at least 31 minutes. If several shorter periods of intensive cardiac rehabilitation services are furnished on a given day, the minutes of service during those periods must be added together for reporting in 1-hour session increments.

Example: If the patient receives 20 minutes of intensive cardiac rehabilitation services in the day, no intensive cardiac rehabilitation session may be reported because less than 31 minutes of services were furnished.

Example: If a patient receives 20 minutes of intensive cardiac rehabilitation services in the morning and 35 minutes of intensive cardiac rehabilitation services in the afternoon of a single day, the hospital or practitioner would report 1 session of intensive cardiac rehabilitation services under 1 unit of the appropriate HCPCS G-code for the total duration of 55 minutes of intensive cardiac rehabilitation services on that day.

Example: If the patient receives 70 minutes of intensive cardiac rehabilitation services in the morning and 25 minutes of intensive cardiac rehabilitation services in the afternoon of a single day, the hospital or practitioner would report two sessions of intensive cardiac rehabilitation services under the appropriate HCPCS G-code(s) because the total duration of intensive cardiac rehabilitation services on that day of 95 minutes exceeds 90 minutes.

Example: If the patient receives 70 minutes of intensive cardiac rehabilitation services in the morning and 85 minutes of intensive cardiac rehabilitation services in the afternoon of a single day, the hospital or practitioner would report three sessions of intensive cardiac rehabilitation services under the appropriate HCPCS G-code(s) because the total duration of intensive cardiac rehabilitation services on that day is 155 minutes, which exceeds 150 minutes and is less than 211 minutes.

100-4, Chapter-32, 140.4

Pulmonary Rehabilitation Program Services Furnished On or After January 1, 2010

As specified in 42 CFR 410.47, Medicare covers pulmonary rehabilitation items and services for patients with moderate to very severe COPD (defined as GOLD classification II, III and IV), when referred by the physician treating the chronic respiratory disease.

Pulmonary rehabilitation programs must include the following components:

- Physician-prescribed exercise. Some aerobic exercise must be included in each pulmonary rehabilitation session;
- Education or training closely and clearly related to the individual's care and treatment which is tailored to the individual's needs, including information on respiratory problem management and, if appropriate, brief smoking cessation counseling;
- Psychosocial assessment;
- Outcomes assessment; and,
- An individualized treatment plan detailing how components are utilized for each patient.

Pulmonary rehabilitation items and services must be furnished in a physician's office or a hospital outpatient setting. All settings must have a physician immediately available and accessible for medical consultations and emergencies at all time items and services are being furnished under the program. This provision is satisfied if the physician meets the requirements for direct supervision of physician office services as specified at 42 CFR 410.26 and for hospital outpatient therapeutic services as specified at 42 CFR 410.27.

As specified at 42 CFR 410.47(f), pulmonary rehabilitation program sessions are limited to a maximum of 2 1-hour sessions per day for up to 36 sessions, with the option for an additional 36 sessions if medically necessary. Contractors shall accept the inclusion of the KX modifier on the claim lines as an attestation by the provider of the service that documentation is on file verifying that further treatment beyond the 36 sessions is medically necessary up to a total of 72 sessions for that beneficiary.

100-4, Chapter-32, 140.4.1

Coding Requirements for Pulmonary Rehabilitation Services Furnished On or After January 1, 2010

The following is the applicable HCPCS code for pulmonary rehabilitation services:

G0424 (Pulmonary rehabilitation, including exercise (includes monitoring), per hour, per session)

Effective for dates of service on or after January 1, 2010, hospitals and practitioners may report a maximum of 2 1-hour sessions per day. In order to report one session of pulmonary rehabilitation services in a day, the duration of treatment must be at least 31 minutes. Two sessions of pulmonary rehabilitation services may only be reported in the same day if the duration of treatment is at least 91 minutes. In other words, the first session would account for 60 minutes and the second session would account for at least 31 minutes, if two sessions are reported. If several shorter periods of pulmonary rehabilitation services are furnished on a given day, the minutes of service during those periods must be added together for reporting in 1-hour session increments.

Example: If the patient receives 20 minutes of pulmonary rehabilitation services in the day, no pulmonary rehabilitation session may be reported because less than 31 minutes of services were furnished.

Example: If a patient receives 20 minutes of pulmonary rehabilitation services in the morning and 35 minutes of pulmonary rehabilitation services in the afternoon of a single day, the hospital or practitioner would report 1 session of pulmonary rehabilitation services under 1 unit of the HCPCS G-code for the total duration of 55 minutes of pulmonary rehabilitation services on that day.

Example: If the patient receives 70 minutes of pulmonary rehabilitation services in the morning and 25 minutes of pulmonary rehabilitation services in the afternoon of a single day, the hospital or practitioner would report two sessions of pulmonary rehabilitation services under the HCPCS G-code because the total duration of pulmonary rehabilitation services on that day of 95 minutes exceeds 90 minutes.

Example: If the patient receives 70 minutes of pulmonary rehabilitation services in the morning and 85 minutes of pulmonary rehabilitation services in the afternoon of a single day, the hospital or practitioner would report two sessions of pulmonary rehabilitation services under the HCPCS G-code for the total duration of pulmonary rehabilitation services of 155 minutes. A maximum of two sessions per day may be reported, regardless of the total duration of pulmonary rehabilitation services.

100-4, Chapter-32, 250.1

Coverage Requirements

Effective August 3, 2009, pharmacogenomic testing to predict warfarin responsiveness is covered only when provided to Medicare beneficiaries who are candidates for anticoagulation therapy with warfarin; i.e., have not been previously tested for CYP2C9 or VKORC1 alleles; and have received fewer than five days of warfarin in the anticoagulation regimen for which the testing is ordered; and only then in the context of a prospective, randomized, controlled clinical study when that study meets certain criteria as outlined in Pub 100-03, section 90.1, of the NCD Manual.

NOTE: A new temporary HCPCS Level II code effective August 3, 2009, G9143, warfarin responsiveness testing by genetic technique using any method, any number of specimen(s), was developed to enable implementation of CED for this purpose.

100-4, Chapter-32, 250.2

Billing Requirements

Institutional clinical trial claims for pharmacogenomic testing for warfarin response are identified through the presence of all of the following elements:

- Value Code D4 and 8-digit clinical trial number (when present on the claim) -Refer to Transmittal 310, Change Request 5790, dated January 18, 2008;
- ICD-9 diagnosis code V70.7 -Refer to Transmittal 310, Change Request 5790, dated January 18, 2008;
- Condition Code 30 -Refer to Transmittal 310, Change Request 5790, dated January 18, 2008;

- HCPCS modifier Q0: outpatient claims only -Refer to Transmittal 1418, Change Request 5805, dated January18, 2008; and,
- HCPCS code G9143 (mandatory with the April 2010 Integrated Outpatient Code Editor (IOCE) and the January 2011 Clinical Laboratory Fee Schedule (CLFS) updates. Prior to these times, any trials should bill FIs for this test as they currently do absent these instructions, and the FIs should process and pay those claims accordingly.)

Practitioner clinical trial claims for pharmacogenomic testing for warfarin response are identified through the presence of all of the following elements:

- ICD-9 diagnosis code V70.7;
- 8-digit clinical trial number(when present on the claim);
- HCPCS modifier Q0; and
- HCPCS code G9143 (to be carrier priced for claims with dates of service on and after August 3, 2009, that are processed prior to the January 2011 CLFS update.)

100-4, Chapter-32, 260.1

Policy

The Centers for Medicare & Medicaid Services (CMS) received a request for national coverage of treatments for facial lipodystrophy syndrome (LDS) for human immunodeficiency virus (HIV)-infected Medicare beneficiaries. Facial LDS is often characterized by a loss of fat that results in a facial abnormality such as severely sunken cheeks. This fat loss can arise as a complication of HIV and/or highly active antiretroviral therapy. Due to their appearance and stigma of the condition, patients with facial LDS may become depressed, socially isolated, and in some cases may stop their HIV treatments in an attempt to halt or reverse this complication.

Effective for claims with dates of service on and after March 23, 2010, dermal injections for facial LDS are only reasonable and necessary using dermal fillers approved by the Food and Drug Administration for this purpose, and then only in HIV-infected beneficiaries who manifest depression secondary to the physical stigmata of HIV treatment.

See Pub. 100-03, National Coverage Decision manual, section 250.5, for detailed policy information concerning treatment of LDS.

100-4, Chapter-32, 260.2.1

Hospital Billing Instructions

A -Hospital Outpatient Claims

For hospital outpatient claims, hospitals must bill covered dermal injections for treatment of facial LDS by having all of the required elements on the claim:

- A line with HCPCS codes Q2026 or Q2027 with a Line Item Date of service (LIDOS) on or after March 23, 2010,
- A line with HCPCS code G0429 with a LIDOS on or after March 23, 2010,
- If ICD-9-CM is applicable,ICD-9-CM diagnosis codes 042 (HIV) and 272.6 (Lipodystrophy)or,
- If ICD-10-CM is applicable, ICD-10-CM diagnosis codes B20 Human Immunodeficiency Virus (HIV) disease and E88.1 Lipodystrophy, not elsewhere classified

The applicable NCD is 250.5 Facial Lipodystrophy.

B - Outpatient Prospective Payment System (OPPS) Hospitals or Ambulatory Surgical Centers (ASCs):

For line item dates of service on or after March 23, 2010, and until HCPCS codes Q2026 and Q2027 are billable, facial LDS claims shall contain a temporary HCPCS code C9800 (this code has been deleted in 2017), instead of HCPCS G0429 and HCPCS Q2026/Q2027, as shown above.

C -Hospital Inpatient Claims

Hospitals must bill covered dermal injections for treatment of facial LDS by having all of the required elements on the claim:

- Discharge date on or after March 23, 2010,

If ICD-9-CM is applicable,

- ICD-9-CM procedure code 86.99 (other operations on skin and subcutaneous tissue, i.e., injection of filler material), or
- ICD-9-CM diagnosis codes 042 (HIV) and 272.6 (Lipodystrophy)
- If ICD-10-PCS is applicable,
- ICD-10-PCS procedure code 3E00XGC Introduction of Other Therapeutic Substance into Skin and Mucous Membranes, External Approach, or
- ICD-10-CM diagnosis codes B20 Human Immunodeficiency Virus [HIV] disease and E88.1 Lipodystrophy not elsewhere classified.

A diagnosis code for a comorbidity of depression may also be required for coverage on an outpatient and/or inpatient basis as determined by the individual Medicare contractor's policy.

100-4, Chapter-32, 260.2.2

Practitioner Billing Instructions

Practitioners must bill covered claims for dermal injections for treatment of facial LDS by having all of the required elements on the claim:

Performed in a non-facility setting:

- A line with HCPCS codes Q2026 or Q2027 with a LIDOS on or after March 23, 2010,
- A line with HCPCS code G0429 with a LIDOS on or after March 23, 2010,
- If ICD-9-CM applies, diagnosis codes 042 (HIV) and 272.6 (Lipodystrophy) or,
- If ICD-10-CM applies, diagnosis codes B20 Human Immunodeficiency Virus (HIV) disease and E88.1 (Lipodystrophy not elsewhere classified).

NOTE: A diagnosis code for a comorbidity of depression may also be required for coverage based on the individual Medicare contractor's policy.

Performed in a facility setting:

- A line with HCPCS code G0429 with a LIDOS on or after March 23, 2010,
- If ICD-9 applies,ICD-9-CM diagnosis codes 042 (HIV) and 272.6 (Lipodystrophy)or
- If ICD-10 applies, ICD-10-CM diagnosis codes B20 Human Immunodeficiency Virus (HIV) disease and E88.1 (Lipodystrophy not elsewhere classified).

NOTE: A diagnosis code for a comorbidity of depression may also be required for coverage based on the individual Medicare contractor's policy.

100-4, Chapter-32, 280.1

Policy

Effective for services furnished on or after June 30, 2011, a National Coverage Determination (NCD) provides coverage of sipuleucel-T (PROVENGE®) for patients with asymptomatic or minimally symptomatic metastatic, castrate-resistant (hormone refractory) prostate cancer. Conditions of Medicare Part A and Medicare Part B coverage for sipuleucel-T are located in the Medicare NCD Manual, Publication 100-03, section 110.22.

100-4, Chapter-32, 280.2

Healthcare Common Procedure Coding System (HCPCS) Codes and Diagnosis Coding
HCPCS Codes

Effective for claims with dates of service on June 30, 2011, Medicare providers shall report one of the following HCPCS codes for PROVENGE®:

- C9273 - Sipuleucel-T, minimum of 50 million autologous CD54+ cells activated with PAP-GM-CSF, including leukapheresis and all other preparatory procedures, per infusion, or
- J3490 –Unclassified Drugs, or
- J3590 –Unclassified Biologics.

NOTE: Contractors shall continue to process claims for HCPCS code C9273, J3490, and J3590, with dates of service June 30, 2011, as they do currently.

Effective for claims with dates of service on and after July 1, 2011, Medicare providers shall report the following HCPCS code:

Q2043 – Sipuleucel-T, minimum of 50 million autologous CD54+ cells activated with PAP-

GM-CSF, including leukapheresis and all other preparatory procedures, per infusion; short descriptor, Sipuleucel-T auto CD54+.

ICD-9 Diagnosis Coding

For claims with dates of service on and after July 1, 2011, for PROVENGE®, the on-label indication of asymptomatic or minimally symptomatic metastatic, castrate-resistant (hormone refractory) prostate cancer, must be billed using ICD-9 code 185 (malignant neoplasm of prostate) and at least one of the following ICD-9 codes:

ICD-9 Code	Description
196.1	Secondary and unspecified malignant neoplasm of intrathoracic lymph nodes
196.2	Secondary and unspecified malignant neoplasm of intra-abdominal lymph nodes
196.5	Secondary and unspecified malignant neoplasm of lymph nodes of inguinal region and lower limb
196.6	Secondary and unspecified malignant neoplasm of intrapelvic lymph nodes
196.8	Secondary and unspecified malignant neoplasm of lymph nodes of multiple sites
196.9	Secondary and unspecified malignant neoplasm of lymph node site unspecified -The spread of cancer to and establishment in the lymph nodes.
197.0	Secondary malignant neoplasm of lung –Cancer that has spread from the original (primary) tumor to the lung. The spread of cancer to the lung. This may be from a primary lung cancer, or from a cancer at a distant site.

ICD-9 Code	Description
197.7	Malignant neoplasm of liver secondary -Cancer that has spread from the original (primary) tumor to the liver. A malignant neoplasm that has spread to the liver from another (primary) anatomic site. Such malignant neoplasms may be carcinomas (e.g., breast, colon), lymphomas, melanomas, or sarcomas.
198.0	Secondary malignant neoplasm of kidney -The spread of the cancer to the kidney. This may be from a primary kidney cancer involving the opposite kidney, or from a cancer at a distant site.
198.1	Secondary malignant neoplasm of other urinary organs
198.5	Secondary malignant neoplasm of bone and bone marrow –Cancer that has spread from the original (primary) tumor to the bone. The spread of a malignant neoplasm from a primary site to the skeletal system. The majority of metastatic neoplasms to the bone are carcinomas.
198.7	Secondary malignant neoplasm of bone and bone marrow –Cancer that has spread from the original (primary) tumor to the bone. The spread of a malignant neoplasm from a primary site to the skeletal system. The majority of metastatic neoplasms to the bone are carcinomas.
198.82	Secondary malignant neoplasm of genital organs

Coding for Off-Label PROVENGE® Services

The use of PROVENGE® off-label for the treatment of prostate cancer is left to the discretion of the Medicare Administrative Contractors. Claims with dates of service on and after July 1, 2011, for PROVENGE® paid off-label for the treatment of prostate cancer must be billed using either ICD-9 code 233.4 (carcinoma in situ of prostate), or ICD-9 code 185 (malignant neoplasm of prostate) in addition to HCPCS Q2043. Effective with the implementation date for ICD-10 codes, off-label PROVENGE® services must be billed with either ICD-10 code D075(carcinoma in situ of prostate), or C61 (malignant neoplasm of prostate) in addition to HCPCS Q2043.

ICD-10 Diagnosis Coding

Contractors shall note the appropriate ICD-10 code(s) that are listed below for future implementation. Contractors shall track the ICD-10 codes and ensure that the updated edit is turned on as part of the ICD-10 implementation effective October 1, 2013.

ICD-10	Description
C61	Malignant neoplasm of prostate (for on-label or off-label indications)
D075	Carcinoma in situ of prostate (for off-label indications only)
C77.1	Secondary and unspecified malignant neoplasm of intrathoracic lymph nodes
C77.2	Secondary and unspecified malignant neoplasm of intra-abdominal lymph nodes
C77.4	Secondary and unspecified malignant neoplasm of inguinal and lower limb lymph nodes
C77.5	Secondary and unspecified malignant neoplasm of intrapelvic lymph nodes
C77.8	Secondary and unspecified malignant neoplasm of lymph nodes of multiple regions
C77.9	Secondary and unspecified malignant neoplasm of lymph node, unspecified
C78.00	Secondary malignant neoplasm of unspecified lung
C78.01	Secondary malignant neoplasm of right lung
C78.02	Secondary malignant neoplasm of left lung
C78.7	Secondary malignant neoplasm of liver
C79.00	Secondary malignant neoplasm of unspecified kidney and renal pelvis

ICD-10	Description
C79.01	Secondary malignant neoplasm of right kidney and renal pelvis
C79.02	Secondary malignant neoplasm of left kidney and renal pelvis
C79.10	Secondary malignant neoplasm of unspecified urinary organs
C79.11	Secondary malignant neoplasm of bladder
C79.19	Secondary malignant neoplasm of other urinary organs
C79.51	Secondary malignant neoplasm of bone
C79.52	Secondary malignant neoplasm of bone marrow
C79.70	Secondary malignant neoplasm of unspecified adrenal gland
C79.71	Secondary malignant neoplasm of right adrenal gland
C79.72	Secondary malignant neoplasm of left adrenal gland
C79.82	Secondary malignant neoplasm of genital organs

100-4, Chapter-32, 280.4

Payment Method

Payment for PROVENGE® is as follows:

- TOBs 12X, 13X, 22X and 23X -based on the Average Sales Price (ASP) + 6%,
- TOB 85X –based on reasonable cost,
- TOBs 71X and 77X –based on all-inclusive rate.

For Medicare Part B practitioner claims, payment for PROVENGE® is based on ASP + 6%.

Contractors shall not pay separately for routine costs associated with PROVENGE®, HCPCS Q2043, except for the cost of administration. (Q2043 is all-inclusive and represents all routine costs except for its cost of administration).

100-4, Chapter-32, 280.5

Medicare Summary Notices (MSNs), Remittance Advice Remark Codes (RARCs), Claim Adjustment Reason Codes (CARCs), and Group Codes

Contractors shall use the following messages when denying claims for the on-label indication for PROVENGE®, HCPCS Q2043, submitted without ICD-9-CM diagnosis code 185 and at least one diagnosis code from the ICD-9 table in Section 280.2 above:

MSN 14.9 - Medicare cannot pay for this service for the diagnosis shown on the claim.

Spanish Version -Medicare no puede pagar por este servicio debido al diagnóstico indicado en la reclamación.

RARC 167 - This (these) diagnosis (es) are not covered.

NOTE: Refer to the 835 Healthcare Policy Identification segment (loop 2110 Service Payment Information REF), if present.

Group Code – CO (Contractual Obligation)

Contractors shall use the following messages when denying claims for the off-label indication for PROVENGE®, HCPCS Q2043, submitted without ICD-9-CM diagnosis code 233.4:

MSN 14.9 - Medicare cannot pay for this service for the diagnosis shown on the claim.

Spanish Version - Medicare no puede pagar por este servicio debido al diagnóstico indicado en la reclamación.

RARC 167 - This (these) diagnosis (es) are not covered.

NOTE: Refer to the 835 Healthcare Policy Identification segment (loop 2110 Service Payment Information REF), if present.

Group Code –CO (Contractual Obligation)

For claims with dates of service on or after July 1, 2012, processed on or after July 2, 2012, when denying claims for PROVENGE®, HCPCS Q2043 that exceed three (3) services in a patient's lifetime, contractors shall use the following messages:

MSN 20.5 - These services cannot be paid because your benefits are exhausted at this time.

Spanish Version - Estos servicios no pueden ser pagados porque sus beneficios se han agotado.

RARC N362 - The number of Days or Units of Service exceeds our acceptable maximum.

CARC 149 -Lifetime benefit maximum has been reached for this service/benefit category.

Group Code – CO (Contractual Obligation)

100-4, Chapter-32, 300

Billing Requirements for Ocular Photodynamic Therapy (OPT) with Verteporfin

Ocular Photodynamic Therapy (OPT) is used in the treatment of ophthalmologic diseases; specifically, for age-related macular degeneration (AMD), a common eye disease among the elderly. OPT involves the infusion of an intravenous photosensitizing drug called Verteporfin, followed by exposure to a laser. For complete Medical coverage guidelines, see National Coverage Determinations (NCD) Manual (Pub 100-03) § 80.2 through 80.3.1.

100-4, Chapter-32, 300.1

Coding Requirements for OPT with Verteporfin

The following are applicable Current Procedural Terminology (CPT®) codes for OPT with Verteporfin:

67221- Destruction of localized lesion of choroid (e.g. choroidal neovascularization); photodynamic therapy (includes intravenous infusion)

67225- Destruction of localized lesion of choroid (e.g. choroidal neovascularization); photodynamic therapy, second eye, at single session (List separately in addition to code for primary eye treatment)

The following are applicable Healthcare Common Procedure Coding System (HCPCS) code for OPT with Verteporfin:

J3396- Injection, Verteporfin, 0.1 mg

100-4, Chapter-32, 300.2

Claims Processing Requirements for OPT with Verteporfin Services on Professional Claims and Outpatient Facility Claims

OPT with Verteporfin is a covered service when billed with ICD-9-CM code 362.52 (Exudative Senile Macular Degeneration of Retina (Wet)) or ICD-10-CM code H35.32 (Exudative Age-related Macular Degeneration).

Coverage is denied when billed with either ICD-9-CM code 362.50 (Macular Degeneration (Senile), Unspecified) or 362.51 (Non-exudative Senile Macular Degeneration) or their equivalent ICD-10-CM code H35.30 (Unspecified Macular Degeneration) or H35.31 (Non-exudative Age-Related Macular Degeneration).

OPT with Verteporfin for other ocular indications are eligible for local coverage determinations through individual contractor discretion.

Payment for OPT service (CPT® code 67221/67225) must be billed on the same claim as the drug (J3396) for the same date of service.

Claims for OPT with Verteporfin for dates of service prior to April 3,2013 are covered at the initial visit as determined by a fluorescein angiogram (FA) CPT® code 92235. Subsequent follow-up visits also require a FA prior to treatment.

For claims with dates of service on or after April 3, 2013, contractors shall accept and process claims for subsequent follow-up visits with either a FA, CPT® code 92235, or optical coherence tomography (OCT), CPT® codes 92133 or 92134, prior to treatment.

Regardless of the date of service of the claim, the FA or OCT is not required to be submitted on the claim for OPT and can be maintained in the patient's file for audit purposes.

100-4, Chapter-32, 310

Transesophageal Doppler Used for Cardiac Monitoring

Effective May 17, 2007, Transesophageal Doppler used for cardiac monitoring is covered for ventilated patients in the ICU and operative patients with a need for intra-operative fluid optimization was deemed reasonable and necessary. See National Coverage Determinations Manual (Pub. 100-03)§220.5, for complete coverage guidelines.

A new Healthcare Common Procedure Coding System (HCPCS) code, G9157, Transesophageal Doppler used for cardiac monitoring, will be made effective for use for dates of service on or after January 1, 2013.

100-4, Chapter-32, 310.2

Coding Requirements for Transesophageal Doppler Cardiac Monitoring Furnished On or After January 1, 2013

After January 1, 2013, the applicable HCPCS code for Transesophageal Doppler cardiac monitoring is:

HCPCS G9157: Transesophageal Doppler used for cardiac monitoring

Contractors shall allow HCPCS G9157 to be billed when services are provided in POS 21 for ventilated patients in the ICU or for operative patients with a need for intra-operative fluid optimization.

Contractors shall deny HCPCS 76999 when billed for Esophageal Doppler for ventilated patients in the ICU or for operative patients with a need for intra-operative fluid optimization using the following messages:

CARC 189: "'Not otherwise classified' or 'unlisted' procedure code (CPT®/HCPCS) was billed when there is a specific procedure code for this procedure/service."

RARC M20: "Missing/incomplete/invalid HCPCS."

MSN 16.13: "The code(s) your provider used is/are not valid for the date of service billed." (English version) or "El/los código(s) que usó su proveedor no es/son válido(s) en la fecha de servicio facturada." (Spanish version).

Group Code: Contractual Obligation (CO)

100-4, Chapter-32, 310.3

Correct Place of Service (POS) Code for Transesophageal Doppler Cardiac Monitoring Services on Professional Claims

Contractors shall pay for Transesophageal Doppler cardiac monitoring, G9157, only when services are provided at POS 21.

Contractors shall deny HCPCS G9157 when billed globally in any POS other than 21 for ventilated patients in the ICU or for operative patients with a need for intra-operative fluid optimization using the following messages:

CARC 58:"Treatment was deemed by the payer to have been rendered in an inappropriate or invalid place of service. *NOTE:* Refer to the 835 Healthcare Policy Identification Segment (loop 2110 Service Payment Information REF), if present.

MSN 16.2: This service cannot be paid when provided in this location/facility.

Group Code: CO

100-4, Chapter-36, 50.14

Purchased Accessories & Supplies for Use With Grandfathered Equipment

Non-contract grandfathered suppliers must use the KY modifier on claims for CBA-residing beneficiaries with dates of service on or after January 1, 2011, for purchased, covered accessories or supplies furnished for use with rented grandfathered equipment. The following HCPCS codes are the codes for which use of the KY modifier is authorized:

- Continuous Positive Airway Pressure Devices, Respiratory Assistive Devices, and Related Supplies and Accessories – A4604, A7030, A7031, A7032, A7033, A7034, A7035, A7036, A7037, A7038, A7039, A7044, A7045, A7046, E0561, and E0562
- Hospital Beds and Related Accessories – E0271, E0272, E0280, and E0310
- Walkers and Related Accessories – E0154, E0156, E0157 and E0158

Grandfathered suppliers that submit claims for the payment of the aforementioned purchased accessories and supplies for use with grandfathered equipment should submit the applicable single payment amount for the accessory or supply as their submitted charge on the claim. Non-contract grandfathered suppliers should be aware that purchase claims submitted for these codes without the KY modifier will be denied. In addition, claims submitted with the KY modifier for HCPCS codes other than those listed above will be denied.

After the rental payment cap for the grandfathered equipment is reached, the beneficiary must obtain replacement supplies and accessories from a contract supplier. The supplier of the grandfathered equipment is no longer permitted to furnish the supplies and accessories once the rental payment cap is reached.

100-4, Chapter-36, 50.15

Hospitals Providing Walkers and Related Accessories to Their Patients on the Date of Discharge

Hospitals may furnish walkers and related accessories to their own patients for use in the home during an admission or on the date of discharge and receive payment at the applicable single payment amount, regardless of whether the hospital is a contract supplier or not. Separate payment is not made for walkers furnished by a hospital for use in the hospital, as payment for these items is included in the Part A payment for inpatient hospital services.

To be paid for walkers as a non-contract supplier, the hospital must use the modifier J4 in combination with the following HCPCS codes: A4636; A4637; E0130; E0135; E0140; E0141; E0143; E0144; E0147; E0148; E0149; E0154; E0155; E0156; E0157; E0158; and E0159. Under this exception, hospitals are advised to submit the claim for the hospital stay before or on the same day that they submit the claim for the walker to ensure timely and accurate claims processing.

Hospitals that are located outside a CBA that furnish walkers and/or related accessories to travelling beneficiaries who live in a CBA must affix the J4 modifier to claims submitted for these items.

The J4 modifier should not be used by contract suppliers.

100-8, Chapter-4, 4.26.1

Proof of Delivery and Delivery Methods

This section applies to UPICs. This section is applicable to DME MACs, RACs, SMRC, and CERT medical review contractors, as noted in Ch. 5, Section 5.8.

For the purpose of the delivery methods noted below, designee is defined as:

"Any person who can sign and accept the delivery of durable medical equipment on behalf of the beneficiary."

Suppliers, their employees, or anyone else having a financial interest in the delivery of the item are prohibited from signing and accepting an item on behalf of a beneficiary (i.e., acting as a designee on behalf of the beneficiary). The signature of the designee should be legible. If the signature of the designee is not legible, the supplier/shipping service should note the name of the designee on the delivery slip.

Three methods of delivery are:

- Supplier delivering directly to the beneficiary or designee;
- Supplier utilizing a delivery/shipping service to deliver items; and
- Delivery of items to a nursing facility on behalf of the beneficiary.

The date of delivery may be entered by the beneficiary, designee or the supplier. As a general Medicare rule, the date of service shall be the date of delivery. Exceptions are made for suppliers who use a delivery/shipping service. If the supplier uses a delivery/shipping service, the supplier may use the shipping date as the date of service on the claim. The shipping date may be defined as the date the delivery/shipping service label is created or the date the item is retrieved for delivery; however, such dates should not demonstrate significant variation. (See Pub. 100-08, chapter 5, section 5.2.4 for further information on written orders prior to delivery.)

NOTES

Get the guidance you need for CMS coding compliance.

TCI's 25+ specialty-specific newsletters feature:

- Analysis of latest codes and regulatory changes
- Must-have advice for day-to-day scenarios
- How-to articles and archives
- Reader questions with expert answers

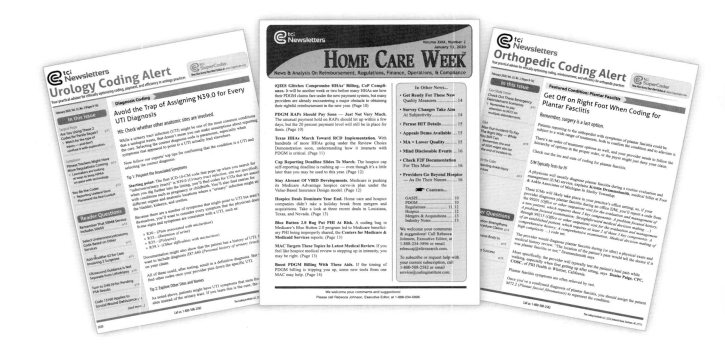

Save time, increase coding accuracy, and earn CEU opportunities!

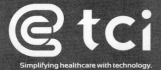

Simplifying healthcare with technology.

Subscribe Now
Visit **www.aapc.com/newsletters** or call **844.334.2816** to get started

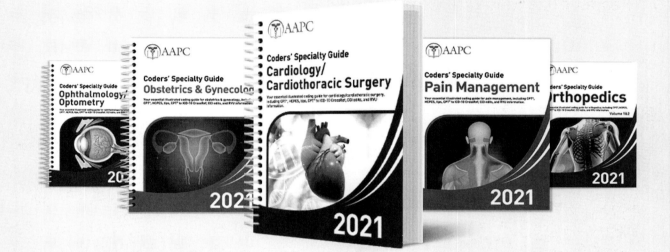

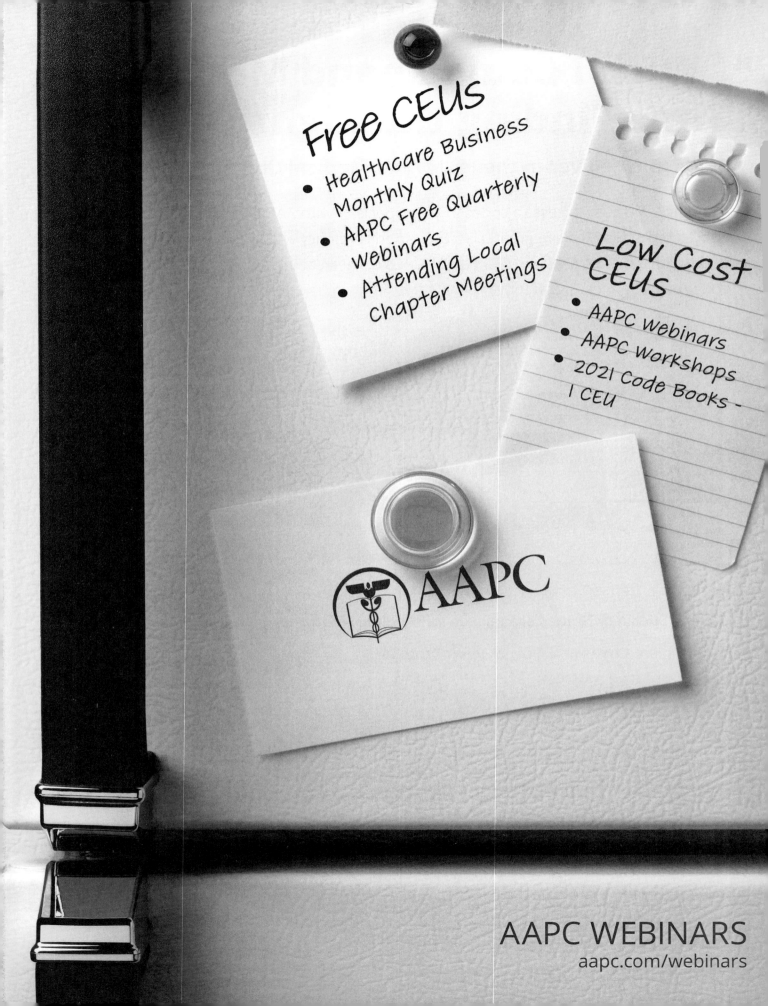

NOTES

NOTES